An anthology of psychiatric ethics

An anthology of psychiatric ethics

Stephen A. Green
Clinical Professor of Psychiatry, Georgetown University, Washington D.C.

Sidney Bloch
Professor of Psychiatry, Department of Psychiatry and Centre for Health & Society, University of Melbourne, Australia

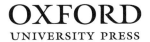

OXFORD
UNIVERSITY PRESS

OXFORD
UNIVERSITY PRESS

Great Clarendon Street, Oxford OX2 6DP

Oxford University Press is a department of the University of Oxford.
It furthers the University's objective of excellence in research, scholarship,
and education by publishing worldwide in

Oxford New York

Auckland Cape Town Dar es Salaam Hong Kong Karachi
Kuala Lumpur Madrid Melbourne Mexico City Nairobi
New Delhi Shanghai Taipei Toronto

With offices in

Argentina Austria Brazil Chile Czech Republic France Greece
Guatemala Hungary Italy Japan Poland Portugal Singapore
South Korea Switzerland Thailand Turkey Ukraine Vietnam

Oxford is a registered trade mark of Oxford University Press
in the UK and in certain other countries

Published in the United States
by Oxford University Press Inc., New York

© Oxford University Press, 2006

British Library Cataloguing in Publication Data
Data available

Library of Congress Cataloging in Publication Data
An anthology of psychiatric ethics / [edited by] Stephen Green, Sidney Bloch.
 p. ; cm.
 Includes bibliographical references and index.
 1. Psychiatric ethics.
[DNLM: 1. Psychiatry—ethics—Collected Works. 2. Ethics, Clinical—
Collected Works. 3. Mental Health Services—ethics—Collected Works.
WM 5 A628 2006] I. Green, Stephen A., 1945–ⅠⅠ. Bloch, Sidney.
 RC455.2.E8A58 2006
 174.2—dc22
                                                        2006003818

Typeset by Newgen Imaging Systems (P) Ltd., Chennai, India
Printed in Italy
on acid-free paper by Lito Terrazi

ISBN 0–19–856–487–2 (Hbk)   978–0–19–856–487–4 (Hbk)
     0–19–856–488–0 (Pbk)   978–0–19–856–488–1 (Pbk)

10 9 8 7 6 5 4 3 2 1

Foreword

Paul Chodoff

When *homo sapiens* climbed the evolutionary ladder from hominid status, a defining characteristic of the new breed was an interest in matters of right and wrong. And, as soon as our ancestors acquired the ability to record their thoughts in some durable form, discussions of such issues have proliferated endlessly in almost every human culture and field of human endeavor, both theoretical and practical. This has certainly been the case as the activities of some people offering help to others with psychological and emotional problems gradually became professionalized into psychiatry, psychology and social work.

Psychiatric ethics[1] was an attempt to delineate and summarize systematically the differing views about the various ethical issues of concern to psychiatrists principally, but also to members of the other helping professions. The initial impetus for its publication was the editors' recognition that ethical issues in their profession could no longer be subsumed under general moral theory or within the confines of medical ethics, but would require more specific consideration of the complexities and interrelationships that characterize psychiatric practice. Each chapter dealt with important, complex ethical issues within particular areas of psychiatry. Topics selected by the editors were assigned to an expert for discussion, and each chapter contained a list of references that guided further reading. Subsequent editions added to or omitted chapters from the original volume as their importance waxed or waned in the judgment of the editors.

An *Anthology of psychiatric ethics* can be seen as a further step in fulfilling the purposes responsible for publication of *Psychiatric ethics*. Drs. Green and Bloch [with some help from me] have undertaken to provide interested readers with a volume-the first of its kind – containing a comprehensive and integrated set of readings in the field. They are presented in nine sections, each introduced by an essay that outlines and summarizes ethical issues and debates central to the area and includes a reference list of associated relevant readings. The selections were judged by the editors to best represent the field, to be of outstanding merit, or to have stimulated ongoing, valuable debate [e.g., *The myth of mental illness* by Szasz].

The anthology's first chapter explores theoretical-philosophical foundations of moral decision making as they apply to ethical questions in psychiatry. Succeeding chapters deal with a broad spectrum of issues, addressing such questions as: How does the therapeutic role relate to the social setting within which it operates? What ethical responsibilities does the power to make diagnostic judgments bestow on practitioners? To what extent can (and should) the therapist be able to offer confidentiality to his patient? How should limited psychiatric resources be allocated among various populations, and to what degree should factors such as age, gender, race and economic status guide that process? How should we cope with the age old dilemma concerning the effects of disordered mental functioning on criminal responsibility? How should the possible beneficial effects of research for the mentally ill be reconciled with the need to employ experimental subjects whose ability to give informed consent is compromised?

How important are ethical issues in the practice of psychiatry? Based on my long experience I have come to the conviction that almost everything one does in treating people with mental, emotional, and psychological problems is inextricably entwined with questions about right and wrong. This is because psychiatry, to a greater extent than other branches of medicine, cannot be separated from, and is inevitably influenced by, the moral norms associated with the social, cultural and religious context within which it operates. It is the intent of *An anthology of psychiatric ethics* to illuminate thorny ethical issues that confront the practitioner, and thus facilitate conscientious, clinical decision-making. Obviously, no single volume can explore all the ethical issues related to psychiatry, but I am confident that the reader will find *An anthology of psychiatric ethics* covers a major portion of the territory.

[1] Bloch, S. and Chodoff, P. (eds): *Psychiatric ethics*, Oxford University Press, 1981.

Contents

Foreword *v*

Preface *xi*

Acknowledgements *xiii*

1 Theoretical foundations *1*

The Virtuous Physician, and the Ethics
of Medicine *7*
Edmund D. Pellegrino

Getting Down to Cases *13*
John D. Arras

Grounding for the Metaphysics of Morals *20*
Immanuel Kant

Utilitarianism *28*
John Stuart Mill

The 'Four-principles' Approach *34*
Tom L. Beauchamp

The 'Voice of Care' *38*
Alisa L. Carse

2 The Therapeutic Relationship and
the Social Domain *45*

The Dynamics of the Transference (1912) *50*
Sigmund Freud

The Exploitation Index *53*
Richard S. Epstein and Robert I. Simon

The Concept of Boundaries in Clinical Practice *60*
Thomas G. Gutheil and Glen O. Gabbard

Psychotherapists Who Transgress Sexual
Boundaries with Patients *67*
Glen O. Gabbard

In the Service of the State *71*
*A Conference on Conflicting Loyalties cosponsored
by the American Psychiatric Association and
The Hastings Center, March 24–26, 1977*

The Psychiatrist as Double Agent *88*
Daniel Callahan and Willard Gaylin

The Effect of Third-Party Payment on the
Practice of Psychotherapy *90*
Paul Chodoff

3 Diagnosis *93*

A Woman's View of DSM-III *99*
Marcie Kaplan

The Myth of Mental Illness *104*
Thomas S. Szasz

What a Theory of Mental Health
Should Be *108*
Christopher Boorse

A Symposium: Should Homosexuality be
in the APA Nomenclature? *116*
*Robert J. Stoller, Judd Marmor, Irving Bieber,
Ronald Gold, Charles W. Socarides, Richard Green
and Robert L. Spitzer*

On Being Sane in Insane Places *123*
D. L. Rosenhan

The Concept of Mental Disorder *130*
Jerome C. Wakefield

A Psychiatric Dialogue on the Mind-Body
Problem *142*
Kenneth S. Kendler

4 Confidentiality *151*

The Limits of Confidentiality *156*
Sissela Bok

Absolute Confidentiality? *163*
Sir Douglas Black

Tarasoff v. Regents of the University
of California *167*

Family Involvement in the Care of People
with Psychoses *171*
George I. Szmukler and Sidney Bloch

Secrets of the Couch and the Grave *175*
Edmund D. Pellegrino

5 Psychiatric Treatment and Services *181*

Involuntary Hospitalization of the Mentally
Ill as a Moral Issue *192*
Paul Chodoff

The Case Against Suicide Prevention *196*
Thomas Szasz

Incapacity to give informed consent owing to
mental disorder *201*
C. W. Van Staden, C. Krüger

The Ethics of Mandatory Community
Treatment *204*
*Mark R. Munetz, Patricia A. Galon and
Frederick J. Frese III*

Donaldson v. O'Connor *210*

The Psychiatric Patient's Right to Effective
Treatment *219*
Gerald L. Klerman

Law, Science, and Psychiatric Malpractice *226*
Alan A. Stone

Effect of Joint Crisis Plans on use of Compulsory
Treatment in Psychiatry *232*
*Claire Henderson, Chris Flood, Morven Leese,
Graham Thornicroft, Kim Sutherby and
George Szmukler*

Ethical and Pragmatic Issues in the Use of
Psychotropic Agents in Young Children *236*
Peter S Jensen

Antidepressants for Children *239*
Rhoda L. Fisher and Seymour Fisher

The Valorization of Sadness *242*
Peter D. Kramer

Pursued by Happiness and Beaten
Senseless *246*
Carl Elliott

Ethical Aspects of Research and Practice
of ECT *250*
Jan-Otto Ottosson

Values in Psychotherapy *254*
Jeremy Holmes

Psychoanalysis and Ethics – Avowed
and Unavowed *259*
Erik H. Erikson

Advocacy and Corruption in the
Healing Professions *263*
Robert Jay Lifton

Psychotherapy and Religious Values *270*
Allen E. Bergin

The Negotiation of Values in Therapy *276*
Harry J. Aponte

6 Special Clinical Populations *283*

Consent to Treatment During Childhood *290*
John Pearce

Autonomy and the Demented Self *293*
Ronald Dworkin

Dworkin on Dementia *297*
Rebecca Dresser

Autonomy in Long Term Care: Some Crucial
Distinctions *302*
Bart J. Collopy

Racism in Psychiatry: Paradigm Lost – Paradigm
Regained *308*
Dinesh Bhugra and Kamaldeep Bhui

Some Central Ideas in the 'Just Therapy'
Approach *313*
Charles Waldegrave and Kiwi Tamasese

7 Forensic Psychiatry *319*

The Parable of the Forensic Psychiatrist *325*
Paul S. Appelbaum

The Ethics of Forensic Psychiatry *330*
Alan A. Stone

A Theory of Ethics for Forensic
Psychiatry *336*
Paul S. Appelbaum

The Role of Traditional Medical Ethics in
Forensic Psychiatry *342*
*Robert Weinstock, Gregory B. Leong and
J. Arturo Silva*

Principles and Narrative in Forensic
Psychiatry: Toward a Robust View of
Professional Role *350*
*Philip J. Candilis, Richard Martinez,
and Christina Dording*

On Wearing Two Hats: Role Conflict in
Serving as Both Psychotherapist and Expert
Witness *354*
Larry H. Strasburger, Thomas G. Gutheil, and
Archie Brodsky

Ethical Issues Involved in the Dual Role of
Treater and Evaluator *360*
Robert D. Miller

The Ethical Dilemmas of Forensic
Psychiatry *369*
Seymour L. Halleck

The Moral Basis of the Insanity Defense *373*
Richard J. Bonnie

Forum – Psychiatrists and the Death Penalty:
Some Ethical Dilemmas *376*
Alfred M. Freedman, Abraham L. Halpern,
John Gunn, Lawrence Hartmann, Edmund
D. Pellegrino, Richard J. Bonnie, M. Gregg Bloche,
Paul S. Appelbaum, Marianne Kastrup, Ahmed
Okasha and Juan J. López-Ibor

8 Resource Allocation *385*

Two Wrongs Don't Make a Right *390*
M. Jellinek and B. Nurcombe

Rights to Health Care, Social Justice, and Fairness
in Health Care Allocations *393*
H. Tristram Engelhardt

Determining 'Medical Necessity' in Mental
Health Practice *398*
James E. Sabin and Norman Daniels

Caring About Patients and Caring
About Money *405*
James E. Sabin

Setting Mental Health Priorities *411*
Daniel Callahan

Minds and Hearts *417*
Philip J. Boyle and Daniel Callahan

Prioritization of Mental Health Services
in Oregon *431*
David A. Pollack, Bentson H. Mcfarland,
Robert A. George, and Richard H. Angell

9 Research *443*

The Nuremberg Statement *448*

Declaration of Helsinki *449*

Competency to Consent to Research *451*
Paul S. Appelbaum and Loren H. Roth

Decisional Capacity for Informed Consent
in Schizophrenia Research *458*
William T. Carpenter, Jr, James M. Gold,
Adrienne C. Lahti, Caleb A. Queern,
Robert R. Conley, John J. Bartko, Jeffrey Kovnick,
and Paul S. Appelbaum

Caring About Risks *463*
Carl Elliott

Informed Consent and the Capacity
for Voluntarism *466*
Laura Weiss Roberts

Placebo-Controlled Trials in Psychiatric
Research *472*
Franklin G. Miller

The Rationale and Ethics of Medication-Free
Research in Schizophrenia *478*
William T. Carpenter, Jr, Nina R. Schooler and
John M. Kane

Preventing Severe Mental Illnesses – New
Prospects and Ethical Challenges *484*
Kenneth F. Schaffner and Patrick D. McGorry

Index *491*

Preface

The origins of this volume can be traced back to 1977. At the international congress of the World Psychiatric Association held in Honolulu that year, the organization was buffeted by allegations that psychiatry had been abused for political purposes in the former Soviet Union. A resolution before the governing body of the WPA condemning such a flagrant violation of psychiatric ethics was passed by the narrowest of margins. Ironically, it was at the same congress that the first international code of ethics specifically formulated for psychiatrists was adopted—the Declaration of Hawaii. Paul Chodoff and Sidney Bloch, who were at the congress, did their utmost to ensure that the Soviet issue was not fudged as it had been at the WPA's previous international gathering in 1971 in Mexico City.

They also concluded that psychiatry was in need of moral consciousness-raising, and that a pivotal means to advance that objective would be to produce a book on psychiatric ethics. When they proceeded to examine the pertinent literature they were not at all surprised at how scanty it was – no books on the subject and very few articles and chapters of substance. It was as if the psychiatric profession had not recognized the need to focus on the ethical dimension of its practice. Chodoff and Bloch took it upon themselves to identify potential authors to a volume to fill the void. Thus it was that the first edition of *Psychiatric Ethics* was published in 1981. Over the next decade, the subject attracted considerably more attention. A second edition appeared in 1991. Although comprising a similar number of chapters, it would have been possible to double the length but it was decided that the volume be concise enough to attract a wide readership rather than become an occasionally used reference source. A similar policy was adopted when preparing the third edition in 1999; on this occasion the editors were joined by Stephen A. Green.

In the two decades since Chodoff and Bloch concluded that a text on psychiatric ethics was required for the field, the picture has altered radically. More and more psychiatrists and ethicists have contributed, both conceptually and empirically, to the literature. Indeed, ample evidence has accumulated to confirm that psychiatric ethics has come of age. Regular conferences on the subject have been held, ethical themes have often been incorporated into the programs of general psychiatry and subspecialty conferences, journal articles and book chapters have been published on diverse facets of the field, a new journal *Philosophy, Psychiatry and Psychology* has become an influential forum, and special interest groups in national psychiatric associations like the Royal College of Psychiatrists have been established. As we commented in our introduction to the third edition of *Psychiatric Ethics*: 'Psychiatric ethics has attained a firm place in the affairs of psychiatrists universally; its future is secure, and this prospect is a source of immense encouragement to those who see the subject as paramount for the ongoing welfare of the profession'.

The precise trigger for the birth of the idea for a specific anthology on the ethics of psychiatry was the invitation to Sidney Bloch to review an anthology of bioethics. To his astonishment, there were virtually no papers on mental health ethics among the several dozen selections. On perusing other anthologies in bioethics, similar neglect of this area was manifest. Indeed, it seemed as if the compilers were oblivious of the lively picture that we described earlier. On this occasion, it dawned upon Bloch and Green that

the need for a specific anthology on psychiatric ethics was timely. We therefore began to read the relevant literature and found to our pleasure that there was material of good quality to proceed. We were delighted when Oxford University Press, which had supported *Psychiatric Ethics* for over two decades, agreed that our proposal had merit.

Our purpose in launching this project has been to assemble published articles and chapters which facilitate the study of psychiatric ethics by mental health professionals, both trained and in training, so that our patients and their families will benefit from a hope for enhanced moral sensitivity and capacity to reach well reasoned ethical decisions. We opted for a selection procedure whose results would complement the third edition of *Psychiatric Ethics*. The twenty-four chapters in that text had been carefully mapped out over the years and represented, as far as we could ascertain, the central themes pertinent to psychiatric practice and research. Nine domains emerged from this exercise and these constitute the sections of our anthology. They are philosophical underpinnings, the therapeutic relationship and its social context, diagnosis, confidentiality, treatment and mental health services, special clinical populations, forensic psychiatry, resource allocation and research.

Our next task was to read the published literature in these areas. Our key objective in this exercise was to select articles and chapters (and occasionally excerpts from books) that stand out as landmarks in as much as they have contributed consequentially to the field. Criteria we have applied range from material that advances a thesis in an innovative way and provokes mental health professionals into thinking about critical aspects of their practice to contributions that promote discourse challenging the reader to deliberate about the issues involved.

The word anthology derives from the Greek *anthos*, meaning flower. We have been as diligent as we could possibly be in searching for the flowers in the field of psychiatric ethics. In so doing, we have sought material that achieves clarity of presentation, adds to our knowledge, is of value to students in their study of psychiatric ethics and is relevant to the practicing clinician. We have not always found 'good enough' contributions in terms of quality and originality. This reflects the need for further development in certain spheres. We may have missed the pearl although we have strived to avoid this by consulting with professional colleagues and searching all relevant databases.

The nine domains represent one 'cut'. Colleagues may prefer to divide the pie in other ways. Nonetheless, we hope that these areas are sufficiently delineated from one another and constitute the major areas of interest for the contemporary psychiatrist. We have prepared introductory essays for each domain. These are mainly in the form of an orientation, not a detailed review. If we were to review, we would be treading on ground already covered in our sister volume *Psychiatric Ethics*. We also use the introductions to identify the selections we have made, justify our judgments (in mostly implicit ways) and present a list of referenced readings that guides the reader to an appreciation of each domain.

We hope we have done justice to the particular areas of study. We anticipate that *An Anthology of Psychiatric Ethics* will, like *Psychiatric Ethics*, be a dynamic volume in the sense that future editions will be published, containing new material and, possibly, articles or chapters we may have overlooked. We ask the reader to bear this in mind, and advise us of any work that might merit inclusion in a new edition. We urge readers not to hesitate to let us know about their own publications.

Selection has proved an enormously unnerving task. Given that we are generalists with limited expertise in the subspecialties of psychiatry, we have consulted with colleagues throughout the world whom we would like to thank for their recommendations as well as their encouragement and support. We have valued the advice offered to us by mental health professionals and philosophers who have shared their knowledge of specific areas.

Paul Chodoff played a vital role as wise adviser in the early phase of our thinking about how to proceed and also read drafts of some of the introductions. Our gratitude to him knows no bounds. We also thank Tony Hope, Julian Hughes, Jennifer Radden, Gary Walter, George Halasz, Bill Fulford, Vikram Patel, Gwen Adshead, David Joseph, Allen Dyer, Franklin Miller, Sarah Romans, Paul Brodwin, John Sadler, Robert Simon, Robert Okin, Norman Daniels and Tom Beauchamp. Our task would have been immeasurably more difficult without the enthusiastic support of the librarians at the Kennedy Institute of Bioethics in Washington D.C., the Victorian Mental Health Library based at the Royal Melbourne Hospital and the medical library at St Vincent's Hospital in Melbourne. Our warmest thanks to all the staff who have helped us so assiduously.

We also wish to highlight the contribution of our postgraduate students who through their feedback over the years have helped us to identify useful teaching material. There is nothing better than an eager and curious student to challenge one to determine what sources are of value.

As we mentioned earlier, Oxford University Press has been outstanding in its support of the subject of psychiatric ethics. We were extremely encouraged on hearing their first response to our proposal for this volume and realized that we could not have approached a more suitable publisher. We thank Martin Baum and Carol Maxwell for their continuing support. We are most grateful to Catherine Roberts and Renee Best for their secretarial help–they were most patient with the many revisions.

We thank our respective families – Madeleine, Jessica, Julia, Felicity, Leah, David and Aaron – for their support and for their appreciation of the significance of the project itself.

Finally, we would like to repeat the tribute we made in the third edition of *Psychiatric Ethics* to our colleagues who have recognized that the ethical dimension of psychiatry is as critical as the science and the art of the discipline. Happily, psychiatric ethics has come into its own since the 1980's. We hope this anthology will promote its status even further.

Washington D.C. and Melbourne, April 2005   SG and SB

Acknowledgements

Chapter 1

Pellegrino, E.: The virtuous physician and the ethics of medicine, in *Virtue and Medicine*, ed. Earl Shelp. Dordrecht, Holland, D. Reidel Publishing, 1985, pp 237–255. Reprinted with permission from Springer and the author.

Arras, J.: Getting down to cases: the revival of casuistry in bioethics. *The Journal of Medicine and Philosophy* **16**:29–51, 1991. Reprinted with permission from Taylor & Francis.

Kant, I.: Grounding for the Metaphysics of Morals, in *Ethical Philosophy*, trans. James Ellington, Indianapolis, Hackett Publishing Company, 1983, pp 7–17; 19–27; 30–32; 40–41. Reprinted with permission from Hackett Publishing.

Mill, J.S.: *Utilitarianism, 2nd edn*, ed. G Sher. Indianapolis, Hackett Publishing Company, 2001, chs 1 & 2. Reprinted with permission from Hackett Publishing.

Beauchamp, T.: "The 'four principles' approach." In R. Gillon (ed.), *Principles of health care ethics*, Chichester, Wiley and Sons, 1994, pp 3–12. Reprinted with permission of John Wiley & Sons Ltd.

Carse, A.: The 'voice of care': implications for bioethical education. *Journal of Medicine and Philosophy* **16**:5–28, 1991. Reprinted with permission from Taylor & Francis.

Chapter 2

Freud, S.: The dynamics of the transference, in *The standard edition of the complete psychological works of Sigmund Freud* (Vol 12), ed. J. Strachey. London: Hogarth Press, 1958. (Original work published in 1912).

Epstein, R.S. & Simon, R.I.: The exploitation index: an early warning indicator of boundary violations in psychotherapy. *Bulletin of the Menninger Clinic* **54**: 450–465, 1990.

Gutheil, T.H. & Gabbard, G.O.: The concept of boundaries in clinical practice: theoretical and risk management dimensions. *American Journal of Psychiatry* **150**:188–196, 1993. Reprinted with permission from the American Journal of Psychiatry, Copyright 1993. American Psychiatric Association.

Gabbard, G.O.: Psychotherapists who transgress sexual boundaries with patients. *Bulletin of the Menninger Clinic* **58**:124–135, 1994.

In the service of the state: the psychiatrist as double agent. *Hastings Center Reports, Special Supplement*, April 1978, S1–23. Reprinted with permission from the Hastings Center.

Callahan, D. & Gaylin, W.: The psychiatrist as double agent. *Hastings Center Reports* **4**:12–14, 1974. Reprinted with permission from the Hastings Center and the author

Chodoff, P.: The effect of third-party payment on the practice of psychotherapy. *American Journal of Psychiatry* **129**:540–545, 1972. Reprinted with permission from the American Journal of Psychiatry, copyright 1972. American Psychiatric Association.

Chapter 3

Kaplan, M.: A woman's view of DSM-III. *American Psychologist* **38**:786–792, 1983.

Szasz, T.: The myth of mental illness. *American Psychologist* **15**:113–118, 1960. Copyright © 1960 by the American Psychological Association. Reprinted with permission.

Boorse, C.: What a theory of mental health should be. *Journal for the Theory of Social Behavior* **6**:61–84, 1976. Reprinted with permission from Blackwell Publishing.

Stoller, R. et al.: A symposium: should homosexuality be in the APA nomenclature. *American Journal of Psychiatry* **130**:1207–1216, 1973. Reprinted with permission from the American Journal of Psychiatry, copyright 1973. American Psychiatric Association

Rosenhan, D.: On being sane in insane places. *Science* **179**:250–258, 1973.

Wakefield, J.: The concept of mental disorder: on the boundary between biological facts and social values. *American Psychologist* **47**:373–388, 1992. Copyright © 1992 by the American Psychological Association. Reprinted with permission.

Kendler, K.: A psychiatric dialogue on the mind-body problem. *American Journal of Psychiatry* **158**:989–1000, 2001. Reprinted with permission from the American Journal of Psychiatry, copyright © 2001. American Psychiatric Association.

Chapter 4

Bok, S.: *Secrets: on the ethics of concealment and revelation*. Oxford, Oxford University Press, 1996, pp 116–135. Copyright © 1982 by Sissela Bok. Reprinted with permission from Pantheon Books, a division of Random House, Inc.

Black, D.: Absolute confidentiality, in *Principles of health care ethics*, ed. R. Gillon. Chichester, Wiley, 1994, pp 479–488. Reprinted with permission from John Wiley & Sons Ltd.

Tarasoff v. Regents of the University of California. 131 Cal Rptr 14, 17 Cal. 3d 425, 551P. 2d 334, 1976.

Szmukler, G. and Bloch, S.: Family involvement in the care of people with psychoses. *British Journal of Psychiatry* **171**:401–405, 1997. Reprinted with permission.

Pellegrino, E.: Secrets of the couch and the grave: the Anne Sexton case. *Cambridge Quarterly of Healthcare Ethics* **5**:189–203, 1996.

Chapter 5

Chodoff, P.: Involuntary hospitalisation of the mentally ill as a moral issue. *American Journal of Psychiatry* **141**:384–389, 1984. Reprinted with permission from the American Journal of Psychiatry, copyright © 1984. American Psychiatric Association.

Szasz, T.: The case against suicide prevention. *American Psychologist* **41**:806–812, 1986. Copyright © 1986 by the American Psychological Association. Reprinted with permission.

Van Staden, C. and Kruger, C. Incapacity to give informed consent owing to mental disorder. *Journal of Medical Ethics* **29**:41–43, 2003. Reprinted with permission from the BMJ Publishing Group.

Munetz, M., Galon, P. and Frese, F.: The ethics of mandatory community treatment. *Journal of the American Academy of Psychiatry and the Law* **31**:173–183, 2003. © American Academy of Psychiatry and the Law. Reprinted with permission.

Donaldson v O'Connor, F.2d 5th Cir, decided Apr. 26, 1974,*O'Connor v Donaldson 422US. 563, 1975.

Klerman, G.: The psychiatric patient's right to effective treatment: Implications of Osheroff v Chestnut Lodge. *American Journal of Psychiatry* **147**:419–427, 1990. Reprinted with permission from the American Journal of Psychiatry, Copyright 1990. American Psychiatric Association.

Stone, A.: Law, Science, and psychiatric malpractice: A response to Klerman's indictment on psychoanalytic psychiatry. *American Journal of Psychiatry* **147**:419–427, 1990. Reprinted with permission from the American Journal of Psychiatry, Copyright 1990. American Psychiatric Association.

Henderson, C., Flood, C., Leese, M., Thornicroft, G., Sutherby, K. and Szmukler, G. Effect of joint crisis plans on the use of compulsory treatment in psychiatry: single blind randomized controlled trial. *British Medical Journal* **329**:136–138, 2004. Reprinted with permission from the BMJ Publishing Group.

Jensen, P. Ethical and pragmatic issues in the use of psychotropic agents in young children. *Canadian Journal of Psychiatry* **43**:585–88, 1998. Reprinted with permission.

Fisher, R. L. and Fisher, S.: Antidepressants for children. Is scientific support necessary? *Journal of Nervous and Mental Disease* **184**:99–102, 1996.

Kramer, P. The valorisation of sadness. *Hastings Center Report* **30**:13–18, 2000. Copyright the Hastings Center. Reprinted with permission.

Elliott, C. Pursued by happiness and beaten senseless. *Hastings Center Report* **30**: 7–12, 2000. Copyright the Hastings Center. Reprinted with permission.

Ottosson, J-O. Ethical aspects of research and practice of ECT. *Convulsive Therapy* **11**:288–299, 1995. Reprinted with permission from Lippincott Williams & Wilkins.

Holmes, J. Values in psychotherapy. *American Journal of Psychotherapy* **50**:259–273, 1996.

Erikson, E. Psychoanalysis and ethics-avowed and unavowed. *International Review of Psychoanalysis* **3**:409–15, 1976. Reprinted with permission from the *International Review of Psychoanalysis*.

Lifton, R. J. Advocacy and corruption in the healing professions. *International Review of Psychoanalysis* **3**:385–98, 1976. © Institute of Psychoanalysis, London, UK. Reprinted with permission.

Bergin, A. Psychotherapy and religious values. *Journal of Consulting and Clinical Psychology* **48**:95–105, 1980. Copyright © 1992 by the American Psychological Association. Reprinted with permission.

Aponte, H. J. The negotiation of values in therapy. *Family Process* **24**:323–338, 1985. Reprinted with permission from Blackwell Publishing.

Chapter 6

Pearce, J. Consent to treatment during childhood. The assessment of competence and avoidance of conflict. *British Journal of Psychiatry* **165**:713–716, 1994. Reprinted with permission from the Royal College of Psychiatrists.

Dworkin, R. Autonomy and the demented self. *Milbank Quarterly* **64**:4–16, 1986. Reprinted with permission from the Milbank Memorial Fund.

Dresser, R. Dworkin on dementia: Elegant theory, questionable policy. *Hastings Center Report* **25**:32–38, 1995. © The Hastings Center. Reprinted with permission.

Collopy, B. Autonomy in long term care: Some crucial distinctions. *Gerontologist.* **28**:10–17, 1988. Reprinted with permission.

Bhugra, D. and Bhui, K. Racism in psychiatry: paradigm lost – paradigm regained. *International Review of Psychiatry* **11**:236–243, 1999. Reprinted with kind permission of Professor Dinesh Bhugra.

Waldegrave C. and Tamasese, K. Some central ideas in the "Just Therapy" approach. *Australian and New Zealand Journal of Family Therapy* **14**:1–8, 1993. Reprinted with permission from the Australian and New Zealand Journal of Family Therapy.

Chapter 7

Appelbaum, P.: The parable of the forensic psychiatrist: ethics and the problem of doing harm. *International Journal of Law and Psychiatry* **13**:249–259, 1990. © 1990, reprinted with permission from Elsevier.

Stone, A.: The ethics of forensic psychiatry: a view from the ivory tower, in *Law, Psychiatry and Morality*. Washington, D.C., American Psychiatric Press, Inc., 1984, pp 57–75. Reprinted with permission from the American Psychiatric Association.

Appelbaum, P.: A theory of ethics for forensic psychiatry. *Journal of the Academy of Psychiatry and Law* **25**:233–247, 1997. Reprinted with permission.

Weinstock, R., Leong, G. and Silva, J.: The role of traditional medical ethics in forensic psychiatry, in *Ethical practice in psychiatry and the law*, eds. R. Rosner & R. Weinstock. New York, Plenum Press, 1990, pp 31–51. Reprinted with permission from Springer NL.

Candilis, P., Martinez, R. and Dording, C.: Principles and narrative in forensic psychiatry: towards a robust view of professional role. *Journal of the American Academy of Psychiatry and the Law* **29**:167–173, 2001. © American Academy of Psychiatry and the Law. Reprinted with permission.

Strasburger, L., Gutheil, T. and Brodsky, A.: On wearing two hats: role conflict in serving as both psychotherapist and expert witness. *American Journal of Psychiatry* **154**:448–456, 1997. Reprinted with permission from the American Journal of Psychiatry, copyright 1997. American Psychiatric Association.

Miller, R.D.: Ethical issues involved in the dual role of treater and evaluator, in *Ethical practice in psychiatry and the law*, eds. R. Rosner and R. Weinstock. New York, Plenum Press, 1990, pp 129–150. Reprinted with permission from Springer NL.

Halleck, S.: The ethical dilemmas of forensic psychiatry: a utilitarian approach. *Bulletin of the American Academy of Psychiatry and Law* **12**:279–288, 1984. © American Academy of Psychiatry and the Law. Reprinted with permission.

Bonnie, R.: The moral basis of the insanity defense. *American Bar Association Journal* **69**:194–197, 1983. Reprinted with permission.

Freedman, A. and Halpern, A.: A crisis in the ethical and moral behaviours of psychiatrist. *Current Opinion in Psychiatry* **11**:1–2, 1998. Reprinted with permission from Lippincott williams & Wilkins.

Chapter 8

Jellinek, M. and Nurcombe, B.: Two wrongs don't make a right: managed care, mental health, and the marketplace. *Journal of the American Medical Association* **14**:1737–9, 1993. Reprinted with permission from the American Medical Association.

Engelhardt, H. T.: "Rights to health care, social justice, and fairness in health care allocations: frustrations in the face of finitude" in *The foundation of bioethics 2edn*. New York, NY, Oxford University Press, 1996, pp 376–387. Reprinted with permission of Oxford University Press Inc.

Sabin, J. and Daniels, N.: Determining "medical necessity" in mental health practice. *Hastings Center Report* **24**(6):5–13, 1994. © The Hastings Center. Reprinted with permission.

Sabin, J.: Caring about patients and caring about money: the American Psychiatric Association Code of Ethics meets managed care. *Behavioural Sciences and the Law* **12**:317–330, 1994. Reprinted with permission from John Wiley & Sons Ltd.

Callahan, D.: Setting mental health priorities: problems and possibilities. *Milbank Quarterly* **72**:451–470, 1994. Reprinted with permission from the Milbank Memorial Fund.

Boyle, P. and Callahan, D.: Mind and hearts: priorities in mental health services. *Special supplement, Hastings Center Report* **23**:S1–S23, 1993. © The Hastings Center. Reprinted with permission.

Pollack, D., McFarland, B., George, R. and Angell, R.: Prioritization of mental health services in Oregon. *Milbank Quarterly* **72**:515–551, 1994. Reprinted with permission from the Milbank Memorial Fund.

Chapter 9

The Nuremberg Statement. Appendix, in Psychiatric Ethics, *3rd edn*, ed. Bloch, S., Chodoff, P. and Green, S. Oxford, Oxford University Press, 1999, pp 512–514. With permission from Oxford University Press.

The Declaration of Helsinki. Appendix, in *Psychiatric Ethics, 3rd edn.* ed. Bloch, S., Chodoff, P. and Green, S. Oxford, Oxford University Press, 1999, pp 514–517. With permission from Oxford University Press.

Appelbaum, P. and Roth, L.: Competency to consent to research: a psychiatric overview. *Archives of General Psychiatry* **39**:951–958, 1982. Reprinted with permission from the American Medical Association.

Carpenter, W., Gold, J., Lahti, A., Queern, C., Conley, R., Bartko, J., Kovnick, J. and Appelbaum, P.: Decisional capacity for informed consent in schizophrenia research. *Archives of General Psychiatry* **57**:533–538, 2000. Reprinted with permission from the American Medical Association.

Elliot, C. Caring about risks. Are severely depressed patients competent to consent to research? *Archives of General Psychiatry* **54**:113–116, 1997. Reprinted with permission from the American Medical Association.

Roberts, L.: Informed consent and the capacity for voluntarism. *American Journal of Psychiatry* **159**:705–712, 2002. Reprinted with permission from the American Journal of Psychiatry, copyright 2002. American Psychiatric Association.

Miller, F.: Placebo-controlled trials in psychiatric research: an ethical perspective. *Biological Psychiatry* **47**:707–716, 2000. Reprinted with permission of the Society of Biological Psychiatry.

Carpenter, W., Schooler, N. and Kane J.: The rationale and ethics of medication-free research in schizophrenia. *Archives of General Psychiatry* **54**: 401–407, 1997. Reprinted with permission from the American Medical Association.

Schaffner, K. and McGorry, P.: Preventing severe mental illnesses – new prospects and ethical challenges. *Schizophrenia Research* **51**:3–15, 2001. Copyright 2001. Reprinted with permission from Elsevier.

1 Theoretical foundations

Introduction

Moral decision-making is concerned with analysis of human conduct regarding right and wrong actions. Moral theories formulate presumed judgments about right and wrong in an attempt to facilitate objective application of those precepts to particular circumstances and thereby guard against inconsistency and relativism. The primary goal of this section is to provide an understanding of the various theories utilized in the broader context of bioethics as preparation for applying them to the ethical dilemmas arising in psychiatric practice and research that are explored in this volume.

The inherent complexity of matters subject to moral deliberation suggests that resolution by a single theoretical approach is unlikely. To illustrate this point consider physician-assisted suicide. It is not hard to imagine that different practitioners and varied clinical circumstances might yield reasonable, though contradictory, judgments as to whether or not assisted suicide is ethically justified. Opponents might invoke a core obligation to 'do no harm' as an absolute prohibition against promoting a patient's death, whereas proponents might invoke a similar justification, claiming that they would be imposing harm if they failed to end a patient's unremitting pain. Respect for autonomy is another widely held principle for responding to a person's request for assisted suicide, while the same principle supports the belief that physicians should never act to deprive autonomous human beings of their life. Yet another line of moral reasoning, based on consequences, may proscribe physician-assisted suicide because a 'slippery slope' is inevitable, and may culminate in policies like the Nazi euthanasia project in which 70,000 chronically mentally ill people were gassed to death.[1] On the other hand, a consequential argument can also embrace the notion that a greater benefit will ensue for patients suffering unbearable pain if their wish to hasten death is honoured. This moral debate may also revolve around character, in that promoting death involves a trait some consider inconsistent with an ethical doctor, though others may see it as a virtuous course given the degree of a patient's suffering.

Moral decision-making, then, is grounded in an amalgam of obligations, rights, virtues and consequences, in conjunction with other values, such as religious convictions, communitarian concerns and the caring dimension of relationships. Analysis of clinical situations from these varied perspectives helps guide psychiatrists towards ethically sound judgments. This section discusses a range of moral theories, an overview that suggests they are more complementary than mutually exclusive, and that some approaches may be especially relevant to psychiatry.

Virtue ethics

Virtue theory emerged from a Greek philosophical tradition and is most closely identified with Aristotle.[2] A person's character is regarded as the core feature of moral deliberation. The prerequisite to living an ethical life is, therefore, to develop character traits that promote virtuous behaviour. People manifest their own goodness in this way and, through relationships with members of society, advance a common morality. Aristotle's catalogue of virtues, reflecting his conception of proper conduct (as practiced by the male Athenian aristocracy) ranged from magnanimity, agreeableness and friendship to scientific knowledge, prudence, technical skill and wisdom.

Aristotelian theory is teleological – concerned with achieving the *good* towards which things move. To strive for *telos* (the Greek word for end) is to pursue virtue. Aristotle held that the end towards which human beings move was intelligence; pursuit of reason was the most elevated virtue. He was not, however, referring only to the intellectual wisdom that derives from teaching, but also of *phronesis*, or practical wisdom, which results from habit and training and serves as the basis of moral virtue. For Aristotle study and experience informed people about which ends should be defined as good, whereas *phronesis* was achieved by pursuing those ends continually. The virtuous person thus cultivates such right motives as honesty, courage, faithfulness, integrity and trustworthiness, in order to pursue the correct course in particular situations. One *develops* morally by acquiring an increasingly habitual correct motivation that leads to virtue, a state of character 'that makes a human being good and makes him perform his function well' (2, 1106a, 23–25).

Aristotelian theory exerted an influence on ethical thinking during the Middle Ages. The Thomastic philosophy of Aquinas combined theological belief with virtue ethics, and valued *phronesis* over the intellectual understanding of good and evil. Aquinas viewed human acts as teological, and believed that the good for man was fulfilment of activities peculiar to humans. Guidelines of good and evil which no one could fail to know were inherent in human nature. Actions of the type known to be good were the product of character; repeatedly performing these acts produced good character.

Aristotelian ethics, in modern times, is championed by Alasdair MacIntyre, who avers that virtue-grounded moral deliberation is the only approach that has retained relevance and legitimacy over the course of history.[3] Pursuit of virtue promotes the right and good in 'any coherent and complex form of socially established cooperative human activity,' which he terms a 'practice,' regardless of its historical context. He defines virtue as 'an acquired human quality the possession and exercise of which tends to enable us to achieve those goods which are internal to practices', such as the medical profession, by attaining excellence in our work.[4]

This Aristotelian perspective is applied to the modern medical setting by Edmond Pellegrino.[5] In the selection 'The virtuous physician, and the ethics of medicine,' he describes the virtuous doctor as one inclined to promote the good of the patient and to hold that good above his own good. Reiterating the precepts of virtue theory, namely that virtues are habits enabling one to reason well and act in accordance with right reason, Pellegrino argues for its primacy over approaches governed by rules. He views the latter as 'too abstract, too rationalistic, and too removed from the psychological milieu in which moral choices are actually made' in that they 'ignore a person's character, life story, cultural background, and gender'. Moreover, he asserts that despite rules duties ultimately 'turn on the disposition and character traits' of the doctor since decisions affecting patients are always filtered through the individual practitioner.

One appeal of virtue theory is its powerful link to an ancient ethos that is more than merely traditional. McCullough,[6] for example, highlights how widespread attention to virtues in the care of patients has typified the evolution of modern Western medicine. This is evident in the continuing influence of the Oath of Hippocrates,[7] such as its applicability to confidentiality and relationship boundaries between patient and physician. Virtue theory also appeals by regarding a place for emotions in moral deliberation, thereby emphasizing human relating in the ethical life. Morality is, after all, concerned with the interpersonal, yet this can be easily overlooked when rules dominate ethical theory. For example, a moral obligation never to lie could justify revealing the whereabouts of a friend to an assassin, resulting in a wrongful death. Virtue theory helps to circumvent an absolutist application of rules that may generate such counterintuitive results. Advocates of virtue theory believe its benefits render it particularly relevant to such issues as micro- and macro-allocation of mental health care resources (see Chapter 8), conducting research on psychiatric patients (see Chapter 9) and as a guiding ethic of the psychotherapeutic relationship (see Chapter 2).

Criticisms of virtue theory centre around the requirement that it be linked to a disposition to habitually do good. Although articulating the nature of that good has spanned centuries of philosophical debate, no consensus prevails regarding the attributes essential to become a virtuous person. Can the good be determined according to a person's idiosyncratic interests? Undoubtedly we all have a personal conception of virtue, but is it a concern that virtue may not have a distinctive meaning? Veatch[8] notes that in the realm of medicine a 'variety of conceivably professional and lay roles testifies against the existence of a unique set of character traits which we could call *the* virtue of medicine'. If the conception of the good is so elusive guidelines may be required to set a minimum ethical standard, which, in turn, may blur boundaries between virtue and rule-based theories.

Another objection to virtue theory is reflected in the dialogue written centuries ago by Plato when he has Meno pose the key question of Socrates: 'Can you tell me Socrates – is virtue something that can be taught? Or does it come by practice? Or is it neither teaching nor practice that gives it to a man but natural aptitude or something else?'[9] Plato's question remains definitively unanswered although many attempts have been made. Pellegrino,[5] for instance, describes virtue as 'a character trait, an internal disposition, habitually to seek moral perfection, to live one's life in accord with the moral law, and to attain balance between noble intention and just action'. From a psychoanalytic perspective, pursuit of the 'ego ideal' may facilitate moral development, but certainly cannot guarantee it. Whether one needs a core nature to cultivate virtue remains an open question, and one that has implications for the applicability of virtue theory.

Casuistry

Casuistry, as described in the selection by Arras[10] 'Getting down to cases: the revival of casuistry in bioethics,' is concerned with the appraisal of individual cases in order to resolve questions of right or wrong. Its roots extend back to Greek philosophy, as reflected in the Sophists' contention that moral matters depend on the analysis of particular circumstances, and on the Aristotelian concept of *phronesis*, namely the application of practical wisdom in specific situations. Casuistry is most closely identified with religious dogma of the Middle Ages, as embodied in the practice of determining punishment for particular sins. In numerous volumes thinkers like Thomas Aquinas and William of Ockham catalogued moral behaviours and penitential guidelines appropriate to the seriousness of offences committed. The approach was continued by the Jesuits who critically teased out moral issues and formulated guidelines of proper conduct.

Casuistry is a 'bottom-up' process that contrasts markedly with the 'top-down' quality of rule-based theory where general guidelines are applied to particular situations. Casuistry stands more as a method of *how* to conduct

moral deliberation, than as an ethical theory, as revealed in Jonsen's account of the casuistic approach:

> . . . The interpretation of moral issues, using procedures of reasoning based on paradigms and analogies, leading to the formulation of expert opinion about the existence and stringency of particular moral obligations, framed in terms of rules or maxims that are general but not universal or invariable, since they hold good with certainty only in typical conditions of the agent and circumstances of action.[11]

Jonsen proceeds to explicate three interrelated features of casuistry: morphology, taxonomy and kinetics. Morphology refers to the form of a case, as determined by its circumstances, the rules that usually prevail in that situation, and the ethical arguments traditionally applied in that type of case. For example, when requested to withdraw life support in a terminally ill patient, the clinician reflects on a body of similar cases and standards against which decision-making can be refined. Taxonomy refers to placing cases along a spectrum, according to the strength of their association, in order to facilitate comparison of a specific case against established paradigms. Aggregating cases in this manner of 'family resemblance' can clarify ethical analysis. For example, in end of life situations noted above, classification focuses consideration of the issues of withholding versus withdrawing treatment, physician-assisted suicide and euthanasia. By grouping issues accordingly, ethical deliberation is expedited and pragmatic outcomes are derived. Finally, kinetics refers to the impact of a particular case on others in a way that shifts moral perspective. This has clearly been at play in right-to-die cases, where a growing influence of respect for autonomy has advanced societal values towards accepting physician-assisted suicide and, in a few jurisdictions, legalized euthanasia.

Casuistry and case law are similar in that each uses past judgments to resolve current, related questions. The analogy highlights an issue contested among advocates of casuistry, namely, the degree to which theoretical principles should influence consideration of a particular case. Legal debate is undoubtedly affected by overarching doctrine, such as guarantees of a Constitution (e.g., freedom of speech), which influences analysis of a particular issue across a series of related cases. Many casuists hold that similarly established ethical principles have a normative effect and that paradigmatic cases serve as contexts within which to explicate the principle. Relevance of this position to the practice of forensic psychiatry is discussed in Chapter 7. However, more radical casuists reject this argument by maintaining that principles are too abstract to provide reality-based cases with normative force.

An advantage of casuistry is its practicality, in that it allows debate of mid-level ethical principles (e.g., informed consent) in the framework of a specific case, in contrast to requiring that a distinctive, often complex, clinical situation conform to a more demanding high-level principle (e.g., respect for autonomy). This pragmatism is relevant to medical ethics, which requires discretionary judgments about a particular patient resulting from the confluence of his unique biopsychosocial background, a specific medical state, and the binding power of an applicable ethical principle. The approach is well suited to psychiatry. For example, as discussed in Chapter 4, confidentiality is not absolute, but often depends on assessing a family's needs to know if a relative is a serious threat to himself or others.

The criticisms of casuistry are threefold. First, since case-based analysis begins with debate about a current belief or practice, it risks undue influence from a social context that might support unethical practices. Indeed, casuistry's decline in the seventeenth century largely resulted from consideration of hypothetical situations that often produced guidelines absolving the influential few from recognized wrongs, a practice that fostered widespread criticism of the Church. A second, related objection is the narrow scope of casuistry compared to ethical theory. If moral deliberation is confined to specific cases the potential to explore larger issues, like the euthanasia policies of Nazi Germany, is sharply curtailed. Third, casuistry is considered ill suited to the pluralistic values inherent in contemporary society. Whereas case law yields legal precedent, case-based moral deliberation does not establish an analogous moral authority. Rather, it often reflects conflicting ethical orientations of different groups. For example, abortion is justified by some on the basis of a woman's autonomous right to choose and condemned by others as taking an innocent life, two positions that have produced a raging social debate that underscores casuistry's limitations for moral consensus-building.

Deontological theory

The limitations of casuistry, combined with the growing intellectualism of the Enlightenment, spurred pursuit of alternative modes of moral deliberation. Deontological theory, which emerged during the eighteenth century, grounds ethical decision-making in a framework of duty. ('Deontology' is derived from the Greek *deon*, a necessary obligation.) The theory holds that the right action is justified by a person's intrinsic values, such as motivation, in contrast to an extrinsic value, like the results of a judgment. Deontological theory claims that one must do the morally right thing in and of itself (e.g., tell the truth) and not because of some other reason (e.g., lying might bring about negative consequences). The mainstay of deontological theory is the requirement that the motive for any action is the genuine moral obligation of an individual, which then qualifies that person as possessing 'good will'.

Deontological theory evolved from the work of the German moral philosopher Immanuel Kant (1724–1804), whose rule-oriented approach is based on the rational determination of universal moral principles. His overriding canon, the categorical imperative, is a conception of a moral obligation that is universalizable, as discussed in the selection from his 'Grounding for the metaphysics of morals'.[12] Kant expresses the categorical imperative as follows: 'I ought never to act except in such a way that I can also will that my maxim should become a universal law.' The principle is categorical in that it is absolutely binding and establishes what is right and wrong by virtue of its generalized effect. For example, a universal rule that endorsed lying would be incongruous with moral obligation as it would undermine legitimate interaction among members of a society by negating the value of truth-telling. Another formulation of the categorical imperative concerns the principle of respect for autonomy. By directing that '[o]ne must act to treat every person as an end and never as a means only', Kant posits that moral relationships are grounded in the respect people hold for others' autonomous goals, and in the dignity they show one another.

Kantian theory embraces pure reason as the sole basis for determining moral rules. Intuition, consideration of the consequences of moral action, or convictions of conscience may promote ethically correct judgments, but they do not provide their moral justification. That rests in autonomous will derived from rationally formulated principles that apply to human beings regardless of their individual interests.

An appeal of deontological theory is the clarity and consistency it purportedly brings to moral deliberation. A categorical imperative, once established, is always and absolutely binding, and its application to a given circumstance indicates adherence to the imperative in similar circumstances. This seemingly is a highly valued approach for defining ethical guidelines of psychiatric practice. However, as illustrated by most sections of this volume, the absolutist feature of a categorical imperative is also a shortcoming, since it prevents nuanced determinations required in many interactions with patients. For example, if it is never acceptable to abridge the autonomy of a patient, how does the clinician respond to psychotically driven behaviours, including suicidal or homicidal actions?

A second, basic difficulty with deontological theory is the notion that pure reason can actually yield universally binding moral maxims. Formulating a rule applicable to *all* situations may be more problematic than acknowledged, as illustrated by factors that may override a maxim advocating absolute respect for autonomy when conducting psychiatric research (see Chapter 9) or making determinations concerning the degree of confidentiality that should be afforded some patients with serious mental and/or substance abuse disorders. (see Chapter 4).

A third criticism is the dilemma of resolving conflicting moral obligations. Consider a patient with advanced cancer who has informed her doctor that she does not wish to know the truth about her state as it would cause her unbearable distress. How does the clinician obligated to not causing harm *and* to truth-telling determine the ethically correct response? If it is *always* morally imperative to do no harm *and* to tell the truth, the physician is trapped in a moral dilemma that seems irresolvable by deontological theory. W. D. Ross[13] responded to this criticism by proposing a means to deal with pluralist values within a deontological framework. In *The right and the good* he argues that moral reasoning often requires a determination as to the most pressing among conflictual obligations in order to establish the most compelling balance of right over wrong. To accomplish this task Ross introduced the concept of *prima facie* duty, one that is always right and binding all other things being equal. *Prima facie* obligations are therefore not absolute, but responsive to circumstance. For example, lying to the hypothetical patient is a *prima facie* wrong, unless the doctor believes more moral weight should be given to protecting the patient from distress through withholding the truth. In this situation of two competing *prima facie* obligations, reasoning about one's ethical duty determines what Ross considers to be an *actual duty*, the moral obligation considered the most binding. Ross thus challenges the notion of absolutism of a moral rule. His method has been embraced for its pragmatism, but criticized for its vulnerability to subjectivity. However, as noted in Chapter 8, deontological theory can incorporate objective ordering of obligations, as illustrated by John Rawls's principles of justice.[14]

Utilitarianism

First espoused by Jeremy Bentham (1748–1832), utilitarianism was refined in the latter part of the eighteenth century by John Stuart Mill, who argued that the primary purpose of morality is to promote the harmony desired by human beings via conduct that secures 'the agent's own happiness and that of all concerned'. Utilitarianism's basic tenet is consequentialism, the belief that an act is morally right if, when compared to alternative acts, it produces the greatest possible balance of good consequences or the least possible balance of bad consequences – that is, the greatest happiness. The intrinsic value of an action is morally irrelevant since right and wrong conduct is solely dependent on consequences. For example, a law that benefits the many while depriving a few is morally right since it promotes human welfare by maximizing benefits and minimizing harms. Consideration of other criteria to determine right and wrong, such as obligations of duty or individual rights, are secondary. These points are expounded by Mill in the selected excerpt from his book *Utilitarianism*.[15]

Utilitarianism revolves around the Principle of Utility, which holds that the degree of happiness and pain caused by an action determines its moral value. The principle is absolute. For instance, it can justify breaching confidentiality when a patient threatens a specific person, as in the *Tarasoff* judgments[16] (see Chapter 4) or lying to a patient with a grave prognosis in order to spare anguish.[17] Another feature of this ethical theory, flowing directly from the Principle of Utility, is the task of weighing benefit against harm as part of understanding what does and does not constitute a benefit or good. A third feature is impartiality, that is, maintaining a perspective that regards all relevant parties in an unbiased, non-partisan way. Each calculation of benefits and harms must afford equal attention to the preferences of every individual and group of individuals affected by that determination. (These basic aspects of Utilitarianism are explicated by Scheffler.)[18]

At least four criticisms can be levelled against utilitarianism. First, determining what is a benefit or harm is obviously a difficult task, and one that has divided proponents of this moral theory. Some define a benefit solely in terms of happiness and pleasure, whereas others argue for a pluralist approach that aggregates diverse values, such as intelligence and friendship. Yet another group believes the 'good' is accomplished by satisfying personal preferences. How to accommodate these different conceptions highlights a key limitation of utilitarianism. Similarly, given the pluralist nature of society, impartiality may be an ideal rather than a useful goal. The values of underrepresented groups, such as the socio-economically deprived, are often neglected in a formula that favours the goals of certain groups at the expense of others. One has only to reflect on how the efficiency arguments of managed care organizations affect certain patients, such as the chronically mentally ill, to appreciate the elusiveness of impartiality. Chapter 8 further explores the issue when describing how the utilitarian conception of justice affects the distribution of health care resources.

Third, utilitarian theory can make excessive demands on individuals. If the balance of happiness and pain determines an action's moral value, utilitarianism can be faulted for pressing people to pursue inordinate good, a demand that could segue into an expectation of supererogatory behaviour associated with exceptional altruism. A fourth criticism concerns the principle of utility and autonomy. Maximizing the ratio of benefits to harms may force an individual to act in a way inconsistent with his personal beliefs and, as discussed by Williams,[19] result in his integrity being undermined. If, for example, utilitarianism stipulates that physician-assisted suicide maximizes utility by relieving suffering as well as conserving medical resources, physicians would be expected to comply with that policy even if they believed strongly in the sanctity of life.

Principle-based ethics (Principlism)

Criticism of utilitarianism and the deontological approach suggests a need to refine these theories in order to make them relevant to contemporary bioethics, including psychiatric ethics. Because medicine is increasingly challenged by complex issues that call for sophisticated analysis (e.g., repercussions of genomic research for the diagnosis and treatment of illness), ethical theories constrained by universal rules may not be sufficient. Moreover, utilitarianism and deontological theory are so divergent they each challenge the other's legitimacy, fostering a scepticism that binding principles may 'obscure the nature of moral thinking rather than illuminate it'.[20] Because duty and utility may be mutually exclusive, an appeal to universal rules may aggravate, rather than facilitate, moral debate. The *Tarasoff* decision[16] illustrates the point. The court espoused a utilitarian view whereas a dissenting opinion argued that the decisions jeopardized professionals' obligation to fidelity and, correspondingly, patients' trust in the privacy of the psychotherapeutic relationship. One response is to link moral decision-making to principles that are subject to modification (e.g., in the face of new scientific data); principle-based ethics seeks to achieve this goal.

As noted at the outset, an ethical theory is a comprehensive, coherent formulation of presumed moral judgments with specific guidelines to apply those judgments to particular circumstances. Principle-based ethics, as described by its leading proponents Beauchamp and Childress,[21] does not satisfy these criteria. Rather, it stands as 'an analytic framework' through which moral problems in general, and bioethical problems in particular, can be identified and reflected upon. Principlism is based in the belief that widely held ethical principles, too general to address the particulars of diverse circumstances, provide a starting point for moral judgment in tandem with input pertinent to a particular issue, such as established health policy. The synthesis of general principles and other such guiding information permits moral deliberation well suited to bioethics. The result is principlism's current pre-eminent status in bioethics, and the widespread application of its quartet of principles – nonmaleficence, beneficence, respect for autonomy, and justice-explicated in the selection, 'The four-principles approach'.[22]

Nonmaleficence has its roots in the Hippocratic directive *primum non nocere* – 'First, do no harm'. Intentionally or inadvertently causing harm is a moral wrong justifying the restriction of certain actions. This has been embodied in a variety of rules (and codes) in medicine, like not inflicting unnecessary pain, not killing patients, not exploiting them, not undermining the pledge of fidelity, not withholding information and not lying.

Beneficence, also derived from the Hippocratic tradition, entails the advancement of a person's interests and/or protecting them from harm and suffering. Beneficent care involves promoting the health of patients by preventing, treating and (hopefully) curing illness. The activity may require a measure of paternalism, a reflection of the doctor's concern that stops short of compromising the patient's own decision-making.

Respect for autonomy stems from one aspect of the Kantian categorical imperative, namely that people should be regarded as ends and not solely as means. The principle is grounded in the acceptance that we all espouse personal values and beliefs that motivate our life choices. As a corollary, people are granted control over their own decision-making in order to seek those personal ends. Infringing autonomy may be justified in specific clinical situations, as when a patient shows significant deficits in mental capacity. In general, however, respect for autonomy commands enormous power in contemporary medicine, in large measure a legacy of social movements of the 1960s.

The principle of justice generally refers to fair treatment of individuals as established by conventions and normative social values. A person is treated justly if afforded the guarantees due to all members of society, such as political rights, and treated unjustly if denied what he is owed in that regard. Distributive justice, which has a related but more limited meaning, refers to the fair allocation of social benefits (e.g., health care resources) and burdens (e.g., taxes). Justice has become an increasingly prominent ethical issue in response to disparities in the availability of health services. An ethical responsibility rests on society to examine policies that restrict health care to the needy, and on health care professionals who may function in settings that implicitly or explicitly ration care in a manner that may harm patients (see Chapter 8).

Beauchamp and Childress's approach includes a methodology for applying their four core principles. When principles inevitably clash in many clinical situations, moral action requires weighing up the respective merit of each one. For example, a clinician's ethical responsibility when a patient requests termination of life-sustaining treatment requires balancing the principles of respect for autonomy and beneficence, and considering the distinctive features of the case. Respect for autonomy is the likely guiding principle when a patient close to death is suffering intensely, whereas beneficence is likely to prevail when a patient is psychotically depressed and adamantly refusing an antibiotic that would cure a life-threatening pneumonia. These examples highlight several strengths of principle-based ethics. First, since it is compatible with, and embraces tenets of both utilitarian and deontological theories, it can lay claim to a broad grounding for moral deliberation. Second, it is typified by a pragmatism influenced by input from relevant empirical data and, consequently, more flexible than classical ethical theories, like utilitarianism. Third, it provides specific guidelines for resolving dilemmas, in contrast to the complexities of deriving a categorical imperative from pure reasoning or assessing the benefits and harms in particular circumstances. Finally, it is readily applicable to most bioethical dilemmas.

Principle-based ethics is prone to the same criticism as deontological theory concerning its methodology – weighing up principles relies on Ross's procedure of establishing the most pressing among a conflicting set, an approach regarded by some as vague and subjective. Principlism seeks to overcome these purported limitations by articulating particular requirements, such as aiming for the least possible infringement in a given situation of one principle by another. The approach, however, fails to offer a hierarchical ordering of principles. In their critique of principlism, Clouser and Gert[23] present a more fundamental challenge to principle-based ethics which they view as an inadequate method applied to a set of mid-level principles that 'obscure[s] and confuse[s] moral reasoning'. The criticism seems unduly harsh in light of Beauchamp and Childress's acknowledgment that they do not regard principlism as a general theory, but rather an analytical approach that helps focus on the shortcomings of classical theories.

Ethics of care

Emergence of a framework that values the human capacity to extend care to people in need is the most recent contribution to moral deliberation. This care ethic blends components of virtue theory with feminist ideology, psychological concepts and an emphasis on emotions. The family serves as the model for moral behaviour; for example, fidelity is interpreted as the kind held by a parent towards a child, and perceived quite differently from fidelity owed to an unknown member of society. Ethical decision-making is thereby grounded in aspects of individual character and interpersonal relationships, a *perspective* of moral deliberation (more than an explicit theory) well suited to most issues of psychiatric ethics addressed in this volume.

In *In a different voice*,[24] Carol Gilligan highlights the disparity in patterns of interaction of groups of boys and groups of girls; the former are apt to relate to one another following set guidelines, while girls place much greater store on emotions they engender. For example, boys generally resolve disagreements in play by resorting to rules, whereas girls invest in maintaining human links and are likely to resolve a conflict by merely ending the game. The difference is pertinent in terms of the moral development of boys and girls, and elaboration of the distinction has evolved into an ethical framework whose core properties are set forth in the selection by Carse, 'The voice of care: implications for bioethical education'.[25]

The appeal of care ethics reflects several of its strengths. First, universal rules for moral guidelines are eschewed since they are abstractions detached from the real world. Reasoning is unacceptable as the pivotal method to general moral guidelines, given its inability to fully capture what occurs in moral life. Moreover, utilitarian impartiality and deontological theory's stress on autonomy are based on a perception that misrepresents actual links among people wrestling with day-to-day moral questions. The world is not atomistic. Dealing with moral conflicts requires focus on distinctive interpersonal relationships in conjunction with regard for interests of a broader community, not the interaction of autonomous human beings.

This emphasis on the interpersonal is matched by the importance care ethics assigns to 'moral emotion' like fidelity, compassion, friendship and love. Grappling with moral conflict must occur contextually and consider psychological attachments among people. Baier[26] highlights the role of emotion in moral development, which she sees as deriving from 'the risky adventure of interdependence' between parent and child. An analogous pattern applies to the doctor-patient relationship, as clinicians assess patients' emotions in order to understand their distinctive fears, wishes and needs. Bioethical decisions are then guided accordingly in the context of a person's unique life narrative.

Third, the ethics of care draws heavily on Aristotelian theory in calling forth cultivation of virtuous personal traits, such as sympathy, compassion and patience. These qualities embody a goodness that facilitates ethical behaviour. Thus, care ethics combines virtue theory with a focus on emotions in order to sort out ethical complications of human relationships.

A criticism of the approach is that it is much more a method than it is a theory. Baier[27] considers this an irrelevant objection, given her position that overarching theories are superfluous and impede meaningful moral action. Rather, care ethicists advocate for what they regard as an appropriate perspective to explore mid-level principles, an approach not dissimilar to casuistry.

Care-based ethics is also charged with subjectivity. As moral rules can be faulted for their constrictiveness, so their absence may facilitate a relativism that undermines claims of reasonable ethical debate. It is argued that contemporary cultural diversity, and the range of setpoints for emotional awareness and expression that characterize different communities, could result in contradictory and, consequently, inconsistent appraisal of moral matters.

Conclusion

Pellegrino[28] reviews the wide array of theoretical underpinnings of moral deliberation in a thirty-year retrospective view of medical ethics. He suggests that none holds primacy and argues that clinicians must therefore complement philosophical reflection with their own insight and experience in order to advance ethical practice. The preceding overview of moral theory will hopefully facilitate that task, by helping the reader to critically assess issues discussed in subsequent chapters of this volume, and thereby promote thoughtful, proficient moral reflection.

References

1   Proctor, R.: *Racial hygiene*. Cambridge, MA, Harvard University Press, 1988.

2   Aristotle: *Nicomachean ethics*, trans. T. Irwin. Indianapolis, IN, Hackett, 1985.

3   MacIntyre, A.: *After virtue*. Notre Dame, IN, University of Notre Dame Press, 1981.

4   MacIntyre, A.: The nature of the virtues. *The Hastings Center* 11:27–34, 1981.

*5 Pellegrino, E.: The virtuous physician, and the ethics of medicine, in *Virtue and medicine*, ed. E. Shelp. Dordrecht, Holland, D. Reidel Publishing, 1985, pp. 237–255.

6   McCullough, L.: Virtues, etiquette, and Anglo-American medical ethics in the eighteenth and nineteenth centuries, in *Virtue and Medicine*, ed. E. Shelp. Dordrecht, Holland, D. Reidel Publishing, 1985, pp. 81–92.

7   Oath of Hippocrates in *Ancient medicine: selected papers of Ludwig Edelstein*, eds. O. Temkin and C. Temkin. Baltimore, MD, Johns Hopkins University Press, 1967.

8   Veatch, R.: Against virtue: a deontological critique of virtue theory in medical ethics, in *Virtue and medicine*, ed. E. Shelp. Dordrecht, Holland, D. Reidel Publishing, 1985, pp. 329–345.

9   Plato: Meno, in *Greek philosophy: Thales to Aristotle*, 3rd edn, ed. R. Allen. New York: The Free Press, 1991, pp. 110–141.

*10 Arras, J.: Getting down to cases: the revival of casuistry in bioethics. *The Journal of Medicine and Philosophy* 16:29–51, 1991.

11 Jonsen, A.: Casuistry as methodology in clinical ethics. *Theoretical Medicine* 12:295–307, 1991.

*12 Kant, I.: Grounding for the metaphysics of morals, in *Ethical philosophy*, trans. J. Ellington. Indianapolis, IN, Hackett Publishing Company, 1983, pp. 7–17; 19–27; 30–32; 40–41.

13 Ross, W.D.: *The right and the good*. Oxford, England, Clarendon Press, 1930, pp. 16–47.

14 Rawls, J.: *A theory of justice*. Cambridge, MA, Harvard University Press, 1971.

*15 Mill, J.S.: *Utilitarianism*, 2nd edn, ed. G. Sher. Indianapolis, IN, Hackett, 2001, Chapters 1 and 2.

16 *Tarasoff v Regents of the University of California*. 529 P.2d 553 (Cal 1974); 551 p. 2d 533 (Cal 1976).

17 Oken, D.: What to tell cancer patients: a study of medical attitudes. *Journal of the American Medical Association* 175:1120–1128, 1963.

18 Scheffler S. (ed.): *Consequentialism and its critics*. Oxford, Oxford University Press, 1988, pp. 1–13.

19 Williams B.: Consequentialism and integrity, in *Consequentialism and its critics*, ed. S. Scheffler. Oxford, Oxford University Press, 1988, pp. 29–50.

20 Mackie, J.: *Ethics: inventing right and wrong*. London, Penguin Books, 1977, pp. 1–49.

21 Beauchamp, T. and Childress, J.: *Principles of biomedical ethics*, 4th edn. Oxford, Oxford University Press, 1994. (Chapters 3 through 6 present a detailed exploration of each principle, along with discussion of their relevance to clinical medicine, health policy, and health law.)

*22 Beauchamp, T.: The 'four principles' approach, in *Principles of health care ethics*, ed. R. Gillon. Chichester, Wiley and Sons, 1994, pp. 3–12.

23   **Clouser, K.** and **Gert, B.**: A critique of principlism. *Journal of Medicine and Philosophy* **15**:219–236, 1990.

24   **Gilligan, C.**: *In a different voice*. Cambridge, MA, Harvard University Press, 1982.

*25   **Carse, A.**: The 'voice of care': implications for bioethical education. *Journal of Medicine and Philosophy* **16**:5–28, 1991.

26   **Baier, A.**: Theory and reflective practices, in *Postures of the mind*. Minneapolis, MN, University of Minnesota Press, 1985, pp. 207–227.

27   **Baier, A.**: Doing without moral theory, in *Postures of the mind*. Minneapolis, MN, University of Minnesota Press, 1985, pp. 228–243.

28   **Pellegrino, E.**: The metamorphosis of medical ethics: a 30-year retrospective. *Journal of the American Medical Association* **269**: 1158–1162, 1993.

The Virtuous Physician, and the Ethics of Medicine*

Edmund D. Pellegrino

> Consider from what noble seed you spring: You were created not to live like beasts, but for pursuit of virtue and of knowledge.
>
> Dante, *Inferno* 26, 118–120

Introduction

In the opening pages of his *Dominations and Powers*, Santayana asserts that 'Human society owes all its warmth and vitality to the intrinsic virtue of its members' and that the virtues therefore are always 'hovering silently' over his pages ([32], p. 3). And, indeed, the virtues have always hovered over any theory of morals. They give credibility to the moral life; they assure that it will be something more than a catalogue of rights, duties, and rules. Virtue adds that extra 'cubit' that lifts ethics out of its legalisms to the higher reaches of moral sensitivity.

Yet, as MacIntyre's brilliant treatise so ably attests, virtue-ethics since the Enlightenment has become a dubious enterprise [19]. We have lost consensus on a definition of virtue, and without moral consensus there is no vantage point from which to judge what is right and good. Virtue becomes confused with conformity to the conventions of social and institutional life. The accolades go to those who get along and get ahead. Without agreeing on the nature of the good, moreover, we can hardly know what a 'disposition' to do the right and good may mean.

These uncertainties force us to rely on ethical systems built upon specific rights, duties, and the application of rules and principles. Their concreteness seems to promise protection against capricious and antithetical interpretations of vice and virtue. But that concreteness turns to illusion once we try to agree on what is the right and good thing to do, in a given circumstance.

Despite the erosion of the concept of virtue, it remains an inescapable reality in moral transactions. We know there are people we can trust to temper self-interest, to be honest, truthful, faithful, or just, even in the face of the omnipresence of evil. Sadly, we also know that there are others who cannot be trusted habitually to act well. We may not be virtuous ourselves, we may even sneer at the folly of the virtuous man in our age, yet we can recognize him nonetheless. It is as Marcus Aurelius said, '. . . no thing delights as much as the examples of the virtues when they are exhibited in the morals of those who live with us and present themselves in abundance as far as possible. Wherefore we must keep these before us' [23].

And, in fact, the virtues are again being brought before us in the resurgence, among moral philosophers, of an interest in virtue-based ethics [9, 11, 13, 17, 21, 29, 33, 34, 35, 38, 39]. For the most part the resurgence is based in a re-examination, clarification, and refurbishment of the classical-medieval concept of virtue. On the whole, the contemporary reappraisal is not an abnegation of rights or duty-based ethics, but a recognition that rights and duties notwithstanding, their moral effectiveness still turns on the disposition and character traits of our fellow men and women.

This is preeminently true in medical ethics where the vulnerability and dependance of the sick person forces him to trust not just in his rights but in the kind of person the physician *is*. The variability with which this trust is honored, and at times its outright violation, account for the current decline in the moral credibililty of the profession. It accounts, too, for the trend toward asserting patients' rights more forcefully in contract as opposed to covenantal models of the physician–patient relationship. In illness, when we are most exploitable, we are most dependent upon the kind of person who will intend, and do, the right and the good thing, because he cannot really do otherwise.

MacIntyre has expressed his pessimism about the possibilities of an ethic of virtue in our times. He ends his tightly reasoned treatise with a surprisingly romantic hope for '. . . a local form of community within which civility and the intellectual and moral life can be sustained in the rough new dark ages which are already upon us' ([19], p. 245). One can accept MacIntyre's astute historical diagnoses without waiting too quietistically for the appearance of his new and 'doubtless very different' St. Benedict to lead us into some new moral consensus. Even in this 'dark age', it may be possible to incorporate the remnants of the classical-medieval idea of virtue into a more satisfactory moral structure that also includes rights and duties.

This essay examines that possibility in the limited domain of professional medical ethics. Using the classical-medieval concept of virtue, it attempts to define the virtuous physician, to relate his virtue to the ends of medicine and to the usual principles applied in medical ethics, as well as to the prevailing rights and duty-based systems of professional ethics.

This essay is part of a larger effort to link a theory of the patient-physician relationship, a theory of patient good, and theory of virtue in a unified conceptual substructure for the professional ethics of medicine [24, 25].

The Classical medieval concept of virtue

What is virtue? What are the virtues? Are they one or many? Can they be taught? These are still the fundamental first order questions for any virtue-based ethical theory. And, as with so many of the perennial philosophical questions, they were first examined in an orderly way in the Platonic dialogues. In the first dialogues, Socrates raises them with his characteristic to, and fro, probing. Given his circumambulation of definitions, and the difficulties of translating from ancient languages, Socrates' precise meanings remain somewhat problematic.

Most commentators, however, focus on his equilibration in the *Meno*, *Protagoras*, and *Gorgias* of virtue (*aretè*) with knowledge (*epistemè*) [5, 13, 36, 37]. Virtue is here synonymous with excellence in living the good life. This excellence depends upon knowledge of good, evil, and self. It is not specialized knowledge directed to any one activity but rather to living one's whole life well. It must, like an art, be perfected through practice. The individual virtues – courage, justice, temperance, wisdom, and piety – order life towards excellence. But they too depend on knowledge so that, on this view, vice is the result primarily of ignorance.

How much of this intellectualist definition of virtue is Socrates' and how much Plato's is debatable. In the later dialogues, the *Laws* and the *Republic*,

* Pellegrino, E.: The virtuous physician, and the ethics of medicine, in *Virtue and medicine*, ed. E. Shelp. Dordrecht, Holland, D. Reidel Publishing, 1985, pp. 237–255.

more attention is given to justice as a central virtue and to proper ordering of the state [12]. Wisdom is still a virtue but for the statesman it is knowledge of what is good not just for the individual good life but the good of the whole state. The aim of laws should be virtue but the chief of these is wisdom, so that wisdom is the knowledge that 'presides' over justice (*Republic*, Bk. IV).

In the *Republic*, still exploring definitions, Plato draws the analogy of virtue with bodily health – 'Virtue then as it sees would be a certain health, beauty and good condition of a soul and vice a sickness, ugliness and weakness' (*Republic*, Bk. IV). He likens virtue to the order and balance between the parts of the body that characterize health. For Socrates that, ordering results from intellectual perfection of the art of living a good life. Plato, as Aristotle pointed out, paid more attention than Socrates to the non-rational elements in human life. Virtue, for him is as much a matter of disposition to act in the right way, as it is a desire for the good, arising from knowledge of the good.

Aristotle reacted to Socrates' over-intellectualization of virtue. He devoted large portions of the *Nicomachean Ethics* to his concept of virtue. His own work, Aristotle said, '. . . does not aim at theoretical knowledge like the others (for we are inquiring not in order to know what virtue is, but in order to become good, since otherwise our inquiry would have been of no use), we must examine the nature of actions, namely, how we ought to do them' (*Nicomachean Ethics*, 1099a, 10–11). He does not reject the role of intellect; he judges it a proper part of virtue, but not its whole. Thus he emphasizes that virtue is also concerned with feelings and actions – '. . . just acts are pleasant to the lover of justice and in general virtuous acts to the lover of virtue' (*Nicomachean Ethics*, 1099a, 10–11).

But virtue is not just feeling. It is of two kinds: intellectual and moral – 'Intellectual virtue in the main owes both its birth and growth to teaching (for which reasons it requires experience and time) while moral virtue comes about as a result of habit, whence also its name *ethikè* that is formed by a slight variation of the word *ethos* (habit)' (*Nicomachean Ethics*, 1103a, 14–18). Virtue is not simply a passion, or a function, but a '. . . state of character' (*Nicomachean Ethics*, 1106a, 11). Virtue is that state of character, which makes a man good and which makes him do his own work well' (*Nicomachean Ethics*, 1106a, 22–24).

But states of character must be in accord with the 'right rule.' Hence the intellectual virtues play a part in making a man virtuous. Practical wisdom is that aspect of intellect that enables a man to direct his life to its *chief* good. The 'right rule' is reached, as Ross says, 'by the deliberative analysis' of the practically wise man and telling him that the end of human life is to be best attained by certain actions which are intermediate between extremes. Obedience to such a rule is moral virtue' [31].

Aristotle's doctrine of the mean and his divisions and subdivisions of the intellectual and moral virtues are too complex to engage us here [31]. What is significant for the present discussion is the balance Aristotle strikes between moral virtue and reason, feelings, dispositions, and right action. These are Aristotle's modifications and extensions of the Socratic notion of virtue.

Aristotle made more explicit the Socratic orientation of virtue to ends. Thus '. . . very virtue or excellence both brings into good condition the thing of which it is the excellence and makes the work of that thing to be done well . . .' (*Nicomachean Ethics*, 2, 5, 1106a, 15–17). The end of virtue for both Socrates and Aristotle is the good life. What constitutes the good life is for both of them the fulfillment of the potentiality of human nature.

Aristotle summarizes the essential elements which distinguish the virtuous man: '. . . in the first place he must have knowledge, secondly, he must choose the acts and choose them for their own sakes, and thirdly his actions must proceed from a firm and unchangeable character' (*Nicomachean Ethics*, 11, 4, 1104, 6, 31–34). This combination of character, knowledge, and deliberate choice makes for a virtuous person. Actions themselves are virtuous when they emanate from just such a person (*Nicomachean Ethics*, 1105b, 5–6). For Aristotle, then, virtue resides not only in the act or in the knowledge of virtue, but the act itself must also be done virtuously, as a virtuous man would do it. '. . . But as a condition of the possession of the virtues knowledge has little or no weight, while the

other conditions count not for a little, but for everything. Nor does virtue reside in the act itself' (*Nicomachean Ethics*, 1105b, 1–4).

Aquinas' treatment of the virtues is best understood in the context of his total enterprise, to reconcile, emend, and amend the ancient philosophers through the revealed truths of the Christian experience. Precisely to what extent his emphasis on the cardinal virtues coincides with, or departs from, Artistotle is difficult to say. Aquinas too had to surmount the problem of trying to apprehend the nuances of words in an ancient language no longer in daily use. MacIntyre calls him a 'marginal figure' not representing the general opinion of the virtues extant in his time. He does, however, recognize that Aquinas' interpretation of the *Nicomachean Ethics* 'has never been better' ([19], p. 166).

For Aristotle, the intellectual and moral virtues were requisite for the full development of man's natural capacities. But for Aquinas, man's natural end was itself insufficient because he had a spiritual destiny that transcends the merely natural [4]. Man is destined to union with God. To this end not only the natural virtues but the supernatural are needed, and these can be known only through the Christian revelation. For the Christian the perfection of the natural virutes is not sufficient [4].

Like Aristotle, Aquinas held virtue to be grounded in good habits, in dispositions to do the right and good thing, but always in association with the right reason. Thus he says, 'It belongs to human virtue to make a man good and his work according to reason' [2]. 'Through virtue man is ordered to the utmost limit of his capacity' [5]. It is a condition of the perfection of human life. Or said another way, 'Virtue is called the limit of potentiality . . . because it causes an inclination to the highest act which a faculty can perform' [1].

Virtues for Aquinas are habits and dispositions that enable a man to reason well (the intellectual virtues) and to act in accordance with a right reason (moral virtues) – *recta ratio agibilium* [20]. These two kinds of virtue can be independent of each other, but in the virtuous man, who strives for the perfection of his human potentiality, they are joined. And they are joined most firmly in the one virtue from which the others derive – prudence, the standard of right willing and acting, the form and mold for the other virtues [29].

Josef Pieper among modern commentators has most clearly expounded Aquinas' teaching on prudence and the other cardinal virtues [29]. Without attempting to restate that teaching here, suffice it to say that for Aquinas all virtue is necessarily prudent, acting in accord with right reason in conformity with the reality of things. This is not prudence in the pejorative modern sense of caution, timidity, rationalized cowardice, cunning, or casuistic deviousness. Rather, it is the analogue of Aristotle's wisdom, the capacity and disposition to will and act rightly in particular, practical, and uncertain circumstances. As such, prudence informs, measures, guides, shapes, and generates the other virtues, by inclining us to choose good means to good ends for man.

The post-medieval transformations of the classical concepts were many: Rousseau opposed virtue to society; for Shaftesbury virtue lay in the pursuit of public interest; Hutcheson and Hume identified it with a 'moral sense'; to Montaigne virtue was 'an innocence, accidental and fortuitous'; for Descartes, strength of soul; for Malebranche, love of order; and for Spinoza, the soul directing itself by a universal and clear idea; Mandeville paradoxically defended the utility of the vices. MacIntyre shows with a wealth of detail the continuing emotivist and intuitionist trends of philosophies of virtue since the Enlightenment.

In the last several years the classical concept has been reexamined by a growing number of moral philosophers. They have underscored such things as the differences in meanings of the word *arete* in Greek, *virtus* in Latin and 'virtue' in English, the distinctions between virtues and skills, the difficulties in defining such words, as 'disposition' and 'habit' as used in the traditional definitions, the relationships between the natural and the supernatural virtues, the relations of virtue, values and concepts of the good, the unity or non-unity of the virtues, whether they are teachable or not, their relevance to health and medical care, and their relationship with duties, rights, and obligations [11, 17, 19, 21, 23, 29].

MacIntyre, for example, extends the Aristotelian concept from qualities internal to practices, to role reference and to community good [19]. Hauerwas relates them to the narrative of a particular people [14]. Some commentators are more critical, some more accepting of the classical concepts. In the end, the great majority say almost the same thing as the ancients but in more modern language. One is tempted to say of virtue, as it has been said of *pornography*. 'I can't define it but I know it when I see it.'

The Virtuous person, the virtuous physician

Through these multitudinous definitions a set of common themes seems discernible. Virtue implies a character trait, an internal disposition, habitually to seek moral perfection, to live one's life in accord with the moral law, and to attain a balance between noble intention and just action. Perhaps C. S. Lewis has captured the idea best by likening the virtuous man to the good tennis player:

What you mean by a good player is the man whose eye and muscles and nerves have been so trained by making innumerable good shots that they can now be relied upon. . . . They have a certain tone or quality which is there even when he is not playing . . . . In the same way a man who perseveres in doing just actions gets in the end a certain quality of character. Now it is that quality rather than the particular actions that we mean when we talk of virtue [18].

On almost any view, the virtuous person is someone we can trust to act habitually in a 'good' way – courageously, honestly, justly, wisely, and temperately. He is committed to *being* a good person and to the pursuit of perfection in his private, professional and communal life. He is someone who will act well even when there is no one to applaud, simply because to act otherwise is a violation of what it is to be a good person. No civilized society could endure without a significant number of citizens committed to this concept of virtue. Without such persons no system of general ethics could succeed, and no system of professional ethics could transcend the dangers of self interest. That is why, even while rights, duties, obligations may be emphasized, the concept of virtue has 'hovered' so persistently over every system of ethics.

Is the virtuous physician simply the virtuous person practicing medicine? Are there virtues peculiar to medicine as a practice? Are certain of the individual virtues more applicable to medicine than elsewhere in human activities? Is virtue more important in some branches of medicine than others? How do professional skills differ from virtue? These are pertinent questions propaedeutic to the later questions of the place of virtue in professional medical ethics.

I believe these questions are best answered by drawing on the Aristotelian-Thomist notion of virtues and its relationship to the ends and purposes of human life. The virtuous physician on this view is defined in terms of the ends of medicine. To be sure, the physician, before he is anything else, must be a virtuous person. To be a virtuous physician he must also be the kind of person we can confidently expect will be disposed to the right and good intrinsic to the practice he professes. What are those dispositions?

To answer this question requires some exposition of what we mean by the good in medicine, or more specifically the good of the patient – for that is the end the patient and the physician ostensibly seek. Any theory of virtue must be linked with a theory of the good because virtue is a disposition habitually to do the good. Must we therefore know the nature of the good the virtuous man is disposed to do? As with the definition of virtue we are caught here in another perennial philosophical question – what is the nature of the Good? Is the good whatever we make it to be or does it have validity independent of our desires or interest? Is the good one, or many? Is it reducible to riches, honors, pleasures, glory, happiness, or something else?

I make no pretense to a discussion of a general theory of the good. But any attempt to define the virtuous physician or a virtue-based ethic for medicine must offer some definition of the good of the patient. The patient's good is the end of medicine, that which shapes the particular virtues required for its attainment. That end is central to any notion of the virtues peculiar to medicine as a practice.

I have argued elsewhere that the architectonic principle of medicine is the good of the patient as expressed in a particular right and good healing action [26]. This is the immediate good end of the clinical encounter. Health, healing, caring, coping are all good ends dependent upon the more immediate end of a right and good decision. On this view, the virtuous physician is one so habitually disposed to act in the patient's good, to place that good in ordinary instances above his own, that he can reliably be expected to do so.

But we must fact the fact that the 'patient's good' is itself a compound notion. Elsewhere I have examined four components of the patient's good: (1) clinical or biomedical good; (2) the good as perceived by the patient; (3) the good of the patient as a human person; and (4) the Good, or ultimate good. Each of these components of patient good must be served. They must also be placed in some hierarchical order when they conflict within the same person, or between persons involved in clinical decisions [27].

Some would consider patient good, so far as the physician is concerned, as limited to what applied medical knowledge can achieve in *this* patient. On this view the virtues specific to medicine would be objectivity, scientific probity, and conscientiousness with regard to professional skill. One could perform the technical tasks of medicine well, be faithful to the skills of good technical medicine per se, but without being a virtuous person. Would one then be a virtuous physician? One would have to answer affirmatively if technical skill were all there is to medicine.

Some of the more expansionist models of medicine – like Engel's biopsychosocial model, or that of the World Health Organization (total well-being) would require compassion, empathy, advocacy, benevolence, and beneficence, i.e., an expanded sense of the affective responses to patient need [8]. Some might argue that what is required, therefore, is not virtue, but simply greater skill in the social and behavioral sciences applied to particular patients. On this view the physician's habitual dispositions might be incidental to his skills in communication or his empathy. He could achieve the ends of medicine without necessarily being a virtuous person in the generic sense.

It is important at this juncture to distinguish the virtues from technical or professional skills, as MacIntyre and, more clearly, Von Wright do. The latter defines a skill as 'technical goodness' – excellence in some particular activity – while virtues are not tied to any one activity but are necessary for 'the good of man' ([38], pp. 139–140). The virtues are not 'characterized in terms of their results' ([38]), p. 141). On this view, the technical skills of medicine are not virtues and could be practiced by a non-virtuous person. Aristotle held *technè* (technical skills) to be one of the five intellectual virtues but not one of the moral virtues.

The virtues enable the physician to act with regard to things that are good for man, when man is in the specific existential state of illness. They are dispositions always to seek the good intent inherent in healing. Within medicine, the virtues do become in MacIntyre's sense acquired human qualities '. . . the possession and exercise of which tends to enable us to achieve those goods which are internal to practices and the lack of which effectively prevents us from achieving any such goods' ([19], p. 178).

We can come closer to the relationships of virtue to clinical actions if we look to the more immediate ends of medical encounters, to those moments of clinical truth when specific decisions and actions are chosen and carried out. The good the patient seeks is to be healed – to be restored to his prior, or to a better, state of function, to be made 'whole' again. If this is not possible, the patient expects to be helped, to be assisted in coping with the pain, disability or dying that illness may entail. The immediate end of medicine is not simply a technically proficient performance but the use of that performance to attain a good end – the good of the patient – his medical or biomedical good to the extent possible but also his good as he the patient perceives it, his good as a human person who can make his own life plan, and his good as a person with a spiritual destiny if this is his belief [24, 25]. It is the sensitive balancing of these senses of the patient's good which the virtuous physician pursues to perfection.

To achieve the end of medicine thus conceived, to practice medicine virtuously, requires certain dispositions: conscientious attention to technical knowledge and skill to be sure, but also compassion – a capacity to feel something of the patient's experience of illness and his perceptions of what is worthwhile; beneficence and benevolence – doing and wishing to do good for the patient; honesty, fidelity to promises, perhaps at times courage as well – the whole list of virtues spelled out by Aristotle: '. . . justice, courage, temperance, magnificence, magnanimity, liberality, placability, prudence, wisdom' (*Rhetoric*, 1, c, 13666, 1–3). Not every one of these virtues is required in every decision. What we expect of the virtuous physician is that he will exhibit them when they are required and that he will be so habitually disposed to do so that we can depend upon it. He will place the good of the patient above his own and to seek that good unless its pursuit imposes an injustice upon him, or his family, or requires a violation of his own conscience.

While the virtues are necessary to attain the good internal to medicine as a practice, they exist independently of medicine. They are necessary for the practice of a good life, no matter in what activities that life may express itself. Certain of the virtues may become duties in the Stoic sense, duties because of the nature of medicine as a practice. Medicine calls forth benevolence, beneficence, truth telling, honesty, fidelity, and justice more than physical courage, for example. Yet even physical courage may be necessary when caring for the wounded on battlefields, in plagues, earthquakes, or other disasters. On a more ordinary scale courage is necessary in treating contagious diseases, violent patients, or battlefield casualties. Doing the right and good thing in medicine calls for a more regular, intensive, and selective practice of the virtues than many other callings.

A person who is a virtuous person can cultivate the technical skills of medicine for reasons other than the good of the patient – his own pride, profit, prestige, power. Such a physician can make technically right decisions and perform skillfully. He could not be depended upon, however, to act against his own self-interest for the good of his patient.

In the virtuous physician, explicit fulfillment of rights and duties is an outward expression of an inner disposition to do the right and the good. He is virtuous not because he has conformed to the letter of the law, or his moral duties, but because that is what a good person does. He starts always with his commitment to be a certain kind of person, and he approaches clinical quandaries, conflicts of values, and his patient's interests as a good person should.

Some branches of medicine would seem to demand a stricter and broader adherence to virtue than others. Generalists, for example, who deal with the more sensitive facets and nuances of a patient's life and humanity must exercise the virtues more diligently than technique-oriented specialists. The narrower the specialty the more easily the patient's good can be safeguarded by rules, regulations rights and duties; the broader the specialty the more significant are the physician's character traits. No branch of medicine, however, can be practiced without some dedication to some of the virtues [21].

Unfortunately, physicians can compartmentalize their lives. Some practice medicine virtuously, yet are guilty of vice in their private lives. Examples are common of physicians who appear sincerely to seek the good of their patients and neglect obligations to family or friends. Some boast of being 'married' to medicine and use this excuse to justify all sorts of failures in their own human relationships. We could not call such a person virtuous. Nor could we be secure in, or trust, his disposition to act in a right and good way even in medicine. After all, one of the essential virtues is balancing conflicting obligations judiciously.

As Socrates pointed out to Meno, one cannot really be virtuous in part:

Why did not I ask you to tell me the nature of virtue as a whole? And you are very far from telling me this; but declare every action to be virtue which is done with a part of virtue; as though you had told me and I must already know the whole of virtue, and this too when frittered away into little pieces. And therefore my dear Meno, I fear that I must begin again, and repeat the same question: what is virtue? For otherwise, I can only say that every action' done with a part of virtue is virtue; what else is the meaning of saying that every action done with justice is virtue? Ought I not to ask the question over again; for can any one who does not know virtue know a part of virtue?

(Meno, 79)

Virtues, rights and duties in medical ethics

Frankena has neatly summarized the distinctions between virtue-based and rights- and duty-based ethics as follows:

In an ED (ethics of duty) then, the basic concept is that a certain kind of external act (or doing) ought to be done in certain circumstances; and that of a certain disposition being a virtue is a dependent one. In an EV (ethics of virtue) the basic concept is that of a disposition or way of being – something one has, or is not does – as a virtue, as morally good; and that of an action's being virtuous or good or even right, is a dependent one [10].

There are some logical difficulties with a virtue-based ethic. For one thing, there must be some consensus on a definition of virtue. For another there is a circularity in the assertion that virtue is what the good man habitually does, and that at the same time one becomes virtuous by doing good. Virtue and good are defined in terms of each other and the definitions of both may vary among sincere people in actual practice when there is no consensus. A virtue-based ethic is difficult to defend as the sole basis for normative judgments.

But there is a deficiency in rights- and duty-ethics as well. They too must be linked to a theory of the good. In contemporary ethics, theories of good are rarely explicitly linked to theories of the right and good. Von Wright, commendably, is one of the few contemporary authorities who explicitly connects his theory of good with his theory of virtue. This essay, together with three previous ones, is part of the author's effort in that direction [25–27].

In most professional ethical codes, virtue and duty-based ethics are intermingled. The Hippocratic Oath, for example, imposes certain duties like protection of confidentiality; avoiding abortion, not harming the patient. But the Hippocratic physician also pledges: '. . . in purity and holiness I will guard my life and my art.' This is an exhortation to be a good person and a virtuous physician, in order to serve patients in an ethically responsible way.

Likewise, in one of the most humanistic statements in medical literature, the first century A.D. writer, Scribonius Largus, made *humanitas* (compassion) an essential virtue. It is thus really a role-specific duty. In doing so he was applying the Stoic doctrine of virtue to medicine [3, 28].

The latest version (1980) of the AMA 'Principles of Medical Ethics' similarly intermingles duties, rights, and exhortations to virtue. It speaks of 'standards of behavior', 'essentials of honorable behavior', dealing 'honestly' with patients and colleagues and exposing colleagues 'deficient in character'. *The Declaration of Geneva*, which must meet the challenge of the widest array of value systems, nonetheless calls for practice 'with conscience and dignity' in keeping with 'the honor and noble traditions of the profession'. Though their first allegiance must be to the Communist ethos, even the Soviet physician is urged to preserve 'the high title of physician', 'to keep and develop the beneficial traditions of medicine' and to 'dedicate' all his 'knowledge and strength to the care of the sick'.

Those who are cynical of any protestation of virtue on the part of physicians will interpret these excerpts as the last remnants of a dying tradition of altruistic benevolence. But at the very least, they attest to the recognition that the good of the patient cannot be fully protected by rights and duties alone. Some degree of supererogation is built into the nature of the relationship of those who are ill and those who profess to help them.

This too may be why many graduating classes, still idealistic about their calling, choose the Prayer of Maimonides (not by Maimonides at all) over the more deontological Oath of Hippocrates. In that 'prayer' the physician asks:

... may neither avarice nor miserliness, nor thirst for glory or for a great reputation engage my mind; for the enemies of truth and philanthropy may easily deceive me and make me forgetful of my lofty aim of doing good to thy children.

This is an unequivocal call to virtue and it is hard to imagine even the most cynical graduate failing to comprehend its message.

All professional medical codes, then, are built of a three-tiered system of obligations related to the special roles of physicians in society. In the ascending order of ethical sensitivity they are: observance of the laws of the land, then observance of rights and fulfillment of duties, and finally the practice of virtue.

A legally based ethic concentrates on the minimum requirements – the duties imposed by human laws which protect against the grosser aberrations of personal rights. Licensure, the laws of torts and contracts, prohibitions against discrimination, good Samaritan laws, definitions of death, and the protection of human subjects of experimentation are elements of a legalistic ethic.

At the next level is the ethics of rights and duties which spells out obligations beyond what law defines. Here, benevolence and beneficence take on more than their legal meaning. The ideal of service, of responsiveness to the special needs of those who are ill, some degree of compassion, kindliness, promise-keeping, truth-telling, and non-maleficence and specific obligations like confidentiality and autonomy, are included. How these principles are applied, and conflicts among them resolved in the patient's best interests, are subjects of widely varying interpretation. How sensitively these issues are confronted depends more on the physician's character than his capability at ethical discourse or moral casuistry.

Virtue-based ethics goes beyond these first two levels. We expect the virtuous person to do the right and the good even at the expense of personal sacrifice and legitimate self-interest. Virtue ethics expands the notions of benevolence, beneficence, conscientiousness, compassion, and fidelity well beyond what strict duty might require. It makes some degree of supererogation mandatory because it calls for standards of ethical performance that exceed those prevalent in the rest of society [30].

At each of these three levels there are certain dangers from over-zealous or misguided observance. Legalistic ethical systems tend toward a justification for minimalistic ethics, a narrow definition of benevolence or beneficence, and a contract-minded physician-patient relationship. Duty- and rights-based ethics may be distorted by too strict adherence to the letter of ethical principles without the modulations and nuances the spirit of those principles implies. Virtue-based ethics, being the least specific, can more easily lapse into self-righteous paternalism or an unwelcome over-involvement in the personal life of the patient. Misapplication of any moral system even with good intent converts benevolence into maleficence. The virtuous person might be expected to be more sensitive to these aberrations than someone whose ethics is more deontologically or legally flavored.

The more we yearn for ethical sensitivity the less we lean on rights, duties, rules, and principles, and the more we lean on the character traits of the moral agent. Paradoxically, without rules, rights, and duties specifically spelled out, we cannot predict what form a particular person's expression of virtue will take. In a pluralistic society, we need laws, rules, and principles to assure a dependable minimum level of moral conduct. But that minimal level is insufficient in the complex and often unpredictable circumstances of decision-making, where technical and value desiderata intersect so inextricably.

The virtuous physician does not act from unreasoned, uncritical intuitions about what feels good. His dispositions are ordered in accord with that 'right reason' which both Aristotle and Aquinas considered essential to virtue. Medicine is itself ultimately an exercise of practical wisdom – a right way of acting in difficult and uncertain circumstances for a specific end, i.e., the good of a particular person who is ill. It is when the choice of a right

and good action becomes more difficult, when the temptations to self interest are most insistent, when unexpected nuances of good and evil arise and no one is looking, that the differences between an ethics based in virtue and an ethics based in law and/or duty can most clearly be distinguished.

Virtue-based professional ethics distinguishes itself, therefore, less in the avoidance of overtly immoral practices than in avoidance of those at the margin of moral responsibility. Physicians are confronted, in today's morally relaxed climate, with an increasing number of new practices that pit altruism against self interest. Most are not illegal, or, strictly speaking, immoral in a rights- or duty-based ethic. But they are not consistent with the higher levels of moral sensitivity that a virtue-ethics demands. These practices usually involve opportunities for profit from the illness of others, narrowing the concept of service for personal convenience, taking a proprietary attitude with respect to medical knowledge, and placing loyalty to the profession above loyalty to patients.

Under the first heading, we might include such things as investment in and ownership of for-profit hospitals, hospital chains, nursing homes, dialysis units, tie-in arrangements with radiological or laboratory services, escalation of fees for repetitive, high-volume procedures, and lax indications for their use, especially when third party payers 'allow' such charges.

The second heading might include the ever decreasing availability and accessibility of physicians, the diffusion of individual patient responsibility in group practice so that the patient never knows whom he will see or who is on call, the itinerant emergency room physician who works two days and skips three with little commitment to hospital or community, and the growing over-indulgence of physicians in vacations, recreation, and 'self-development'.

The third category might include such things as 'selling one's services' for whatever the market will bear, providing what the market demands and not necessarily what the community needs, patenting new procedures or keeping them secret from potential competitor-colleagues, looking at the investment of time, effort, and capital in a medical education as justification for 'making it back', or forgetting that medical knowledge is drawn from the cumulative experience of a multitude of patients, clinicians, and investigators.

Under the last category might be included referrals on the basis of friendship and reciprocity rather than skill, resisting consultations and second opinions as affronts to one's competence, placing the interest of the referring physician above those of the patients, looking the other way in the face of incompetence or even dishonesty in one's professional colleagues.

These and many other practices are defended today by sincere physicians and even encouraged in this era of competition, legalism, and self-indulgence. Some can be rationalized even in a deontological ethic. But it would be impossible to envision the physician committed to the virtues assenting to these practices. A virtue-based ethics simply does not fluctuate with what the dominant social mores will tolerate. It must interpret benevolence, beneficence, and responsibility in a way that reduces self interest and enhances altruism. It is the only convicing answer the profession can give to the growing perception clearly manifest in the legal commentaries in the FTC ruling that medicine is nothing more than business and should be regulated as such.

A virtue-based ethic is inherently elitist, in the best sense, because its adherents demand more of themselves than the prevailing morality. It calls forth that extra measure of dedication that has made the best physicians in every era exemplars of what the human spirit can achieve. No matter to what depths a society may fall, virtuous persons will always be the beacons that light the way back to moral sensitivity; virtuous physicians are the beacons that show the way back to moral credibility for the whole profession.

Albert Jonsen, rightly I believe, diagnoses the central paradox in medicine as the tension between self-interest and altrusim [15]. No amount of deft juggling of rights, duties, or principles will suffice to resolve that tension. We are all too good at rationalizing what we want to do so that personal gain can be converted from vice to virtue. Only a character formed by the virtues can feel the nausea of such intellectual hypocrisy.

To be sure, the twin themes of self-interest and altruism have been inextricably joined in the history of medicine. There have always been physicians who reject the virtues or, more often, claim them falsely. But, in addition, there have been physicians, more often than the critics of medicine would allow, who have been truly virtuous both in intent and act. They have been, and remain, the leaven of the profession and the hope of all who are ill. They form the sea-wall that will not be eroded even by the powerful forces of commercialization, bureaucratization, and mechanization inevitable in modern medicine.

We cannot, need not, and indeed must not, wait for a medical analogue of MacIntyre's 'new St. Benedict' to show us the way. There is no new concept of virtue waiting to be discovered that is peculiarly suited to the dilemmas of our own dark age. We must recapture the courage to speak of character, virtue, and perfection in living a good life. We must encourage those who are willing to dedicate themselves to a 'higher standard of self effacement' [6].

We need the courage, too, to accept the obvious split in the profession between those who see and feel the altruistic imperatives in medicine, and those who do not. Those who at heart believe that the pursuit of private self-interest serves the public good are very different from those who believe in the restraint of self-interest. We forget that physicians since the beginnings of the profession have subscribed to different values and virtues. We need only recall that the Hippocratic Oath was the Oath of physicians of the Pythagorean school at a time when most Greek physicians followed essentially a craft ethic [7]. A perusal of the Hippocratic Corpus itself, which intersperses ethics and etiquette, will show how differently its treatises deal with fees, the care of incurable patients, and the business aspects of the craft.

The illusion that all physicians share a common devotion to a high-flown set of ethical principles has done damage to medicine by raising expectations some members of the profession could not, or will not, fulfill. Today, we must be more forthright about the differences in value commitment among physicians. Professional codes must be more explicit about the relationships between duties, rights, and virtues. Such explicitness encourages a more honest relationship between physicians and patients and removes the hypocrisy of verbal assent to a general code, to which an individual physician may not really subscribe. Explicitness enables patients to choose among physicians on the basis of their ethical commitments as well as their reputations for technical expertise.

Conceptual clarity will not assure virtuous behavior. Indeed, virtues are usually distorted if they are the subject of too conscious a design. But conceptual clarity will distinguish between motives and provide criteria for judging the moral commitment one can expect from the profession and from its individual members. It can also inspire those whose virtuous inclinations need re-enforcement in the current climate of commercialization of the healing relationship.

To this end the current resurgence of interest in virtue-based ethics is altogether salubrious. Linked to a theory of patient good and a theory of rights and duties, it could provide the needed groundwork for a reconstruction of professional medical ethics as that work matures. Perhaps even more progress can be made if we take Shakespeare's advice in *Hamlet*: 'Assume the virtue if you have it not . . . . For use almost can change the stamp of nature.'

Bibliography

1   Aquinas, T.: 1875, 'De Virtutibus in Communi', in S. Fretté (ed.), *Opera Omnia*, Louis Virés, Paris, Vol. 14, pp. 178–229.

2   Aquinas, T.: 1964, *Summa Theologica*, Blackfriars, Cambridge, England, Vol. **23**.

3   Cicero: 1967, *Moral Obligations*, J. Higginbotham (trans.), University of California Press, Berkeley and Los Angeles.

4   Copleston, F.: 1959, *Aquinas*, Penguin Books, New York.

5   Cornford, F.: 1932, *Before and After Socrates*, Cambridge University Press, Cambridge, England.

6   Cushing, H.: 1929, *Consecratio Medici and Other Papers*, Little, Brown and Co., Boston.

7   Edelstein, L.: 1967, 'The Professional Ethics of the Greek Physician', in O. Temkin (ed.), *Ancient Medicine: Selected Papers of Ludwig Edelstein*, Johns Hopkins University Press, Baltimore.

8   Engel, G.: 1980, 'The Clinical Application of the Biopsychosocial Model', *American Journal of Psychiatry* **137**: 2, 535–544.

9   Foot, P.: 1978, *Virtues and Vices*, University of California Press, Berkeley and Los Angeles.

10   Frankena, W.: 1982, 'Beneficence in an Ethics of Virtue', in E. Shelp (ed.), *Beneficence and Health Care*, D. Reidel, Dordrecht, Holland, pp. 63–81.

11   Geach, P.: 1977, *The Virtues*, Cambridge University Press, Cambridge, England.

12   Gould, J.: 1972, *The Development of Plato's Ethics*, Russell and Russell, New York.

13   Guthrie, W.: 1971, *Socrates*, Cambridge University Press, Cambridge, England.

14   Hauerwas, S.: 1981, *A Community of Character*, University of Notre Dame Press, Notre Dame, Indiana.

15   Jonsen, A.: 1983, 'Watching the Doctor', *New England Journal of Medicine* 308:25,1531–1535.

16   Jowett, B.: 1953, *The Dialogues of Plato*, Random House, New York.

17   Kenny, A.: 1978, *The Aristotelian Ethics*, Clarendon Press, Oxford, England.

18   Lewis, C.: 1952, *Mere Christianity*, MacMillan Co., New York.

19   MacIntyre, A.: 1981, *After Virtue*, University of Notre Dame Press, Notre Dame, Indiana.

20   Maritain, J.: 1962, *Art and Scholasticism With Other Essays*, Charles Scribner and Sons, New York.

21   May, W.: Personal communication, 'Virtues in a Professional Setting', unpublished.

22   McKeon, R. (ed.): 1968, *The Basic Works of Aristotle*, Random House, New York.

23   Oates, W. (ed.): 1957, *The Stoic and Epicurean Philosophers*, Modern Library, New York.

24   Pellegrino, E.: 1979, 'The Anatomy of Clinical Judgments: Some Notes on Right Reason and Right Action', in H. T. Engelhardt, Jr., *et al.* (eds.), *Clinical Judgment: A Critical Appraisal*, D. Reidel, Dordrecht, Holland, pp. 169–194.

25   Pellegrino, E.: 1979, 'Toward a Reconstruction of Medical Morality: The Primacy of the Act of Profession and the Fact of Illness', *Journal of Medicine and Philosophy* 4: 1,32–56.

26   Pellegrino, E.: 1983, The Healing Relationship: The Architectonics of Clinical Medicine', in E. Shelp (ed.), *The Clinical Encounter*, D. Reidel, Dordrecht, Holland, pp. 153–172.

27   Pellegrino, E.: 1983, 'Moral Choice, The Good of the Patient and the Patient Good', in J. Moskop and L. Kopelman (eds.), *Moral Choice and Medical Crisis*, D. Reidel, Dordrecht, Holland.

28   Pellegrino, E.: 1983, '*Scribonius Largus* and the Origins of Medical Humanism', address to the American Osler Society.

29   Pieper, J.: 1966, *The Four Cardinal Virtues*, University of Notre Dame Press, Notre Dame, Indiana.

30   Reader, J.: 1982, 'Beneficence, Supererogation, and Role Duty', in E. Shelp (ed.), *Beneficence and Health Care*, D. Reidel, Dordrecht, Holland, pp. 83–108.

31   Ross, W.: 1959, *Aristotle: A Complete Exposition of His Works and Thoughts*, Meridian Books, New York.

32   Santayana, G.: 1951, *Dominations and Powers: Reflections on Liberty, Society and Government*, Charles Scribner and Sons, New York.

33   Shelp, E. (ed.): 1982, *Beneficence and Health Care*, D. Reidel, Dordrecht, Holland.

34   Shelp, E. (ed.): 1981, *Justice and Health Care*, D. Reidel, Dordrecht, Holland.

35   Sokolowski, R.: 1982, *The Good Faith and Reason*, University of Notre Dame Press, Notre Dame, Indiana.

36   Taylor, A.: 1953, *Socrates: The Man and His Thought*, Doubleday and Co., New York.

37   Versanyi, L.: 1963, *Socratic Humanism*, Yale University Press, New Haven, Connecticut.

38   Von Wright, G.: 1965, *The Varieties of Goodness*, The Humanities Press, New York.

39   Wallace, J.: 1978, *Virtues and Vices*, University of California Press, Berkeley and Los Angeles.

Getting down to cases

*The revival of casuistry in bioethics**

John D. Arras

The Revival of Casuistry

Developed in the early Middle Ages as a method of bringing abstract and universal ethico-religious precepts to bear on particular moral situations, casuistry has had a checkered history (Jonsen and Toulmin, 1988). In the hands of expert practitioners during its salad days in the 16th and 17th centuries, casuistry generated a rich and morally sensitive literature devoted to numerous real-life ethical problems, such as truth-telling, usury, and the limits of revenge. By the late 17th century, however, casuistical reasoning had degenerated into a notoriously sordid form of logic-chopping in the service of personal expediency (Pascal, 1981). To this day, the very term 'casuistry' conjures up pejorative images of disingenuous argument and moral laxity.

In spite of casuistry's tarnished reputation, some philosophers have claimed that casuistry, shorn of its unfortunate excesses, has much to teach us about the resolution of moral problems in medicine. Indeed, through the work of Albert Jonsen (1980, 1986a, 1986b, 1988) and Stephen Toulmin (1981; Jonsen and Toulmin, 1988) this 'new casuistry' has emerged as a definite alternative to the hegemony of the so-called 'applied ethics' method of moral analysis that has dominated most bioethical scholarship and teaching since the early 1970s (Beauchamp and Childress, 1989). In stark contrast to methods that begin from 'on high' with the working out of a moral theory and culminate in the deductivistic application of norms to particular factual situations, this new casuistry works from the 'bottom up', emphasizing practical problem-solving by means of nuanced interpretations of individual cases.

This paper will assess the promise of this reborn casuistry for bioethics education. In order to do that, however, it will be necessary to say quite a bit in general about the nature of this form of moral analysis and its strengths and weaknesses as a method of practical thinking. Indeed, a general catalogue of the promise and potential pitfalls of the casuistical method should be directly applicable to the assessment of casuistry in educational settings.

Before we can exhibit the salient features of this rival bioethical methodology, we must first confront an initial ambiguity in the definition of casuistry. As Jonsen describes it, 'casuistry' is the art or skill of applying abstract or general principles to particular cases (1986b). In this context, Jonsen notes that the major monotheistic religions were likely sources for casuistic ethics, since they all combined a strong sense of duty with a definite set of moral precepts couched in universal terms. The pre-eminent task for devout Christians, Jews and Muslims was thus to learn how to apply these universal precepts to particular situations, where their stringency or applicability might well be affected by particular factual conditions.

Defined as the art of applying abstract principles to particular cases, the new casuistry could appropriately be viewed, not so much as a rival to the applied ethics model, but rather as a necessary complement to any and all moral theories that would guide our conduct in specific situations. So long as we take some general principles or maxims to be ethically binding, no matter what their source, we must learn through the casuist's art to fit them to particular cases. But on this gloss of 'casuistry', even the most hidebound adherent of the applied ethics model, someone who held that answers to particular moral dilemmas can be deduced from universal theories and principles, would have to count as a casuist. So defined, casuistry might appear to be little more than the handmaiden of applied ethics.

There is, however, another interpretation of casuistry in the writings of Jonsen and Toulmin that provides a distinct alternative to the applied ethics model. Instead of focusing on the need to fit principles to cases, this interpretation stresses the particular nature, derivation, and function of the principles manipulated by the new casuists. Through this alternative theory of principles, we begin to discern a morality that develops, not from the top down as in most interpretations of Roman law, but rather from case to case (or from the bottom up) as in the common law. What differentiates the new casuistry from applied ethics, then, is not the mere recognition that principles must eventually be applied, but rather a particular account of the logic and derivation of the principles that we deploy in moral discourse.

A 'case driven' method

Contrary to 'theory driven' methodologies, which approach particular situations already equipped with a full complement of moral principles, the new casuistry insists that our moral knowledge must develop incrementally through the analysis of concrete cases. From this perspective, the very notion of 'applied ethics' embodies a redundancy, while the correlative notion of 'theoretical ethics' conveys an illusory and counterproductive ideal for ethical thought.

If ethics is done properly, the new casuists imply, it will already have been immersed in concrete cases from the very start. To be sure, one can always apply the results of previous ethical inquiries to fresh problems, but to the casuists good ethics is always 'applied' in the sense that it grows out of the analysis of individual cases. It's not as though one could or should first develop a pristine ethical theory planing above the world of moral particulars, and then, having put the finishing touches on the theory, point it in the direction of particular cases. Rejecting the idea that there are such things as 'essences' in the domain of ethics, Toulmin (1981), citing Aristotle and Dewey, argues that this pursuit of rigorous theory is unhinged from the realities of the moral life and animated by an illusory quest for moral certainty. Thus, whereas many academic philosophers scorn 'applied ethics' as a pale shadow of the real thing (viz., ethical theory), the new casuists insist that good ethics is always immersed in the messy reality of cases, and that the philosophers' penchant for abstract and rigorous theory is a misleading fetish.

According to both Jonsen and Toulmin, the work of the National Commission for the Protection of Human Subjects of Biomedical and Behavioral Research provides an excellent example of this case driven method in bioethics (1988, pp. 16–19, 264, 305, 338). Although the various commissioners represented different academic, religious and philosophical perspectives, Jonsen and Toulmin (who both served, respectively, as Commissioner and consultant to the Commission) attest that the commissioners could still reach consensus by discussing the issues 'taxonomically'.

* Arras, J.: Getting down to cases: the revival of casuistry in bioethics. *The Journal of Medicine and Philosophy* **16**:29–51, 1991.

Bracketing their differences on 'matters of principle', the commissioners would begin with an analysis of paradigmatic cases of harm, cruelty, fairness and generosity, and then branch out to more complex and difficult cases posed by biomedical research. The commissioners thus 'triangulate[d] their way across the complex terrain of moral life', (Toulmin, 1981) gradually extending their analysis of relatively straightforward problems to issues requiring a much more delicate balancing of competing values.

Thus, instead of looking for ethical progress in the theoretical equivalent of the Second Coming – i.e., the establishment of *the* correct ethical theory – Jonsen and Toulmin contend that a more realistic and attainable notion of progress is afforded by this notion of moral 'triangulation', an incremental approach to problems whose model can be found in the history of our common law. Just as English-speaking peoples have developed highly complex and sophisticated legal frameworks for thinking about tort liability and criminal guilt without the benefit of pre-established legal principles, so (Jonsen and Toulmin argue) ought we to develop a 'common morality' or 'morisprudence' on the basis of case analysis – without recourse to some pre-established moral theory or moral principles.

The role of principles in the new Casuistry

Contrary to common interpretations of Roman law and to deductivist ethical theories, wherein principles are said to preexist the actual cases to which they apply, the new casuistry contends that ethical principles are 'discovered' in the cases themselves, just as common law legal principles are developed in and through judicial decisions on particular legal cases (Jonsen, 1986a). To be sure, common law and 'common law morality' (or 'morisprudence') contain a body of principles too; but the way these principles are derived, articulated, used, and taught is very different from the Roman law and deductivist ethical approach (Pitkin, 1972).

The derivation and meaning of principles

Jonsen and Toulmin have sent mixed messages regarding their views of the derivation of moral maxims and principles. In some places they appear to incline towards a weaker interpretation of casuistry as the art of applying whatever moral maxims happen to be lying around at hand in one's culture. At other places, however, Jonsen and Toulmin suggest a much stronger and more controversial view, according to which moral principles of 'common law morality' are entirely derived from (or abstracted out of) particular cases. Rather than stemming originally from some ethical theory, such as utilitarianism or Rawls's theory of justice, these principles are said to emerge gradually from reflection upon our responses to particular cases.

Whichever view of the derivation of principles modern casuistry ultimately embraces, both are fully compatible with the casuistical thesis that the full articulation of those principles cannot be determined in isolation from particular factual contexts. In order to fully understand any principle or maxim, one has to ask, through a process of interpretation, how it might apply to a variety of situations. Thus, whereas 'privacy' might simply mean an undifferentiated interest in 'liberty' to a theorist unfamiliar with the cases, to the casuist the meaning and scope of personal privacy is delimited and shaped by the features of the cases that have called for a public response. Thus, whether or not consensual sodomy is protected by a moral right of privacy will depend upon how the casuist interprets the features of previous controversial cases dealing with such issues as family life, contraception and abortion.

The priority of practice

In the applied ethics model, principles not only 'come before' our practices in the sense of being antecedently derived from theory before being applied to cases; they also have priority over practices in the sense that their function is to justify (or criticize) practices. Indeed, it is precisely through this logical priority of principles over practice that the applied ethics model derives its critical edge. It is just the reverse for the new casuists, who sometimes imply that ethical principles are nothing more than mere *summaries* of meanings already embedded in our actual practices (Toulmin, 1981). Rather than serving as a justification for certain practices, principles within the new casuistry often merely seem to report in summary fashion what we have already decided.

This logical priority of practice to principles is clearly evident in Jonsen's and Toulmin's ruminations on the experience of the National Commission for the Protection of Human Subjects. In attempting to carry out the mandate of Congress to develop principles for the ethical conduct of research on humans, the commissioners could have straightforwardly drafted a set of principles and then applied them to problematic cases. Instead, note Jonsen and Toulmin, the commissioners acted like good casuists, plunging immediately into nuanced discussions of cases. Progress in these discussions was achieved, not by applying agreed-upon principles, but rather by seeking agreement on responses to particular cases. Indeed, according to this account, the *Belmont Report* which articulated the Commission's moral principles and serves to this day as a major source of the 'applied ethics' approach to moral reasoning, was written at the end of the Commission's deliberations, long after its members had already reached consensus on the issues (Jonsen, 1986a, p. 71).

The Open texture of principles

In contrast to the deductivist method, whose principles glide unsullied over the facts, the principles of the new casuistry are always subject to further revision and articulation in light of new cases. This is true not only because casuistical principles are inextricably enmeshed in their factual surroundings, but also because the determination of the decisive or morally relevant features of this factual web is often a highly uncertain and controversial business.

By way of example, consider the question of withdrawing artificial feeding as presented in the case of Claire Conroy.[1] One of the crucial precedents for this case, both legally and morally, was the Quinlan[2] decision. What were the morally relevant features of Karen Quinlan's situation, and what might they teach us about our responsibilities to Claire Conroy? Was it crucial that Ms. Quinlan was described as being in a persistent vegetative state? Or that she was being maintained by a mechanical respirator? If so, then one might well conclude that Claire Conroy's situation – i.e., that of a patient with severe dementia being maintained by a plastic, nasogastric feeding tube–is sufficiently disanalogous to Quinlan's to compel continued treatment. On the other hand, a re-reading of Quinlan might reveal other features of that case that tell in favor of withdrawing Conroy's feeding tube, such as the unlikelihood of Karen ever recovering sapient life, the bleakness of her prognosis, and the questionable proportion of benefits to burdens derived from the treatment.

Although the Quinlan case may have begun by standing for the patient's right to refuse treatment, subsequent readings of that case in light of later cases have fastened onto other aspects of the case, thereby giving rise to modifications of the original principle, or perhaps even to the wholesale substitution of new principles for the old. The principles of casuistic analysis might thus be said to exhibit an 'open texture' (Hart, 1961, pp. 120ff.). Somewhat in the manner of Thomas Kuhn's 'paradigms' of scientific research (Kuhn, 1970), each significant case in bioethics stands as an object for further articulation and specification under new or more complex conditions. Viewed this way, casuistical analysis might be summarized as a form of reasoning by means of examples that always point beyond themselves. Both the examples and the principles derived from them are always subject to reinterpretation and gradual modification in light of subsequent examples.

Teaching and learning

In contrast to legal systems derived from Roman law, where jurors are governed by a systematic legal code, common law systems derive from the particular judicial decisions of particular judges. As a result of these radically differing approaches to the nature and derivation of law, common law and Roman law are taught and learned in correspondingly different ways. Students of Roman law need only refer to the code itself, and perhaps to the scholarly literature explicating the meaning of the code's various provisions; whereas students of the common law must refer directly to prior judical opinions. Consequently, the so-called 'case method' of legal study is naturally suited to common law jurisdictions, for it is only through a study of the cases that one can learn the concrete meaning of legal principles and learn to apply them correctly to future cases (Patterson, 1951).

What is true of the common law is equally true of 'common law morality'. According to the casuists, bioethical principles are best learned by the case method, not by appeals to abstract theoretical notions. Indeed, anyone at all experienced in teaching bioethics in clinical settings must know (often by means of painful experience) that physicians, nurses, and other health care providers learn best by means of case discussions. (The best way to put them to sleep, in fact, is to begin one's talk with a recitation of the 'principles of bioethics'). This is explained not simply by the fact that case presentations are intrinsically more gripping than abstract discussions of the moral philosophies of Mill, Kant, and Rawls; they are, in addition, the best vehicle for conveying the concrete meaning and scope of whatever principles and maxims one wishes to teach. Contrary to ethical deductivism and Roman law, whose principles could conceivably be taught in a practical vacuum, casuistry demands a case-driven method of instruction. For casuists, cases are much more than mere illustrated rules or handy mnemonic devices for the 'abstracting impaired'. They are, as Jonsen and Toulmin argue, the very locus of moral meaning and moral certainty.

Although Jonsen and Toulmin have yet to consider the concrete pedagogical implications of their casuistical method, we can venture a few suggestions. First, it would appear that a casuistical approach would encourage the use, whenever possible, of real as opposed to hypothetical cases. This is because hypothetical cases, so beloved of academic philosophers, tend to be theory-driven; that is, they are usually designed to advance some explicitly theoretical point. Real cases, on the other hand, are more likely to display the sort of moral complexity and untidiness that demand the (non-deductive) weighing and balancing of competing moral considerations and the casuistical virtues of discernment and practical judgment (*phronesis*).

Second, a casuistical pedagogy would call for lengthy and richly detailed case studies. If the purpose of moral education is to prepare on for action in the real world, the cases discussed should reflect the degree of complexity, uncertainty, and ambiguity encountered there. If for casuistry moral truth resides 'in the details', if the meaning and scope of moral principles is determined contextually through an interpretation of factual situations in their relationship to paradigm cases, then cases must be presented in rich detail. It won't do, as is so often done in our textbooks and anthologies, to cram the rich moral fabric of cases into a couple of paragraphs.

Third, a casuistical pedagogy would encourage the use, not simply of the occasional isolated case study, but rather of whole sequences of cases bearing on a related principle or theme. Thus, instead of simply 'illustrating' the debate over the termination of life-sustaining treatments with, say, the single case of Karen Quinlan, teachers and students should read and interpret a sequence of cases (including, e.g., Quinlan, Saikewicz, Spring, Conroy, and Cruzan) in order to see just how reasoning by paradigm and analogy takes place and how the so-called 'principles of bioethics' are actually shaped in their effective meaning by the details of successive cases.

Fourth, a casuistically-driven pedagogy will give much more emphasis than currently allotted to what might be called the problem of 'moral diagnosis'. Given any particular controversy, exactly what kind of issues does it raise? What, in other words, is the case really about? As opposed to the anthologies, where each case comes neatly labelled under a discrete rubric, real life does not announce the nature of problems in advance. It requires interpretation, imagination and discernment to figure out what is going on, especially when (as is usually the case) a number of discussable issues are usually extractable from any given controversy.

Problems with the casuistical method

Since the new casuistry attempts to define itself by turning applied ethics on its head, working from cases to principles rather than vice-versa, it should come as no surprise to find that its strengths correlate perfectly with the weaknesses of applied ethics. Thus, whereas applied ethics, and especially deductivism, are often criticized for their remoteness from clinical realities and for their consequent irrelevance (Fox *et al.*, 1984; Noble, 1982) casuistry prides itself on its concreteness and on its ability to render useful advice to caregivers in the medical trenches. Likewise, if the applied ethics model appears rather narrow in its single-minded emphasis on the application of principles and in its corresponding neglect of moral interpretation and practical discernment, the new casuistry can be viewed as a defense of the Aristotelian virtue of *phronesis* (or sound, practical judgment).

Conversely, it should not be surprising to find certain problems with the casuistical method that correspond to strengths of the applied ethics model. I shall devote the second half of this essay to an inventory of some of these problems. It should be stressed, however, that not all of these problems are unique to casuistry, nor does applied ethics fare much better with regard to some of them.

What is 'a case'?

For all of their emphasis upon the interpretation of particular cases, casuists have not said much, if anything, about how to select problems for moral interpretation. What, in other words, gets placed on the 'moral agenda' in the first place, and why? This is a problem because it is quite possible that the current method of selecting agenda items, whatever that may be, systematically ignores genuine issues equally worthy of discussion and debate (O'Neil, 1988).

I think it safe to say that problems currently make it onto the bioethical agenda largely because health practitioners and policy makers put them there. While there is usually nothing problematic in this, and while it always pays to be scrupulously attentive to the expressed concerns of people working in the trenches, practitioners may be bound to conventional ways of thinking and of conceiving problems that tend to filter out other, equally valid experiences and problems. As feminists have recently argued, for example, much of the current bioethics agenda reflects an excessively narrow, professionally driven, and male outlook on the nature of ethics (Carse, 1989). As a result, a whole range of important ethical problems – including the unequal treatment of women in health care settings, sexist occupational roles, personal relationships, and strategies of *avoiding* crisis situations – have been either downplayed or ignored completely (Warren, 1989, pp. 77–82). It is not enough, then, for casuistry to tell us *how* to interpret cases; rather than simply carrying out the agenda dictated by health professionals, all of us (casuists and applied ethicists alike) must begin to think more about the problem of *which* cases ought to be selected for moral scrutiny.

An additional problem, which I can only flag here, concerns not the identification of 'a case' – i.e., what gets placed on the public agenda – but rather the specification of 'the case' – i.e., what description of a case shall count as an adequate and sufficiently complete account of the issues, the participants and the context. One of the problems with many case presentations, especially in the clinical context, is their relative neglect of alternative perspectives on the case held by other participants. Quite often, we get the attending's (or the house officer's) point of view on what constitutes 'the case', while missing out on the perspectives of nurses, social workers and others. Since most cases are complicated and enriched by such alternative medical, psychological and social interpretations, our casuistical analyses will remain incomplete without them. Thus, in addition to being long, the cases that we employ should reflect the usually complementary (but often conflicting) perspectives of all the involved participants.

Is casuistry really theory-free?

The casuists claim that they make moral progress by moving from one class of cases to another without the benefit of any ethical principles or theoretical apparatus. Solutions generated for obvious or easy categories of cases adumbrate solutions for the more difficult cases. In a manner somewhat reminiscent of pre-Kuhnian philosophers of science clinging to the possibility of 'theory free' factual observations, to a belief in a kind of epistemological 'immaculate perception', the casuists appear to be claiming that the cases simply speak for themselves.

As we have seen, one problem with this suggestion is that it does not acknowledge or account for the way in which different theoretical preconceptions help determine which cases and problems get selected for study in the first place. Another problem is that it does not explain what allows us to group different cases into distinct categories or to proceed from one category to another. In other words, the casuists' account of case analysis fails to supply us with principles of relevance that explain what binds the cases together and how the meaning of one case points beyond itself toward the resolution of subsequent cases. The casuists obviously cannot do without such principles of relevance; they are a necessary condition of any kind of moral taxonomy. Without principles of relevance, the cases would fly apart in all directions, rendering coherent speech, thought, and action about them impossible.

But if the casuists rise to this challenge and convert their implicit principles of relevance into explicit principles, it is certainly reasonable to expect that these will be heavily 'theory laden'. Take, for example, the novel suggestion that anencephalic infants should be used as organ donors for children born with fatal heart defects. What is the relevant line of cases in our developed 'morisprudence' for analyzing this problem? To the proponents of this suggestion, the brain death debates provide the appropriate context of discussion. According to this line of argument, anencephalic infants most closely resemble the brain dead; and since we already harvest vital organs from the latter category, we have a moral warrant for harvesting organs from anencephalics (Harrison, 1986). But to some of those opposed to any change in the status quo, the most relevant line of cases is provided by the literature on fetal experimentation. Our treatment of the anencephalic newborn should, they claim, reflect our practices regarding nonviable fetuses. If we agree with the judgment of the National Commission that research which would shorten the already doomed child's life should not be permitted, then we should oppose the use of equally doomed anencephalic infants as heart donors (Meilaender, 1986).

How ought the casuist to triangulate the moral problem of the anencephalic newborn as organ donor? What principles of relevance will lead him to opt for one line of cases instead of another? Whatever principles he might eventually articulate, they will undoubtedly have something definite to say about such matters as the concept of death, the moral status of fetuses, the meaning and scope of respect, the nature of personhood, and the relative importance of achieving good consequences in the world versus treating other human beings as ends in themselves. Although one's position on such issues perhaps need not implicate any full-blown ethical theory, in the strictest sense of the term, they are sufficiently theory-laden to cast grave doubt on the new casuists' ability to move from case to case without recourse to mediating ethical principles or other theoretical notions.

Although the early work of Jonsen and Toulxnin can easily be read as advocating a theory-free methodology comprised of mere 'summary principles', their recent work appears to acknowledge the point of the above criticism. Indeed, it would be fair to say that they now seek to articulate a method that is, if not 'theory free', then at least 'theory modest'. Drawing on the approach of the classical casuists, they now concede an indisputably normative role for principles and maxims drawn from a variety of sources, including theology, common law, historical tradition, and ethical theories. Rather than viewing ethical theories as mutually exclusive, reductionists attempts to provide an apodictic *foundation* for ethical thought, Jonsen and Toulmin now view theories as limited and complementary *perspectives* that might enrich a more pragmatic and pluralistic approach to the ethical life (1988, Chapter 15). They thus appear reconciled to the usefulness, both in research and education, of a severely chastened conception of moral principles and theories.

One lesson of all this for bioethics education is that casuistry, for all its usefulness as a method, is nothing more than (and nothing less) than an 'engine of thought' that must receive *direction* from values, concepts and theories outside of itself. Given the important role such 'external' sources of moral direction must play even in the most case-bound approaches, teachers and students need to be self-conscious about which traditions and theories are in effect driving their casuistical interpretations. This means that they need to devote time and energy to studying and criticizing the values, concepts and rank-orderings implicitly or explicitly conveyed by the various traditions and theories from which they derive their overall direction and tools of moral analysis. In short, it means that adopting the casuistical method will not absolve teachers and students from studying and evaluating either ethical theories or the history of ethics.

Indeterminacy and consensus

One need not believe in the existence of uniquely correct answers to all moral questions to be concerned about the casuistical method's capacity to yield determinate answers to problematical moral questions. Indeed, anyone familiar with Alastair MacIntyre's (1981) disturbing diagnosis of our contemporary moral culture might well tend to greet the casuists' announcement of moral consensus with a good deal of skepticism. According to MacIntyre, our moral culture is in a grave state of disorder: lacking any comprehensive and coherent understanding of morality and human nature, we subsist on scattered shards and remnants of past moral frameworks. It is no wonder, then, according to MacIntyre, that our moral debates and disagreements are often marked by the clash of incommensurable premises derived from disparate moral cultures. Nor is it any wonder that our debates over highly controversial issues such as abortion and affirmative action take the form of a tedious, interminable cycle of assertion and counter-assertion. In this disordered and contentious moral setting, which MacIntyre claims is *our* moral predicament, the casuists' goal of consensus based upon intuitive responses to cases might well appear to be a Panglossian dream.

One need not endorse MacIntyre's pessimistic diagnosis in its entirety to notice that many of our moral practices and policies bear a multiplicity of meanings; they often embody a variety of different, and sometimes conflicting, values. An ethical methodology based exclusively, on the casuistical analysis of these practices can reasonably be expected to express these different values in the form of conflicting ethical conclusions.

Political theorist Michael Walzer's remarks on health care in the United States provide an illuminating case in point. Although Walzer might not recognize himself as a modern day casuist, his vigorous anti-theoretical stance and reliance upon established social meanings and norms certainly make him an ally of the methodological approach espoused by Jonsen and Toulmin (Walzer, 1983 1987). According to Walzer, if we look carefully at our current values and practices regarding health care and its distribution – if we look, in other words, at the choices we as a people have already made, at the programs we have already put into place, etc. – we will conclude that health care services are a crucially important social good, that they should be allocated solely on the basis of need; and that they must be made equally available to all citizens, presumably through something like a national health service (1983, pp. 86ff.).

One could argue, however, that current disparities – both in access to care and in quality of care – between the poor, the middle class and the rich reflect equally 'deep' (or even deeper) political choices that we have made regarding the relative importance of individual freedom, social security, and the health needs of the 'non-deserving' poor. In this vein, one could claim that our collective decisions bearing on Medicaid, Medicare, and access to emergency rooms – the same decisions that Walzer uses to argue for a national health service – are more accurately interpreted as grudging aberrations from our free market ideology. According to this opposing view, our stratified health care system pretty well reflects our values and commitments in this area: a 'decent minimum' (read 'understaffed, ill-equipped, impersonal urban clinics') for the medically indigent, decent health insurance and HMOs for the working middle class; and first cabin care for the well-to-do (Dworkin, 1983; Warnke, 1989).

Viewed in the light of Walzer's democratic socialist commitments, which I happen to share, this arrangement may indeed look like an 'indefensible triage'; but placed in the context of American history and culture, it could just as easily be viewed as business as usual. Thus, on one reading our current practices point toward the establishment of a thoroughly egalitarian health care system; viewed from a different angle, however, these same 'choices we have already made' justify pervasive inequalities in access to care and quality of care. The problem for the casuistical method is that, barring any and all appeals to abstract principles of justice, it cannot decisively adjudicate between such competing interpretations of our common practices (Dworkin, 1983). When these do not convey a univocal message, or when they carry conflicting messages of more or less equal plausibility, casuistry cannot help us to develop a uniquely correct interpretation upon which a widespread social consensus might be based. Contrary to the assurances of Jonsen and Toulmin, the new casuistry is an unlikely instrument for generating consensus in a moral world fractured by conflicting values and intuitions.

In Jonsen and Toulmin's defense, it should be noted that abstract theories of justice divorced from the conventions of our society are equally unlikely sources of uniquely correct answers. If philosophers cannot agree amongst themselves upon the true nature of abstract justice – indeed, if criticizing our foremost theoretician of justice, John Rawls, has become something of a philosophical national pastime (Daniels, 1989; Arneson, 1998) – it is unclear how their theorizing could decisively resolve the ongoing debate among competing interpretations of our common social practices.

It might also be noted in passing that even Rawls has become increasingly loathe in his recent writings to appeal to an abstract, timeless, and deracinated notion of justice as the ultimate court of appeal from conflicting social interpretations. Eschewing any pretense of having established a theory of justice 'sub specie aeternitatis', Rawls now claims that his theory of 'justice as fairness' is only applicable in modern democracies like our own (Rawls, 1980, p. 318). He claims, moreover, that the justification of his theory is derived, not from neutral data, but from its 'congruence with our deeper understanding of ourselves and our aspirations, and our realization that, given our history and the traditions embedded in our public life, it is the most reasonable doctrine for us' (Rawls, 1980, p. 519; see also Rawls, 1985, p. 228). Notwithstanding the many differences that distinguish their respective views, it thus appears that Rawls, Walzer, and Jonsen and Toulmin could all agree that there is no escape from the task of interpreting the meanings embedded in our social practices, institutions and history. Given the complexity and tensions that characterize this moral 'data', the search for uniquely correct interpretations must be seen as misguided. The best we can do, it seems, is to argue for our own determinate but contestable interpretations of who we are as a people and who we want to become. Neither theory nor casuistry is a guarantor of consensus.

Conventionalism and critique

The stronger, more controversial version of casuistry and its 'summary view' of ethical principles gives rise to worries about the nature of moral truth and justification. Eschewing any theoretical derivation of principles and insisting that the locus of moral certainty is the particular, the casuist asks 'What principles best organize and account for what we have already decided?' Viewed from this angle, the casuistic project amounts to nothing more than an elaborate refinement of our intuitions regarding cases. As such, it begins to resemble the kind of relativistic conventionalism recently articulated by Richard Rorty (Rorty, 1989).

Obviously, one problem with this is that our intuitions have often been shown to be wildly wrong, if not downright prejudicial and superstitious. To the extent that this is true of *our own* intuitions about ethical matters, then casuistry will merely refine our prejudices. Any casuistry that modestly restricts itself to interpreting and cataloguing the flickering shadows on the cave wall can easily be accused of lacking a critical edge. If applied ethics might rightly be said to have purchased critical leverage at the expense of the concrete moral situation, then casuistry might be charged with having purchased concreteness and relevance at the expense of philosophical criticism. This charge might take either of two forms. First, one could claim that the casuist is a mere expositor of *established* social meanings and thus lacks the requisite critical distance to formulate telling critiques of regnant social understandings. Second, casuistry could be accused of ignoring the power relations that shape and inform the social meanings that its practitioners interpret.

In response to the issue of critical distance, Jonsen and Toulmin could point out that the social world of established meanings is by no means monolithic and usually harbors alternative values that offer plenty of critical leverage against the regnant social consensus. As Michael Walzer has recently argued, even such thundering social critics as the prophet Amos have usually been fully committed to their societies, rather than 'objective' and detached; and the values to which they appeal are often fundamental to the self-understanding of a people or group (Walzer, 1987). (How else could they accuse their fellows of hypocrisy?) The lesson for casuists here is not to become so identified with the point of view of health care professionals that they lose sight of other important values in our culture.

The second claim, while not necessarily fatal to the casuistical enterprise, is harder to rebut. As Habermas has contended in his longstanding debate with Gadamer, interpretive approaches to ethics [such as casuistry] can articulate our shared social meanings but ignore the economic and power relations that shape social consensus. His point is that the very conversation through which cases, social practices and institutions are interpreted is itself subject to what he calls 'systematically distorted communication' (Habermas, 1980). In order to avoid merely legitimizing social understandings conditioned on power and domination – for example, our conception of the appropriate relationship between nurses and physicians – casuistry will have to supplement its interpretations with a critical theory of social relationships, or with what Paul Ricoeur has called a 'hermeneutics of suspicion'. (Ricoeur, 1986).

Reinforcing the individualism of bioethics

Analytical philosophers working as applied ethicists have often been criticized for the ahistorical, reductionist, and excessively individualistic character of their work in bioethics (Fox et al., 1984; Noble, 1982; MacIntyre, 1982). While the casuistical method cannot thus be justly accused of importing a short-sighted individualism into the field of bioethics – that honor already belonging to analytical philosophy – it cannot be said either that casuistry offers anything like a promising remedy for this deficiency. On the contrary, it seems that the casuists' method of reasoning by analogy only promises to exacerbate the individualism and reductionism already characteristic of much bioethical scholarship.

Consider, for example, how a casuist might address the problem of heart transplants. He or she might reason like this: Our society is already deeply committed to paying for all kinds of 'half-way technologies' for those in need. We already pay for renal dialysis and transplantation, chronic ventilatory support for children and adults, expensive open-heart surgery, and many other 'high tech' therapies, some of which might well be even more expensive than heart transplants. Therefore, so long as heart transplants qualify medically as a proven therapy, there is no reason why Medicaid and Medicare should not fund them (Overcast et al., 1985).

Notwithstanding the evident fruitfulness of such analogical reasoning in many contexts of bioethics, and notwithstanding the possibility that these particular examples of it might well prevail against the competing arguments on heart transplantation, it remains true that such contested practices raise troubling questions that tend not to be asked, let alone illuminated, by casuistical reasoning by analogy. The extent of our willingness to fund heart transplantation has great bearing on the kind of society in which we wish to live and on our priorities for spending within (and without) the health care budget. Even if we already fund many high technology procedures that cost as much or more than heart transplants, it is possible that this new round of transplantation could threaten other forms of care that provide greater benefits to more people; and we might therefore wish to draw the line here (Massachusetts Task Force, 1984; Annas, 1985).

The point is that, no matter where we stand on the particular issue of heart transplants, we *might* think it important to raise such 'big questions', depending on the nature of the problem at hand. We might want to ask, to borrow from a recent title, 'What kind of life?' (Callahan, 1990). But the kind of reasoning by analogy championed by the new casuists tends to reduce our field of ethical vision down to the proximate moral precedents, and thereby suppresses the important global questions bearing on who we are and what kind of society we want. The result is likely to be a method of moral reasoning that graciously accommodates us to any and all technological innovations, no matter what their potential long-term threat to fundamental and cherished institutions and values.

Conclusions

The revival of casuistry, both in practice and in Jonsen and Toulmin's (1988) recent defense, is a welcome development in the field of bioethics. Its account of moral reasoning (emphasizing the pivotal role of paradigms, analogical thinking, and the prudential weighing of competing factors) is far superior, both as a description of how we actually think and as a prescription of how we ought to think, to the tiresome invocation of the applied ethics mantra (i.e., the principles of respect for autonomy, beneficence and justice). By insisting on a *modest* role for ethical theory in a pragmatic, non-deductivist approach to ethical interpretation, Jonsen and Toulmin join an important chorus of contemporary thinkers troubled by the reductionism inherent in most analytical ethics (Williams, 1985; Hampshire, 1983; Taylor, 1982).

As for its role in bioethics education, no one needs to tell teachers about the importance of cases in the classroom. It's pretty obvious that discussing cases is fun, interesting, and certainly more memorable than any philosophical theory, which for the average student usually has a half-life of about two weeks. Moreover, a casuistical education gives students the methodological tools they are most likely to need when they later encounter bioethical problems in the 'real world', whether as health care professionals, clergy, lawyers, journalists or informed citizens. For all of the obviousness of these points, however, it remains true that all of us teachers could profit from sound advice on how better to use cases, and some such advice can be extrapolated from the work of Jonsen and Toulmin.

For all its virtues *vis-à-vis* the sclerotic invocation of 'bioethical principles', the casuistical method is not, however, without problems of its own. First, we found that the very principles of relevance that drive the casuistical method need to be made explicit; and we surmised that, once unveiled, these principles will turn out to be heavily theory laden. Second, we showed that the casuistical method is an unlikely source of uniquely correct interpretations of social meanings and therefore an unlikely source of societal consensus. Third we have seen that, because of the casuists' view of ethical principles as mere summaries of our intuitive responses to paradigmatic cases, their method might suffer from ideological distortions and lack a critical edge. Moreover, relying so heavily on the perceptions and agenda of health care professionals, casuists might tend to ignore the existence of important issues that could be revealed by other theoretical perspectives, such as feminism. Finally, we saw that casuistry, focusing as it does on analogical resemblances, might tend to ignore certain difficult but inescapable 'big questions' (e.g., 'What kind of society do we want?'), and thereby reinforce the individualistic tendencies already at work in contemporary bioethics.

It remains to be seen whether casuistry, as a program in practical ethics, will be able to marshall sufficient internal resources to respond to these criticisms. Whatever the outcome of that attempt, however, an equally promising approach might be to incorporate the insights and tools of casuistry into the methodological approach known as 'reflective equilibrium' (Rawls, 1971; Daniels, 1979). According to this method, the casuistical interpretation of cases, on the one hand, and moral theories,

principles and maxims, on the other, exist in a symbiotic relationship. Our intuitions on cases will thus be guided, and perhaps criticized, by theory; while our theories and moral principles will themselves be shaped, and perhaps reformulated, by our responses to paradigmatic moral situations. Whether we attempt to flesh out this method of reflective equilibrium or further develop the casuistical program, it should be clear by now that the methodological issue between theory and cases is not a dichotomous 'either/or' but rather an encompassing 'both-and'.

In closing I would like to gather together my various recommendations, strewn throughout this paper, for the use of casuistry in bioethics education:

1   Use real cases rather than hypotheticals whenever possible.

2   Avoid schematic case presentations. Make them long, richly detailed, messy, and comprehensive. Make sure that the perspectives of all the major players (including nurses and social workers) are represented.

3   Present complex sequences of cases that sharpen students' analogical reasoning skills.

4   Engage students in the process of 'moral diagnosis'.

5   Be mindful of the limits of casuistical analysis. As a mere engine of moral argument, casuistry must be supplemented and guided by appeals to ethical theory, the history of ethics, and moral norms embedded in our traditions and social practices. It must also be supplemented by critical social analyses that unmask the power behind much social consensus and raise larger questions about the kind of society we want and the kind of people we to be.

Acknowledgements

This article is based upon a presentation at a conference on 'Bioethics as an Intellectual Field', sponsored by the University of Texas Medical Branch, Galveston, Texas. The author would like to thank Ronald Carson and Thomas Murray for their encouragement.

Notes

1   Matter of Claire C. Conroy, Supreme Court of New Jersey, 486 A. 2d 1209 (1985).

2   Matter of Quinlan, Supreme Court of New Jersey, 355 A. 2d 647 (1976).

Bibliography

Annas, G.: 1985, 'Regulating heart and liver transplants in Massachusetts', *Law, Medicine and Health Care* **13**(1), 4–7.

Arneson, R.J. (ed.): 1989, 'Symposium on Rawlsian theory of justice: Recent developments', *Ethics* 99 (4), 695–944.

Beauchamp, T.L. and **Childress J.F.**: 1989, *Principles of Biomedical Ethics*, 3rd edition, Oxford University Press, New York, New York.

Callahan, D.: 1990, *What Kind of Life?*, Simon and Schuster, New York, New York.

Carse, A.L.: 1991, 'The "voice of care", Implications for bioethics education', *Journal of Philosophy and Medicine* **16**, 5–28.

Daniels, N.: 1979, 'Wide reflective equilibrium and theory acceptance in ethics', *The Journal of Philosophy* **76**, 256–82.

Daniels, N.: 1989, *Reading Rawls*, 2nd edition, Stanford University Press, Stanford, California.

Dworkin, R.: 1983: '*Spheres of Justice*: An exchange', *New York Review of Books*, 30 (12), 44.

Dworkin, R.: 1985, *A Matter of Principle*, Harvard University Press, Cambridge.

Fox, R.C. and **Swazey, J.P.**: 1984, 'Medical morality is not bioethics – medical ethics in China and the United States', *Perspectives in Biology and Medicine* **27**, 336–360.

Habermas, J.: 1980, 'The hermeneutic claim to universality' in J. Bleicher (ed.), *Contemporary Hermeneutics*, Routledge & Kegan Paul, London, pp. 181–211.

Hampshire, S.: 1983, *Morality and Conflict*, Harvard University Press, Cambridge, Massachusetts.

Harrison, M.R.: 1986, 'The anencephalic newborn as organ donor: Commentary', *Hastings Center Report* **16**, 21–22.

Hart, H.L.A.: 1961, *The Concept of Law*, Oxford University Press, Oxford, England.

Jonsen, A.R.: 1980, 'Can an ethicist be a consultant?', in V. Abernethy (ed.), *Frontiers in Medical Ethics*, Ballinger Publishing Company, Cambridge, Massuchsetts, pp. 157–171.

Jonsen, A.R.: 1986a, 'Casuistry and clinical ethics', *Theoretical Medicine* **7**, 65–74.

Jonsen, A.R.: 1986b, 'Casuistry', in J.F. Childress and J. Macgvarrie (eds.), *Westminster Dictionary of Christian Ethics*, Westminster Press, Philadelphia, Pennsylvania, pp. 78–80.

Jonsen, A.R. and Toulmin, S.: 1988, *The Abuse of Casuistry*, University of California Press, Berkeley, California.

Kuhn, T.: 1970, *The Structure of Scientific Revolutions*, 2nd edition, University of Chicago Press, Chicago, Illinois.

MacIntyre, A.: 1981, *After Virtue*, University of Notre Dame Press, Notre Dame, Indiana.

Massachusetts Task Force on Organ Transplantation: 1984, *Report of the Massachusetts Task Force on Organ Transplantation*, Boston, Massachusetts.

Meilaender, G.: 1986, 'The anencephalic newborn as organ donor: Commentary', *Hastings Center Report* **16**, 22–23.

Noble, C.: 1982, 'Ethics and experts', *Hastings Center Report* **12**, 7–9.

O'Neill, O.: 1988, 'How can we individuate moral problems?' in D.M. Rosenthal and F. Shehadi (eds.), *Applied Ethics and Ethical Theory*, University of Utah Press, Salt Lake City, pp. 84–99.

Overcast, D. *et al.*: 1985, 'Technology assessment, public policy and transplantation', *Law, Medicine and Health Care* **13**(3), 106–111.

Pascal, B.: 1981, *Lettres écrites à un provincial*, A. Adam (ed.), Flammarion, Paris.

Patterson, E.W.: 1951, The case method in American legal education: Its origins and objectives', *Journal of Legal Education* **4**, 1–24.

Pitkin, H.: 1972, *Wittgenstein and Justice*, University of California Press, Berkeley, California.

Rawls, J.: 1971, *A Theory of Justice*, Harvard University Press, Cambridge Massachusetts.

Rawls, J.: 1980, 'Kantian constructivism in moral theory: The Dewey Lectures 1980', *The Journal of Philosophy* **77**, 515–572.

Rawls, J.: 1985, 'Justice as fairness: Political not metaphysical', *Philosophy and Public Affairs* **14**, 223–251.

Ricoeur, P.: 1986, 'Hermeneutics and the critique of ideology', in B.R. Wachterhauser (ed.), *Hermeneutics and Modern Philosophy*, State University of New York Press, Albany, New York, pp. 300–339.

Rorty, R.: 1989, *Contingency, Irony, and Solidarity*, Cambridge University Press, Cambridge, England.

Taylor, C.: 1982, The diversity of goods', in A. Sen and B. Williams (eds.), *Utilitarianism and Beyond*, Cambridge University Press, Cambridge, England, pp. 129–144.

Toulmin, S., 1981: 'The tyranny of principles', *Hastings Center Report* **11**, 31–39.

Walzer, M.: 1983, *Spheres of Justice*, Basic Books, New York, New York.

Walzer, M.: 1987, *Interpretation and Social Criticism*, Harvard University Press, Cambridge, Massachusetts.

Warnke, G.: 1989–1990, 'Social interpretation and political theory: Walzer and his critics', *The Philosophical Forum* **21** (1–2), 204–226.

Warren, V.: 1989, 'Feminist directions in medical ethics', *Hypatia* **4**, 73–87.

Williams, B.: 1985, *Ethics and the Limits of Philosophy*, Harvard University Press, Cambridge, Massachusetts.

Grounding for the Metaphysics of Morals: First and Second Sections*

Immanuel Kant

First section

Transition from the ordinary rational knowledge of morality to the philosophical

393 There is no possibility of thinking of anything at all in the world, or even out of it, which can be regarded as good without qualification, except a *good will*. Intelligence, wit, judgment, and whatever talents of the mind one might want to name are doubtless in many respects good and desirable, as are such qualities of temperament as courage, resolution, perseverance. But they can also become extremely bad and harmful if the will, which is to make use of these gifts of nature and which in its special constitution is called character, is not good. The same holds with gifts of fortune; power, riches, honor, even health, and that complete well-being and contentment with one's condition which is called happiness make for pride and often hereby even arrogance, unless there is a good will to correct their influence on the mind and herewith also to rectify the whole principle of action and make it universally conformable to its end. The sight of a being who is not graced by any touch of a pure and good will but who yet enjoys an uninterrupted prosperity can never delight a rational and impartial spectator. Thus a good will seems to constitute the indispensable condition of being even worthy of happiness.

394 Some qualities are even conducive to this good will itself and can facilitate its work. Nevertheless, they have no intrinsic unconditional worth; but they always presuppose, rather, a good will, which restricts the high esteem in which they are otherwise rightly held, and does not permit them to be regarded as absolutely good. Moderation in emotions and passions, self-control, and calm deliberation are not only good in many respects but even seem to constitute part of the intrinsic worth of a person. But they are far from being rightly called good without qualification (however unconditionally they were commended by the ancients). For without the principles of a good will, they can become extremely bad; the coolness of a villain makes him not only much more dangerous but also immediately more abominable in our eyes than he would have been regarded by us without it.

A good will is good not because of what it effects or accomplishes, nor because of its fitness to attain some proposed end; it is good only through its willing, i.e., it is good in itself. When it is considered in itself, then it is to be esteemed very much higher than anything which it might ever bring about merely in order to favor some inclination, or even the sum total of all inclinations. Even if, by some especially unfortunate fate or by the niggardly provision of stepmotherly nature, this will should be wholly lacking in the power to accomplish its purpose; if with the greatest effort it should yet achieve nothing, and only the good will should remain (not, to be sure, as a mere wish but as the summoning of all the means in our power), yet would it, like a jewel, still shine by its own light as something which has its full value in itself. Its usefulness or fruitlessness can neither augment nor diminish this value. Its usefulness would be, as it were, only the setting to enable us to handle it in ordinary dealings or to attract to it the attention of those who are not yet experts, but not to recommend it to real experts or to determine its value.

But there is something so strange in this idea of the absolute value of a   395 mere will, in which no account is taken of any useful results, that in spite of all the agreement received even from ordinary reason, yet there must arise the suspicion that such an idea may perhaps have as its hidden basis merely some high-flown fancy, and that we may have misunderstood the purpose of nature in assigning to reason the governing of our will. Therefore, this idea will be examined from this point of view.

In the natural constitution of an organized being, i.e., one suitably adapted to the purpose of life, let there be taken as a principle that in such a being no organ is to be found for any end unless it be the most fit and the best adapted for that end. Now if that being's preservation, welfare, or in a word its happiness, were the real end of nature in the case of a being having reason and will, then nature would have hit upon a very poor arrangement in having the reason of the creature carry out this purpose. For all the actions which such a creature has to perform with this purpose in view, and the whole rule of his conduct would have been prescribed much more exactly by instinct; and the purpose in question could have been attained much more certainly by instinct than it ever can be by reason. And if in addition reason had been imparted to this favored creature, then it would have had to serve him only to contemplate the happy constitution of his nature, to admire that nature, to rejoice in it, and to feel grateful to the cause that bestowed it; but reason would not have served him to subject his faculty of desire to its weak and delusive guidance nor would it have served him to meddle incompetently with the purpose of nature. In a word, nature would have taken care that reason did not strike out into a practical use nor presume, with its weak insight, to think out for itself a plan for happiness and the means for attaining it. Nature would have taken upon herself not only the choice of ends but also that of the means, and would with wise foresight have entrusted both to instinct alone.

And, in fact, we find that the more a cultivated reason devotes itself to the   396 aim of enjoying life and happiness, the further does man get away from true contentment. Because of this there arises in many persons, if only they are candid enough to admit it, a certain degree of misology, i.e., hatred of reason. This is especially so in the case of those who are the most experienced in the use of reason, because after calculating all the advantages they derive, I say not from the invention of all the arts of common luxury, but even from the sciences (which in the end seem to them to be also a luxury of the understanding), they yet find that they have in fact only brought more trouble on their heads than they have gained in happiness. Therefore, they come to envy, rather than despise, the more common Mon run of men who are closer to the guidance of mere natural instinct and who do not allow their reason much influence on their conduct. And we must admit that the judgment of those who would temper, or even reduce below zero, the boastful eulogies on behalf of the advantages which reason is supposed to provide as regards the happiness and contentment of life is by no means morose or ungrateful to the goodness with which the world is governed. There lies at the root of such judgments, rather, the idea that existence has another and much more

* Kant, I.: Grounding for the metaphysics of morals, in *Ethical philosophy*, trans. J. Ellington. Indianapolis, IN, Hackett Publishing Company, 1983, pp. 7–17; 19–27; 30–32; 40–41.

worthy purpose, for which, and not for happiness, reason is quite properly intended, and which must, therefore, be regarded as the supreme condition to which the private purpose of men must, for the most part, defer.

Reason, however, is not competent enough to guide the will safely as regards its objects and the satisfaction of all our needs (which it in part even multiplies); to this end would an implanted natural instinct have led much more certainly. But inasmuch as reason has been imparted to us as a practical faculty, i.e., as one which is to have influence on the will, its true function must be to produce a will which is not merely good as a means to some further end, but is good in itself. To produce a will good in itself reason was absolutely necessary, inasmuch as nature in distributing her capacities has everywhere gone to work in a purposive manner. While such a will may not indeed be the sole and complete good, it must, nevertheless, be the highest good and the condition of all the rest, even of the desire for happiness. In this case there is nothing inconsistent with the wisdom of nature that the cultivation of reason, which is requisite for the first and unconditioned purpose, may in many ways restrict, at least in this life, the attainment of the second purpose, viz., happiness, which is always conditioned. Indeed happiness can even be reduced to less than nothing, without nature's failing thereby in her purpose; for reason recognizes as its highest practical function the establishment of a good will, whereby in the attainment of this end reason is capable only of its own kind of satisfaction, viz., that of fulfilling a purpose which is in turn determined only by reason, even though such fulfilment were often to interfere with the purposes of inclination.

397 The concept of a will estimable in itself and good without regard to any further end must now be developed. This concept already dwells in the natural sound understanding and needs not so much to be taught as merely to be elucidated. It always holds first place in estimating the total worth of our actions and constitutes the condition of all the rest. Therefore, we shall take up the concept of *duty*, which includes that of a good will, though with certain subjective restrictions and hindrances, which far from hiding a good will or rendering it unrecognizable, rather bring it out by contrast and make it shine forth more brightly.

I here omit all actions already recognized as contrary to duty, even though they may be useful for this or that end; for in the case of these the question does not arise at all as to whether they might be done from duty, since they even conflict with duty. I also set aside those actions which are really in accordance with duty, yet to which men have no immediate inclination, but perform them because they are impelled thereto by some other inclination. For in this [second] case to decide whether the action which is in accord with duty has been done from duty or from some selfish purpose is easy. This difference is far more difficult to note in the [third] case where the action accords with duty and the subject has in addition an immediate inclination to do the action. For example, that a dealer should not overcharge an inexperienced purchaser certainly accords with duty; and where there is much commerce, the prudent merchant does not overcharge but keeps to a fixed price for everyone in general, so that a child may buy from him just as well as everyone else may. Thus customers are honestly served, but this is not nearly enough for making us believe that the merchant has acted this way from duty and from principles of honesty; his own advantage required him to do it. He cannot, however, be assumed to have in addition [as in the third case] an immediate inclination toward his buyers, causing him, as it were, out of love to give no one as far as price is concerned any advantage over another. Hence the action was done neither from duty nor from immediate inclination, but merely for a selfish purpose.

398 On the other hand, to preserve one's life is a duty; and, furthermore, everyone has also an immediate inclination to do so. But on this account the often anxious care taken by most men for it has no intrinsic worth, and the maxim of their action has no moral content. They preserve their lives, to be sure, in accordance with duty, but not from duty. On the other hand, if adversity and hopeless sorrow have completely taken away the taste for life, if an unfortunate man, strong in soul and more indignant at his fate than despondent or dejected, wishes for death and yet preserves his life

without loving it – not from inclination or fear, but from duty – then his maxim indeed has a moral content.

[. . .]

To be beneficent where one can is a duty; and besides this, there are many persons who are so sympathetically constituted that, without any further motive of vanity or self-interest, they find an inner pleasure in spreading joy around them and can rejoice in the satisfaction of others as their own work. But I maintain that in such a case an action of this kind, however dutiful and amiable it may be, has nevertheless no true moral worth. It is on a level with such actions as arise from other inclinations, e.g., the inclination for honor, which if fortunately directed to what is in fact beneficial and accords with duty and is thus honorable, deserves praise and encouragement, but not esteem; for its maxim lacks the moral content of an action done not from inclination but from duty. Suppose then the mind of this friend of mankind to be clouded over with his own sorrow so that all sympathy with the lot of others is extinguished, and suppose him still to have the power to benefit others in distress, even though is not touched by their trouble because he is sufficiently absorbed with his own; and now suppose that, even though no inclination moves him any longer, he nevertheless tears himself from this deadly insensibility and performs the action without any inclination at all, but solely from duty – then for the first time his action has genuine moral worth. Further still, if nature has put little sympathy in this or that man's heart, if (while being an honest man in other respects) he is by temperament cold and indifferent to the sufferings of others, perhaps because as regards his own sufferings he is endowed with the special gift of patience and fortitude and expects or even requires that others should have the same; if such a man (who would truly not be nature's worst product) had not been exactly fashioned by her to be a philanthropist, would he not yet find in himself a source from which he might give himself a worth far higher than any that a good-natured temperament might have? By all means, because just here does the worth of the character come out; this worth is moral and incomparably the highest of all, viz., that he is beneficent, not from inclination, but from duty.

To secure one's own happiness is a duty (at least indirectly); for discontent with one's condition under many pressing cares and amid unsatisfied wants might easily become a great temptation to transgress one's duties. But here also do men of themselves already have, irrespective of duty, the strongest and deepest inclination toward happiness, because just in this idea are all inclinations combined into a sum total. But the precept of happiness is often so constituted as greatly to interfere with some inclinations, and yet men cannot form any definite and certain concept of the sum of satisfaction of all inclinations that is called happiness. Hence there is no wonder that a single inclination which is determinate both as to what it promises and as to the time within which it can be satisfied may outweigh a fluctuating idea; and there is no wonder that a man, e.g., a gouty patient, can choose to enjoy what he likes and to suffer what he may, since by his calculation he has here at least not sacrificed the enjoyment of the present moment to some possibly groundless expectations of the good fortune that is supposed to be found in health. But even in this case, if the universal inclination to happiness did not determine his will and if health, at least for him, did not figure as so necessary an element in his calculations; there still remains here, as in all other cases, a law, viz., that he should promote his happiness not from inclination but from duty, and thereby for the first time does his conduct have real moral worth.

Undoubtedly in this way also are to be understood those passages of Scripture which command us to love our neighbor and even our enemy. For love as an inclination cannot be commanded; but beneficence from duty, when no inclination impels us and even when a natural and unconquerable aversion opposes such beneficence, is practical, and not pathological, love. Such love resides in the will and not in the propensities of feeling, in principles of action and not in tender sympathy; and only this practical love can be commanded.

The second proposition[12] is this: An action done from duty has its moral worth, not in the purpose that is to be attained by it, but in the maxim

399

400

according to which the action is determined. The moral worth depends, therefore, not on the realization of the object of the action, but merely on the principle of volition according to which, without regard to any objects of the faculty of desire, the action has been done. From what has gone before it is clear that the purposes which we may have in our actions, as well as their effects regarded as ends and incentives of the will, cannot give to actions any unconditioned and moral worth. Where, then, can this worth lie if it is not to be found in the will's relation to the expected effect? Nowhere but in the principle of the will, with no regard to the ends that can be brought about through such action. For the will stands, as it were, at a crossroads between its a priori principle, which is formal, and its a posteriori incentive, which is material; and since it must be determined by something, it must be determined by the formal principle of volition, if the action is done from duty – and in that case every material principle is taken away from it.

401   The third proposition, which follows from the other two, can be expressed thus: Duty is the necessity of an action done not of respect for the law. I can indeed have an inclination for an object as the effect of my proposed action; but I can never have respect for such an object, just because it is merely an effect and is not an activity of the will. Similarly, I can have no respect for inclination as such, whether my own or that of another. I can at most, if my own inclination, approve it; and, if that of another, even love it, i.e., consider it to be favorable to my own advantage. An object of respect can only be what is connected with my will solely as ground and never as effect – something that does not serve my inclination but, rather, outweighs it, or at least excludes it from consideration when some choice is made – in other words, only the law itself can be an object of respect and hence can be a command. Now an action done from duty must altogether exclude the influence of inclination and therewith every object of the will. Hence there is nothing left which can determine the will except objectively the law and subjectively pure respect for this practical law, i.e., the will can be subjectively determined by the maxim[13] that I should follow such a law even if all my inclinations are thereby thwarted.

Thus the moral worth of an action does not lie in the effect expected from it nor in any principle of action that needs to borrow its motive from this expected effect. For all these effects (agreeableness of one's condition and even the furtherance of other people's happiness) could have been brought about also through other causes and would not have required the will of a rational being, in which the highest and unconditioned good can alone be found. Therefore, the pre-eminent good which is called moral can consist in nothing but the representation of the law, in itself, and such a representation can admittedly be found only in a rational being insofar as this representation, and not some expected effect, is the determining ground of the will. This good is already present in the person who acts according to this representation, and such good need not be awaited merely from the effect.

402   But what sort of law can that be the thought of which must determine the will without reference to any expected effect, so that the will can be called absolutely good without qualification? Since I have deprived the will of every impulse that might arise for it from obeying any particular law, there is nothing left to serve the will as principle except the universal conformity of its actions to law as such, i.e., I should never act except in such a way that I can also will that my maxim should become a universal law.[15] Here mere conformity to law as such (without having as its basis any law determining particular actions) serves the will as principle and must so serve it if duty is not to be a vain delusion and a chimerical concept. The ordinary reason of mankind in its practical judgments agrees completely with this, and always has in view the aforementioned principle.

403   For example, take this question. When I am in distress, may I make a promise with the intention of not keeping it? I readily distinguish here the two meanings which the question may have; whether making a false promise conforms with prudence or with duty. Doubtless the former can often be the case. Indeed I clearly see that escape from some present difficulty by means of such a promise is not enough. In addition I must carefully consider whether from this lie there may later arise far greater inconvenience for me

than from what I now try to escape. Furthermore, the consequences of my false promise are not easy to foresee, even with all my supposed cunning; loss of confidence in me might prove to be far more disadvantageous than the misfortune which I now try to avoid. The more prudent way might be to act according to a universal maxim and to make it a habit not to promise anything without intending to keep it. But that such a maxim is, nevertheless, always based on nothing but a fear of consequences becomes clear to me at once. To be truthful from duty is, however, quite different from being truthful from fear of disadvantageous consequences; in the first case the concept of the action itself contains a law for me, while in the second I must first look around elsewhere to see what are the results for me that might be connected with the action. For to deviate from the principle of duty is quite certainly bad; but to abandon my maxim of prudence can often be very advantageous for me, though to abide by it is certainly safer. The most direct and infallible way, however, to answer the question as to whether a lying promise accords with duty is to ask myself whether I would really be content if my maxim (of extricating myself from difficulty by means of a false promise) were to hold as a universal law for myself as well as for others, and could I really say to myself that everyone may promise falsely when he finds himself in a difficulty from which he can find no other way to extricate himself. Then I immediately become aware that I can indeed will the lie but can not at all will a universal law to lie. For by such a law there would really be no promises at all, since in vain would my willing future actions be professed to other people who would not believe what I professed, or if they over-hastily did believe, then they would pay me back in like coin. Therefore, my maxim would necessarily destroy itself just as soon as it was made a universal law.

Therefore, I need no far-reaching acuteness to discern what I have to do in order that my will may be morally good. Inexperienced in the course of the world and incapable of being prepared for all its contingencies, I only ask myself whether I can also will that my maxim should become a universal law. If not, then the maxim must be rejected, not because of any disadvantage accruing to me or even to others, but because it cannot be fitting as a principle in a possible legislation of universal law, and reason exacts from me immediate respect for such legislation. Indeed I have as yet no insight into the grounds of such respect (which the philosopher may investigate). But I at least understand that respect is an estimation of a worth that far outweighs any worth of what is recommended by inclination, and that the necessity of acting from pure respect for the practical law is what constitutes duty, to which every other motive must give way because duty is the condition of a will good in itself, whose worth is above all else.

Thus within the moral cognition of ordinary human reason we have   404 arrived at its principle. To be sure, such reason does not think of this principle abstractly in its universal form, but does always have it actually in view and does use it as the standard of judgment. It would here be easy to show how ordinary reason, with this compass in hand, is well able to distinguish, in every case that occurs, what is good or evil, in accord with duty or contrary to duty, if we do not in the least try to teach reason anything new but only make it attend, as Socrates did, to its own principle – and thereby do we show that neither science nor philosophy is needed in order to know what one must do to be honest and good, and even wise and virtuous. Indeed we might even have conjectured beforehand that cognizance of what every man is obligated to do, and hence also to know, would be available to every man, even the most ordinary. Yet we cannot but observe with admiration how great an advantage the power of practical judgment has over the theoretical in ordinary human understanding. In the theoretical, when ordinary reason ventures to depart from the laws of experience and the perceptions of sense, it falls into sheer inconceivabilities and self-contradictions, or at least into a chaos of uncertainty, obscurity, and instability. In the practical, however, the power of judgment first begins to show itself to advantage when ordinary understanding excludes all sensuous incentives from practical laws. Such understanding then becomes even subtle, whether in quibbling with its own conscience or with other claims regarding what is to be called right, or whether in wanting to determine correctly for its own instruction the worth of various actions. And the most extraordinary thing is that ordinary understanding in this practical case may have just as good a hope of hitting the mark as that which any philosopher may promise himself. Indeed it is almost more certain in this than even a philosopher is, because he can have no principle other than what ordinary understanding has, but he may easily confuse his judgment by a multitude of foreign and irrelevant considerations and thereby cause it to swerve from the right way. Would it not, therefore, be wiser in moral matters to abide by the ordinary rational judgment or at most to bring in philosophy merely for the purpose of rendering the system of morals more complete and intelligible and of presenting its rules in a way that is more convenient for use (especially in disputation), but not for the purpose of leading ordinary human understanding away from its happy simplicity in practical matters and of bringing it by means of philosophy into a new path of inquiry and instruction?

405   Innocence is indeed a glorious thing; but, unfortunately, it does not keep very well and is easily led astray. Consequently, even wisdom – which consists more in doing and not doing than in knowing – needs science, not in order to learn from it, but in order that wisdom's precepts may gain acceptance and permanence. Man feels within himself a powerful counterweight to all the commands of duty, which are presented to him by reason as being so pre-eminently worthy of respect; this counterweight consists of his needs and inclinations, whose total satisfaction is summed up under the name of happiness. Now reason irremissibly commands its precepts, without thereby promising the inclinations anything; hence it disregards and neglects these impetuous and at the same time so seemingly plausible claims (which do not allow themselves to be suppressed by any command). Hereby arises a natural dialectic, i.e., a propensity to quibble with these strict laws of duty, to cast doubt upon their validity, or at least upon their purity and strictness, and to make them, where possible, more compatible with our wishes and inclinations. Thereby are such laws corrupted in their very foundations and their whole dignity is destroyed – something which even ordinary practical reason cannot in the end call good.

Thus is ordinary human reason forced to go outside its sphere and take a step into the field of practical philosophy, not by any need for speculation (which never befalls such reason so long as it is content to be mere sound reason) but on practical grounds themselves. There it tries to obtain information and clear instruction regarding the source of its own principle and the correct determination of this principle in its opposition to maxims based on need and inclination, so that reason may escape from the perplexity of opposite claims and may avoid the risk of losing all genuine moral principles through the ambiguity into which it easily falls. Thus when ordinary practical reason cultivates itself, there imperceptibly arises in it a dialectic which compels it to seek help in philosophy. The same thing happens in reason's theoretical use; in this case, just as in the other, peace will be found only in a thorough critical examination of our reason.

Notes

12   [The first proposition of morality says that an action must be done from duty in order to have any moral worth. It is implicit in the preceding examples but was never explicitly stated.]

13   A maxim is the subjective principle of volition. The objective principle (i.e., one which would serve all rational beings also subjectively as a practical principle if reason had full control over the faculty of desire) is the practical law.

Grounding for the Metaphysics of Morals: First and Second Sections*

Immanuel Kant

Second section

Transition from popular moral philosophy to a metaphysics of morals

If we have so far drawn our concept of duty from the ordinary use of our practical reason, one is by no means to infer that we have treated it as a concept of experience. On the contrary, when we pay attention to our experience of the way human beings act, we meet frequent and – as we ourselves admit – justified complaints that there cannot be cited a single certain example of the disposition to act from pure duty; and we meet complaints that although much may be done that is in accordance with what duty commands, yet there are always doubts as to whether what occurs has really been done from duty and so has moral worth. Hence there have always been philosophers who have absolutely denied the reality of this disposition in human actions and have ascribed everything to a more or less refined self-love. Yet in so doing they have not cast doubt upon the rightness of the concept of morality. Rather, they have spoken with sincere regret as to the frailty and impurity of human nature, which they think is noble enough to take as its precept an idea so worthy of respect but yet is too weak to follow this idea: reason, which should legislate for human nature, is used only to look after the interest of inclinations, whether singly or, at best, in their greatest possible harmony with one another.

407 In fact there is absolutely no possibility by means of experience to make out with complete certainty a single case in which the maxim of an action that may in other respects conform to duty has rested solely on moral grounds and on the representation of one's duty. It is indeed sometimes the case that after the keenest self-examination we can find nothing except the moral ground of duty that could have been strong enough to move us to this or that good action and to such great sacrifice. But there cannot with certainty be at all inferred from this that some secret impulse of self-love, merely appearing as the idea of duty, was not the actual determining cause of the will. We like to flatter ourselves with the false claim to a more noble motive; but in fact we can never, even by the strictest examination, completely plumb the depths of the secret incentives of our actions. For when moral value is being considered, the concern is not with the actions, which are seen, but rather with their inner principles, which are not seen.

408 Moreover, one cannot better serve the wishes of those who ridicule all morality as being a mere phantom of human imagination getting above itself because of self-conceit than by conceding to them that the concepts of duty must be drawn solely from experience (just as from indolence one willingly persuades himself that such is the case as regards all other concepts as well). For by so conceding, one prepares for them a sure triumph. I am willing to admit out of love for humanity that most of our actions are in accordance with duty; but if we look more closely at our planning and striving, we everywhere come upon the dear self, which is always turning up, and upon which the intent of our actions is based rather than upon the

---

* Kant, I.: Grounding for the metaphysics of morals, in *Ethical philosophy*, trans. J. Ellington. Indianapolis, IN, Hackett Publishing Company, 1983, pp. 7–17; 19–27; 30–2; 40–41.

strict command of duty (which would often require self-denial). One need not be exactly an enemy of virtue, but only a cool observer who does not take the liveliest wish for the good to be straight off its realization, in order to become doubtful at times whether any true virtue is actually to be found in the world. Such is especially the case when years increase and one's power of judgment is made shrewder by experience and keener in observation. Because of these things nothing can protect us from a complete falling away from our ideas of duty and preserve in the soul a well-grounded respect for duty's law except the clear conviction that, even if there never have been actions springing from such pure sources, the question at issue here is not whether this or that has happened but that reason of itself and independently of all experience commands what ought to happen. Consequently, reason unrelentingly commands actions of which the world has perhaps hitherto never provided an example and whose feasibility might well be doubted by one who bases everything upon experience; for instance, even though there might never yet have been a sincere friend, still pure sincerity in friendship is nonetheless required of every man, because this duty, prior to all experience, is contained as duty in general in the idea of a reason that determines the will by means of a priori grounds.

There may be noted further that unless we want to deny to the concept of morality all truth and all reference to a possible object, we cannot but admit that the moral law is of such widespread significance that it must hold not merely for men but for all rational beings generally, and that it must be valid not merely under contingent conditions and with exceptions but must be absolutely necessary. Clearly, therefore, no experience can give occasion for inferring even the possibility of such apodeictic laws. For with what right could we bring into unlimited respect as a universal precept for every rational nature what is perhaps valid only under the contingent conditions of humanity? And how could laws for the determination of our will be regarded as laws for the determination of a rational being in general and of ourselves only insofar as we are rational beings, if these laws were merely empirical and did not have their source completely a priori in pure, but practical, reason?

409 Moreover, worse service cannot be rendered morality than that an attempt be made to derive it from examples. For every example of morality presented to me must itself first be judged according to principles of morality in order to see whether it is fit to serve as an original example, i.e., as a model. But in no way can it authoritatively furnish the concept of morality. Even the Holy One of the gospel must first be compared with our ideal of moral perfection before he is recognized as such. Even he says of himself, 'Why do you call me (whom you see) good? None is good (the archetype of the good) except God only (whom you do not see).' But whence have we the concept of God as the highest good? Solely from the idea of moral perfection, which reason frames a priori and connects inseparably with the concept of a free will. Imitation has no place at all in moral matters. And examples serve only for encouragement, i.e., they put beyond doubt the feasibility of what the law commands and they make visible what the practical rule expresses more generally. But examples can never justify us in setting aside their true original, which lies in reason, and letting ourselves be guided by them.

If there is then no genuine supreme principle of morality that must rest merely on pure reason, independently of all experience, I think it is unnecessary even to ask whether it is a good thing to exhibit these concepts generally '*in abstracto*', which, along with the principles that belong to them, hold a priori, so far as the knowledge involved is to be distinguished from ordinary knowledge and is to be called philosophical. But in our times it may well be necessary to do so. For if one were to take a vote as to whether pure rational knowledge separated from everything empirical, i.e., metaphysics of morals, or whether popular practical philosophy is to be preferred, one can easily guess which side would be preponderant.

410 This descent to popular thought is certainly very commendable once the ascent to the principles of pure reason has occurred and has been satisfactorily accomplished. That would mean that the doctrine of morals has first been grounded on metaphysics and that subsequently acceptance for morals has been won by giving it a popular character after it has been firmly established. But it is quite absurd to try for popularity in the first inquiry, upon which depends the total correctness of the principles. Not only can such a procedure never lay claim to the very rare merit of a true philosophical popularity, inasmuch as there is really no art involved at all in being generally intelligible if one thereby renounces all basic insight but such a procedure turns out a disgusting mishmash of patchwork observations and half-reasoned principles.

[. . .]

One need only look at the attempts to deal with morality in the way favored by popular taste. What he will find in an amazing mixture is at one time the particular constitution of human nature (but along with this also the idea of a rational nature in general), at another time perfection, at another happiness; here moral feeling, and there the fear of God; something of this, and also something of that. But the thought never occurs to ask whether the principles of morality are to be sought at all in the knowledge of human nature (which can be had only from experience). Nor does the thought occur that if these principles are not to be sought here but to be found, rather, completely a priori and free from everything empirical in pure rational concepts only, and are to be found nowhere else even to the slightest extent – then there had better be adopted the plan of undertaking this investigation as a separate inquiry, i.e., as pure practical philosophy or (if one may use a name so much decried) as a metaphysics of morals. It is better to bring this investigation to full completeness entirely by itself and to bid the public, which demands popularity, to await the outcome of this undertaking.

411 But such a completely isolated metaphysics of morals, not mixed with any anthropology, theology, physics, or hyperphysics, and still less with occult qualities (which might be called hypophysical), is not only an indispensable substratum of all theoretical and precisely defined knowledge of duties, but is at the same time a desideratum of the highest importance for the actual fulfillment of their precepts. For the pure thought of duty and of the moral law generally, unmixed with any extraneous addition of empirical inducements, has by the way of reason alone (which first becomes aware hereby that it can of itself be practical) an influence on the human heart so much more powerful than all other incentives which may be derived from the empirical field that reason in the consciousness of its dignity despises such incentives and is able gradually to become their master. On the other hand, a mixed moral philosophy, compounded both of incentives drawn from feelings and inclinations and at the same time of rational concepts, must make the mind waver between motives that cannot be brought under any principle and that can only by accident lead to the good but often can also lead to the bad.

412 It is clear from the foregoing that all moral concepts have their seat and origin completely a priori in reason, and indeed in the most ordinary human reason just as much as in the most highly speculative. They cannot be abstracted from any empirical, and hence merely contingent, cognition. In this purity of their origin lies their very worthiness to serve us as supreme practical principles; and to the extent that something empirical is added to them, just so much is taken away from their genuine influence and from the absolute worth of the corresponding actions. Moreover, it is not only a requirement of the greatest necessity from a theoretical point of view, when it is a question of speculation, but also of the greatest practical importance,

to draw these concepts and laws from pure reason, to present them pure and unmixed, and indeed to determine the extent of this entire practical and pure rational cognition, i.e., to determine the whole faculty of pure practical reason. The principles should not be made to depend on the particular nature of human reason, as speculative philosophy may permit and even sometimes finds necessary; but, rather, the principles should be derived from the universal concept of a rational being in general, since moral laws should hold for every rational being as such.

[. . .]

Everything in nature works according to laws. Only a rational being 413 has the power to act according to his conception of laws, i.e., according to principles, and thereby has he a will. Since the derivation of actions from laws requires reason, the will is nothing but practical reason. If reason infallibly determines the will, then in the case of such a being actions which are recognized to be objectively necessary are also subjectively necessary, i.e., the will is a faculty of choosing only that which reason, independently of inclination, recognizes as being practically necessary, i.e., as good. But if reason of itself does not sufficiently determine the will, and if the will submits also to subjective conditions (certain incentives) which do not always agree with objective conditions; in a word, if the will does not in itself completely accord with reason (as is actually the case with men), then actions which are recognized as objectively necessary are subjectively contingent, and the determination of such a will according to objective laws is necessitation. That is to say that the relation of objective laws to a will not thoroughly good is represented as the determination of the will of a rational being by principles of reason which the will does not necessarily follow because of its own nature.

The representation of an objective principle insofar as it necessitates the will is called a command (of reason), and the formula of the command is called an imperative.

[. . .]

Now all imperatives command either hypothetically or categorically. The former represent the practical necessity of a possible action as a means for attaining something else that one wants (or may possibly want). The categorical imperative would be one which represented an action as objectively necessary in itself, without reference to another end.

Every practical law represents a possible action as good and hence as necessary for a subject who is practically determinable by reason; therefore all imperatives are formulas for determining an action which is necessary according to the principle of a will that is good in some way. Now if the action would be good merely as a means to something else, so is the imperative hypothetical. But if the action is represented as good in itself, and hence as necessary in a will which of itself conforms to reason as the principle of the will, then the imperative is categorical.

An imperative thus says what action possible by me would be good, and it presents the practical rule in relation to a will which does not forthwith perform an action simply because it is good, partly because the subject does not always know that the action is good and partly because (even if he does know it is good) his maxims might yet be opposed to the objective principles of practical reason.

A hypothetical imperative thus says only that an action is good for some 415 purpose, either possible or actual. In the first case it is a problematic practical principle; in the second case an assertoric one. A categorical imperative, which declares an action to be of itself objectively necessary without reference to any purpose, i.e., without any other end, holds as an apodeictic practical principle.

Whatever is possible only through the powers of some rational being can be thought of as a possible purpose of some will. Consequently, there are in fact infinitely many principles of action insofar as they are represented as necessary for attaining a possible purpose achievable by them. All sciences have a practical part consisting of problems saying that some end is possible for us and of imperatives telling us how it can be attained. These can, therefore, be called in general imperatives of skill. Here there is no question at all whether the end is reasonable and good, but there is only a question as to what must be done to attain it. The prescriptions needed by a doctor in order to make his patient thoroughly healthy and by a poisoner in order to make sure of killing his victim are of equal value so far as each serves to bring about its purpose perfectly. Since there cannot be known in early youth what ends may be presented to us in the course of life, parents especially seek to have their children learn many different kinds of things, and they provide for skill in the use of means to all sorts of arbitrary ends, among which they cannot determine whether any one of them could in the future become an actual purpose for their ward, though there is always the possibility that he might adopt it. Their concern is so great that they commonly neglect to form and correct their children's judgment regarding the worth of things which might be chosen as ends.

416   There is, however, one end that can be presupposed as actual for all rational beings (so far as they are dependent beings to whom imperatives apply); and thus there is one purpose which they not merely can have but which can certainly be assumed to be such that they all do have by a natural necessity, and this is happiness. A hypothetical imperative which represents the practical necessity of an action as means for the promotion of happiness is assertoric. It may be expounded not simply as necessary to an uncertain, merely possible purpose, but as necessary to a purpose which can be presupposed a priori and with certainty as being present in everyone because it belongs to his essence. Now skill in the choice of means to one's own greatest well-being can be called prudence in the narrowest sense. And thus the imperative that refers to the choice of means to one's own happiness, i.e., the precept of prudence, still remains hypothetical; the action is commanded not absolutely but only as a means to a further purpose.

Finally, there is one imperative which immediately commands a certain conduct without having as its condition any other purpose to be attained by it. This imperative is categorical. It is not concerned with the matter of the action and its intended result, but rather with the form of the action and the principle from which it follows; what is essentially good in the action consists in the mental disposition, let the consequences be what they may. This imperative may be called that of morality.

417   Willing according to these three kinds of principles is also clearly distinguished by dissimilarity in the necessitation of the will. To make this dissimilarity clear I think that they are most suitably named in their order when they are said to be either *rules of skill, counsels of prudence, or commands (laws) of morality.* For law alone involves the concept of a necessity that is unconditioned and indeed objective and hence universally valid, and commands are laws which must be obeyed, i.e., must be followed even in opposition to inclination. Counsel does indeed involve necessity, but involves such necessity as is valid only under a subjectively contingent condition, viz., whether this or that man counts this or that as belonging to his happiness. On the other hand, the categorical imperative is limited by no condition, and can quite properly be called a command since it is absolutely, though practically, necessary. The first kind of imperatives might also be called technical (belonging to art), the second kind pragmatic (belonging to welfare), the third kind moral (belonging to free conduct as such, i.e., to morals).

[. . .]

Hence there is only one categorical imperative and it is this: Act only according to that maxim whereby you can at the same time will that it should become a universal law.

Now if all imperatives of duty can be derived from this one imperative as their principle, then there can at least be shown what is understood by the concept of duty and what it means, even though there is left undecided whether what is called duty may not be an empty concept.

The universality of law according to which effects are produced constitutes what is properly called nature in the most general sense (as to form), i.e., the existence of things as far as determined by universal laws. Accordingly, the universal imperative of duty may be expressed thus: Act as if the maxim of your action were to become through your will a universal law of nature.

We shall now enumerate some duties, following the usual division of them into duties to ourselves and to others and into perfect and imperfect duties.

1. A man reduced to despair by a series of misfortunes feels sick of life   422 but is still so far in possession of his reason that he can ask himself whether taking his own life would not be contrary to his duty to himself. Now he asks whether the maxim of his action could become a universal law of nature. But his maxim is this: from self-love I make as my principle to shorten my life when its continued duration threatens more evil than it promises satisfaction. There only remains the question as to whether this principle of self-love can become a universal law of nature. One sees at once a contradiction in a system of nature whose law would destroy life by means of the very same feeling that acts so as to stimulate the furtherance of life, and hence there could be no existence as a system of nature. Therefore, such a maxim cannot possibly hold as a universal law of nature and is, consequently, wholly opposed to the supreme principle of all duty.

2. Another man in need finds himself forced to borrow money. He knows well that he won't be able to repay it, but he sees also that he will not get any loan unless he firmly promises to repay it within a fixed time. He wants to make such a promise, but he still has conscience enough to ask himself whether it is not permissible and is contrary to duty to get out of difficulty in this way. Suppose, however, that he decides to do so. The maxim of his action would then be expressed as follows: when I believe myself to be in need of money, I will borrow money and promise to pay it back, although I know that I can never do so. Now this principle of self-love or personal advantage may perhaps be quite compatible with one's entire future welfare, but the questions is now whether it is right.[1] I then transform the requirement of self-love into a universal law and put the question thus: how would things stand if my maxim were to become a universal law? He then sees at once that such a maxim could never hold as a universal law of nature and be consistent with itself, but must necessarily be self-contradictory. For the universality of a law which says that anyone believing himself to be in difficulty could promise whatever he pleases with the intention of not keeping it would make promising itself and the end to be attained thereby quite impossible, inasmuch as no one would believe what was promised him but would merely laugh at all such utterances as being vain pretenses.

3. A third finds in himself a talent whose cultivation could make him   423 a man useful in many respects. But he finds himself in comfortable circumstances and prefers to indulge in pleasure rather than to bother himself about broadening and improving his fortunate natural aptitudes. But he asks himself further whether his maxim of neglecting his natural gifts, besides agreeing of itself with his propensity to indulgence, might agree also with what is called duty.[2] He then sees that a system of nature could indeed always subsist according to such a universal law, even though every man (like South Sea Islanders) should let his talents rust and resolve to devote his life entirely to idleness, indulgence, propagation, and, in a word, to enjoyment. But he cannot possibly will that this should become a universal law of nature or be implanted in us as such a law by a natural instinct. For as a rational being he necessarily wills that all his faculties should be developed, inasmuch as they are given him for all sorts of possible purposes.

4. A fourth man finds things going well for himself but sees others (whom he could help) struggling with great hardships; and he thinks: what does it matter to me? Let everybody be as happy as Heaven wills or as he can make himself; I shall take nothing from him nor even envy him; but I have no desire to contribute anything to his well-being or to his assistance when in need. If such a way of thinking were to become a universal law of nature, the human race admittedly could very well subsist and doubtless could subsist even better than when everyone prates about sympathy and benevolence and even on occasion exerts himself to practice them but, on the other hand, also cheats when he can, betrays the rights of man, or otherwise violates them. But even though it is possible that a universal law of nature could subsist in accordance with that maxim, still it is impossible to will

that such a principle should hold everywhere as a law of nature.[3] For a will which resolved in this way would contradict itself, inasmuch as cases **424** might often arise in which one would have need of the love and sympathy of others and in which he would deprive himself, by such a law of nature springing from his own will, of all hope of the aid he wants for himself.

These are some of the many actual duties, or at least what are taken to be such, whose derivation from the single principle cited above is clear. We must be able to will that a maxim of our action become a universal law; this is the canon for morally estimating any of our actions. Some actions are so constituted that their maxims cannot without contradiction even be thought as a universal law of nature, much less be willed as what should become one. In the case of others this internal impossibility is indeed not found, but there is still no possibility of willing that their maxim should be raised to the universality of a law of nature, because such a will would contradict itself. There is no difficulty in seeing that the former kind of action conflicts with strict or narrow [perfect] (irremissible) duty, while the second kind conflicts only with broad [imperfect] (meritorious) duty. By means of these examples there has thus been fully set forth how all duties depend as regards the kind of obligation (not the object of their action) upon the one principle.

[. . .]

434 A rational being must always regard himself as legislator in a kingdom of ends rendered possible by freedom of the will, whether as member or as sovereign. The position of the latter can be maintained not merely through the maxims of his will but only if he is a compeletely independent being without needs and with unlimited power adequate to his will.

Hence morality consists in the relation of all action to that legislation, whereby alone a kingdom of ends is possible. This legislation must be found in every rational being and must be able to arise from his will, whose principle then is never to act on any maxim except such as can also be a universal law and hence such as the will can thereby regard itself as at the same time the legislator of universal law. If now the maxims do not by their very nature already necessarily conform with this objective principle of rational beings as legislating universal laws, then the necessity of acting on that principle is called practical necessitation, i.e., duty. Duty does not apply to the sovereign in the kingdom of ends, but it does apply to every member and to each in the same degree.

The practical necessity of acting according to this principle, i.e., duty, does not rest at all on feelings, impulses, and inclinations, but only on they relation of rational beings to one anther, a relation in which the will of a rational being must always be regarded at the same time as legislative, because otherwise he could not be thought of as an end in himself. Reason, therefore, relates every maxim of the will as legislating universal laws to every other will and also to every action toward oneself; it does so not on account of any other practical motive or future advantage but rather from the idea of the dignity of a rational being who obeys no law except what he at the same time enacts himself.

In the kingdom of ends everything has either a price or a dignity. Whatever has a price can be replaced by something else as its equivalent; on the other hand, whatever is above all price, and therefore admits of no equivalent, has a dignity.

Whatever has reference to general human inclinations and needs has **435** a market price; whatever, without presupposing any need, accords with a certain taste, i.e., a delight in the mere unpurposive play of our mental powers, has an affective price; but that which constitutes the condition under which alone something can be end in itself has not merely a relative worth, i.e., a price, but has an intrinsic worth, i.e., dignity.

Now morality is the condition under which alone a rational being can be an end in himself, for only thereby can he be a legislating member in the kingdom of ends. Hence morality and humanity, insofar as it is capable of morality, alone have dignity. Skill and diligence in work have a market price; wit, lively imagination, and humor have an affective price; but fidelity to promises and benevolence based on principles (not on instinct) have intrinsic worth. Neither nature nor art contain anything which in default of these could be put in their place; for their worth consists, not in the effects which arise from them, nor in the advantage and profit which they provide, but in mental dispositions, i.e., in the maxims of the will which are ready in this way to manifest themselves in action, even if they are not favored with success. Such actions also need no recommendation from any subjective disposition or taste so as to meet with immediate favor and delight; there is no need of any immediate propensity or feeling toward them. They exhibit the will performing them as an object of immediate respect; and nothing but reason is required to impose them upon the will, which is not to be cajoled into them, since in the case of duties such cajoling would be a contradiction. This estimation, therefore, lets the worth of such a disposition be recognized as dignity and puts it infinitely beyond all price, with which it cannot in the least be brought into competition or comparison without, as it were, violating its sanctity.

What then is it that entitles the morally good disposition, or virtue, to **436** make such lofty claims? It is nothing less than the share which such a disposition affords the rational being of legislating universal laws, so that he is fit to be a member in a possible kingdom of ends, for which his own nature realism has already determined him as an end in himself and therefore as a legislator in the kingdom of ends. Thereby is he free as regards all laws of nature, and he obeys only those laws which he gives to himself. Accordingly, his maxims can belong to a universal legislation to which heat the same time subjects himself. For nothing can have any worth other than what the law determines. But the legislation itself which determines all worth must for that very reason have dignity, i.e., unconditional and incomparable worth; and the word 'respect' alone provides a suitable expression for the esteem which a rational being must have for it. Hence autonomy is the ground of the dignity of human nature and of every rational nature.

[. . .]

Notes

1 [Keeping promises is an example of a perfect duty to others.

2 [Cultivating one's talents is an example of an imperfect duty to oneself.

3 [Benefiting others is an example of an imperfect duty to others.

Utilitarianism*

John Stuart Mill

General remarks

There are few circumstances among those which make up the present condition of human knowledge more unlike what might have been expected, or more significant of the backward state in which speculation on the most important subjects still lingers, than the little progress which has been made in the decision of the controversy respecting the criterion of right and wrong. From the dawn of philosophy, the question concerning the *summum bonum*, or, what is the same thing, concerning the foundation of morality, has been accounted the main problem in speculative thought, has occupied the most gifted intellects and divided them into sects and schools carrying on a vigorous warfare against one another.

[. . .]

It is true that similar confusion and uncertainty and, in some cases, similar discordance exist respecting the first principles of all the sciences, not excepting that which is deemed the most certain of them – mathematics, without much impairing, generally indeed without impairing at all, the trust worthiness of the conclusions of those sciences. An apparent anomaly, the explanation of which is that the detailed doctrines of a science are not usually deduced from, nor depend for their evidence upon, what are called its first principles. Were it not so, there would be no science more precarious, or whose conclusions were more insufficiently made out, than algebra, which derives none of its certainty from what are commonly taught to learners as its elements, since these, as laid down by some of its most eminent teachers, are as full of fictions as English law, and of mysteries as theology. The truths which are ultimately accepted as the first principles of a science are really the last results of metaphysical analysis practiced on the elementary notions with which the science is conversant; and their relation to the science is not that of foundations to an edifice, but of roots to a tree, which may perform their office equally well though they be never dug down to and exposed to light. But though in science the particular truths precede the general theory, the contrary might be expected to be the case with a practical art, such as morals or legislation. All action is for the sake of some end, and rules of action, it seems natural to suppose, must take their whole character and color from the end to which they are subservient. When we engage in pursuit, a clear and precise conception of what we are pursuing would seem to be the first thing we need, instead of the last we are to look forward to. A test of right and wrong must be the means, one would think, of ascertaining what is right or wrong, and not a consequence of having already ascertained it.

The difficulty is not avoided by having recourse to the popular theory of a natural faculty, a sense of instinct, informing us of right and wrong. For – besides that the existence of such a moral instinct is itself one of the matters in dispute – those believers in it who hare any pretensions to philosophy have been obliged to abandon the idea that it discerns what is right or wrong in the particular case in hand, as our other senses discern the sight or sound actually present. Our moral faculty, according to all those of its interpreters who are-entitled to the name of thinkers, supplies us only with the general principles of moral judgments; it is a branch of our reason, not of our sensitive faculty, and must be looked to for the abstract doctrines of morality, not for perception of it in the concrete. The intuitive, no less than what may be termed the inductive, school of ethics insists on the necessity of general laws. They both agree that the morality of an individual action is not a question of direct perception, but of the application of a law to an individual case. They recognize also, to a great extent, the same moral laws, but differ as to their evidence and the source from which they derive their authority. According to the one opinion, the principles of morals are evident *a priori*, requiring nothing to command assent except that the meaning of the terms be understood. According to the other doctrine, right and wrong, as well as truth and falsehood, are questions of observation and experience, But both hold equally that morality must be deduced from principles; and the intuitive school affirm as strongly as the inductive that there is a science of morals. Yet they seldom attempt to make out a list of the *a priori* principles which are to serve as the premises of the science; still more rarely do they make any effort to reduce those various principles to one first principle or common ground of obligation. They either assume the ordinary precepts of morals as of *a priori* authority, or I they lay down as the common groundwork of those maxims some generality much less obviously authoritative than the maxims themselves, and which has never succeeded in gaining popular acceptance. Yet to support their pretensions there ought either to be some one fundamental principle or law at the root of all morality, or, if there be several, there should be a determinate order of precedence among them; and the one principle, or the rule for deciding between the various principles when they conflict, ought to be self-evident.

To inquire how far the bad effects of this deficiency have been mitigated in practice, or to what extent the moral beliefs of mankind have been vitiated or made uncertain by the absence of any distinct recognition of an ultimate standard, would imply a complete survey and criticism of past and present ethical doctrine. It would, however, be easy to show that whatever steadiness or consistency these moral beliefs have attained has been mainly due to the tacit influence of a standard not recognized. Although the nonexistence of an acknowledged first principle has made ethics not so much a guide as a consecration of men's actual sentiments, still, as men's sentiments, both of favor and of aversion, are greatly influenced by what they suppose to be the effects of things upon their happiness, the principle of utility, or, as Bentham latterly called it, the greatest happiness principle, has had a large share in forming the moral doctrines even of those who most scornfully reject its authority. Nor is there any school of thought which refuses to admit that the influence of actions on happiness is a most material and even predominant consideration in many of the details of morals, however unwilling to acknowledge it as the fundamental principle of morality and the source of moral obligation. I might go much further and say that to all those *a priori* moralists who deem it necessary to argue at all, utilitarian arguments are indispensable. It is not my present purpose to criticize these thinkers; but I cannot help referring, for illustration, to a systematic treatise by one of the most illustrious of them, the *Metaphysics*

* Mill, J.S.: *Utilitarianism*, 2nd edn, ed. G. Sher. Indianapolis, IN, Hackett, 2001, Chapters 1 and 2.

of Ethics by Kant. This remarkable man, whose system of thought will long remain one of the landmarks in the history of philosophical speculation, does, in the treatise in question, lay down a universal first principle as the origin and ground of moral obligation; it is this: 'So act that the rule on which thou actest would admit of being adopted as a law by all rational beings.' But when he begins to deduce from this precept any of the actual duties of morality, he fails, almost grotesquely, to show that there would be any contradiction, any logical (not to say physical) impossibility, in the adoption by all rational beings of the most outrageously immoral rules of conduct. All he shows is that the *consequences* of their universal adoption would be such as no one would choose to incur.

On the present occasion, I shall, without further discussion of the other theories, attempt to contribute something toward the understanding and appreciation of the 'utilitarian' or 'happiness' theory, and toward such proof as it is susceptible of. It is evident that this cannot be proof in the ordinary and popular meaning of the term. Questions of ultimate ends are not amenable to direct proof. Whatever can be proved to be good must be so by being shown to be a means to something admitted to be good without proof. The medical art is proved to be good by its conducing to health; but how is it possible to prove that health is good? The art of music is good, for the reason, among others, that it produces pleasure; but what proof is it possible to give that pleasure is good? If, then, it is asserted that there is a comprehensive formula, including all things which are in themselves good, and that whatever else is good is not so as an end but as a means, the formula may be accepted orrejected, but is not a subject of what is commonly understood by proof. We are not, however, to infer that its acceptance or rejection must depend on blind impulse or arbitrary choice. There is a larger meaning of the word 'proof,' in which this question is as amenable to it as any other of the disputed questions of philosophy. The subject is within the cognizance of the rational faculty; and neither does that faculty deal with it solely in the way of intuition. Considerations may be presented capable of determining the intellect either to give or withhold its assent to the doctrine; and this is equivalent to proof.

We shall examine presently of what nature are these considerations; in what manner they apply to the case, and what rational grounds, therefore, can be given for accepting or rejecting the utilitarian formula. But it is a preliminary condition of rational acceptance or rejection that the formula should be correctly understood. I believe that the very imperfect notion ordinarily formed of its meaning is the chief obstacle which impedes its reception, and that, could it be cleared even from only the grosser misconceptions, the question would be greatly simplified and a large proportion of its difficulties removed. Before, therefore, I attempt to enter into the philosophical grounds which can be given for assenting to the utilitarian standard, I shall offer some illustrations of the doctrine itself, with the view of showing more clearly what it is, distinguishing it from what it is not, and disposing of such of the practical objections to it as either originate in, or are closely connected with, mistaken interpretations of its meaning. Having thus prepared the ground, I shall afterwards endeavor to throw such light as I can upon the question considered as one of philosophical theory.

[. . .]

Chapter II: What Utalitariansims Is

The creed which accepts as the foundation of morals 'utility' or the 'greatest happiness principle' holds that actions are right in proportion as they tend to promote happiness; wrong as they tend to produce the reverse of happiness. By happiness is intended pleasure and the absence of pain; by unhappiness, pain and the privation of pleasure. To give a clear view of the moral standard set up by the theory, much more requires to be said; in particular, what things it includes in the ideas of pain and pleasure, and to what extent this is left an open question. But these supplementary explanations do not affect the theory of life on which this theory of morality is grounded – namely, that pleasure and freedom from pain are the only things desirable as ends; and that all desirable things (which are as numerous in the utilitarian as in any other scheme) are desirable either for pleasure inherent in themselves or as means to the promotion of pleasure and the prevention of pain.

Now such a theory of life excites in many minds, and among them in some of the most estimable in feeling and purpose, inveterate dislike. To suppose that life has (as they express it) no higher end than pleasure – no better and nobler object of desire and pursuit – they designate as utterly mean and groveling, as a doctrine worthy only of swine, to whom the followers of Epicurus were, at a very early period, contemptuously likened; and modern holders of the doctrine are occasionally made the subject of equally polite comparisons by its German, French, and English assailants.

When thus attacked, the Epicureans have always answered that it is not they, but their accusers, who represent human nature in a degrading light, since the accusation supposes human beings to be capable of no pleasures except those of which swine are capable. If this supposition were true, the charge could not be gainsaid, but would then be no longer an imputation; for if the sources of pleasure were precisely the same to human beings and to swine, the rule of life which is good enough for the one would be good enough for the other. The comparison of the Epicurean life to that of beasts is felt as degrading, precisely because a beast's pleasures do not satisfy a human being's conceptions of happiness. Human beings have faculties more elevated than the animal appetites and, when once made conscious of them, do not regard anything as happiness which does not include their gratification. I do not, indeed, consider the Epicureans to have been by any means faultless in drawing out their scheme of consequences from the utilitarian principle. To do this in any sufficient manner, many Stoic, as well as Christian, elements require to be included. But there is no known Epicurean theory of life which does not assign to the pleasures of the intellect, of the feelings and imagination, and of the moral sentiments a much higher value as pleasures than to those of mere sensation. It must be admitted, however, that utilitarian writers in general have placed the superiority of mental over bodily pleasures chiefly in the greater permanency, safety, uncostliness, etc., of the former – that is, in their circumstantial advantages rather than in their intrinsic nature. And on all these points utilitarians have fully proved their case; but they might have taken the other and, as it may be called, higher ground with entire consistency. It is quite compatible with the principle of utility to recognize the fact that some kinds of pleasure are more desirable and more valuable than others. It would be absurd that, while in estimating all other things quality is considered as well as quantity, the estimation of pleasure should be supposed to depend on quantity alone.

If I am asked what I mean by difference of quality in pleasures, or what makes one pleasure more valuable than another, merely as a pleasure, except its being greater in amount, there is but one possible answer. Of two pleasures, if there be one to which all or almost all who have experience of both give a decided preference, irrespective of any feeling of moral obligation to prefer it, that is the more desirable pleasure. If one of the two is, by those who are competently acquainted with both, placed so far above the other that they prefer it, even though knowing it to be attended with a greater amount of discontent, and would not resign it for any quantity of the other pleasure which their nature is capable of, we are justified in ascribing to the preferred enjoyment a superiority in quality so far outweighing quantity as to render it, in comparison, of small account.

Now it is an unquestionable fact that those who are equally acquainted with and equally capable of appreciating and enjoying both do give a most marked preference to the manner of existence which employs their higher faculties. Few human creatures would consent to be changed into any of the lower animals for a promise of the fullest allowance of a beast's pleasures; no intelligent human being would consent to be a fool, no instructed person would be an ignoramus, no person of feeling and conscience would be selfish and base, even though they should be persuaded that the fool, the dunce, or the rascal is better satisfied with his lot than they are with theirs. They would not resign what they possess more than he for the most complete satisfaction of all the desires which they have in common with him. If they ever fancy they would, it is only in cases of unhappiness so extreme that to escape from it they would exchange their lot for almost any other, however undesirable in their own eyes. A being of higher faculties requires more to make him happy, is capable probably of more acute suffering, and certainly accessible to it at more points, than one of an inferior type; but in spite of these liabilities, he can never really wish to sink into what he feels to be a lower grade of existence. We may give what explanation we please of this unwillingness; we may attribute it to pride, a name which is given indiscriminately to some of the most and to some of the least estimable feelings of which mankind are capable; we may refer it to the love of liberty and personal independence, an appeal to which was with the Stoics one of the most effective means for the inculcation of it; to the love of power or to the love of excitement, both of which do really enter into and contribute to it; but its most appropriate appellation is a sense of dignity, which all human beings possess in one form or other, and in some, though by no means in exact, proportion to their higher faculties, and which is so essential a part of the happiness of those in whom it is strong that nothing which conflicts with it could be otherwise than momentarily an object of desire to them. Whoever supposes that this preference takes place at a sacrifice of happiness – that the superior being, in anything like equal circumstances, is not happier than the inferior – confounds the two very different ideas of happiness and content. It is indisputable that the being whose capacities of enjoyment are low has the greatest chance of having them fully satisfied; and a highly endowed being will always feel that any happiness which he can look for, as the world is constituted, is imperfect. But he can learn to bear its imperfections, if they are at all bearable; and they will not make him envy the being who is indeed unconscious of the imperfections, but only because he feels not at all the good which those imperfections qualify. It is better to be a human being dissatisfied than a pig satisfied; better to be Socrates dissatisfied than a fool satisfied. And if the fool, or the pig, are of a different opinion, it is because they only know their own side of the question. The other party to the comparison knows both sides.

[. . .]

From this verdict of the only competent judges, I apprehend there can be no appeal. On a question which is the best worth having of two pleasures, or which of two modes of existence is the most grateful to the feelings, apart from its moral attributes and from its consequences, the judgment of those who are qualified by knowledge of both, or, if they differ, that of the majority among them, must be admitted as final. And there needs be the less hesitation to accept this judgment respecting the quality of pleasures, since there is no other tribunal to be referred to even on the question of quantity. What means are there of determining which is the acutest of two pains, or the intensest of two pleasurable sensations, except the general suffrage of those who are familiar with both? Neither pains nor pleasures are homogeneous, and pain is always heterogeneous with pleasure. What is there to decide whether a particular pleasure is worth purchasing at the cost of a particular pain, except the feelings and judgment of the experienced? When, therefore, those feelings and judgment declare the pleasures derived from the higher faculties to be preferable *in kind*, apart from the question of intensity, to those of which the animal nature, disjoined from the higher faculties, is susceptible, they are entitled on this subject to the same regard.

I have dwelt on this point as being a necessary part of a perfectly just conception of utility or happiness considered as the directive rule of human conduct. But it is by no means an indispensable condition to the acceptance of the utilitarian standard; for that standard is not the agent's own greatest happiness, but the greatest amount of happiness altogether; and if it may possibly be doubted whether a noble character is always the happier for its nobleness, there can be no doubt that it makes other people happier, and that the world in general is immensely a gainer by it. Utilitarianism, therefore, could only attain its end by the general cultivation of nobleness of character, even if each individual were only benefited by the nobleness of others, and his own, so far as happiness is concerned, were a sheer deduction from the benefit. But the bare enunciation of such an absurdity as this last renders refutation superfluous.

According to the greatest happiness principle, as above explained, the ultimate end, with reference to and for the sake of which all other things are desirable – whether we are considering our own good or that of other people – is an existence exempt as far as possible from pain, and as rich as possible in enjoyments, both in point of quantity and quality; the test of quality and the rule of measuring it against quantity being the preference felt by those who, in their opportunities of experience, to which must be added their habits of self-consciousness and self-observation, are best furnished with the means of comparison. This, being according to the utilitarian opinion the end of human action, is necessarily also the standard of morality, which may accordingly be defined 'the rules and precepts for human conduct,' by the observance of which an existence such as has been described might be, to the greatest extent possible, secured to all mankind; and not to them only, but, so far as the nature of things admits, to the whole sentient creation.

Against this doctrine, however, arises another class of objectors who say that happiness, in any form, cannot be the rational purpose of human life and action; because, in the first place, it is unattainable; and they contemptuously ask, What right hast thou to be happy? – a question which Mr. Carlyle clinches by the addition, What right, a short time ago, hadst thou even to *be*? Next they say that men can do *without* happiness; that all noble human beings have felt this, and could not have become noble but by learning the lesson of *Entsagen*, or renunciation; which lesson, thoroughly learned and submitted to, they affirm to be the beginning and necessary condition of all virtue.

The first of these objections would go to the root of the matter were it well founded; for if no happiness is to be had at all by human beings, the attainment of it cannot be the end of morality or of any rational conduct. Though, even in that case, something might still be said for the utilitarian theory, since utility includes not solely the pursuit of happiness, but the prevention or mitigation of unhappiness; and if the former aim be chimerical, there will be all the greater scope and more imperative need for the latter, so long at least as mankind think fit to live and do not take refuge in the simultaneous act of suicide recommended under certain conditions by Novalis. When, however, it is thus positively asserted to be impossible that human life should be happy, the assertion, if not something like a verbal quibble, is at least an exaggeration. If by happiness be meant a continuity of highly pleasurable excitement, it is evident enough that this is impossible. A state of exalted pleasure lasts only moments or in some cases, and with some intermissions, hours or days, and is the occasional brilliant flash of enjoyment, not its permanent and steady flame. Of this the philosophers who have taught that happiness is the end of life were as fully aware as those who taunt them. The happiness which they meant was not a life of rapture, but moments of such, in an existence made up of few and transitory pains, many and various pleasures, with a decided predominance of the active over the passive, and having as the foundation of the whole not to expect more from life than it is capable of bestowing. A life thus composed, to those who have been fortunate enough to obtain it, has always appeared worthy of the name of happiness. And such an existence is even now the lot of many during some considerable portion of their lives. The present wretched education and wretched social arrangements are the only real hindrance to its being attainable by almost all.

The objectors perhaps may doubt whether human beings, if taught to consider happiness as the end of life, would be satisfied with such a moderate share of it. But great numbers of mankind have been satisfied with much less. The main constituents of a satisfied life appear to be two, either of which by itself is often found sufficient for the purpose: tranquillity and excitement. With much tranquillity, many find that they can be content with very little pleasure; with much excitement, many can reconcile themselves to a considerable quantity of pain. There is assuredly no inherent impossibility of enabling even the mass of mankind to unite both, since the two are so far from being incompatible that they are in natural alliance, the prolongation of either being a preparation for, and exciting a wish for, the other. It is only those in whom indolence amounts to a vice that do not desire excitement after an interval of repose; it is only those in whom the need of excitement is a disease that feel the tranquillity which follows excitement dull and insipid, instead of pleasurable in direct proportion to the excitement which preceded it. When people who are tolerably fortunate in their outward lot do not find in life sufficient enjoyment to make it valuable to them, the cause generally is caring for nobody but themselves. To those who have neither public nor private affections, the excitements of life are much curtailed, and in any case dwindle in value as the time approaches when all selfish interests must be terminated by death; while those who leave after them objects of personal affection, and especially those who have also cultivated a fellow-feeling with the collective interests of mankind, retain as lively an interest in life on the eve of death as in the vigor of youth and health. Next to selfishness, the principal cause which makes life unsatisfactory is want of mental cultivation. A cultivated mind – I do not mean that of a philosopher, but any mind to which the fountains of knowledge have been opened, and which has been taught, in any tolerable degree, to exercise its faculties – finds sources of inexhaustible interest in all that surrounds it: in the objects of nature, the achievements of art, the imaginations of poetry, the incidents of history, the ways of mankind, past and present, and their prospects in the future. It is possible, indeed, to become indifferent to all this, and that too without having exhausted a thousandth part of it, but only when one has had from the beginning no moral or human interest in these things and has sought in them only the gratification of curiosity.

Now there is absolutely no reason in the nature of things why an amount of mental culture sufficient to give an intelligent interest in these objects of contemplation should not be the inheritance of everyone born in a civilized country. As little is there an inherent necessity that any human being should be a selfish egotist, devoid of every feeling or care but those which center in his own miserable individuality. Something far superior to this is sufficiently common even now, to give ample earnest of what the human species may be made. Genuine private affections and a sincere interest in the public good are possible, though in unequal degrees, to every rightly brought up human being. In a world in which there is so much to interest, so much to enjoy, and so much also to correct and improve, everyone who has this moderate amount of moral and intellectual requisites is capable of an existence which may be called enviable; and unless such a person, through bad laws or subjection to the will of others, is denied the liberty to use the sources of happiness within his reach, he will not fail to find this enviable existence, if he escapes the positive evils of life, the great sources of physical and mental suffering – such as indigence, disease, and the unkindness, worthlessness, or premature loss of objects of affection. The main stress of the problem lies, therefore, in the contest with these calamities from which it is a rare good fortune entirely to escape; which, as things now are, cannot be obviated, and often cannot be in any material degree mitigated. Yet no one whose opinion deserves a moment's consideration can doubt that most of the great positive evils of the world are in themselves removable, and will, if human affairs continue to improve, be in the end reduced within narrow limits. Poverty, in any sense implying suffering, may be completely extinguished by the wisdom of society combined with the good sense and providence of individuals. Even that most intractable of enemies, disease, may be indefinitely reduced in dimensions by good physical and moral education and proper control of noxious influences, while the progress of science holds out a promise for the future of still more direct conquests over this detestable foe. And every advance in that direction relieves us from some, not only of the chances which cut short our own lives, but, what concerns us still more, which deprive us of those in whom our happiness is wrapt up. As for vicissitudes of fortune and other disappointments connected with worldly circumstances, these are principally the effect either of gross imprudence, of ill-regulated desires, or of bad or imperfect social institutions. All the grand sources, in short, of human suffering are in a great degree, many of them almost entirely, conquerable by human care and effort; and though their removal is grievously slow – though a long succession of generations will perish in the breach before the conquest is completed, and this world becomes all that, if will and knowledge were not wanting, it might easily be made – yet every mind sufficiently intelligent and generous to bear a part, however small and inconspicuous, in the endeavor will draw a noble enjoyment from the contest itself, which he

would not for any bribe in the form of selfish indulgence consent to be without.

And this leads to the true estimation of what is said by the objectors concerning the possibility and the obligation of learning to do without happiness. Unquestionably it is possible to do without happiness; it is done involuntarily by nineteen-twentieths of mankind, even in those parts of our present world which are least deep in barbarism; and it often has to be done voluntarily by the hero or the martyr, for the sake of something which he prizes more than his individual happiness. But this something, what is it, unless the happiness of others or some of the requisites of happiness? It is noble to be capable of resigning entirely one's own portion of happiness, or chances of it; but, after all, this self-sacrifice must be for some end; it is not its own end; and if we are told that its end is not happiness but virtue, which is better than happiness,. I ask, would the sacrifice be made if the hero or martyr did not believe that it would earn for others immunity from similar sacrifices? Would it be made if he thought that his renunciation of happiness for himself would produce no fruit for any of his fellow creatures, but to make their lot like his and place them also in the condition of persons who have renounced happiness? All honor to those who can abnegate for themselves the personal enjoyment of life when by such renunciation they contribute worthily to increase the amount of happiness in the world; but he who does it or professes to do it for any other purpose is no more deserving of admiration than the ascetic mounted on his pillar. He may be an inspiring proof of what men *can* do, but assuredly not an example of what they *should*.

Though it is only in a very imperfect state of the world's arrangements that anyone can best serve the happiness of others by the absolute sacrifice of his own, yet, so long as the world is in that imperfect state, I fully acknowledge that the readiness to make such a sacrifice is the highest virtue which can be found in man. I will add that in this condition of the world, paradoxical as the assertion may be, the conscious ability to do without happiness gives the best prospect of realizing such happiness as is attainable. For nothing except that consciousness can raise a person above the chances of life by making him feel that, let fate and fortune do their worst, they have not power to subdue him; which, once felt, frees him from excess of anxiety concerning the evils of life and enables him, like many a Stoic in the worst times of the Roman Empire, to cultivate in tranquillity the sources of satisfaction accessible to him, without concerning himself about the uncertainty of their duration any more than about their inevitable end.

Meanwhile, let utilitarians never cease to claim the morality of self-devotion as a possession which belongs by as good a right to them as either to the Stoic or to the Transcendentalist. The utilitarian morality does recognize in human beings the power of sacrificing their own greatest good for the good of others. It only refuses to admit that the sacrifice is itself a good. A sacrifice which does not increase or tend to increase the sum total of happiness, it considers as wasted. The only self-renunciation which it applauds is devotion to the happiness, or to some of the means of happiness, of others, either of mankind collectively or of individuals within the limits imposed by the collective interests of mankind.

I must again repeat what the assailants of utilitarianism seldom have the justice to acknowledge, that the happiness which forms the utilitarian standard of what is right in conduct is not the agent's own happiness but that of all concerned. As between his own happiness and that of others, utilitarianism requires him to be as strictly impartial as a disinterested and benevolent spectator. In the golden rule of Jesus of Nazareth, we read the complete spirit of the ethics of utility. 'To do as you would be done by,' and 'to love your neighbor as yourself,' constitute the ideal perfection of utilitarian morality. As the means of making the nearest approach to this ideal, utility would enjoin, first, that laws and social arrangements should place the happiness or (as, speaking practically, it may be called) the interest of every individual as nearly as possible in harmony with the interest of the whole; and, secondly, that education and opinion, which have so vast a power over human character, should so use that power as to establish in the mind of every individual an indissoluble association between his own happiness and the good of the whole, especially between his own happiness and the practice of such modes of conduct, negative and positive, as regard for the universal happiness prescribes; so that not only he may be unable to conceive the possibility of happiness to himself, consistently with conduct opposed to the general good, but also that a direct impulse to promote the general good may be in every individual one of the habitual motives of action, and the sentiments connected therewith may fill a large and prominent place in every human being's sentient existence. If the impugners of the utilitarian morality represented it to their own minds in this its true character, I know not what recommendation possessed by any other morality they could possibly affirm to be wanting to it; what more beautiful or more exalted developments of human nature any other ethical system can be supposed to foster, or what springs of action, not accessible to the utilitarian, such systems rely on for giving effect to their mandates.

The objectors to utilitarianism cannot always be charged with representing it in a discreditable light. On the contrary, those among them who entertain anything like a just idea of its disinterested character sometimes find fault with its standard as being too high for humanity. They say it is exacting too much to require that people shall always act from the inducement of promoting the general interests of society. But this is to mistake the very meaning of a standard of morals and confound the rule of action with the motive of it. It is the business of ethics to tell us what are our duties, or by what test we may know them; but no system of ethics requires that the sole motive of all we do shall be a feeling of duty; on the contrary, ninety-nine hundredths of all our actions are done from other motives, and rightly so done if the rule of duty does not condemn them. It is the more unjust to utilitarianism that this particular misapprehension should be made a ground of objection to it, inasmuch as utilitarian moralists have gone beyond almost all others in affirming that the motive has nothing to do with the morality of the action, though much with the worth of the agent. He who saves a fellow creature from drowning does what is morally right, whether his motive be duty or the hope of being paid for his trouble; he who betrays the friend that trusts him is guilty of a crime, even if his object be to serve another friend to whom he is under greater obligations. But to speak only of actions done from the motive of duty and in direct obedience to principle: it is a misapprehension of the utilitarian mode of thought to conceive it as implying that people should fix their minds upon so wide a generality as the world, or society at large. The great majority of good actions are intended not for the benefit of the world, but for that of individuals, of which the good of the world is made up; and the thoughts of the most virtuous man need not on these occasions travel beyond the particular persons concerned, except so far as is necessary to assure himself that in benefiting them he is not violating the rights, that is, the legitimate and authorized expectations, of anyone else. The multiplication of happiness is, according to the utilitarian ethics, the object of virtue: the occasions on which any person (except one in a thousand) has it in his power to do this on an extended scale – in other words, to be a public benefactor – are but exceptional; and on these occasions alone is he called on to consider public utility; in every other case, private utility, the interest or happiness of some few persons, is all he has to attend to. Those alone the influence of whose actions extends to society in general need concern themselves habitually about so large an object. In the case of abstinences indeed – of things which people forbear to do from moral considerations, though the consequences in the particular case might be beneficial – it would be unworthy of an intelligent agent not to be consciously aware that the action is of a class which, if practiced generally, would be generally injurious, and that this is the ground of the obligation to abstain from it. The amount of regard for the public interest implied in this recognition is no greater than is demanded by every system of morals, for they all enjoin to abstain from whatever is manifestly pernicious to society.

The same considerations dispose of another reproach against the doctrine of utility, founded on a still grosser misconception of the purpose of a standard of morality and of the very meaning of the words 'right' and 'wrong.' It is often affirmed that utilitarianism renders men cold and unsympathizing; that it chills their moral feelings toward individuals; that it makes them regard only the dry and hard consideration of the consequences of actions, not taking into their moral estimate the qualities from which those actions emanate. If the assertion means that they do not allow their judgment respecting the rightness or wrongness of an action to be influenced by their opinion of the qualities of the person who does it, this is a complaint not against utilitarianism, but against any standard or morality at all; for certainly no known ethical standard decides an action to be good or bad because it is done by a good or bad man, still less because done by an amiable, a brave, or a benevolent man, or the contrary. These considerations are relevant, not to the estimation of actions, but of persons; and there is nothing in the utilitarian theory inconsistent with the fact that there are other things which interest us in persons besides the rightness and wrongness of their actions. The Stoics, indeed, with the paradoxical misuse of language which was part of their system, and by which they strove to raise themselves above all concern about anything but virtue, were fond of saying that he who has that has everything; that he, and only he, is rich, is beautiful, is a king. But no claim of this description is made for the virtuous man by the utilitarian doctrine. Utilitarians are quite aware that there are other desirable possessions and qualities besides virtue, and are perfectly willing to allow to all of them their full worth. They are also aware that a right action does not necessarily indicate a virtuous character, and that actions which are blamable often proceed from qualities entitled to praise. When this is apparent in any particular case, it modifies their estimation, no certainly of the act, but of the agent. I grant that they are, notwithstanding, of opinion that in the long run the best proof of a good character is good actions; and resolutely refuse to consider any mental disposition as good of which the predominant tendency is to produce bad conduct. This makes them unpopular with many people, but it is an unpopularity which they must share with everyone who regards the distinction between right and wrong in a serious light; and the reproach is not one which a conscientious utilitarian need be anxious to repel.

If no more be meant by the objection than that many utilitarians look on the morality of actions, as measured by the utilitarian standards, with too exclusive a regard, and do not lay sufficient stress upon the other beauties of character which go toward making a human being lovable or admirable, this may be admitted. Utilitarians who have cultivated their moral feelings, but not their sympathies, nor their artistic perceptions, do fall into this mistake; and so do all other moralists under the same conditions. What can be said in excuse for other moralists is equally available for them, namely, that, if there is to be any error, it is better that it should be on that side. As a matter of fact, we may affirm that among utilitarians, as among adherents of other systems, there is every imaginable degree of rigidity and of laxity in the application of their standard; some are even puritanically rigorous, while others are as indulgent as can possibly be desired by sinner or by sentimentalist. But on the whole, a doctrine which brings prominently forward the interest that mankind have in the repression and prevention of conduct which violates the moral law is likely to be inferior to no other in turning the sanctions of opinion against such violations. It is true, the question 'What does violate the moral law?' is one on which those who recognize different standards of morality are likely now and then to differ. But difference of opinion on moral questions was not first introduced into the world by utilitarianism, while that doctrine does supply, if not always an easy, at all events a tangible and intelligible, mode of deciding such differences.

[. . .]

Again, utility is often summarily stigmatized as an immoral doctrine by giving it the name of 'expediency,' and taking advantage of the popular use of that term to contrast it with principle. But the expedient, in the sense in which it is opposed to the right, generally means that which is expedient for the particular interest of the agent himself; as when a minister sacrifices the interests of his country to keep himself in place. When it means anything better than this, it means that which is expedient for some immediate object, some temporary purpose, but which violates a rule whose observance is expedient in a much higher degree. The expedient, in this sense, instead of being the same thing with the useful, is a branch of the hurtful.

Thus it would often be expedient, for the purpose of getting over some momentary embarrassment, or attaining some object immediately useful to ourselves or others, to tell a lie. But inasmuch as the cultivation in ourselves of a sensitive feeling on the subject of veracity is one of the most useful, and the enfeeblement of that feeling one of the most hurtful, things to which our conduct can be instrumental; and inasmuch as any, even unintentional, deviation from truth does that much toward weakening the trustworthiness of human assertion, which is not only the principal support of all present social well-being, but the insufficiency of which does more than any one thing that can be named to keep back civilization, virtue, everything on which human happiness on the largest scale depends – we feel that the violation, for a present advantage, of a rule of such transcendent expediency is not expedient, and that he who, for the sake of convenience to himself or to some other individual, does what depends on him to deprive mankind of the good, and inflict upon them the evil, involved in the greater or less reliance which they can place in each other's word, acts the part of one of their worst enemies. Yet that even this rule, sacred as it is, admits of possible exceptions is acknowledged by all moralists; the chief of which is when the withholding of some fact (as of information from a malefactor, or of bad news from a person dangerously ill) would save an individual (especially an individual other than oneself) from great and unmerited evil, and when the withholding can only be effected by denial. But in order that the exception may not extend itself beyond the need, and may have the least possible effect in weakening reliance on veracity, it ought to be recognized and, if possible, its limits defined; and, if the principle of utility is good for anything, it must be good for weighing these conflicting utilities against one another and marking out the region within which one or the other preponderates.

Again, defenders of utility often find themselves called upon to reply to such objections as this – that there is not time, previous to action, for calculating and weighing the effects of any line of conduct on the general happiness. This is exactly as if anyone were to say that it is impossible to guide our conduct by Christianity because there is not time, on every occasion on which anything has to be done, to read through the Old and New Testaments. The answer to the objection is that there has been ample time, namely, the whole past duration of the human species. During all that time mankind have been learning by experience the tendencies of actions; on which experience all the prudence as well as all the morality of life are dependent. People talk as if the commencement of this course of experience had hitherto been put off, and as if, at the moment when some man feels tempted to meddle with the property or life of another, he had to begin considering for the first time whether murder and theft are injurious to human happiness. Even then I do not think that he would find the question very puzzling; but, at all events, the matter is now done to his hand. It is

truly a whimsical supposition that, if mankind were agreed in considering utility to be the test of morality, they would remain without any agreement as to what *is* useful, and would take no measures for having their notions on the subject taught to the young and enforced by law and opinion. There is no difficulty in proving any ethical standard whatever to work ill if we suppose universal idiocy to be conjoined with it; but on any hypothesis short of that, mankind must by this time have acquired positive beliefs as to the effects of some actions on their happiness; and the beliefs which have thus come down are the rules of morality for the multitude, and for the philosopher until he has succeeded in finding better. That philosophers might easily do this, even now, on many subjects; that the received code of ethics is by no means of divine right; and that mankind have still much to learn as to the effects of actions on the general happiness, I admit or rather earnestly maintain. The corollaries from the principle of utility, like the precepts of every practical art, admit of indefinite improvement, and, in a progressive state of the human mind, their improvement is perpetually going on. But to consider the rules of morality as improvable is one thing; to pass over the intermediate generalization entirely and endeavor to test each individual action directly by the first principle is another. It is a strange notion that the acknowledgment of a first principle is inconsistent with the admission of secondary ones. To inform a traveler respecting the place of his ultimate destination is not to forbid the use of landmarks and direction-posts on the way. The proposition that happiness is the end and aim of morality does not mean that no road ought to be laid down to that goal, or that persons going thither should not be advised to take one direction rather than another. Men really ought to leave off talking a kind of nonsense on this subject, which they would neither talk nor listen to on other matters of practical concernment. Nobody argues that the art of navigation is not founded on astronomy because sailors cannot wait to calculate the Nautical Almanac. Being rational creatures, they go to sea with it ready calculated; and all rational creatures go out upon the sea of life with their minds made up on the common questions of right and wrong, as well as on many of the far more difficult questions of wise and foolish. And this, as long as foresight is a human quality, it is to be presumed they will continue to do. Whatever we adopt as the fundamental principle of morality, we require subordinate principles to apply it by; the impossibility of doing without them, being common to all systems, can afford no argument against any one in particular; but gravely to argue as if no such secondary principles could be had, and as if mankind had remained till now, and always must remain, without drawing any general conclusions from the experience of human life is as high a pitch, I think, as absurdity has ever reached in philosophical controversy.

[...]

The 'Four-principles' Approach*

Tom L. Beauchamp

This essay presents and supports the four-principles approach to health care ethics that Jim Childress and I developed almost two decades ago[1]. The principles included in the framework are:

1 Beneficence (the obligation to provide benefits and balance benefits against risks).

2 Non-maleficence (the obligation to avoid the causation of harm).

3 Respect for autonomy (the obligation to respect the decision-making capacities of autonomous persons).

4 Justice (obligations of fairness in the distribution of benefits and risks).

Rules for health care ethics can be formulated by reference to these four principles, together with other moral considerations, although these rules cannot be straightforwardly *deduced* from the principles, because additional interpretation and specification is needed. Such rules include rules of truth-telling, confidentiality, privacy and fidelity, as well as more specific guidelines pertaining to problems such as physician-assisted suicide, informed consent, withdrawing treatment, using randomized clinical trials.

In the four-principles approach, moral principles in their bare form as principles are little more than abstract rallying points for reflection. Principles are starting, foundational points in health care ethics, not solely sufficient or final appeals. The four principles, as well as rules such as 'Don't kill' and 'Tell the truth', do not give us much more information about how to lead our lives than such admonitions as 'Be competent' or 'Act virtuously'. All skeletal moral norms must be embedded in and then interpreted for specific contexts; that is, there must be some means to clothe them with a specific content that develops their meaning, implications, complexity, limits, exceptions, and the like.

In the first section I motivate the analysis of the four principles by arguing that some of the principles have played an important historical role, whereas others came into prominence because of distinctively modern problems. In the second section I connect the principles to models of moral responsibility in medicine. In the third section I discuss the normative character of principles, particularly their status as *prima-facie* moral principles. Then, in the fourth section, I discuss some recent criticisms of the four-principles approach to health care ethics, especially those who refer to the account as *principlism* and reject it altogether. In the penultimate section I discuss the need to interpret and specify these principles for particular contexts, and also the need for a method known as 'reflective equilibrium'. Finally, in the Conclusion, I connect the previous five sections to the thesis that there is no canon of principles for biomedical ethics.

I cannot here engage in extended philosophical argument about the meaning and commitments of these principles. Instead, I try to express why principles are important and why these particular principles provide a useful, but not canonical, framework for health care ethics.

* Beauchamp, T.: The 'four principles' approach, in *Principles of health care ethics*, ed. R. Gillon. Chichester, Wiley and Sons, 1994, pp. 3–12.

The framework and its roots in health care

Recent systematic and theoretical work in health care ethics tends to converge to the conclusion that moral responsibility in medicine ideally should be conceived in terms of fundamental principles, rules, rights, and virtues. Many controversies in health care ethics turn on the precise moral content of these guidelines, as well as on how much weight they have in particular contexts, how conflicts among the notions are to be handled, and how to specify their precise significance for particular circumstances.

Some moral guidelines seem to be best framed as rules, others as standards of virtue, others as rights, and others as principles. Although rules, rights, and virtues are unquestionably of the highest importance for health care ethics, I believe principles provide the most comprehensive starting point, for reasons I shall try to make clear as we proceed. Other principles may be relevant to moral judgement. Nothing in the four-principles approach makes a claim to have assembled the only worthwhile listing of relevant principles.

The justification for choosing the particular four moral guidelines I am defending is in part historical – that is, some of the principles are deeply embedded in medical traditions of health care ethics – and in part that the principles point to an important part of morality that has been traditionally neglected in health care ethics but now needs to be placed at the foreground. To defend these claims I shall first briefly discuss some aspects of the history of health care ethics.

Throughout the centuries the health professional's obligations, rights, and virtues, as found in codes and learned writings on ethics, have been conceived through professional commitments to shield patients from harm and provide medical care, expressed in ethical terms as fundamental obligations of non-maleficence and beneficence. Medical beneficence has long been viewed as the proper goal of medicine, and professional dedication to this goal has been viewed as essential to being a physician.

The principle of beneficence expresses an obligation to help others further their important and legitimate interests by preventing and removing harms; no less important is the obligation to weigh and balance possible goods against the possible harms of an action. This principle of beneficence potentially demands more than the principle of non-maleficence because it requires positive steps to help others, not merely the omission of harm-causing activities.

The principle of non-maleficence has long been associated in medicine with the injunction *primum non nocere*: 'Above all [or first] do no harm'. This maxim has been mistakenly attributed to the Hippocratic tradition, but the Hippocratic corpus does proclaim both a duty of non-maleficence and a duty of beneficence; together they carve out a conception of medical ethics in which the overriding principle is acting for the patient's best medical best interest[2,3]. This Hippocratic tradition was carried forward from medieval to modern medicine as an ideal of moral commitment and behavior.

From the perspective of the English-speaking world it was British physician Thomas Percival who furnished the first well-shaped doctrine of health care ethics. Easily the dominant influence in both British and American health care ethics of the period, Percival argued that non-maleficence and beneficence fix the physician's primary obligations and triumph over the patient's rights of autonomy in any serious circumstance of conflict:

To a patient . . . who makes inquiries which, if faithfully answered, might prove fatal to him, it would be a gross and unfeeling wrong to reveal the truth. His right to it is suspended, and even annihilated; because, its beneficial nature being reversed, it would be deeply injurious to himself, to his family, and to the public. And he has the strongest claim, from the trust reposed in his physician, as well as from the common principles of humanity, to be guarded against whatever would be detrimental to him. . . . The only point at issue is, whether the practitioner shall sacrifice that delicate sense of veracity, which is so ornamental to, and indeed forms a characteristic excellence of the virtuous man, to this claim of professional justice and social duty [4].

Like the Hippocratic physicians, Percival moved from the premise of the patient's best medical interest as the proper goal of the physician's actions to descriptions of the physician's proper deportment, including traits of character such as benevolence and sympathetic tenderness that maximize the patient's welfare.

Percival's work served as the pattern for the American Medical Association's (AMA) first code of ethics in 1847. Many passages were taken verbatim from his book. But much more than Percival's language survived in America: his beneficence-based viewpoint on ethics gradually became the creed of professional conduct in the United States. Beneficence and non-maleficence became through his delineations the landmark principles that gave shape to health care ethics. These two principles remained until very recently the most prominent values in the major writings on medical ethics in the patient – physician relationship.

In recent years, however, the idea has emerged – largely from writings in law and philosophy – that the proper model of the physician's moral responsibility should be understood less in terms of traditional ideals of medical benefit, and more in terms of the rights of patients, including autonomy-based rights to truthfulness, confidentiality, privacy, disclosure and consent, as well as welfare rights rooted in claims of justice. These proposals have jolted medicine from its traditional preoccupation with a beneficence-based model of health care ethics in the direction of an autonomy model, as well as into a confrontation with a wider set of social concerns.

The principle of respect for autonomy is rooted in the liberal western tradition of the importance of individual freedom, both for political life and for personal development. 'Autonomy' and 'respect for autonomy' are terms loosely associated with several ideas, such as privacy, voluntariness, choosing freely, and accepting responsibility for one's choices.

Finally, *the principle of justice* is really many principles about the distribution of benefits and burdens, not a single principle. Several distributive theories of justice have been put forth, and to a limited extent these theories give us anchors in health care ethics. To cite one example, an egalitarian theory of justice implies that if there is a departure from equality in the distribution of health care benefits and burdens, such a departure must serve the common good and enhance the position of those who are least advantaged in society.

Of course there are other theories of justice than the egalitarian theory. For example, utilitarian theories emphasize a mixture of criteria so that public utility is maximized, comparable to the way public health policy has often been formulated in western nations. In the distribution of health care utilitarians see justice as involving trade-offs and balances. In devising a system of public funding for health care the utilitarian believes we must balance public and private benefit, predicted cost savings, the probability of failure, the magnitude of risks, etc. Under this theory a just distribution of the benefits and burdens of research is to be determined by the utility of research to all affected by the research.

The arrival of a new health care ethics emphasizing autonomy rights and justice-based rights is not surprising, in light of recent social history. It seems likely that both increased legal interest and increased ethical interest in the professional–patient relationship and in a variety of topics of social justice are but instances of a new civil-rights orientation that various social movements of the past 30 years introduced. The issues raised by minority rights, women's rights, the consumer movement, and the rights of prisoners, the homeless, and the mentally ill often included health care components such as reproductive rights, rights of access to abortion and contraception, the right to health care information, access to care, and rights to be protected against unwarranted human experimentation.

One result of these developments has been to introduce both confusion and constructive change into medicine and health care institutions, which continue to struggle with unprecedented challenges to their authority in the control and treatment of patients. Several justice-based controversies in contemporary public policy have added to the confusion in the attempt to determine what is fair or owed when scarce medical resources must be rationed, or when third parties have interests and rights in the treatment or non-treatment of an individual.

These problems in health care ethics cannot be addressed here. The point of this section has simply been to explain the background and motivation for the acceptance of four moral principles.

Models and their underlying principles

I spoke above of 'models' of health care ethics (or of responsibility in providing health care). These are philosophically loaded ideas that give shape to what is only inchoate and unsystematically formed in the history of medical practice and health care ethics.* The 'autonomy model' refers to the view that responsibilities to the patient of disclosure, confidentiality, privacy, and consent-seeking are established primarily (perhaps exclusively) by the moral principle of respect for autonomy. The conflict between this principle and the principle of beneficence, of course the mainstay behind the beneficence model, can be expressed as follows: the physician's responsibilities are conceived in terms of the physician's primary obligation to provide medical benefits. The management of information is therefore understood in terms of the management of patients ('due care') generally. That is, the physician's primary obligation in handling information and in making recommendations is understood in terms of maximizing the patient's medical benefits, not in terms of respecting the patient's autonomous choices.

The central problem of authority in these discussions has become whether an autonomy model of medical practice should be given practical priority over the beneficence model, and whether even some combination of the two is adequate to address many problems of social justice to which health care finds itself inextricably linked. Major conflicts of value occur between autonomy and beneficence. For example, some health care professionals will accept a patient's refusal as valid, whereas others will ignore the fact that no consent has been given, and so try to 'benefit' the patient through a medical intervention. The difference between these two models can be understood in terms of the underlying principled justifications at work. The premise that authority rests with patients or subjects should be justified, according to proponents of the autonomy model, *not* by arguments from beneficence to the effect that decisional autonomy by patients enables them to survive, heal, or otherwise improve their own health, but solely by the principle of respect for autonomy. Similarly in research settings, a proponent of the autonomy model holds that requiring the consent of subjects must be based on the principle of respect for autonomy, and never solely on the premise that consent protects subjects from risks.

Both respect for autonomy and beneficence are valid moral principles, and both are of the highest importance for health care ethics. I shall return

---

* See ref. 5, esp. pp. 26–27.

momentarily to the problem of how to handle conflicts between the two principles.

The normative nature of principles

Principles in the four-principles approach should be conceived neither as rules of thumb nor as absolute prescriptions. Rather, they are *prima facie*: they are always binding *unless* they conflict with obligations expressed in another moral principle, in which case a balancing of the demands of the two principles is necessary. In this event, further specification is required of the precise commitments of the guidelines for the special circumstance(s). Which principle overrides in a case of conflict will depend on the particular context, which is likely to have unique features.

This method of 'overriding' duties by other duties might seem precariously flexible, as if moral guidelines in the end lack mettle and mainstay. But this is a misunderstanding. It is true that in ethics, as in all walks of life, there is no escape from the exercise of judgement in circumstances of uncertainty; but not just any judgement will be acceptable. For an infringement of a moral principle or rule to be justified the infringement must be necessary in the circumstances, in the sense that there are no morally preferable alternative actions that could be substituted, and the form of infringement selected must constitute the least infringement possible.

Recent critiques of principlism

Not everyone agrees that these four principles, or any principles, provide the best framework for health care ethics. Some have severely criticized the four-principles approach as a 'mantra of principles', meaning that the principles have functioned for some adherents like a ritual incantation of norms repeated with little reflection or analysis. The most sustained and best-argued attack on principle-based ethics has come from K. Danner Clouser and Bernard Gert in a critique of 'principlism'[6], a term they use to designate all theories that rely on a plural body of potentially conflicting *prima facie* principles (but especially ours and William Frankena's).

In particular, Gert and Clouser bring the following accusations against our four-principle system: (1) the 'principles' are little more than checklists or headings for lists of values worth remembering, and so the principles have no deep moral substance and do not produce directive guidelines for moral conduct; (2) principle analyses fail to provide a theory of justification or a theory that ties the principles together so as to generate clear, coherent, specific rules, with the consequence that the principles and so-called derivative rules are *ad hoc* constructions without systematic order; (3) these *prima facie* principles must often compete in difficult circumstances, yet the underlying account is unable to decide how to adjudicate the conflict in particular cases and unable theoretically to deal with a conflict of principles.

I do not deny that these are important problems, worthy of the most careful and sustained reflection in moral theory. I do deny, however, that Clouser and Gert – or anyone else who uses either a principle-based or rule-based theory (as they do) – have surmounted the very problems they list for our four-principles approach. The primary difference between what Childress and I call principles and they call rules is that their rules tend (as they point out) to have a more directive and specific content than our principles, thereby superficially seeming to give more guidance in the moral life. But we have pointed out this very fact since our first edition (in 1979). We have always accepted specific rules, not merely principles, as essential for health care ethics. There is also not more and not less normative content between their rules and our rules; not more and not less direction in the moral life. It is true that principles order and classify more than they lay down directive moral law, and therefore principles do have more of a 'heading'-like character, but what we say about rules is noticeably similar to what Clouser and Gert say about rules, and with a similar content.

The principles Childress and I defend are not constructed with an eye to eliminating possible conflicts among the principles, because no system of guidelines could reasonably anticipate the full range of conflicts. No set of principles or general guidelines can provide mechanical solutions or definitive procedures for decision-making about moral problems in medicine. Experience and sound judgement are indispensable allies.

So far as I can see, the major difference between our theory and the Clouser/Gert approach has nothing to do with whether principles or rules are the primary normative guides in a theory, but rather with several aspects of their theory that I, at least, would reject. First, they assume that there is or at least can be what they call a 'well-developed unified theory' that removes conflicting principles and consistently expresses the grounds of correct judgement – in effect, a canon of rules that expresses the 'unity and universality of morality'. They fault us heavily for believing that more than one kind of ethical theory can justify a moral belief. They insist that to avoid relativism there can only be 'a single unified ethical theory', and that there cannot be 'several sources of final justification' (ref. 6, pp. 231–232). These are all claims that I would reject, although there is no space to engage in such tussles here.

I must now bring this discussion of Gert and Clouser's criticism to a conclusion, in order to deal with two problems that grow out of their criticisms. First, a major problem in health care ethics, for our critics as well as for us, is how to interpret and make more specific the principles and rules in the system – so as to give them more determinative content for practice and help in the resolution of particular problems. I will sketch a solution to this problem in the next section. Second, Gert and Clouser say that

In formulating theory we start with particular moral judgments about which we are certain, and we abstract and formulate the relevant features of those cases to help us in turn to decide the unclear cases (ref. 6, p. 232).

This is precisely the model Childress and I have supported since the first edition. I will also discuss this problem of methodology in the next section.

The need for specification and reflective equilibrium

The philosopher G. W. F. Hegel properly criticized Immanuel Kant for developing a moral theory of 'empty formalism' that preached obligation for obligation's sake, without any power to develop what Hegel called an 'immanent doctrine of duties'. He thought all 'content and specification' in a living code of ethics had been replaced by abstractness in Kant's account[7]. The four-principles analysis has been similarly accused,* and I believe the criticism does rightly point to a serious gap in contemporary health care ethics. Every ethical theory, and indeed morality itself, contain regions of indeterminacy that need to be reduced through further development of principles, augmenting them with a more specific moral content.

Here is an example of the problem: if non-maleficence is the principle that we ought not to inflict evil or harm, this principle does little to give specific guidance for the moral problem of whether active voluntary euthanasia can be morally justified. If we question whether physicians ought to be allowed to be the agents of euthanasia, we again get no real guidance. Although abstract guidelines provide relevant considerations, they must be developed into concrete action-guides, taking into consideration such factors as efficiency, institutional rules, law, clientele acceptance, and the like. That is, in addition to abstract principles there must be mediating rules that translate an ethical theory into a practical strategy and set of meaningful guidelines for real-world problems involving demands of efficiency, political procedures, legal constraints, uncertainty about risk, and the like.

In light of indeterminacy at the heart of principles, I follow Henry Richardson[9] in arguing that the specification of principles and related rules involves a filling in of details so as to overcome apparent moral conflicts. The process of specification is the progressive, substantive delineation of principles, pulling them out of abstractness and making them into concrete rules.

---

* In addition to Clouser and Gert (6), see Toulmin (8), pp. 31–39.

The following is a simple example of specification. The principle 'doctors should always* put their patients' interests first' has long been advanced as foundational for medical ethics. But suppose the only way to advance the patient's interest is to act illegally by purchasing a kidney from someone who needs the money. It hardly follows from the principle of patient-priority that a physician should act illegally by purchasing or using someone's organ. The original principle needs specification so as to give better, more fully stated moral advice. We might start on this project by replacing the principle of patient-priority, in its spare form, with the following more concrete rule: 'physicians should place their patients' interests first using all means that are both morally and legally acceptable'.

This principle itself will need further specification in other circumstances of conflict; in fact, progressive specification usually must take place, gradually eliminating the dilemmas and circumstances of conflict that the abstract principle itself has insufficient content to resolve. All moral norms are, in principle, subject to such further revision and specification. The reason, as Richardson nicely puts it, is that 'the complexity of the moral phenomena always outruns our ability to capture them in general norms'.

There are, however, tangled problems about the best method to use in order to achieve specification, and how we know whether any particular proposed specification is justified. The model of analysis for reaching specification and justification in health care ethics that Childress and I have long used is that of a dialectical balancing of principles against other encountered moral considerations, in an attempt to achieve general coherence and a mutual support among the accepted norms. As Joel Feinberg suggests, moral reasoning is analogous to the dialectical process that occurs in courts of law. If a legal principle commits a judge to some unacceptable judgement, the judge needs to modify or supplement the principle in a way that does the least damage to the judge's beliefs about the law. Yet, if a well-founded principle demands a change in a particular judgement, the overriding claims of consistency with precedent may require that the judgement be adjusted, not the principle. Sometimes both judgements and principles need revision[11].

One method of special importance for the specification of principles is 'reflective equilibrium', a method formulated by John Rawls for use in general ethical theory. It views the acceptance of principles in ethics as properly beginning with our 'considered judgements', those moral convictions in which we have the highest confidence, and which we believe to have the lowest level of bias. The goal of reflective equilibrium is to match, prune, and develop considered judgements and principles in an attempt to make them coherent. We start with the paradigms of what is morally proper or morally improper. We then search for principles that are consistent with these paradigms and consistent with each other[12].

'Considered judgements' is in effect a technical term referring to 'judgements in which our moral capacities are most likely to be displayed without distortion'. Examples are judgements about the wrongness of racial discrimination, religious intolerance, and political conflict of interest. But, as Rawls puts it, considered judgements occur at all levels of generality in our moral thinking: 'from those about particular situations and institutions through broad standards and first principles to formal and abstract conditions'[13]. Widely accepted principles of right action (moral beliefs) are thus taken, as Rawls puts it, 'provisionally as fixed points', but also as 'liable to revision'.

By using reflective equilibrium, general ethical principles and particular judgements can be brought into equilibrium. From this perspective, moral thinking is like other forms of theorizing in that hypotheses must be tested, buried, or modified through experimental thinking. A specified principle, then, is acceptable in the system if it heightens the mutual support of the guidelines in the system that have themselves been found acceptable using reflective equilibrium.

Conclusion

Health care ethics is often said to be an 'applied ethics', but this metaphor may be as misleading as it is helpful. There is no such thing as a simple 'application' of a principle so as to resolve a complicated moral problem. It is no less misleading to suggest that those who engage in ethical theory can produce all relevant moral guidelines or crank out conclusions that immediately follow from principles. Ethical theory using principles invites us to reason through our moral dilemmas and offers some ways of doing so. But general ethical theory has long contained within its own fabric a sustained body of controversies, and it needs careful development to serve the needs of health care ethics.

Among the advantages of 'principlism' is that it disavows the idea that there is a single ultimate principle of ethics or some rules that are either absolute or that receive a priority ranking. The four-principles approach supports a method of content-expansion into more specific normative rules, rather than a system layered in terms of priorities among rules. In this respect the four principles are the point at which the real work begins, rather than a system of norms ready-to-hand for reaching moral conclusions of concern in health care. Moreover, it is insupportably optimistic to think we will ever attain a fully specified system of norms for health care ethics.

Not surprisingly, the four-principles approach rejects the view that there is a canon for bioethics, including a canon of four principles. There is no scripture, no authoritative interpretation of anything analogous to scripture, and no authoritative interpretation of that large mass of judgements, rules, standards of virtue, and the like that we often collectively sum up by use of the word 'morality'. Nonetheless, much work in health care ethics and in ethical theory is an attempt to articulate basic, pre-existing values with a philosophical sophistication and polish that provides a solid basis for the specification of norms. This is the most that can reasonably be expected of general philosophical ethics.

References

1 Beauchamp. T. L. and Childress, J. F. 1989. *Principles of biomedical ethics*, 3rd edn. Oxford University Press, New York.

2 Jones, W. H. S. 1923. *Hippocrates*, vol. 1, p. 165. Harvard University Press, Cambridge, MA.

3 Jonsen, A. R. 1977. Do no harm: axiom of medical ethics. pp. 27–41, *in* Spicker, S. F. and Tristram Engelhardt, jr, H. (Eds), *Philosophical and medical ethics: its nature and significance*. Reidel, Dordrecht.

4 Percival, T. 1803. *Medical ethics; or a code of institutes and precepts, adapted to the professional conduct of physicians and surgeons*, pp. 165–166. S. Russell, Manchester.

5 Beauchamp, T. L. and McCullough, L. 1984. *Medical ethics*. Prentice Hall, Englewood Cliffs, NJ.

6 Clouser, K. D. and Gert, B. 1990. A critique of principlism. *Journal of Medicine and Philosophy* 15: 219–236.

7 Hegel, G. W. F. (trans. T. M. Knox) 1942. *Philosophy of right*, pp. 89–90, 106–107. Clarendon Press, Oxford.

8 Toulmin, S. 1981. The tyranny of principles. *Hastings Center Report* 11.

9 Richardson, H. S. 1990. Specifying norms as a way to resolve concrete ethical problems. *Philosophy and Public Affairs* 19: 279–310.

10 Gillon, R. 1986. Doctors and patients. *British Medical Journal* 292: 466–469.

11 Feinberg, J. 1973. *Social philosophy*, p. 34. Prentice Hall, Englewood Cliffs, NJ.

12 Rawls, J. 1971. *A theory of justice*, pp. 20ff., 46–49, 195–201, 577ff. Harvard University Press, Cambridge, MA.

13 Rawls, J. 1974–5. The independence of moral theory. *Proceedings and Addresses of the American Philosophical Association* 48: 8.

---

* Richardson (9), p. 294. ('Always' in this formulation should perhaps be understood to mean 'in principle always'; specification may, in some cases, reach a final form.) For an example of elementary specification (but not so called) using the four-principles approach, see Raanan Gillon (10).

The 'Voice of Care':

Implications for bioethical education *

Alisa L. Carse

Introduction

When Carol Gilligan published *In a Different Voice* in 1982, she claimed to hear a 'distinct moral voice' in the reflections of the women subjects she interviewed for her research on moral development. Gilligan dubbed this 'voice' the 'voice of care' and contrasted it with the 'voice of justice' expressed in standard ethical theories rooted in Kant and the contractarians. Gilligan's research was designed in part as a corrective to the research of Piaget (1932) and Kohlberg (1981, 1984), whose studies of moral development initially excluded women, and later found women to be 'less developed' morally than men and who, in their research, equated morality with the 'justice' approach simpliciter. Gilligan's research and the work it has inspired in psychology and philosophy have given rise to a set of challenges, both to orthodox theories of moral development and to dominant strains in ethical theory. I want to examine and motivate a number of those challenges to ethical theory and to identify their implications for bioethics and education.[1]

'Justice', 'Care', and Gender

It is most helpful to understand the two moral 'voices' as distinct *orientations* within morality. These orientations are distinguished by differences in the reasoning strategies employed and the moral themes emphasized in the interpretation and resolution of moral problems; they represent distinct moral sensibilities and 'different moral concerns' (Gilligan, 1987, pp. 22–23; Gilligan *et al.*, 1988, p. 82).

According to Gilligan, the justice orientation construes the moral point of view as an impartial point of view, understands particular moral judgments as derived from abstract and universal principles, sees moral judgment as essentially dispassionate rather than passionate, and emphasizes individual rights and norms of formal equality and reciprocity in modelling our moral relationships. By contrast, the care orientation rejects impartiality as an essential mark of the moral, understands moral judgments as situation-attuned perceptions sensitive to others' needs and to the dynamics of particular relationships, construes moral reasoning as involving empathy and concern, and emphasizes norms of responsiveness and responsibility in our relationships with others. Whereas we are, on the justice orientation, viewed as individuals first, and in relationship to each other only secondarily, through choice, we are, on the care orientation, understood as *essentially in relationship*, though no single kind of relationship is endorsed as alone morally paradigmatic.[2]

Now it is important to note, first, that Gilligan herself denies that the justice and care orientations correlate strictly with gender. She reports that recent studies show both women and men capable of shifting easily from one orientation to the other when asked to do so, though it is women who are most likely to exhibit a dominant care orientation – a tendency, that is, for the terms of care to take precedence over those of justice in their approach to moral problems (Gilligan *et al.*, 1988).

Second, Gilligan claims that the justice-and care orientations are not mutually exclusive: 'Like the figure-ground shift in ambiguous figure perception, the perspectives of justice and care are not,' she says, 'opposites or mirror-images of one another, with justice uncaring and care unjust. Instead, these perspectives denote different ways of organizing the basic elements of moral judgment: self, others, and the relationship between them' (1987, pp. 22–23). I will investigate this claim critically later, because it appears to underestimate the degree of tension between the two orientations as Gilligan describes them.

My concern in this discussion is with the implications for ethical theory generally, and for bioethics in particular, of Gilligan's characterization of these two moral orientations. It is not on the empirical status of the differences Gilligan claims to have found between male and female moral reasoners that I will focus, but on the different modes of moral judgment her work has highlighted. As Marilyn Friedman has aptly put it, 'the different voice hypothesis has a significance for ethical theory and ethics which would survive the demise of the gender difference hypothesis. At least part of its significance lies in revealing the lopsided obsession of . . . contemporary theories of morality with universal and impartial conceptions of justice and rights' (1987, p. 92).

Along these lines, I want to emphasize that we must steadfastly reject any suggestion that women speak in one moral voice; such a claim would be preposterous at best. And we must be wary of the tendency toward gender-essentialism that the language of gender difference can, even unwillingly, invite.[3] Moreover, we need not, in the end, deny the crucial importance of justice and rights in affirming the wisdom and value of the voice of care. We might, that is, defend the need to retain a sturdy rights conception within ethics, but affirm at the same time the need for an ethic more demanding than the ethic of justice – one which gives an essential place to 'care' through norms of character and citizenship (for all people), traditionally thought more appropriate for women than for men.

Most deeply at stake in the care-oriented challenge is the conception of the moral subject, of the capacities and skills constitutive of moral maturity. The question thus naturally arises what implications the challenge has for ethical education, which aims to nurture and encourage moral capacities and skills. My aim is first to set out the broad contours of the challenge and then to explore a number of implications the challenge has for bioethical education.

What are the chief criticisms leveled against the justice orientation by care theorists? There are four that get to the heart of the matter, corresponding to the four points of contrast listed above.

Impartiality as the Mark of the Moral

Recall that a first feature of the justice perspective is its commitment to impartiality as the hallmark of the moral point of view (the point of view from which moral judgment is rendered, moral choice is made). On the justice orientation, we are to refrain from giving special weight to our particular values and preferences, personal attributes, relationships, and

* Carse, A.: The 'voice of care': implications for bioethical education. *Journal of Medicine and Philosophy* **16**:5–28, 1991.

situations, or for that matter to anyone else's either, in determining what morality demands. On this construal of impartiality, the benefit a course of action might have for me, my child, or my neighborhood, for example, is not itself deemed relevant to the moral justification of that course of action. The impartiality requirement, so understood, captures the intuition that what is morally required of one person is morally required of any person relevantly similarly situated. Moral demands don't favor any one in particular, or any particular relationship as such. We can see the relationship between the impartiality requirement, so understood, and the conception of moral principles as abstract and universal in scope (Rawls, 1972; Kohlberg, 1981).

Seyla Benhabib has called the impartial moral standpoint the standpoint of the 'generalized other' (1987, p. 163). From this standpoint we view every individual as an independent, rational agent entitled to the very same rights to which we ourselves are entitled as independent, rational agents. In taking this standpoint, I might acknowledge that the other has a unique life history, particular affections, attachments, commitments, and aspirations; however, what grounds the other's moral claim on me is not any of these particular identifying features, but the fact of his or her personhood itself. Thus, from the impartial point of view, I can acknowledge the other's *personhood*, in an abstract sense, but not his or her distinctive identity as a person.

Now, the impartiality requirement is seen by feminist critics as morally problematic precisely because it requires abstraction away from the concrete identity of others and our relationships to them. Gilligan writes: 'As a framework for moral decision, care is grounded in the assumption that . . . detachment, whether from self or from others is morally problematic, since it breeds moral blindness or indifference – a failure to discern or respond to need' (1987, p. 24). The worry is that in taking an impartial standpoint, I become unable to see into the other's position, to imagine myself in the other's place, and thus to understand the other's concerns or needs; 'the other as different from the self disappears' (Benhabib, 1987, p. 165). The care orientation champions a close attentiveness to particularities of identity and relationship as a crucial feature of moral understanding, claiming that without such attentiveness we are, in many cases, in no position to render moral judgment or make a moral choice at all. The impartial observer is *disqualified* rather than *legitimated* as a competent moral judge (cf. Gilligan, 1984; Held, 1987; Murdoch, 1970; Ruddick, 1989).

One might attempt to defend the traditional commitment to impartiality by arguing that it is properly to be understood as a *justificational* constraint, not a constraint on all moral deliberation. We might, that is, hold that impartiality is crucial to the evaluation and justification of moral requirements (or recommendations), without thereby holding that impartially justified moral requirements (or recommendations) always enjoin moral agents to take an impartial point of view in going about their lives (Hill, 1987). Both deontologists and consequentialists have standardly required that moral prescriptions be justified from an impartial standpoint. But nothing prohibits prescriptions so justified from acknowledging partial duties and special obligations, pertaining, for example, to people in virtue of the roles they inhabit (e.g., physician, nurse, teacher, or governor) or the specific relationships in which they stand to others (e.g., spouse, parent, friend, or fellow patriot).

An adequate response to this line of thought is impossible here. Let me just say, first, that the feminist criticism of impartiality is best understood as the claim that there is no single or privileged justificational standpoint in morality. If one is contemplating what responsibilities one has generally as a teacher to one's students or as a physician to one's patients, appeal to impartially justified principles may be illuminating and appropriate. If one is trying to decide how to respond to a particular student's truancy, or to a particular patient's refusal of treatment, attunement to the peculiarities of individual need and to the vagaries of circumstance may be essential to sound moral judgment. The *broad* requirement that we attend to the particularities of others and our relationships to them can itself be validated from an impartial point of view – one which privileges no one in particular and no particular group or relationship as such (Sher 1987). However the justifiability of impartially justified prescriptions must be subject to assessment with an eye to particulars. The suggestion, then, is that impartial prescriptions cannot always inform us sufficiently about how to respond to others, and morally relevant features of particular situations will sometimes be obscured through an overzealous reliance on impartial prescriptions, even those that recognize special obligations and duties. This is not to deny that impartial deliberation is sometimes appropriate to moral justification; it is rather to claim that the impartial point of view has no special authority as such in determining the moral validity of our judgments or the assessment of moral requirements and recommendations.

More broadly, the rejection of impartiality as the mark of the moral is a rejection of the prevailing tendency in ethical theory to construe, as morally paradigmatic, forms of judgment that abstract away from concrete identity and relational context, and to view moral maturity and skill as residing essentially in the capacity for abstract judgment so construed. The focus on impartiality as the hallmark of moral judgment has had the effect of ascribing a derivative, secondary status to forms of epistemic skill – involving attention to nuance and peculiarity – that are, from the perspective of care, often of the first importance.

Moral judgment as principle-derived

This first challenge to the justice orientation leads us to a second. Recall the conception of moral judgment within the justice perspective as principled judgment. Moral conclusions about what to do in particular cases are depicted as derived from general principles or rules of conduct. The care orientation is characterized by a general antipathy to moral principles. At one point, Gilligan describes a moral judgment as 'a contextual judgment, bound to the particulars of time and place . . . and thus resisting all categorical formulation' (1982, pp. 58–59). The resistance to principles coincides with the rejection of impartiality as a (necessary) mark of moral judgment; to act on principles is just to act for reasons that are taken to hold with the same force for all others who are similarly situated. But there is some confusion about the nature of principles and the role principles can (and cannot) play in moral judgment. Thus, I want to try to motivate the movement away from a conceptions of moral judgment as essentially principle-driven while in the end acknowledging a reduced, but important, role for moral principles, properly understood.

An extreme conception of principled judgment asserts, with Kant, that principles admit of no exceptions. Let us consider, however, a less extreme conception of principles according to which they have *prima facie* status, for this is the conception generally used in bioethics (cf. Ross, 1930; Beauchamp and Childress, 1989; Beauchamp and McCullough, 1984). On this conception, no single principle is granted absolute priority in cases of conflict. Rather, the weight of principles must be assessed as cases arise, and any principle can on some conditions be overridden. On this construal of principled reasoning, an apprehension of contextual detail and a willingness to tailor moral judgments to the particulars of context does not amount to an abandonment of principles. Quite the contrary, sensitivity to contextual detail is necessary in order to apply principles to particular situations.

The question thus arises, Why not maintain a conception of moral judgment as principle-driven, even within a care orientation? The answer lies in the limited usefulness of principles in informing and guiding a caring response. This can be seen in several ways.

First, there arises a general point about principle application. Recognizing that a general principle or rule is relevant to the situation at hand, and knowing how it is fittingly to be acted upon requires a capacity for discernment that is *distinct from*, and *presupposed by*, the application of principles themselves. Consider the apparently simple injunction to be kind to other people. What does meeting this injunction amount to? Being kind is no mechanical matter. A kind response in one situation could be an intrusive or meddlesome response in another. Now we might generalize about what kind people do: kind people, for example, tend to try to cheer up their friends when their friends are sad, to help people pick up the groceries they have dropped, to comfort others who are suffering, and the like. But there are no principles or rules to guide such actions; those judging must be responsive to particular nuances of situations as they arise. Being a kind person is, among other things, being disposed to 'see' that one's friend needs cheering up or that, in *this* case offering a hand with the groceries would be helpful rather than meddlesome. To be kind is, among other things, to be capable of interpreting when a situation is one in which kindness is called for and what being kind amounts to in that situation.[4] An account of moral judgment according to which it consists in the deductive application of general principles (even *prima facie* ones) to particular cases does not alone provide an adequate picture of how we come properly to interpret situations and judge what we ought to do (Nussbaum, 1985; Sherman, 1990b).

Moreover, as the kindness example illustrates, it is, within the care orientation, not just a sensitivity to the particular features of context that is integral to moral judgment, but more specifically, a sensitivity to *other people*, a capacity to perceive (as best we can) how others feel, and how they understand themselves and their circumstances. Attention must be given to the unique and unrepeatable features of other persons, our relationship to them, and the circumstances in which we find ourselves with them. This attention, and the discernment of particulars it involves, is itself a *moral capacity* which can be developed and exercised with greater or lesser success and which, crucially, is not itself principle-governed.

Because the injunction to give care generally requires that we be attuned in certain (caring) ways to the particular and unique contours of situations as they come up, and more particularly, to *other people*, an account of moral judgment as principle or rule-derived cannot, in an ethic of care, provide a full picture of how we come properly to judge what we ought to do.

This is not to say, however, that there is no role for principles to play in a care orientation; principles may prove indispensable. For they can help to activate virtuous perception by calling to mind broad norms of conduct and thereby aid us in articulating at least some of the moral stakes of our decisions. They can also provide crucial checks on our pursuit of others' welfare. But an appeal to principle can not alone establish the moral validity of particular judgments, for the appeal to principle is itself valid only insofar as decisions based on the principle are good ones. Establishing this will require a discernment of the particulars (Nussbaum, 1985; Aristotle, Nichomachean Ethics 11137b13ff. in McKeon, 1941). And properly discerning the particulars will require the exercise of specific forms of affective and cognitive skill – of emotional attunement and sympathetic insight which are not themselves principle-governed.

This brings us to another, related point. When we 'see' that the child crouched in the corner wants to be approached and touched rather than called to or left alone, when we speak more softly to quell someone's fear or comfort someone in pain, or look away from someone who has just been humiliated, our response to the other may be direct and dispositional rather than indirect and deliberative. Though I may come to avert my eyes from someone through a process of principled deliberation, I might also avert my eyes spontaneously, in direct (non-deliberative) response to his distress. Similarly, I might approach and touch someone or modulate my voice 'without even thinking'. Practically attuned responses to situations are not always grounded in forms of explicit awareness or undertaken as a result of principled deliberation. They can be the result of practical insight that is dispositional and non-interferential, a *sympathetic attunement* to others' needs or concerns which directly informs our response to them.

This suggests that it is not only the case that principled moral deliberation involves the exercise of discernment that is not itself principle-directed, but also that principled deliberation is not itself always integral to generating a caring response to others.

Moral intellectualism

This brings us to a third feature of the feminist challenge, namely, the challenge to the intellectualism of the justice orientation and a correlative assertion of the centrality to the moral personality of well-cultivated emotion. This general challenge raises complex and highly controversial issues which I can only touch on here. It is useful to understand the challenge as having two dimensions: the first concerns the importance of the emotions to moral discernment; the second concerns the importance of emotion, and in particular, the expression of emotion, to moral response (Nussbaum, 1985, esp. pp. 183–193; Sherman, 1990a, 1990b).

How are the emotions important to moral discernment? The suggestion is that it is often through our emotions that we discern the condition of others; insight into the feelings and concerns of others is not a deliverance of the intellect alone. Our own capacity for humiliation can, for example, tune us in to the fact that someone else is being humiliated, rather than merely ribbed or teased. Through empathy or compassion, we may recognize another's pain or discomfort, even when its manifestations are subtle or masked. Similarly, anger, suprise, anguish, fear, embarrassment, grief, joy, yearning, and sympathetic versions of these, are ways of being attuned to situations, *modes of attention*, in virtue of which certain features of a situation stand out for us and others recede from our attention.

To view the emotions, as they often are viewed in ethical theory, as agitations or disturbances of moral judgment – messy encumbrances of the moral self that need not concern us so long as they are kept subject to the control of a rational will – is to overlook the crucial role emotions can play, when properly cultivated, in alerting us to morally salient dimensions of situations (Murdoch, 1970; McDowell, 1979; Blum, 1980).

In addition to their role in moral discernment, the emotions play an important expressive role in moral response. As the example of kindness illustrates, it is not just *what* we do, but also *how* we do what we do, that can make a moral difference in giving care; and this is reflected in our gestures, our tone of voice, where and how we stand or move, how we listen – crucially, the emotions we do (or don't) express. Expressing the right emotions at the right time in the right way is, on this view, an integral feature of moral agency (Aristotle, *Nicomachean Ethics* 1106b21–23 in McKeon, 1941). It is important to distinguish this point from the claim that we ought to act *out* of good motives, out of interest and concern for the other. The emotional quality of our response to another is not just a matter of the motivation out of which we act; it is also a matter of the *manner* in which we act. This is an important distinction, for the treatment of emotion in ethics is standardly confined to an assessment of the motives of action. Yet it can be morally significant not just that one acts, for example, from sympathetic, considerate, or kind motives, but that one acts sympathetically, considerately, or kindly, that is, in such a way as to *express* sympathy, consideration, or kindness in acting (Sherman, 1990b).

It appears, then, that we are not simply in need of an enriched normative vocabulary in terms of which to address those skills and capacities agents require in order effectively to *apply* general principles or rules of conduct to particular cases. We are also in need of an account of those skills and capacities agents need in order effectively to *discern* what morality demands, encourages, or recommends and, having done so, to conduct themselves in the proper *manner*, to express themselves effectively and appropriately.

Thus, it is clear that the emphasis on impartial, principled, and dispassionate judgment that marks the traditional justice orientation will fall short of providing adequate guidance within an ethic of care. A key element of the care orientation in ethics, as the philosophical analysis of care is further developed, will need to be an account of the skills and character traits – the virtues – which constitute the caring person. Insofar as care theory infuses bioethical theory, more attention will need to be given in bioethical theory to the virtues relevant to caretaking within medical and nursing practice. And among the virtues will be certain cultivated emotional capacities.

Modelling our relationships

Let us turn now to a fourth feature of the justice orientation to which the challenge of care theory has been directed, namely, the emphasis within this orientation on norms of formal equality and reciprocity in treating the morality of human relationships. Annette Baier writes,

It is a typical feature of the dominant moral theories and traditions, since Kant, or perhaps since Hobbes, that relationships between equals or those who are deemed equal in some important sense, have been the relationships that morality is concerned primarily to regulate. Relationships between those who are clearly unequal in power, such as parents and children, earlier and later generations in relation to one another, states and citizens, doctors and patients, the well and the ill, large states and small states, have had to be shunted to the bottom of the agenda, and then dealt with by some sort of 'promotion' of the weaker so that an appearance of virtual equality is achieved. Citizens collectively become equal to states, children are treated as adults-to-be, the ill and dying are treated as continuers of their earlier more potent selves, so that their 'rights' could be seen as the rights of equals (1987a, p. 53).

The commitment to equality can sometimes be indispensable in ensuring that those more vulnerable and less powerful are protected against forms of harm, for example, exploitation or neglect. But as Baier notes, this commitment also covers over, 'masks', the nuances of those relationships between people of unequal power or one-sided dependence, and the special moral demands weakness or dependency can introduce into a relationship:

A more realistic acceptance of the fact that we begin as helpless children, that at almost every point of our lives we deal with both the more and the less helpless, that equality of power and interdependency, between two persons or groups, is rare and hard to recognize when it does occur, might lead us to a more direct approach to questions concerning the design of institutions structuring these relationships between unequals (families, schools, hospitals, armies) and of the morality of our dealings with the more and the less powerful (1987a, p. 53).

The relative weight given to relations among 'equals' has led to *silence* in moral theory about good and bad kinds of engagement in relationships characterized by material inequality – of power, of knowledge, of vulnerability (as with the sick or young or dependent).

This criticism is related to a second, directed to the rights-based model of moral relationship and the individualistic conception of the self. In particular, the centrality of the right to non-interference in many justice models is based in a commitment to the value of autonomy, and thus of social frameworks within which individuals are ensured the liberty to pursue their (autonomously affirmed) conceptions of the good, consistent with the equal liberty of others. On this view, if you have a right to something, then I have the duty not to impede your pursuit of it. In meeting this requirement, I respect your right to non-interference and I have a legitimate right to demand that you will respect mine. Our interactions are thus marked by a norm of mutual non-interference. What does the emphasis on individual autonomy and the right to non-interference have to do with the individualistic conception of the self? What objections have been raised against these features of the justice orientation?

One worry is that a moral model of our relationships which construes them as paradigmatically structured by rights to mutual non-interference, except when more robust association has been voluntarily assumed, can address very few of our relationships. Just as detachment was seen, from the perspective of care, to threaten us with moral blindness, so non-interference is seen, from the perspective of care, to threaten us with neglect and isolation, especially if we are dependent or relatively powerless, like the very young, the very old, or the sick.

This brings us back to the individualism of the self on the justice perspective. On this perspective, it isn't assumed that we are in relationship, or that human relationship *per se* has value. The existence and value of particular relationships and of human relationship more generally are treated as resting in individual choice. Relationships are construed as among the autonomously affirmed goods we are, as individuals, to be at liberty to pursue.

Now we do, as individuals, choose *some* of our relationships. We tend, for example, to choose who (if anyone) we will marry or divorce; we sometimes choose friends and often choose the clubs we join. But many of our relationships, and more importantly, of our caring relationships, are not undertaken through choice; we don't choose our parents or siblings, nor do they choose us; and though we might choose to have children, we don't choose the children we have. This holds true of many of our students and patients as well. And though we can reflect critically on the *terms* of our relationships – *how* we relate to others or they to us – we can not, as individuals, independently choose or dictate these terms. Relationships require flexibility and responsiveness on the part of those in the relationship.

Gilligan writes: 'As a framework for moral decision, care is grounded in the assumption that the other and self are interdependent' (1982, p. 24); that a good life is one which involves a 'progress of affiliative relationship' (1982, p. 170); that ' "the concept of identity . . . includes the experience of interconnection" ' (1982, p. 173; cf. Baier, 1987a, 1987b; Bishop, 1987; Ruddick, 1984, 1989). A more adequate moral model of us as individuals would more realistically recognize the full extent of our mutual *interdependence*; it would attend more actively to modes of relating to and being with others that help to sustain good relationships among individuals who are not equal in power and relative dependence (cf. May, 1977, 1983; Pellegrino and Thomasma, 1988).

The ethic of care

Where do these criticisms, if taken seriously, point us? The care critique has both methodological implications, for the *process* of moral reasoning and judgment by which we are to come to understand what morality demands of us, and normative implications, for what it is that morality demands of us.

On the methodological front we have seen that 'care' reasoning is concrete and contextual rather than abstract; it is sometimes principle-guided, rather than always principle-derived, and it involves sympathy and compassion rather than dispassion. This introduces a conception of moral psychology much thicker and richer in its skills and capacities than the conception needed on the justice perspective and suggests a movement in a more virtue-theoretic direction, in which not only our actions, but also our characters, are a focus of moral attention.

On the normative front, we have seen that the ethic of care asserts the importance of a concern for the good of others and of community with them, of a capacity for imaginative projection into the position of others, and of situation-attuned responses to others' needs. We have also seen moral importance extended from *what* we do, to *how* we do what we do – the manner in which we act, where this includes the emotional quality or tone of our actions as integral to moral response. Finally, we have seen a call for more moral acknowledgement of our mutual interdependence, of the actual limitations of material equality, and of the special responsibilities vulnerability and dependence can introduce into our relationships.

Both the methodological and normative implications of the care critique suggest that the differences dividing the two perspectives concern much more than emphasis; they concern our conception of the most fundamental elements of moral life: moral judgment, the nature of the moral self, and our responsibilities as individuals to each other.

There are strong theoretical precedents for the care perspective, so understood. A historical alternative to the deductive, principle-driven account of moral judgement is found in Aristotle, for example, for whom moral deliberation involves practical wisdom, which is understood to outrun any general rules or principles one might possibly devise (*Nichomachean Ethics* 1104a1–9 in McKeon, 1941). Moreover, Aristotelian virtue consists in dispositions to passion as well as action, feeling the right emotions 'at the right times, with reference to the right objects, towards the right people, with the right motive, and in the right way' (*Nichomachean Ethics* 1106b21–3, 1109b30 in McKeon, 1941). The care orientation also finds a kindred spirit in David Hume, who criticizes Hobbes and Locke for what he calls their ' "selfish systems of morals" ' and who views corrected sympathy, not principled reason, as our basic moral capacity (Baier, 1987b).

Bioethics and education

I want, in this section, to identify some implications for bioethics and education of the preceding challenges to the justice orientation in ethical theory. There are some clear affinities between standard approaches taken in bioethics and the justice orientation that care theorists characterize. Bioethical theories tend to take a principle-based approach on which moral judgments are construed to be directed paradigmatically to the question 'What ought morally to be done?' and thus to be concerned primarily with right action, rather than good character or virtue. Bioethical theories tend largely to emphasize, as fundamental, the impartial principles of respect for autonomy, justice, and beneficence. Much current debate in bioethics is between deontologists and utilitarians, and concerns how we are to understand and rank the importance of these principles.

It is true that the importance placed on beneficence in some bioethical theories may seem to make these theories morally richer than the justice orientation challenged by care theorists. For the principle of beneficence requires us to do more than recognize others' rights to non-interference; it requires us actively to promote the welfare of others. Nonetheless, there is a notable difference: the care orientation emphasizes sympathy and compassion as modes of concerned attention to concrete and particular others, whereas the principle of beneficence urges a 'love of humanity', an abstract concern for others in virtue of our common humanity.[5]

The fact that case studies are a central focus of bioethical discussion, that discussions of standard bioethical issues such as euthanasia, confidentiality, informed consent, or resource allocation often involve paying attention to the concrete details of particular contexts in which those issues arise, may reinforce in a second way a sense that there are strong similarities between standard bioethical approaches and the ethic of care. It is important to emphasize, therefore, that while bioethics discussions, in virtue of focusing on applied issues, tend to be more concrete than some discussions in theoretical ethics, standard bioethical approaches continue to be abstract in a crucial sense: they rely on a language of abstract rights and principles, and on conceptions of obligation formulated independently of particular contexts. Details of context are consulted only in order to apply abstract, general principles to particular cases.

The care-oriented challenge thus has implications for the ethical theory taught, the issues addressed, and the skills and sensitivities encouraged through bioethical education. Let me set out seven implications here, as suggestions for further discussion and inquiry.

1. One issue the care-oriented challenge raises for bioethical education is the possible tendency of a bioethical approach that pictures moral judgment as essentially principle-driven to emphasize institutionally developed rights-based codes and procedures and to underemphasize the personal skills and capacities that go into good caretaking. Too much rule-dependence may run the risk of encouraging a courseness of feeling and a lack of care and compassion necessary to fostering hope and ensuring that a patient's good is served in the healing process.

An example of a change in bioethics which is a change in the direction of an ethic of care, is found in more recent treatments of the issue of informed consent – in particular, the shift away from an emphasis on institutional rules of information disclosure toward greater attention to the quality of the patient's understanding and of the communicative exchange. What this shift in emphasis demonstrates is that in a properly caring context, respect for autonomy – the principle which grounds informed consent, will involve not only negative prohibitions against coercion, manipulation and the like, but also positive duties, to nurture and sustain the patient's capacity to exercise autonomous choices. This process requires much more than procedurally correct forms of information disclosure; it requires sensitivity to the individual patient – to his or her fears, hopes, values, and capacities in the decision-making process (cf. Faden and Beauchamp, 1986, esp.,

Chapter 7; Beauchamp and Childress, 1989, esp., Chapter 3; Pellegrino and Thomasma, 1988).

2. This suggests that more effort should be made to attune students to their own and others' values, fears, capacities and commitments, and to encourage the consideration of such factors in the interpretation and resolution of ethical conflicts. Along these lines, the care-oriented challenge raises the question for educators how we can, through education, widen and expand emotional knowledge and imaginative power, and encourage in our students the capacity to enter into the feelings and perspectives of others. Iris Murdoch recommends the study of literature as a way to learn to 'picture and understand human situations' (1970, p. 34). A bioethical education might include exposure, through readings, testimonials, and films to the health care problems and healing practices of different cultures, religions, and peoples, thereby enhancing students' awareness and sensitivity to others. It might also provide examples of real or fictional people who can inspire or serve as role models, and encourage discussion of both these particular lives and of cultural ideals.

3. On the care orientation, what is sought in ethical debate is not so much theoretically neat, universally justifiable solutions to moral conflicts as shared interpretations of problems and collective success in mediating and balancing the different moral claims and concerns various parties to a case express. If we accept this picture of moral conflict-resolution, more emphasis would need to be placed in bioethical education – particularly of those who will work in the clinical setting (such as physicians, nurses, clinical ethicists, and the like) – on the development of communication skills. We need to ask ourselves as educators what sorts of skills facilitate people in expressing themselves and listening to others, in interpreting what others say or do with insight and understanding. We might pay more explicit attention to the implications of manner, tone, forms of demeanor and expression – for the ability to communicate effectively.

4. A broad implication of the care-oriented challenge – particularly the worries voiced about impartiality – is that bioethical issues ought not to be addressed in a social and political vacuum. Bioethical education should encourage critical reflection on the gender patterned occupational roles among health care providers, on the way in which the roles of physician and nurse, for example, have historically been construed as male and female roles, respectively, and on the effect this has had on the division of labor and authority in health care practice (cf. Warren, 1989, p. 77; Winslow, 1984). This becomes particularly important as more women enter medicine and the nursing shortage becomes an ever greater problem. Bioethical education should also include an examination of the broad social and economic implications of particular medical practices and technologies, such as reproductive technologies, and address the implications both for our access to health care and for our health care needs of factors such as age, gender, class, religion, and sexual orientation (Overall, 1987; 1989, p. 182; Sherwin, 1987, 1989). Ignoring these factors in our ethical reflections can desensitize us to the very real differences in the health care needs particular individuals and groups face.

5. Related to this point, more attention might be paid to the nature and dynamics of particular relationships and relationship-types as significant feature of ethical analysis. The interpretation of cases can involve an acknowledgement of the inequalities of dependency, vulnerability, and knowledge within the relationships that actually structure our lives. Recognition of the inequalities and articulation of the positive duties of care and empowerment they introduce can be an important dimension or bioethical analysis. Students might be encouraged to reflect on various normative models of human relationship that have been proposed in the bioethical literature (e.g., the contract model, the covenant model) and their suitability given the different forms of interdependency and responsibility that characterize relationships between patients and health care providers.[6]

6. Bioethical education must, in the end, affirm the very real moral ambivalence often experienced by all of us, especially by those who wield

power in helping others, and guide students in learning to cope constructively with their own and others' sources of moral ambivalence through open dialogue, role-playing, and essay and journal writing (Warren, 1989, p. 84). Along these lines, the scope of moral discourse might be self-consciously and explicitly expanded to include not only what is morally obligatory, but also what is recommended, urged, advised, or encouraged by morality. Invoking a richer moral psychological vocabulary and paying greater attention to contextual peculiarity and social-economic patterns in our analyses of cases and issues, can facilitate the process of articulation and analysis in a way that remains true to the intricate moral and psychological stakes present.

7. Finally, what becomes clear is that from the perspective of the care orientation, moral maturity involves a wide range of perceptual, imaginative, emotional and expressive capacities. This suggests that bioethical discussions should be addressed not only to the question 'What is the moral status of this action (or policy for action)?' but also 'What kind of person ought I to be?' and 'What traits and capacities ought I to develop?'. As we have seen, this introduces the need for a richer moral vocabulary, for the ability to address issues of character and virtue as well as right action. But it also suggests that bioethical education would, at its best, be aimed at developing not only intellectual skills and moral theoretical knowledge but the whole character of the moral agent. It would itself be a kind of 'fitness program' (Solomon, 1988, p. 437) intended to sharpen verbal tools and analytical skill *but also* to foster moral virtue.

Conclusion

There are, of course, many worries that might be raised for the care orientation in the context of bioethics. Let me look at three that are particularly germane to the present discussion.

It might, first, be objected that there are important moral issues which fall outside the reach of an ethic of care, even if it is caring that leads us to be concerned about them. The worry is that an ethic of care will have nothing to say about certain forms of injustice, that we might, as Virginia Held has put it, 'decide that the rich will care for the rich and the poor for the poor, with the gap between them, however unjustifiably wide, remaining what it is' (1987, p. 120). It is important to stress, first, that what is in question in the challenge we have reviewed is not the importance of justice but the sufficiency of justice and the primacy that has been granted the justice orientation in moral theory. An adequate moral theoretical approach may well involve an integration of the justice and care orientations so as to retain their respective strengths through rehabilitated notions of 'justice' and 'care'.

Second, there might be a perceived need for detachment on the part of good physicians and nurses that is incompatible with the emphasis on compassion and sympathy on the care orientation. As Beauchamp and Childress write: 'A physician who lacked compassion would generally be viewed as deficient; yet compassion also may cloud judgment and preclude rational and effective responses. Constant contact with suffering can overwhelm and even paralyze a compassionate physician' (1989, p. 383). The important point to make in response to this worry is that there is nothing intrinsic to the care perspective which excludes appropriately detached forms of concern and compassion. A good health care professional should be able to summon the appropriate. degree of emotional detachment, or equanimity, when this is crucial to serving the well-being of the patient.

The third difficulty concerns the possible tendency of an ethic of care to allow, on the one hand, too much self-sacrifice on the part of the health care professional, and on the other, overzealous caretaking, leading to too much involvement with patients, or to paternalism. In response, let me note first that a full account of the virtues of caretaking would need to spell out conceptions of proper self-regard – or care for oneself – as protection against self-effacement or problematic self-denial and as a precondition of sound caring for others (cf. Ruddick, 1984, pp. 217–218; Gilligan, 1982,

p. 149). Secondly, it is important, in light of worries about paternalism, to build into our very conception of caretaking the requirement that the caretaker respect the person cared for.[7] A principal aim of a medical ethics informed by an ethic of care would need to be to address how our institutions and practices of health care can further empower patients and in general encourage more active participation on the part of non-experts in their own health care. This would involve a critical exploration of traditional construals of medical authority and reflection on the effects of power dynamics within 'healing' relationships (cf. Warren, 1989, p. 81; May, 1983).

In conclusion, we are still in need of a clear and systematic account of the modes of feeling, of thought, and of action that characterize the care orientation. And we still need to articulate a dear set of standards by which we can distinguish morally good from morally problematic (or even morally debased) forms of 'care'. We also have a need for boundaries which exclude conceptions of care that serve to justify relations of domination and subordination or which threaten to bolster, rather than to challenge, existing forms of gender division and stratification.

But the strength of the care-oriented approach lies in its most basic recommendation: that we reflect upon the moral voices employed in health care practice and bioethics – the values and ideals that are highlighted, the forms of discourse used, and the models and paradigms that are central to attempts to make sense of medical and moral questions which arise. That challenge urges that we become self-conscious about how the dominant models shape our conception of what morality demands and invites us to question the assumption that there is only one legitimate mode of moral reasoning, only one moral voice. That challenge suggests that part of our job in coming to understand our moral world will involve coming to be reflective about the voices in which we ourselves speak and to listen to and learn from the voices of others. These skills can be made an integral part of a bioethical education.[8]

Notes

1 A complex and important question that I cannot go into here is whether and to what extent Kantian and contractarian theories, generally constituting the target of attack in this feminist movement, can accommodate the care orientation. My own position is that they can to some extent, but not fully. Whatever position one takes on this issue, however, one thing remains true: the focus of traditional theories rooted in Kant and the contractarians is quite different from that of the care orientation. I hope that my discussion suggests some ways in which the difference is not one of focus alone.

2 This is not to say that all *de facto* relationships are morally acceptable on the care orientation; the care orientation can be understood as striving, among other things, to articulate norms of relationship that more adequately acknowledge the broad facts of human interdependency.

3 Though we must reject the suggestion that there is a distinctive voice that is *woman's as such*, we might understand this recent project in feminist ethics as unveiling – making visible and explicit – in our ethical theories and ethical practices *one* of the important moral orientations emerging out of women's distinctive experiences in our society, given the sexual division of labor and the social significance, of gender generally as it affects identity-formation. This project does *not*, however, affirm the care orientation as most appropriate for women; quite the contrary, it affirms its importance in general – for women and men – and thus highlights forms of moral skill and moral maturity that have been overlooked or granted only secondary status in many of our preeminent ethical theories.

4 This is not to deny that uncaring people or scoundrels can on occasion show genuine kindness for others. It is to suggest that being concerned about others' well-being, being a kind person, is a condition for having the required sensitivity and sympathetic insight into others that is a further condition of effectively promoting others' well-being in general.

5 A notable exception is found in the treatment given the principle of beneficence by Pellegrino and Thomasma (1988).

6   William May (1977, 1983) recommends that the relationship between the health care provider and the patient be viewed as a covenant rather than a contract, because it lacks a specific *quid pro quo*. Warren Reich (1987) argues that contract models and rights language are 'too adversarial' and fail adequately to capture the need for 'acceptance, trust, affection, and care' which can in effect constitute the moral status of others within relationships. He emphasizes the need to encourage bonding and loyalty to those in need of care, not just respect for rights. Pellegrino and Thomasma (1988) explore the limitations of contractual models of relationship in medical ethics, stressing the unequal power and vulnerability introduced through illness. Annette Baier (1986) recommends that a language of trust and anti-trust be introduced into our ethical reflections to supplement if not supplant contract models. All of these proposals and others might be critically evaluated and contrasted with standard contractual models.

7   Pellegrino and Thomasma (1988) develop an account of beneficence which invokes, as an integral part, respect for the autonomy of the one whose good is served.

8   An early version of this paper was first presented in the Intensive Bioethics Course at the Kennedy Institute of ethics at Georgetown University in June 1989. I am grateful to those present in the audience for their challenging questions. In addition, I am especially indebted to Tom Beauchamp's helpful comments and suggestions on an earlier draft of this paper.

Bibliography

Baier, A.: 1986, 'Trust and antitrust', *Ethics* **96**, 231–260.

Baier, A.: 1987a, 'The need for more than justice', in M. Hanen and K. Nielsen (eds.), *Science, Morality and Feminist Theory*, Supplementary Volume 13 of *Canadian Journal of Philosophy*, pp. 41–56.

Baier, A.: 1987b, 'Hume, the women's moral theorist?' in E. Feder Kittay and D.T. Meyers (eds.), *Women and Moral Theory*, Rowman and Littlefield Publishers, Totawa, New Jersey, pp. 37–55.

Beauchamp, T.L. and Childress, J.F.: 1989, *Principles of Biomedical Ethics*, 3rd edition, Oxford University Press, New York, New York.

Beauchamp, T.L. and McCullough, L.B.: 1984, *Medical Ethics: The Moral Responsibilities of Physicians*, Prentice-Hall, Englewood Cliffs, New Jersey.

Benhabib, S.: 1987, 'The generalized and the concrete other: The Kohlberg-Gilligan controversy and moral theory', in E. Feder Kittay and D.T. Meyers (eds.), *Women and Moral Theory*, Rowman and Littlefield Publishers, Totawa, New Jersey, pp. 154–177.

Bishop, S.: 1987, 'Connections and guilt', *Hypatia* **2** (1), 7–23.

Blum, L.: 1980, *Friendship, Altruism, and Morality*, Routledge and Kegan Paul, Boston, Massachusetts.

Faden, R.R. and Beauchamp, T.L.: 1986, *A History and Theory of Informed Consent*, Oxford University Press, New York, New York.

Friedman, M.: 1987, 'Beyond caring: The de-moralization of gender', in M. Hanen and K. Nielsen (eds.), Supplemental Volume 13 of *Canadian Journal of Philosophy*, pp. 87–110.

Gilligan, C.: 1982, *In a Different Voice: Psychological Theory and Women's Development*, Harvard University Press, Cambridge, Massachusetts.

Gilligan, C.: 1984, 'The conquistador and the dark continent: Reflections on the psychology of love', *Daedalus* **113**, 75–95.

Gilligan, C.: 1987, 'Moral orientation and moral development', in E. Feder Kittay and D.T. Meyers (eds.), *Women and Moral Theory*, Rowman and Littlefield Publishers, Totawa, New Jersey, pp. 19–33.

Gilligan, C, Ward, J. and Taylor, J. (eds.): 1988, *Mapping the Moral Domain*, Harvard University Press, Cambridge, Massachusetts.

Held, V.: 1987, 'Feminism and moral theory', in E. Feder Kittay and D.T. Meyers (eds.), *Women and Moral Theory*, Rowman and Littlefield Publishers, Totawa, New Jersey, pp. 111–128.

Hill, T.E., jr.: 1987, 'The importance of autonomy', in E. Feder Kittay and D.T. Meyers (eds.), *Women and Moral Theory*, Rowman and Littlefield Publishers, Totawa, New Jersey, pp. 129–138.

Kohlberg, L.: 1981, *The Philosophy of Moral Development: Moral Stages and the Idea of Justice: Essays on Moral Development*, *1*, Harper and Row, San Francisco, California.

Kohlberg, L.: 1984, *The Psychology of Moral Development: Essays on Moral Development*, *2*, Harper and Row, San Francisco, California.

May, W.: 1977, 'Code and covenant or philanthropy and contract?' in S.J. Reiser, A.J. Dyck, and W.J. Curran (eds.) *Ethics in Medicine*, MIT Press, Cambridge, Massachusetts, pp. 65–76.

May, W.: 1983, *The Physician's Covenant: Images of the Healer in Medical Ethics*, Westminster Press, Philadelphia, Pennsylvania.

McDowell, J.: 1979, 'Virtue and reason', *The Monist* **62**, 331–351.

McKeon, R. (trans.): 1941, *The Basic Works of Aristotle*, Random House, New York, New York.

Murdoch, I.: 1970, *The Sovereignty of Good*, Routledge and Kegan Paul, London, England.

Nussbaum, M.: 1985, 'The discernment of perception: An aristotelian conception of private and public rationality', *Proceedings of the Boston Area Colloquium in Ancient Philosophy*, 151–207.

Overall, C.: 1987, 'Surrogate motherhood', in M. Hanen and K. Nielsen (eds.), *Science, Morality, and Feminist Theory*, Supplemental Volume 13 of *Canadian Journal of Philosophy*, pp. 285–305.

Overall, C.: 1989, 'The politics of communities', *Hypatia* **4**(2), 179–185.

Pellegrino, E. and Thomasma, D.C.: 1988, *For the Patient's Good*, Oxford University Press, New York, New York.

Piaget, J.: 1932, *The Moral Judgment of the Child*, Free Press, New York, New York.

Rawls, J.: 1971, *A Theory of Justice*, The Belknap Press of Harvard University, Cambridge, Massachusetts.

Reich, W.T.: 1987, 'Caring for life in the first of it: Moral paradigms for perinatal and neonatal ethics', *Seminars in Perinatology* **11**, 279–287.

Ross, W.D.: 1930, *The Right and the Good*, Clarendon Press, Oxford, England.

Ruddick, S.: 1984, 'Maternal thinking', in J. Treblicot (ed.), *Mothering*, Rowman and Allanheld, Totawa, New Jersey, pp. 213–230.

Ruddick, S.: 1989, *Maternal Thinking*, Beacon Press, Boston, Massachusetts.

Sher, G.: 1987, 'Other voices, other rooms? Women's psychology and moral theory', in E. Feder Kittay and D.T. Meyers (eds.) *Women and Moral Theory*, Rowman and Littlefield, Publishers, Totawa, New Jersey, pp. 178–189.

Sherman, N.: 1990a (in press), 'The place of emotions in kantian morality', in O. Flanagan and A.O. Rorty (eds.), *Identity, Character, and Morality*, MIT Press, Cambridge, Massachusetts.

Sherman, N.: 1990b (unpublished manuscript), 'The place of emotions in morality'.

Sherwin, S.: 1987, 'Feminist ethics and *in vitro* fertilization', in M. Hanen and K. Nielsen (eds.), *Science, Morality, and Feminist Theory*, Supplemental Volume 13 of *Canadian Journal of Philosophy*, pp. 265–284.

Sherwin, S.: 1989, 'Feminist and medical ethics: Two different approaches to contextual ethics', *Hypatia* **4**(2), 57–72.

Solomon, D.: 1988, 'Internal objections to virtue ethics', in P. French, T.E. Uehling, jr., and H.K. Wettstein (eds.), *Midwest Studies in Philosophy Volume XIII: Ethical Theory: Character and Virtue*, University of Notre Dame Press, Notre Dame, Indiana, pp. 428–441.

Warren, V.L.: 1989, 'Feminist directions in medical ethics', *Hypatia*, 4 (2), 73–87.

Winslow, G.: 1984, 'From loyalty to advocacy: A new metaphor for nursing' in T.L. Beauchamp and L. Walters (eds.), *Contemporary Issues in Bioethics*, Wadsworth Publishing Company, Belmont, California, pp. 323–333.

2 The Therapeutic Relationship and the Social Domain

The source of ethical guidelines governing the relationship between psychiatrists and patients can be traced to the Hippocratic tradition of fourth-century Greece. Though the oath of the Pythagorean School makes no reference to treatment of the mentally ill, it has nevertheless shaped the concept of right and wrong conduct for contemporary physicians, including psychiatrists, by defining two fundamental goals of the medical profession: (i) establishing values that guide its work; and (ii) promoting guild interests by advancing scholarship and technical skills for the purpose of applying 'specific knowledge to the needs of fellow citizens'.[1]

In terms of values the Hippocratic Oath[2] (see Appendices) specifies explicitly ethical standards of practice, such as safeguarding confidences, proscribing certain procedures, (e.g., abortion and euthanasia) and barring behaviours of 'intentional injustice' or 'mischief' (e.g., sexual relations with patients). These guidelines have in turn spawned a benevolent paternalism that has long been invoked by doctors in order to promote patients' interests and well-being.

As to the second goal, the Hippocratic Oath fosters advances in the field of medicine by instructing doctors to hold their teachers 'equal to my parents' and to share learning with 'my sons and . . . the sons of him who has instructed me'. Expertise is thus promoted for use within a self-defined group, and mutual support is prized for its role in enhancing professional skills that, in turn, benefit society.

In this section we explore ethical issues inherent in the psychiatrist's relationship with the patient, illustrating how they derive from contemporary interpretation of the two pillars of the Hippocratic Oath, and the attempt to handle the tension between them.

Values and the doctor-patient relationship

The ethical core of the doctor-patient relationship is the safeguarding of patients' welfare by determining how doctors best satisfy their particular interests. As discussed by Beauchamp and Childress,[3] essential characteristics of the relationship include fidelity to patients, truth-telling, confidentiality and privacy. These principles may be justified by diverse ethical theories (see Chapter 1) and, as demonstrated by history, subjected to varied interpretations by the medical practitioners.

Paternalism was the dominant paradigm from the ancient Greek tradition to the mid-twentieth century, but as Bloch and Pargiter[4] have observed, 'the period extending from Greco-Roman civilization to the Enlightenment was relatively barren' with respect to ethical considerations of psychiatric care. The mental hospitals of seventeenth- and eighteenth-century Europe were cruel and degrading, used more to isolate their charges than to provide succour and treatment, and in seventeenth century New England women who probably suffered from mental illness were accused of witchcraft and executed by stoning and hanging.[5] The beginning of the nineteenth century witnessed a return to benevolent paternalism for psychiatric patients, after Phillipe Pinel removed the chains at the

Saltpêtriére and Bicetre in Paris, and the Quakers established the York Asylum in England.[6] In 1791 Thomas Percival drafted a code of medical practice that included specific mention of desirable attitudes towards the insane, probably the first work of the modern era to deal with the relationship between doctor and psychiatric patient[7]. The mentally ill, he recommended, should be treated with 'tenderness and indulgence', and doctors should advocate on their behalf. His precepts were essentially replicated in the American Medical Association's inaugural code of 1847, and subsequently formed the basis of the American Psychiatric Association's current code of ethics.[8]

Until the twentieth century, delivery of mental health care was oblivious to the moral complexities of the therapeutic interaction. During the early phase of the psychoanalytic movement Freud's papers began to shed light on ethical parameters of the relationship between psychiatrists and patients. In the selection 'The dynamics of the transference'[9] he discusses psychoanalytic aspects of transference, explaining how patients' unresolved attitudes and fantasies are acted out emotionally rather than comprehended intellectually. Observing that these feelings may be 'turned towards the person of the physician' instead of the pertinent people in the patient's life, he highlights how such 'transferring' can distort interpersonal relationships, as well as the one forged with the analyst. The therapeutic task requires a patient 'to fit [transference] emotions into their place in the treatment and in his life-history, subject them to rational consideration, and apprise them at their true psychical value'. The method for realizing this goal is by gaining the insight derived from analysis of transference feelings.

'The dynamics of the transference' was a seminal work guiding analysts to preserve the integrity of the doctor-patient relationship when it was threatened by forces that arise inevitably in the course of treatment. An observation about why contemporary therapists become embroiled in boundary violations, including sexually, is their lack of training in this sphere. Gartrell et al.[10] found many educational programs in the US 'deficient in educating residents about psychiatric ethics and/or countertransference conflicts'. Gabbard and Nadelson[11] similarly emphasize education as the necessary 'key to preventing boundary violations'. Epstein and Simon[12] designed a self-administered instrument to extend the educational process regarding transference and countertransference beyond training. In the selection 'The exploitation index: an early warning indicator of boundary violations in psychotherapy', they map out exploitative behaviours therapists fail to recognize in themselves, often due to narcissistic traits that undermine the trust required for treatment. Their questionnaire aims to sensitize therapists to any vulnerabilities they may have that could progress to boundary violations by having them ask themselves about the potentially exploitative character of their actions (e.g., Do you tell patients personal things about yourself in order to impress them? Do you ask your patient to do personal favours for you?). A report on the effectiveness of the instrument[13] revealed how respondents often became aware of at least one behaviour they recognized as counterproductive to treatment. As Borys and Pope[14] report, these behaviours can progress to boundary violations, such as becoming friends with a patient after the end of treatment, inviting them to a personal social event, employing a patient or buying goods or services from them.

Relatively benign actions may be the first steps towards sexual exploitation of the patient.[15] Freud was cognizant of the potential for this progression, drawing attention to it in his essay on transference-love.[16] He elaborates on earlier thoughts about transference, specifically addressing patients' sexual feelings towards their therapists and how the latter should respond. He stresses the need to 'work through' intense, persistent erotic feelings in order to prevent them from being visited on others, including subsequent therapists. The clinician should 'never in any circumstance accept or return the tender passion proffered him', but rather pursue a 'middle course' that guards 'against ignoring the transference-love, scaring it away or making the patient disgusted with it' and 'just as resolutely . . . withhold[ing] any response to it'. The task in treatment is to trace a sexualized transference to its unconscious roots, thereby 'bringing to light all that is most hidden in the development of the patient's erotic life and helping her learn to control it'. He cautions against taking advantage of the patient through transference love – a harkening back to the Hippocratic Oath – invoking 'ethical motives which combine with the technical reason to hinder [the therapist] from according the patient his love'.

Freud's observations about 'technique and ethics' underpin contemporary understanding of the boundary between psychiatrist and patient regarding sexual matters. Gutheil and Gabbard, in the selection 'The concept of boundaries in clinical practice: theoretical and risk-management dimension',[17] and in 'Misuses and misunderstandings of boundary theory in clinical and regulatory settings',[18] elaborate on Freud's contribution. Echoing Langs'[19] notion of the 'therapeutic frame', the specific parameters that seek to maintain the integrity of the doctor-patient relationship, Gutheil and Gabbard offer related guidelines such as establishing therapeutic neutrality, providing a consistent, private and professional setting, defining the time and duration of sessions, and minimizing physical contact. Adhering to these precepts promotes 'an atmosphere of safety and predictability within which treatment can thrive'.

Their concept of the therapeutic boundary builds on the classical psychoanalytic position, but is not intended to define the limits of psychiatrist-patient interaction as rigidly. Rather, it acknowledges grades of behaviour, ranging from therapeutic to destructive and unethical. 'Boundary violations' are distinguished from a benign variant, 'boundary crossings'. The latter, deviations from orthodox interpretations of unconscious material (e.g., embracing a sobbing mother who announces she has just learned of her child's death) benefit the patient. It would be difficult to construe that comforting action as a harmful boundary violation. Indeed, not responding in a warm, empathic way could be detrimental to the woman and jeopardize the therapeutic alliance. Gutheil and Gabbard note that boundary crossings may also stem from countertransference reactions; for example, clinicians may reveal details about themselves as unconscious responses to the therapeutic process, but ultimately turn the situation to the patient's advantage.

Boundary violations, in contrast, exclusively fulfil the therapist's needs. As such they are exploitative and convey harmful consequences to the patient. These multifarious behaviours may include using abusive language that is rationalized as therapeutic confrontation, acting to elicit complements or gifts, and explicit sexual exploitation. Such transgressions tend to be repetitive and habitual and, unlike boundary crossings, are never the subject of a constructive dialogue between therapist and patient.

Two central points emerge from Gutheil and Gabbard's observations. The first is the role of context in determining whether a boundary crossing reaches the threshold of unethical behaviour. For example, offering a patient a ride home in a blizzard would be variously judged depending on where therapy occurred (in a prairie town or some city with a subway), whether the patient felt coerced to accept the ride, and if the therapist assisted the patient in this way in mild weather. Second, frequent benign boundary crossings are likely to progress to sexual misconduct. It is readily imaginable that a routine hug at the end of a session or setting an appointment late in the evening might encourage growing intimacy that ultimately culminates in a sexual liaison.[15]

Sexual misconduct by psychiatrists occurs at an alarming rate[10,20]. Offenders offer an array of explanations for their behaviour, including pursuit of love or pleasure, a means to enhance patients' self-esteem by providing a restitutive emotional experience, loss of control, lapse in judgment and fulfilment of personal need. The selection by Gabbard, 'Psychotherapists who transgress sexual boundaries with patients',[21] examines these motivations and identifies subgroups – predators manifesting psychopathy and/or paraphilia, 'lovesick' therapists whose impulse is to surrender masochistically within the treatment setting, and the psychotically disturbed – in order to facilitate their treatment. However, it should be noted that sexual misconduct is but one effect an impaired psychiatrist can have on patients.[22]

A related concern is reflected in the debate about a sexual tie between a therapist and a former patient. A survey of 4,800 psychiatrists, psychologists and social workers revealed a consensus that it was unethical to engage sexually with a current patient, but a third felt it permissible after termination of treatment.[14] In another survey a third of the psychiatrist sample believed sex with a former patient might be appropriate.[23] Heated debate in the 1980s prompted an amendment to *The principles of medical ethics with annotations especially applicable to psychiatry* of the APA[24] to declare sexual involvement with a former patient as 'almost always unethical'. However, the revision proved unsatisfactory to many who advocated a total ban on the grounds that 'neither transference nor the real inequality in the power relationship between patient and therapist ends with the termination of therapy'.[23] They maintained that such behaviour reflected naiveté and/or poor appreciation of the essence of the therapeutic relationship. Shopland and VandeCreek[25] concurred, presenting three theoretical justifications for an absolute ban grounded in psychoanalytic, feminist and family systems perspectives. The argument for a less stringent standard – a twelve month waiting period – is justified on the premise that the vast majority of sexual contacts with former patients occurs within a year of termination; as reported by Applebaum and Jorgenson, only in one of 100 cases they reviewed did a sexual liaison begin more than a year after treatment ended.[26] The debate was finally resolved in 1992 in the US when sex between a psychiatrist and former patient was deemed to be always unethical by the American Psychiatric Association,[27] and the *Principles of medical ethics with annotations especially applicable to psychiatry*[24] were subsequently amended accordingly. Similarly, the 1992 code of ethics of the Royal Australian and New Zealand College of Psychiatrists was amended in 1998 by inclusion of the statement:

Furthermore, it is generally improper for psychiatrists to have sexual relationships with former patients unless the circumstances of the professional relationship have not rendered the patient vulnerable to a subsequent approach. The more deeply the psychiatrist becomes involved in the patient's emotional life the more certain is the impossibility of a subsequent equal relationship. Mutual termination of a therapeutic relationship does not ensure the resumption of an equal relationship. Following long -term psychiatric treatment, this is never possible.[28]

A final issue concerning the ethical basis of the relationship between psychiatrist and patient is in the context of clinical research, a topic also dealt with in Chapter 9. We stress here that atrocities committed in the name of medical research, such as those conducted by the Nazis,[29] played a prominent role in sensitizing psychiatrists to the ethical character of clinical interactions. Principles that emerged from the Nuremberg tribunal, particularly fully informed consent, were codified two years later in the Declaration of Geneva of the World Medical Association, a twentieth-century version of the Hippocratic Oath. They ultimately served as standards of professional conduct for ethical codes of many national medical bodies.[4]

The role of guild interests

Fullinwider[30] has defined a profession in terms of three features. First, members of a profession undergo specialized training, revolving around research and the acquisition of explicit skills. Given this expertise, its bearers anticipate their recommendations will be adhered to, the basis for a degree of paternalism. Second, professionals assist people who are inherently vulnerable and dependent. Third, and less consistent, 'a trustworthy and effective' group of knowledgeable and skilled experts serve the common good, thus enhancing aggregate well-being. In addition to requiring respect for ethical principles (as discussed above), each of these components underscores the notion of professionals as members of a guild that facilitates mutual support, protection, and continued learning. Such interests have long influenced physicians' relationship with patients in ways that often convey ethical repercussions.

First, for centuries the medical profession has determined exclusively the degree to which paternalism pervades their work. A shared conviction that patients lacked understanding of pertinent knowledge promoted what Katz[31] dubbed 'a silent world' that fosters an enormous power differential between patients and physicians. Katz has criticized the medical profession for its neglect of this unwarranted asymmetry, disputing its claim that the 'esoteric' quality of medical knowledge justifies freedom from lay control. Moreover, he rejects the assertion that 'altruism protects patients from abuse of that authority', a persuasive position in the historical context of psychiatric abuses.[29, 32–34] Patients are not 'blissfully ignorant children who must be led by the hand', but people with distinctive '[p]ersonal values, considerations of life style, and other competing preferences' that culminate in idiosyncratic treatment choices. Conceding that physicians know more about disease, he avers that 'patients know more about their own needs . . . [and] neither knows at the outset [of their transaction] what each can do for the other'. Katz therefore espouses a model of conversation in which professionals promote patients' autonomy through the process of informed consent.

Goldberg[35] echoes Katz with specific observations about the 'unspoken power of the psychotherapist'. He contends that the predominant ethical concern in the therapeutic relationship should be an 'explicit agreement' between patient and psychiatrist as to 'why they have come together' in order to appreciate the 'existential concerns' that brings one to treatment. The subsequent therapeutic dialogue provides to a person understanding of his normative relationships with significant others and, in turn, facilitates 'equity and balance' within those relationships. Goldberg argues that a paternalistic attitude impedes this fundamental goal by granting the clinician excessive and unjustified influence in defining the therapeutic goals.

Second, a profession is largely self-regulating. By retaining a substantive degree of independence, even while part of overarching societal structures as governments, a profession promulgates distinctive values that bear ethical consequences for clients. For example, control over entry into the group sets standards of competence and character. The impact on the public is obvious if entry standards allow for mediocrity, or more insidious if, for instance, admission criteria are subject to prejudicial policies. The latter circumstance can lead to inappropriate care for certain ethnic groups that are underrepresented in the profession, as Lawson,[36] documents regarding treatment of African-Americans suffering from affective illnesses.

Selection of educational goals also conveys values that can affect patients directly. The re-medicalization of psychiatry in the 1970s, typified by a cleavage between 'psychological' and 'biological' positions, markedly influenced training programs and the form of care administered by their graduates. This was vividly captured in the Osheroff debate,[37, 38] which centered on the extended, ineffective psychotherapeutic treatment of a patient suffering from major depression who ultimately improved with antidepressants. (This issue is discussed in detail in Chapter 5, where the two essays are included as selections.) Conversely, training heavily invested in drug treatment at the expense of psychotherapy tuition arguably limits proficiency treating certain people, such as those afflicted with disorders of personality functioning. Another educational issue concerns psychiatry's movement to subspecialization. Advances gained in obtaining such expertise must be balanced against the risks for reduced appreciation of the 'whole' person[39] and lack of respect for autonomy.

Fourth, a vital professional responsibility concerns monitoring members by enforcing standards of practice and, in the extreme, expelling those who do not adhere to the principles underpinning its work. Since a profession's established values for acceptable and unethical behaviour may vary with those held by non-professionals, its guild-based goal to maintain public trust is grounded in internal procedures designed to preserve organizational integrity. For example, discriminating between a boundary crossing and violation rests on psychiatric expertise beyond the reach of the general public, thereby requiring a paternalistic posture in order to guarantee ethical norms.

Finally, a profession must advocate for policies that favourably influence its interests and those of the public. In the case of psychiatry these activities can have significant ethical implications for the therapeutic relationship. In the United States, the struggle to secure parity in the distribution of health resources between general medical and mental health care has had both direct and indirect effects on the psychiatrist-patient dyad, directly influencing the level of clinical care while generally underscoring a commitment to advocate for the welfare of the mentally ill.[40] Activism for ethical mental health care also takes the form of criticism of inadequate systems of care and proposals for their improvement,[41, 42] including testimony before national governmental agencies.[43]

In sum, psychiatry maintains a guild-like insularism, employing self-defined guidelines that involve ethics in all aspects of professional development – entry, governance, standards of training and practice, criteria for enforced exit and public policy goals. Whether or not ethical issues are formally addressed in psychiatric training, Dyer is correct to observe that they are implicitly but persuasively involved in 'socialization to the norms of the profession'.[1]

The tension between values and guild interests within the doctor-patient relationship

Through much of the twentieth century medicine remained a self-regulated profession guided by the Hippocratic ethic, barring some duties of the modern state such as licensing or prosecuting physicians engaged in criminal practices. Responsibility for monitoring ethical standards has basically occurred within the profession in the context of the dyadic interaction between physicians and patients. However, medicine's more recent and complex association with third parties (e.g., HMOs, prepaid health plans, government agencies and corporate entities), has progressively transformed the therapeutic relationship into one that also includes aspects of the interaction between consumers and providers. The transition to a triadic configuration – psychiatrist/patient/third party – highlights a tension between the professional goals of maintaining ethical values and promoting guild interests that imposes considerable stress on the therapeutic relationship.

Psychiatrists' conflicted allegiance to patients and concerned third parties is discussed extensively in the selection 'In the service of the state: the psychiatrist as double agent',[44] which reports on a landmark conference co-sponsored by the American Psychiatric Association and The Hastings Center. Exploring the role of practitioners in such settings as the military, the criminal justice system and schools, the study group acknowledged decreasing relevance of a traditional private practitioner model based on Freudian guidelines, given obligations contemporary psychiatrists owe to organizations directly affected by their clinical work. For example, questions were raised about clinicians' fidelity to incarcerated patients when they hear information that could be legally damaging to an inmate or germane to the security of prison personnel or other inmates. Concerns about conflicting responsibilities were also discussed in the context of a military psychiatrist who believed his patient was best served by discharge from active duty, despite a commander's desire that he be treated acutely and returned to combat. Hines et al.[45] offer a detailed analysis of dual agency in a military setting as it relates to boundary crossings and violations.

Participants disagreed as to how clinicians should 'serve two masters'. Some felt psychiatrists should only work for individuals or the profession, 'and if institutions want to buy psychiatrists, they must buy them from the profession'. The approach applies the Hippocratic tradition to contemporary settings by relying solely on the profession to regulate its ethical standards in order to protect patients and its reputation. Several members doubted psychiatry 'can have a life separate from that of the social matrix in which it develops', while others felt resolution of ethical issues that arise from the interaction with third parties requires the profession to become more powerful in ways that 'mak[e] it more like a trade association' (e.g., a guild). The participants did reach general agreement on the importance of enunciating the difficult moral issue about conflicting obligations to practitioners 'who may arrogantly or innocently deny' them, devising mechanisms for transparency that educate patients about the rules and practices that prevail in specific institutional situations, and moving the profession towards responsibility for resolving some of the more difficult moral dilemmas. The selection 'The psychiatrist as double agent'[46] articulates these issues in the context of a case study about a medical student suffering from schizophrenia attempting to return to his studies following a leave of absence.

The growing triadic nature of the therapeutic relationship prompts Dyer's[1] question as to whether knowledge, technology, and expertise are commodities to be bartered in the marketplace or professional skills that should be employed to reach ethical ends. Angell[47] and Burnum[48] address the issue of balancing physicians' fidelity to individual patients against the goal of conserving resources in the name of social utility. Shortell et al.[49] pursue a similar task, but specifically in the context of formulating policy that reflects the 'new moral fabric' of a doctor-patient relationship in the era of population-based medicine.

In the selection 'The effect of third-party payment on the practice of psychotherapy', Chodoff[50] discusses the issue specifically in terms of its impact on individual psychotherapy. Acknowledging that most therapists concede a legitimate claim by insurance carriers for certain clinical information about the cases for which they are authorizing payment, he observes how the requirement can progressively undermine patients' trust in therapists not to disclose privileged information – a worry confirmed in later years when patients in the US left treatment after learning their records were subject to audits by managed care organizations.[51] Exploring such issues as confidentiality, the reporting of diagnostic and treatment information, and transference-countertransference interactions, he expresses concern about a growing confusion regarding professional identity as 'the therapist becomes less a priest and more a businessman and the organizations to which he belongs become involved increasingly with guild and political concerns'.

Chodoff's statement was prescient, foreshadowing a slippery slope that has resulted in a fundamental change in the therapist-patient interaction in recent years. Growing incursions into the traditional nature of the relationship has curtailed fully informed consent by imposing 'gag rules' on clinicians, and impeded delivery of appropriate care when 'gatekeepers', usually general practitioners, refuse to authorize mental health treatment.[52, 53] Confidentiality has been breached by managed care organizations that require patients to sign blanket disclosure forms making them (and their therapists) unaware as to who has access to their medical records.[54] These practices underscore the profession's drift towards an enhanced guild-like orientation that has infringed on basic bioethical principles governing the therapeutic relationship.

A final, and extreme, manifestation of dual agency relates to the role of psychiatry in a political context. As illustrated by the Nazi experience, compromise of fundamental bioethical principles that guide the doctor-patient relationship can culminate in horror. Proctor's[29] study of 'racial hygiene' describes the situation as it applied to medicine in general, promoting a philosophy that 'medicalized' anti-Semitism, and psychiatry specifically, resulting in widespread euthanasia of adults suffering from mental illness. Cocks[55] provides a detailed study of psychiatric care during the Third Reich, revealing how patient care and health policies were both corrupted by governmental pressure and influenced by clinicians' personal beliefs. As a result certain treatments that benefited the patient *and* the Reich were emphasized; for example, attention to psychogenic infertility and homosexuality was intended to alleviate personal distress and simultaneously help increase the valued gene pool of the Fatherland.

Conclusion

In 2000, the organizing theme of the American Psychiatric Association's Annual Meeting was the doctor-patient relationship, selected by then President Tasman because of its core importance to patient care and clinical research. He noted the growing understanding 'of this unique relationship to the process of treatment and recovery from illness', as well how it has been affected by recent trends in psychiatry.[56] Changes in the health care delivery system, evolving educational priorities for trainees, neuroscientific advances, and the impact of technology have had diverse effects on the profession, largely because of their impact on the interaction between patients and their caretakers. Tasman's remarks serve as a useful review of this section's intertwining themes: reconciling scientific pursuits and business-related issues within the profession in a manner that preserves ethical integrity of the fundamental unit of psychiatric care, the relationship between patients and therapists.

References

1　**Dyer, A.**: Psychiatry as a profession, in *Psychiatric ethics*, 3rd edn, ed. S. Bloch, P. Chodoff and S. Green. Oxford, Oxford University Press, 1999, pp. 67–79.

2　Oath of Hippocrates, in *Ancient Medicine: Selected Papers of Ludwig Edelstein*, eds. O. Temkin and C. Temkin. Baltimore, MO, Johns Hopkins University Press, 1967.

3　**Beauchamp, T.** and **Childress, J.**: *Principles of Biomedical Ethics*, 4th edn. Oxford, Oxford University Press, 1994, pp. 395–461.

4　**Bloch, S.** and **Pargiter, R.**: A history of psychiatric ethics. *Psychiatric Clinics of North America* **25**:509–524, 2002.

5　**Green, S.**: Salem witchcraft: a biopsychosocial analysis. *Pharos*, Summer 1982, pp 9–13.

6　**Tuke, S.** *Description of the Retreat, an institution near York for insane persons.* London, Process, 1813, 1964.

7　**Percival, T.**: *Codes of institutes and precepts adapted to the professional conduct of physicians and surgeons.* Birmingham, AL, Classics of Medicine Library, 1985.

8　*Principles of medical ethics with annotations especially applicable to psychiatry.* Washington, DC, American Psychiatric Association, 2001.

*9　**Freud, S.**: The dynamics of the transference, in *The standard edition of the complete psychological works of Sigmund Freud* (Vol. 12, pp. 98–107), ed. and trans. J. Strachey. London, Hogarth Press, 1958. (Original work published in 1912).

10　**Gartrell, N.**, **Herman, J.**, **Olarte, S.**, and **Feldstein, M.**: Psychiatrist-patient sexual contact: results of a national survey – I. prevalence. *American Journal Psychiatry* **143**:1126–1131, 1986.

11　**Gabbard, G.O.** and **Nadelson, C.**:Professional boundaries in the physician-patient relationship. *Journal of the American Medical Association* **273**: 1445–1449, 1995.

*12　**Epstein, R.S.** and **Simon, R.I.**: The exploitation index: an early warning indicator of boundary violations in psychotherapy. *Bulletin of the Menninger Clinic* **54**:450–465, 1990.

13　**Epstein, R.S.**, **Simon, R.I.** and **Kay, G.G.**: Assessing boundary violations in psychotherapy: survey results with the Exploitation Index. *Bulletin of the Menninger Clinic* **56**:150–166, 1992.

14　**Borys, D.** and **Pope, K.**: Dual relationships between therapist and client: a national study of psychologists, psychiatrists, and social workers. *Professional Psychology: Research and Practice* **20**:283–293, 1989.

15　**Simon, R.**: Sexual exploitation of patients: how it begins before it happens. *Psychiatric Annals* **19**:104–112, 1989.

16　**Freud, S.**: Further recommendations on the technique of psycho-analysis. Observations on transference-love, in *The standard edition of the complete* *psychological works of Sigmund Freud* (Vol. 12, pp. 157–173), ed. and trans. J. Strachey. London, Hogarth Press, 1958. (Original work published in 1915).

*17 **Gutheil T.H.** and **Gabbard, G.O.**: The concept of boundaries in clinical practice: theoretical and risk-management dimensions. *American Journal of Psychiatry* **150**:188–196, 1993.

18 **Gutheil, T.H.** and **Gabbard, G.O.**: Misuses and misunderstandings of boundary theory in clinical and regulatory settings. *American Journal of Psychiatry* **155**:409–414, 1998.

19 **Langs, R.**:*Psychotherapy: a basic text.* Northvale, NJ, Jason Aronson, 1990.

20 **Perry, J**: Physicians' erotic and nonerotic physical involvement with patients. *American Journal of Psychiatry* **133**:838–840, 1976.

*21 **Gabbard, G.O.**: Psychotherapists who transgress sexual boundaries with patients. *Bulletin of the Menninger Clinic* **58**:124–135, 1994.

22 **Swearingen, C.**: The impaired psychiatrist. *Psychiatric Clinics of North America* **13**:1–11, 1990.

23 **Herman, J., Gartrell, N., Olarte, S., Feldstein, M.,** and **Localio, R.**: Psychiatrist-patient sexual contact: results of a national survey, II: psychiatrists' attitudes. *American Journal Psychiatry* **144**:164–169, 1987.

24 *Principles of medical ethics with annotations especially applicable to psychiatry.* Washington, DC, American Psychiatric Association, 1989.

25 **Shopland, S.** and **VandeCreek, L.**: Sex with ex-clients: theoretical rationales for prohibition. *Ethics and Behavior* **1**:35–44, 1991.

26 **Appelbaum, P.** and **Jorgenson, L.**: Psychotherapist-patient sexual contact after termination of treatment: an analysis and a proposal. *American Journal of Psychiatry* **148**:1466–1473, 1991.

27 Assembly Takes Strong Stand on Patient-Doctor Sex. *Psychiatric News* 27 (23):1, 20.

28 *Code of Ethics.* Melbourne, Royal Australian and New Zealand College of Psychiatrists, 1988, No. 8.

29 **Proctor, R.**: *Racial hygiene.* Cambridge, MA, Harvard University Press, 1988.

30 **Fullinwider, R.**: Professional codes and moral understanding, in *Codes of ethics and the professions*, ed. M. Coady and S. Bloch. Victoria, Australia: Melbourne University Press, 1996.

31 **Katz, J.**:*The silent world of doctor and patient.* New York, The Free Press, 1984.

32 **Bloch, S.** and **Reddaway, P.**: *Psychiatric terror: the abuse of psychiatry in the Soviet Union.* New York, Basic Books, 1977.

33 **Chodoff, P.**: Misuse and abuse of psychiatry: an overview, in *Psychiatric ethics*, 3rd edn, ed. S. Bloch, P. Chodoff and S. Green. Oxford, Oxford University Press, 1999.

34 **Reich, W.**: Psychiatric diagnosis as an ethical problem, in *Psychiatric ethics*, 3rd edn, ed. S. Bloch, P. Chodoff and S. Green. Oxford, Oxford University Press, 1999.

35 **Goldberg, C.**: *Therapeutic partnership: ethical concerns in psychiatry.* New York, Springer, 1977.

36 **Lawson W.**: The art and science of the psychopharmacotherapy of African Americans. *Mount Sinai Journal of Medicine* **63**:301–305, 1996.

37 **Stone, A.**: Law, science, and psychiatric malpractice: a response to Klerman's indictment of psychoanalytic psychiatry. *American Journal Psychiatry* **147**:419–427, 1990.

38 **Klerman, G.**: The psychiatric patient's right to effective treatment: implications of *Osheroff v. Chestnut Lodge. American Journal of Psychiatry* **147**:409–418, 1990.

39 **Engle, G.**: The need for a new medical model: a challenge for biomedicine. *Science* **196**:129–136, 1977.

40 *Psychiatric Times*, 20(5): 1, May, 2003. The mental health care parity debate continues.

41 **Green, S.** and **Bloch, S.**: Working in a flawed mental health care system: an ethical challenge. *American Journal of Psychiatry* **158**:1378–1383, 2001.

42 **Appelbaum, P.**: The 'quiet' crisis in mental health services. *Health Affairs* **22**:110–116, 2003.

43 Appelbaum outlines strategy to fix system in crisis. *Psychiatric News* 7 November 2003, 23. American Psychiatric Association, Washington DC.

*44 In the service of the state: the psychiatrist as double agent. *Hastings Center Reports, Special Supplement*, April 1978, S1–23.

45 **Hines, A., Ader, D., Chang, A.** and **Rundell, J.**: Dual agency, dual relationships, boundary crossing, and associated boundary violations: a survey of military and civilian psychiatrists. *Military Medicine* **163**: 826–833, 1998.

*46 **Callahan, D.** and **Gaylin, W.**: The psychiatrist as double agent. *Hastings Center Report* **4**:12–14, 1974.

47 **Angell, M.**: The doctor as double agent. *Kennedy Institute of Ethics Journal* **3**:279–286, 1993.

48 **Burnum, J.**: The physician as double agent. *New England Journal of Medicine* **297**:278–279, 1977.

49 **Shortell, S., Waters, M., Clarke, K.** and **Budetti, P.**: Physicians as double agents: maintaining trust in an era of multiple accountabilities. *Journal of the American Medical Association* **280**:1102–1108, 1998.

*50 **Chodoff, P.**: The effect of third-party payment on the practice of psychotherapy. *American Journal of Psychiatry* **129**:540–545, 1972.

51 Questions of privacy roil arena of psychotherapy. *New York Times*, 22 May, 1996, A1.

52 **Wells, K., Hays, R., Burnam, M.,** et al: Detection of depressive disorder for patients receiving prepaid or fee-for-service care: results from the medical outcomes study. *Journal of the American Medical Association* **262**:3298–3302, 1989.

53 **Eisenberg, L**: Treating depression and anxiety in the primary care setting. *Health Affairs* **11**:149–156, 1992.

54 **Lazarus, J.** and **Sharfstein, S.**: Changes in the economics and ethics of health and mental health, in *Review of Psychiatry*, vol. 13, ed. J. Oldham and M. Riba. Washington, DC, American Psychiatric Press, 1994, pp. 389–413.

55 **Cocks, G.**: *Psychotherapy in the Third Reich: the Goring institute.* New York, Oxford University Press, 1985.

56 **Tasman, A.**: Presidential address: the doctor-patient relationship. *American Journal Psychiatry* **157**:1763–1768, 2000.

The Dynamics of the Transference*[1] (1912)

Sigmund Freud

The almost inexhaustible subject of 'transference' has recently been dealt with in this Journal by W. Stekel in a descriptive manner.[2] I wish to add a few remarks in order to make clear how it happens that the transference inevitably arises during the analysis and comes to play its well-known part in the treatment.

Let us bear clearly in mind that every human being has acquired, by the combined operation of inherent disposition and of external influences in childhood, a special individuality in the exercise of his capacity to love – that is, in the conditions which he sets up for loving, in the impulses he gratifies by it, and in the aims he sets out to achieve in it.[3] This forms a *cliché* or stereotype in him, so to speak (or even several), which perpetually repeats and reproduces itself as life goes on, in so far as external circumstances and the nature of the accessible love-objects permit, and is indeed itself to some extent modifiable by later impressions. Now our experience has shown that of these feelings which determine the capacity to love only a part has undergone full psychical development; this part is directed towards reality, and can be made use of by the conscious personality, of which it forms part. The other part of these libidinal impulses has been held up in development, withheld from the conscious personality and from reality, and may either expend itself only in phantasy, or may remain completely buried in the unconscious so that the conscious personality is unaware of its existence. Expectant libidinal impulses will inevitably be roused, in anyone whose need for love is not being satisfactorily gratified in reality, by each new person coming upon the scene, and it is more than probable that both parts of the libido, the conscious and the unconscious, will participate in this attitude.

It is therefore entirely normal and comprehensible that the libido-cathexes, expectant and in readiness as they are in those who have not adequate gratification, should be turned also towards the person of the physician.

As we should expect, this accumulation of libido will be attached to prototypes, bound up with one of the *clichés* already established in the mind of the person concerned, or, to put it in another way, the patient will weave the figure of the physician into one of the 'series' already constructed in his mind. If the physician should be specially connected in this way with the father-imago (as Jung has happily named[4] it) it is quite in accordance with his actual relationship to the patient; but the transference is not bound to this prototype; it can also proceed from the mother-or brother-imago and so on. The peculiarity of the transference to the physician lies in its excess, in both character and degree, over what is rational and justifiable – a pecularity which becomes comprehensible when we consider that in this situation the transference is effected not merely by the conscious ideas and expectations of the patient, but also by those that are under suppression, or unconscious.

Nothing more would need to be said or would perplex us concerning this characteristic of the transference, if it were not that two points which are of particular interest to psycho-analysts still remain unexplained by it. First, it is not clear why neurotic subjects under analysis develop the transference so much more intensely than those who are not being analysed; and secondly, it remains a mystery why in analysis the transference provides the *strongest resistance* to the cure, whereas in other forms of treatment we recognize it as the vehicle of the healing process, the necessary condition for success. Experience shows, and a test will always confirm it, that when the patient's free associations fail[5] the obstacle can be removed every time by an assurance that he is now possessed by a thought which concerns the person of the physician or something relating to him. No sooner is this explanation given than the obstacle is removed, or at least the absence of thoughts has been transformed into a refusal to speak.

It appears at the first glance to be an enormous disadvantage in psycho-analysis as compared with other methods that in it the transference, elsewhere such a powerful instrument for success, should become here the most formidable ally of the resistance. On closer consideration, however, the first of these difficulties at least will disappear. It is not the fact that the transference in psycho-analysis develops more intensely and immoderately than outside it. Institutions and homes for the treatment of nervous patients by methods other than analysis provide instances of transference in its most excessive and unworthy forms, extending even to complete subjection, which also show its erotic character unmistakably. A sensitive observer, Gabriele Reuters, depicted these facts at a time when psycho-analysis hardly existed, in a remarkable book[6] which altogether reveals great insight into the nature and causes of the neuroses. This peculiarity of the transference is not, therefore, to be placed to the account of psycho-analysis but is to be ascribed to the neurosis itself. The second problem still remains unexplained.

* Freud, S.: The dynamics of the transference, in *The standard edition of the complete psychological works of Sigmund Freud* (Vol. 12, pp. 98–107), ed. and trans. J. Strachey. London, Hogarth Press, 1958. (Original work published in 1912).

1 First published in the *Zentralblatt*, Bd. II., 1912; reprinted in *Sammlung*, Vierte Folge. [Translated by Joan Riviere.]

2 *Zentralblatt*, Bd. II., Nr. II. S. 26.

3 We will here provide against misconceptions and reproaches to the effect that we have denied the importance of the inborn (constitutional) factor because we have emphasized the importance of infantile impressions. Such an accusation arises out of the narrowness with which mankind looks for causes, inasmuch as one single causal factor satisfies him, in spite of the many commonly underlying the face of reality. Psycho-Analysis has said much about the 'accidental' component in ætiology and little about the constitutional, but only because it could throw new light upon the former, whereas of the latter it knows no more so far than is already known. We deprecate the assumption of an essential opposition between the two series of ætiological factors; we presume rather a perpetual interchange of both in producing the results observed. δαίμων καὶ τύχη determine the fate of man; seldom, perhaps never, one of these powers alone. The relative ætiological effectiveness of each is only to be measured individually and in single instances. In a series comprising varying degrees of both factors extreme cases will certainly also be found. According to the knowledge we possess we shall estimate the parts played by the forces of heredity and of environment differently in each case, and retain the right to modify our opinion in consequence of new knowledge. Further, we may venture to regard the constitution itself as a residue from the effects of accidental influences upon the endless procession of our forefathers.

4 *Symbole and Wandlungen der Libido.*

5 I mean here, when really nothing comes to his mind, and not when he keeps silence on account of some slight disagreeable feeling.

6 *Aus guter Familie*, 1895.

This problem must now be tackled at close quarters: Why does the transference in analysis confront us as resistance? Let us call to mind the psychological situation in the treatment. One of the invariable and indispensable preliminary conditions in *every* case of psychoneurosis is the process which Jung has aptly named *introversion* of the libido.[7] This means that the quantity got libido which is capable of becoming conscious, and is directed towards reality, has become diminished, while the part which is unconscious and turned away from reality (and, although it may still nourish phantasies in the person concerned, belongs to the unconscious) is by so much increased. The libido (entirely or in part) has found its way back into regression and has re-animated the infantile imagos[8]; and thither we pursue it in the analytic treatment, aiming always at unearthing it, making it accessible to consciousness and at last serviceable to reality. Wherever in our analytic delving we come upon one of the hiding-places of the withdrawn libido, there ensues a battle; all the forces which have brought about the regression of the libido will rise up as 'resistances' against our efforts in order to maintain the new condition. For if the introversion or regression of the libido had not been justified by some relation to the outer world (in the broadest terms, by a frustration of some desired gratification) and at the time been even expedient, it would never have taken place at all. Yet the resistances which have this origin are not the only ones, nor even the most powerful. The libido at the disposal of the personality had always been exposed to the attraction of unconscious complexes (strictly speaking, of that part of those complexes which belongs to the unconscious), and underwent regression because the attraction of reality had weakened. In order to free it, this attraction of the unconscious must now be overcome; that is, the repression of the unconscious impulses and their derivatives, which has subsequently developed in the mind of the person concerned, must be lifted. Here arises by far the greater part of the resistances, which so often succeed in upholding the illness, even though the original grounds for the recoil from reality have now disappeared. From both these sources come the resistances with which the analysis has to struggle. Every step of the treatment is accompanied by resistance; every single thought, every mental act of the patient's must pay toll to the resistance, and represents a compromise between the forces urging towards the cure and those gathered to oppose it.

Now as we follow a pathogenic complex from its representative in consciousness (whether this be a conspicuous symptom or something apparently quite harmless) back to its root in the unconscious, we soon come to a place where the resistance makes itself felt so strongly that it affects the next association, which has to appear as a compromise between the demands of this resistance and those of the work of exploration. Experience shows that this is where the transference enters on the scene. When there is anything in the complex-material (the content of the complex) which can at all suitably be transferred on to the person of the physician such a transference will be effected, and from it will arise the next association; it will then manifest itself by the signs of resistance – for instance, a cessation in the flow of associations. We conclude from such experiences that this transferred idea is able to force itself through to consciousness in preference to all other possible associations, just *because* it also satisfies resistance. This type of incident is repeated innumerable times during an analysis. Over and over again, when one draws near to a pathogenic complex, that part of it which is first thrust forward into

consciousness, will be some aspect of it which can be transferred; having been so, it will then be defended with the utmost obstinacy by the patient.[9]

Once this point is won, the elements of that complex which are still unresolved cause little further difficulty. The longer the analysis lasts, and the more clearly the patient has recognized that distortions of the pathogenic material in themselves offer no protection against disclosure, the more consistently he makes use of that variety of distortion which obviously brings him the greatest advantage, the distortion by transference. These incidents all converge towards a situation in which eventually all the conflicts must be fought out on the field of transference.

Transference in analysis thus always seems at first to be only the strongest weapon of the resistance, and we are entitled to draw the inference that the intensity and duration of the transference are an effect and expression of the resistance. The mechanism of transference is indeed explained by the state of readiness in which the libido that has remained accumulated about the infantile images exists, but the part played by it in the process of cure is only intelligible in the light of its relation, to the resistance.

How does it come about that the transference is so pre-eminently suitable as a weapon of resistance? One might think that this could easily be answered. It is surely clear enough that it must become peculiarly difficult to own up to any particular reprehended wish when the confession must be made to the very person with whom that feeling is most concerned. To proceed at all in such situations as this necessity produces would appear hardly possible in real life. This impossibility is precisely what the patient is aiming at when he merges the physician with the object of his emotions. Yet on closer consideration we see that this apparent gain cannot supply the answer to the riddle, for, on the contrary, an attitude of affectionate and devoted attachment can surmount any difficulty in confession; in analogous situations in real life we say; 'I don't feel ashamed with you; I can tell you everything'. The transference to the physician might quite as well relieve the difficulties of confession, and we still do not understand why it aggravates them.

The answer to this reiterated problem will not be found by pondering it any further, but must be sought in the experience gained by examination of individual instances of transference-resistance occurring in the course of an analysis. From these one perceives eventually that the use of the transference for resistance cannot be understood so long as one thinks simply of 'transference'. One is forced to distinguish 'positive' transference from 'negative' transference, the transference of affectionate feeling from that of hostile feeling, and to deal separately with the two varieties of the transference to the physician. Positive transference can then be divided further into such friendly or affectionate feelings as are capable of becoming conscious and the extensions of these in the unconscious. Of these last, analysis shows that they invariably rest ultimately on an erotic basis; so that we have to conclude that all the feelings of sympathy, friendship, trust and so forth which we expend in life are genetically connected with sexuality and have developed out of purely sexual desires by an enfeebling of their sexual aim, however pure and non-sensual they may appear in the forms they take on to our conscious self-perception. To begin with we knew none but sexual objects; psycho-analysis shows us that those persons whom in real life we merely respect or are fond of may be sexual objects to us in our unconscious minds still.

So the answer to the riddle is this, that the transference to the physician is only suited for resistance in so far as it consists in *negative* feeling or in the repressed *erotic* elements of positive feeling. As we 'raise' the transference by making it conscious we detach only these two components of the emotional relationship from the person of the physician; the conscious and unobjectionable component of it remains, and brings about the successful

---

7 Although many of Jung's utterances give the impression that he sees introversion as something characteristic of dementia præcox and not observable to the same extent in the other neuroses.

8 It would be easy to say: the libido has re-invested the infantile 'complexes'. But this would be erroneous; it would be correct only if expressed thus: 'the unconscious part of these complexes'. The exceptional intricacy of the theme dealt with in this essay tempts one to discuss further a number of adjunct problems, which require elucidation before one can speak definitely enough about the psychical processes here described. Such problems are: The definition of the boundary between introversion and regression; the incorporation of the complex-doctrine into the libido-theory; the relationship of phantasy-creation to the conscious, the unconscious, and to reality; etc. I need not apologize for having resisted these temptations here.

9 From which, however, one need not infer in general any very particular pathogenic importance in the point selected for resistance by transference. In warfare, when a bitter fight is raging over the possession of some little chapel or a single farmhouse, we do not necessarily assume that the church is a national monument, or that the barns contain the military funds. Their value may be merely tactical; in the next onslaught they will very likely be of no importance.

result in psycho-analysis as in all other remedial methods. In so far we readily admit that the results of psycho-analysis rest upon a basis of suggestion; only by suggestion we must be understood to mean that which we, with Ferenczi,[10] find that it consists of – influence on a person through and by means of the transference-manifestations of which he is capable. The eventual independence of the patient is our ultimate object when we use suggestion to bring him to carry out a mental operation that will necessarily result in a lasting improvement in his mental condition.

The next question is, Why do these manifestations of transference-resistance appear only in psychoanalysis and not in other forms of treatment, in institutions, for example? The answer is that they do appear there also, but they need to be recognized for what they are. The outbreak of negative transference is a very common occurrence in institutions; as soon as he is seized by it the patient leaves, uncured or worse. The erotic transference has not such an inhibitory effect in institutions, since there, as otherwise in life, it is decorously glossed over, instead of being exposed; nevertheless, it betrays itself unequivocally as resistance to the cure, not, indeed, by driving the patient out of the place – on the contrary, it binds him to the spot – but just as certainly by keeping him away from real life. Actually it is quite unimportant for his cure whether or not the patient can overcome this or that anxiety or inhibition in the institution; what is of importance, on the contrary, is whether or not he will be free from them in real life.

The negative transference requires a more thorough elucidation than is possible within the limits of this paper. It is found in the curable forms of the psychoneuroses alongside the affectionate transference, often both directed on to the same person at the same time, a condition for which Bleuler has coined the useful term ambivalence.[11] This ambivalence of the feelings appears to be normal up to a point, but a high degree of it is certainly a special peculiarity of neurotics. In the obsessional neurosis an early 'splitting of the pairs of opposites' seems to characterize the instinctual life and to form one of the constitutional conditions of this disease. The ability of neurotics to make the transference a form of resistance is most easily

accounted for by ambivalence in the flow of feelings. Where the capacity to transfer feeling has come to be of an essentially negative order, as with paranoids, the possibility of influence or cure ceases.

After all this investigation we have so far considered one aspect only of transference-phenomena; some attention must be given to another side of this question. Those who have formed a true impression of the effect of an extreme transference-resistance on the patient, of the way in which as soon as he comes under its influence he is hurled out of all reality in his relation to the physician – how he then arrogates to himself freedom to ignore the psycho-analytic rule (to communicate without reserve whatever goes through his mind), how all the resolutions with which he entered upon the analysis then become obliterated, and how the logical connections and conclusions which just before had impressed him deeply then become matters of indifference to him – will need some further explanation than that supplied by the factors mentioned above to account for this effect, and these other factors are, indeed, not far to seek; they lie again in the psychological situation in which the analysis has placed the patient.

In following up the libido that is withdrawn from consciousness we penetrate into the region of the unconscious, and this provokes reactions which bring with them to light many of the characteristics of unconscious processes as we have learnt to know them from the study of dreams. The unconscious feelings strive to avoid the recognition which the cure demands; they seek instead for reproduction, with all the power of hallucination and the inappreciation of time characteristic of the unconscious. The patient ascribes, just as in dreams, currency and reality to what results from the awakening of his unconscious feelings; he seeks to discharge his emotions, regardless of the reality of the situation. The physician requires of him that he shall fit these emotions into their place in the treatment and in his life-history, subject them to rational consideration, and appraise them at their true psychical value. This struggle between physician and patient, between intellect and the forces of instinct, between recognition and the striving for discharge, is fought out almost entirely over the transference-manifestations. This is the ground on which the victory must be won, the final expression of which is lasting recovery from the neurosis. It is undeniable that the subjugation of the transference-manifestations provides the greatest difficulties for the psycho-analyst; but it must not be forgotten that they, and they only, render the invaluable service of making the patient's buried and forgotten love-emotions actual and manifest; for in the last resort no one can be slain *in absentia* or *in effigie*.

---

10 Ferenczi, *Introjection and Transference.*
11 E. Bleuler, *Dementia Praecox oder Gruppe der Schizophrenien*, in Aschaffenburg's *Handbuch der Psychiatrie*, 1911; also a Lecture on Ambivalence in Berne, 1910, abstracted in *Zentralblatt für Psychoanalyse*, Bd. I., S. 266. W. Stekel had previously suggested the term *bipolarity* for the same phenomenon.

The Exploitation Index

An early warning indicator of boundary violations in psychotherophy*

Richard S. Epstein and Robert I. Simon

Exploitive behavior by therapists is highly disruptive in psychotherapy because it violates the sense of trust derived from a coherent treatment boundary. Such behavior may be difficult to detect because it is often associated with self-deception. The compensatory need to feel 'special,' a state of mind often associated with exploitiveness, suggests that narcissistic mechanisms play a significant role. The authors present an 'Exploitation Index' (EI), a self-assessment questionnaire for therapists that is designed to serve as an early warning indicator of boundary violations.

(Bulletin of the Menninger Clinic, 54, 450–465)

In the course of conducting treatment, conscientious psychotherapists must continually struggle with the task of maintaining the treatment boundary, and must withstand any temptation to use patients for their own advantage. Although the great majority of clinicians earnestly seek to avoid exploiting patients or being exploited by them, not all succeed, judging from studies suggesting a 7–12% incidence of sexual behavior between therapist and patient (Gartrell, Herman, Olarte, Feldstein, & Localio, 1986; Gutheil, 1989; Kardener, Fuller, & Mensh, 1973; Pope & Bouhoutsus, 1986; Simon, 1987, 1989). Most of these data were obtained by survey studies that probably underestimated the true incidence.

Gross violations of the treatment boundary, such as sexual activity with a patient, can be quite damaging both to patients and to therapists (Feldman-Summers & Jones, 1984; Pope, 1989; Stone, 1976) and may result in a syndrome similar to that seen in child abuse and rape victims (Summit, 1983). More recent data suggest that the incidence of sexual violations may be diminishing (Borys & Pope, 1989). Increased awareness on the part of patients, therapists, and professional licensing boards, and a spate of well-publicized malpractice awards, may explain this trend. It is possible, however, that exploitive therapists are less likely to admit to such behavior on survey studies, even with adequate protection of confidentiality, now that violations are more likely to result in severe penalties.

Unfortunately, other studies of ethical *attitudes* – as opposed to ethical *behaviors* – suggest that many practicing therapists may harbor a potential to exploit their patients if the 'circumstances are right.' For example, Conte, Plutchik, Picard, and Karasu (1989) found that a sizable fraction of respondents thought that marriage to one's patient after termination of therapy was within the realm of appropriate practice. Similarly, in Borys and Pope's (1989) study, 28% of the respondents thought that it was ethically acceptable to engage in sexual activity with a client after termination. A potentially disastrous 'shell game' can result when a therapist maintains such an attitude, because it is likely to be signaled to the patient before the formal ending of treatment. Gabbard and Pope (1989) presented an excellent review of the destructive potential inherent in the illusion that termination permits a relaxation of the treatment boundary.

Less extreme forms of exploitation, such as excessive familiarity, seductiveness, nonclinical business dealings, and breaches of confidentiality, are much more common than overt sexual activity. Borys and Pope (1989) demonstrated this fact in their national survey of psychiatrists, psychologists, and social workers. They found that those clinicians most likely to engage in nonsexual boundary violations with patients were male therapists (as compared with female therapists), practitioners living and working in the same small town (as compared with practitioners in suburban or urban setting), and nonpsychodynamically oriented therapists (as compared with those who are psychodynamically oriented). In a different sample, ethical attitudes alone revealed a similar pattern. The finding of a gender differential is consistent with earlier reports that women are less likely than men to exploit the therapeutic relationship by using erotic contact (Gartrell, Herman, Olarte, Feldstein, & Localio, 1986; Perry, 1976).

Because of its disruptive potential, the tendency to exploit or be exploited must be recognized, whether it originates with the therapists or with the patient. Regardless of the origin of this tendency, failure to detect such activity and to intervene in a timely fashion can result in a range of destructive phenomena within the treatment process, including therapeutic impasse, exacerbation of the underlying disorder, and escalating violation of the treatment boundary.

Thorough training, ongoing supervision, continuing education, consultation with peers, and personal psychotherapy are some of the time-honored methods by which therapists have addressed the issue of exploitive behavior during treatment. Menninger and Holzman (1973) prepared a list to help therapists detect the cognitive, affective, and behavioral manifestations of countertransferential impulses that reveal 'surreptitious satisfactions for infantile needs' (p. 92). The list includes repeatedly experiencing erotic or affectionate feelings towards a patient; permitting or encouraging acting out; trying to impress the patient; trying to impress colleagues about the patient's importance; deriving conscious satisfaction from the patient's praise, appreciation, or affection; experiencing recurrent impulses to ask favors of the patient; manifesting sadistic sharpness in formulating interpretations; and displaying laxness when the patient is late in paying the fee.

Langs (1973) outlined a series of behaviors by therapists that may emanate in part from a patient's unconscious effort to test the therapist's ability to avoid reenacting a misalliance similar to the patient's experience of childhood exploitation. These behaviors include accepting referrals from relatives or from current or former patients, making devious fee arrangements involving false reporting to insurance companies, failing to deal with delinquent payment, and giving gifts to or accepting them from a patient.

Averill *et al.* (1989) and Collins (1989) have stressed a preventive education program as a way of sensitizing and alerting inpatient treatment staff members to these issues. Their efforts were founded on an endeavor to establish clear guidelines and to dispel 'secrets' between staff members and patients. Averill *et al.* and Collins developed profiles of 'vulnerable' patients and staff members who are likely to be at greatest risk for erotic behavior. Male patients were dependent and extremely dysphoric. Female staff members who became sexually involved with patients did so in an effort to 'rescue' them from their despair by healing them with love. Typical female patients suffered from borderline personality disorder and manifested 'emptiness' and marked object hunger. Staff members likely to be involved with such patients fell into two groups: young individuals whose activity with patients appeared to be a continued manifestation of their general exploitive behavior pattern, and middle-aged men who were isolated,

* Epstein, R.S. and Simon, R.I.: The exploitation index: an early warning indicator of boundary violations in psychotherapy. *Bulletin of the Menninger Clinic* 54:450–465, 1990.

needed nurturing, and felt generally devalued or slighted by the hospital organization.

Simon (1989) found that the breach of the treatment boundary in cases of therapist-patient sexual activity usually occurred after a prodromal period involving lesser forms of exploitive behavior. He cautioned that patients and therapists should be alert to possible boundary violations if the therapist suggests tasks for the patient that primarily benefit the therapist, or if sessions or other activities are scheduled outside regular hours. Gutheil (1989) stressed the danger that minor irregularities in procedure may progress to more serious activity, such as sexual behavior with patients. He emphasized that a 'red flag' should be raised when the therapist is tempted to make any 'exceptions' to the usual treatment format.

Brodsky (1989) formulated similar observations about the typical therapist who became sexually involved with a patient. The typical therapist was likely to be a male individual who violated other boundaries, such as employing the patient in his office or seeking financial advice from the patient. Such a therapist often disclosed details of his current life problems to patients and treated them as if they were personal friends. A therapist's experience in terms of years of practice appeared to lead to overconfidence, a reluctance to seek help from colleagues, and a defensive belief in personal superiority and 'innovativeness.'

Gartrell, Herman, Olarte, Feldstein, and Localio (1986) noted that highly trained professionals were capable of gross denial regarding the consequences of therapist-patient sexual contact, which many of them rationalized as beneficial. Gartrell and her colleagues suggested that psychopathology in the therapist, particularly sociopathic traits, and adverse modeling based on previous sex with a supervisor during training could explain this denial. Their concern is justified by studies showing a high incidence (5–10%) of sexual contact between educators and students in mental health training programs (Gartrell, Herman, Olarte, Localio, & Feldstein, 1988; Pope, Levenson, & Schover, 1979). Another study found that 32% of female medical students were subjected to sexual advances by members of the clinical faculty (Sheehan, Sheehan, White, Leibowitz, & Baldwin, 1990).

Narcissistic pathology and exploitation

The way that exploitation is facilitated by and thrives on self-deception was lucidly described in Tolstoy's (1911/1971) fictional account of the abuse of power: 'Yet though convinced that he had acted rightly, some kind of unpleasant after-taste remained, and to stifle that feeling he dwelt on a thought that always tranquilized him – the thought of his own greatness' (p. 317). This soothing sense of 'specialness' may help to explain why well-meaning and well-trained therapists permit exploitive behavior to occur in the treatment setting. Although narcissistic conflicts are ubiquitous and do not necessarily indicate psychopathology, a discussion of narcissism in its most extreme forms may provide a better understanding of how exploitiveness operates in the psychotherapy setting.

In case histories of individuals with severe narcissistic pathology, Kohut (1971) and Kernberg (1975) found that the parents suffered an impaired ability to relate to their children in terms of the children's own dependency needs, yet at the same time the parents became overinvested in the pleasure they received from their children's 'special' performances, attractiveness, or talents. Based on this experience of being used as a part-object for their parents' gratification, these children came to see either themselves or others as objects to be used rather than as complete individuals – the essence of exploitation. Such a child's 'specialness' (whether based on good looks, fame, money, talent, or power) becomes a booby prize – a shallow compensation to cover inner feelings of low self-worth and hollowness.

According to Kernberg (1975), 'pathological narcissism,' or self-esteem that is defensively and artificially inflated, involves a 'libidinal investment in a pathological self structure' (p. 271). Kernberg contrasted this pathological manifestation with 'normal narcissism,' which is a healthy sense of self-regard 'related to real needs' (p. 273), combined with a capacity to be genuinely interested in others.

At the level of a pathological defense, 'specialness' is unlikely to be easily dislodged by exhortation or education. If one is 'special,' the need to follow the rules that govern ordinary mortals can be ignored more easily. 'Specialness' becomes a self-reinforcing, defensive method of feeling better, a way of screening out all external disappointment or injury. It can imbue a person with a sense of entitlement and can facilitate self-justification for using others as part-objects. Even when relatively subdued, such mechanisms operating in a therapist could easily facilitate exploitive behavior and impair insight into its occurrence. These tendencies are often augmented by similar traits in patients, particularly those with borderline personality disorder, who are likely to evoke a mutual mirroring of exploitive behavior in the course of transference reenactments (Gutheil, 1989).

Claman (1987), following Kohut's concepts, emphasized the 'mirror hunger' manifested in therapists who engage in sexual activity with their patients. He described several instances of a therapist with a 'predilection for feelings of dominance and paternalism (i.e., grandiosity) in relation to an idealizing patient with whom the therapist seems inexplicably to "fall in love" ' (p. 38). This 'romance' is often triggered by a narcissistic injury suffered by the therapist, such as marital dissatisfaction or separation. Claman also pointed out that the narcissistic aspect of romantic love, as it occurs naturally, consists of a *mutual* mirroring and idealization between the lovers. He postulated that when erotic love arises out of the misuse of the treatment situation, it is an 'unbalanced process' whereby a dominating, grandiose therapist commands all the mirroring from an awe-stricken, idealizing, and object-hungry patient.

Twemlow and Gabbard (1989) detailed how the 'lovesick,' usually male, therapist can fall in love with a grandiose and idealized image of himself, which is then projected onto the patient. This process involves a pathological narcissistic mechanism leading to an impaired sense of ego boundaries between therapist and patient, in which the therapist is saying, 'I like you to the extent that you are like I want you to be, and like I want to be myself. Provided we do not allow mundane external reality to intervene and spoil what we have . . . as long as we maintain this special and unique relationship' (Twemlow & Gabbard, 1989, p. 82). This position serves as a narcissistic defense against a realistic perception of social reality, and against the underlying aggressive nature of what the therapist is actually projecting. In a process similar to a perversion, the lovesick therapist projects an aspect of his injured self onto the patient, whom he tries to love in a romanticized way on one level while he devalues and destroys her on another, projecting onto her his *own* disavowed self-perception of having been used.

In most circumstances where exploitiveness surfaces in the treatment setting, a narcissistic mechanism is operating in the therapist or patient, although this narcissistic tendency does not necessarily exceed the threshold of clinically recognizable pathology. In some cases, other factors may also impair therapists' ability to detect their own exploitive behavior (e.g., loss of judgment due to manic excitement, antisocial personality traits, substance abuse, dementia, or frontal lobe disorder).

The Exploitation Index (EI)

Many of the recommendations of the previously cited authors should be restated, recirculated, and repeatedly discussed in an open forum among therapists as a reminder of the perils involved in the course of our work, and as a preventive safeguard. This need exists regardless of one's level of experience or training. In fact, extensive clinical experience may lead to over-confidence, rationalization, and carelessness in regard to boundary violations (Brodsky, 1989). Research data bolster this clinical observation. Conte *et al.* (1989), for example, found that therapists with more than 14 years of experience were slightly but significantly less likely, on average, than therapists with fewer than 14 years of experience to see socializing with a patient outside the treatment session as unethical.

Although our questionnaire is still in the process of quantitative validation, we hope that the 'Exploitation Index' (EI) will be of value to therapists who wish to assess their behavior and attitudes in their own practice. We have also found it useful in leading group discussions among professional colleagues, in supervising residents, and in teaching. By themselves, teaching aids and self-assessment checklists such as the EI are unlikely to be of much direct help for therapists possessed of the more malignant forms of denial described in the sexual exploitation literature (Pope, 1989; Twemlow & Gabbard, 1989). It will probably be of more assistance to the majority of individuals whose behavior and attitudes fall in the transitional or pro-dromal category – exploitive activity that may seriously interfere with the efficacy of treatment but that has not yet (and may never) become gross abuse. Some individuals in Twemlow and Gabbards (1989) 'lovesick' cate-gory may benefit by recognizing the early warning signs of presexual boundary violation.

In addition, the more malignant forms of behavior that arise among a small minority of professional psychotherapists should be considered in the context of the underlying attitudes and behavior of the great majority. Analogous to the behavior of Johnson and Szurek's (1952) adolescent patients, who cheerfully acted out their parent's unconscious but forbidden wishes, the floridly errant behavior on the part of a few therapists may be viewed as facilitated by laxness in the collective ethical attitudes of the profession at large. For example, might the pattern of abusive faculty role modeling in professional training be a relevant factor? The studies we have cited indicate that a relatively large percentage of therapists have difficulty maintaining boundaries in their therapeutic and teaching roles. Continued discussion and review of these issues may thus exert, an indirect but beneficial peer pressure on all mental health professionals, similar to Averill et al. 's (1989) experience with hospital personnel.

With these goals in mind, we present the EI (see Tables 1–7). For ease of presentation, it has been divided into sections. It is derived from actual examples of exploitive behavior found in published case reports in the literature (Gartrell, Herman, Olarte, Feldstein, & Localio, 1986; Gutheil, 1989; pope & Bouhoutsus, 1986; Simon 1987, 1989; Stone, 1976), forensic records from cases involving litigation against psychiatrists and other mental health professionals, and personal clinical observation. Each example was formulated into a question that clinicians can ask themselves, and that can be answered concretely based on frequency of occurrence.

The EI questions can be divided into various subcategories of exploitive-ness. As characterized from the therapists viewpoint, they include general-ized boundary violations (Table 1), eroticism (Table 2), exhibitionism (Table 3), dependency (Table 4), power seeking (Table 5), greed (Table 6), and enabling (Table 7). The specific instruction for completing each part of this self-assessment questionnaire is as follows:

Rate yourself according to the frequency that the following statements reflect your behavior, thoughts, or feelings with regard to any particular patients you have seen in psychotherapy within the past 2 years, by placing a check in the appropriate box.

Approximate frequency as follows: rarely = *about once a year or less;* some-times = *about once every 3 months;* often = *once a month or more.*

Generalized boundary violations (Table 1, questions 1–7)

Maintenance of the treatment boundary is the foundation of coherent ther-apy. Trespassing this boundary is tantamount to exploitation because it vio-lates a treatment contract based on both overt and implied agreement that the therapist's sole purpose is to treat the patient's disorder in return for monetary compensation. Changing this contract, whether by subterfuge or consent, amounts to a 'bait-and-switch' tactic. The only direct and specific material gratification appropriate to receive from the patient is straightfor-ward monetary compensation. The therapist may also obtain satisfaction from being involved in an interesting and helpful profession. This benefit, which probably reflects 'normal narcissism,' relates to socially adaptive pride in personal achievement. It is derived, however, from ones practice in general and should not be *imposed* on a specific patient in the same manner as monetary compensation.

Questions 1–7 include items such as therapist and patient addressing each other by first name, participating in social contact outside scheduled visits, accepting mediums of exchange other than money, accepting referrals from previous patients, accepting patients from one's social sphere, and treating one's family members of friends in the same manner as patients. These items address a general problem of adherence to the original task of the therapy.

Sidetracking a patient's initial request for treatment into another endeavor, however friendly and pleasant, is closely analogous to parents' invalidating their children's desires and using them instead for self-gratifi-cation. Similarly, routinely playing the role of therapist for family members and friends subverts personal relationships. In our experience, such misuse of professional skills is frequently associated with other boundary violations.

Although it might be appropriate in certain clinical situations to address a patient by first name (e.g., when treating a child or a regressed adolescent, or in a clinical setting where the use of first names is customary), permit-ting or encouraging a first-name basis between therapist and patient is a form of false advertising in which a professional relationship designed to offer treatment is misrepresented as a social friendship. Patients accus-tomed to catering to the needs of others will readily accept pseudointimacy to defend against the hurtful rage emanating from early suppression of their personal needs. Placating a patient in these circumstances may result from the therapist's desire to avoid arousing this hidden rage, even though such an awakening may be therapeutically required. Similarly, revealing personal information may be appropriate at times (e.g., with a disorganized

Table 1 Generalized boundary violations

	Never	Rarely (yearly)	Sometimes (quarterly)	Often (monthly)
1. Do you seek social contact with patients outside of clinically scheduled visits?				
2. Do you tell patients personal things about yourself in order to impress them?				
3. Do you and your patients address each other on a first-name basis?				
4. Do you accept a medium of exchange other than money for your services? (e.g., work on your office or home, trading of professional services)				
5. Have you accepted for treatment individuals known to be referred by a current or former patient?				
6. Have you accepted for treatment persons with whom you have had social involvement or whom you knew to be in your social or family sphere?				
7. Do you find yourself doing any of the following for your family members or social acquaintances: prescribing medication, making diagnoses, offering psychodynamic explanations for their behavior?				

patient requiring reality testing), but it can be harmful and exploitive when used to create an atmosphere of pseudointimacy.

Accepting referrals from present or former patients breaches the boundary of limiting compensation to money alone, and can facilitate the belief in *both* the referring and the referred patient that the therapist is amenable to subtle forms of bribery (Langs, 1973). We are aware that this subject is controversial, and that most therapists do not consider it a breach of boundaries to accept referrals from a former patient. However, the same reasons for not having sex with a patient who has terminated treatment (Gabbard & Pope, 1989) can be applied to a relaxation of the posttermination treatment boundary with regard to referral sources. Is patient referral less a breach because it seems so harmless, so commonplace, so in keeping with the custom of practitioners outside the field of mental health? How much do economic concerns cloud our assessment of the risks to the new patient? What happens if the referring patient needs to resume treatment?

Eroticism (Table 2, questions 8–14)

Freud (1915/1958) cautioned that transference love was a by-product of the therapeutic situation 'like the exposure of a patient's body,' and that the therapist 'must not derive any personal advantage from it' (p. 169). He advised that 'the treatment must be carried out in abstinence' (p. 165) so that the patient's underlying impulses might be available for understanding. Questions 8–14 see to elicit early warning signs indicating unresolved conflict in the therapist that might impair the ability to prevent erotic feelings from contaminating treatment.

Question 14 addresses the issue of whether it is exploitive for a therapist *ever* to have a personal relationship with a patient, even after the completion of treatment. For example, prolonged fantasizing of, or planning for, a sexual relationship with a patient should alert the therapist to a desire to convert the treatment into a situation where by, like Pygmalion, the therapist is consciously or unconsciously molding the patient into an ideal sexual partner. This hidden agenda would subvert any original intent to facilitate health and independence. Therapists must accept the stipulation that their fee or salary is the *only* specific material gratification they can ever receive from any patient.

Exhibitionism (Table 3, questions 15–17)

Unfortunately, the phenomenon of therapists' bragging about the accomplishments, notoriety, or special qualities of their patients is extremely common (see question 17), even among the most highly trained and experienced mental health professionals. Therapists often rationalize such exploitive discussion by saying that it takes place only among colleagues, is adequately disguised, or is already public knowledge. Disguise of the patient in these instances rarely meets adequate requirements for protecting confidentiality (Clifft, 1986) because that would defeat the exhibitionistic purpose behind the revelation. Such overvaluation or envy of patients may be accompanied by covert signals that keep therapists from helping patients with their exhibitionistic defenses.

Dependency (Table 4, questions 18–20)

Question 20 asks whether the therapist is being gratified by the patient's chronic lateness or silence, a situation in which manifestations of the patient's illness provide a tempting gift that could satisfy the therapist's infantile dependency wishes (i.e., getting something for nothing). Although helping the patient overcome such resistive behavior may not be immediately possible, resolution of the illness may be hampered if the therapist derives too much pleasure from the resistance. Openly acknowledging this potential with the patient may help the therapist elucidate the patient's unconscious desire for unconditional infantile love, which the therapist enjoys vicariously.

Table 2 Eroticism

	Never	Rarely (yearly)	Sometimes (quarterly)	Often (monthly)
8. Do you find yourself comparing the gratifying qualities you observe in a patient with the less gratifying qualities in your spouse or significant other? (e.g., thinking: 'Where have you been all my life?')				
9. Do you feel that your patient's problem would be immeasurably helped if only he/she had a positive romantic involvement with you?				
10. Do you feel a sense of excitement or longing when you think of a patient or anticipate her/his visit?				
11. Do you take pleasure in romantic daydreams about a patient?				
12. When a patient has been seductive with you, do you experience this as a gratifying sign of your own sex appeal?				
13. Do you touch your patients? (Exclude handshake)				
14. Have you engaged in a personal relationship with patients after treatment was terminated?				

Table 3 Exhibitionism

	Never	Rarely (yearly)	Sometimes (quarterly)	Often (monthly)
15. Do you feel that you can obtain personal gratification by helping to develop your patient's great potential for fame or unusual achievement?				
16. Do you take great pride in the fact that such an attractive, wealthy, powerful, or important patient is seeking your help?				
17. Do you disclose sensational aspects of your patient's life to others? (even when you are protecting the patient's identity)				

Power seeking (Table 5, questions 21–23)

Questions 21–23 address the therapist's need to feel a sense of mastery and control over the patient. All patients are potentially vulnerable to this need because of the nature of the transference, and because of the still-common expectation that doctors order patients around 'for their own good.' Certain patients, such as those with passive-dependent traits or those who have been abused, are particularly vulnerable. The willingness of patients to be controlled may tempt therapists to deny the significance of their own behavior. These patients may relinquish control to therapists because adaptation to habitual abuse has become a mechanism for bonding with parental figures (Summit, 1983). Many patients actively encourage and derive a perverse enjoyment from such exploitation, which may be a way to master severe feelings of helplessness associated with victimization.

Greediness (Table 6, questions 24–28)

Contractual fee arrangements are a formal part of the treatment boundary. Devious monetary arrangements will obviously contaminate the foundation of therapy. When a patient seeks help, the overt agreement is that the patient will pay a fee, which is the therapist's *only* compensation. In return, the patient expects the therapist's best recommendations. If the clinician refers the patient to Dr. A, with whom the referring clinician has a financial arrangement (or other quid pro quo), while knowing that another available professional, Dr. B, would be more effective for this particular problem, the referring clinician is exploiting the patient. The referring clinician who rationalizes that Dr. A is, after all, also highly competent is denying the betrayal of the patient, whose trust requires the *best* recommendation, not one that gives the doctor an additional benefit that violates the original treatment covenant (question 28).

Enabling (Table 7, questions 29–32)

As a way of validating their own self-worth, mental health professionals are vulnerable to the occupational hazard of becoming entwined in attempts to 'cure' their patients. The 'rescue fantasy' and the high social value placed on helping others can serve as a tenacious defense against recognizing this form of using patients. Ironically, the therapist almost always winds up being victimized in turn. Fear of experiencing the patient's spiteful rage and of losing the 'special' admiration of the 'rescued' patient forces the therapist into an intimidated and often helpless stance. Such a situation often evolves into a 'mutual exploitation society?' similar to Gutheil's (1989) 'magic bubble.'

Table 4 Dependency

	Never	Rarely (yearly)	Sometimes (quarterly)	Often (monthly)
18. Do you find yourself talking about your own personal problems with a patient and expecting her/him to be sympathetic to you?				
19. Do you find it painfully difficult to agree to a patient's desire to cut down on the frequency of therapy, or to work on termination?				
20. Do you find the chronic silence or tardiness of a patient a satisfying way of getting paid for doing nothing?				

Table 5 Power seeking

	Never	Rarely (yearly)	Sometimes (quarterly)	Often (monthly)
21. Are you gratified by a sense of power when you are able to control a patient's activity through advice, medication, or behavioral restraint? (e.g., hospitalization, seclusion)				
22. Do you ask your patient to do personal favors for you? (e.g., get you lunch, mail a letter)				
23. Do you find yourself trying to influence your patients to support political causes or positions in which you have a personal interest?				

Table 6 Greediness

	Never	Rarely (yearly)	Sometimes (quarterly)	Often (monthly)
24. Do you ever use information learned from patients, such as business tips or political information, for your own financial or career gain?				
25. Do you join in any activity with patients that may serve to deceive a third party? (e.g., insurance company)				
26. Do you undertake business deals with patients?				
27. Do you accept gifts or bequests from patients?				
28. Do you recommend treatment procedures or referrals that you do not believe to be necessarily in your patient's best interests, but that may instead be to your direct orindirect financial benefit?				

Table 7 Enabling

	Never	Rarely (yearly)	Sometimes (quarterly)	Often (monthly)
29. Do you fail to deal with the following patient behavior(s): paying the fee late, missing appointments on short notice and refusing to pay for the time (as agreed), seeking to extend the length of sessions?				
30. Do you make exceptions for your patients, such as providing special scheduling or reducing fees, because you find the patient attractive, appealing, or impressive?				
31. Do you make exceptions in the conduct of treatment because you feel sorry for your patient, or because you believe he/she is in such distress or so disturbed that you have no other choice?				
32. Do you make exceptions for your patient because you are afraid she/he will otherwise become extremely angry or self-destructive?				

The patient's victimization of the therapist also represents a violation of the treatment boundary. Common clinical manifestations of such behavior include failing to pay the fee, paying the fee late, attempting to interfere in the therapist's personal life, or threatening the therapist's safety. If the therapist allows such actions to continue, it raises the question of whether the therapist has some inner personal need that may be contrary to the needs of the patient.

Frequent activity that involves making exceptions for a patient (see question 30), combined with any romantic feelings for the patient, may be prodromal symptoms of 'falling in love.' Such episodes can serve as a warning that the therapist may have already become blind to the patient's short comings, to say nothing of the patient's psychopathology. For this reason, a healthy self-regard on the therapist's part is essential not only for protective purposes and for demonstrating a proper role model, but also for helping detect and deal with cases of patient exploitiveness. Some leeway for empathic flexibility should be allowed (Grunes, 1984), for example, giving an acutely suicidal patient a special appointment, but any exploitive issues should be discussed if this behavior becomes a regular pattern. Like Gutheil (1989), we believe that making exceptions for a patient should raise serious warnings of boundary violation, because treating the patient as 'special' is likely to recapitulate the etiological antecedents of narcissistic pathology.

Conclusion

The therapist's ability to deal with exploitive enticement, whether emanating from within or from without, is a fundamental component of the treatment process and a vital aspect of maintaining its integrity. The complexity and subtlety of conducting treatment can easily lead to therapeutic lapses in this regard. If detected and properly understood, minor errors are usually helpful in understanding the patient's problem, especially when the therapist is responding to transferentially derived cues (Langs, 1973). Even in instances where exploitation originates from the therapist alone, recognition and empathic acknowledgment of its occurrence to the patient may be appropriate and can facilitate substantial therapeutic benefit.

The Exploitation Index can be used as a learning instrument to promote open discussion and increased awareness among mental health practitioners of boundary issues in psychotherapy, and as an additional aid in detecting activity that can derail an otherwise effective therapeutic encounter. Quantitative validation of this questionnaire is currently in process.

References

Averill, S. C., Beale, D., Benfer, B., Collins,D. T., Kennedy, L., Myers, J., pope, D., Rosen, I., & Zoble, E. (1989). Preventing staff-patient sexual relationships. *Bulletin of the Manning Clinic*, **53**, 384–393.

Borys, D. S., & Pope, K. S. (1989). Dual relationships between therapist and client: A national study of psychologists, psychiatrists, and social workers. *Professional Psychology; Research and Practice*, 20, 283–293. Brodsky, A. F. (1989). Sex between patient and therapist: Psychology's data and response. In G. O. Gabbard (Ed.), *Sexual exploitation in professional relationships* (pp. 15–25). Washington, DC: American Psychiatric Press.

Claman, J. M. (1987). Mirror hunger in the psychodynamics of sexually abusing therapists. *American Journal of Psychoanalysis*, **47**, 35–40.

Clifft, M. A. (1986). Writing about psychiatric patients: Guidelines for disguising case material. *Bulletin of the Menninger Clinic*, **50**, 511–524.

Collins, D. T. (1989). Sexual involvement between psychiatric hospital staff and their patients. In G. O. Gabbard (Ed.), *Sexual exploitation in professional relationships* (pp. 151–162). Washington, DC: American Psychiatric Press.

Conte, H. R., Plutchik, R., Picard, S., & Karasu, T. B. (1989). Ethics in the practice of psychotherapy: A survey. *American Journal of Psychotherapy*, **43**, 32–42.

Feldman-Summers, S., & Jones, G. (1984). Psychological impacts of sexual contact between therapists or other health care practitioners and their clients. *Journal of Consulting and Clinical Psychology*, **52**, 1054–1061.

Freud, S. (1958). Observations on transference-love (Further recommendations on the technique of psycho-analysis III). In J. starchey (Ed. and Trans.), *The standard edition of the complete psychological works of Sigmund Freud* (Vol. 12, pp. 157–173). London; Hogarth Press. (Original work published 1915).

Gabbard, G. O., & Pope, K. S. (1989). Sexual intimacies after termination: Clinical, ethical, and legal aspects. In G. O. Gabbard (Ed.), *Sexual exploitation in professional relationships*, (pp. 115–127). Washington, DC: American Psychiatric Press.

Gartrell, N., Herman, J., Olarte, S., Feldstein. M., & Localio, R. (1986). Psychiatrist-patient sexual contact: Results of a national survey: I. Prevalence. *American Journal of Psychiatry*, **143**, 1126–1131.

Gartrell, N., Herman, J., Olarte, S., Localio, R., & Fcldstein, M. (1988). Psychiatric residents' sexual contact with educators and patients: Results of a national survey. *American Journal of Psychiatry*, **145**, 690–694.

Gruels, M. (1984). The therapeutic object relationship. *Psychoanalytic Review*, **71**, 123–143.

Gutheil, T. G. (1989). Borderline personality disorder, boundary violations, and parient-therapist sex: Medicolegal pitfalls. *American Journal of Psychiatry*, **146**, 597–602.

Johnson, A. M., & Szurek, S. A. (1952). The genesis of antisocial acting out in children and adults. *Psychoanalytic Quarterly*, **21**,323–343.

Kardener, S. H., Fuller, M., & Mensh, I. N. (1973). A survey of physicians' attitudes and practices regarding erotic and nonerotic contact with patients. *American Journal of Psychiatry*, **130**, 1077–1081.

Kernberg, O. F. (1975). *Borderline conditions and pathological narcissism*. New York: Aronson.

Kohut, H. (1971). *Analysis of the self: A systematic approach to the treatment of narcissistic personality disorders*. NewYork: International Universities Press.

Langs. R. (1973) *The technique of psychoanalytic psychotherapy* (Vol. 1). New York: Aronson.

Menninger, K., & Holzman, P. (1973). *Theory of psychoanalytic technique* (2nd ed.). New York: Basic Books.

Perry, J. A. (1976). Physicians' erotic and nonerotic physical involvement with patients. *American Journal of Psychiatry*, **133**, 838–840.

Pope, K. S. (1989). Therapist-patient sex syndrome: A guide for attorneys and subsequent therapists to assessing damage. In G. O. Gabbard (Ed.), *Sexual exploitation in professional relationships.* (pp. 39–55). Washington, DC: American Psychiatric Press.

Pope, K. S., & Bouhoutsus, J. L. (1986). *Sexual intimacy between therapists and patients.* New York: Praeger.

Pope, K. S., Levenson, H., & Schoyer, L. R. (1979). Sexual intimacy in psychology training: Results and implications of a national survey. *American Psychologist*, **34**, 682–689.

Sheehan, K. H., Sheehan, D. V., White, K., Leibowitz, A., & Baldwin, D. C., Jr. (1990). A pilot study of medical student 'abuse': Student perceptions of mistreatment and misconduct in medical school. *Journal of the American Medical Association*, **263**, 533–537.

Simon, R. I. (1987). *Clinical psychiatry and the law.* Washington, DC: American Psychiatric Press.

Simon, R. I. (1989). Sexual exploitation of patients: How it begins before it happens. *Psychiatric Annals*, **19**, 104–112.

Stone, M. H. (1976). Boundary violations between therapist and patient, *Psychiatric Annals*, **6**, 670–677.

Summit, R. C. (1983). The child sexual abuse accommodation syndrome. *Child Abuse and Neglect.* **7**, 177–193.

Tolstoy, L. (1971). *Hadji Muraád.* In L. Maude & A. Maude (Trans.), *The death of Ivaán Ilých and other stories* (pp. 227–384). London: Oxford University Press. (Original work published 1911)

Twemlow, S. W., & Gabbard, G. O. (1989). The lovesick therapist. In G. O. Gabbard (Ed.), *Sexual exploitation in professional relationships* (pp. 71–87). Washington, DC: American Psychiatric Press.

The Concept of Boundaries in Clinical Practice:

Theoretical and Risk-Management Dimensions*

Thomas G. Gutheil and Glen O. Gabbard

Role boundaries may be crisp or flexible or fuzzy, depending on the role under consideration and on the cultural climate.

-Ingram[1]

The concept of boundaries, particularly in the sense of boundary crossings and boundary violations, has come under increased scrutiny in relation to the wave of sexual misconduct cases[2] arising in litigation, ethics committee hearings, and complaints to boards of licensure. Like many concepts in psychotherapy, such as 'therapy,' 'transference,' and 'alliance,' the term proves slippery on closer observation. The literature tends to focus on patient-therapist sexual misconduct[3] as an extreme violation and not on the wide variety of lesser and more complex boundary crossings, many of which are, at first glance, less obvious but pose difficulties of their own for clinicians.

Clinicians tend to feel that they understand the concept of boundaries instinctively, but using it in practice or explaining it to others is often challenging. This latter problem is rendered more difficult by the tendency of the legal system, particularly plaintiffs' attorneys, to apply it mechanically: any boundary crossing is bad, wrong, and harmful. Empirical evidence suggests that boundary violations frequently accompany or precede sexual misconduct[2,4,5], but the violations themselves do not always constitute malpractice or misconduct or even bad technique. However, modern clinicians should be aware of three principles that govern the relationship among boundaries, boundary crossing, boundary violations, and sexual misconduct.

First, *sexual misconduct usually begins with relatively minor boundary violations*, which often show a crescendo pattern of increasing intrusion into the patient's space that culminates in sexual contact. A direct shift from talking to intercourse is quite rare; the 'slippery slope' is the characteristic scenario. As Gabbard[4] and Simon[6] have pointed out, a common sequence involves a transition from last-name to first-name basis; then personal conversation intruding on the clinical work; then some body contact (e.g., pats on the shoulder, massages, progressing to hugs); then trips outside the office; then sessions during lunch, sometimes with alcoholic beverages; then dinner; then movies or other social events; and finally sexual intercourse.

Second *not all boundary crossings or even boundary violations lead to or represent evidence of sexual misconduct*. A clear boundary violation from one ideological perspective may be standard professional practice from another. For example, the so-called 'Christian psychiatry movement' might condone the therapist's attendance at a church service with one or more patients, and various group therapeutic approaches or therapeutic communities may involve inherent boundary violations, as when some behaviorist schools permit hiring patients in therapy to do work in the treatment setting. Bad training, sloppy practice, lapses of judgment, idiosyncratic treatment philosophies, regional variations, and social and cultural conditioning may all be reflected in behavior that violates boundaries but that may not necessarily lead to sexual misconduct, be harmful, or deviate from the relevant standard of care.

Third, despite this complexity, *fact finders* – civil or criminal juries, judges, ethics committees of professional organizations, or state licensing boards – *often believe that the presence of boundary violations (or even crossings) is presumptive evidence of, or corroborates allegations of, sexual misconduct.*

To summarize the foregoing more concisely, albeit metaphorically, smoke usually leads to fire; one can, however, find smoke where there is no fire, and yet fact finders may assume that where there's smoke, there's fire. This metaphor is not trivial. In a notorious Massachusetts case (in which the doctor accused of sexual misconduct was eventually exonerated), the Board of Registration in Medicine, the state licensing authority, noted in the course of the process, 'There was an undisputed level of intimacy between the two [patient and doctor] that supports the inference of sexual relations' (transcript of board proceedings, citation withheld). In its language here, the board clearly articulated its 'inference' of fire from the 'undisputed' presence of smoke. Moreover, recent court decisions suggest a trend toward findings of liability for boundary violations even in the absence of sexual contact.[7] On this basis, the risk-management value of avoiding even the appearance of boundary violations should be self-evident.

This communication has three goals: 1) to review the subject in order to define, describe, and illustrate the range of boundary issues, 2) to demonstrate that crossing certain boundaries may at times be salutary, at times neutral, and at times harmful, and 3) to suggest preventive and reparative measures for clinicians dealing with boundary violations in themselves and their patients.

Definitions

What is a boundary? Is it too amorphous, protean, and abstract to define at all? Should we take refuge by saying, as St. Augustine was supposed to have said about time, 'Time? I know what time is, provided you do not ask me'?

Part of the difficulty encountered in defining appropriate boundaries can be related to the historical tradition that modern therapists have inherited. The great figures in the field gave out mixed messages on the issue. Freud, for example, used metaphors involving the opacity of a mirror and the dispassionate objectivity of a surgeon to describe the analyst's role, but his own behavior in the analytic setting did not necessarily reflect the abstinence and anonymity that he advocated in his writings. He sent patients postcards, lent them books, gave them gifts, corrected them when they spoke in a misinformed manner about his family members, provided them with extensive financial support in some cases, and on at least one occasion gave a patient a meal[8]. Moreover, the line between professional and personal relationships in Freud's analytic practice was difficult to pinpoint. During vacations he would analyze Ferenczi while walking through the countryside. In one of his letters to Ferenczi, which were often addressed 'Dear Son,' he indicated that during his holiday he planned to analyze him in two sessions a day but also invited him to share at least one meal with him each day (unpublished manuscript by A. Hoffer). For Freud the analytic relationship could be circumscribed by the time boundaries of the analytic

* Gutheil T.H. and Gabbard, G.O.: The concept of boundaries in clinical practice: theoretical and risk-management dimensions. *American Journal of Psychiatry* 150:188–196, 1993.

sessions, and other relationships were possible outside the analytic hours. The most striking illustration of this conception of boundaries is Freud's analysis of his own daughter, Anna.

Freud was not alone in establishing ambiguous analytic boundaries. When Melanie Klein was analyzing Clifford Scott, she encouraged him to follow her to the Black Forest for her holiday. Each day during this vacation, Scott underwent analysis for a 2-hour session while reclining on Klein's bed in her hotel room[9]. D.W. Winnicott, another therapist of considerable stature, occasionally took young patients into his home as part of his treatment of them[10]. In Margaret Little's report of her analysis with Winnicott[11], she recalled how Winnicott held her hands clasped between his through many hours as she lay on the couch in a near-psychotic state. On one occasion he told her about another patient of his who had committed suicide and went into considerable detail about his countertransference reactions to the patient. He also ended each session with coffee and biscuits. These boundary transgressions by highly revered figures have occasionally been cited in ethics hearings as justification for unethical behavior. We wish to stress that these behaviors are no longer acceptable practice regardless of their place in the history of our field.

The problem of the contradiction between what the master therapists wrote and how they actually behaved in the clinical setting was compounded because psychoanalysis and psychotherapy are treatments that occur in a highly private context. The boundaries of the therapeutic relationship and the characteristics of acceptable technique were thus highly subjective and lacked standardization. This lack of clarity was partially addressed by Eissler's classic 1953 paper[12] in which he suggested that in the ideal situation, the analyst's activity should be confined to interpretation. Any deviation from that model technique was defined by Eissler as a parameter. As examples of parameters, he cited Freud's setting a termination date for the Wolf Man and proposed a hypothetical situation in which an analyst might command a phobic patient to expose himself to the feared situation. By this standard of technique, Freud's own behavior, such as offering a meal to the Rat Man, has been regarded as indicative of an earlier technique that Freud subsequently abandoned[13] or a human failing rather than a technical recommendation[14].

Lipton[8] took a strikingly different view of Freud's apparently unorthodox behavior with the Rat Man. He insisted that Freud's providing a meal for the patient should not be considered part of his psychoanalytic technique. Instead, it should be regarded as part of the nontechnical personal relationship that Freud had with this patient. He pointed out that in every analysis, the analyst is called upon to offer assistance in a personal way from time to time. While the ramifications and fantasies produced by such behavior should be thoroughly analyzed, it would be erroneous, in Lipton's view, to expand the concept of technique to include all aspects of the analyst's relationship with the patient. Lipton expressed the following concern: 'Modern technique tends to move from the position from which the analyst's technique is judged according to his purpose to one from which the analyst's technique is judged according to his behavior'[8], p. 262. He pointed out that following Eissler's model of analytic technique in its literal terms would cause any noninterpretive comment or action on the part of the analyst to be construed as a parameter.

Another major problem with any attempt to derive definitions of boundaries from psychoanalytic concepts of technique is that technique changes with treatments that are less expressive than analysis. As one moves along the expressive-supportive continuum of psychotherapy[15], one relies less on interpretation and more on alternative interventions such as clarification, confrontation, advice and praise, suggestion, and affirmation. Similarly, partial gratification of transference wishes is associated with supportive psychotherapy, whereas it is generally eschewed in psychoanalysis or highly expressive psychotherapy. Hence, there may be a built-in confusion between the notion of therapeutic boundaries and adjusting the technique to the ego organization of the patient.

Another approach to defining therapeutic boundaries is to conceptualize a therapeutic framp,[16,17] i.e., an envelope or membrane around the therapeutic role that defines the characteristics of the therapeutic relationship.

The analyst or therapist constructs the elements or the frame partly consciously and partly unconsciously. These elements include the regular scheduling of appointments, the duration of the appointments, arrangements for payment of the fee, and the office setting itself.

Does the patient's role have a boundary? Spruiell[17] has noted that although the frame is deliberately unbalanced, the patient invariably joins the analyst in elaborating the frame. Most clinicians would agrees basing this answer on recollected violations they have witnessed, such as the patient who refers to the therapist as 'Shrinkie' or springs from the chair and tries without warning to sit on the therapist's lap. It is clear, however, that the patient's boundary is a more forgiving and flexible one. The patient cannot be stopped from calling the therapist names, and that is part of the therapeutic process. The patient can be late and that can be discussed, but the therapist should not be late, and so on. In any case our focus here is on the clinician's boundary.

Let us also agree that the role of therapist embraces the structural aspects of therapy in addition to the content; these include time, place, and money, which may, together with other aspects discussed below, represent possible sites for boundary crossings or violations to occur. If this exploration is to be useful, we should adopt the convention that 'boundary crossing' in this article is descriptive term, neither laudatory nor pejorative. An assessor could then determine the impact of a boundary crossing on a case-by-case basis that takes into account the context and situation-specific facts, such as the possible harmfulness of this crossing to this patient. A violation, then, represent a *harmful* crossing, a transgression, of a boundary. An example might be the case of a patient who had experienced severe or traumatic boundary violations in childhood and who might consequently be highly sensitive to later violations, even those usually considered benign. Note also that the difference between a harmful and a nonharmful boundary crossing may lie in whether it is discussed or discussable; clinical exploration of a violation often defuses its potential for harm.

To organize the discussion we consider the matter of boundaries, boundary crossings, and boundary violations under a series of headings: role; time; place and space; money; gifts, services, and related matters; clothing; language; self-disclosure and related matters; and physical contact. Sexual misconduct as an extreme boundary violation has been extensively addressed elsewhere[2,4,6,18] and is not separately reviewed here. We should also point out that in addition to serving a antecedents to sexual misconduct, some of these area's of boundary crossing may represent ethical violations in and of themselves.

Role

Role boundaries constitute the essential boundary issue. To conceptualize this entity, one might ask, 'Is this what a therapist does?' Although subject to ideological variations, this touchstone question not only identifies the question of clinical role but serves as a useful orienting device for avoiding the pitfalls of role violations.

A middle-aged borderline patient, attempting to convey how deeply distressed she felt about her situation, leaped from her chair in the therapist's office and threw herself to her knees at the therapist's feet, clasping his hand in both of her own and crying, 'Do you understand how awful it's been for me?' The therapist said gently, 'You know, this is really interesting, what's happening here – but it isn't therapy; please go back to your chair.' The patient did so, and the incident was explored verbally.

Although such limit setting may appear brusque to some clinicians, it may be the only appropriate response to halt boundary-violating 'acting in' (especially of the impulsive or precipitous kind) and to make the behavior available for analysis as part of the therapy.

Almost all patients who enter into a psychotherapeutic process struggle with the unconscious wish to view the therapist as the ideal parent who, unlike the real parents, will gratify all their childhood wishes[19]. As a result of the longings stirred up by the basic transference situation of psychotherapy or psychoanalysis, it is imperative that some degree of abstinence be maintained[20]. However, strict abstinence is neither desirable nor possible, and total frustration of all the patient's wishes creates a powerful influence on the patient in its own right.[8,19]

In attempting to delineate the appropriate role for the therapist vis-à-vis the patient's wishes and longings to be loved and held, it is useful to differentiate between 'libidinal demands,' which cannot be gratified without entering into ethical transgressions and damaging enactments, and 'growth needs,' which prevent growth if not gratified to some extent[21]. Greenson[22] made a similar distinction when he noted that the rule of abstinence was constructed to avoid the gratification of a patient's neurotic and infantile wishes, not to lead to a sterile form of treatment in which all the patient's wishes are frustrated.

Efforts to delineate the two varieties of needs often lead to problems in the area of defining the appropriate role for the therapist. Certainly, the patient may have legitimate wishes to be empathically understood, but when the therapist goes too far in the direction of trying to provide parental functions that were not supplied by the original parents, the patient may experience the therapist as making false promises. Casement[21] expressed reservations about Freud's providing a meal to the Rat Man because of the possibility that the patient may have experienced Freud's taking responsibility for a particular part of his life as an implicit promise that Freud was prepared to take over responsibility for other areas of the patient's life as well. Clearly, a therapist cannot become the 'good mother' or 'good father' in a literal sense and attempt to make up for all the deprivations of childhood. Even when therapists feel as though they are being coerced into a parental role by their patients, they must strive not to conform to the patients' expectations. Spruiell[17] made the following observation: 'It is as disastrous for analysts to actually treat their patients like children as it is for analysts to treat their own children as patients' (p. 12).

The therapist's role is subject to some variation, of course. While most therapy is talking, there may be times when it is appropriate, for example, to write a letter on a patient's behalf. Under some circumstances, such a 'breach of the frame'[16] might constitute a boundary violation, as when the therapist attempts to intervene in some extratherapeutic realm of the patient's life (e.g., a therapist wrote a stern letter to a patient's employer rebuking the latter for giving the patient excessively burdensome tasks on the job). In addition, since different modalities of therapy are commonly combined, the 'talking therapist' might appropriately give medications, conceivably by injection at times – a clear boundary crossing but presumably therapeutic and benign.

Time

Time is, of course, a boundary, defining the limits of the session itself while providing structure and even containment for many patients, who derive reassurance because they will have to experience the various stresses of reminiscing, reliving, and so forth for a set time only. The beginnings and endings of sessions – starting or stopping late or early – are both susceptible to crossings of this boundary. Such crossings may be subtle or stark.

A male psychiatrist came in to the hospital to see his female inpatient for marathon sessions at odd times, such as from 2:00 to 6:00 in the morning, rationalizing that this procedure was dictated by scheduling problems. This relationship eventually became overtly sexual.

An interesting prejudice about violating the boundary of time has evolved in sexual misconduct cases, a prejudice deriving from the fact that a clinician interested in having a sexual relationship with a patient might well schedule that patient for the last hour of the day (although, of course, after-work time slots have always been popular). In the fog of uncertainty surrounding sexual misconduct (usually a conflict of credibilities without witnesses), this factor has gleamed with so illusory a brightness that some attorneys seem to presume that because the patient had the last appointment of the day, sexual misconduct occurred! Short of seeing patients straight through the night, this problem does not seem to have a

clear solution. Admittedly, however, from a risk-management standpoint, a patient in the midst of an intense erotic transference to the therapist might best be seen, when possible, during high-traffic times when other people (e.g., secretaries, receptionists, and even other patients) are around.

Langs[23] noted that the boundary of time may be psychologically violated when the therapist brings up material from a previous session. Some patients, indeed, feel that this practice is disruptive and is a departure by the therapist from the here and now. However, most clinicians would regard this view as extreme, since effective therapy depends on continuity from session to session.

The issue of the appropriateness of phone calls between psychotherapy sessions is a controversial one, particularly when the patient suffers from borderline personality disorder. Some therapists view such phone calls as necessary and expectable in light of the borderline patient's difficulties with evocative memory[24,25]. In other words, the patient's inability to evoke a holding, soothing introject causes anxiety of catastrophic proportions related to the fear that the therapist has disappeared. Phone calls are a way of reestablishing contact with the therapist and soothing this anxiety, which might otherwise lead to ill-advised self-destructive behavior. On the other hand, other therapists view such calls as unnecessary and countertherapeutic[26,27]. These therapists go to great lengths in the initial contractual period, at the beginning of therapy, to extract an agreement from the patient that phone calls will be used only in emergency situations. This controversy reflects how a boundary violation may be defined according to the extent to which the appropriate treatment is viewed as having an expressive versus a supportive emphasis.

Place and Space

The therapist's office or a room on a hospital unit is obviously the locale for almost all therapy; some exceptions are noted in the next section. Exceptions usually constitute boundary crossings but are not always harmful. Some examples include accompanying a patient to court for a hearing, visiting a patient at home, and seeing a patient in the intensive care unit after an overdose or in jail after an arrest.

Some boundary crossings of place can have a constructive effect. As with medication, the timing and dosage are critical.

After initially agreeing to attend his analysand's wedding, the analyst later declined, reasoning that his presence would be inappropriately distracting. Later, after the death of the analysand's first child, he attended the funeral service. Both his absence at the first occasion and his presence at the second were felt as helpful and supportive by the analysand. They both agreed later that the initial plan to attend the wedding was an error.

A relevant lesson from this example is that boundary violations can be reversed or undone with further consideration and discussion. At times, an apology by the therapist is appropriate and even necessary.

Some sexual misconduct cases reveal space violations that seem to manifest wishes for fusion on the part of the therapist, as in the following case.

A lesbian therapist treating a female patient would contrive to use the bathroom at the clinic whenever the patient did so and, entering the adjoining stall, would attempt to continue the conversation. The relationship became overtly and exploitatively sexual, with the therapist often wearing the patient's clothes to work the next day after they had spent the night together.

Sorties out of the office usually merit special scrutiny. While home visits were a central component of the community psychiatry movement, the shift in the professional climate is such that the modern clinician is best advised to perform this valuable service with an opposite-sex chaperon and to document the event in some detail.

Sessions during lunch are an extremely common form of boundary violation. This event appears to be a common way station along the path of increasing boundary crossings culminating in sexual misconduct. Although clinicians often advance the claim that therapy is going on, so, inevitably, is much purely social behavior; it does not *look* like therapy, at least to a jury. Lunch sessions are not uncommonly followed by sessions during dinner, then just dinners, then other dating behavior, eventually including intercourse.

Sessions in cars represent another violation of place. Typically, the clinician gives the patient a ride home under various circumstances. Clinician and patient then park (e.g., in front of the patient's house) and finish up the presumably therapeutic conversation. From a fact finder's viewpoint, many exciting things happen in cars, but therapy is usually not one of them.

The complexity of the matter increases, however, when we consider other therapeutic ideologies. For example, it would not be a boundary violation for a behaviorist, under certain circumstances, to accompany a patient in a car, to an elevator, to an airplane, or even to a public restroom (in the treatment of paruresis, the fear of urinating in a public restroom) as part of the treatment plan for a particular phobia. The existence of a body of professional literature, a clinical rationale, and risk-benefit documentation will be useful in protecting the clinician in such a situation from misconstruction of the therapeutic efforts.

Money

Money is a boundary in the sense of defining the business nature of the therapeutic relationship. This is not love, it's work. Indeed, some would argue that the fee received by the therapist is the only appropriate and allowable material gratification to be derived from clinical work[28]. Patient and clinician may each have conflicts about this distinction[29], but consultative experience makes clear that trouble begins precisely when the therapist stops thinking of therapy as work.

On the other hand, most clinicians learned their trade by working with indigent patients and feel that some attempt should be made to pay back this debt by seeing some patients for free – a form of 'tithing,' if you will. Note that this *decision* – to see a patient for free and to discuss that with the patient – is quite different from simply letting the billing lapse or allowing the debt to mount. The latter examples are boundary crossings, perhaps violations.

Consultative experience also suggests that the usual problem underlying a patient's mounting debt is the clinician's conflict about money and its dynamic meanings. Initially reluctant to bring up the unpaid bill, the clinician may soon become too angry to discuss it. Explorations of the dynamic meaning of the bill are more convincing when they do not take place through clenched teeth. A clinician stuck at this countertransference point may simply let it slide. In the minds of fact finders, this raises a question: 'The clinician seems curiously indifferent to making a living; could the patient be paying in some other currency?' – a line of speculation one does not wish to foster.

In rural areas even today, payments to physicians may take the form of barter: when the doctor delivers your child, you pay with two chickens and the new calf. For the dynamic therapist this practice poses some problems, because it blurs the boundary between payment and gift (covered in the next section). The clinician should take a case at a reasonable fee or make a *decision* to see the patient for a low fee (e.g., one dollar) or none. Barter is confusing and probably ill-advised today. Of course, all such decisions require documentation.

Gifts, Services, and Related Matters

A client became very upset during an interview with her therapist and began to cry. The therapist, proffering a tissue, held out a hand-tooled Florentine leather case in which a pocket pack of tissues had been placed. After the patient had withdrawn a tissue, the therapist impulsively said, 'Why don't you keep the case?' In subsequent supervision the therapist came to understand that this 'gift' to the patient was an unconscious bribe designed to avert the anger that the therapist sensed just below the surface of the patient's sorrow.

This gift was also a boundary violation, placing unidentified obligations on the patient and constituting a form of impulsive acting in. A related boundary violation is the use of favors or services from the patient for the benefit of the therapist, as Simon's startling vignette illustrates:

Within a few months of starting . . . psychotherapy, the patient was returning the therapist's library books for him 'as a favor.' . . . The patient began having trouble paying her treatment bill, so she agreed – at the therapist's suggestion – to clean the therapist's office once a week in partial payment . . . .The patient also agreed to get the therapist's lunch at a nearby delicatessen before each session. (6, p. 106)

The obvious exploitive nature of these boundary violations destroys even the semblance of therapy for the patient's benefit.

When Freud heard that one of his patients was planning to buy a set of his complete works, he gave the patient the set as a gift[30]. Immediately following the receipt of this gift, Freud's patient found that he was unable to use his dreams productively in the analysis as he had before. Freud related this 'drying up' to the gift and noted, 'You will see from this what difficulties gifts in analysis always make'.(p. 42)

Other boundary crossings can be relatively minor but can promote a chain of subsequent crossings, as in this example:

A patient walked into the room while her therapist was pouring coffee from a carafe. He later described how he had felt socially incapable of not offering some coffee to the patient and had indeed offered some. At the next session, the patient brought doughnuts.

As the vignette shows, many boundary problems may arise at the interface between manners and technique.

In contrast to the potentially harmful or at least confusing effects of the preceding examples, compare the practice (not uncommon among psychopharmacologists) of giving patients, as part of treatment, educational texts designed for laypersons (e.g., giving *Mood-swing*[31] to a patient with bipolar disorder). Such a boundary crossing may foster mastery of the illness through information – a positive result. A similar point might be made for judicious 'gifts' of medication samples for indigent patients. These two instances represent clear boundary crossings that have some justification. Ideally, even these should be discussed with an ear to any possible negative effects.

A patient in long-term therapy had struggled for years with apparent infertility and eventually, with great difficulty, arranged for adoption of a child. Two years later she unexpectedly conceived and finally gave birth. Her therapist, appreciating the power and meaning of this event, sent congratulatory flowers to the hospital.

In this case, the therapist followed social convention in a way that – though technically a boundary crossing – represented a response appropriate to the real relationship. Offering a tissue to a crying patient and expressing condolences to a bereaved one are similar examples of appropriate responses outside the classic boundaries of the therapeutic relationship.

Clothing

Clothing represents a social boundary the transgression of which is usually inappropriate to the therapeutic situation, yet a patient may appropriately be asked to roll up a sleeve to permit measurement of blood pressure. Excessively revealing or frankly seductive clothing worn by the therapist may represent a boundary violation with potentially harmful effects to patients, but the issue can also be overdone, as in the following case.

A patient in a western state, as part of a sexual misconduct allegation that a jury later found to be false, accused the therapist (among other things) of conducting therapy sessions with the top two buttons of his shirt undone. While such a phenomenon might conceivably represent a violation for a very sensitive patient, evidence was introduced that revealed the exaggerated nature of this claim in *this* case.

Berne[32] noted the technical error of the male clinician who, confronting a patient whose skirt was pulled up high, began to explain to the patient his sexual fantasies in response to this event. Berne suggested instead saying to the patient, 'Pull your skirt down.' Similar directness of limit setting appears to be suited to the patient who – either from psychosis or the wish to provoke – begins to take off her clothes in the office. As before, the comment, 'This behavior is inappropriate, and it isn't therapy; please put your clothes back on,' said in a calm voice, is a reasonable response.

Language

As part of the otherwise laudable efforts to humanize and demystify psychiatry a few decades back, the use of a patient's first name was very much in vogue. While this may indeed convey greater warmth and closeness, such usage is a two-edged sword. There is always the possibility that patients may experience the use of first names as misrepresenting the professional relationship as a social friendship[28]. There may well be instances when using first names is appropriate, but therapists must carefully consider whether they are creating a false sense of intimacy that may subsequently backfire.

A middle-aged woman tried for more than a year to get her therapist to use her first name, but the requests were denied, and exploration of the issue took place instead. After some time the patient recovered memories of previously repressed material, in part because of increased trust in the therapist. The patient spontaneously related her trust to the use of last names as a boundary issue; boundaries had been badly blurred in her family and this had included sexual abuse.

There are distinct advantages to addressing the adult in the patient, in terms of fostering the adult observing ego for the alliance. Trainees often do not see the paradox of expecting adult behavior on the ward from someone they themselves call 'Jimmy,' which is what people called the patient when he was much younger. Last names also emphasize that this process is work or business, an atmosphere which may promote a valuable mature perspective and minimize acting out. In addition, calling someone by the name used by primary objects may foster transference perceptions of the therapist when they are not desirable, as with a borderline patient prone to forming severe psychotic transferences. For balance, however, recall that use of last names may also sound excessively distant, formal, and aloof.

Tone is also a part of language. A patient won a settlement in an allegation of sexual misconduct when the tape recording she had made of a phone call from her therapist revealed his, intimate, seductive tone. The therapist's attorney urged the settlement for fear that the jury would hear the intimate tone as evidence of a sexual relationship.

Word choice can also be violative, as when the therapist inquires, 'What are you feeling now in your vagina?' Note that this inquiry might be proper in analytic therapy after appropriate preparation. Clinical utility aside, the way in which such explorations may violate boundaries should be kept in mind.

Finally, psychotherapy may be a forum for sadomasochistic enactments in which aggressive verbal abuse grows out of countertransference sadism. Cruel and contemptuous comments by the therapist may be rationalized as therapeutic confrontation.

Self-disclosure and Related Matters

Few clinicians would argue that the therapist's self-disclosure is always a boundary crossing. Psychoanalysis and intensive psychotherapy involve intense personal relationships. A useful therapeutic alliance may be forged by the therapist's willingness to acknowledge that a painful experience of the patient is familiar to himself[19]. However, when a therapist begins to indulge in even mild forms of self-disclosure, it is an indication for careful self-scrutiny regarding the motivations for departure from the usual therapeutic stance. Gorkin[33] observed that many therapists harbor a wish to be known by their patients as a 'real person,' especially as the termination of

the therapy approaches. While it may be technically correct for a therapist to become more spontaneous at the end of the therapeutic process, therapists who become more self-disclosing as the therapy ends must be sure that their reasons for doing so are not related to their own unfulfilled needs in their private lives but, rather, are based on an objective assessment that increased focus on the real relationship is useful for the patient in the termination process.

Self-disclosure, however, represents a complex issue. Clearly, therapists may occasionally use a neutral example from their own lives to illustrate a point. Sharing the impact of a borderline patient's behavior on the therapist may also be useful. The therapist's self-revelation, however, of personal fantasies or dreams; of social, sexual, or financial details; of specific vacation plans; or of expected births or deaths in the family is usually, burdening the patient with information, whereas it is the patient's fantasies that might best be explored. The issue is somewhat controversial: a number of patients (and, surprisingly, some therapists) believe that the patient is somehow entitled to this kind of information. In any case, it is a boundary violation and as such may be used by the legal system to advance or support a claim of sexual misconduct. The reasoning is that the patient knows so much about the therapist's personal life that they must have been intimate (compare the remark by a board of registration, quoted earlier).

Subtler variations on the information theme may occur, as when a therapist sees members of a couple in parallel treatment but separately alludes in one member's session to material from the other's. Sensitivity in this area may run quite high.

A patient had a dream involving Nazis. In the interpretation the therapist suggested that this detail referred to himself. The patient seemed doubtful. The therapist noted that the interpretation was based in part on the fact that other patients of his had dreamed of Nazis in response to the therapist's German last name. The patient's mood changed; only later was she able to tell the therapist how violated she had felt at his 'intruding' other patients into the session.

Although the intrusion was at a verbal level only, the impact was clear for this patient, who had been subjected to some disregard of her boundaries in previous therapy.

Finally, the boundary can be violated from the other side. An example would be the therapist's using data from the therapy session for personal gain, such as insider information on stock trading, huge profits to be made in real estate, and the like.

Physical Contact

To place the issue of physical contact in context, it should be noted that psychiatrists traditionally performed their own physical examinations. This practice has declined so markedly that a senior psychiatrist recently wrote about examining a patient's bruised leg as a major return to the past. Hospitals commonly use internists for this purpose. Psychiatric residents still do their own physical examinations but commonly maintain distance by examining each other's patients. Abnormal Involuntary Movement Scale examinations for tardive dyskinesia are often the only routine physical contact.

There is room here for regrets. Physicians working with a patient with AIDS or HIV seropositivity often describe wishing to touch the patient in some benign manner (pat the back, squeeze an arm, pat a hand) in every session. They reason that such patients feel like lepers, and therapeutic touch is called for in these cases. But even such humane interventions must be scrutinized and, indeed, be documented to prevent their misconstruction in today's climate.

From the viewpoint of current risk-management principles, a handshake is about the limit of social physical contact at this time. Of course, a patient who attempts a hug in the last session after 7 years of intense, intensive, and successful therapy should probably not be hurled across the room. However, most hugs from patients should be discouraged in tactful, gentle ways by words, body language, positioning, and so forth. Patients who deliberately or provocatively throw their arms around the therapist despite repeated efforts at discouragement should be stopped. An appropriate response is to step back, catch both wrists in your hands, cross the patient's wrists in front of you, so that the crossed arms form a barrier between bodies, and say firmly, 'Therapy is a talking relationship; please sit down so we can discuss your not doing this any more.' If the work degenerates into grabbing, consider seriously termination and referral, perhaps to a therapist of a different gender.

What is one to make of the brands of therapy that include physical contact, such as Rolfing? Presumably, the boundary extends to that limited physical contact, and the patient expects it and grants consent; thus, no actual violation occurs. Massage therapists may struggle with similar issues, however. In other ideologies the issue may again be the impact of the appearance of a violation:

A therapist – who claimed that her school of practice involved hugging her female patient at the beginning and end of every session, without apparent harm – eventually had to terminate therapy with the patient for noncompliance with the therapeutic plan. The enraged patient filed a sexual misconduct claim against the therapist. Despite the evidence showing that this claim was probably false (a specious suit triggered by rage at the therapist), the insurer settled because of the likelihood that a jury would not accept the principle of 'hug at the start and hug at the end but no hugs in between.' If the claim was indeed false, this is a settlement based on boundary violations alone.

At another level this vignette nicely suggests how nonsexual boundary violations may be harmful to a patient in much the same way that actual sexual misconduct is. Instead of engaging the patient in a mourning process to deal with the resentment and grief about the deprivations of her childhood, the therapist who hugs a patient is often attempting to provide the physical contact normally offered by a parent. The patient then feels entitled to more demonstrations of caring and assumes that if gratification in the form of hugs is available, other wishes will be granted as well (compare Smith's concept of the 'golden fantasy' that all needs will be met by therapy[34]). When actual physical contact occurs, the crucial psychotherapeutic distinction between the symbolic and the concrete is lost[21], and the patient may feel that powerful infantile longings within will finally be satisfied.

Conclusions

Boundary crossings may be benign or harmful, may take many forms, and may pose problems related to both treatment and potential liability. The differences in impact may depend on whether clinical judgment has been used to make the decision, whether adequate discussion and exploration have taken place, and whether documentation adequately records the details. The complexity of the subject and the variability of results from case-by-case analysis merit empirical study. Educational materials are available through the Office of Public Affairs of the American Psychiatric Association. Heightened awareness of the concepts of boundaries, boundary crossings, and boundary violations will both improve patient care and contribute to effective risk management.

In an effort to prevent more serious boundary violations of a sexual nature, Epstein and Simon[28] have developed an exploitation index which comprises a list of questions that therapists can ask themselves about their current behavior with patients. In this manner these authors have attempted to provide an ongoing self-monitoring system. While such approaches may be useful for some clinicians, we must acknowledge that considerable personal variation exists in our field. The relationships between therapist and patient vary from one therapist to another, and there are even variations across patients in the practice of one therapist. As Lipton[8] observed, it is ultimately impossible to codify or prescribe a personal relationship between therapist and patient in a precise manner. Perhaps the best risk management involves careful consideration of any departures from one's usual practice accompanied by careful documentation of the reasons for the departure. Finally, the value of consultation with a respected colleague should be a built-in part of every practitioner's risk-management program.

References

1   Ingram DH: Intimacy in the psychoanalytic relationship: a preliminary sketch. *Am J Psychoanal* 1991; **51**:403–411

2   Gutheil TG: Borderline personality disorder, boundary violations, and patient-therapist sex: medicolegal pitfalls. *Am J Psychiatry* 1989; **146**: 597–602

3   Stone MH: Boundary violations between therapist and patient. *Psychiatr Annals* 1976; **6**:670–677

4   Gabbard GO (ed): *Sexual Exploitation in Professional Relationships*. Washington, DC, American Psychiatric Press, 1989

5   Borys DS, Pope KS: Dual relationships between therapist and client: a national study of psychologists, psychiatrists, and social workers. *Professional Psychol: Research and Practice* 1989; **20**: 280–293

6   Simon RI: Sexual exploitation of patients: how it begins before it happens. *Psychiatr Annals* 1989; **19**:104–122

7   Jorgenson L: Consultation forum. *Psychodynamic Letter* 1991; 1(10):7–8

8   Lipton SD: The advantages of Freud's technique as shown in his analysis of the Rat Man. *Int J Psychoanal* 1977; **58**:255–273

9   Grosskurth P: *Melanie Klein: Her World and Her Work*. New York, Alfred A Knopf, 1986

10 Winnicott DW: Hate in the counter-transference. *Int J Psychoanal* 1949; **30**:69–74

11 Little MI: *Psychotic Anxieties and Containment: A Personal Record of an Analysis With Winnicott*. Northvale, NJ, Jason Aronson, 1990

12 Eissler KR: The effect of the structure of the ego on psychoanalytic technique. *J Am Psychoanal Assoc* 1953; **1**:104–143

13 Zetzel ER: 1965: Additional notes upon a case of obsessional neurosis: Freud 1909. *Int J Psychoanal* 1966; **47**:123–129

14 Shapiro T: On neutrality. *J Am Psychoanal Assoc* 1984; **32**:269–282

15 Gabbard GO: *Psychodynamic Psychiatry in Clinical Practice*. Washington, DC, American Psychiatric Press, 1990

16 Langs R: *The Bipersonal Field*. New York, Jason Aronson, 1976

17 Spruiell V: The rules and frames of the psychoanalytic situation. *Psychoanal Q* 1983; **52**:1–33

18 Appelbaum PS, Gutheil TG: *Clinical Handbook of Psychiatry and the Law*, 2nd ed. Baltimore, Williams & Wilkins, 1991

19 Viederman M: The real person of the analyst and his role in the process of psychoanalytic cure. *J Am Psychoanal Assoc* 1991; **39**:451–489

20 Novey R: The abstinence of the psychoanalyst. *Bull Menninger Clin* 1991; **55**:344–362

21 Casement PJ: The meeting of needs in psychoanalysis. *Psychoanal Inquiry* 1990; **10**:325–346

22 Greenson RR: *The Technique of Psychoanalysis*, vol 1. New York, International Universities Press, 1967

23 Langs R: *Psychotherapy: A Basic Text*. New York, Jason Aronson, 1982

24 Adler G: *Borderline Psychopathology and Its Treatment*. New York, Jason Aronson, 1985

25 Adler G, Buie DH Jr: Aloneness and borderline psychopathology: the possible relevance of child development issues. *Int J Psychoanal* 1979; **60**:83–96

26 Kernberg OF: *Severe Personality Disorders: Psychotherapeutic Strategies*. New Haven, Conn, Yale University Press, 1984

27 Kernberg OF, Selzer MA, Koenigsberg HW, Carr AC, Appelbaum HA: *Psychodynamic Psychotherapy of Borderline Patients*. New York, Basic Books, 1989

28 Epstein RS, Simon RI: The exploitation index: an early warning indreator of boundary violations in psychotherapy. *Bull Menninger Clin* 1990; **54**:450–465

29 **Krueger DW** (ed): *The Last Taboo: Money As Symbol and Reality in Psychotherapy and Psychoanalysis.* New York, Brunner Mazel, 1986

30 **Blanton S:** *Diary of My Analysis With Sigmund Freud.* New York, Hawthorn Books, 1971

31 **Fieve R:** *Moodswing: The Third Revolution in Psychiatry.* New York, Bantam Books, 1976

32 **Berne E:** *What Do You Say After You Say Hello? The Psychology of Human Destiny.* New York, Grove Press, 1972

33 **Gorkin M:** *The Uses of Countertransference.* Northvale, NJ, Jason Aronson, 1987

34 **Smith S:** The golden fantasy: a regressive reaction to separation anxiety. *Int J Psychoanal* 1977; **58**:311–324

Psychotherapists who transgress sexual boundaries with patients*

Glen O. Gabbard

With sexual misconduct rapidly becoming the number-one liability concern for the mental health professions, the field has been struggling to understand the phenomenon (Apfel & Simon, 1985; Gabbard, 1989; Gartrell, Herman, Olarte, Feldstein, & Localio, 1986; Pope & Bouhoutsos, 1986; Schoener, Milgrom, Gonsiorek, Luepker, & Conroe, 1989). Among these efforts have been several attempts to develop typologies of therapists who transgress sexual boundaries with patients (Averill et al., 1989; Gonsiorek, 1989; Olarte, 1991; Pope & Bouhoutsos, 1986; Twemlow & Gabbard, 1989). A psychodynamic understanding of these therapists and the forces that lead them to resort to such highly self-destructive behavior is more difficult to ascertain.

Part of the difficulty has been a tendency in recent years to politicize therapist-patient sex in such a way as to discourage systematic psychodynamic understanding. The 'politically correct' view of the phenomenon in some venues is that thoroughly evil male therapists prey on helpless female patients (Gutheil & Gabbard, 1992). In this model, the problem can be solved simply by eradicating the 'bad apples' from the profession. This reductionistic view has the appeal of reassuring therapists that those who engage in sexual misconduct are vastly different from them. Therapists involved in this inappropriate activity are a group of 'impaired professionals' who can be differentiated from everyone else by their utterly corrupt superegos and their morally reprehensible behavior.

Another aspect of this narrow view of therapist-patient sex is that it lends itself to sexual stereotypes in the culture (Gutheil & Gabbard, 1992). Men are the seducers, and women are the seduced. In one study of sexual transgressions; when female therapists were involved with male patients, the male patients were regarded as responsible and blameworthy for the behavior, while the female therapists were viewed as their victims (Averill et al., 1989). Although most studies suggest that males are the perpetrators in the vast majority of cases, substantial evidence now demonstrates that females are also involved in sexual misconduct. Moreover, same-sex pairings represent a significant problem, even though they are less frequently reported than opposite-sex pairings (Benowitz, 1991; Gonsiorek, 1989; Gutheil & Gabbard, 1992; Lyn, 1990).

The fact that sexual misconduct is a complex problem involving a variety of different scenarios becomes apparent to anyone who studies a sufficient number of cases. Systematic examination of data often yields results that do not conform to politically correct formulas. At The Menninger Clinic, where therapists who have transgressed sexual boundaries with patients have been evaluated and treated for many years, this diversity of psychodynamic themes has emerged in the work with these individuals. In this article, I will report on a series of pastoral counselors, social workers, psychiatrists, and psychologists whom I have seen in psychoanalysis, psychotherapy, hospital treatment, or consultation, in addition to other cases in which I have been indirectly involved as a supervisor or consultant to other clinicians. In trying to explicate the psychodynamic themes in these therapists, I have encountered a problem related to confidentiality that others in the field have shared. Because I am discussing the psychology

of colleagues who may be recognizable to readers of this article, I am not at liberty to describe the details of individual cases. Instead, I am forced for ethical reasons to talk about the psychodynamic themes I have observed in broad brushstrokes that paint a general picture but leave out the idiosyncratic and specific details of any one therapist.

A psychodynamic classification

It is heuristically useful to group these therapists in rubrics that are psychodynamically based rather than limited to specific diagnostic categories. The vast majority of therapists who become sexually involved with patients will manifest psychopathology that falls into one of four categories: (1) psychotic disorders, (2) predatory psychopathy and paraphilias, (3) lovesickness, and (4) masochistic surrender. The first category, psychotic disorders, is definitely the smallest group, consisting of therapists who suffer from such disorders as bipolar affective disorder, paranoid psychosis, schizophrenia, and psychotic organic brain syndrome. These therapists generally require extensive treatment that includes pharmacotherapy and vocational counseling to discourage them from continuing in the career of psychotherapist. Because the other three categories are more common and more complex from a dynamic perspective, I will consider each of them in substantially more detail.

Predatory psychopathy and paraphilias

Within this rubric I am including not only antisocial personality disorders but also severe narcissistic personality disorders with prominent antisocial features. Although all persons suffering from paraphilias are certainly not psychopathic predators, those who act on their paraphiliac impulses with patients under their care generally have a severely compromised superego and character pathology on the narcissistic to antisocial continuum.

These therapists are generally male, but female practitioners have also been reported to fit this category. Benowitz (1991) described two female therapists who engaged in violent behavior during sex with clients, such as urging a patient to perform violent acts with sharp objects on herself. Another female therapist asked a patient to perform the same behaviors that had been degrading to her in past sexually abusive relationships, a common form of sadistic humiliation in this category of therapists. Male offenders in this group tend to have been involved with a long string of clients and are notoriously refractory to rehabilitation of any kind. When caught, they may pretend to be remorseful and claim that they were in love with the patient. They may be masters at manipulating the legal system as well, so they often escape any severe legal or ethical sanctions.

For therapists in this category, patients are regarded merely as objects to be used for their own sexual gratification. Because these therapists lack empathy or concern for the victim, they are incapable of feeling remorse or guilt about any harm they might have done the patient. This massive failure of superego development appears to be related to profound impairment of internalization during childhood development. The only form of object-relatedness they appear to know is sadistic bonding with others through the exercise of destructiveness and power (Meloy, 1988). Some of these therapists have a childhood history of profound neglect or abuse, and

* Gabbard, G.O.: Psychotherapists who transgress sexual boundaries with patients. *Bulletin of the Menninger Clinic* **58**:124–135, 1994.

some clinicians have understood their exploitation of others as an effort to achieve active mastery of passively experienced trauma (Schwartz, 1992).

One particular variant operating in same-sex dyads involves split-off homo erotic feelings. Therapists who may ordinarily regard themselves as heterosexual may split off and protectively disavow both their own self-loathing and their sexual feelings toward persons of the same sex (Gonsiorek, 1989). They then act out such feelings secretly with their patients, often with cruel and sadistic methods, as a way of compartmentalizing ego-dysgenic homosexual feelings.

Lovesickness

Most therapists who become sexually involved with patients are either predatory or lovesick. In one survey of psychiatrists (Gartrell *et al.*, 1986), 65% of those who had been in a sexual relationship with a patient described themselves as being in love with the patient. Lovesick therapists may be associated with a variety of different diagnostic categories (Gabbard, 1991a; Twemlow & Gabbard, 1989). In some cases, they suffer from less severe forms of narcissistic personality disorder that lack the antisocial features typical of the predatory group. The narcissistic themes in these therapists involve a desperate need for validation by their patients, a hunger to be loved and idealized, and a tendency to use patients to regulate their own self-esteem. Some lovesick therapists may have borderline personality disorder that leads them to quickly idealize patients and impulsively act on their feelings of infatuation. Still others in this category have neurotic problems, while some are essentially normal, from a diagnostic standpoint, but are in the midst of a life crisis.

The most common scenario is that of a middle-aged male therapist who falls in love with a much younger female patient while he is experiencing divorce, separation, disillusionment with his own marriage, or the loss of a significant person in his life (Gabbard, 1991a; Twemlow & Gabbard, 1989). He may begin to share his own problems with his patient and present himself in psychotherapy sessions as needy and vulnerable. This role reversal is a common precursor to sexual transgressions.

One way of viewing this development in a psychotherapy process is to describe the countertransference as having become ebonized in the same way that certain incest victims and borderline patients develop ebonized *transference* (Blum, 1973; Gabbard, 1991a). The ability to distinguish a countertransference wish from the reality of the situation is compromised, so that the loving feelings toward the patient lose the 'as if' quality characteristic of milder forms of transference. The therapist can no longer appreciate that something from the past is being repeated and that feelings for significant persons from the therapist's past are displaced onto the patient. In light of this loss of insight, a form of 'nonpsychotic loss of reality testing' can be observed (Twemlow & Gabbard, 1989, p. 83). Outside the particular *folie à deux* that involves the therapist-patient dyad, the therapist's reality testing appears to be intact. Within the dyad, however, a loss of judgment and reality testing makes it difficult for the therapist to see how self-destructive and harmful the relationship has become. Indeed, many lovesick therapists, when confronted, will insist that the relationship transcends any considerations of transference and counter transference.

A variety of psycho dynamic themes can be identified in cases of lovesickness. In any single case, one or several of the following issues may figure prominently in the therapist's transgression:

Unconscious reenactment of incestuous longings. There can be little doubt that therapist-patient sex is symbolically incestuous to both therapist and patient. Each member of the dyad is a forbidden object to the other. For the therapist, the psychological proscription is intensified by ethical and legal prohibitions. One way of viewing the development of a sexual relationship in the context of psychotherapy is that it is a re-creation of an earlier incestuous situation for both persons. As Klutz (1989) has noted, incest victims tend to put themselves in situations where they become revictimized and therefore are 'sitting ducks' for therapist-patient sex. As Freud (1905/1953) observed, 'The finding of an object is in fact a refining of it' (p. 222). Both therapist and patient are refining forbidden objects from the

past, and the therapist colludes in an enactment rather than interpreting the unconscious wish to repeat past trauma, all under the guise of 'true love.'

Misperception of wish for maternal nurturing as sexual overture. With incest victims in particular, receiving care may be inextricably bound up with sexuality. To be reassured that they are cared for and valued, they may explicitly demand some form of physical contact. The professional boundaries of the relationship may be regarded with contempt, and the longing to be loved and held may be repeated again and again until the therapist acquiesces (Gabbard & Wilkinson, 1994). Therapists often misconstrue the patient's wish for maternal nurturance as a sexual overture and act accordingly. A pre-genital need is misunderstood as a demand for genital sexual activity.

Interlocking enactments of rescue fantasies. Apfel and Simon (1985) have noted that the patient's tendency to repeat his or her past may, in fact, be mirrored by the therapist's need to repeat. A female patient may have harbored a childhood fantasy that she was somehow ministering to a father who-was despairing over his marriage. Similarly, a male therapist may be unconsciously rescuing his depressed mother. Hence, the therapist-patient dyad is involved in interlocking rescue enactments.

Patient seen as idealized version of the self. Lovesick therapists with narcissistic problems may project aspects of themselves into the patient. This projected ego ideal or idealized self-representation may then obscure the patient's real qualities. Just as Narcissus fell in love with his own image in the water, these therapists are infatuated with an idealized reflection of themselves.

Confusion of therapist's needs with patient's needs. Sullivan (1954) once noted that psychotherapy is a truly unique profession because practitioners must put aside their own needs in the interest of addressing the needs of the patient. An occupational hazard for all therapists is to inadvertently or unconsciously gratify their own needs while they think they are meeting the patient's needs. In cases of sexual misconduct, this dynamic is particularly problematic. Because many therapists grew up in homes where they felt unloved, they may attempt to elicit from their patients the love they did not receive from their parents (Gabbard, in press; Sussman, 1992). Longings to be loved are defended against by giving to others. Many lovesick therapists genuinely feel they are giving something wonderful to their patients, even though they are involved in an ethical transgression. In this manner, they defend against acknowledging their own dependency longings and their use of the patient for their own gratification.

Fantasy that love in and of itself is curative. This theme is also closely related to conscious or unconscious childhood fantasies that persist in adult therapists. They may feel a deep conviction that they would have been much happier as adults if they had been loved as children. Similarly, therapists who transgress sexual boundaries with patients often harbor a belief that they can love the patient better than the patient's own parents did. Many films that feature sexual relationships between therapists and patients suggest that love itself is much more curative than any technique acquired through professional training. In Barbra Sterisand's 1991 film, *The Prince of Tides*, for example, the audience is left with the impression that Tom's improvement is primarily related to his love affair with his therapist, rather than to any insight or understanding related to the therapist's professional expertise.

Repression or disavowal of rage at patient's persistent thwarting of therapeutic efforts. For some therapists, the patient's improvement is essential to the therapist's self-esteem. When certain patients continue to deteriorate despite the therapist's most zealous efforts, some therapists may resort to sexual relationships out of despair at the frustration of their omnipotent strivings to heal (Searles, 1979). Their rage at the patient for failing to respond is buried beneath professions of love and caring.

Anger at organization, institute, or training analyst. When therapists work in institutional settings, they may develop bitterness and resentment based on their perception that the institution has mistreated them. Investigations of therapist-patient sex in such settings commonly reveal that anger has been acted out at the organization through the ethical transgression. In cases of pastoral counselors, resentment toward the church or a particular church official may be a fertile field for sexual misconduct. When an analyst is the transgressor anger at the training analyst or institute is often involved. Such behavior may also represent an unconscious fantasy of revenge against one's parents.

Manic defense against mourning and grief at termination. In every psychotherapy relationship, there is an inevitable loss. A paradox of the process is that if treatment goes well, the relationship must end. Neither the therapist nor the patient looks forward to dealing with feelings of grief and mourning at the time of termination. One defensive way to avoid such feelings is to deny the ending by beginning a new, personal relationship (Gabbard, 1990). Indeed, many cases of therapist-patient sex-begin as therapy is ending.

The exception fantasy. Some lovesick therapists convince themselves that their sexual relationship with a patient is somehow an exception to accepted ethical guidelines. Often these therapists will view the relationship as having transcended transference or counter-transference. They may view themselves and the patient as 'soulmates' who were destined to find each other and just happened to have done so in the context of a psychotherapy relationship. The love is regarded as so extraordinary that mundane ethical codes are irrelevant.

Insecurity regarding masculine identity. Male therapists who engage in sex with patients are often insecure about their maleness. Some may be seeking affirmation and validation for themselves as men because they feel they did not receive that sort of affirmation from their mother or father while growing up. The sexual gratification in such cases is secondary to a validation of their gender identity.

Patient as transformational object. Although it is tempting to draw parallels between the forbidden aspects of the oedipal situation in childhood and the boundary violations between therapist and patient as adults, clinical work with such therapists suggests that primitive preoedipal themes are prominent (Twemlow & Gabbard, 1989). One is the wish to be transformed by the patient. Bollas (1987) noted that the mother is initially experienced not so much as a separate person as a process of transformation: 'In adult life, the quest is not to possess the object; rather the object is pursued in order to surrender to it as a medium that alters the self' (p. 14). Hence, at the most fundamental level, the therapist may harbor the fantasy that the patient will be a love object that serves as an agent of magical change.

Settling down the 'rowdy' man. Although most of the literature on the dynamics of. therapist-patient sex has been focused on a male therapist involved with a female patient, female therapists are also prone to attempt misguided efforts to rescue male patients. In such scenarios, the patient tends to be a young man with a personality disorder diagnosis characterized by impulsivity, action orientation, and substance abuse (Gabbard, 1991a). Despite these characterologica symptoms, however, the young man usually possesses considerable interpersonal charm and may have a knack for engaging females in a treatment capacity. A female clinician is often drawn to such men with an unconscious fantasy that her love and attention will somehow influence this essentially decent young man to give up his wayward tendencies and 'straighten up' (Gabbard, 1991 b).

In American literature and film, there is a pervasive cultural myth that a 'rowdy' young man simply needs a 'good woman' to settle him down. At the beginning of Clint Eastwood's 1992 film, *Unforgiven*, for example, the protagonist repeatedly comments on how he was a cold-blooded murderer and a drunk until the right woman transformed him into a decent husband, father, and breadwinner. Another theme in these female therapist-male patient dyads relates to the woman's vicarious enjoyment of the danger and risk typified by her male patient's life-style.

Conflicts around sexual orientation. In same-sex dyads, some therapists will use a relationship with a patient as a way of acting out conflicts around their own sexual orientation. In the Benowitz (1991) study of 15 female therapist-female patient liaisons, 20% of the therapists identified themselves to patients as heterosexual, 20% as bisexual, and only 40% as clearly lesbian. Twenty percent said they had not been sexually involved with a woman before, and 33.3% demonstrated internal conflict around their sexual orientation or sexual behavior with women. Gonsiorek (1989) has noted a similar pattern in male therapist-male patient dyads.

Masochistic surrender

The last category involves certain therapists with fundamentally masochistic and self-destructive tendencies who allow themselves to be intimidated and controlled by a patient, even though they know the deleterious consequences of their actions. I am not using 'masochistic' here in the Freudian sense of deriving pleasure from pain. Rather, I am describing a relational mode in which the therapist, usually male, allows himself to be tormented by the patient. In the typical scenario, these therapists feel badgered into increasingly escalating boundary violations as a way to prevent suicide (Eyman & Gabbard, 1991). The patient, often an incest victim, may suffer from syndromes such as posttraumatic stress disorder, dissociative disorder, or borderline personality disorder. As a result, the patient may demand some concrete demonstration of love so that the therapist extends hours, holds the patient during sessions, accepts frequent late-night telephone calls, and even gives free therapy. Therapists who fit this category attempt to accommodate these demands, even though they know better. They often feel that they have no choice. The therapist soon learns that the patient's demands are bottomless and endless and begins to feel tormented. Demands to be held escalate to demands for sexual contact that the therapist feels compelled to oblige.

These therapists characteristically have problems dealing with their own aggression. Setting limits on the patient feels as though it is sadistic. As the patient's demands escalate, the therapist uses reaction formation to defend against growing resentment and hatred toward the patient. Just at the point when the therapist's resentment is reaching monumental proportions, the patient may accuse the therapist of not caring. In such confrontations, therapists often feel that their negative feelings have been exposed. The ensuing guilt feelings lead them to accede to the patient's demands, so that aggression in either member of the dyad is kept at bay.

Clinical work with such therapists commonly reveals an over-identification of the therapist with the patient. In many cases, both parties have childhood histories of abuse. Because of this over-identification, these therapists. try to gratify the patient's entitlement to be compensated for suffering as a child. Like lovesick therapists, masochistic therapists may be reenacting their own childhood abuse in addition to the patient's. Unlike lovesick therapists, however, they are not in love with the patient and often feel that they are being 'dragged down' by the patient. Some therapists who have masochistically surrendered in this manner describe dissociation or depersonalization during the sexual episode. They feel as though they are just going through the motions of sex or are doing so in an altered state of consciousness.

Many of these therapists recognize the unethical nature of the sexual activity after it has happened, and they attempt to stop the therapy and seek help for themselves. In hope of receiving help, they may masochistically turn themselves in to licensing boards or ethics committees. When litigation enters the picture, they often fare far worse than therapists who are psychopathic predators because they are much less manipulative and. they deal with the proceedings in a straightforward and honest manner.

Conclusion

These categories and the psychodynamic themes that accompany them should be considered tentative hypotheses that require further confirmation. There may well be other sexually exploitative therapists who 'fall through the cracks' and who require new categories to describe them. In addition to the heuristic value of attempting to classify such therapists, these groupings are useful in identifying which of the sexually transgressing therapists are likely to benefit from treatment and rehabilitation.

The psychopathic predators are almost always refractory to treatment because they either deny the patient's allegations or do not view them as problematic and requiring treatment. These therapists clearly should not continue in the mental health field. Although *some* persons suffering from paraphilias may be treatable in *some* settings, they, too, should not work in a field in which intense and highly intimate relationships are part of the daily practice.

Certain lovesick therapists are also unlikely to be treatable when they are in the throes of infatuation with their patient. They may be puzzled that anybody would suggest treatment for such an ecstatic mutual experience. Because they regard their love as unrelated to transference or countertransference issues, they view psychotherapy as having no purpose. When the infatuation dissipates, however, many of the lovesick therapists then have greater insight into their folly and may be amenable to psychotherapy or psychoanalysis as a way of helping them understand what intrapsychic issues made them vulnerable to such an unethical transgression. Those therapists who have been involved in a masochistic surrender scenario generally are filled with remorse and eager to receive treatment so that they do not repeat such self-destructive behavior.

Even with successful treatment, therapists who have acted on sexual feelings with patients should consider themselves at high risk for repeating the transgression. In most cases, they, should probably avoid, conducting psychotherapy and instead should confinetheir work to less intense forms of clinical practice.

References

Apfel, R.J., & Simon, B. (1985). Patient-therapist contact: I. Psychodynamic perspectives on the causes and results. *Psychotherapy and Psychosomatics, 43,* 57–62.

Averill, S.A., Beale, D., Benfer, B., Collins, D.T., Kennedy, L., Myers, J., Pope, D., Rosen, I., & Zoble, E. (1989). Preventing staff-patient sexual relationships. *Bulletin of the Menninger Clinic, 53,* 384–393.

Benowitz. M.S. (1991. May). *Sexual exploitation of female clients by female. psychotherapists: Interviews with clients and a comparison to women exploited by male psychotherapists.* Unpublished doctoral dissertation, University of Minnesota, Minneapolis.

Blum, H.P (1973). The concept of erotized transference. *Journal of the American Psychoanalytic Association. 21,* 61–76.

Bollas, C. (1987). *The shadow of the object: Psychoanalysis of the unthought known.* New York: Columbia University Press.

Eastwood, C. (Director). (1992). *Unforgiven.* Warner Brothers.

Eyman, J.R., & Gabbard, G.O. (1991). Will therapist-patient sex prevent suicide? *Psychiatric Annals, 21,* 669–674.

Freud, S. (1953). Three essays on the theory of sexuality. In J. Strachey (Ed. and Trans.), *The standard edition of the complete psychological works of Sigmund Freud* (Vol. 7, pp. 123–245). London: Hogarth Press. (Original work published in 1905)

Gabbard, G.O. (Ed.). (1989). *Sexual exploitation in professional relationships.* (Washington, DC: American Psychiatric Press.

Gabbard, G.O. (1990). *Psychodynamic psychiatry in clinical practice.* Washington, DC: American Psychiatric Press.

Gabbard, G.O. (1991a). Psychodynamics of sexual boundary violations. *Psychiatric Annals, 21,* 651–655.

Gabbard, G.O. (1991b). Sexual misconduct by female therapists: The love cure fantasy. *The Psychodynamic Letter, 1(6),* 1–3.

Gabbard, G.O. (in press). When the therapist is a patient: Special challenges in the psychoanalytic treatment of mental health professionals. *Psychoanalytic Review.*

Gabbard, G.O., & Wilkinson, S.M. (1994). *Management of countertransference borderline patients.* Washington, DC: American Psychiatric Press.

Gartrell, N., Herman, J., Olarte, S., Feldstein, M., & Localio, R. (1986). Psychiatrist-patient sexual contact: Results of a national survey, I: Prevalence. *American Journal of Psychiatry, 143,* 1126–1131.

Gonsiorek, J. (1989). Sexual exploitation by psychotherapists: Male victims. In G.R. Schoener, J.H. Milgrom, J.C. Gonsiorek, E.T. Luepker, & R.M. Conroe (Eds.), *Psychotherapists' sexual involvement with clients; Intervention and prevention* (pp. 113–119). Minneapolis, MN: Walk-in Counseling Center.

Gutheil, T.G., & Gabbard, G.O. (1992). Obstacles to the dynamic understanding of therapist-patient sexual relations. *American Journal of Psychotherapy, 46,* 515–525.

Kluft, R.P. (1989). Treating the patient who has been sexually exploited by a previous therapist. *Psychiatric Clinics of North America, 12,* 483–500.

Lyn, L. (1990, September). *Life in the fishbowl: Lesbian and gay therapists' social interactions with clients.* Unpublished master's thesis, Southern Illinois University, Carbondale.

Meloy, J.R. (1988). *The psychopathic mind: Origins, dynamics, and treatment.* Northvale, NJ:Aronson.

Olarte, S.W. (1991). Characteristics of therapists who become involved in sexual boundary violations. *psychiatric Annals, 21,* 657–660.

Pope, K.S., & Bouhoutsos, J. (1986). *Sexual intimacy between therapists and patients.* New York:Praeger.

Schoener, G.R., Milgrom, J.H., Gonsiorek, J.C, Luepker, E.T., & Conroe, R.M. (Eds.). (1989). *Psychotherapists' sexual involvement with clients: Interventions and prevention.* Minneapolis, MN: Walk-in Counseling Center.

Schwartz, M.F. (1992). Sexual compulsivity as post-traumatic stress disorder: Treatment perspectives. *Psychiatric Annals, 22,* 333–338.

Searles, H.F. (1979). *Countertransference and related subjects.* New York: International Universities Press.

Streisand, B. (Director), (1991). *The prince of tides.* Columbia Pictures.

Sullivan, H.S. (1954). *The psychiatric interview.* New York: Norton.

Sussman, M.B. (1992). *A curious calling: Unconscious motivations for practicing psychotherapy.* Northvale, NJ: Aronson.

Twemlow, S.W., & Gabbard, G.O. (1989). The lovesick therapist. In G.O. Gabbard (Ed.), *Sexual exploitation in professional relationships* (pp. 71–87). Washington, DC: American Psychiatric Press.

In the Service of the State:

*The Psychiatrist as Double Agent**

A Conference on Conflicting Loyalties cosponsored by the American Psychiatric Association and The Hastings Center, March 24–26, 1977

Introduction

This conference had its origin five years ago when the misuse of Soviet psychiatry in relationship to political dissenters was brought to the attention of the Board of Trustees of the American Psychiatric Association. In the course of Board discussion, however, it became clear that the fundamental problem was a much deeper one, cutting across national boundaries and entering into many different aspects of psychiatric practice in our own country as well as elsewhere.

For example, consider military psychiatrists – are their primary loyalties to the soldier or to the armed forces? Psychiatrists in prisons – whom do they serve, the prison officials, society, or the prisoner? Psychiatrists in schools – whose interests are they serving, those of the children, parents, or of the school administration? Psychiatrists in mental hospitals – do they not also get caught in conflicts between the interests of the patient, those of the institution, and those of society? Even psychiatrists in private practice are caught in conflicting roles with to regard confidentiality – when does loyalty to society transcend loyalty to the issues of privacy and confidentiality?

Indeed, the issue of conflicting loyalties is by no means confined to the psychiatrist. It is an issue that confronts lawyers, accountants, internists, surgeons, and many other professionals.

The APA Board finally decided to sponsor a research project to investigate the conflicting roles of psychiatirsts in mental institutions. This was to be a broad-based exploration focused upon but not necessarily limited to processes in our own country. However, when the research project was presented to the Board, it became clear from the composition of the investigating team that the project was designed to be an adversarial muckraking investigation rather than an objective scientific exploration. Thus, when the Board rejected the proposal it was not, as asserted at the time, by our good friend Judge David Bazelon, out of psychiatry's fear of investigating itself. Rather, it was out of a more fundamental concern that the research proposal that was offered would simply add to the troubles of an already beleaguered profession without contributing significantly to the basic underlying issues.

To put the matter in other terms, there is no disagreement about the fact that conflicting role behavior does exist in our profession as well as in others. The real question in documenting such conflicts is to explore the underlying matrix that contributes to such conflicts and to try to answer the questions of how and if such conflicts can be resolved. This conference is a first step in the process.

Judd Marmor

From its inception, The Hastings Center has been concerned with the moral problems inherent in the capacity to influence and change human behavior. Modern technology – the development of drugs, electrode implantations, psychosurgery, the use, of operant conditioning, and the like – has dramatized problems that have lain dormant in the traditional methods of controlling and changing human behavior.

Under the comfortable illusion of being a value-free discipline in a period that still accepted the concept of a value-free science, psychiatry ignored the immense ethical and moral implications of its activity. We were therapists, ministers of medicine, not of the soul; servants of the body and its extension, 'the mind' – divorced from both ethical and political concerns. Had these views ever been put into explicit language, their incredibly naive assumptions would have immediately been exposed.

In the past, the psychiatrist examined the question of whom he served only in rare and extreme cases – 'of course' he served the intentions and purposes of his patient except in such extreme cases as potential suicide or violence. Even under these circumstances, the psychiatrist confronted the problems reluctantly and as a last resort, assuming he still served the 'real' desires of his temporarily aberrant charge.

He assumed, for the most part, that his practice was free of moral dilemma. But, by building a body of psychology that defined normalcy in all areas of behavior and action, he had constructed a coercive tool beyond electrodes and surgical scalpels, and was using that tool to fashion a model of behavior for others.

We have, however, entered a new period in the relationship between society and science. It is a general period of reassessment. While this conference focuses on the central position of the psychiatrist, he is not alone. It is the reevaluation of the whole practice of medicine that brings these issues of conflicting loyalties before the psychiatrist.

When the exploitation of Russian psychiatry by the Soviet state became obvious, the first response of American psychiatry was disbelief, and then outrage. With condemnation, however, came the recognition that a reevaluation of American psychiatry's own confused role in relationship to the society in which it exists and to the values of that society was long overdue.

The problem that we at The Hastines Center had traditionally called the 'double agent problem' is really a problem of multiple agentry, of conflicting responsibilities and confused loyalties, of undefined purposes and contradictory goals. It is important and significant tnat the American Psychiatric Association has decided to examine its own role in this area. Whatever its dilemmas, they are not unique. Psychiatry can become, therefore, a paradigm, an example, and a guide for other medical specialties to reexamine the tacit conditions, the hidden scenarios, and the unsigned contracts that exist in the dramatically changing world of patient and physician.

Willard Gaylin

Moral Dilemmas in Military Practice

Arlene Kaplan Daniels: Any helping profession in which advice and control functions are entwined will have many moral dilemmas. One of the problems in studying those moral dilemmas is that practitioners find it difficult

* In the service of the state: the psychiatrist as double agent. *Hastings Center Reports, Special Supplement*, April 1978, S1–23.

perceive a conflict between advice and control, and to understand the amount and extent of their coercive powers and functions over clients.

Waldo Burchard, a fellow sociologist, has written on the role conflicts of the military chaplain. How did military chaplains resolve the conflict between their assignments and the Ten Commandments that they were nominally expected to support? Chaplains in effect told Burchard, 'I don't see any problem here. There is no inflict. Young men must go to war and fight for their country.' Burchard created a problem where none existed. The chaplains saw no real conflict between military service and the injunction 'Thou shall not kill.' In consequence, chaplains saw no responsibility to encourage recruits to escape from service through reasons of conscience. The same sort of situation arises for the military psychiatrist. The dedicated military psychiatrist can explain why he believes that there are no conflicts between responsibility as a physician to preserve life and his duties as an officer, requiring soldiers to risk life.

One barrier to recognizing the conflict is the founding myth of psychiatry. For the psychiatrist, that myth is focused not on great administrative or institutional psychiatrists, but on Freud – the private practitioner helping, consoling, advising, and offering interpretations. When a psychiatrist enters the field, he is following the private practitioner model. Even those in veterans' hospitals and military residencies think of themselves in that kind of practice. And that is an advisory model, not a coercive one. Operating on such a model, psychiatrists usually do not see evidence of the difficulties or strains in their who work in prisons, in state mental hospitals, and the military have a tendency, to ignore or minimize the amount of time they spend at coercive functions and in helping institutions control others.

Thomas Scheff pointed out in his book *Being Mentally III* that psychiatrists participating in lunacy commission hearings always complained that the state did not give them enough money to do their investigations. They said, 'I can't spend an hour with each client examining the case. I'd be lucky if I could spend as much as a half hour or forty-five minutes.' But when Scheff timed them, psychiatrists were spending less than ten minutes on each client to discover signs of mental illness. Now when that little time is spent investigating a case, there is an enormous temptation to follow the bent of the agency (here, to remove' troublesome persons from the society); for such decisions will remain unquestioned. In the military, my informants could find patients not mentally ill in about same amount of time because the needs of *their* institution (to retain soldiers rather than excuse them from duty) forces such a direction.

The difficulties facing psychiatrists in understanding their role (as agents of social control) when they make decisions for institutions are compounded by their place in medicine – a profession with exalted status. The aura surrounding the physician extends to the psychiatric specialty and encourages people to come to the psychiatrist for help rather than to go, say, to faith healers. When they do consult the psychiatrist, clients are in a desperate state and do not have the same kind of power as clients consulting other professionals. A client who comes to a CPA for help with tax returns does not relinquish the same kind of control over his affairs as a client who comes to a psychiatrist. No matter how enlightened we are now about mental illness, a patient's judgment is under question when consulting a psychiatrist. If not crazy, the patient is, at the least, not in a condition to show good judgment. Thus a psychiatrist's view is likely to be more powerful in opposition to a patient, particularly in institutional settings where the countervailing power of the private patient (who may refuse payment) is absent. In this context, even efforts to protect patients can have adverse consequences.

Confidentiality is one practice designed to safeguard patient rights in either private or institutional care. The good thing about confidentiality is that it preserves the secrets of clients. The bad part is that it protects the psychiatrist from the kind of independent observation important to any system of accountability. And the problem is exacerbated in a field where little agreement exists about the standards every therapist should meet.

I asked a panel of experts in one of my studies to suggest techniques they thought the majority of the field would agree to as acceptable. They agreed on a set of conditions under which electro-convulsive therapy should be used. Yet in my study of 100 psychiatrists, I found that a third agreed about

use of this therapy, a third disagreed, and a third weren't sure. Even with the help of a panel of experts, I could not discover any practices about which there was substantial agreement in the field.

Against this background, what are the dilemmas of the military psychiatrist? The greatest dilemma is that this agent of social control is himself controlled. Yet the military psychiatrist holds the illusion that except for the areas where the military component requires certain decisions, he is really quite independent. The combination of service to the institution and his own discretionary activity in the time remaining is entirely up to him.

One of the bad things about professional training is that it creates the belief that professional discretion can be used in a wide variety of areas that, in fact, are quite questionable. During the Vietnam war, psychiatrists supportive of the government often told me that they refused to find young men mentally ill when asked for excuses to avoid service. And these psychiatrists would say, 'I don't have the right to make these decisions'; in effect, they were making judgments just as were psychiatrists opposing the government who said, 'Every young man who comes to me will get an excuse to get out of service'. There is a great difference in being a conscientious objector and using the cloak of expertise to flout and evade the law. I would consider that a real moral dilemma which these men, though I questioned them about it closely, did not see. In sum, I have the same problem Waldo Burchard had; I expected to find professional concerned about moral conflicts and I did not.

Willard Gaylin: Would you outline for us the conclusions of your studies on the military so that some of us who are not familiar with them can learn what the military psychiatrist sees the moral dilemmas to be, what he sees they are not, and what in reality they are?

Daniels: The conflict centers on being an agent of the military – an agent who forces men into a service they do not want to face. Let me mention one of the difficulties about even describing this conflict. I wrote a paper about these moral conflicts with a military psychiatrist. We wanted to list them in a series. I said the chief one was sending men back to possible death. He said, 'No, you can't put that in the paper, you must call it arduous duty.' I said, 'No, Colonel, to me arduous duty means cleaning the garbage cans all night or having a bivouac in the middle of winter in Alaska.' That was our last collaboration. The problem was to get the military psychiatrists to look squarely at the issue, and that in itself is a moral dilemma.

Gaylin: What does the military psychiatrist owe to the army, the government, the just war, and what does he owe to the patient? Do you think there should be no military psychiatrists, surgeons, internists, chaplains? Do you think they should exist? If so, then what ought to be their responsibility?

Daniels: Let me put it this way: once the psychiatrist is in the military, he has very little leeway. He can perform his duties more or less humanely or conscientiously, and that is his personal choice. The dilemma is whether or not psychiatry should be used for these kinds of purposes. Psychiatrists had this kind of conflict over the abortion issue before the 1973 Supreme Court ruling. It is a good parallel to the issue of whether the psychiatrist should serve in the military and be used to diagnose men well enough to return to battle. If it wished, the profession could say it was not in the position to make those kinds of decisions. I am not arguing that this is necessarily a good idea; I am saying that these are the kinds of questions psychiatry could face.

David Mechanic: One principle that could be applied is consistency. Indeed, if psychiatrists have a role and a position independent of any institution they serve, consistency of practice is understood as part of the role. I don't know military psychiatry except through the literature, but I understand that it has one policy that is particularly inconsistent. Psychiatrists identify potential troublemakers in a very early stage of military service, people who have caused more trouble than provided functional service. They are removed from service not to help them, not to diminish their despair, but to make that organization more efficient.

Once these people have been excluded from the organization, the military then moves to a contrasting policy: now there is a body of men who are likely to provide more performance than cost. No longer is the policy to remove them quickly; the emphasis is now on maintaining their functioning. Policies are designed to keep the soldier performing by telling him that everyone else experiences distress, that everyone else has symptoms like his.

Alan Stone: Fifteen years ago the military operated the way David describes, but not now. It is clear that the army had an interest in preventing people from developing a service connected disability. They want to spot these people and get them out as soon as possible because after a designated time the presumption is that a disability is service-connected.

When there is a war and psychiatry becomes a way out of the war, there are conflicts because the psychiatrist controls the gates to a scarce resource, and it is fraught with conflict It would be useful to look at the constraints on the psychiatrist in that situation. When the constraint is that the country is at war, and the psychiatrist is concerned about a problem being used as a way to avoid military service, there is a tremendous conflict between that constraint and the idea doctor-patient relationship.

Gerald Klerman: The psychiatrist or any other professional in the double-agent situation always has a dilemma when he is not in concordance with the values of the agency. The typical example conjured up is the psychiatrist in the military who feels a tension with the stated grounds of the military at a particular historical moment, like the Vietnam war.

Consider the alternative situation where the psychiatrist is ideologically in agreement with the military, as were many psychiatrists in World War II. For those people there was no doubt that the psychiatrist had a moral obligation to the society; for them that moral obligation may have had a higher moral value than the obligation to the distressed single individual. For the military psychiatrist it was not a question of being an agent of an immoral or non-moral situation, it was a dilemma between two moral commitments: loyalty to a set of values threatened in a wartime situation and loyalty to the value of treating individuals who may or may not be in distress. The double-agent problem is qualitatively different, depending upon whether the psychiatrist is committed to a moral situation. One may disagree with him as to whether he should be in a agreement with the goals of that society at that point, but from his point of view it is not immoral to urge a particular soldier to go back to the front lines. Those are two very different situations and I don't know of any external body of data that would help resolve that dilemma.

Eliot Freidson: Those who practice psychiatry, medicine, law, or the ministry all presume in Western society that they have a relationship with individuals, a relationship in which individuals should trust them because the professional is concerned with their welfare. This trust and confidence is predicated on the assumption that the professionals are on that individual's side. In an institution the professional's loyalties are divided. For me the moral dilemma lies not in the *division* of loyalty, but in relying on the historical assumption of trust. The *Miranda* warning might be a good model for thinking about the problem.

The moral issue is not that a psychiatrist may be committed to sending the troops back to the front line, but that an individual may have an unfounded trust in the professional's *lack* of such a duty. Shouldn't you give them a *Miranda* warning at the very outset, namely, 'Anything you say may be used to send you back to the front lines, or anything you say may keep you in prison'? That is better than allowing them to assume that you are on their side, that they can say anything to you, that what is said will be kept in confidence and will be used only to *their* benefit, and not to the benefit of the institution or organization.

Klerman: Is it possible to separate the clinical role from the administrative one? In general, we in psychiatry have a tremendous propensity to mix these roles. We want to treat people clinically, but we also want to save the world. We do this everywhere: in schools, in prisons in the military. Now if we knew more precisely what some of these conflicts were and could distinguish them, it might be possible to devise distinct roles. For instance, one psychiatrist would treat a schizophrenic in the military and treat him as he would in civilian practice. Somebody else could decide when he goes back to duty or when he is to be discharged. If psychiatrists were clear about the decision they are supposed to make, they would be better off.

Melvin Sabshin: I want to mention the Howard Levy case in the context of concordance versus nonconcordance. Gerald Klerman's classification is useful to look at those situations where the physician's opinion is not in accord with the military code. Levy was said to be in violation of the uniform code of military justice. In the 1960s the AMA stated that there was no conflict between the ethics of the medical profession and the oath which officers must take when sworn into the armed services. It is very interesting to look at that opinion and trace its consequences.

Paul Friedman: I find myself troubled by the argument that if the psychiatrist sees himself as an agent of the military and is in harmony with the agency's values at that time, then he has no moral dilemma. Subjectively, that is true. The psychiatrist doesn't *feel* in moral conflict. But what about the soldier being treated?

Let's say it's World War II. We all think it is a good war and the military wants as many troops as possible on the line. The psychiatrist believes in those values and is not aware of a moral dilemma. But the soldier might well come to the psychiatrist with the expectation that his relationship would be more or less the same kind of exclusive relationship he has been led to expect exists in the private sector. It might be helpful if someone would try to distinguish between moral dilemmas and role conflicts or clashes. The psychiatrist in this hypothetical situation has no role conflict, but the moral dilemma remains because the psychiatrist is giving the soldier what the army wants and not what the soldier wants.

Gaylin: Let me try to summarize the discussion. There is an assumption by nonphysicians that the physician serves the interests, purposes, values, and desires of his patients. The physicians don't see that at all. They believe that they serve the values of their profession. If a patient comes to us and desires ill health, we do not serve that. If he wishes to be mutilated, we don't do that. If he wants amphetamines so he can run faster, we don't serve that. The physician never primarily serves the interests, desires, values of his patient, he serves the interests, desires, values of his profession.

Now that is still not a great problem because, as Eliot Freidson pointed out, the average patient who goes to the average physician also assumes the values of the profession. The problem comes when the values of the profession are in conflict with the values of the institutional setting.

Judd Marmor: Isn't the basic moral dilemma between a relativistic approach to morals and an absolute one? As Arlene pointed out, in certain situations a psychiatrist may not experience any moral conflict because he feels he is serving a particular moral good. Morals in general are not absolute. They serve the purpose of the society in which they have developed. In China the overriding value is to preserve the society and its homogeneity. In a democratic society the moral values seem to serve individual interests. In hierarchical societies in general the values tend to be those of subservience to authority.

The military is a hierarchical society and the dominant value is that of serving the values of the hierarchy. Everyone in the military who is part of the institutional hierarchy is expected to serve that moral value. The psychiatrist who becomes a military physician is part of that system. What we are doing over and over again is posing some kind of unspoken, absolute moral value against this relativism.

Freidson: There is a critical missing element in this discussion. We are talking about abstractions, not human beings. Basically, any practicing professional, no matter what he is – physician, teacher, priest, or psychiatrist – assumes some degree of trust and confidence on the part of an individual so that he can assume he will get reasonably full and accurate information. If somebody connected with an institution is essentially committed to advancing that institution's activities, then the practitioner has no right to expect the individual to be free and open with information.

The *Miranda* warning is important as a model because it is *understood* that the police and state attorneys are there to collect evidence about somebody's guilt. It is their obligation to warn the suspect that anything he says might be held against him, to remind him of their commitment to the goal of law enforcement. The duty of the police is to society, to justice, or to the law, and not to the personal advantage of a suspect; the individual is being weighted in the balance.

Now a psychiatrist in the military has made his choice and serves its goals. We needn't criticize that choice here, at least for the time being. But too often the presumption is made that he can eat his cake and have it too. On the one hand, he expects full and complete information based on trust and has only contempt and hostility for individual who refuse to cooperate with him. But the individual soldier is quite right not to trust him. It is the relationship involved and the presumptions of these relationships that underlie the moral issues, and we must keep that relationship at the forefront of our conversation.

Daniels: Not only am I in complete agreement with Eliot, but I would like to add something about moral issues being lumped together with technical issues. I am concerned with the way uncertainty is related to moral dilemmas. To the extent that it is unclear what the theory or practice ought to be in a particular situation, it becomes that much easier for moral issues to be mingled with factual ones. All kinds of moral judgements are mixed together with what are supposed to be scientific predictions. Though lots of people play God in the professions, psychiatrists, more than many other kinds of practitioners, take upon themselves the task of making certain kinds of predictions with all sorts of fateful outcomes when there is no reason to belive they really can predict.

A lot of this is crystal ball gazing. Psychiatry has brought upon itself some of the moral dilemmas we are looking at; it is willing to make decisions for the society based on assumptions about scientific data which are not there.

Psychiatrists in Prisons

Robert A. Burt: Why might prison psychiatrists feel role conflict or special moral tension in their work? The typical argument is that psychiatrists in prisons are forced to serve two antagonistic interests – society's interest in social control and the criminal/patient's interest in being free from such control – and that this creates a 'role conflict.' But what psychiatrist can take sides with criminal conduct – at least involving violence – not just in his 'personal capacity' but in his professional capacity? What psychiatrist can ever take sides with his patient's violent, infantile psychic elements? A psychiatrist is professionally trained and committed to take sides with the verbalizing, rational, self-controlling adult developmental potentials in his patient, and against the acting out, irrational, dependent, infantile, regressive potential.

Psychiatrists in prisons face special problems, and I believe these problems do cluster around notions of 'role conflict,' but not because of the stereotyped view. The conflict in prison occurs because the psychiatrist has more difficulty than in private practice in fostering 'adult' behavior in his prisoner patient, and therefore siding with society's interests in social control and bringing his patient to embrace this normative postion with him and the rest of society.

In private practice, the psychiatrist rarely 'chooses sides' to favor 'adult behavior' against his patient's interest or self-definition, because the typical patient is conflicted precisely on this question and this conflict is more or less accessible to the patient's conscious awareness. Thus in response to the charge that the psychiatrist is 'taking sides' against his patient, the psychiatrist can quite properly respond, 'How can I take sides against the patient when the patient clearly doesn't know which side he's on?'

But insofar as typical convicted criminals have personality structures that 'have taken sides' – insofar as they do experience any inkling of conflict about their antisocial behavior – the psychiatrist's normative stance is more stark. The viewpoint that criminals are 'sociopathic personalities' who do not feel conflict and thus are necessarily 'untreatable' is much disputed in psychiatric literature. But if this proposition is true, then the source for 'role conflict' of the psychiatrist in prison is clear: there is nothing he can do, in his role as a psychiatrist, in a prison. Thus he must ask himself, if he is not there as a psychiatrist, what is his 'role'?

This clinical view of 'sociopathy' and its 'treatability' may be too rigid, and quite wrong. But this much is clear: successful psychiatrist treatment of

prisoners is very difficult. And this fact inspires feelings of profound demoralization for any psychiatrist practicing in a prison setting.

The basic source for this demoralization, I think, comes from a question that philosophers at least since Plato have posed: is it possible to be a 'just man' in an 'unjust society'? I am not suggesting that our society is unjust and that prisons enforcing the norms of that society are also necessarily unjust, though the popular currency of that notion does play some limited role in creating moral tension for those who work in prisons. I mean this question in two more prosaic senses. First, is it possible to be a 'good man' when you feel you are doing a 'bad job'? Second, is it possible to be a 'good man' when you feel you are 'bad place'?

Whatever one might say about the ultimate justice of the norms that prisons enforce in this society (and I think it indisputable that norms against murder, rape, and arson, for example, are quintessentially just), nonetheless it is hard for any psychiatrist to avoid feeling that he is doing a 'bad job,' because criminal offenders are so difficult to treat and so scorned and feared by society. It is hard for anyone to avoid feeling that prisons are 'bad places' in which to work, because they are frightening, violence-and-hate-filled institutions.

If it is true that prisons are inherently demoralizing work-places for psychiatrists, can psychiatrists preserve their their personal and professional integrity only by withdrawing prison work? Most psychiatrists in this country seem implicitly or explicitly to have reached this conclusion. But I don't think this proposition necessarily follows. Prison work is demoralizing for everybody involved, wardens and guards as well as psychiatrists. For psychiatrists to withdraw in order to protect their moral purity constitutes a chilling judgement, and a somewhat supercilious moral posturing.

But still this problem of role definition remains: What is there for a psychiatrist, as a psychiatrist, to do in a prison? If there is such a professional role, that role must be clearly differentiated from the role of other persons in the prison such as the wardens or the guards (or, I would also say, the inmates). Thus inevitable so-called 'confusion of roles' which may be tolerable in private practice should be more starkly differentiated, however arbitrarily, in prison practice.

Yet even here there are considerable problems. Take the confidentiality rule. Civil commitment statutes provide blatant exceptions to this rule in all psychiatric practice. But one might argue that these statutes are tolerable precisely because the typical private patient rarely thinks about them and they are rarely invoked by private practitioners; whereas in prisons squealing to the warden by the prison psychiatrist is a more palpable and thus more intrusive possibility for both prisoner/patient and psychiatrist.

But adopting a rigid confidentiality rule for prison psychiatrists brings this problems: if a prisoner/patient tells the psychiatrist that he is planning to murder a guard, how is the psychiatrist able to free himself from complicity in the crime – not simply complicity in a general 'moral' sence but also in a specially 'anti-therapeutic' sence (which may be the same thing)? If the psychiatrist keeps silent, will not his patient who has offered this confidence then view the psychiatrist as having taken sides with his infantile, violent, out-of-control psychic elements, and will not the very purpose of the therapeutic encounter be endangered if not defeated? This is what I meant when I said that psychiatrists must have a role definition that differentiates them not only from prison guards but also from inmates, their patients.

Many times in prison settings, prisoners act to test the corruptibility of their psychiatrists and their guards precisely in order to create moral tension in these 'representatives of law and order,' precisely in order to lure them into behaviour that makes *them* feel guilty. Corruption and criminality are 'in the air' in prisons, and these are highly communicable diseases. They bring what may be the worst role conflict for the prison psychiatrist – that he is led to feel he is acting like his patients, rather than as a responsible, morally upright member of the broader society. Though this may sound paradoxical, I believe that the most intolerable feeling of role conflict for a psychiatrist in prison comes precisely when he feels unable to act as society's agent (in the sense of representing law-abiding values) and is trapped into acting as his prisoner/patient's agent (in the sense of acting as this criminal offender's *alter ego*).

I don't want to end on a hopeless note. There is one route for psychiatric professional role redefinition that could significantly ameliorate the role conflict problems of psychiatrist in prisons: reduce the grandiosity of claims for psychiatric capacities in prisons to very modest and readily defensible proportions. Whatever moral tension comes from doing a 'bad job' in a 'bad place,' I belive that even greater tension comes from pretending that things are better than they are. This pretense is clearly expressed, indeed grandiosely expressed, by statutes or other institutional arrangements that give special roles to psychiatrists in prisons.

The recently repealed Maryland stature that created Patuxent as an institution for 'dangerous defective delinquents' is not unique in giving psychiatrists and their behavioral colleagues an explicit 'gatekeepers role' for the prisons. Compare for example, the role of the so-called California Medical Facility at Vacaville in presiding over the indeterminate sentence in that state. The demoralization that comes either from acknowledging or struggling to avoid acknowledging one's hypocrisy is, I think an important underlying explanation for the extraordinary brutality against inmate populations that has been documented in places like Vacaville – brutality inflicted not by so-called 'sadistic and uneducated' guards, but by professional behaviorists, by Ph.D. psychologists, and by M.D. psychiatrist, purporting to act in behalf of scientific norms.

The organized profession of psychiatry can protect the professional and personal integrity of its practitioners in prison work by fighting openly for a self-consciously modest role and for elimination of the statutes and administrative practices that embody these self-defeating claims for psychiatric infallibility. If it is true that all psychiatrists necessarily speak in there dealings with all patients on behalf of societal values such as controlling violence and maintaining respect for others, and are to that extent 'prison wardens' that is still no reason for any psychiatrist to define himself solely and simply as a prison warden. Even if eliminating these statutes will not make prisons a 'good place' for psychiatrists to work, and thus eliminate the basic source for role conflict, this reform will make prisons a 'better place' for psychiatrists. And that in itself is worth doing.

Robert Michels: Although I would not argue that the psychiatrist should be morally purer than the prison guard, there may be an important social reason for the psychiatrist, unlike the prison guard, to be, like Caesar's wife, above suspicion. For that reason, he may need to remove himself from the mess in order to protect the values of professionals outside the prison and the perceived trust psychiatrists must have from the public.

I would like to offer a series of model here. We start with a patient, client, customer, or prisoner who has some psychiatric condition. When they conflict with each other, we get into trouble. One model is the patient's (or client's or customer's) desired state – what he hopes for. Another is the psychiatrist's model of health – what the psychiatrist hopes for. The third is a psychiatrist's reasonable expectation of the results of treatment – where he thinks he will end up regardless of what he hopes for. A fourth is society's model of health – what it hopes for. A fifth is society's potential role available for that individual – what they will tolerate as opposed to what they hope for. In the situations we have been talking about, the army and the prison, those models are very different from each other. Society's potential role for the individual is strikingly different from the psychiatrist's model of health, and both might be strikingly different from the patient's desired state. All kind of conflicts thus occur.

In the idealized (and nonexistent) private practice situation that we are using as our prototype, all these things are so congruent that we don't even notice that they are different: what the patient wants, and what the psychiatrist wants, and what the psychiatrist expects, and what society hopes for, and what society will tolerate are all the same and we happily proceed with treatment without worrying about conflict. What Burt is saying is that prisons are like Klerman's society, in which the social norm is different from the psychiatrist's value system. And it doesn't seem to me that his prison is significantly different on that problem than an evilsociety anywhere. I assume from your comments, Bo Burt, that you think prisons

are evil societies, and that they therefore in microcosm raise the problems Gerry Klerman was talking about. It seems to me that this approach might help generalize the issues to the world outside prison, where psychiatrists really work since they have fled those prisons.

Hannah Levin: There is a definite difference between practicing in an institution and outside, and I don't think that the moral questions are the same. In an institution the psychiatrist has an incredible amount of power and sanction and the patient-client has no freedom at all to make decisions. There is no counterbalance to the power of the mental health professional.

Another potential abuse is the many conflicting roles we attempt to assume in the criminal justice system. Lawyers represent criminals. That is their commitment, and they do the best job they can. Why can't the psychiatrist or any mental health professional accept that same kind of limited role and say, 'My commitment is to be the best representative for this patient.'

We would never accept a society where one person makes all the decisions about our lives, makes the rules and then decides whether we've broken them and then has the power to sentence us. And yet that is what we professionals are doing when we work in prisons.

Fritz Redlich: It has been said that psychiatric practice in a prison or a school is different from private practice. This need not be the case. I think very much the same contract could apply in all these settings. For instance, a serious risk of a crime would have to be reported, whether it is in private practice or in the prison.

The problem comes when a prison psychiatrist is asked for a recommendation by a parole board. He may have to give a recommendation which the prisoner may note like. I think that the psychiatrist should not even get into the situation. The psychiatrist who is treating the patient follows the contract with treatment, and another person should be involved in these administrative decisions. I think in all cases, even in private practice, I really would favor something resembling the *Miranda* doctrine. I would say to a patient, 'Look all you say is confidential, but just in case some very major antisocial behavior comes up, I would report it.' Now obviously you don't say this when a harmless person comes in for treatment and there is no such danger. But if any such danger begins to be detected, I think it is really an absolute rule that such a warning be given.

Stone: I have a student who spent several years in four different penitentiaries as a conscientious objector to the Vietnam war. He has a practical, sensible formula for doing what Professor Redlich has suggested. He says that prisoners should be given Medicaid and allowed to seek whatever medical help or psychiatric help that they want outside the institution. There should be no connection between the medical, the psychiatric, the rehabilitative, and the punitive arm of the prison.

There are people in prisons who might like to tale to a psychiatrist, not about what you're calling their 'infantile' side, but about something that is troubling them. They might not want to talk to the prison doctor, but they might want to go to a psychiatrist, a psychologist a sex therapist, or any one of a number of professionals. The private doctor or psychologist might still be in a situation where they might have a conflict over whether they should tell the warden that their patient is planning to kill a guard, who, by the way, might be a sadistic racist. They might still have a dilemma, but there would be lines drawn so that it is clear that they are not in the warden's pocket or in the parole's.

I feel very strongly that what Professor Redlich is saying is correct. I think that there should be a role distinction. That certain psychiatrists should have an 'I' for inquisitor on their forehead and that they should come with *Miranda* warning and say 'I am the one who talks to you for an administrative decision. I am the one who talks to you for administrative decision. I am the one who talks to you for a legal decision. I am the one who talks to you for a parole decision.' And there ought to be an effect to protect the therapeutic relationship of the others by allowing only such persons who are clearly in it.

Sabshin: Do prisoners have a 'right to treatment' in any way that is different from those outside prisons? The commonwealth of Virginia claimed in a recent suit that there was no obligation for the state to provide such treatment. The circuit court handed down an interesting ruling saying that Virginia is wrong. It does have an obligation under certain circumstances to provide treatment.

Burt: That is a large and complex area. For example, regarding psychosurgery I would differentiate between what a prisoner can request and receive and what would be available to people outside a prison. And I feel it's appropriate to ban experimental psychosurgery in prison not only because of the complexity of the consent issue, but also because of the destructive characteristics of prisons as institutions.

To turn that around, however, and say that there are some special rehabilitative procedures prisoners have a right to demand denied to people outside, is, I think, going too far what is the role of the rehabilitative ideal? Is there more harm than good in encouraging that notion within a prison setting? My initial sense is that, no, outright rejection of the rehabilitative stance is not a useful position regarding convicted criminal population group. On the other hand, I want to qualify that stance in a number of ways because I am troubled by the pretentiousness and the hypocrisy involved in prison rehabilitation.

Friedman: There have been some cases about a prisoner's right to rehabilitation. A couple of years ago in Alabama after Frank Johnson reformed the mental institutions, he wen on to the prisons system. In *Newman* v. *Alabama* he said that prisoners had a constitutional right to some kind of rehabilitation and to minimum adequate medical services which included psychiatric services. That doesn't mean the advocate groups for prisoners' right such as the ACLU National Prison Project won't take a position against this decision if it exposes prisoners to risk. Perhaps it would be better for prisoners not to expect rehabilitation in those settings. What is clear is that a prisoner can either have problems relating to the antisocial criminal behaviors which get him into prison in the first place, or in prison he can develop some phobia or hysterical system. What is the role of psychiatrists in trying to modify or influence the antisocial criminal behavior? That is one set of issues.

Another set of cases concerns providing minimum decent medical or psychiatric care for prisoners, just like anyone else. It is only that first problem that should bring on value conflicts. There the psychiatrist is being asked to be a social control agent and accomplish society's purpose in modifying some criminal or antisocial behavior.

Daniel: I'd like to point out that there are some useful perspectives on this from other professions. Early in the history of certified public accounting it became quite clear that the concept of the independence of the audit needed some review. CPAs were saying, 'Yes, we are professionals and we can keep our different responsibilities clear in our minds so that we can audit companies in which we hold some interest, some stock, without it affecting us in anyway.' The Securities and Exchange Commission, the IRS, and a lot of other government agencies said, 'Well, that may be, but we think we had better set down some rules about that. We will specify very carefully what we mean by independence of the audit.' And the AICPA agreed with those specifications.

It is always much clearer when money is involved in our society than when trust is involved, but we might take that as an example of the principle by which to set up some kind of independence. If there were, for example, outside psychiatric help available to the prison patient there might be some advantage. If you really need psychotherapeutic help in the military, they urge you to get it outside. In fact, sometimes military writers on this subject will bemoan the fact that they cannot get officers into treatment when necessary. Others see this as quite sensible because it would certainly affect the officers' promotion if it were known they were in treatment.

Klerman: A theme has come through this discussion thus far which I think would lend itself to useful empirical study; that is, what are the expectations of individual clients when they seek out psychiatrists or psychologists in various institutional settings: prisons, military, schools, colleges, and even mental hospitals? One paradigm has been the expectation that the psychiatrist will treat clients as though he were the ideal solo practitioner. Therefore, being embedded in the institutional setting undermines the trust and the confidentiality that is essential to the classic doctor-patient relationship.

Now my experience is the exact opposite. My friends who are psychiatrists and work in prisons or in psychiatric services in universities have the opposite problem: they have to convince the inmates and the students that psychiatrists can be trusted. I have served on a committee to the Dean of the Harvard Medical School designed to set up a policy of dealing with medical students who have psychiatric problems, and one of the members of that committee is also a psychiatrist for the medical school. He is caught in a terrible dilemma about what he should tell the students about what he will tell the Dean about their mental illnesses. Furthermore, there are probably ten entering medical students taking lithium who aren't telling him because they feel that than the admissions committee wouldn't let them into medical school.

Do the clients expect the psychiatrists in the prison to behave in the classic model, or is the opposite true? Patients in mental hospitals know that they can't tell the shrink what's going on because he is going to tell the board of administrators that they are going to set a fire tomorrow night, and so on. Some empirical data might be useful as to what patients actually expect when they seek help in these various institutional settings.

Friedman: I think we need some kind of functional analysis: what are the purposes that the psychiatrist thinks he is serving in various institutional settings? Presumably there will be more than one. Having identified them, we may find that one role undermines the other.

Psychiatric Institutions: An Administrator's Perspective

Klerman: As a psychiatrist who has been the head of a mental institution my view is based on a number of premises. First, the practice of psychiatry in an institutional setting such as mental hospital or a mental health center, is different from the ideal doctor-patient dyad. Second, psychiatric institutions perform multiple functions. Third, the mental hospital is different from prisons, schools, and the military because the psychiatrist in those institutions is a guest in someone else's house. In the hospital, the psychiatrist runs the house; this clouds many of the issues because the psychiatrist is in both an administrative and therapeutic situation. Some of the role conflicts as well as some of the moral dilemmas may be more evident in a prison, where the psychiatrist is a guest in another's house, where someone else has the power. There is on question that, as a superintendent of a mental hospital, one has a lot of power; that's part of the fun and also part of the price.

The ideal system has two parties, the patient and the physician-psychiatrist. They exist in some hypothetical vacuum that has no reality other than the transaction between them. In the institution there are many dyads beside the physician and the patient – the patient and the nurse-clinicians, or volunteer-clinicians, or psychologist-clinicians. The director has at least two functions: one is the hierarchical function whereby internal matters are regulated, and the other is the boundary function between the institution and various other extra-institutional powers, like the legislature, police department, university, parents, and civil rights lawyers, all of whom want to have the right to influence what goes on in that institution.

Multiple Functions. what are the multiple functions of the institution? I have catalogued four types, each of which carries various role dilemmas.

1. The classic function of the mental hospital is the care and treatment of sick people. The assumption here is that there are some mentally ill people who fit the sick role and there is a medical technology that is relevant to them. We can have a long debate about whether mental illness is a myth, but, assuming that it exists, there are at least three or four dilemmas within that category.

First, who is the responsible physician in an institution? At least in Massachusetts, in a state-run institution, like a public mental or veterans' hospital, the superintendent is responsible for all the patients, and the staff acts as his or her deputy. This view had a noble history during the moral treatment era; doctors were seen as the fathers and all staff were seen as their assistants. That view sees the institutions as one extended treatment center, different, for example, from the statement of responsibility in a general hospital. In the Massachusetts General Hospital the responsible physician is the individual attending physician and the hospital assumes primarily a hotel management function. To the extent that there exist various degrees of delegation, whether through the chief of service or the superintendent, the decision making about an individual dyad is influenced by various hierarchical arrangements, which may or may not involve persuasion, coercion, or various combinations in practice.

Second, in the public hospital at least, there is conflict about access to scarce resources. Are there enough drugs, enough nurses on night duty or enough spaces in the day program? The ability to treat the individual patient according to the individual practitioner's sense of what would be best is always restrained by access to increasingly scarce resources in the public sector.

The third issue is involuntary treatment, namely, the extent to which individuals in public hospitals, committed or not, have the right to refuse the treatment that is offered to them or prescribed for them. That is now a hot legal issue in many jurisdictions, including Massachusetts.

2. The second function of the mental hospital is a custodial one. In addition to people who are sick in the classic sense, there are lots of people who have various forms of chronic disability and who are handicapped. The handicap may or may not be the result of some mental illness like schizophrenia or manic-depressive illness. The institution provides various kinds of long-term residences for such individuals and that function of the institution has received a great deal of attention from sociologists. These individuals are not only socially handicapped but are often nuisances, though not necessarily dangerous. Society wishes these people taken care of and also removed from usual social interaction.

Even if one believes that these kinds of nuisance behaviors and helpless behaviors are in fact the consequence of a real illness, that still leaves a moral dilemma for someone who's running an institution. If one doesn't believe that there is such a real illness and that these people aren't sick, but are socially handicapped for reasons that have nothing to do with any medical problem, then I'm not sure whether the dilemmas become easier or harder. But they are different.

3. The third function is the asylum function, that is, the protection of the patient, from other people. This is an old function forgotten about in recent discussions. I predict attention is going to come back to this function because of the large number of mentally ill patients in the community who are subject to a good deal of predatory behavior, particularly in urban settings. Here the profession may have failed in its responsibilities to protect these patients from being placed in situations in which they are easily abused. Maybe our desire to deinstitutionalize and to make our statistics look good has allowed us to be less than vigorous in protecting certain kinds of patients.

A subset of the asylum function is the case of the patient who may be in conflict with family or with other groups The classic problem is a manic patient involved in a business endeavor. The family and other people disagree about the patient's judgment. The psychiatrist is then asked to decide whether the patient's judgment is sound. In one case, I saw recently on rounds, the patient had made a down payment on a liquor store and the family disagreed. The party from whom he was purchasing the store said, 'He made the payment, go through with the contract.' My advice was that at least three parties needed a lawyer: the patient, the family, and the hospital, because the patient was there voluntarily.

4. In its fourth function the mental hospital is clearly acting as an agent of social control. Here it has at least three roles. First, it is called upon to assess or to diagnose. When was running the Lynwood center, at any one time we had three or four patients under observation. And there the *Miranda* issue was very clear. We would say to the person 'Look, we are agents of the

court. You are here under a court order and our job is to tell the court as much as we can about you. If in the process we can be helpful to you that might be nice.' I hope the individuals understood Maybe the *Miranda* principle should be applied more forthrightly. Or maybe there should be separate institutions for advising the courts. The courts think that we have a technology that can be helpful. They want assessments about neurologic status or about child development or about unconscious conflicts or about drug effects.

Second, the mental hospital keeps certain people off the streets; they perform an incarceration role. This often comes up as: is this patient ready for discharge? And the discussion that ensues covers not only the clinical state of the patient but what will the community think, or what will Senator so-and-so think when he learns that Mr. X has been released because Mr. X used to call Senator so-and-so and talk about his private parts.

Third, the mental hospital has a therapeutic role. We have technology to change behavior, including drugs, psychotherapy, behavior modification, and of course that's what we are meant to do.

Some Solutions: How can we resolve the conflicts inherent the mental hospital? The first and most common solution, especially among my colleagues, is to say, 'There is no role conflict. These are clinical problems and the rest of the world should leave the doctor alone because we physicians know best.' That is probably the most comfortable solution; but it doesn't work anymore. Even so, a modest percentage of my colleagues still hold to that position.

The second solution is one I call the 'benevolent buffer.' I consoled myself with that when I was running a hospital, but recently I have come to question it. Should the administrative director buffer the institution from the external sources of intrusion so as to protect the classic dyads as much as possible? Is it the function of leadership to mediate between the institution and the legislature, the family and the lawyers, and the medical society, and to thereby preserve wherever possible the ideal dyad? Should the director work for more resources, more nurses on night duty, and keep out the public interest lawyers and the angry relatives?

The third solution, which I come to more and more, is to attempt a balance of power by urging all the parties to have their own advocates. Open the door to lawyers, including lawyers for the institution. Whenever there was a jam, I would say, 'Let's go to the court and try to avoid making the decisions on purely medical grounds.'

The fourth solution is the radical solution, and there are three types:

(a) Eliminate mental hospitals. This admits that the problem arises because there are mental hospitals. One way to solve the problem is deinstitutionalization. Release all the patients and the problems will go away, or create lots of psychiatric units in general hospitals and thus do away with the public mental hospital. That is, not going to work, because we cannot do away with the mental hospital's custodial functions or its control of social deviants.

(b) Stop the physician from controlling the mental hospital But what makes the mental hospital unique is that the physician runs the hospital in which he also attempts to do treatment. He could have a situation where a mental hospital is run by nonphysicians: citizens' groups, patient groups, hospital managers. Then the distinction between power, administrative control, and therapy would be clearer.

(c) Remove the treatment from the mental hospital. We would have mental hospitals, but the treatment function would be performed externally.

Alfred Freedman: Gerry described what he thought was unique for mental hospitals: the psychiatrist is an charge. I suggest that is really a delusion. The seeming control of the physician-psychiatrist-administrator is subject to many other forces; he is really in the middle of a matrix. There has been no discussion of politics, bureaucracy, and the consequent deficiencies that result in unsatisfactory practice. The interrelationship between ethical practice and the material realities of a situation are inextricably interwoven.

What should a psychiatrist do where there is an obvious deficiency of services? We could look for ways of joining and developing links between providers of services, legal professionals, and other critics in order to advance programs. We could resolve certain ethical dilemmas through political action, particularly in focusing on the situation where there isn't a full panoply of services available.

Klerman: I both agree and disagree with you. It is important to distinguish between having legitimate authority and having available resources to exercise that authority. We fight for the authority to be in charge of public mental hospitals, while very few American-trained psychiatrists want to work there; the majority of physicians tend to be foreign-trained. So there is an issue of legitimized medical authority distinct from having the resources to fulfill our mandate.

What would psychiatry be like if there were no involuntary incarceration? As a superintendent of a mental hospital, I would say, life would be a hell of a lot easier. Psychiatry as a profession might enhance its position if we got out of the business of running public mental health hospitals.

Friedman: I am glad we are beginning to get the issue of power into the discussion, because it cannot be separated from the discussion of moral dilemmas and role conflicts. These dilemmas and conflicts occur because psychiatry has been given and has accepted power in some areas in which it is not justified.

To give a concrete example, the Mental Health Law Project has taken a position that psychiatrists should not be allowed to testify at civil commitment hearings that a patient is likely to commit a future dangerous act. Psychiatrists do not have the competence to do that. Traditionally society asked them to fulfill that role and it gave psychiatrists a certain degree of power and influence. I have been struck at how reluctant some psychiatrists seem to be at the notion of giving up power. I do think that is changing now. The notion that psychiatry doesn't have this power of predicting future dangerous conduct has begun to be accepted.

Burt: Gerry's description of the different roles of a psychiatric hospital highlights a tension, if not a contradiction, in my own presentation. At one point I posed the question: what does the psychiatrist as a psychiatrist do with an obviously, unbeatable patient? One of the things a psychiatrist does is offer asylum – a peaceful, decent refuge. Of course, role confusion enters at some point. And that confusion I think has had some destructive consequences. It has had this consequence at least, – that many people who don't need asylum, who are really quite reasonably competent to take care of themselves, are nonetheless confined 'for their own good.'

Is clarifying this confusion the best thing? Will it work to the advantage of most people? What happens in fact if we abandon the fiction of curability for certain groups of people? When said let's abandon that fiction about prisons, a lot of people said, and I thing quite rightly, what's going to happen then? One of the things that will or might happen in a prison setting, for example that people will say, 'If these people are not curable then why not kill them? Why let them out at all?' In a way, the fiction of curability also may help feed the fiction of cure. We release a lot of people from prison, the recidivism statistics notwithstanding. So it is quite possible that the fiction of curability and, rehabilitation is protective in an important way. Let me illustrate this briefly. In *Dixon v. Weinberger*, when the psychiatrists said, 'There is really nothing we can do to help Mr. Dixon in a hospital, so move him elsewhere,' he was horribly abused in a community setting. In this so-called 'unrestrictive setting,' he was incredibly worse off. When he was finally found, he begged to go back to the hospital and never leave again.

Psychiatric Institutions: an Advocate's Perspective

Friedman: As a lawyer representing mental patients, I want to describe some of the conflicts that I have become aware of in institutions, mental hospitals, and psychiatry. I will try to distinguish between value conflicts and duty conflicts. I think the potential for duty or role conflicts is greatest where the psychiatrist, as part of his professional role, sees himself as an agent of social control.

I would like to talk about conflicts in four areas: (1) the civil commitment process; (2) service delivery in an inadequate facility under adverse conditions; (3) treatment decisions and the right to refuse treatment; and (4) the intersection of the criminal justice and mental health systems.

Civil Commitment. Under present civil commitment statutes the standard is that the patient has to be found to be mentally ill and in need of treatment or, more commonly these days, mentally ill and dangerous to himself or others.

The fundamental issue is whether psychiatrists can define the 'mentally ill' part of that standard with reasonable precision. Thomas Szasz has claimed that nobody is mentally ill. I think that is an untenable position. Nonetheless, there are some very difficult problems in defining mental illness and the degree or kind of mental illness that justifies locking somebody up. Psychiatrists are traditionally brought in to give testimony and judgments about this in civil commitment hearings.

The Supreme Court in the *Donaldson* case touched on this issue without really addressing it. There is an important short digression in the majority opinion, however, where the Court recognizes that perhaps mental illness cannot be defined with a sufficient degree of exactness to satisfy constitutional standards.

Another criterion for commitment, the need for treatment, has generally been attacked as unconstitutionally vague and overbroad. The majority of states are moving toward a standard of dangerousness, dangerous to self, dangerous to other, or both. The trend is to be more specific and objective about dangerousness, recognizing that psychiatrists cannot accurately predict dangerousness. Because we don't have the technology or the diagnostic skills to predict, the trend is to rely on overt acts, rather than subjective impressions. This of course brings the process closer to a criminal proceeding where people have to be found guilty beyond a reasonable doubt. But overt acts of violence are not necessarily criminal acts. There are important differences.

A duty conflict rather than a value conflict is coming into play here. Society clearly wants the psychiatric community to provide a preventative detention function and to take out of circulation people who may not be criminal but who, as Gerry Klerman pointed out, are upsetting, smelly, or a nuisance. The psychiatric profession accepted that responsibility in the past and has been willing to give expert testimony about whether someone is mentally ill and dangerous. Is it the psychiatrist's primary duty to remove this annoying class of people, or is the psychiatrist's primary duty to the patient? How dangerous does a patient have to be to himself or to others for commitment to be justified?

The *Donaldson* opinion was very limited. The court found that a man who was capable of surviving in the community, was not dangerous to other people, and who was not receiving treatment in the institution, had a constitutional right to liberty. But what does 'capable of surviving in the community' mean? The Supreme Court seems to have said that a person cannot be committed on the grounds that he is dangerous to himself, if he is capable of surviving in the community. But there are many unanswered questions: What if that person can't get a job, sleeps in the street, eats out of garbage cans? Is that survival in the community? Does that meet the *Donaldson* standard? Or is that a sufficiently low level of survival that the person can be said to be dangerous to himself and be committed? These are the kind of value judgments that have to be clarified.

Service Delivery. If the patients have a right to treatment and the institution is so badly understaffed or underfinanced that it is not possible to provide a reasonable opportunity to have one's condition cured or functioning improved, and to the extent that liberty can be restored, then what is the psychiatrist's responsibility? It becomes a major problem because the psychiatrist has been fulfilling multiple roles, providing asylum, social control, and therapy. Conclusions about what to do in this case are quite different depending on the predominant role or the balance of roles. Everyone at this meeting seems aware of this and the representatives of the psychiatric community here are very sophisticated and articulate, but my impression is that in a number of large public facilities the psychiatrists are not so sophisticated, and all these functions are lumped together. It would be a real service to clarify some of these roles and to offer some guidance about what one should do when they confllict.

Although the legal code of ethics shares many features with the psychological and medical ones, it is much more specific. On the basis of the legal code of ethics, it is possible to pose a very concrete problem and get an answer from your local ethics committee. I think the psychiatric community should pose hypothetical situations, such as: what is a psychiatrist to do if he works in an institution where, because of inadequate financing, treatment is impossible, yet the state statute mandates treatment?

My view is that this is a societal problem for which psychiatrists have been forced to accept responsibility. Under such intolerable conditions, psychiatrists should go back to the a court of law issuing the decisions or back to the legislature which drafted the statute. A psychiatrist should bring a patient back to court and say, 'Your Honor, I don't know what to do. There is a legal obligation to treat. On the one hand, we don't have the resources to treat; on the other hand, if we release this patient, we will be dumping him. He needs something, but there aren't adequate resources in our institution.' Let the court of law make these decisions. They are not *medical* decisions, but rather social policy and legal decisions.

Treatment Decisions.   Does a patient have the right to refuse treatment? I think that there are independent constitutional bases for a right of patients to refuse certain procedures that are hazardous, experimental, or intrusive. Society may have the right to protect itself by removing persons and confining them, but those confined still have a right to refuse to accept certain procedures such as psychosurgery or electro-shock therapy or perhaps drugs. But what should psychiatrists do when the patient refuses a treatment? Do they have the power and is it moral to impose certain procedures on patients against their will? That is a duty conflict, I'd say. With patients of questionable competency there are terrible dilemmas about whether to emphasize autonomy and err on the side of doing what the patient says he wants even if you think it is not in his best interests, or to act paternalistically and do what you think is best for the person whose ability to make such decisions is questionable.

Another treatment issue has to do with treatment of committed children, which multiplies the problems I have just mentioned. Now the family is involved. Perhaps what's good for the child is not what the parent wants. Or the problem may lie within the family, but the psychiatrist has authority only to treat the child who has been committed. What if the child is in conflict with the parents, and the parents approve electro-shock therapy, to which the child objects? This area hasn't been scrutinized at all and will be affected by the forthcoming decision of the Supreme Court in *Bartley v. Kremens.*

Criminal Justice.   Another set of issues clusters around forensics. If the institutional psychiatrist is treating a patient who says something, not about a future dangerous act, but about a murder committed in the past, what is the obligation of the psychiatrist? Does he have to reveal those past crimes or does he owe a duty of confidentiality to the patient? The way to answer a question like that, it seems to me, is with social policy judgments about how to minimize harms and maximize benefits. And if there isn't any morally right or wrong answer, the key is to make explicit the rules of the games. A patient being treated in an institution ought to know that if he happens to mention a past crime, or happens to talk about some dangerous act, that information will or will not be reported. There is a state of confusion right now, both in terms of inconsistent practices and expectations.

Similar conflicts arise when psychiatrists are forced into multiple role that they can't handle, making judgments about whether to label somebody not guilty by reason of insanity. These judgment are made quite apart from any really hard or objective test, because psychiatrists think it would be better for a particular person to be placed in a mental institution than in a prison.

There is throughout society, it seems to me, a questioning about the right of authority figures to make discretionary judgments, and this new skepticism is healthy.

Stone: What We have to begin to do is to think through the limits of discretion. The kind of suggestion Paul Friedman is making, that When we bounce this back to the courts the courts will do better, is wrong. People are increasingly distrustful of courts and their discretionary judgment. I think paul is well aware of the situation of *Memmel v. Mundy*, Where even with all the due process right in place, the judges abused due process and misused discretion at least as much as they had before. We in psychiatry ought to limit the medical model very tightly and get out many of the other kinds of discretionary judgments that have little to do with treatment per se.

Is the psychiatrist a special case? I really don't think so. What has developed over at least the last decade is an increasing suspiciousness toward authorities and all of those who make discretional judgments. That reflects itself in a growing tendency to look at sentencing and to take away the discretion of judges. In turn concern about the rehabilitator's ends in taking away the discretion of the parole board. It manifests itself in the Buckley Amendment questioning the discretion of teachers in their judgments about students. We are now even questioning the discretion of parents to control the lives of their children.

Conflicts and Professional Etiquette

Freidson: Many of the recent ethical issues in medicine have been occasioned by the problems created by new technology, for example, the Karen Ann Quinlan case. With very few exceptions these issues have been put in highly individualistic terms. By and large the issues are treated as personal decisions by responsible physicians on individual cases. I think this is highly unrealistic and I want to stress something quite different.

We have already discussed the social and institutional context that an individual's decision must take into account: the need of the military for troops in wartime, the needs of society for some reasonable freedom from harm from individuals who might be considered dangerous to society, and so on. So insofar as it plays a role in individual ethical decisions, the social and institutional context is extremely important. However, the net outcome seems to be a little like the Ten Commandments: thou shalt do this, or in the face of this dilemma, thou shalt choose this means.

But surely physicians in general, if not psychiatrists in particular, should be aware of the psychological mechanisms, as well as the sociological and institutional ones, that can distort individuals' choices and that can lead them to rationlize their choices even when those choices are doing damage to other people. What the intellectual world has learned from psychiatry over the past hundred years, the various defense mechanisms that individual create, will also be exercised by psychiatrists in the course of their decisions, since they too are human beings.

So, while we can discuss these ethical issues and clarify them, agree on provisional solutions, and perhaps even ultimately list them as codes or commandments, there is no guarantee that individuals will follow them. First, our health care system is predicated on economic advantage with monetary incentives being very strong. No one is immune. Second, the conditions of work in health care make time an extremely precious commodity. Time-consuming deliberations and the searching of conscience are really discouraged by the condition of practice. Thus there is the ever-present danger that economic advantage and time pressure strongly combine to influence decisions, aided and abetted by defense mechanisms like rationalization, feelings of omnipotence, and so on. I would agree that discussing and resolving the subject of ethical issues and teaching awareness of them to individuals is a necessary and a very important step, but it is not a sufficient step to assure a reasonable level of ethical action.

What is equally necessary is a set of norms and commonly accepted practices that would militate against the possibility that ethical decisions be solely individual in character. These norms must be in some sense collectively professional and not individually professional. The norms and commonly accepted practices that I refer to are those that govern collegial relationships within a profession or within any organized group of workers. These norms *should* be employed in stimulating observation of others' choices, as well as in debate, discussion, and consensual correction of these choices where they seem to deviate from what we would generally agree to be proper, or appear to be unduly influenced by an individual's own defense mechanisms, haste, or greed.

In short, a new system of professional etiquette is needed to exercise influence over individual ethical decisions. That etiquette is not merely a matter of being polite. It is an etiquette that requires from the individual important moral decisions about his or her for the conduct of colleagues well as responsibility for those patients for whom colleagues are immediately responsible.

Present notions of etiquette in medicine, it seems to me, sabotage mutual professional influence, in part this can be explained by their historical development. They developed in the nineteenth century as the medical profession, among others, was consolidating itself into a new form of occupational organization. They were designed essentially to protect the profession from outside criticism, rather then to protect individual patients from colleagues who may be mistaken. We may assume that a very small, unimportant proportion of physicians are simply bad. The real question is how good people deceive themselves, certainly a topic on which psychiatrists are experts. Present notions of etiquette are designed to preserve the appearance of professional probity to the outside world while minimizing friction among colleagues. They do this in part by controlling professional competition and in part by reducing intra-professional controversies, disagreements about what is right and wrong.

Present notions of etiquette are predicated on a series of justifying assumptions, and each of them is in some partial sense true. First, no one is immune from making a mistake. Of course, that is true. Second, except for the few obvious cases of gross incompetence or negligence, all difference in performance is based on difference in objective error or thought. Third, only the person who works directly with the patient can accurately judge the issues. And finally, the practitioner in charge of the case is ultimately the only one responsible for it.

The net consequence of these assumptions is that when an individual sees others erring, there is a suspension of judgment and a suspension of action to correct the deviance.

Now the justifying assumptions sustain the basic rules of etiquette, which are: First, do not judge an apparently erring colleague. Only he can really know the case; besides, there but for the grace of God go I. Second, restrict your sense of ethical responsibility to your own cases. Don't tamper with anybody else's. Third, don't talk about an apparently erring colleague to others and don't criticize him. The net result is to create a system in which ethical action can be a function only of individual action, which is at the mercy of individual variation.

There are some rather clear practices in psychiatry perhaps more particularly in institutional psychiatry, where things tend to be more visible. One might cite as an example, the use of electro-shock thereapy at enormously high levels of voltage. What does one do about a colleague who does that? The rule of etiquette is that one shouldn't do anything. I submit that doing nothing is a moral choice not merely a question of 'etiquette.' The ethical relationships between colleagues are as important as the ethical sensitivities of individuals in approaching their 'own' cases.

The relationship between colleagues is changing; in fact, the law is beginning to change. A draft act of the New York legislature states: 'Every physician . . . shall report to the Board [of professional Medical Conduct] any information which such individual may have which appears to show that a physician is or may be guilty of professional misconduct, or is otherwise incompetent to practice medicine safely.' And the act goes on to cover confidentiality, procedure, and immunity from suit. The Education Law of New York State has added a new definition of professional misconduct namely, 'willfully failing to report to the State Board of Professional Medical Conduct any information which the licensee may have which appears to show that a physician is or may be medically incompetent, or is or may be guilty of professional misconduct . . . or is or may be mentally or physically unable [to perform] safely in the practice of medicine.' If it is determined that an individual has willfully failed to report misconduct, that individual physician can lose his license or have it suspended, if this act is passed. [It was passed.]

I am on the legislative advisory committee concerned with revising the law, and, as a matter of fact, I indicated that I could not endorse the draft for a variety of reasons. Independently of how we regard it, however, the point is that enough has gone on in the world to lead legislators to decide that in fact a legal remedy may be necessary to change the rules of etiquette. Now I think that a legal remedy under these terms is, in fact, inappropriate and likely to be counterproductive, but the rules of etiquette are at the bottom of the need for it. My argument is that what seems be superficial etiquette is also an important issue of ethics, of how much responsibility one has for other peoples' patients and how much responsibility one has for protecting one's colleagues.

Ruth Macklin: I agree that there is an intersection between etiquette and ethics, or professional etiquette and ethics, but I think the intersection is relatively small. Now I take it that your view, Professor Freidson, is that what's necessary is a set of norms or commonly accepted practices that should be collectively professional and not individually professional. Whether they are legally enforceable or enforced or not is not at issue. But what happens when individual psychiatrists disagree, when other persons in the community – lay persons or other professionals – disagree? And what happens when that disagreement might be viewed as legitimate on the moral issues, that is, there are good reasons on both sides?

What then does apsychiatrist do when he disagrees with a collectively agreed upon set of norms? Does he engage in a form of civil disobedience against the professional code of etiquette? If these are genuine moral dilemmas rather than merely questions of eqiquette, then what is the mechanism for coming up with such a code of etiquette? Should it be by consensus, by vote, by majority rule? Should it be resolved by those in power in the various professional organizations? I see a lot of problems with conflating ethics and etiquette. In particular, treating them as problems of collective responsibility fails to recognize or to take account of the legitimate disagreements that exist in the moral arena where there are genuine dilemmas between individual liberty and protection of society.

Freidson: Well, if I gave you that impression, I didn't mean to. Etiquette is separate from the moral dilemmas that we are discussing here. And I tried by the examples I gave, namely, somebody giving massive does of electro-shock therapy which can lead to brain damage, to refer to instances in which there is no ethical dilemma so far as I am concerned. The problem is what do you do about it. Do you say, 'Well, it's his patient. It's none of my business and besides he'll yell at me and our professional relationship will deteriorate'? Or is it a matter of feeling that you are ethically responsible for somebody else's patient and not just your own? That is also really an ethical issue of responsibility, not politeness.

Macklin: Within that domain I would agree. What you are doing is selecting examples of what we might call patently immoral conduct or bad practices. But those, I think, are the easy cases which might be handled by the kind of solution you purpose. But those dilemmas that involve value conflicts are not going to be settled by a collective professional approach.

Freidson: The easy cases can be handled a lot better than they are now. And they constitute the vast majority of cases confronting practitioners and the public.

Daniels: In some of my studies on psychiatrists, I have asked them how they feel about issues of control. I was amazed to discover the number, both from the institutional sample and the private practice sample, who said that they thought it was appropriate to control the lives of patients, to make decisions for them, even though this is not considered the most appropriate kind of therapeutic practice. There is an enormous lack of sophistication in the helping profession about what's *comme il faut*, never mind what's ethical. Some of the ethical issues that we have been discussing are easier to see and talk about than trying to regulate one's colleagues. It is the problems of day-to-day practice that are going to be difficult to call to their attention as ethical issues because they do go against professional autonomy.

Michels: There is minor, but nicely tangible issue that cuts across these presentations. Gerry begins by describing his model, and it is delightful to hear the superintendent of a mental hospital talk about his role in such subtle and complex ways. Paul Friedman even compliments us by saying that we are not like psychiatrists out there in the hinterlands. And the professional etiquette Eliot describes really focuses not on the dilemmas of the typical or even good practitioner, but on the inferior deviant, and the control and regulation of him.

The problem that emerges – although it is not inherently unique to psychiatry, it may be more important in psychiatry than in many other areas – is the incredible range of competence, skill, and ability between the good, the average, and the poor practitioner, as compared to orthopedic surgery or internal medicine. The optimal etiquette probably rests on the average expected competence of a typical practitioner and the standard deviation. The optimal amount of peer review and regulation probably depends on the same. The optimal amount of external social control, and the optimal proportion of the practioner's time spent making his efforts publicly reviewable (as opposed to carrying them out) are probably all functions of the likelihood that any given practitioner will be inept, incompetent, dangerous, or seriously deviant from the professional norm.

The problem is that I don't want my psychiatrist to have to spend the amount of time he would have to spend dealing with the civil rights lawyer or the peer review committee of the District Branch of the American Psychiatric Association, although I recognize that the borderline competent psychiatrists ought to spend even more time doing just those things. One solution to the problem is to narrow the range of competence so that the difference between the good ones and the terrible ones would be less than it is now and somewhat more approximate to other areas of medicine. That requires lots of social resources but I think an argument could be made that those resources, are necessary not only because of the desires of the profession, but alsobecause of the social needs for effective regulatory systems.

Psychiatrists and Potentially Dangerous Patients

Claudewell Sidney Thomas: On April 21, 1973, Judge David L. Bazelon delivered an important speech to the Southern California Psychiatry Society, a speech which proved disconcerting to psychiatrists as well as laymen. Bazelon was suspicious of the nonmedical bases on which many socially relevant decisions are being made by psychiatrists. The judge abhorred the fact that 'It takes serious legal and public challenges to bring to light the hidden agendas on which psychiatrists operate.' As a result of the speech and concern within the APA, J.J. Lindenthal, a socilogist, Clyde Sullivan, a clinical psychologist, and I undertook a research project that would begin to provide answers about psychiatry and agentry, that is, who the psychiatrist represents.

We developed a series of ten vignettes, each of which represents a conflict that physicians might confront in their practices. The vignettes treated increasingly serious problems: homicide, suicide, pyromania, incest, and threats to national security, among others. The respondents to the questionnaire could check off three possible responses about their reaction to a patient presenting such a conflict.

For example, a patient comes in and reports having set a series of fires and announces he will set another one. What would the physician do and why? Would he give another appointment? Would be refer to another physician? Would he call the fire department? The physician who would give another appointment is rater as acting as the agent of the patient. The one who would call the fire department is rated as being societally oriented.

We thought that comparing internists to psychiatrists would give us a contrast between two groups in medical practice, differing primarily in terms of instrumentation and orientation. Examining a group of psychologists, on the other hand, would allow us to compare two groups of professionals, one medically trained, the other lacking medical training, but both having similar orientations in terms of patient care.

A total of 436 clinicians responded to the survey, including 144 internists, 200 psychiatrists, and 92 psychologists. The findings indicate that there are highly significant differences in orientation toward patients. Three different curves emerged. The internists start out patient-oriented and very rapidly go up to societal orientation. Psychiatrists start out patient-oriented and stay reasonably patient-oriented until clearly antisocial kinds of behavior are at issue and then swing out toward societal orientation. Psychologists, on the other hand, start out patient-oriented and tend to stay patient-oriented until the vignettes describe extreme acts with extreme social consequences.

The differences between psychiatrists and internists, in terms of patient orientation, are statistically significant, as are differences between psychiatrists and psychologists and between psychologists and internists. If one started out with a null hypothesis, something to the effect that the essential orientation of psychiatric practice is medical, there should be no differences between an internist and a psychiatrist. But there are differences. We could say that it is not the biomedical orientation of the psychiatrist that is most important, but the use of interpersonal relations for therapeutic purposes. There should be no difference between clinical psychologists and psychiatrist who espouse the same instrumentation and much the same values, but this assumption too is not borne out by the data. There are statistical differences between psychologists and psychiatrists. Now if concern for patients is the value we espouse, then psychiatrists look pretty good compared to internists, but psychologists look even better.

What does it mean? We can only speculate. Exposure to the structural, functional hypotheses of medicine may be a conservative influence, pulling the psychiatrist in the direction of the internist's response.

There is another possibility. A number of the psychologists who responded sent notes indicating that they had completed the questionnaire after consulting the Committee on Ethics of the American Psychological Association. No psychiatrist indicated that he had consulted the Committee on Ethics of the American Psychiatric Association, although I believe one exists. Instead, a number of psychiatrists consulted lawyers. It may be that the psychiatrists are not aware of an ethical position taken by the APA Committee on Ethics. It may be that the psychologists were freed, in terms of patient orientation, by the prior existence of such a stand taken by their Committee.

The second preliminary finding is that the demographic variables, by and large, are not associated with orientation.

The third finding is that the nature of the work setting is weakly related to orientation toward patient or society.

The fourth preliminary finding, related to the first, the final disposition of the individual client will depend on what kind of professional the person sees: an internist, a psychologist, or a psychiatrist.

Other findings also attain statistical significance. One important one is that psychoanalytic training is highly associated with a patient orientation. If the value of the system is toward patients, then psychoanalytic training gets grades.

The first preliminary conclusion is that the way in which we design our future medical care institutions will affect the tendencies of the caregivers to embrace patient values or societal values as a primary orientation. The second conclusion is that there is an enormous variation between professional groups. The third conclusion, and I don't know whether this is justified or not, is: professionals are desperately seeking guidance on ethical issues. That tentative conclusion is based on the number of letters that accompanied the questionnaires and, indicating an enormous distress, particularly within psychiatry. These writers asked: do you give a course? what are the right answers? where can we go for guidance? The asssumption that psychiatrists do not perceive their role conflict is simply not borne out. It is acutely perceived. Occasionally we still receive a questionnaire even though the research is virtually ended. We suspect that somebody has been worrying over this questionnaire and has finally gotten around to returning it.

And the fourth conclusion, which is related to the third, is the need for the sharing of information among clinicians about the kind of problems that these questionnaires represented, how the problems were handled, what the implications are, and the the information needs to be shared widely within the counselling field.

Sabshin: One interesting point is that we talk about psychiatrists as if they are some kind of homogeneous group of people and, quite obviously, from your data, there are at least two widely different groups of psychiatrists. My experience is that the hospital-based psychiatrist is much more like a doctor, and some office-practicing psychiatrists have difficulty with classical medical roles.

Thomas: Also office-practicing psychiatrists may be broken up to into other groups, biologically oriented and psychoanalytically oriented, with different value systems.

Michels: Obviously this is a very complicated study. There is one dimension that it would be interesting for this group to think about. One of our interests ought to be, are those responses right or wrong, or how are they different from each other, and how do they come to be? What is the process of socialization that goes into these response patterns and how might it be different? For example, I suspect that the differences between psychoanalysts and non psychoanalytic psychiatrists probably begin before professional training. That is probably a bigger factor than anything that happens to them in psychoanalytic school or in nonpsychoanalytic school.

Gaylin: Having done this research, where do we go from here? Psychiatrists now find out that they are more society-oriented and the psychologists find out that they are more individual-oriented. What does that tell us in terms of moral values? Should we psychiatrists be working to be more like psychologists? Should they be working to be more like us? I sense the conversation circling around a word that has a nasty odor these days. That word is 'paternalism.'

In a model which generated paternalism there was much talk about responsibilities, duties, and obligations, for both doctor and patient. Now we have an antipaternalistic model, bacause paternalism went too far.

Most of us trained in the medical model were trained in a paternalistic fashion. We did not see the patient as a client or a contractor. We did see him as someone to whom we owed a certain moral obligation. I mention paternalism here because in a peculiar way it closes the circle on my mystification about Claude's terminology.

What does he mean by 'patient orientation'? I find it almost exactly the opposite of his lable. Let's take the extreme case. My patient tells me that as soon as she leaves my office she is going to kill herself. By his standard, my shaking her hand and saying, 'See you later,' is being patient-oriented. Now if that is patient-oriented, I suppose that ultra-patient-oriented would be to offer her pills with which to do the job. I find it very difficult to accept Claudewell Thomas' categories, that to be patien-oriented is to facilitate the act of arson, inces, murder, and the like.

Thomas: In interpreting a survey, you can only answer the questions that the instrument has been constructed to ask. You are entitled to construct your own vignettes and your own interpretations. But you really ought to pay attention to the tool that was constructed. I tried to point out that there were at least two things that went into the decision of patient orientation or society orientation. One was the answer that was checked, along a scale of five possibilities.

Daniel Callahan: I can see the need for some more empirical evidence, that is, what are the expectations of the general public on these questions? My own guess is that one will find a rather significant discrepancy between what the professionals think and what a sample of citizens would think.

Second, to what extent to psychiatrists have a right to develop their own value system? Are we going to see them as private individuals who have a right to their own values and consciences as public servants? I would be inclined to say that a psychiatrist by virtue of being licensed has certain social obligaions, one of which is that his values do not simply represent capricious personal values. There should be a very strong attempt to find a good fit between the rights of the public to certain kinds of expectations and the obligation of the psychiatrist to live up to those expectations, if only to prevent the public from being misled about what it is getting. Finally, it would be useful to have a public debate, say, of vignettes of this sort and the

principles that underlie them, to see how in the very course of argumentation, some of the values might shift. My own impression is that these issues are not discussed very much in the professional literature. Practitioners are coming to their conclusions in a very casual fashion.

Klerman: The discussion leaves me dissatisfied; I am not sure that the notions of paternalism and autonomy do justice to my sense of the issue. Psychotherapists, like other healers. claim discreationary power. One aspect of discretionary power is the right to distinguish between the patient's wishes and the patient's best interests. To be patient-oriented is not to accede to the patient's wish to kill himself or to commit incest, but to exercise discretionary power and to make a judgment as to his best interest.

Psychiatrists and other psychotherapists are often accuse of paternalism or imposing values or not going along with a libertarian view. Their assumption is that there are certain conditions where the individual's mental capacities may be imparied and they may not always be able to act in their own best interests. Szasz and other libertarians may feel that there is never any condition, except in coma, where there can be impairment of judgement. That point of view at least ought to be acknowledged.

Redlich: Claude's data suggests that those operating within the medical model are inclined to intervene. In the psychoanalytic model we are taught not to intervene and are less inclined to interevene. In terms of consequences very much will depend on whether we move toward one or the other model. If the trend is to move toward the medical model, there will be more intervention, more reporting to authority, more societal orientation.

Klerman: I have one comment about the psychoanalytic model. If a patient came in and told Sigmund Freud that he was going to Kill Anna, Sigmund would not have been neutral. Actually Freud was not neutral in the way he practiced. But if he has a duty to protect his own daughter, why doesn't he have a duty to protect his neighbor's daughter? Is the analytic model pure simply because it rarely gets tested? It rarely gets tested because the kind of patients who are in it are not the kind of patients who will test this. Is the psychoanalytic model, in fact, generalizable? In terms of Dr. Thomas's data, people who work in a community mental health center do not work within the analytic framework, but within a framework of radical nonintervention. I feel increasingly that this paradigm of radical nonintervention, of not interfering with people's lives, is the direction our society should take and the direction we should take in our own ethics and values.

Stone: One of our tasks is to ask: what are the practical implications of our ethical positions? For a variety of reasons having to do with the legal system and the social system, people who make the difficult ethical decisions are often totally unaccountable to anyone. People decide that somebody should be committed without any sense of personal accountability, of what they are doing to another human being. Doctors say that they are doing something to protect the patient, or to protect society, when in fact they are protecting themselves. A very important motivation in this area is dumping. The doctor in the emergency room sees a patient and wants to dump him, so he writes out a commitment order saying 'This patient is gravely suicidal' to get him into the hospital.

Callahan: I find the notion of accountability rather intriguing; it has become a public ethical concept. I am not always sympathetic with people in power or in the professions, but it seems to me there is a legitimate complaint on the part of many people being called to accountability. They complain that it is no longer clear just what the standards are that they are called to account for. There are lots of ways of being accountable. One can be accountable, presumably, to a moral code, to a professional code, to the public-at-large, to public opinion; One can probably be accountable under certain circumstances to a specific contract that, one has explicitly or implicitly entered into. So in what sense, Alan, did you use accountability? To whom or to what? To values, or to people or to some mixture of both?

Stone: I feel, that our judges and our psychiatrists work in an insane, universe because whatever our judges do is going to be wrong. If prisons are for rehabilitation, they send someone who will probably get socialized to crime. They end up not being able to either rehabilitate or protect society;

they also end up not knowing what they are doing, or being able to avoid knowing what they are doing.

Take another example. I would ask the doctor who commits a patient to be the doctor who also treats the patient. I would make him or her accountable. I would say, 'If you say this person needs to be in the hospital and be treated, you are going to be the one who treats him, and then in three or four weeks or however long you say, you come back into court and tell us how you have done.' The problem is that the judge gets a psychiatrist to testify, that person will leave the scene and not be accountable, nor is the judge accountable. He doesn't worry after he has made the decision. I'd like to hold both people's noses to the grindstone and force them to confront what it is they are doing. That is my sense of accountability. I want to put people's reputation and lives on the line when they control other people's lives. I want them to have a major investment in their decisions.

Daniels: It is clear to me how much we all stick to our own interests. My interests were expressed this morning and the interest that a lot of you who were talking this afternoon have a little different from mine. The way you conceptualize ethical problems and the issues that you want to address are not the ones I see as particularly important. One of the things that interests me is the way the issues Eliot Freidson raised were just dropped. I think these are the key ethical issues.

Gaylin: Arlene seems to feel we are avoiding problems, perhaps we are. I do not feel that way. If we seem to be avoiding some of the questions of the bad apple, it isn't that we don't think that these are important. For instance, when The Hastings Center began to study psychosurgery, we were given reports of neurosurgeons in Mississippi operating on nonpsychotic conditions on prepubescent boys. This may sound brutal, but that wasn't an interesting or important subject for us. It was a crucially important subject for human beings or civilized individuals. But that is only one category of problem, the person doing patently bad things. The other problem is the one the conference is really oriented toward: what do you do when there is a conflict between two goods, so that wherever you move you are in moral pain?

Stone: I personally feel that Professor Freidson touched on a raw nerve. For example, I have seen a residency training program in which one resident's behavior was bizarre if not psychotic. He was sent off to another residency training program. He was dumped on another institution, but no one was told why.

The reluctance among doctors about exposing malpractice and the immoral practice of each other is more powerful than the canons of ethics. Now as a matter of fact, the canons of ethics require the reporting of unethical behavior. I have done it. It makes me quite unpopular. I have taken as a personal responsibility reporting psychiatrists who break patients' confidentiality. And I get a lot of feedback from people who are very angry. The argument can be made, and I am going to make it, that soil has to be planted or tilled before the Association begins to look at this 'other area,' in any kind of way that is going to be meaningful.

Gaylin: I agree that in terms of urgency, equity, justice, morality, you may be right, Alan, but those problems certain ready solutions. What I am saying is that even if those issues are resolved, we are still faced with another important set of issues. Who is the psychiatrist? Whose agent is he? Has he been cast in the role of a social controller rather than a therapist? If so, ought he remove himself from medicine? If not, why?

Sabshin: I'd like to link up some of the discussion about accountability with Eliot's earlier comments. In my judgement, there has been more collegial interaction on responsiblity than perhaps has been apparent. As APA medical director, I tend to see the volume of ethics cases with their implicit as well as explicit effects. Knowing that an APA district branch actually adheres to the process of investigating complaints would fit some of your discussions about collegial responsibility. From the standpoint of psychiatrists, the systems of accountability from which they are currently feeling pressure, have grown rapidly in recent years. Part of the tension and difficulty in response lies in these systems' undeveloped stage. However, look at what's happening in certification and recertification, licensing and relicensing. Sitting in an office like mine I see the letters protesting mandated continuing education requirements and the development of PSROs. Despite these complaints I see a certain kind of confluence moving in the direction of accountability. Part of our reaction, though, is to avoid it because it is so painful to many colleagues.

Marmor: I am concerned that this conference will limit itself to an exposition of the different kinds of role conflicts, and fail to come up with some solutions for resolving these conflicts. I have heard at least two suggestions thus far that are in the direction of trying to come up with a constructive solution. One is that wherever possible the administrative and the therapeutic roles of psychiatrists should be separated in institutions, in prisons, and so forth. Another suggestion was that, wherever we are aware of our values, we should make those values explicit – a kind of *Miranda* role for the practice of psychotherapy. At least our patients would then know where we stand and are not being unwittingly traduced in one way or another.

I still think we have not come to grips with the point that Will Caylin has been making: how do we meet the problem Where there are two rights?

I am hoping that we can discuss that, because we come back to the issue, I think, of whether ethics is essentially a relative problem or whether there are any absolute values. I find myself being far less critical of the decisions of Soviet psychiatrists than I was when I started this conference, even though I consider their practice abhorrent. But I find myself understanding that within a different kind of social context, different values may rule.

Principles and Recommendations

Gaylin: Out of these deliberations so far have come three propositions. One, psychiatry now feels the necessity to face in a systematic way certain difficult moral questions about its conflicting moral obligations. Two, the enunciation of those conflicts by a leadership group serves a useful purpose in educating a rank-and-file who may arrogantly or innocently deny such conflicts. Three, the obligations in the moral sphere rest not just with the individual but with institutions including the profession as an institution.

In addition, two major categories of questions emerged. One, since the psychiatrist is never a single agent, what are some guidelines in establishing the priorities as to which role takes precedence? Two, agreeing that a right to coercion exists, that is, that there is no sanctity in absolute autonomy, what are the limits of the right to coercion?

After discussing specific problems of the military, prisons, and mental hospitals, we arrived at three recommendations. One: separate the roles. Assign different people within the profession to handle the different roles. Two: with a *Miranda* model, announce our priorities and purposes to our patients in advance and indicate to them clearly under which set of obligations and rules we are working and which role we are assuming. Three: actively assume the responsibility to clean our own house. For definitions and guidelines suggesting possible resolution of the role conflicts, I will turn to Dan Callahan.

Callahan: Let me start with mat point Judd has raised, the problem of relativism. Let me put forward a proposition that seems to me relatively easy to justify: in any given society there must be standards and values. One cannot have a culture or a society unless there are well-understood rules and a common core of shared values. We live in a pluralistic society, but pluralism has its limits. People cannot live together unless they have common expectations and share at least some rules regulating their mutual life. In that respect, we are now going through a phase that Alan Stone called a reaction to arbitrary authority. I also think we are experiencing a reaction to rampant individualism; we are finding that we cannot run a society unless we not only recognize human rights but just as importantly recognize the limits of private values systems spread too widely in the marketplace.

The particular problem in the case of psychiatry is that the implicit, tacit working values have to be made explicit and examined. Will Gaylin was correct in saying that a new contract is being worked out between society and medicine and, in particular, between society and psychiatry. The problem is to determine the conditions of that new contract.

Let me propose some very specific priorities: first, the primary obligation of the psychiatrist is to the patient. That obligation may be overridden on occasion only if the conditions for overriding it are publicly explicit in law or in professional codes and those who are in the presence of psychiatrists understand under what circumstances the principle of patient obligation is to overridden. As a subpart of the same proposition, a psychiatrist may be an agent of an institution, or of society at large, as long as that is publicly understood and stated.

Second, some kind of rank ordering of accountability is necessary. Here I want to argue, following the first principle, that the psychiatrist is *first of all* accountable to the patient, but is also accountable to the public at large. Psychiatry is a public profession and has obligations to society as a whole.

And third, the psychiatrist has obligations to the profession.

What should we do when rights and obligations are in conflict? A genuine moral dilemma might be defined as those situations where two fundamental rights or obligations come into conflict. Society has to work at a general policy for resolving dilemmas of that sort and come to some determination on relative priorities. I will not try here to propose what that policy should be, but one might say, even if there are going to be losses in choosing one right or obligation over another, decisions have to be made. In that respect it is probably good to establish very broad principles as to which rights and obligations are comparatively more important.

There will be many situations where a happy resolution will be impossible. If one can establish a general system of preferences for one right or obligation over another, one will probably do so recognizing that there are going to be exceptions. And here one cannot set down a set of *a priori* rules as to how one ought to reslove true dilemmas, but one can keep a record of the way these individual decisions are resolved, so that an historical collection of cases can be made and these cases can, from time to time, be publicly reviewed by the profession. The assumption behind this kind of a review process is that individuals must make hard choices and that where the choice could have gone either way, people will generally differ. But if there are mechanisms to bring out and expose to public view the kinds of decisions made and the reasons for them, then the profession can collectively deliberate over a period of time about which decisions seem to be correct and adjust their general policy concerning the resolution of similar dilemmas.

Michels: In my comments let me take a purely clinical approach. We have a patient, in this case a profession, whose presenting complaint is a felt conflict is described in various ways. At least in one situation it seems to be between some venal drive for money or power or status or security and nobler codes of professional morality and ethics. Now this felt conflict is currently handled by an integrating structure of the professional organization. I think it is intriguing that professor Freidson picks the word 'etiquette' – a very dainty word, very elegant and refined, but somewhat thin – to describe the structure that we have evolved to handle these conflicts. I am not sure that I want substantive major conflicts to be integrated by something called 'etiquette,' and that may be part of the problem we are facing.

We are talking about the kinds of new structures we need that will give us the power and the capacity to deal with these conflicts. We want to have a more powerful profession, but we must convince that outside world somehow or other that that professional autonomy and power won't lead to even further abuses of the type that got us into this conflict in the first place. Let's look at certain very concrete attractions of that solution. One of the problems we kept facing was: what happens when the psychiatrist works for an institution, and therefore, has two masters? That problem stems from the fact that institutions are more powerful than psychiatrists. One answer is that psychiatrist should never work for institutions, but only for individuals or for the profession of psychiatry. And if institutions want to buy psychiatrists, they must buy them from the profession. There fore, when any individual psychiatrist is serving two masters, one will be his patient, the other will be his profession. Negotiations between prisons or the military or schools or other evil subsets of society would have to deal with

another powerful organization, not with an individual practitioner. That has certain interesting possibilities to me. It would mean that the psychiatrist's payoff could never come from being coopted by an evil institution other than his own profession. That still leaves the problem of ensuring that his own profession is not an evil institution.

I would except Paul Friedman to raise some problems about my simple plan for greatly increasing the power and autonomy of the psychiatric profession. The most important is the price that must be paid for doing it. That price would be to to have the professional organization include appropriate representation from the general community to safeguard the values that the profession represents, and to make sure they are not simply trade union values. In effect, if the APA is to be much stronger and more powerful than it is, its board of trustees must include nonpsychiatrists and members of the general public.

I would suggest that the core theme of this conference is: strengthen the profession as a structure which the individual practitioners are only, in a sense, agents or representatives. Dan says that there are three levels of accountability: to the patient, to the public, and to the profession. But I think in fact accountability to the patient and to the public must be monitored through the profession. Accountability to the profession is the means for evaluating, testing, and measuring accountability to the patient and to the public.

The Hippocratic code originated in a problem strangely similar to the one we face today. The Hippocratic physician was peripatetic, wandering from town to town; he treated strangers for the most part. The size and heterogeneity of modem society has brought us back to that practice arrangement. We are probably closer to the Hippocratic ethical problem than was nineteenth-century medicine. One of the important reasons for the Hippocratic code of ethics was that every practitioner had an obligation to his brothers-in-practice to be above any possible suspicion of venality or exploitation. He was an advertisement for all others. It was vital for the efficacy of the, stranger-practitioner arriving in a new town that he be automatically accepted as trustworthy; the only way that could be guaranteed; was that it was widely known that members of this brotherhood were sworn to follow certain rules lest death or some terrible punishment result. We are in a very similar situation: the loyalty to the profession is essential to the maintenance of our credibility and therefore our capacity to practice. The profession serves as the intervening variable in our contract with the public. One change from the days of Hippocrates is that society would no longer trust or allow the brotherhood to carry on without societal representation in the group of elders.

Marmor: What troubles me is Bob Michels's assumption that the profession can have a life separate from that of the social matrix in which it develops. I seriously question this. If we were to go by the dominant values of the psychiatric profession, we would find ourselves going down a rather narrow road. I think part of the struggle in which the leadership of our profession is constantly involved is trying to broaden the values of our profession, and not reduce it to a guildlike orientation. Moreover, as Bob points out, the only way the profession can have this kind of strength is to include the public. But, which members of the public? Society isn't a monolith, and there are different publics and contradictory demands.

I think that Dan's propositions reflect value orientation toward Western democratic society. It happens to be one that I share, but if we are going to look at the problem in global terms, can we escape the issue of ethical relativism? In China it would be unthinkable to place the interests of the individual ahead of the interests of the society. Now, obviously within our pluralistic society, we do not have uniform value systems. I think the value system that places the individual first is probably the prevailing one, but that is sometimes contradicted by social needs, and I think that is why we are caught, perhaps more strongly than in any totalitarian society, with these kinds of role conflicts.

Friedman: But the contrast with China points out how difficult it would be for psychiatrists in our pluralistic society to say anything but that their allegiance is to the patient. They will see many different patients who themselves will have different values and value conflicts. The psychiatrist's role should be to work with patients to resolve their own value conflicts.

Sabshin: Often when cables come from the Soviet Union they are sent to HEW or NIMH, instead of, let's say, to the American Psychiatric Association. In the Soviet Union, one writes to the Ministry of Health to discuss the medical profession. In this country the nature of professions and their regulations have special boundary problems. Not every psychiatrist is a member of the APA. About 5,000 are not. What are the regulatory systems governing them?

Moreover, we have to recognize that there are differences in philosophy in certification. For example, in some countries certification is handled by the profession to self. What is the public interest in that role? Would getting the profession more involved include taking on more regulatory functions, or do these need to be shared? What about those boundaries that also pertain to the ethical cases? To what extent is there an obligation to reduce dissonance and to report to outside agencies rather than keeping problems within the profession?

Redlich: We might consider how little we have talked about money and how money influences rules, regulations, and laws. After all, a lot of our role conflicts occur because certain people get paid for certain functions. A military psychiatrist gets paid as a military officer. A prison psychiatrist gets paid as a prison official. Thinking of an absurd example, if the APA were to decide all therapy from now on should be nude, the members might follow this advice or not. If HEW, Blue cross, and Aetna Life Insurance would decide that only nude therapists get paid, it would be a completely different story.

Klerman: While one a acknowledges different value systems, I think that there is a danger that ethical or cultural relativism disarms one's sense of moral justice. And it seems to me that for a group like the APA, there is a difficult set of problems in dealing with our own organization and strengthening its moral position with respect to our clients and the rest of society, an dealing with the problems of Soviet or Chinese psychiatrists. I would agree. with Paul that one way to handle both is to be sure of what our values are and affirm them in both arenas. We should say that we do place a very high value on the individual. We should be prepared to assert that forcefully if we do get involved in a cross-cultural or cross-national discussion.

One way in which the profession need to be strengthened is to maintain some sense of internal moral strength. Now whether this can be accomplished by the specific administrative reforms that have been suggested, I think is a matter for vigorous debate. I would be interested in hearing whether our consultants from outside the profession, like Arlene and Eliot, would agree that those suggestions are sufficient to strengthen the profession. But there is no doubt in my mind that our position toward our own clients and them Soviet Union and China would be strengthened by affirming the propositions that Dan and Paul put forth and by strengthening the profession without making it a guild.

Sabshin: When we start to think of practical ways of dealing with this problem, we are going to have to face up to the fact that we do not live in splendid isolation. For instance. Professor Freidson's remarks about etiquette. If we look at that issue, it seems to me quite clear that there are forces at work in society, separate from the profession, which are going to have a major impact. How do we work with these forces? I think it is very hard to make an organization the profession, more powerful without making it more like a trade association. If through malpractice and through regulation it becomes increasingly clear that hospitals have to begin to control people who work there, if we are going to have rate-setting in advance all over the United States for heath care, the administration of the hospital is going to have to become more powerful in controlling the individual decision makers who raise costs. If you are going to have the hospitals sued for malpractice of doctors, the hospital and those in regulatory roles vis-a-vis hospitals are going to become involved in this issue of etiquette.

what is the APA's position going to be? I think that we have to relate to those real forces and think through the propositions in those terms.

Friedman: No matter how well-intentioned this group, I think the resolution to build up the prominence or strength of the APA would be misperceived by a lot of people. The result might be counterproductive. So I conclude that if there is going to be some movement in this area, it ought to be building up some Substructure like the Ethics Committee. This committee or some kind of a new panel ought to have some representatives of outside world.

There are two rather different kinds of responsibility called for. One has to do with quality of care and the competency of the deliverers of care, which I thought professor Freidson was primarily speaking about, which I see as essentially being taken care of by in-house discussion. The second has to do with potential conflicts and allegiances to different forces in society or agencies. I see those as being addressed by concerned psychiatrists in concert with other outside representatives. So we may be may be working on two different structures.

Freidson: We cannot visualize professional work as solely the relationship of one individual professional to an individual patient, complicating it perhaps by an institutional context. It is also the individual professional in relationship to his colleagues and his colleagues' patients. As an ethical person, the individual professional assumes, if not responsibility, at least some concern for their well-being, as well as a concern for the well-being of the colleagues. I do want to insist that what I had in mind is a real dilemma and not something separate from all of the other dilemmas.

I use the distinction between 'ethics' and 'etiquette' only because in the history of medicine, the word 'etiquette' has been used separately from the word 'ethics' to refer to those issues involving collegial relationships. Perhaps I did not clearly indicate that to my mind it is not merely politeness, but there are ethical choices involved in most relationships, namely, where your primary responsibility rests, I was using the word 'etiquette' in a technical, not entirely idiosyncratic, but apparently foreign sense here.

Levin: When these moral conflicts go public, they should go public not to psychiatry, but to the people. It seems to me that, no matter what you say we are building, that no matter how big the organization gets, you cannot handle all roles. You can't be advocates for the public and advocates for yourself. The process of protecting the public must be done by the public. One of our responsibilities is to make the public, all publics, aware of these conflicts. Then have confidence in the intelligence of the public to utilize this information and advocate for itself. There are role models in other professions: certainly atomic scientists who sensed the dangers of nuclear power went to the public. And so did the molecular biologists working on recombinant DNA research. Informing the public starts breaking down the mystification of our professionals and the public feels less powerless.

Daniels: As a researcher on the professions, and one who has been particularly interested in codes of ethics and their relationship to certification and autonomy of professions, it is my considered opinion that codes of ethics are window dressing. People who are going to behave well will do so and people who will not are not going to be bound by a code of ethics nor are they going to see that it applies to them particularly. In general, although the APA has done very well in specifying for the areas of therapy, the code of ethics does not tell you about particular instances. As one of my friends said to me, after making a terrible error, 'I knew about the category, but I didn't see this as an instance of it.'

In order to make people understand the categories and their instances, you have to have sanction boards, because professionals are no better men and women than anyone else. They are not more malevolent certainly, by they are not better either, and so they need social controls. I found in reviewing the CPAs, that they are much more ethical than any of the helping professions, because their codes of ethics are all backed up by a rather careful system of sanctions. In medicine, short of removing a license, there is no effective system of penalties or sanctions. What I mean by enforcement procedures is that psychiatrists can be fined, can be held up to public sanction, and can be given a lot of nasty publicity, which is worse than taking away their membership in the APA.

Sabshin: We could do that. All the states are developing those boards of discipline. That is where the action is going to take place. The question is, what relationship should the APA have to those boards of discipline?

Stone: Since I agree that our ethics committees have tended to function as protective, rather than disciplinary boards, I would recommend that they should tell people who complain to them that we have very little power. The first thing that our ethics committee should decide to do is start to refer people to a proper agency. But there will be tremendous resistance for all the reasons that Professor Freidson described.

Freidson: I'd like to register a disagreement, particularly with the implication of Arlene's choice of words, in which the terms 'sanction' and 'punishment' keep occurring. This is likely to be rather ineffective. I also reject Alan's suggestion, namely, that the Ethics Committee of the APA can't handle anything because it has no power; let the state disciplinary committees do it. What is done by state committees is likely to be unjust and subject to all kinds of political and journalistic whims; they are much too remote from where practice is and, furthermore, are punitively oriented. The basic issue is not sanctioning in the sense of punishing but rather interacting with colleagues – educating, persuading and making it damn clear what one's position is, ethically and professionally and that one expects one's colleagues to perform in the same way. The APA could be very creative and constructive in thinking of ways of cleaning house. First consider the kinds of processes that exist in hospitals. One of the deficiencies of presently available processes is that hospital boards are scared to death of being sued by physicians who have been dropped from the staff. Legislation could give immunity to those who provide information to the State Disciplinary Committee. It is possible to recommend legislation in the context of the ordinary processes of self-regulation that take place in institutions where psychiatrists work. Consider the kinds of legislation that would remove some of the legal barriers to exercising educative influence and pressure on colleagues without getting to the point of simply rejecting them, throwing them out, which may or may not solve anything.

Gaylin: I would like to support Eliot's position. I think there is incredible power in the need for approval from one's colleagues.

Macklin: In discussing recommendations and guidelines, one has to make distinctions. What one can do depends on the area in which one wants to do it. These areas are now being conflated, whereas before they were kept separate. We are talking simultaneously about four things. Bad eggs and housecleaning is number one. Bad eggs, I take it, are those who are morally deficient in the practice of psychiatry. Second, we are talking about competence, that is , not coming up exactly to the highest standards of the profession. Professional incompetence is different from moral deficiency, but both might require some housecleaning or some internal monitoring of affairs. Third is duty conflicts in psychiatry, which has been the primary focus of this conference. Those are the insoluble moral dilemmas that anyone faces either in personal life or professional life. Fouth is the social role of psychiatry. Fritz Redlich has raised this question: should psychiatry be controlling deviancy, or should it operate on a strictly therapeutic model? Now those four separate areas have to be looked at carefully, if recommendations are to be developed, study groups are going to go forward, and guidelines are going to be presented.

Levin: No one would agree on the limits of the area of social control. There are some who would say that is what psychiatry is all about. I would suggest that a better way to pursue the question is to examine each area. Take the criminal justice system, take the educational system, and see where one acts as an agent of social control and where one does not. It may be important to have counselling for prisoners, just to alleviate some psychological problem that has nothing to do with their deviant criminal

behavior. One has to look very carefully at what the mental health professions can do as a service, and what we can not do.

Michels: I agree with Professor Freidson that the house-cleaning issue is terribly important, but not particularly because we will get the house much cleaner. Its importance has to do with changing the profession from trade union to representative of public interest, and with the issue of trust of the profession as an agent of public rather than of personal interest. There are, however, problems with house-cleaning. I think that Professor Freidson's solution to it is going to be a very weak solution to a very big problem, because of the peculiarities of psychiatry compared to most other areas of medicine. His solution is a solution that would work in those other areas.

One of psychiatry's peculiarities is that the range of competence is probably greater for the tasks it faces than in most other medical specialities. Another is that psychiatrists often practice in secret, and frequently exclusively in secret. The psychiatrist may bring a patient to the front door of the hospital or more often send him there, but he rarely treats him in that hospital. Some other psychiatrist treats him in the hospital, and so to a considerable extent there are two populations of psychiatrists; those that work outside hospitals and those that work in them. And they rarely have important interactions with each other. A psychiatrist who avoids hospitals could be a drooling idiot for years and unless it showed in a public forum like this, his colleagues would never know from the way he treats his patients. And if his patients complained, we could talk about their negative transference and dismiss them on the basis of their incompetence to judge him.

For the last few years I have been the co-chairman of the American Analytic Association's Committee on Peer Review and we have been trying to deal with this in a number of ways, but we keep running into such problems as the fact that there are no data to review except what analysts tell you they did after they know they are being reviewed. That is not a sort of optimal situation to evaluate. I don't have a solution, but I think it is a problem that is unique to the field.

Robert Moore: One big problem is in the area of out-patient psychiatry. How does one establish a true competency review system for that? We are certainly trying to develop systems to handle that. One other practical problem is that the APA is not one cohesive organization, but an amalgam of 70 local psychiatric societies, each of which has an Ethics Committee. And each one handles complaints in very different ways. Our national Ethics Committee is really an appeals body and also a promulgator of new annotations. The last time we tried to develop a new code the AMA said, 'You can't do it because we are all members of the medical profession, and thus you cannot have a separate code.' Now what we can do is develop new annotations, as Dan suggested. We do that now. Our annotations are historical records of cases.

Freedman: I think we have avoided rather deliberately taking votes or trying to achieve a consensus, which would be rather premature, but I think out of this a good deal can be developed. I will now ask our panelists for final statements.

Gaylin: Our tasks are roughly twofold: One is to take the educative process, which has served 12 or 15 psychiatrists at this conference, and expand that process so that it reaches the larger population. The second is to continue the research, using as our case studies prisons and deviation in general.

Callahan: It seems to me possible to hope for the achievement of an effective working consensus, which, if it does not pretend to be the answer, at least, sets down rules for people to live and work by. In our society we often despair about solving these, large ethical issues, because there are enormous value conflicts, but it seems to me in fact we really do resolve them in rough-and-ready ways and I can see a consensus emerging from this meeting.

Marmor: This conference has helped to clarify a number of important issues, problems of institutional role conflicts. And I think it has some constructive solutions. I think that there are still some obscurities. For example, I think we would all agree that we ought to get out of the social control business, but this is not as simple as we might think. We agree that the issue of what constitutes social control is often very obscure. It is implicit in our norm, in our professional definitions of what constitutes healthy and neurotic behavior.

And I think that the simplest example of this would be our attitudes toward sexual deviants. There are honest differences about whether sexual deviance constitutes psychopathology and therefore falls within the realm of treatment or whether it is simply a variant that is, in itself, not relevant to the issue of psychopathology. There are also elements of social responsibility here that need to be delineated. These exceptions to our therapeutic responsibilities to the patient need to be clarified. I feel what we have accomplished at this conference has been most constructive.

Freedman: We have come a long way. I think there is still a good deal to be done. I want to thank all of you for participating in this very valuable and worthwhile conference. Thank you.

The Psychiatrist as Double Agent*

Daniel Callahan and Willard Gaylin

Case No. 174

A young first year medical student was having a severe emotional crisis. Obviously on the verge of a complete breakdown, he went to a private psychiatrist. He was agitated, anxious, didn't know if he could handle his studies. He had a brilliant college record, and clearly outstanding intellectual capacity.

He was in acute distress and seemingly in the process of disintegration. The psychiatrist, trying very hard to avoid hospitalization, started intensive psychotherapy. The student was already at a point where it looked like he was going to have a schizophrenic break: reality testing was impaired, ideas of reference were occurring, and a hypomanic mood with grandiose ideation, was forming. To relieve the pressures on him the psychiatrist recommended that he take a medical leave of absence from school. He dropped out at the end of the semester in good academic standing. The psychiatrist wrote a letter for him saying that he was treating the student for 'emotional problems' and recommended a medical leave of absence.

The next fall the student attempted to return to medical, school but was refused readmission, even though the psychiatrist had written a letter, as the physician in charge of the treatment, that he was medically able to continue his studies. They gave no reason for not reinstating him except that he was not considered suitable. He then began to apply to other medical schools at his psychiatrist's suggestion and was refused in every case. Before seeing the private psychiatrist the student had consulted the school psychiatrist who made a diagnosis of latent schizophrenia.

When other medical schools wrote to his former school, the reason for discharge was medical leave with latent schizophrenia. It is known that about half of those with schizophrenia in remission will have another break. In the case of this student there was a real risk to future patients. He was planning to become a surgeon. The combination of a grandiose self-appraisal with the power of the surgeon could cause serious harm.

The private psychiatrist recognized that there may be psychiatric conditions which would interfere with a career in medicine and therefore might be grounds for exclusion from medical school. The problem, as he saw it, was whether the school psychiatrist was seeing the student in his role as psychiatrist or in his role as part of the school administration, and whether these two roles could be separated.

Is it acceptable for a physician who is on the staff of a school or a business corporation to simultaneously serve as the agent of the organization employing him and the patient who is the student or employee of that organization?

This case raises questions at two different levels, one general, the other more specific. At the most general level, I have long been troubled by the problem of whether there can be ethically correct decisions within settings which are inherently unjust or immoral, i.e., in those situations where certain kinds of

ethical dilemmas would not ordinarily arise but for the fact of distorted or corrupt institutions. In the era of slavery, for example, acute ethical dilemmas used to arise (for some, at least) over the most moral way of separating children from parents when all were to be sold at auction. Obviously the very institution of slavery was immoral. But does that entail that each and every decision made within the *given* context of such an institution was also and equally immoral, regardless of what the decision was?

I will leave that question hanging for the moment. But it has direct bearing on how one might judge the actions of the various parties in the case at hand. On the face of it, the procedure used in judging the question of readmission for the student was unjust. First, it is highly doubtful that, when the student initially went to the school psychiatrist, he was informed that 'anything you say to me may be held against you,' which was exactly what turned out to be the case. Second, it seems clear that the school psychiatrist acted as the agent of the school, a final, critical moment – the moment of decision about readmission. Third, and worse still, the school psychiatrist acted in effect as the agent for all medical schools, creating a very nasty kind of black-ball system. Fourth, since the case clearly implies that the student, on the advice of his private psychiatrist, initiated the request for leave, and took that leave voluntarily, it seems to me thoroughly unjust that he should be subjected to special conditions in order to regain his place in the school. He had already won his admission to the school. Finally, it is evident that the school provided no formal review mechanism for its procedurally arbitrary decision, and nothing remotely approaching due process.

But did the school make a wrong ethical decision in this particular case? My phrasing of the question implies that a distinction can be made between an unjust system of making decisions and the moral correctness of any given decision within the context of that system. Given the specifics of the case, I think the action of the school can be defended, though hardly praised. Let us charitably assume that, when the student's readmission case came up, those making the decision were at least sensitive enough to recognize that it would be a great blow to the student, a blow made all the harsher by the black-ball system which then ensued. But I would also assume they felt, appropriately enough, that they had obligations not only to the student but also to his potential future patients. The notion of a surgeon incipiently subject to 'grandiose self-appraisal' is hardly reassuring. Even if there were only a risk (though not a negligible one), the consequences for his patients could be enormous. And I would suppose that, given the fact that there are many qualified candidates for medical school (who are not latent schizophrenics and who could be taken but for lack of space), they may well have reasoned that there was no *need* to run the risk to future patients. In a situation where a hard choice had to be made, they chose to worry more about the potential harm to patients than the harm caused by thwarting the student's medical ambitions. It is a defensible choice and, as in many hard cases, that may be all that can be achieved.

Let me return to the question I left hanging in the opening paragraph. My answer is 'no': correct ethical choices *can sometimes* be made in unjust contexts. But the larger ethical question remains that of the unjust context, which requires correction. I am hardly a devotee of the increasing tendency in our society for all institutional disputes to be taken to court. But in

* Callahan, D. and Gaylin, W.: The psychiatrist as double agent. *Hastings Center Report* 4:12–14, 1974.

this instance I wish the student had done so. He may not have been admitted in the end, but others might have been the beneficiaries of a system forced to give up arbitrary exercises of power; and the school psychiatrist might have been forced to protect the confidentiality of his relationship with other students.

Daniel Callahan.

No man serves one master. Not in these complicated times. We are stretched by the conflicting demands – of our various responsibilities; our obligations to children, country, self, spouse, profession, humanity, life, justice, pleasure and conscience.

Certain roles, because they serve needs of such essential importance, have been granted extraordinary privilege and priority. The physician, perceived as preserver of life, has traditionally been a man of great privilege and has pledged himself to honor that privilege with responsibility. In order to sustain a relationship in which one individual places his very life in the hands of another, there must be some assurance that the relationship will be governed by its primary purpose: that is, the good of the patient, the preservation of his life, the protection of his well-being. The physician is under oath to 'do no harm.' It is the basis of trust on which the profession of medicine has survived.

Any infringement on the inviolability of this contract threatens the whole medical structure. Of course nothing in life is inviolate, and there will always be times when the physician will break his word to his patient for higher responsibilities. We will quarantine the contagious, commit the psychotic and confine the dangerous.

A young student, recognizing mental illness in himself, consults the physician assigned by his school to serve those needs. On making the diagnosis the school physician refers him for outside help, and, indeed, he is helped. Then he wishes to continue his career. In the judgment of the treating physician, the patient is qualified to go on with his professional work. Yet he is refused readmission, despite the fact that it is of the nature of most medical leaves to allow for return. Further, it is apparent that a kind of black-ball by diagnosis has been effected. Schizophrenia, a broad category of disease, in psychiatry carries the same often unwarranted dread as cancer in general medicine. Knowing this, the private physician guarded this diagnosis. Had the student only seen the private doctor, he would have been readmitted. The student's problems arose because he assumed that the school psychiatrist was indeed a psychiatrist, bound by the codes of conduct, oath and ethics of his general profession.

Were I an admission officer in a medical school I would discourage the admission of schizophrenic applicants. On the other hand, there is also no question that among the schizophrenic patients I personally have seen have been successful medical students, not to mention political leaders, psychoanalytic candidates, judges, educators, doctors, lawyers and merchant chiefs. Schizophrenia is no asset in any of these professions.

If the physician has a great responsibility to his patient, he also has a responsibility to the future patients of this would-be physician. Nonetheless, the young man in the case approached the school psychiatrist for care, not for professional guidance. Because of cases similar to this, I have repeatedly advised all of my patients and friends to make sure that their children never consults school professionals, whether they be psychiatrists, psychologists, internists, or what have you. I have seen too many cases where the school psychiatrist has adopted the manner, of personal physician, but seen his responsibility as an employee of the institution. And that is precisely the problem. Unless a physician's role is clearly defined as primarily serving the needs of the individual patient rather than the needs of the employer, the trust on which all medicine rests, particularly psychiatric medicine, will be destroyed.

Every occasion when it is decided that responsibility to a greater good must supersede responsibility to the patient is a violation of the medical contract with the patient. It must not be called otherwise. We must not rationalize the dilemma by asserting that we are fulfilling our responsibility to our patient. We are not. We are granting a higher priority to other responsibilities. Never should this violation of contract be a matter of diffidence or routine, as is too often the case with 'company' physicians. To use the diagnostic skills of the physician to the detriment of the patient, albeit for a larger good, should be a decision made with the personal agony that always accompanies a moral dilemma. I wonder if the school psychiatrist in this case suffered much when he committed his casual diagnosis to the public record.

Willard Gaylin

Notes

This is one of a series of case studies raising ethical dilemmas in medicine and the life sciences. It was selected and prepared by Robert M. Veatch from a collection of medical ethics cases being edited by the Institute for book publication.

While the cases are based on actual situations, the content, including names and other identifying material, has been modified sufficiently to assure anonymity and clarity of issues.

The Effect of Third-Party Payment on the Practice of Psychotherapy*

Paul Chodoff

Many issues are raised by the use of third-party mechanisms such as health insurance to pay for psychotherapeutic services. These include such questions as confidentiality, diagnostic and reporting practices, the medical versus the nonmedical model, and transference-countertransference relationships. The role of peer review and other quality control mechanism will undoubtedly increase as psychiatry is asked to document more fully than in the past the criteria for various forms of psychotherapy and to demonstrate their effectiveness.

A recent issue of the *Journal of the American Medical Association*[1] contained a letter from a psychiatrist asking for guidance about a sticky situation with which he had been confronted. He was treating the mistress of a married man who asked the psychiatrist to make out the bill in his name as if he were the patient. It had occurred to the psychiatrist that the married man's purpose was not only to keep the relationship secret but also to collect insurance payment for the services. What, dear editor, the psychiatrist prayed, was his duty in the face of this thorny ethical and legal conundrum?

This tidbit illustrates that when we accept the participation of an otherwise uninvolved third-party in the financial aspects of the psychotherapeutic contract, we have come very far from the simple and uncomplicated situation in which the purveyor of the psychotherapeutic services is paid directly either by the recipient of those services or by some one, usually a relative, who has a personal interest in and responsibility for the patient or client.

However, the issues raised by the increasing use of impersonal third-party payment mechanisms such as health insurance for psychotherapeutic services far transcend in scope and importance the doctor's dilemma described above. In those areas of the country in which this method of payment has become a significant factor in the financial transactions between the two parties involved in psychotherapy, a host of unexpected problems has appeared, either as a direct result of the new mode of payment or because problems previously dormant or glossed over have begun to surface with an urgency demanding answers in terms of dollars and cents rather than theories.

To suggest the range of these problems, I could mention that third-party payment has brought into question such issues as confidentiality, the therapist's allegiance, diagnostic, and reporting practices, and transference-countertransference relationships in the therapy. Professional identity confusions appear as the therapist becomes less a priest and more a businessman and the organizations to which he belongs become involved increasingly with guild and political concerns rather than with purely professional ones. Ultimately the third-party interest raises questions about the applicability of the medical model to psychotherapy.

Third-party payment, of course, occurs not only in the private practice of psychotherapy but also when psychiatric care, including psychotherapy, is provided in state and federal hospitals and in outpatient psychiatric clinics and community mental health centers funded by various means. However, in this discussion I shall confine myself to the setting with which I am most familiar – that is, the office practice of private psychotherapy – and I will draw

to a considerable extent on the experiences of myself and my colleagues in the Washington, D.C., area, where the Federal Employees Health Benefits Program has provided a substantial portion of the income of psychiatrists treating government employees and their families.

Medical Versus Nonmedical Model

For the federal employee in the Washington area whose major medical insurance coverage provides 80 percent payment for outpatient psychotherapy; the third-party influence may first be felt at the point when a prospective patient seeks a therapist. Of course in those cases in which he is referred to or seeks out a physician specializing in psychiatry, the problem I will delineate does not arise. But the potential patient may instead be considering treatment with a nonphysician, such as a psychologist. If, he is paying for the services out of his own pocket he can choose between the psychiatrist and psychologist on the basis of what he knows about the kinds of services these two disciplines provide and his feeling about the particular individual. However, if the insurance carrier is paying a substantial portion of the fee, there will usually be an advantage in choosing the psychiatrist instead of the psychologist since the former will be treated by the insurance carrier like any other doctor and will receive his payments accordingly, as long as he lives up to certain requirements. The psychologist, however, is not an M.D. and he will therefore be in a somewhat ambiguous and unclear position as a potential recipient of payment for medical services. If the patient is insured by the largest local, carrier, the Blue Cross and Blue Shield plan covering federal employees, the psychologist therapist will have to submit himself either nominally or substantially to the supervision of a psychiatrist physician before his services become eligible for insurance payment; this will affect both his self-image and his relationship with the patient.

The magnetism of financial advantage inherent in this situation will have a differing effect on psychiatrists and on nonmedical psychotherapists. The former group includes a substantial number who in the past have not been reluctant to emphasize the ways in which they are dissimilar from other physicians. Such attitudes are likely to be reversed as psychiatrists respond to the economic spur of third-party payment, prodding them to mend their medical fences and reestablish their allegiance to the medical model; this obscures some of the real problems about its applicability to their psychotherapeutic practices. The nonmedical therapist, on the other hand, may find himself on the horns of a dilemma since, although his heart may be with the behavioral change model, his pocketbook may push him toward at least grudging acceptance of the medical model. That is, in order to fall within the purview of medical insurance, he will have to acknowledge that he is treating, disease rather than changing behavior.

He may choose the alternative of seeking a basic change in the criteria used by the insurance companies, that is, to try to convince them that, psychotherapeutic treatment by psychologists should be accepted as parallel and equal to that by psychiatrists.[2] This course, which is being, pursued by the American Psychological Association, raises very fundamental questions about the use of medical insurance for purposes that could be considered nonmedical and may also tend to widen the breach between medical and

* Chodoff, P.: The effect of third-party payment on the practice of psychotherapy. *American Journal of Psychiatry* 129:540–545, 1972.

nonmedical psychotherapists, already illustrated by the recent conflicts within, major psychoanalytic organizations about the admission of certain non-M.D.s as full-fledged members. Although real and substantive differences are involved in this dispute there also appears to be a hidden agenda present in the form of economic guild issues, one of which is the fate of psychoanalysis under present in the form of economic guild issues, one of which is the fate of psychoanalysis under present insurance plans and, even more, under a, future national health insurance program.

Confidentiality

Let us assume now that the therapist has been selected and that he is a physician. The contract between patient and physician must now include provisions for complying with certain requirements of the third-party insurance carrier. With the approval and knowledge of the patient, some facts about the patient will have to be conveyed to the insurance company by the psychiatrist. But if this requirement is complied with, what about the ideal of absolute confidentiality in the psychiatrist-patient relationship? This is an emotionally laden area for many psychiatrists, inducing a great deal of anxiety and resentment and, along with this, certain defensive maneuvers. Some psychiatrists, choosing to disregard the axiom that he who pays the piper calls the tune, may go so far as to deny that the insurance company has the right to any information about the patient for whose treatment it is authorized payment; these psychiatrists may then engage in conflicts or obfuscating maneuvers with the carrier.

Even though the majority of psychiatrists recognize the legitimate need of the insurance carrier to have certain facts about the cases for which they are authorizing payment, they may be troubled by this requirement and by its possible effect in breaching the trust the patient must have that he can say anything at all to his therapist without fear of disclosure. To obviate this uneasiness, psychiatric organizations in the Washington area have worked with the insurance carriers to define and keep to a minimum the information the carriers requires to carry out their obligation to their policy holders and to ensure that such information remains only in authorized hands.

But the uneasiness among psychiatrists, justified or not, remains. One of the ways in which it is manifested is in the diagnostic reporting of the condition for which the patient is being treated. Although I have no data on this matter, it is my impression that the most common diagnoses submitted on insurance company forms are anxiety neurosis and depressive neurosis; such *DSM-II*[3] diagnoses as alcoholism, schizophrenia, and homosexuality are made so infrequently as to suggest that patients suffering from these conditions may be receiving other diagnoses.

If this kind of mislabeling is occurring, two sets of reasons could be advanced for it, both at least partially the result of the influence of third-party payment. The first (already mentioned) is the psychiatrist's uneasiness about the confidentiality of the information he is transmitting to an impersonal bureaucracy, where leakage cannot be ruled out; this leakage, including the diagnoses I have just mentioned, may be harmful to the interests of the patients under his care. In this case, incidentally, there is no doubt that the psychiatrist's allegiance is to his patient rather than to the insurance company, so that conflicts about whose interest he is representing would not arise as they might in other instances of third-party payment such as the military service, where a psychiatrist might have a real conflict between his allegiance to his patient and to the military organization of which he is a member.

But fears that confidentiality may be breached are not the only reason for the diagnostic reporting practices I have suggested. A second factor is the difficulty in conforming some patients to the diagnostic scheme of *DSM-II*.[3] This is not a problem in the case of all or even most psychiatric patients receiving psychotherapy; most fall quite comfortably into medically oriented diagnostic rubrics, whether or not the psychiatrist chooses to employ them. However, especially among patients who are being treated by intensive psychotherapeutic (including psychoanalytic) techniques, there are a certain number whose problems, although real, cannot be adequately described in medically oriented diagnostic terms. These are the people whose difficulties in such interpersonal areas as family, work, and social relationships result in relatively little disability in the ordinary medical use of this term. When such individuals pay for their own psychotherapy, the troublesome question of whether they conform to the medical definition of a 'patient' need not be a matter of concern to themselves or to their therapists. If the need and the suffering are sufficient, treatment will be undertaken regardless of diagnosis or of whether the sufferer is a 'patient.' However, medical insurance requires medical diagnoses, and unless this requirement is altered for certain categories of patients seeking psychotherapy, the psychiatric profession is under the increasing necessity of somehow coming to terms with the problem of diagnosis.

Effect on Treatment Pattern

Having agreed to undertake a psychotherapeutic enterprise together, the two parties involved must now also agree on the frequency of visits, a decision that is of major importance in determining whether the psychotherapy will be at the supportive end or the more intensive, psychoanalytically oriented end of the spectrum of possible approaches. When substantial third-party financial assistance is available, this choice becomes relatively free of financial hindrances so that it may be dictated more by the therapist's judgment about what would be best in this particular case than by the patient's means. Such a payment arrangement provides an opportunity for individuals otherwise not able to afford it to receive skilled and experienced psychotherapeutic help.

However, although substantial help in paying for psychotherapy is clearly beneficial in allowing a freer choice of treatment modality, there may be other consequences. For instance, the absence of clear-cut indications for various types of psychotherapy might influence therapists to choose the kind of therapy they prefer to do rather than to make a decision on the basis of more objective criteria; an increase in the more intensive types of treatment might well result. This danger is not unique to psychiatry; it has been pointed out as a general trend in medicine that the existence of third-party payment provides 'little incentive for efficiency. Instead, the trend is to use the higher cost facilities and services and to make as many of these available as possible'.[4] On the other hand, it is likely that one of the factors stimulating the present popularity of the various varieties of group therapy is the availability of insurance payment.

It is also clear that, as long as there is a discrepancy in the amount of insurance coverage in different geographical areas, more psychotherapeutic services will be dispensed where insurance coverage is substantial. For example, in the Washington, D.C., area the organization previously known as the Baltimore Psychoanalytic Society, has changed its name to the Baltimore-D.C. Psychoanalytic Society, since more of its activities are taking place in Washington than in Baltimore, where insurance coverage of mental disorders is much less extensive. Such a differential will tend to disappear once the uniform provisions of a national health insurance program have been agreed upon and implemented; the effect of third-party payment on the choice of psychotherapeutic modalities will then be determined by the amount of coverage for outpatient psychotherapy contained in such a program.

I will now turn to the effect of third-party payment on the course of the psychotherapy itself, that is, its influence on such treatment dynamics as transference-countertransference issues, resistances, fantasies, defense, motivations for treatment, etc. This subject, which merges with the general effect of payment on psychotherapeutic transactions, although rich in its implications for psychotherapy, has to the best of my knowledge not been sufficiently treated in the relevant literature. Such discussions of the subject as exist are found mainly in regard to intensive psychotherapies, and especially psychoanalysis, since it is in these forms of therapy where a scrutiny of the relationship between therapist and patients is of such importance that these issues find their fullest play and are most likely to be affected by financial transactions.

The Issue of Financial Sacrifice

As far as psychoanalytic psychotherapy is concerned, the paramount question posed by the increasing availability of third-party payment is whether and to what extent such treatments are crippled when regular, direct payments are not made by the patient to the therapist. In a paper written in 1964,[5] I summarized the classical psychoanalytic position as holding that the analyst must require sacrificial fees from his patient because they provide the patient with motivation, generate analytical material, and are beneficial to the countertransference. However, reports of actual experiences with free and low cost analysis available at that time suggested that such a payment milieu was not fatally inimical to treatment; rather, despite theoretical preconceptions and individual examples to the contrary, the evidence indicated that psychoanalysis can proceed successfully in the absence of fees or with low fees. This finding supported the view that motivation for patients to work at psychoanalysis (or in psychotherapy generally) is not simply a function of the willingness to spend money for treatment; such a willingness is an evidence of motivation but it cannot provide motivation. There is ample experience that motivation to work in psychoanalysis may very well be present in high degree even when the treatment does not represent a financial sacrifice. It appears that the fee is a more important source of motivation for the therapist than for the patient.

Since 1964 third-party payment has be come far more common, than formerly, and a considerable; amount of experience has accumulated on the effects of third-party insurance payment of psychoanalytic and other forms of psychotherapy. A recent report by Halpert (6) sounds a warning note, on the basis of two cases, that insurance payment may offer a focus for resistance, making the analytic task more difficult.

There is also a school of thought which holds that no form of psychotherapeutic treatment in which payment is not a private matter between therapist and analysand can be considered psychoanalysis. This represents an example of classification by definition and if it is accepted, one will have to find a new name for what many fully qualified psychoanalysts with impeccable credentials are doing with patients from whom they receive third-party payment under the mistaken notion that they are practicing psychoanalysis.

My own experience and that of the colleagues with whom I have discussed this matter seems to support the view that when payment is made partially through a third party, some problems appear in the psychoanalysis or other intensive psychotherapy that otherwise would not be present. Some are like the ones cited in Halpert's cases, where the narcissistic gratification the patients were reported to have received in the form of fulfillment of fantasies of omnipotence from the fact that they themselves did not have to pay for the treatment was sufficient to interfere with their motivation to work in their analyses.

However, fantasies of this kind often appear in analysis and are subject to interpretation and working through like any other kind of fantasy. It sometimes may even be an advantage to the analysis to have the patient feeling that he is getting something for nothing mobilized by the fact that he does not have to pay, in exactly the same way that other fantasies may be mobilized and must be interpreted when the patients must make regular payments. At any rate, the practice of psychoanalysis and other intensive psychotherapy with third-party payment is flourishing where such payment is available, and there is no reason to believe that the results of such psychotherapy are in any way inferior to those produced in direct-payment settings.

The Trend Toward Greater Accountability

In making the above statement, I am aware that I am venturing on rather shaky ground because of the uncertainty that pertains to the whole field of outcome studies in psychotherapy. The reasons for this state of affairs are complicated. The most important may simply be the extreme difficulty of the task, but it also seems likely that practitioners of psychotherapy have not been particularly motivated to scrutinize their work and that of their colleagues in a manner approaching scientific standards. However, this is a situation that inevitably will change under the economic spur of third-party intervention as the various carriers increasingly supplement the monetary carrot with the stick of accountability. Insurance officials and their actuaries are going to want to know what they are paying for, whether patients are being treated under proper indications, and whether psychotherapeutic practices are being abused. They expect this kind of accountability from surgeons, and although somewhat confused by the differences between psychiatry and the other medical specialties, they are not likely to regard psychiatrists as any more sacrosanct or immune from questioning than other medical specialists.

Also, we are undoubtedly entering an era when organizations of psychiatrists and other psychotherapists are going to have to negotiate contracts with various insurance carriers, and in these negotiations the representatives of psychiatry will have to answer such questions if they wish their services to be included under insurance coverage. Thus we see that an already troublesome problem – the criteria for various forms of psychotherapy and evaluation of their effectiveness – has been given a new urgency by the increase in third-party payment.

A relatively new development in psychiatry is the peer review committee, which makes recommendations about such matters as fees and indications for type and duration of treatment when these are called into question in individual cases. It is difficult to imagine that monitoring agencies of this kind would ever have been considered necessary or useful before the interposition of a third-party payment mechanism between patient and therapist. There is little doubt that the near future will see an increasing use of such quality control methods; the real question is whether they will be adequated and acceptable or whether such functions will be taken out of the sole control of psychotherapists. Whether this latter eventuality, with its far-reaching effects, ever comes to pass is dependent on the attitude of psychiatrists who specialize in psychotherapy not only toward peer review committees but also toward all the other issues involving third-party payment that I have raised.

If they take the position that everything which happens between their patients and themselves is nobody's business but their own, they will be in a difficult and anxiety-providing situation in dealing with third-party requirements, they may be better off refusing to accept patients who pay their bills by such means. If, however, they accept the queen's shilling of insurance payment for part of their patients' financial obligations to them, they will have to come to terms with some of the hard questions I have touched upon.

References

1. Married man asks to be billed for psychiatric care of mistress. *JAMA* **218**:1443, 1971

2. Psychologists bid for inclusion in health insurance legislation. *Psychiatric News*, Dec 1, 1971, p 1

3. **American Psychiatric Association**: *Diagnostic and Statistical Manual of Mental Disorders*, 2nd ed Washington, DC, APA, 1968

4. **Bevan W**: The topsy-turvy world of health care delivery. *Science* **173**:985, Sept 10, 1971

5. **Chodoff P**: Psychoanalysis and fees. *Compr Psychiat* **5**:137–145, 1964

6. **Halpert E**: The effect of insurance on psychoanalytic treatment. *J Amer Psychoanal Ass* **20**:122–133, 1972

3 Diagnosis

Conferring a diagnosis of mental illness on people initiates a process that has the potential to impose profound, adverse effects on their lives. Placed in a group that requires treatment, the person, once labelled a psychiatric patient, commonly encounters prejudice and may well feel stigmatized. Moreover, those deemed at risk of harm to themselves or others may have their fundamental civil rights abridged through legal commitment, often resulting in treatments which have disturbing and/or severe side-effects. These possible consequences justify Reich's[1] call for the most thorough ethical examination of what he terms the clinician's 'prerogative to diagnose'. In this section we will follow his advice and begin with the core question of what constitutes mental illness.

The concept of mental illness

Psychiatrists establish diagnoses by employing objective criteria as much as possible, and relying on knowledge gained from previous clinical encounters. The procedure is relatively straightforward in the face of obvious findings, such as gross defects of memory, persecutory delusions, or the life-threatening withdrawal of severe depression. In other circumstances, however, clinicians determine that persons warrant a diagnosis when suffering from symptoms that go beyond the limits of what is consensually considered to be 'normal'; this is somewhat akin to the depiction of pornography as 'something I know when I see it' by US Supreme Court Justice Stewart. Here, in tandem with objective findings, a psychiatrist's judgment is grounded in appraisal of such phenomena as pervasive anxiety, failure of concentration, depersonalization and existential distress. For example, pronounced turmoil by a bereaved person may incline the clinician towards diagnosing clinical depression rather than attributing her state to the normal process of grieving. Similarly, a person wrestling with the travails of everyday life may be defined as a diagnosable case rather than viewed like other human beings dealing with stressful circumstances. Unquestionably, professional expertise (encompassing both comprehensive training and sound experience), systems of peer review and an attitude of benevolent paternalism combine to provide a degree of protection against arbitrariness, idiosyncrasy or whim. Notwithstanding, it is not difficult to conceive of a clinician who relies unduly on what we may term 'reasoned subjectivism', and applies psychiatric diagnoses to those persons who would not be so regarded by professional colleagues.

Over the past three decades sustained effort has gone into elaborating objective criteria of mental illness that, among other goals, serve to limit the potential for diagnostic inconsistency and the harms to patients that may ensue. The difficulty is that, despite widely respected protocols like the American Psychiatric Association's DSM-IV[2] and World Health Organization's ICD[3], controversy about the nebulousness – and, in some cases, even legitimacy – of certain categories persists. Concerns about scientific methodology and the intrusion of value judgments into contemporary classifications have led to charges that a number of diagnoses reflect pejorative labelling more than science. Kaplan[4] voices this position in the selection, 'A woman's view of DSM-III'. She argues that behaviours considered healthy or pathologic have, according to masculine-based assumptions, been codified into diagnostic criteria that were incorrectly afforded scientific validity. She re-iterates Chesler's[5] assertion that 'woman are diagnosed for both over conforming and under conforming to sex role stereotypes', illustrating the claim via discussion of histrionic and dependent personality disorders. In regard to the latter she summarizes her perceived errors of DSM-II[6] vis-à-vis dependency as follows:

[It's] extreme expression in women is reflective not simply of women's relationship to (e.g., subordinate position in) society but also of women's behavioural, psychological, or biological dysfunction.

She asserts that dependency in women, in contrast to men, has thereby merited 'clinicians' labelling and concern'. Williams and Spitzer[7] reject Kaplan's interpretation of DSM-II and DSM-III out of hand. Criticizing her 'faulty assumption that recognizing a societal problem (e.g., sexism) excludes the utility of clinical diagnosis of the individual', they present data to refute the charge of any sex-based assumptions in either volume.

Claims about sexist influence are but one reflection of the degree to which objective criteria and value-laden judgments are deployed to define what constitutes abnormal mental states. That determination, often a complex task, is at the heart of the debate concerning ethical aspects of psychiatric diagnosis.

The fact-based model

In 'The myth of mental illness', our selection by Thomas Szasz,[8] this *eminence grise* of psychiatry is dismissive of any ethical aspects of psychiatric diagnosis by claiming that mental illness simply does not exist. His argument is grounded in the biomedical model, a reductionistic paradigm that embraces a cause-and-effect approach to medical practice – viewing the diagnostic procedure exclusively in terms of physical aetiology (e.g., arteriosclerosis of the coronary arteries) and defining treatment solely in terms of addressing that pathology (e.g., bypass surgery). Szasz's approach, which spurns the widely accepted biopsychosocial clinical approach,[9] extends the biomedical perspective to mental functioning by claiming that disorders of thinking and behaviour are 'diseases of the brain' caused by structural abnormalities of the central nervous system, while 'diseases of the mind' are merely theoretical concepts that reflect social values. Szasz notes that one cannot 'catch or get a 'mental illness' . . . have or harbor it . . . transmit it to others . . . and get rid of it', and concludes it is therefore a 'myth' created by society in tandem with the medical profession to explain away 'problems of living' that arise from the conflict of diverse human values. To that end he observes,

The belief in mental illness, as something other than man's trouble in getting along with his fellow man, is the proper heir to the belief in demonology and witchcraft. Mental illness exists or is 'real' in exactly the same sense in which witches existed or were 'real'

Szasz's argument has been challenged on philosophical grounds,[10] as well as for its naïve appreciation of the realities of clinical practice.[11,12] Moreover, though he starkly contrasts fact- and value-based conceptions of illness, other advocates of a fact-based biological model challenge his contention that mental illness is mythical because it lacks a definitive physical substrate. In 'The concept of disease and its implications for psychiatry', Kendell[13] is unequivocally critical of value-laden diagnoses of illness based on 'what people complain of' or 'what doctors treat', because diagnoses are thereby 'free to expand or contract with changes in social attitudes and therapeutic optimism and [are] at the mercy of idiosyncratic decisions by doctors or patients'. Thus, he conceptualizes illness as a condition that produces concrete, 'significant biological disadvantage' that, unlike Szasz, includes mental disorders like schizophrenia, manic-depressive illness and drug dependence. Kendall's argument is grounded in the claim that mental illness can diminish life expectancy and fertility, thereby conveying to the patient an intrinsic biological disadvantage, 'the same criteria' required for a physical illness. This challenge to Szasz is limited, in that Kendell also rejects certain 'areas, which psychiatrists have come to regard as illness', and cautions them against presumptuous attempts to treat 'all the woes of mankind'. Nevertheless, his fact-based thesis undercuts Szasz's claim that mental illness is merely a social construct, and allows for a middle ground between the two theoretical positions.

Boorse[14] also adheres to a biological conception of illness but advocates a perspective that responds to criticism of Kendell's circumscribed diagnostic parameters of diminished fertility and longevity. In the selection 'What a theory of mental health should be,' Boorse[15] argues for a *functional* conception of health and disease: disease is a type of internal state that interferes with the performance of one or more natural functions that are age-specific and typical of a species, and necessary for its survival. In terms of mental functioning he contends that certain types of processes (e.g., perception, intelligence and memory) are needed to support adaptive human behaviour; consequently, 'it is hard to see any obstacle to calling unnatural obstructions of these functions mental diseases, exactly as in the physiological case'. Boorse concedes a degree of discrepancy between normal psychological and physical functioning given the characteristic 'plasticity' of the former that allows 'normal psychological functions to be somewhat less specific than their physiological counterparts'. Nevertheless, since 'the functional organization typical of a species is a biological fact', Boorse asserts that the concept of disease, including mental disease, is value-free.

Boorse suggests that *diseases* become *illnesses* when they satisfy normative, value-laden criteria, such as undesirability to their bearers or acceptable excuses for normally criticizable behaviour. As a result, a mental disease may be incorrectly 'classed as a "mental illness" when some accepted explanation of it refers not to the patient's physiology but to feelings, beliefs and experiences' related to that disturbance; this permits an illegitimate conception of mental illness, like establishing as criteria of health a set of personality traits that are valued by a culture but not needed for normal development. In contrast, more objective assessment of mental processes, such as markedly lowered frustration tolerance in psychosis, provide 'good grounds for provisionally calling these conditions pathological' since affected people have impaired functioning relative to others.

Though Boorse purports to advance a value-free model based on biological functioning, his guiding notion of normal versus impaired species-typical functioning has itself been criticized as value-laden for several reasons. First, if impaired functioning is the standard measure of disease, a subjective judgment is required to establish the degree to which impairment impedes species-typical functioning. Consider, for example, 'excessive' obsessional thinking and behaviour. Would the meticulousness, extreme vigilance and the ability to compartmentalize affect when confronting emergencies in the operating room classify a surgeon as professionally advantaged or psychologically impaired? A border between typical and atypical functioning must be delineated; many dispute Boorse's claim that objective assessment of biological functioning can readily define that boundary. Second, Boorse has been faulted for claiming that species-typical functioning is defined by value-free biological norms while actually arguing that disease is present

only when statistical deviance has a negative impact. For example, though people whose intelligence is several standard deviations above and below the normal bell curve are atypical, according to Boorse only those with subnormal intelligence have a pathologic condition.

The value-based model

Boorse's attempt to limit the degree to which psychiatric diagnoses are shaped by value judgments is important but it highlights the difficulty, if not impossibility, of applying objective diagnostic criteria alone. Sedgwick[16] argues that all illness is predominantly value-laden since diagnoses are always made in a moral context, namely that something *bad* is happening to the affected person. Pneumonia, for instance, is an illness not only because it consists of a cluster of signs and symptoms attributable to pathology of the respiratory system but also because it is detrimental to a person's overall well-being. Sedgwick's observations are not sufficient to justify a broader assertion that diagnoses are primarily grounded in value. Nevertheless, the history of psychiatry has revealed a particularly value-laden dimension to the conception of mental disorders. Drapetomania, for example, was supposedly manifest by attempts of American slaves to flee from captivity – an absurd concept of Dr. Samuel Cartwright.[17] A more recent illustration centers on debate among American psychiatrists concerning the legitimacy of homosexuality as an illness.[18]

In the selection, 'A symposium: should homosexuality be in the APA nomenclature?',[19] panelists debate the aetiological role of value in sexual disorders. They position themselves at different points along the fact-value spectrum as justifying diagnostic parameters. At one extreme Socarides[19], pp. 1212–1213 citing data from his own clinical work, advances a pre-Oedipal theory of causation. He argues that separation-individuation is a prerequisite 'to establish gender identity' and that a 'course toward homosexual development' results when a boy fails in this task *vis-à-vis* his mother. Green[19] (pp. 1213–1214) questions the validity of scientific criteria 'based on a theoretical model of human psychological development', while Gold[19] (pp. 1211–1212) regards 'the illness theory of homosexuality [as] a pack of lies, concocted out of the myths of a patriarchal society for a political purpose'. The complexity of determining the degree to which psychiatric diagnosis is influenced by scientific or social forces is well illustrated in this symposium. Spitzer[20] offers a relevant footnote to the panel with a reformulation of his original contribution that discusses the diagnostic status of homosexuality in terms of a value judgment about heterosexuality, as opposed to a factual dispute about homosexuality.

Apart from such social consequences as stigmatization, serious treatment implications flow from the debate concerning homosexuality's legitimacy as an illness. Despite an official action by the APA in 1973 stating that *per se* it is not a diagnosable disorder and the removal of ego-dystonic homosexuality from DSM-III-R, religious and political forces in the US have continued efforts to pathologize homosexuality. Amongst other tacks, they claim it can be cured by 'reparative' therapies. In response, the APA Board of Trustees issued a position statement in 1998,[21] subsequently revised in 2000,[22] that strongly opposed these types of therapies because of their questionable scientific validity, and admonished clinicians for employing coercion or subtle influence to gain patients' acceptance of these treatments.

The thesis that mental illnesses are merely social constructions conveying harmful consequences to those who deviate from societal norms is offered by a group of 'anti-psychiatrists' intent on reversing that trend. Scheff,[23] for example, regards mental illness largely as a response to the effects of being labeled insane, the expectations it produces and the treatments it imposes. He views schizophrenia as an artifice created by professionals who claim it is an illness and construct bureaucracies and institutions to treat it. In a similar vein, Laing[24] regards so-called symptoms of schizophrenia as sane responses to circumstances created by insane environments, such as dysfunctional families. Those labeled 'schizophrenic' are, in his view, 'divided selves' who suffer a 'divorce of the self from the body . . . as the basic means of defence' against noxious circumstances.[25] Laing concludes that adolescents receive incompatible messages from their families and society and respond with behaviours that are, in fact, rational (though deemed pathological by mental health professionals) given their circumstances.

Foucault[26] echoes Laing's conception of mental illness, but much more expansively. He views society as composed of intrusive, controlling associations of citizens, and the medical profession as a dominant force which controls deviations from social norms by adopting the construct of mental illness as a critical, evaluatory category. Foucault's account of the asylum highlights how the inception of moral treatment of the insane liberated patients from the asylum's physical constraints only to deliver them to the surveillance and judgment of society at large. He concludes that madness is subject to arbitrary societal values that define 'its cause, model, and limit'.

The anti-psychiatry movement has been challenged for espousing unsubstantiated dogma and subjected to the same charge it levels against traditional schools of psychiatry, namely claiming a factual basis for findings grounded in values. In the selection 'On being sane in insane places', Rosenhan[27] attempts to counter this challenge with empirical data. Eight 'pseudopatients', people with no history of psychiatric illness, presented to a number of mental health facilities with the sham complaint of auditory hallucinations. Staff failed 'to detect sanity' in any of the cases throughout their hospital stay (a range of 7–52 days), despite the fact that none of these individuals exhibited any behaviour consistent with psychosis once admitted. Because of adverse effects of psychiatric hospitalization – 'powerlessness, depersonalization, segregation, mortification, and self-labelling' – as well as the 'stickiness' of a diagnosis, Rosenhan argues against 'psychiatric labelling', particularly since '[i]t is clear that we cannot distinguish the sane from the insane'.

Though many have challenged these conclusions, some mental health professionals have undoubtedly been guilty of purposefully inventing the disorders they attribute to patients, a phenomenon captured in the extreme by the malignant abuse of psychiatry in the former Soviet Union to suppress political dissent. Once identified as exhibiting the overwhelmingly subjective clinical criteria of 'sluggish schizophrenia',[28] people were forcibly hospitalized and many subjected to coercive treatments.[1,29,30] In addition to stigmatization emanating from self-perceptions and reactions by members of society to a person labeled ill, the force of manipulated public opinion can result in 'patients' outright ostracism. Proctor[31] offers chilling examples of this phenomenon when describing Nazi social policy towards citizens leading 'lives not worth living' due to physical and mental handicaps.

Fact-value synthesis

At this point it seems reasonable to conclude that a conception of mental illness grounded in either value or fact alone is uninformed, since each position is absolutist to a degree that undermines its relevance and legitimacy in the face of clinical realities. It may be, as Szasz avers, that travails of life are too readily regarded as mental disorders – but perhaps only *certain* problems of living are pertinent in this regard. The difficulty lies in delineating the boundary between the distress of ordinary life and psychopathological states. How, for example, does the clinician tease out the customary emotional distress arising from marital discord from a level of disturbance that warrants the diagnosis of an adjustment disorder? At what point along that spectrum should a person receive a diagnosis, which, as a result, would justify the need and permissibility to seek professional help in the eyes of society? These questions suggest that psychiatric disorders are defined by components of both fact and value.

In the selection by Wakefield[32] the concept of a mental illness, defined as the perception of mental disturbance largely shared by professionals and the lay public, is positioned 'on the boundary between the given natural world and the constructed social world' by grounding diagnosis in the notion of 'harmful dysfunction'. For Wakefield, 'dysfunction' is a scientific and factual

term based in biology that refers to the failure of an internal evolutionary mechanism to perform a natural function for which it is designed, whereas 'harmful' is a value-oriented term which refers to the consequences of the dysfunction for the person that are deemed detrimental in terms of sociocultural norms. Applying this notion to mental functioning, he describes the beneficial effects of natural mental mechanisms, like those mediating cognition and emotional regulation, and judges their dysfunction harmful when it yields consequences disvalued by society (e.g., aphasia or self-destructive acts). Only at that point do such behaviours merit classification as disorders because the inability of an internal mechanism to perform its natural function causes harm to the person. Consequently, someone with elevated anxiety whose symptoms are not disabling is considered not to have a psychiatric disorder in the same way that a person lacking a kidney who retains normal renal function is not seen to have a physical disorder. Failure of an internal mechanism and the element of harm are required to constitute a disorder, which 'shows only that values are part of the concept of disorder, not that disorder is composed only of values'.

The implications of this formulation are several. First, while acknowledging that the DSM classification embraces the thesis of harmful dysfunction, Wakefield is critical of the way the notion of dysfunction 'diverges substantially from the . . . requirement that it is meant to capture' in that a disorder is defined roughly as 'unexpected distress or disability'. This approach, Wakefield claims, can too easily degenerate into the justification of diagnosis on the basis of statistical norms which conflicts with his point that the dysfunction of an adjustment disorder, for example, requires 'a breakdown in the way the coping mechanisms were designed to function and not merely a greater than average response to stress'.

Wakefield also argues that the 'harmful dysfunction' paradigm is justified by theories that propose psychological and genetic causes of psychiatric disorders. In terms of the former, dysfunction of ego mechanisms facilitates harms that bolster claims for a disorder. Repression, for example, normally helps ward off painful feelings that may disrupt usual functioning. Impairment of this ego function, either enduringly or secondary to a situation that leads to acute de-repression, can pave the way for symptoms (e.g., panic) that qualify as psychiatric diagnoses.

Wakefield does not illustrate his claim that a psychiatric disorder can derive from a genetic cause but correctly notes that dysfunction of genetic mechanisms may lead to harm. Kandel[33] explores this issue in his account of psychiatry's 'new intellectual framework', concerned with the genetic component of psychiatric disorders. Multigenic dysfunction and a requisite degree of penetrance of each gene are needed to produce symptoms that reach the threshold of a disorder. Kandel also argues that the role of environmental factors is mediated genetically, as social influences become 'biologically incorporated in the altered expressions of specific genes in specific nerve cells of specific regions of the brain' through genetic transcriptional control.

In the *Encyclopaedia of applied ethics*, Fulford[34] discusses Wakefield's concept of harmful dysfunction in a clinical context, reserving the term mental illness

[F]or those mental disorders . . . nowadays widely assumed to be generically linked with physical illness [including] disturbances of higher mental functions, such as thought, belief, perception, volition, and emotion . . . e.g., respectively, obsessional disorder, delusion, hallucination, addiction and depression.

His account of the conception of psychiatric disorder calls for the legitimacy of a 'fact-plus-value' model (akin to Wakefield's thesis). Fulford's conceptual map integrates primarily 'physical illnesses' (e.g., dementia, alcohol addiction) and primarily 'life/moral problems' (e.g., acute stress reaction, conduct disorder), in a thought-provoking schema that underscores the inextricable link between mind and body in disordered mental functioning. Its obvious value is its challenge to an either/or paradigm (represented by Szasz's contrast between 'diseases of the brain' and 'problems of living') and support of a moderate position as reflected in Kandel's account.

While 'fact-plus-value' allows for informed deliberation about diagnosis, it does not guarantee the resolution of ethical dilemmas that arise in clinical and research settings. Consider this example: Is a person diagnosed with an impulse-control disorder expressed as kleptomania legally culpable for shop lifting if the behaviour is viewed as having a predominantly physical, as opposed to psychological, cause?[35] This type of question yields another complex question: Is aberrant behaviour a disorder of the brain (a bottom-up process stemming from neurobiological sources) or a fundamental disorder of consciousness (a top-down process derived from the subjective expression of idiosyncratic thoughts and feelings)?

The latter question concerns the degree to which harmful dysfunction is constrained by conscious decision-making or unaffected by will. The issue is taken up in the selection 'A psychiatric dialogue of the mind-body problem',[36] a thought-provoking analysis of the 'fact-plus-value' conception of mental illness in the context of a specific patient. Kendler examines the case of a severely depressed man in terms of objective brain functioning (e.g., serotonin dysfunction) and subjective experiences (e.g., unresolved anger towards, and competitiveness with, his father). A physician/philosopher leads his students in a debate about whether mind and brain are synonymous, a position that equates synaptic firings with thoughts and feelings and ignores the distinction between the physical nature of the brain (e.g., mass, temperature) and the fact that mind is typified by intangibles (e.g., wishes, intentions, fears). Beginning with an explanation of the concept of 'identity relationship', Kendler explores key concepts of the philosophy of mind in order to understand the relationship between the mind–body dichotomy and mental functioning. His 'explanatory dualism' suggests that 'it is possible to believe that mind and brain are the same thing and yet not deny the unique status of mental experiences'.

Conclusion

The preceding has explored the central issue of what constitutes mental illness, and addressed implications of the fact-value basis of diagnosis, such as whether homosexuality and 'slow schizophrenia' are mental disorders or simply stigmatizing labels invoked for social and political purposes? In closing we present some contemporary issues that pose ethical dilemmas to clinicians because of uncertainties regarding diagnostic legitimacy.

First, controversy about addictive behaviours abounds, considered to be illnesses by some clinicians and willful actions by others. The extensive argument about whether or not alcohol dependence is an illness[37] has largely been abandoned, with acceptance of a disease model that recognizes biological, psychological, social and cultural determinants of addictive behaviour.[38,39] However, debate persists as to whether hyperactive sexual activity or excessive gambling represent diagnosable disorders. Implications of the disease perspective (e.g., viewing these behaviours as variants of an obsessive-compulsive disorder) might include justifying treatments subsidized by health insurance, as well as potentially mitigating legal and personal consequences of a person's actions. On the other hand, the belief that biological causes do not necessarily and sufficiently 'negate agency'[40] diminishes the ability to respond to these behaviours exclusively from the perspective of the sick role.

Diagnostic legitimacy also had considerable consequences in terms of pharmacological treatment. Reviewing 'mistaken diagnosis' of ADHD in Australia, Halasz[41] argues that 'valid diagnosis' requires observation of the child in the family context, as well as additional input from school and related social settings. He worries that clinicians too readily ascribe certain behaviours to ADHD absent a comprehensive assessment that might reveal other aetiological causation, such as anxiety, panic, grief or frustration. Halasz believes a trend towards over-diagnosis is motivated by inadequate clinical evaluation, as well as by efforts of the pharmaceutical industry to proselytize the considerable benefits of their products. He presents data concerning regional prescribing trends of dexamphetamine in Australia to support his claim.

A related issue about the relationship between diagnosis and use of medications concerns the debate about treatment versus enhancement. Kramer[42] explores the subject in his landmark book about Prozac's ability to

modulate affect, and the charge that it thereby could rob us of 'uniquely human' emotions, such as anxiety, guilt, shame, grief, and self-consciousness. The discussion is counterpoised to a Walker Percy novel[43] in which a variant of the element sodium is introduced into the water supply of a town, transforming shy and anxious persons into bold, ambitious and, ultimately, un-self-conscious, insensitive creatures. In contrast to these dire consequences, Kramer describes Prozac's ability to influence responses to uniquely human emotions in a way that changes 'the sort of evidence we attend to', altering our observing, as opposed to fundamental, selves. He concedes that moral implications of Prozac have not been worked out, as the implications of allowing one to possess 'two senses of self' are ethically complex. However, he does not frame the issue in terms of whether or not this is a good thing, likening that enquiry to judging the morality of Freud's discovery of the unconscious. Others are not as cavalier. Elliott,[44] for example, worries that Prozac 'treats the self rather than proper disease', altering personality and offering 'a mechanistic cure for spiritual problems'. He believes that humankind suffers primarily from alienation, the 'incongruity between the self and external structure of meaning', and that 'neither pills nor psychotherapy can fix metaphysics'. To Elliot, assigning a name to existential distress does not establish a legitimate diagnosis and, more importantly, facilitates the use of 'Prozac and its ilk' in a manner that does little more than distract us from the 'unbearably sad place where we live'. The current debate about treatment versus enhancement incorporates consequences of pharmacological interventions into Szasz's earlier concerns about confusing legitimate problems of living with constructed mental disorders.

The impact of diagnosis on the family warrants comment given that it may rend its members apart, starkly reflected in the heated debate about false memory syndrome. (1, p. 216) Presumed recovery of memories of childhood abuse have alienated patients from their relatives and even resulted in lawsuits.[45] Controversy over the issue spawned the False Memory Syndrome Foundation, organized by relatives accused of child abuse presumably recalled by patients during the course of treatment, and supported by a number of prominent psychiatrists. The organization seeks to challenge the legitimacy of the recovered memory diagnosis, alleging that therapists simply suggested these memories to patients.

Financial implications of psychiatric diagnoses persist. As Chodoff[46] notes, an inexorable intrusion of third parties into the therapeutic relationship has provided greater incentive for clinicians to assign diagnostic labels to patients in order 'to qualify [them] for insurance reimbursement'. (His essay is included as a selection in Chapter 2.) General medical practitioners have acknowledged the 'gamesmanship' of manipulating diagnoses and exaggerating symptom severity in reports to insurers.[47,48] They invoked consequences to justify their actions, judging patients' welfare of greater value than truth-telling to third-party payers. Given that insurance coverage has been curtailed for persons suffering from certain mental illnesses,[49] it is reasonable to assume psychiatrists – both for their patients' benefit and their own livelihood – may also employ diagnostic labelling as a way of extracting maximum amounts from ever-declining sources of re imbursement. Chodoff worries that translating patients' legitimate problems of living into diagnosable disorders will cause them harmful consequences, such as incorrectly perceiving themselves as 'sick' and/or being permanently labelled as such by society.

Chodoff[50] also disputes the objectivity of psychiatric diagnosis in what he terms borderline areas, such as differentiating social phobia from the shyness and timidity that falls within a person's normal range of functioning. He emphasizes that 'no subjective checklist of a patient's history and complaints can infallibly separate clinical syndromes that qualify as disorders from various kinds of human discomfort of lesser intensity', nor is there a biologic marker of tissue or serologic abnormality that can do so. For these reasons, as well as his concerns about the economic motivation of making a diagnosis, he argues for psychodynamic formulation as more legitimate than DSM's 'atheoretical, symptom-based' diagnostic scheme that enjoys favour internationally.

In a similar vein, Spitzer[51] argues that psychiatric diagnoses are not based in checklist criteria of diagnostic manuals, but 'on the interaction of two people'. He views diagnostic evaluation as a process – a dialogue that enables the clinician to sort relevant from irrelevant verbal and nonverbal data, organize it in a meaningful way, establish tentative hypotheses, test them out, and ultimately come to understand the unique pathology of a person. To him, accurate diagnosis rests in the clinician's appreciation of 'the most coherent story' about a patient.

Spitzer's thinking suggests a final issue concerning ethical parameters of establishing a psychiatric diagnosis, namely the influence of cultural values. Wallace[52] explores the topic from a theoretical perspective, noting that psychopathology is clearly shaped by a culture's 'prevailing schemata and categories for abnormal experiences, cognitions, and behaviours'. He offers historical illustrations to support his argument, including the belief by some that borderline personality disorder is 'specific to the recent West or even America'. Wallace essentially presents a detailed description of the biopsychosocial model and discusses how all its components 'converge to pattern modes of human being in health and sickness' that can be quite distinctive despite 'elements of temporal and geographic continuity' in conditions of significant illness (e.g., schizophrenia and major affective disorders). Leff's[53] substantive text on transcultural psychiatry presents case studies supporting this view. For example, study of the West Indian population in the UK revealed a lack of understanding on the part of British clinicians regarding culture-specific abnormalities of bodily activity that dominated the clinical presentation of psychosis. As a consequence they experienced difficulty distinguishing between schizophrenia and affective illness, particularly among females, which complicated appropriate treatment in some cases.

References

1   Reich, W.: Psychiatric diagnosis as an ethical problem, in Psychiatric ethics, 3rd edn, ed. S. Bloch, P. Chodoff and S. Green. Oxford, Oxford University Press, 1999, p. 193–224.

2   Diagnostic and statistical manual of mental disorders, 4th edn, Washington, D.C., American Psychiatric Association, 1994.

3   International statistical classification of diseases and related health problems, 1989 revision. Geneva, World Health Organization, 1992.

*4   Kaplan, M.: A woman's view of DSM-III. American Psychologist 38: 786–792, 1983.

5   Chesler, P.: Women and madness. New York: Avon Books, 1972.

6   Diagnostic and statistical manual of mental disorders, 3rd edn, Washington, D.C., American Psychiatric Press, 1968.

7   Williams, J. and Spitzer, R.: The issue of sex bias in DSM-III. A critique of 'A woman's view of DSM-III' by Marcie Kaplan. American Psychologist 38: 793–798, 1983.

*8   Szasz, T.: The myth of mental illness. American Psychologist 15: 113–118, 1960.

9   Engel, G: The need for a new medical model: a challenge for biomedicine. Science 196:129–136, 1977.

10   Moore, M.: Some myths about 'mental illness'. Archives of General Psychiatry 32:1483–1497, 1975.

11   Schaler, J. (ed.): Szasz under fire: the psychiatric abolitionist faces his critics. Chicago, Illinois, Open Court, 2004.

12   Engel, G.: The clinical application of the biopsychosocial model. American Journal of Psychiatry 137: 535–544, 1980.

13   Kendell, R.: The concept of disease and its implications for psychiatry. British Journal of Psychiatry 127: 305–315, 1975.

14   Boorse, C.: Concepts of health, in Health care ethics: an introduction, ed. D. VanDeVeer and T. Regan. Philadelphia, Pennsylvania, Temple University Press, 1987, pp. 359–393.

*15   Boorse, C: What a theory of mental health should be. Journal for the Theory of Social Behaviour 6: 61–84, 1976.

16   Sedgwick, P: Psycho politics. New York, Harper and Row, 1982.

17   Cartwright, S.: Report on the diseases and physical peculiarities of the Negro race, in Concepts of health and disease: interdisciplinary perspectives, ed.

A. Caplan, H. Engelhardt, Jr., and J. McCartney. Reading, Massachusetts, Addison-Wesley, 1981, pp. 305–326. (Original work published 1851).

18   Bayer, R.: Homosexuality and American psychiatry: the politics of diagnosis. New York, Basic Books, 1981.

*19   Stoller, R., Marmor, J., Bieber, I., Gold, R. et al.: A symposium: should homosexuality be in the APA nomenclature. American Journal of Psychiatry 130: 1207–1216, 1973.

20   Spitzer, R. and Williams, J.: The diagnostic status of homosexuality in DSM-III. A reformulation of the issues. American Journal of Psychiatry 138: 210–215, 1981.

21   American Psychiatric Association: Position statement on psychiatric treatment and sexual orientation. American Journal of Psychiatry 156: 1131, 1999.

22   American Psychiatric Association: Position statement on therapies focused on attempts to change sexual orientation (reparative or conversion therapies). American Journal of Psychiatry 157: 1719–1721, 2000.

23   Scheff, T.: Being mentally ill: a sociological theory. Chicago, Illinois, Aldine, 1966.

24   Laing, R.: Sanity, madness and the family. Penguin Books, Harmondsworth, 1970.

25   Laing, R.: The divided self. New York, Pantheon Books, 1969.

26   Foucault, M.: Madness and civilization: a history of insanity in the age of reason, trans. R. Howard. New York, Vintage Books, 1965, pp. 241–278.

*27   Rosenhan, D.: On being sane in insane places. Science 179: 250–258, 1973.

28   Snezhnevsky, A.: The symptomatology, clinical forms and nosology of schizophrenia, in Modern perspectives in world psychiatry, ed. J. Howells. New York, Brunner-Mazel, 1971, pp. 423–47.

29   Bloch, S. and Reddaway, P.: Psychiatric terror: the abuse of psychiatry in the Soviet Union. New York, Basic Books, 1977.

30   Chodoff, P.: Misuse and abuse of psychiatry: an overview, in Psychiatric ethics, 3rd edn, ed. S. Bloch, P. Chodoff and S. Green. Oxford, Oxford University Press, 1999, pp 49–66.

31   Proctor, R.: Racial hygiene. Cambridge, Massachusetts, Harvard University Press, 1988.

*32   Wakefield, J. C.: The concept of mental disorder: on the boundary between biological facts and social values. American Psychologist 47:373–388, 1992.

33   Kandel, E.: A new intellectual framework for psychiatry. American Journal of Psychiatry 155: 457–69, 1998.

34   Fulford, K. W.: Mental illness, concept of, in Encyclopaedia of Applied Ethics, Volume 3, ed. R. Chadwick. Academic Press, San Diego, California, 1998, pp. 213–233.

35   Aboujaoude, E., Gamel, N. and Koran, L.: A case of kleptomania correlating with premenstrual dysphoria. Journal of Clinical Psychiatry 65: 725–726, 2004.

*36   Kendler, K.: A psychiatric dialogue on the mind–body problem. American Journal Psychiatry 158: 989–1000, 2001.

37   LaVigne, G. and Hassenfeld, N.: The ethics of alcoholism treatment and rehabilitation. Advances in Bioethics 3: 81–101, 1997.

38   Vaillant, G.: We should retain the disease concept of alcoholism. Harvard Medical School Mental Health Letter 6: 4–6, 1990.

39   Vaillant, G.: Is alcoholism more often the cause or the result of depression? Harvard Review of Psychiatry 1: 94–99, 1993.

40   Morse, S.: Hooked on hype: addiction and responsibility. Law and Philosophy 19: 3–49, 2000.

41   Halasz, G.: A symposium of attention deficit hyperactivity disorder (ADHD): an ethical perspective. Australian and New Zealand Journal of Psychiatry 36: 472–475, 2002.

42   Kramer, P.: Listening to Prozac. New York, Viking, 1993.

43   Percy, W.: The thanatos syndrome. New York, Farrar, Strauss & Giroux, 1987.

44   Elliott, C.: Pursued by happiness and beaten senseless: Prozac and the American dream. Hastings Center Report March-April 2000, 7–12, 2000.

45   Simon, R. and Gutheil, T.: Ethical and clinical risk management principle in recurrent memory cases: maintaining therapist neutrality, in Trauma and memory: clinical and legal controversies, ed. P. Applebaum, L. Uyehara and M. Elin. New York, Oxford University Press, 1997, Chapter 20.

46   Chodoff, P.: The effect of third-party payment on the practice of psychotherapy. American Journal of Psychiatry 129: 540–545, 1972.

47 Healing vs. honesty: for doctors, managed care's cost controls pose moral dilemma. *The Washington Post* 15 March 1998, H-1.

48 **Novack, D., Deterring, B., Arnold, R., Forrow, L.** *et al.*: Physicians' attitudes toward using deception to resolve difficult ethical problems. *Journal American Medical Association* **261**: 2980–2985, 1989.

49 **Schlesinger, M.**: On the limits of expanding health care reform: chronic care in prepaid settings. *The Milbank Quarterly* **64**: 189–215, 1986.

50 **Chodoff, P.**: The medicalization of the human condition. *Psychiatric Services* **53**: 627–628, 2002.

51 **Spitzer, M.**: The basis of psychiatric diagnosis, in *Philosophical perspectives on psychiatric diagnostic classification*, ed. J. Sadler, O. Wiggins and M. Schwartz. Baltimore, Maryland, Johns Hopkins University Press, 1994, pp. 163–177.

52 **Wallace, E.**: Psychiatry and its nosology: a historico-philosophical overview, in *Philosophical perspectives on psychiatric diagnostic classification*. ed. J. Sadler, O., Wiggins and M. Schwartz. Baltimore, Maryland, Johns Hopkins University Press, 1994, pp. 16–88.

53 **Leff, J.**: *Psychiatry around the globe: a transcultural view*. London, Royal College of Psychiatrists, 1988.

A Woman's View of DSM-III*

Marcie Kaplan

More adult women than adult men are treated for mental illness (e.g., Gove & Tudor, 1973; Rohrbaugh, 1979). There are a variety of theories, most of which concern sex roles, that account for this sex difference. There is good reason for the sex role related explanation. According to Bem (1974) and Berzins, Welling, and Wetter (1978), most females are feminine typed and most males are masculine typed. Kelly (1983) concludes that sex differences in behavioral disorders may be associated not with sex but with sex role typing.

In this article I will review several of the popular sex role related theories on sex differences in mental illness treatment rates and then posit an additional one: A contributor to the sex differences in treatment rates is clinicians' diagnostic criteria – that is in DSM-II (American Psychiatric Association, 1968) and now DSM-III (American Psychiatric Association, 1980). In other words, masculine-biased assumptions about what behaviors are healthy and what behaviors are crazy are codified in diagnostic criteria; these criteria then influence diagnosis and treatment rates and patterns. In my discussion of the influence of diagnostic criteria on sex differences in treatment patterns, I will look at some criteria for specific diagnoses.

Theories About Sex Differences in Treatment Rates

One theory (which has not adequately been supported by data) that accounts for the sex difference in treatment rates is that women are not sicker, they are just more willing to express symptomatology (Phillips & Segal, 1969). Another (more data-supported) theory is that women actually are sicker; their disadvantaged status in society makes them more at risk for mental illness. For instance, the Subpanel on the Mental Health of Women of the President's Commission on Mental Health (1978) documented ways in which inequality creates dilemmas for women in certain contexts (e.g., marriage, child rearing, aging, work). Carmen, Russo, and Miller (1981) add that this same inequality facilitates the occurrence of events (e.g., incest, rape, and marital violence) that heighten women's vulnerability to mental illness. They also point out the link between alienation, powerlessness, and poverty – many women's lot – and impaired mental health.

The theories that women are more willing to express symptomatology and that women's disadvantaged status makes them more vulnerable to mental illness are broad ones. Gove (1979) and Gove and Tudor (1973) formulated several more specific sex role related explanations for gender differences in disordered behavior. First they refined the finding that adult women have higher rates of mental illness and reported that women's higher rate is primarily due to the higher rate of mental illness among married women than among married men. (Widowered, divorced, and never-married men have higher rates of mental illness, respectively, than widowed, divorced, and never-married women [Gove, 1972].) Gove and Tudor offer several sex role related explanations for married women's greater vulnerability to mental illness. These are: (a) Whereas men have two sources of gratification (family and work), traditional married women have

only one source of gratification (family); (b) even when a married woman works, she is discriminated against in the workplace and expected to work and be a homemaker, whereas the man is only expected to work; (c) homemaking is a frustrating, low-prestige job, unconsonant with the education and intellectual attainment of a large number of women; (d) the role of housewife is unstructured and invisible, allowing the individual time to brood alone; (e) expectations confronting women are unclear; for instance, women are supposed to adjust to and prepare for contingencies (Gove, 1979). (Data supporting these explanations are not supplied.)

Another sex role related theory accounting specifically for married women's higher treatment rates is based on Gilligan's (1979) work. Gilligan claims that whereas for men identity precedes intimacy (Erikson, 1950), sex roles dictate that for women identity and intimacy tasks are simultaneous. In other words, women claim an identity through intimate relationships. Bernard (1975) and Mischel (1966) suggest that women are thus more dependent on others than are men. Nadelson and Notman (1981) mention some resulting difficulties for women (and for men who marry early). For instance, those who marry before establishing identities may find their marital choices inappropriate later, and those who are 'burdened by excessive dependency needs, unrealistic expectations of their partners, or unresolved psychological issues' (p. 1355) may find their intimate relationships difficult and stressful and their mental health at risk.

Sex Ratios of Specific Disorders

I turn now from the subject of women's higher treatment rates for disordered behavior in general to the subject of specific behavioral disorders. Table 1 divides those adult disorders for which (according to DSM-III) there are data on sex ratio into two categories: those more commonly diagnosed in adult women and those more commonly diagnosed in adult men. (Disorders whose onset is in adolescence are not included in the table; thus, Anorexia and Bulimia, primarily diagnosed in females, are not listed.) Inspecting Table 1 might lead one to the conclusion that women internalize conflict and that men act it out or, to use Allport's (1958) terms, that women are intropunitive and men, extropunitive.

What are some of the more specific sex role related explanations for so-called female disorders? There are two popular sex role related theories that account for depression (Weissman, 1980). One is the social status hypothesis: Sex discrimination results in 'legal and economic helplessness, dependency on others, chronically low self-esteem, low aspirations, and, ultimately, clinical depression' (Weissman & Klerman, 1977, p. 106). The second sex role related popular theory that accounts for depression is the learned helplessness hypothesis (Seligman, 1973, 1975). Another theory less frequently cited than the above two is drawn from Lewinsohn (1974): Women have sex role related deficits in their capacity to obtain reinforcement from the environment. Thus, according to Kelly (1983), feminine-typed responses such as kindness, emotionality, self-subordination, and gentleness may not obtain reinforcement as effectively as masculine-typed responses such as assertiveness and forcefulness. Thus, those limited to feminine-typed

* Kaplan, M.: A woman's view of DSM-III. *American Psychologist* **38**: 786–792, 1983.

Table 1 Disorders for which there are data on sex ratio

More commonly diagnosed in women	More commonly diagnosed in men
Primary degenerative dementia	Multi-infarct dementia
Depression	Alcohol hallucinosis
Cyclothymic disorder	Substance use disorders
Dysthymic disorder	Transsexualism
Agoraphobia	Paraphilias
Simple phobia	Factitious disorder
Panic disorder	Impulse control disorder
Somatization disorder	Paranoid personality disorder
Psychogenic pain disorder	Antisocial personality disorder
Multiple personality	Compulsive personality disorder
Inhibited sexual desire	
Inhibited orgasm	
Histrionic personality disorder	
Borderline personality disorder	
Dependent personality disorder	

Note. Information adapted from DSM-III.

responses might reach fewer goals than others might reach and thus would be more vulnerable to depression.

That Dependent and Histrionic Personality Disorders, Agoraphobia, and Anorexia are more commonly diagnosed in females has been explained as follows: These disorders represent caricatures of the traditional female role. In other words, as Chesler (1972) claimed, women's high treatment rates for mental illness reflect partially a labeling of women who overconform to sex role stereotypes as pathological. Thus, the individual with Dependent Personality Disorder is passive and subordinate; the individual with Histrionic Personality Disorder is vain, dependent, and given to exaggerated expression of emotions; the agoraphobic may fear entering and coping with a man's world (Chambless & Goldstein, 1980); and the anorexic may have faithfully followed her model – the fashion model – to a society-condoned anorexic weight level.

Many of the sex role related theories accounting for female disorders have some basis in data, but that data may be tangentially related. For instance, Hare-Mustin (1983) connected Linehan's (Note 1) study on the prevalence of behavior modification that teaches women to be thin with the prevalence of Anorexia in women. Another example of an indirect relationship between clinical and research data is the application of Seligman's (1974) learned helplessness studies to depressed women (an example of analogue studies). Most sex role related theories about women's higher treatment rates await empirical validation. Kelly (1983) suggests that a goal for the 1980s is to 'integrate more directly sex role 'personality' research with research on clinical disorders' (p. 24).

Overconforming and Underconforming: A Theory Supported by Data

One might say that of all the sex role explanations for women's higher treatment rates, one explanation is more directly supported by data than the others: Chesler's (1972) assertion that women are diagnosed for both overconforming and underconforming to sex role stereotypes. Data supporting this assertion are supplied by Broverman, Broverman, Clarkson, Rosenkrantz, and Vogel's (1970) study and similar subsequent studies. Broverman *et al.* found that therapists' criteria for healthiness in men and

healthiness in adults were the same, but their criteria for healthiness in women were different:

healthy women differ from healthy men [and thus healthy adults] by being more submissive, less independent, less adventurous, more easily influenced, less aggressive, less competitive, more excitable in minor crises, having their feelings more easily hurt, being more emotional, more conceited about their appearance, less objective, and disliking math and science. (p. 4)

Sherman (1980) reviewed 10 studies of therapists' and counselors' attitudes toward women that have been conducted since the Broverman study and found that despite the publicity of the Broverman findings and supposed changes in society's attitude toward women, stereotyping, albeit less severe than 10 years ago, still exists. Many studies showed that men stereotyped more than women; and some studies showed that older people and those with Freudian orientations stereotyped more than others.

The implications of the stereotyping described by Broverman *et al.* (1970) and the other researchers are that to be considered an unhealthy adult, women must act as women are supposed to act (conform too much to the female sex role stereotype); to be considered an unhealthy woman, women must act as men are supposed to act (not conform enough to the female sex role stereotype). Not only does this Catch-22 predict that women are bound to be labeled unhealthy one way or another, but also the double bind itself could drive a woman crazy.

DSM-III

Bearing in mind this discussion of sex role explanations for women's higher treatment rates, I point to my own argument, which I advance not as an alternative to the above explanations but an additional explanation. As previously mentioned, the thesis is that masculine-based assumptions as to what behaviors are healthy and what behaviors are crazy were codified in DSM-II and are now in DSM-III, and thus influenced and will continue to influence diagnosis and treatment rates. The masculine based assumptions are codified most explicitly in diagnostic criteria for Personality Disorders, which will be discussed in detail below. However, for the record, the assumptions are also codified in criteria for disorders other than Personality Disorders. For instance, classical Freudians would find Gender Identity Disorder of Childhood in every little girl and Atypical Gender Identity Disorder in many women, according to the Freudians' and DSM-III's (p. 263) respective assumptions about penis envy.

Definitions

DSM-III's definition of Mental Disorder and creteria for Personality Disorders is as follows:

a clinically significant behavioral or psychological syndrome or pattern that occurs in an individual and that is typically associated with either a painful symptom (distress) or impairment in one or more important areas of functioning (disability). In addition, there is an interference that there is a behavioral, psychological, or biological dysfunction, and that the disturbance is not only in the relationship between the individual and society. (When a disturbance is *limited* to a conflict between an individual and society, this may represent social deviance, which may or may not be commendable, but is not by itself a Mental Disorder.) (p. 6)

According to DSM-III, all Personality Disorders entail 'either significant impairment in social or occupational functioning or subjective distress' (p. 305), which spells out one of the criteria for Mental Disorder: 'impairment in one or more important areas of functioning (disability)' (p. 6).

Problems

What does impairment in social or occupational functioning mean? I believe these criteria contain assumptions and then generate diagnoses accordingly. For instance, is a woman unemployed outside the home impaired in occupational functioning? Is a man who is employed outside the home and never there when his children come home school impaired in social functioning? Evidently users of DSM-III assume not, or many 'healthy' individuals who assume traditional sex roles would have diagnoses; yet a woman who neglects her children and a man who can't hold down a job – perhaps healthy individuals who assume nontraditional roles – may be labeled *impaired* by a diagnostician.

The above examples of potential diagnoses concern individuals who may experience no primary subjective distress, that is, no distress related directly to these behaviors mentioned (although they may experience distress related to society's and thus to their own reactions to these behaviors). These nondistressed, perhaps healthy, people are labeled *unhealthy*. What about individuals who perhaps are healthy and are subjectively distressed? Through arbitrary assumptions implicit in diagnostic criteria, do they too win diagnoses? For instance, consider the woman who experiences subjective distress because of the double bind inherent in wanting to be a healthy adult – self sufficient – and also in wanting to be a healthy woman – dependent on a man. She may have very real symptoms of unhappiness; according to DSM-III she may have Major Depression. But in her unhappiness, she may be reacting to an impossible situation the way any normal, healthy person would. Her unhappiness and her label of *depressed* may be manifestations that she is a scapegoat for society's illness, its unjust sex role imperatives. In other words, in terms of DSM-III's definitions of Mental Disorder and social deviance, it is difficult, if not impossible, to say when a disturbance is only brought about by a conflict between an individual and society. It is difficult to say when society should be labeled as *unjust* and when an individual should be labeled as *crazy*. This difficulty makes one wonder what assumptions clinicians make – and which diagnostic criteria encourage and support those assumptions – when they designate the individual, as opposed to society, as the problem.

Histrionic Personality Disorder ('Hysterical Personality' in DSM-II)

To make more specific this discussion of assumptions about what is healthy and what is crazy, I will turn to a specific DMS-III diagnosis – Histrionic Personality Disorder. Compare the criteria for that diagnosis with the findings of the Broverman *et al.* (1970) study concerning clinicians' criteria for healthiness in women. To earn the label of Histrionic Personality Disorder, which according to DSM-III is 'diagnosed far more frequently in females than in males' (p. 314), an individual must satisfy three out of five criteria in Category A and two out of five criteria in Category B (p. 315). Three Category A criteria are 'self-dramatization, e.g., exaggerated expression of emotions' (cf. Broverman *et al.*'s [p. 3] 'being more emotional'), 'overreaction to minor events' (cf. Broverman *et al.*'s 'more excitable in minor crises'), and 'irrational, angry outbursts or tantrums' (cf. Broverman *et al.*'s 'more excitable,' 'more emotional,' 'less objective,' i.e., less rational). Two Category B criteria are 'vain and demanding' (cf. Broverman *et al.*'s 'more conceited about their appearance') and 'dependent, helpless, constantly seeking reassurance' (cf. Broverman *et al.*'s 'more submissive, less independent, less adventurous, more easily influenced'). It appears then that via assumptions about sex roles made by clinicians, a healthy woman automatically earns the diagnosis of Histrionic Personality Disorder or, to help female clients, clinicians encourage them to get sick.

Dependent Personality Disorder ('Passive-Dependent Personality' in DSM-II)

Look at another set of assumptions codified in DSM-III about what is healthy and what is crazy. These assumptions result in the selective application of the label *dependency*. Why is dependency considered so subjectively distressing or impairment causing that it earns in its extreme expression the diagnosis of a Personality Disorder? The diagnosed individual

passively allows others to assume responsibility for major areas of life because of inability to function independently, . . . subordinates own needs to those of

persons on whom he or she depends in order to avoid any possibility of having to rely on self . . . [and] lacks self-confidence. (pp. 325, 326)

Again, these criteria echo the clinicians' idea of healthy women as described in the Broverman *et al.* (1970) study; they also echo Miller's (1976) description of subordinate-group members (women) in situations of inequality (society). Thus as in the Histrionic Personality Disorder, clinicians help individuals to attain a diagnosis, or clinicians label the individual *ill* in lieu of labeling society *unjust*.

As regards dependency, there is another means, besides the assumption that women should act more dependently than men, by which DSM-III guides clinicians to label women. That is, DSM-III singles out for scrutiny and therefore diagnosis the ways in which women express dependency but not the ways in which men express dependency. For instance, DSM-III does not mention the dependency of individuals – usually men – who rely on others to maintain their houses and take care of their children. (These are the others *from whom the individuals are independent.*) DSM-III does not mention the dependency of individuals – usually men – who, when widowed, seek a new spouse to take care of them (widowed women seek a new spouse to take care of [Troll, 1979]). DSM-III does not mention the dependency of individuals – usually men – whose mental illness rates are higher when they are alone than when they are married (women's rates are higher when they are married than when they are alone [Gove, 1972]). In short, men's dependency, like women's dependency, exists and is supported and sanctioned by society; but men's dependency is not labeled as such, and men's dependency is not considered sick, whereas women's dependency is.

To summarize, DSM-III makes three major assumptions about dependency. One is that there is something unhealthy about it. Another is that dependency's extreme expression in women is reflective not simply of women's relationship to (e.g., subordinate position in) society but also of women's behavioral, psychological, or biological dysfunction. A third assumption is that whereas women's expression of dependency merits clinicians' labeling and concern, men's expression of dependency does not.

DSM-III makes similar assumptions regarding histrionicness (as did DSM-II regarding hysteria). For instance, DSM-III assumes that the constellation of histrionic personality traits is not mostly reflective of women's subordinate position in society; however, contrast Miller's (1976) discussion of subordinate-group members carrying unsolved aspects of human experience such as childishness. Another DSM-III and DSM-II assumption is that histrionicness (hysteria) is unhealthy, but its opposite (see Restricted Personality below) is not.

Independent Personality Disorder and Restricted Personality Disorder

To underscore the above points regarding DSM-III's assumptions about dependency and histrionics, consider the following two fictitious diagnostic categories (presented in the DSM-III's format) and compare the first to the diagnosis of Dependent Personality Disorder and the second to the diagnosis of Histrionic Personality Disorder.

Diagnostic criteria for Independent Personality Disorder

The following are characteristic of the individual's current and long-term functioning, are not limited to episodes of illness, and cause either significant impairment in social functioning or subjective distress.

A Puts work (career) above relationships with loved ones (e.g., travels a lot on business, works late at night and on weekends).

B Is reluctant to take into account the others' needs when making decisions, especially concerning the individual's career or use of leisure time, e.g., expects spouse and children to relocate to another city because of individual's career plans.

C Passively allows others to assume responsibility for major areas of social life because of inability to express necessary emotion (e.g., lets spouse assume most child-care responsibilities).

Differential diagnosis. In Compulsive Personality Disorder, there is a perfectionism and an in decisiveness that are lacking in the Independent Personality Disorder. In Avoidant Personality Disorder there is more social withdrawal; the individual with Independent Personality Disorder has relationships with people but behaves as if she or he were independent of those people. However all three of these disorders may coexist. Restricted Personality Disorder might coexist with Independent Personality Disorder.

Diagnostic criteria for Restricted Personality Disorder

The following are characteristic of the individual's current and long-term functioning, are not limited to episodes of illness, and cause either significant impairment in social or occupational functioning (though usually not the latter) or subjective distress.

A   Behavior that is overly restrained, unresponsive, and barely expressed, as indicated by a least three of the following:

   (1) limited expression of emotions, e.g., absence of crying at sad moments

   (2) repeated denial of emotional needs, e.g. of feeling hurt

   (3) constant appearance of self-assurance

   (4) apparent underreaction to major events e.g., is often described as stoic

   (5) repeatedly choosing physical or intellectual activities over emotional experience

B   Characteristic disturbances in interpersonal relationships as indicated by at least two of the following:

   (1) perceived by others as distant; e.g., in individual's presence others feel uncomfort able disclosing their feelings

   (2) engages others (especially spouse) to perform emotional behaviors such as writing the individual's thank-you notes or telephoning to express the individual's concern

   (3) engages in subject-changing, silence, annoyance, physical behavior, or leave taking when others introduce feeling-related conversation topics

   (4) indirectly expresses resistance to answering others' expressed needs (e.g., by forgetting, falling asleep, claiming need to tend to alternate responsibilities).

The above two diagnoses share criteria with DSM-III's Compulsive Personality Disorder. For instance, three criteria for Compulsive Personality Disorder are: 'restricted ability to express warm and tender emotions,' . . . 'insistence that others submit to his or her way of doing things, . . . [and] excessive devotion to work and productivity to the exclusion of pleasure and the value of interpersonal relationships' (pp. 327–328). But satisfying those criteria alone will not win a DSM-III diagnosis. An individual must also be a perfectionist (e.g., preoccupied with details, lists, etc.) or be indecisive. In other words, whereas behaving in a feminine stereotyped manner alone will earn a DSM-III diagnosis (e.g., Dependent or Histrionic Personality Disorder), behaving in a masculine stereotyped manner alone will not. A masculine stereotyped individual, to be diagnosed, cannot just be remarkably masculine. Masculinity alone is not clinically suspect; femininity alone is.

Women's Sexuality

As a final illustration of my argument that masculine-biased assumptions shape diagnosis and treatment patterns, I turn to the past literature on and conceptions of women's sexuality. Freud's classic theory that vaginal orgasms are different from and more mature than clitoral orgasms caused clinicians, their clients, and the public to believe that women who experienced clitoral orgasms were arrested in their psychological development. It was not until Masters and Johnson published *Human Sexual Response* in 1966 and claimed that there is only one female orgasm, and it is clitoral, that women who experienced clitoral orgasms were considered cured. In other words, women who before 1966 were immature or even dysfunctional were suddenly, in 1966, mature and functional. The women's sexual behavior did not change, but diagnostic criteria did. The DSM-III is compiled mostly by men, and the Psychosexual Disorder Advisory Committee is made up of approximately two-thirds men. That the DSM-III currently identifies Inhibited Orgasm and Inhibited Sexual Desire as (a) disorders, and (b) disorders more commonly found in females, in the light of psychiatry's past mistake regarding women's sexuality, should encourage some thought when one is considering women's sexual pathology. (The diagnostic criteria of Inhibited Female Orgasm acknowledge that diagnosis requires a 'difficult judgment' [p. 279].)

Conclusion

Evidence discussed in this article should give one pause when one is considering women's pathology in general, sexual or otherwise. Our diagnostic system, like the society it serves, is male centered. In a female-centered system and society, the public mental health profile might be different. All young macho males seeking psychotherapy might tempt clinicians to award a diagnosis of restricted Personality Disorder (cf. clinicians' current generosity with the labels *histrionic* or *hysterical*). A Broverman study might discover the belief that healthy adult traits were dependence and emotionality; men might be caught in the double bind of choosing between male and adult healthiness; men's treatment rates might be higher than women's.

What is the significance of women's higher rates? As discussed earlier, Chesler (1972) asserts (and the Broverman *et al.* [1970] study supports the assertion) that one reason healthy women are labeled disordered is that they refuse to play the traditional female role. But Franks and Rothblum (1983) claim that women are disordered; that is, they are depressed, agoraphobic, and experience sexual dysfunction. If Franks and Rothblum are correct, then the demands of traditional sex roles may be more maladaptive for women than they are for men. Another explanation and the one explored in this article is that adaptiveness and maladaptiveness are arbitrarily defined. In other words, not only are women being punished (by being diagnosed) for acting out of line (not acting like women) and not only are traditional roles driving women crazy, but also male-centered assumptions – the sunglasses through which we view each other – are causing clinicians to see normal females as abnormal.

Note

1.   Linehan, M. Behavior therapy for women: When equal treatment is unequal. In S. B. Sobel (Chair), *Clinical psychology of women: Old concerns and new approaches*. Symposium presented at the meeting of the American Psychological Association, Montreal, September 1980.

References

Allport, G. W. *The nature of prejudice*. Garden City, N.Y.: Doubleday, 1958.

American Psychiatric Association. *Diagnostic and statistical manual of mental disorders* (2nd ed.). Washington, D.C.: Author, 1968.

American Psychiatric Association. *Diagnostic and statistical manual of mental disorders* (3rd ed.). Washington, D.C.: Author, 1980.

Bem, S. L. The measurement of psychological androgyny. *Journal of Consulting and Clinical Psychology*, 1974, **42**, 155–162.

Bernard, J. *Women, wives and mothers: Values and options*. Chicago: Aldine, 1975.

Berzins, J. I., Welling, M. A., & Wetter, R. E. A new measure of psychological androgyny based on the Personality Research Form. *Journal of Consulting and Clinical Psychology*. 1978, **46**, 126–138.

Broverman, I. D., Broverman, D. M., Clarkson, F. E., Rosenkrantz, P. S., & Vogel, S. R. Sex-role stereotypes and clinical judgments of mental health. *Journal of Consulting and Clinical Psychology* 1970, **34**, 1–7.

Carmen, E. H., Russo, N. F., & Miller, J. B. Inequality and women's mental health: An overview. *American Journal of Psychiatry*, 1981, **138**(10), 1319–1330.

Chambless, D. L., & Goldstein, A. J. Anxieties: Agoraphobia and hysteria. In A. M. Brodsky & R. T. Hare-Mustin (Eds.), *Women and psychotherapy: An assessment of research and practice*. New York: Guilford, 1980.

Chesler. P. *Women and madness*. New York: Avon Books, 1972.

Erikson, E. *Childhood and society*. New York: W. W. Norton, 1950.

Franks, V., & Rothblum, E. D. Concluding comments, criticism and caution: Consistent conservatism or constructive change? In V. Franks & E. D. Rothblum (Eds.), *The stereotyping of women: Its effects on mental health*. New York: Springer. 1983.

Gilligan, C. Woman's place in a man's life cycle. *Harvard Educational Review*, 1979, **49**, 431–446.

Gove, W. R. The relationship between sex roles, mental illness and marital status. *Social Forces*, 1972, **51**, 34–44.

Gove, W. R. Sex differences in the epidemiology of mental disorder: Evidence and explanations. In E. S. Gomberg & V. Franks (Eds.), *Gender and disordered behavior: Sex differences in psychopathology*. New York: Brunner/Mazel, 1979.

Gove, W. R., & Tudor, J. Adult sex roles and mental illness. *American Journal of Sociology*, 1973, **73**, 812–835.

Hare-Mustin, R. T. An appraisal of the relationship between women and psychotherapy: 80 years after the case of Dora. *American Psychologist*, 1983, **38**, 593–601.

Kelly, J. A. Sex role stereotypes and mental health: Conceptual models in the 1970's and issues for the 1980's. In V. Franks & E. D. Rothblum (Eds.), *The stereotyping of women: Its effects on mental health*. New York: Springer. 1983.

Lewinsohn, P. H. A behavioral approach to depression. In R. J. Friedman & M. M. Katz (Eds.), *The psychology of depression: Contemporary theory and research*. Washington, D.C.: Winston-Wiley, 1974.

Masters, W. H., & Johnson, V. E. *Human sexual response*. Boston: Little, Brown, 1966.

Miller, J. B. *Toward a new psychology of women*. Boston: Beacon Press, 1976.

Mischel, W. A social learning view of sex differences and behavior. In E. Maccoby (Ed.), *The development of sex differences*. Stanford, Calif.: Stanford University Press, 1966.

Nadelson, C. C., & Notman, M. T. To marry or not to marry: A choice. *American Journal of Psychiatry*, 1981, **138**(10), 1352–1356.

Phillips, D., & Segal, B. E. Sexual status and psychiatric symptoms. *American Sociological Review*, 1969, **34**(1), 58–72.

President's Commission on Mental Health: Subpanel on the Mental Health of Women. In *Report to the President* (Vol. 3). Washington, D.C.: U.S. Government Printing Office, 1978.

Rohrbaugh, J. B. *Women; Psychology's puzzle*. New York: Basic Books, 1979.

Seligman, M. E. P. Depression: Fall into helplessness. *Psychology Today* June 1973, pp. 43–46, 48.

Seligman, M. E. P. Depression and learned helplessness. In R. J. Friedman & M. M. Katz (Eds.), *The psychology of depression: Contemporary theory and research*. Washington, D.C.: Winston-Wiley, 1974.

Seligman, M. E. P. *Helplessness: On depression, development and death*. San Francisco: Freeman, 1975.

Sherman, J. A. Therapist attitudes and sex-role stereotyping. In A. M. Brodsky & R. T. Hare-Mustin (Eds.), *Women and psychotherapy: An assessment of research and practice*. New York: Guilford, 1980.

Troll, L. Sex differences in aging. In E. S. Gomberg & V. Franks (Eds.), *Gender and disordered behavior: Sex differences in psychopathology*. New York: Brunner/Mazel, 1979.

Weissman, M. M. Depression. In A. M. Brodsky & R. T. Hare-Mustin (Eds.), *Women and psychotherapy: An assessment of research and practice*. New York: Guilford, 1980.

Weissman, M. M., & Klerman, G. L. Sex differences and the epidemiology of depression. *Archives of General Psychiatry*, 1977, **34**, 98–111.

The Myth of Mental Illness*

Thomas S. Szasz

My aim in this essay is to raise the question 'Is there such a thing as mental illness?' and to argue that there is not. Since the notion of mental illness is extremely widely used nowadays, inquiry into the ways in which this term is employed would seem to be especially indicated. Mental illness, of course, is not literally a 'thing' – or physical object – and hence it can 'exist' only in the same sort of way in which other theoretical concepts exist. Yet, familiar theories are in the habit of posing, sooner or later – at least to those who come to believe in them – as 'objective truths' (or 'facts'). During certain historical periods, explanatory conceptions such as deities, witches, and microorganisms appeared not only as theories but as self-evident *causes* of a vast number of events. I submit that today mental illness is widely regarded in a somewhat similar fashion, that is, as the cause of innumerable diverse happenings. As an antidote to the complacent use of the notion of mental illness – whether as a self-evident phenomenon, theory, or cause – let us ask this question: What is meant when it is asserted that someone is mentally ill?

In what follows I shall describe briefly the main uses to which the concept of mental illness has been put. I shall argue that this notion has outlived whatever usefulness it might have had and that it now functions merely as a convenient myth.

Mental Illness as a Sign of Brain Disease

The notion of mental illness derives its main support from such phenomena as syphilis of the brain or delirious conditions – intoxications, for instance – in which persons are known to manifest various peculiarities or disorders of thinking and behavior. Correctly speaking, however, these are diseases of the brain, not of the mind. According to one school of thought, *all* so-called mental-illness is of this type. The assumption is made that some neurological defect, perhaps a very subtle one, will ultimately be found for all the disorders of thinking and behavior. Many contemporary psychiatrists, physicians, and other scientists hold this view. This position implies that people *cannot* have troubles – expressed in what are *now called* 'mental illnesses' – because of differences in personal needs, opinions, social aspirations, values, and so on. *All problems in living* are attributed to physicochemical processes which in due time will be discovered by medical research.

'Mental illnesses' are thus regarded as basically no different than all other diseases (that is, of the body). The only difference, in this view, between mental and bodily diseases is that the former, affecting the brain, manifest themselves by means of mental symptoms; whereas the latter, affecting other organ systems (for example, the skin, liver, etc.), manifest themselves by means of symptoms referable to those parts of the body. This view rests on and expresses what are, in my opinion, two fundamental errors.

In the first place, what central nervous system symptoms would correspond to a skin eruption or a fracture? It would *not* be some emotion or complex bit of behavior. Rather, it would be blindness or a paralysis of some part of the body. The crux of the matter is that a disease of the brain, analogous to a disease of the skin or bone, is a neurological defect, and not

a problem in living. For example, a *defect* in a person's visual field may be satisfactorily explained by correlating it with certain definite lesions in the nervous system. On the other hand, a person's *belief* – whether this be a belief in Christianity, in Communism, or in the idea that his internal organs are 'rotting' and that his body is, in fact, already 'dead' – cannot be explained by a defect or disease of the nervous system. Explanations of this sort of occurrence – assuming that one is interested in the belief itself and does not regard it simply as a 'symptom' or expression of something else that is *more interesting* – must be sought along different lines.

The second error in regarding complex psychosocial behavior, consisting of communications about ourselves and the world about us, as mere symptoms of neurological functioning is *epistemological*. In other words, it is an error pertaining not to any mistakes in observation or reasoning, as such, but rather to the way in which we organize and express our knowledge. In the present case, the error lies in making a symmetrical dualism between mental and physical (or bodily) symptoms, a dualism which is merely a habit of speech and to which no known observations can be found to correspond. Let us see if this is so. In medical practice, when we speak of physical disturbances, we mean either signs (for example, a fever) or symptoms (for example, pain). We speak of mental symptoms, on the other hand, when we refer to a patient's *communications about himself, others, and the world about him*. He might state that he is Napoleon or that he is being persecuted by the Communists. These would be considered mental symptoms *only* if the observer believed that the patient was *not* Napoleon or that he was *not* being persecuted by the Communists. This makes it apparent that the statement that '*X* is a mental symptom' involves rendering a judgment. The judgment entails, moreover, a covert comparison or matching of the patient's ideas, concepts, or beliefs with those of the observer and the society in which they live. The notion of mental symptom is therefore inextricably tied to the *social* (including *ethical*) *context* in which it is made in much the same way as the notion of bodily symptom is tied to an *anatomical* and *genetic context* (Szasz, 1957a, 1957b).

To sum up what has been said thus far: I have tried to show that for those who regard mental symptoms as signs of brain disease, the concept of mental illness is unnecessary and misleading. For what they mean is that people so labeled suffer from diseases of the brain; and, if that is what they mean, it would seem better for the sake of clarity to say that and not something else.

Mental Illness as a Name for Problems in Living

The term 'mental illness' is widely used to describe something which is very different than a disease of the brain. Many people today take it for granted that living is an arduous process. Its hardship for modern man, moreover, derives not so much from a struggle for biological survival as from the stresses and strains inherent in the social intercourse of complex human personalities. In this context, the notion of mental illness is used to identify or describe some feature of an individual's so-called personality. Mental illness – as a deformity of the personality, so to speak – is then regarded as the

* Szasz, T.: The myth of mental illness. American Psychologist 15: 113–118, 1960.

cause of the human disharmony. It is implicit in this view that social intercourse between people is regarded as something *inherently harmonious*, its disturbance being due solely to the presence of 'mental illness' in many people. This is obviously fallacious reasoning, for it makes the abstraction 'mental illness' into a *cause* even though this abstraction was created in the first place to serve only as a shorthand expression for certain types of human behavior. It now becomes necessary to ask: 'What kinds of behavior are regarded as indicative of mental illness, and by whom?'

The concept of illness, whether bodily or mental, implies *deviation from some clearly defined norm*. In the case of physical illness, the norm is the structural and functional integrity of the human body. Thus, although the desirability of physical health, as such, is an ethical value, what health *is* can be stated in anatomical and physiological terms. What is the norm deviation from which is regarded as mental illness? This question cannot be easily answered. But whatever this norm might be, we can be certain of only one thing: namely, that it is a norm that must be stated in terms of *psychosocial, ethical, and legal concepts*. For example, notions such as 'excessive repression' or 'acting out an unconscious impulse' illustrate the use of psychological concepts for judging (so-called) mental health and illness. The idea that chronic hostility, vengefulness, or divorce are indicative of mental illness would be illustrations of the use of ethical norms (that is, the desirability of love, kindness, and a stable marriage relationship). Finally, the widespread psychiatric opinion that only a mentally ill person would commit homicide illustrates the use of a legal concept as a norm of mental health. The norm from which deviation is measured whenever one speaks of a mental illness is a *psychosocial and ethical one*. Yet, the remedy is sought in terms of *medical* measures which – it is hoped and assumed – are free from wide differences of ethical value. The definition of the disorder and the terms in which its remedy are sought are therefore at serious odds with one another. The practical significance of this covert conflict between the alleged nature of the defect and the remedy can hardly be exaggerated.

Having identified the norms used to measure deviations in cases of mental illness, we will now turn to the question: 'Who defines the norms and hence the deviation?' Two basic answers may be offered: (*a*) It may be the person himself (that is, the patient) who decides that he deviates from a norm. For example, an artist may believe that he suffers from a work inhibition; and he may implement this conclusion by seeking help *for* himself from a psychotherapist. (*b*) It may be someone other than the patient who decides that the latter is deviant (for example, relatives, physicians, legal authorities, society generally, etc.). In such a case a psychiatrist may be hired by others to do something *to* the patient in order to correct the deviation.

These considerations underscore the importance of asking the question 'Whose agent is the psychiatrist?' and of giving a candid answer to it (Szasz, 1956, 1958). The psychiatrist (psychologist or nonmedical psychotherapist), it now develops, may be the agent of the patient, of the relatives, of the school, of the military services, of a business organization, of a court of law, and so forth. In speaking of the psychiatrist as the agent of these persons or organizations, it is not implied that his values concerning norms, or his ideas and aims concerning the proper nature of remedial action, need to coincide exactly with those of his employer. For example, a patient in individual psychotherapy may believe that his salvation lies in a new marriage; his psychotherapist need not share this hypothesis. As the patient's agent, however, he must abstain from bringing social or legal force to bear on the patient which would prevent him from putting his beliefs into action. If his *contract* is with the patient, the psychiatrist (psychotherapist) may disagree with him or stop his treatment; but he cannot engage others to obstruct the patient's aspirations. Similarly, if a psychiatrist is engaged by a court to determine the sanity of a criminal, he need not fully share the legal authorities' values and intentions in regard to the criminal and the means available for dealing with him. But the psychiatrist is expressly barred from stating, for example, that it is not the criminal who is 'insane' but the men who wrote the law on the basis of which the very actions that are being judged are regarded as 'criminal.' Such an opinion could be voiced, of course, but not in a courtroom, and not by a psychiatrist who makes it his practice to assist the court in performing its daily work.

To recapitulate: In actual contemporary social usage, the finding of a mental illness is made by establishing a deviance in behavior from certain psychosocial, ethical, or legal norms. The judgment may be made, as in medicine, by the patient, the physician (psychiatrist), or others. Remedial action, finally, tends to be sought in a therapeutic – or covertly medical – framework, thus creating a situation in which *psychosocial, ethical*, and/or *legal deviations* are claimed to be correctible by (so-called) *medical action*. Since medical action is designed to correct only medical deviations, it seems logically absurd to expect that it will help solve problems whose very existence had been defined and established on nonmedical grounds. I think that these considerations may be fruitfully applied to the present use of tranquilizers and, more generally, to what might be expected of drugs of whatever type in regard to the amelioration or solution of problems in human living.

The Role of Ethics in Psychiatry

Anything that people *do* – in contrast to things that *happen* to them (Peters, 1958) – takes place in a context of value. In this broad sense, no human activity is devoid of ethical implications. When the values underlying certain activities are widely shared, those who participate in their pursuit may lose sight of them altogether. The discipline of medicine, both as a pure science (for example, research) and as a technology (for example, therapy), contains many ethical considerations and judgments. Unfortunately, these are often denied, minimized, or merely kept out of focus; for the ideal of the medical profession as well as of the people whom it serves seems to be having a system of medicine (allegedly) free of ethical value. This sentimental notion is expressed by such things as the doctor's willingness to treat and help patients irrespective of their religious or political beliefs, whether they are rich or poor, etc. While there may be some grounds for this belief – albeit it is a view that is not impressively true even in these regards – the fact remains that ethical considerations encompass a vast range of human affairs. By making the practice of medicine neutral in regard to some special issues of value need not, and cannot, mean that it can be kept free from all such values. The practice of medicine is intimately tied to ethics; and the first thing that we must do, it seems to me, is to try to make this clear and explicit. I shall let this matter rest here, for it does not concern us specifically in this essay. Lest there be any vagueness, however, about how or where ethics and medicine meet, let me remind the reader of such issues as birth control, abortion, suicide, and euthanasia as only a few of the major areas of current ethicomedical controversy.

Psychiatry, I submit, is very much more intimately tied to problems of ethics than is medicine. I use the word 'psychiatry' here to refer to that contemporary discipline which is concerned with *problems in living* (and not with diseases of the brain, which are problems for neurology). Problems in human relations can be analyzed, interpreted, and given meaning only within given social and ethical contexts. Accordingly, it *does* make a difference – arguments to the contrary notwithstanding – what the psychiatrist's socioethical orientations happen to be; for these will influence his ideas on what is wrong with the patient, what deserves comment or interpretation, in what possible directions change might be desirable, and so forth. Even in medicine proper, these factors play a role, as for instance, in the divergent orientations which physicians, depending on their religious affiliations, have toward such things as birth control and therapeutic abortion. Can anyone really believe that a psychotherapist's ideas concerning religious belief, slavery, or other similar issues play no role in his practical work? If they do make a difference, what are we to infer from it? Does it not seem reasonable that we ought to have different psychiatric therapies – each expressly recognized for the ethical positions which they embody – for, say, Catholics and Jews, religious persons and agnostics, democrats and communists, white supremacists and Negroes, and so on? Indeed, if we look at how psychiatry is actually practiced today (especially in the United States) we find that people do seek psychiatric help in accordance with their social status and ethical beliefs (Hollingshead & Redlich, 1958). This should really not surprise us more than being told that practicing Catholics rarely frequent birth control clinics.

The foregoing position which holds that contemporary psychotherapists deal with problems in living, rather than with mental illnesses and their cures, stands in opposition to a currently prevalent claim, according to which mental illness is just as 'real' and 'objective' as bodily illness. This is a confusing claim since it is never known exactly what is meant by such words as 'real' and 'objective.' I suspect, however, that what is intended by the proponents of this view is to create the idea in the popular mind that mental illness is some sort of disease entity, like an infection or a malignancy. If this were true, one could *catch* or *get* a 'mental illness,' one might *have* or *harbor* it, one might *transmit* it to others, and finally one could get *rid* of it. In my opinion, there is not a shred of evidence to support this idea. To the contrary, all the evidence is the other way and supports the view that what people now call mental illnesses are for the most part *communications* expressing unacceptable ideas, often framed, moreover, in an unusual idiom. The scope of this essay allows me to do no more than mention this alternative theoretical approach to this problem (Szasz, 1957c).

This is not the place to consider in detail the similarities and differences between bodily and mental illnesses. It shall suffice for us here to emphasize only one important difference between them: namely, that whereas bodily disease refers to public, physicochemical occurrences, the notion of mental illness is used to codify relatively more private, sociopsychological happenings of which the observer (diagnostician) forms a part. In other words, the psychiatrist does not stand *apart* from what he observes, but is, in Harry Stack Sullivan's apt words, a 'participant observer.' This means that he is *committed* to some picture of what he considers reality – and to what he thinks society considers reality – and he observes and judges the patient's behavior in the light of these considerations. This touches on our earlier observation that the notion of mental symptom itself implies a comparison between observer and observed, psychiatrist and patient. This is so obvious that I may be charged with belaboring trivialities. Let me therefore say once more that my aim in presenting this argument was expressly to criticize and counter a prevailing contemporary tendency to deny the moral aspects of psychiatry (and psychotherapy) and to substitute for them allegedly value-free medical considerations. Psychotherapy, for example, is being widely practiced as though it entailed nothing other than restoring the patient from a state of mental sickness to one of mental health. While it is generally accepted that mental illness has something to do with man's social (or interpersonal) relations, it is paradoxically maintained that problems of values (that is, of ethics) do not arise in this process.[1] Yet, in one sense, much of psychotherapy may revolve around nothing other than the elucidation and weighing of goals and values – many of which may be mutually contradictory – and the means whereby they might best be harmonized, realized, or relinquished.

The diversity of human values and the methods by means of which they may be realized is so vast, and many of them remain so unacknowledged, that they cannot fail but lead to conflicts in human relations. Indeed, to say that human relations at all levels – from mother to child, through husband and wife, to nation and nation – are fraught with stress, strain, and disharmony is, once again, making the obvious explicit. Yet, what may be obvious may be also poorly understood. This I think is the case here. For it seems to me that – at least in our scientific theories of behavior – we have failed to *accept* the simple fact that human relations are inherently fraught with difficulties and that to make them even relatively harmonious requires much patience and hard work. I submit that the idea of mental illness is now being put to work to obscure certain difficulties which at present may be inherent – not that they need be unmodifiable – in the social intercourse of persons. If this is true, the concept functions as a disguise; for instead of calling attention to conflicting human needs, aspirations, and values, the notion of mental illness provides an amoral and impersonal 'thing' (an 'illness') as an explanation for *problems in living* (Szasz, 1959). We may recall in this connection that not so long ago it was devils and witches who were held responsible for men's problems in social living. The belief in mental illness, as something other than man's trouble in getting along with his fellow man, is the proper heir to the belief in demonology and witchcraft. Mental illness exists or is 'real' in exactly the same sense in which witches existed or were 'real.'

Choice, Responsibility, and Psychiatry

While I have argued that mental illnesses do not exist, I obviously did not imply that the social and psychological occurrences to which this label is currently being attached also do not exist. Like the personal and social troubles which people had in the Middle Ages, they are real enough. It is the labels we give them that concerns us and, having labelled them, what we do about them. While I cannot go into the ramified implications of this problem here, it is worth noting that a demonologic conception of problems in living gave rise to therapy along theological lines. Today, a belief in mental illness implies – nay, requires – therapy along medical or psychotherapeutic lines.

What is implied in the line of thought set forth here is something quite different. I do not intend to offer a new conception of 'psychiatric illness' nor a new form of 'therapy.' My aim is more modest and yet also more ambitious. It is to suggest that the phenomena now called mental illnesses be looked at afresh and more simply, that they be removed from the category of illnesses, and that they be regarded as the expressions of man's struggle with the problem of *how* he should live. The last mentioned problem is obviously a vast one, its enormity reflecting not only man's inability to cope with his environment, but even more his increasing self-reflectiveness.

By problems in living, then, I refer to that truly explosive chain reaction which began with man's fall from divine grace by partaking of the fruit of the tree of knowledge. Man's awareness of himself and of the world about him seems to be a steadily expanding one, bringing in its wake an ever larger *burden of understanding* (an expression borrowed from Susanne Langer, 1953). *This burden*, then, *is to be expected and must not be misinterpreted.* Our only *rational* means for lightening it is *more understanding*, and appropriate *action* based on such understanding. The main alternative lies in acting as though the burden were not what in fact we perceive it to be and taking refuge in an outmoded theological view of man. In the latter view, man does not fashion his life and much of his world about him, but merely lives out his fate in a world created by superior beings. This may logically lead to pleading nonresponsibility in the face of seemingly unfathomable problems and difficulties. Yet, if man fails to take increasing responsibility for his actions, individually as well as collectively, it seems unlikely that some higher power or being would assume this task and carry this burden for him. Moreover, this seems hardly the proper time in human history for obscuring the issue of man's responsibility for his actions by hiding it behind the skirt of an all-explaining conception of mental illness.

Conclusions

I have tried to show that the notion of mental illness has outlived whatever usefulness it might have had and that it now functions merely as a convenient myth. As such, it is a true heir to religious myths in general, and to the belief in witchcraft in particular; the role of all these belief-systems was to act as *social tranquilizers*, thus encouraging the hope that mastery of certain specific problems may be achieved by means of substitutive (symbolic-magical) operations. The notion of mental illness thus serves mainly to obscure the everyday fact that life for most people is a continuous struggle, not for biological survival, but for a 'place in the sun,' 'peace of mind,' or some other human value. For man aware of himself and of the world about him, once the needs for preserving the body (and perhaps the race) are more or less satisfied, the problem arises as to what he should do with himself. Sustained adherence to the myth of mental illness allows people to avoid facing this problem, believing that mental health, conceived as the absence of mental illness, automatically insures the making of right and safe choices in one's conduct of life. But the facts are all the other way. It is the making of good choices in life that others regard, retrospectively, as good mental health!

The myth of mental illness encourages us, moreover, to believe in its logical corollary: that social intercourse would be harmonious, satisfying, and the secure basis of a 'good life' were it not for the disrupting influences of mental illness or 'psychopathology.' The potentiality for universal human happiness, in this form at least, seems to me but another example of the

I-wish-it-were-true type of fantasy. I do not believe that human happiness or well-being on a hitherto unimaginably large scale, and not just for a select few, is possible. This goal could be achieved, however, only at the cost of many men, and not just a few being willing and able to tackle their personal, social, and ethical conflicts. This means having the courage and integrity to forego waging battles on false fronts, finding solutions for substitute problems – for instance, fighting the battle of stomach acid and chronic fatigue instead of facing up to a marital conflict.

Our adversaries are not demons, witches, fate, or mental illness. We have no enemy whom we can fight, exorcise, or dispel by 'cure.' What we do have are *problems in living* – whether these be biologic, economic, political, or sociopsychological. In this essay I was concerned only with problems belonging in the last mentioned category, and within this group mainly with those pertaining to moral values. The field to which modern psychiatry addresses itself is vast, and I made no effort to encompass it all. My argument was limited to the proposition that mental illness is a myth, whose function it is to disguise and thus render more palatable the bitter pill of moral conflicts in human relations.

Note

1   Freud went so far as to say that: 'I consider ethics to be taken for granted. Actually I have never done a mean thing' (Jones, 1957, p. 247). This surely is a strange thing to say for someone who has studied man as a social being as closely as did Freud. I mention it here to show how the notion of 'illness' (in the case of psychoanalysis, 'psychopathology,' or 'mental illness') was used by Freud – and by most of his followers – as a means for classifying certain forms of human behavior as falling within the scope of medicine, and hence (by *fiat*) outside that of ethics!

References

Hollingshead, A. B., and Redlich, F. G. *Social class and mental illness.* New York: Wiley, 1958.

Jones, E. *The life and work of Sigmund Freud.* Vol. III. New York: Basic Books, 1957.

Langer, S. K. *Philosophy in a new key.* New York: Mentor Books, 1953.

Peters, R. S. *The concept of motivation.* London: Routledge & Kegan Paul, 1958.

Szasz, T. S. Malingering: 'Diagnosis' or social condemnation? *AMA Arch Neurol. Psychiat.*, 1956, 76, 432–443.

Szasz, T. S. *Pain and pleasure: A study of bodily feelings.* New York: Basic Books, 1957. (a)

Szasz, T. S. The problem of psychiatric nosology: A contribution to a situational analysis of psychiatric operations. *Amer. J. Psychiat.*, 1957, **114**, 405–413. (b)

Szasz, T. S. On the theory of psychoanalytic treatment. *Int. J. Psycho-Anal.*, **38**, 166–182. (c)

Szasz, T. S. Psychiatry, ethics and the criminal law. *Columbia law Rev.*, 1958, **58**, 183–198.

Szasz, T. S. Moral conflict and psychiatry, *Yale Rev.* [1960, **49**, 555–566.]

What a Theory of Mental Health Should Be*

Christopher Boorse

Among mental-health professionals there is wide agreement that the concept of mental health is a web of obscurity. One growing body of opinion, ably led by Szasz (1961, 1963, 1970a, 1970b), Sarbin (1967, 1969), and the behaviour-modification theorists, maintains that the whole idea of mental illness has outlived its usefulness and become both 'scientifically worthless and socially harmful' (Szasz, 1961, p. ix). This remains a minority view; but those writers who continue to believe in mental health disagree sharply about what it is and even about how one might find out. At the bottom of this impasse, I think, are two causes. One is the lack of 'a completely acceptable supertheory on which psychiatry can . . . rest its work' (Redlich & Freedman, 1966, p. 79). Until general psychology can achieve the broad theoretical consensus characteristic of other sciences, deep controversies over mental health seem inevitable. But these controversies are likely to remain irresolvable until a second obstacle is removed as well. I refer to the unwillingness of mental-health theorists to take physiology as a paradigm.

Reluctance to require any analogy between mental and physical health tends to cripple clinical discussion, from high-level theory to the analysis of particular conditions like homosexuality (e.g., Stoller *et al.*, 1973). The reason is that mental-health theory and practice have not sprung up in a vacuum. On the contrary, they originally rose within physiological medicine, a mature and fairly well-articulated body of thought. From this established discipline they borrowed both the root notion of health and the many unspoken assumptions that surround it: that health is worth promoting, for example, and that well-informed observers ought in principle to agree on the norms of the healthy personality. We are by now so familiar with the 'medical model' that any use of the term 'health' brings these and other assumptions irresistibly in its train. In consequence, I think, there are only two terminological options consistent with clarity and social responsibility. One may abandon the medical vocabulary altogether, as Szasz and the behaviour modifiers have urged, and found clinical psychology and psychiatry on something other than the model of health and disease. Or one may continue to use the health vocabulary in the same way in which it is used in physiological medicine – and accept the implications of such use in the psychological domain.

To explore and defend the second option is the purpose of this essay. In the first section I shall argue that the functional idea of health in physical medicine applies as straightforwardly to the mind as to the body. Section II examines accepted procedures for obtaining mental-health ideals, and concludes that all of them are inappropriate to a theory of health. Despite this methodological failure, section III suggests that current clinical criteria may have something to tell us about mental health after all.

I

Most discussions of the 'medical model' of mental illness are vitiated by confusion about what this model involves.[1] One reason for this confusion is that physical medicine itself has never felt the need to produce any clear

philosophical analysis of its notions of health and disease. I am going to presuppose the results of my own attempt at such an analysis, which might be summarized as follows:

An organism is healthy at any moment in proportion as it is not diseased; and a disease is a type of internal state of the organism which:

(i) interferes with the performance of some natural function – i.e., some species-typical contribution to survival and reproduction – characteristic of the organism's age; and

(ii) is not simply in the nature of the species, i.e. is either atypical of the species or, if typical, mainly due to environmental causes.[2]

The crucial points about this analysis are two. First, diseases are interferences with natural-functions. Second, since the functional organization typical of a species is a biological fact, the concept of disease is value-free. Whether or not an organism is diseased can be settled in principle by the methods of natural science. The popularity of the opposite view is, I think, due to a failure to distinguish between the idea of a disease and the much narrower idea of an illness. Diseases become illnesses only when they satisfy certain further, and normative, conditions:

A disease is an *illness* only if it is serious enough to be incapacitating, and therefore is

(i) undesirable for its bearer;

(ii) a title to special treatment; and

(iii) a valid excuse for normally criticizable behaviour. (Boorse, 1975)

Thus we must distinguish, as Szasz and others usually do not, between two questions: whether 'mental illness' makes sense, and whether 'mental disease' makes sense. I shall consider only the latter question here.[3]

The analysis of health just given, though derived from physiology, shows no obvious partiality to body over mind. Physical health is simply the special case obtained by focusing on the functions of physiological processes. Mental health, then, would be the special case obtained by focusing on the functions of mental processes; and so there is such a thing as mental health if there are mental functions. For this, two conditions must be satisfied. First, some mental processes must play a causal role in action. Since philosophers are divided over whether mental events can be causes, the issue cannot readily be treated here. I agree with Davidson (1963) that the arguments against mental causation are weak and will conduct the discussion on that assumption. The second condition required for mental health is that mental processes contribute to action in a sufficiently species-uniform way to have natural functions. This thesis also seems plausible. Freud aside, the work of Chomsky and Piaget suggests that there are complicated patterns of mental functioning invariant in the species. No doubt it is generally assumed, outside the orbit of learning theory, that the human mind has *some* characteristic organization and operation. It is something of a historical accident that the term 'biological function' calls to mind sex and excretion rather than intelligence and drive; Darwin, for one, was deeply interested in the evolution of the human mental apparatus. If certain types of mental processes perform standard functions in human behaviour, it is hard to see any obstacle to calling unnatural obstructions of these functions

* Boorse, C: What a theory of mental health should be. *Journal for the Theory of Social Behaviour* 6: 61–84, 1976.

mental diseases, exactly as in the physiological case. So far the analogy between physical and mental health is unproblematic.

One source of disanalogy is that we may expect normal psychological functions to be somewhat less specific than their physiological counterparts. The outstanding feature of human mentality is its plasticity. There is an enormous range of physical and cultural environments to which the human mind can adapt its functioning. This adaptability, as a characteristic of the individual as well as of the group, is without parallel in the biological kingdom. Even so, however, and without relying on any controversial psychological theory, it is easy to draw some of the outlines of human mental functioning. Perceptual processing, intelligence, and memory clearly serve to provide information about the world that can guide effective action. Drives serve to motivate it. Anxiety and pain function as signals of danger, language as a device for cultural co-operation and cognitive enrichment, and so on. If these and other mental processes play standard functional roles throughout the species, we seem to have everything requisite for the possibility of mental health. Why then do Szasz and Sarbin reject this possibility?

These authors object to the idea of mental health on two grounds. One is that it involves Cartesian dualism; the other is that it involves explaining behaviour causally as due to disease entities in this immaterial soul, rather than explaining it by a 'rule-following' or 'communication' or 'social systems' model. As one would expect from this compressed description, Ryle and Peters are the philosophical mainstays of this line of criticism of the medical model in psychiatry. Sarbin writes:

The basic Galenic model was not rejected by psychiatry and its immediate antecedents. Microbes, toxins, and growths, which were material and operated according to mechanical principles, were appropriate "causes" for diseases of the body. They were *inside* the body. The appropriate causes for abnormal *behavior* had to be sought along different lines. Since the dualistic mind-body concept was everyone's heritage, the hypothesis could be entertained that the causes of abnormal conduct, conduct already considered as nonsomatic disease, were *in the mind*. . . .

Through historical and linguistic processes, the postulation was reified. Contemporary users of the mental illness concept are guilty of illicitly shifting from metaphor to myth. Instead of maintaining the metaphorical rhetoric 'it is as if there were states of mind' and 'it is as if such states of mind could be characterized as sickness,' the contemporary mentalist conducts much of his work as if he believes that minds are 'real' entities and that, like bodies, they can be sick or healthy (1969, pp. 15, 19).

Sarbin's discussion, though fascinating, is not an accurate reconstruction of the origin of the mental-illness concept. In many respects Freud is the beginning of the tradition Sarbin is criticizing, but he was far from being a Cartesian. Instead he seems to have anticipated a full physiological reduction of his theoretical apparatus.[4] As we have seen, the part of everyone's heritage on which the mental-illness idea depends is not Cartesian dualism, but just the mentalistic framework of beliefs, perceptions, wishes, fantasies, dreams, etc. One need not be a Cartesian to believe that people have such mental states as these, and Sarbin is surely not questioning their existence in questioning the reality of the mind. Rather, he is disputing whether they are states of an incorporeal substance, and further whether they can be causes of behaviour. We can agree that the mental-health concept stands or falls with mental causation. The interesting question is why Sarbin supposes that dualism is the only mind-body view that can support such a notion of mental health. I suspect the answer is that he implicitly accepts the following argument. If mental states are states of the body rather than of a soul, then mental diseases must be diseases of the brain or nerves. In that case there is no need for a concept of mental health distinct from physical health, and we are back with pre-Freudian neuropathology. This reasoning is defective, and I shall now explain why.

Consider the relation between mental and physical health according to one familiar variant of the identity theory, which is a fusion of ideas of Putnam and Davidson.[5] This view holds that every mental event is a physical event. Taking mental states as degenerate mental events, consisting merely of the persistence of some psychological property over time, a parallel claim can be made about states. Every mental state is a physical state. But the states thus claimed identical are to be particulars, i.e. dated conditions of specific persons, rather than universals, i.e. types of conditions. Not *the* desire for a lobster dinner, but *Smith's* desire for a lobster dinner as felt between 4 and 5 p.m. on 13 February 1975, is claimed to be identical to his being in some neural configuration during this period.[6] The distinction is crucial, for if types of mental states are defined by their functional properties, type-type identity statements are unlikely to hold. If Smith's current neural state is a desire for a lobster dinner, that is probably not because of any anatomical feature, such as its containing a lobster-shaped nerve net. Rather, on the view we are considering, it is because of the motivational role this state plays in producing a search for seafood restaurants or other lobster-obtaining behaviour. Now the same motivational role might be played by quite different neural configurations in different people. Hence the neural state in Smith that is his desire for a lobster dinner may bear no anatomical resemblance to the neural state in Jones that is his desire for a lobster dinner. And so there may be no set of anatomical properties that could define the mentalistic term 'desire for a lobster dinner'; the mentalistic vocabulary, even for a materialist, may not be neurologically definable.

My purpose in rehearsing this view is to show why it is in no way obvious that psychiatrists who reject Cartesian dualism thereby destroy the autonomy of their discipline. On the version of the identity theory just summarized, they must concede that any particular person's mental disease is a physical state. But this is a very limited admission. It is not the same as saying that every mental disease is a physical disease. Diseases, e.g. tuberculosis or cancer or schizophrenia, are essentially universals rather than particulars. They are types of states which are instantiated in particular patients. But there is no guarantee that a mentalistically defined disease-type will coincide with any physiologically defined disease-type. Suppose, for example, that a type of mental disorder is marked by ambivalent feelings toward the patient's father. As in the lobster case, there may be no anatomical criterion by which one could examine the patient's brain and discover the idea of the father. The brains of the various patients who share this disorder may show no distinctive neural similarity. Thus mental diseases, in spite of being everywhere instantiated by neural states, may fail to be physical diseases by failing to be physiologically definable.

Further support for this suggestion emerges if one asks what makes a patient's condition a mental disease in the first place. It is not the presence of mental symptoms. Pain, delirium, and depression are mental symptoms that occur in many physical diseases. Nor does it seem to be true that a disease is classed as a mental illness when it has mental symptoms and is assumed to have a physical aetiology currently unknown. 'Mental illness' is not just a shorthand for 'obscure brain disease,' since various conditions with obscure neural bases – dyslexia, aphasia, retardation – are not usually called mental illnesses. Rather, a mental disturbance gets classed as 'mental illness' when some accepted explanation of it refers not to the patient's physiology but to his feelings, beliefs, and experiences. The defining property of mental disease is mental causation.[7] Now on the version of the identity theory just discussed, the causal chain of mental events leading to a disease condition must be equally a chain of physical events. But this chain figures in a causal *explanation* only in so far as it can be brought under causal laws (Hempel, 1965, pp. 347 ff.). If the mentalistic vocabulary is not neurologically definable, there will be no way to reduce causal laws of the mind to causal laws of the body. If so, the distinction between conditions that receive one kind of causal explanation and those that receive the other may be a permanent one, justifying an autonomous science of mental health.

In practice the issue of materialism tends to be confused with the separate issue of how to treat mental diseases. If mental states are brain states, it is assumed that mental diseases must yield to such physical methods as drugs and surgery. This conclusion is doubly unfounded. In the first place, according to our version of the identity theory, it is as unreasonable as expecting a computer expert called in for consultation on a botched program to locate the trouble by going into the machine with a flashlight and a screwdriver. Whether and how a computer program, or a mental state, is dysfunctional need not be evident from any of its physical properties. In the second place, physical medicine itself includes conditions, e.g. partial paralysis of a limb following nerve damage, that can be treated only by molar like exercise. Of course, nothing that I have said proves that physical medicine *cannot* find an explanation and treatment for familiar mental disorders; what I am arguing is that materialism *per se* gives no guarantee that it can. A psychiatrist who rejects dualism can consistently regard mental diseases as a theoretical category distinct from physical diseases and calling for unique molar treatment, e.g. psychotherapy. What threatens the concept of mental disease is not materialism, but the denial of mental causation.

II

So far we have seen that given a few plausible assumptions, the idea of mental health not only makes perfect sense but generates an autonomous field of clinical theory. We now encounter a striking paradox. It is quite likely that there is such a thing as mental health; yet the majority of 'mental-health' theorists use methodologies that offer no assurance of finding out the first thing about it. They do not set out to investigate the normal functional organization of the human mind, as they ought to do if their subject is mental health. Instead they arrive at their mental-health criteria by one of three unsatisfactory routes.

The first route is to select some set of personality traits that are highly valued, either by the theorist or by our culture, and call them 'mental health.' The view that health judgments are at bottom nothing but value judgments has in fact come to be a sort of orthodoxy among clinicians.[8] But it is a mistaken view. In physical medicine the health of a body is not at all the same as its worth. One does not expect physicians to call anything they dislike about a person's body, e.g. its ugliness, a disease and proceed to shape it to their own standards. Whether the subject is disease or illness, all judgments of physical health involve factual claims about the conformity of the individual to the species design, i.e., to the inherited adaptive organization which is the basic subject matter of biology (Boorse, 1975). The doctrines of physiology about this functional design rest on empirical evidence and are either true or false. Where this factual component is wholly lacking, then, as in much psychological and psychiatric discussion, we do not have a *health* concept at all but one of moral acceptability or the good life for man.[9]

It is easy to notice that a mental-health theorist's criteria rests on nothing but a personal affirmation of values when one disagrees with the values. The Victorian flavour of such a statement as the following now inspires amusement:

Wholesome-minded people are not averse to frank consideration of sex under proper conditions and right motives, but they do not enjoy having it dragged into prominence on every possible pretext and occasion. Dignity and decency are the marks of successful sex adjustment.[10]

But we might not be so quick to realize that we have a right to ask for evidence for the claim that

the crucial consideration in determining human normality is whether the individual is an asset or a burden to society and whether he is or is not contributing to the progressive development of man.[11]

No doubt most people, like Adler, admire individuals who contribute to the development of man more than individuals who do not. But that in itself gives us no reason whatever to suppose that individuals who do not are unhealthy, i.e. suffer from psychological dysfunction.

Even no less an authority than Karl Menninger leaves room for similar worries about the provenance of his idea of health:

Let us define mental health as the adjustment of human beings to the world and to each other with a maximum of effectiveness and happiness. Not just efficiency, or just contentment – or the grace of obeying the rules of the game cheerfully. It is all of these together. It is the ability to maintain an even temper, an alert intelligence, socially considerate behavior, and a happy disposition. This, I think, is a healthy mind. (1930, 2)

I would not suggest that Menninger has no evidence that he has correctly described the healthy mind. Nevertheless the opening phrase and inspirational tone of this proposal, as well as its position at the beginning of his discussion, tend to obscure the fact that what the healthy mind is like is an empirical question that can be answered correctly or incorrectly. We are no more free to define mental health as the constellation of qualities we most admire than we would be for physical health. Mental health must be a constellation of qualities displayed in the standard functional organization of members of our species. Only empirical inquiry can show whether normal human beings have an even temper, engage in socially considerate behaviour, and advance the species – or make love with 'dignity and decency.' Some animals are naturally irascible and treat their peers with unbroken hostility. Most copulate with utter abandon. Perhaps we are not so constituted; perhaps we are. The point is that a theory of health should be a description of how we are constituted and not how we would like to be.

Besides the affirmation of values, a second popular route to mental-health criteria is to abstract them from a set of agreed instances of disease. Presupposing that some class of mental conditions, e.g. psychoses, are unhealthy, the theorist looks for their common features and takes these as a negative definition of mental health. A good illustration is Kubie's view that mental health consists in a low level of unconscious motivation:

The implicit ideal of normality that emerges . . . is an individual in whom the creative alliance between the conscious and preconscious systems is not constantly subject to blocking and distortion by the counterplay of preponderant unconscious forces . . . (1954, p. 187).

Kubie presents this view as a general account of mental health. His title confirms, however, that the core class of instances from which he has abstracted it is the neuroses. To see some practical difficulties with this abstraction route, one needs only ask whether, say, character disorders are unhealthy. Some character disorders are not marked by psychic conflict; thus by Kubie's criterion one would not be inclined to call them diseases. On the other hand, one could equally well abstract other criteria from Kubie's class of instances – e.g., capacity for accurate empathy for others – by which these character disorders *would* count as unhealthy. Any class of agreed instances may have various common features that imply different verdicts on problematic cases outside the class. And this first problem is intensified by two more. From a class of cases all defective in some quality, one cannot tell how much of the quality would be required in a healthy specimen. If psychotics are alike in, say, a lack of self-knowledge, how much self-knowledge is required for health? The abstraction method is incapable of giving any answer. Worst of all, the class of disorders on which almost all mental-health theorists would agree is severely limited. At best it includes psychoses and fairly spectacular neuroses, psychopathic personalities, etc. Certainly persons whom Kubie would call neurotic and therefore unhealthy, such as compulsively ambitious politicians, would not be called unhealthy by everyone. One writer's character neurosis is another writer's model of successful adjustment. Not surprisingly, then, the abstraction method invariably fails in practice to produce any wide consensus.

From the theoretical standpoint, an equally telling objection to the abstraction route is its presupposition that any given cases are unhealthy ones. As Szasz insists, the fact that a condition involves incapacitation and suffering is no proof that it is an illness.[12] It is even less obvious that every neurosis or character disorder is a defect of health. Conceptually speaking, neuroses could easily be what biologists call facultative adaptations to life circumstances, like the calluses on a workman's fingertips. That there is adaptive value in unconscious processes seems evident enough, from dreams to the syntax of spoken language and the symphonies of Mozart. Why then should we think that the unconscious motivation of the neurotic deviates from species design? No doubt we would be more creative, more flexible, and happier without our neuroses; but would we be healthier? However we may disvalue neurosis and seek to eradicate it, we cannot call it unhealthy until we know that the mind is not supposed to work that way. It is in no way obvious, and requires empirical support, that what clinicians see in their offices are usually cases of biological dysfunction.

It is surely in part a desire to avoid the hazards of these first two routes that leads many mental-health theorists to follow the third one. The opening move in this final strategy is to discard mental processes altogether in favour of behaviour. The aim of providing criteria of mental health is replaced by the aim of providing criteria of normal behaviour. Redlich and Freedman justify this move as follows:

In older texts and in current lay parlance, psychiatry is often defined as the science dealing with mental diseases and illnesses of the mind or psyche. Since these are terms reminiscent of the metaphysical concepts of soul and spirit, we prefer to speak of behavior disorder. Behavior refers to objective data that are accessible to observation, plausible inference, hypothesis-making, and experimentation. The term disorder, although vague, is descriptive of malfunctioning of behavior without specifying etiology or underlying mechanism (1966, p. 2).

This quotation, like the earlier one from Sarbin, suggests the misconception that a true 'mental disease' would have to be a sort of gangrene on the Cartesian ego. It does not have to be, as we have seen; it need only be a psychogenic disturbance of mental functions. But the great popularity of this behavioural approach merits continued analysis.

Health in physiology is primarily a feature of the internal state of an organism rather than of its behaviour. One can imagine extending the concept to label behaviour itself as healthy or unhealthy. Behaviour as well as internal processes may have a biological function (cf. Roe & Simpson, 1958), as long as the behaviour is uniform in the species. Indeed, it is *via* their contributions to behaviour that internal processes have functions. One might call behaviour healthy or unhealthy, then, accordingly as it is biologically functional or dysfunctional. This new concept would apply most clearly to the fixed motor patterns studied by animal ethologists; whether anything of interest to clinicians would emerge in the human case is open to question. But an immediate problem is that this resort to behaviour does nothing to mark off a domain of 'mental' health as distinguished from physical health (Macklin, 1972, p. 342). If something we might call biologically dysfunctional behaviour can result from psychosis, it can certainly also result from multiple sclerosis or epilepsy or blindness. Unless one wishes psychiatry to swallow up medicine, therefore, some criterion must be given to distinguish those 'behaviour disorders' that fall within the province of psychiatry from those that do not. The most natural suggestion is unavailable: that psychiatry studies behaviour disorders that are produced by disfunctional mental processes. Avoiding mental processes was the motivation for the behavioural approach in the first place. As soon as they are reinstated, it is not more obvious why mental disease has to show up in overt behaviour than physical disease. The proper domain of psychiatry will then consist of disorders of the mind rather than disorders of behaviour, and we will return to square one.

Given that one is determined to avoid mental processes, the best move might be to hold that, psychiatry deals with dysfunctional behaviour in which there is no physiological abnormality. This position is not the one adopted by theorists of our third group. Instead they almost universally make a fatal error: they desert biological dysfunction in favour of social deviance. Redlich and Freedman have this to say about the term 'behaviour disorder':

Defying easy definition, the term refers to the presence of certain behavioral patterns – variously described as abnormal, subnormal, undesirable, inadequate, inappropriate, maladaptive, or maladjusted – that are not compatible with the norms and expectations of the patient's social and cultural system (1966, p. 1).

Since deviant behaviour can result from physical disease, presumably the intended view is that psychiatry deals with those behavioural patterns deemed deviant by society which are not physiologically explainable.

This move to social deviance makes Szasz's criticisms quite unanswerable. As long as the physiological paradigm is to be given any weight at all, society can have no title to decree what states of organisms are unhealthy. Tuberculosis and epilepsy are diseases not because society disvalues them, but because they are cases of biological malfunction. They would not cease

to be disease if some culture developed an admiration for epileptics or consumptives; like anything else, diseases can be assigned to a high social status. Within the realm of physiology social judgments of illness are no more infallible than social judgments of the shape of the earth or the number of planets, for they involve claims about the biological constitution of man. When, therefore, psychiatric theorists discard this biological constitution altogether in favour of the norms of a 'social and cultural system,' it seems fair to say that they have stopped talking about health. To reject the straightforward extension of the health vocabulary to the psychological domain, while giving it instead a new meaning grossly disanalogous to its established use, is hardly a responsible terminological policy.

One can indeed admit the conceptual gulf between biologically dysfunctional behaviour and socially disvalued behaviour and nevertheless assume that the two happen to coincide. In other words, one can hold it to be an *empirical* fact that behaviour is healthy only if society approves of it. But as an empirical hypothesis the view seems most implausible when clearly understood. It is true that man is a social animal. Our biological design, both mental and physical, seems to be adapted to life in a social group. But which social group? When judgments of deviance are made, the usual reference class is society at large. By this standard homosexuals, drug addicts, women's liberationists, Vietnam protesters, and fornicators are among the paradigm American deviants. But it is notorious that these and other nonconformists can flourish within non-conforming subcultures. As long as a person's behaviour is consistent with adjustment to some social group, one cannot call it unhealthy on the grounds that man is a social animal. As ordinarily understood, then, behavioural deviance seems too wide to be a sufficient condition of mental disorder. A narrower notion of deviance would count behaviour deviant only when it is considered deviant by all social groups. But this account will be clinically unsatisfactory for the opposite reason. Psychotics may be thoroughly accepted by their fellow patients in a psychiatric hospital, but they are surely not thereby healthy. Deviance from every conceivable standard is not a necessary condition for mental disorder.

Whether or not there is some middle ground, finally, seems irrelevant simply because deviants are not usually wholly ostracized even from the group that considers them deviant. Neither sexual swingers nor unwed mothers nor radical feminists are biologically incompetent in the sense of being totally excluded from the group way of life. They are merely disapproved of. And it would be fantastic to suggest that biological normality requires complete approval by one's peers, rather than just enough approval to satisfy whether needs of ours involve the medium of a group. It is not as though existing social structures reward conforming members with ideal opportunities for human fulfilment. Social agitation of a sort that is unpopular and even illegal is often morally justified; and there is no reason to suppose that the moral sensitivity and individual autonomy which can drive such behaviour is unnatural to the species. So Wootton's comments on 'adjustment,' i.e. social acceptance, again seem right on target:

In the literature of mental health generally, this concept of adjustment is particularly prominent. Fine phrases cannot, however, obscure the fact that adjustment means adjustment to a particular culture or to a particular set of institutions; and that to conceive adjustment and maladjustment in medical terms is in effect to identify health with the ability to come to terms with that culture or with those institutions – be they totalitarian methods of government, the dingy culture of an urban slum, the contemporary English law of marriage, or what I have elsewhere called the standards of an 'acquisitive, competitive, hierarchical, envious' society.[13]

There is in the end so little evidence for any general connection between social deviance and biological dysfunction that one is tempted to class the 'behaviour disorder' view as one more affirmation of values on the part of some conservative clinicians.

Thus Redlich and Freedman, along with the many other psychiatric authors who take the social-deviance route, are in fact doing what the behaviour modifiers are doing more openly. They are *abandoning* the 'medical model,' i.e. the model of health and disease. In this charge Szasz is perfectly correct. Since social deviance does not define any health concept, it would be preferable to introduce a new vocabulary. For example, one might speak with Ullmann and Krasner of 'maladaptive behaviour':

Maladaptive behavior is behavior that is considered inappropriate by those key people in a person's life who control reinforcers (1966, p. 20).

This definition suggests a refreshing lack of pretence that non-conformity is sickness. However, the value of the new terminology depends on our constantly remembering – as behaviour-modification theorists often do not – that 'maladaptive' so defined cannot be used interchangeably with 'pathological' or 'abnormal' or any other term meaning 'unhealthy.' It is both dishonest and dangerous to throw the health concept out at the front door and then let it in at the back. If one wishes to avoid the theoretical inconveniences of the medical model, one must constantly relinquish its practical implications as well. There is no objection to advocating the use of techniques like behaviour modification on clinical populations. But if the aim of such techniques is to be 'adaptive behavior' rather than mental health, one should candidly admit that many of our assumptions about health – in particular, its desirability – may not carry over to adaptive behaviour at all.

III

We have been directing heavy criticism upon the three main sources of contemporary mental-health criteria: affirmations of values, abstraction from established diagnostic classes, and social judgments of behaviour. We have seen that there is no reason, in principle, why any of these methods that mental-health theorists typically follow should generate an accurate account of mental health. It is time for some conciliatory remarks.

Apart from the inherent difficulties of all psychological research, there are several reasons why theorists overlook their obligation to describe the system of normal mental functions in which mental health must consist. One reason is that the functional conception of health in physiological medicine has gone largely unrecognized, both by philosophers and by physicians. A second reason is that contemporary biology has not, for the most part, continued Darwin's interests in the adaptive functions of mental abilities (Montague, 1962). Psychologists influenced by a narrowly physiological view of biology will tend to discount any possibility of transferring its functional model to the mental domain.

Perhaps a third reason, however, is the most important of all. Early physical medicine itself undoubtedly began with a primitive notion of illness lacking all reference to natural physiological functions. Patients were presumably classified as ill by a criterion of observable suffering or incapacitation alone. In time, with the rise of empirical thinking, supernatural explanations of these conditions were gradually replaced by the idea of internal malfunction. Contemporary psychiatry has not yet reached the stage of agreement on a substantive theory of the mind. In default of such a theory, it has, not unnaturally, reverted to the primitive conception of illness, although it must be said that it has also immeasurably extended its scope. Once again medical professionals are calling people 'ill' without any thought of internal malfunctioning, but solely on the grounds of emotional turmoil or social maladjustment.

The trouble with this procedure, however understandable, is that it is two thousand years too late. Physiological medicine has in the interim undergone a particular historical development. That development has culminated in the functional conception of disease with which we are thoroughly familiar. Not everyone is willing to assume that psychiatry can follow the same course of development, which is the assumption we defended earlier in connection with the functional notion of mental health. But to revert at this point to the archaic usage of the health vocabulary is to invite unbearable cognitive strain. My proof for this statement is simply the opacity of current controversies over mental health. In the interests of conceptual clarity, psychiatry must either conform its usage of 'health' to the functional paradigm or else devise new ways of speaking of the conditions with which it deals. And my final suggestion is that in spite

of the methodological defects of current mental-health theory, it would be a mistake for the clinical disciplines to follow Szasz *et al.* in discarding mental health. Regardless of the origin of existing clinical criteria, there is reason to take many of them seriously as hypotheses about the normal human design. I will conclude with a series of points in defence of this suggestion.

Consider first some broad categories of traditional psychopathology. It seems certain that a few of the recognized mental disorders are genuine diseases, whether mental or physical. Even without any knowledge of the relevant functional systems, one can sometimes infer internal malfunction immediately from biologically incompetent behaviour. Functions in physiology are species-typical contributions of a part to survival and reproduction. Some mental patients, e.g. catatonic schizophrenics, are clearly incompetent with respect to these biological goals and would remain so under almost any circumstances. Whatever the detailed functional organization of the human mind and body may be, then, these people depart from it and so are authentically unhealthy. Of course, the class of conditions that supports this kind of inference is only a fraction of the domain of standard clinical theory. Even some psychotic people, as well as the great mass of those with neuroses and character disorders, function successfully at the minimal level required for basic biological goals. Since different cultures achieve these goals by an astonishing variety of life-styles anyway, any further defence of established clinical categories seems to require some specific functional assumptions about the mind.

One should not underestimate the mileage that can be got out of elementary functional assumptions that are scarcely controversial. We may surely assume, for example, that the main function of perceptual and intellectual processes is to give us knowledge of the world. The imperfection of this cognitive apparatus is obvious. Since there are limits both to human intelligence and to the evidence on which it works, it would be wrong to suppose that every false belief is a functional abnormality. Nevertheless, one could plausibly suggest that the perceptions and beliefs of a healthy mind must at least show, in Jahoda's words, 'relative freedom from need-distortion' (1958, 51). That is, if my cognitive functions are disrupted to a highly unusual degree by my wishes, it seems safe to call my condition an unnatural dysfunction, i.e. a disease. By this standard schizophrenia and all other psychoses with thought disorders look objectively unhealthy. Moreover, if one accepts the traditional analytic description of the neurotic process, very limited functional assumptions will suffice to construe serious neurosis as a disease. Since opposite desires are common in human beings, there must be some normal mechanism for resolving them without permanent and paralysing conflict. If some of the neurotic's strongest desires remain locked in combat without freely releasing their motivational force in behaviour, it is not an implausible hypothesis that the conflict-resolution mechanism is functioning incorrectly.

These arguments show that some elementary functional claims about the species, together with a small body of widely accepted descriptive information about the mental processes of psychotics and neurotics, may give good ground for provisionally calling these conditions pathological. Any stronger vindication of current clinical categories would require a detailed and well-confirmed theory of the functions of a normal human mind. But a further reason for clinical professionals to cast their lot with mental health is that a well-developed example of the right kind of theory is already in the field. Formally speaking, psychoanalytic theory is the best account of mental health we have. It closely follows the physiological model by positing three mental substructures, the id, ego, and superego, and assigning fixed functions to each. It is not entirely clear that the mental functions psychoanalysts describe are functions in the biological sense. One sometimes has the impression in psychoanalytic writing that the function of a mental process is the gratification it can secure for the id.[14] From the biological standpoint, the function of a mental process is its contribution, not to our pleasure, but to our behaviour; pleasure itself has a function in producing behaviour. But it would not be difficult to construe psychoanalytic theory as a set of theses about biological functions of the mind. On this view the id might emerge as a reservoir of motivation, the ego as an instrument of rational integration and cognitive competence, and the superego as a device for socialization.[15] One could then give a straightforward argument that neurosis is disease by appealing to its disturbance of the integrative and motivational functions of the ego and the id. In any case, it is this sort of structural detail that is necessary to raise claims about psychopathology above the level of plausible conjecture.

I am recommending psychoanalytic theory as our best model, apart from physiology, of what a theory of mental health should be. Hence I will also mention a recurrent failure in its exposition. This is the uncritical assumption that neurosis is always unhealthy. Freud was willing to call religion a 'universal neurosis' (1927, p. 44). It is also often suggested that a mild childhood neurosis is a typical developmental stage. This evidence does not lead psychoanalytic writers to abandon the assumption. For example, Hartmann writes:

Typical conflicts are a part and parcel of 'normal' development, and disturbances in adaptation are included in its scope. . . . Here health clearly includes pathological reactions as a means to its attainment.[16]

Although I am not sure what Hartmann means here, it is hard to imagine how a standard developmental stage can be pathological. The normal functional organization for an organism is always relative to its age. If the functional organization of children of a certain age includes neurotic conflict, the correct conclusion is that neurosis is not always unhealthy. In general, according to the analysis I gave at the outset, a nearly universal condition can be unhealthy only if it can be viewed as an environmental injury. It is just possible that Freud had environmental injuries in mind when he said that 'a normal ego . . . is, like normality in general, an ideal fiction' (1937, p. 235). But it seems more likely that he was employing the same rigorous standard Ernest Jones uses as a definition of health: 'the fullest possible development of the organism' (1932, p. 80).

What these quotations reveal is a clear tendency among psychoanalytic writers to make of the concept of health something more grandiose than it is in physical medicine. To have a healthy heart or biceps, I need not subject them to their fullest possible development. Health never requires ideal functioning, but only the functioning of each part at a species-normal level unimpeded by atypical or environmentally induced obstructions. Apart from the trivial injuries of a hostile environment, a normal biceps is far from an 'ideal function.' Along with many other writers, some psychoanalytic theorists are confusing the healthy personality with the *ideal* personality – a much more demanding goal – and presenting their notions of 'vital perfection' (Hartmann, 1964, p. 5) or the good life for man as if they were norms of health. It would be better to admit that what is undesirable, including neurosis, is not necessarily pathological. If it standardly happens that the child ego is presented with impulses it is too immature to master, that is surely a design defect in the species rather than a disease. How strong or lasting a neurotic process must be to be a disease is a question I cannot discuss here. But it seems evident that psychoanalysts could prevent considerable misunderstanding by avoiding such claims as that 'we have no experience of a completely normal mind' (Jones, 1932, p. 81), when what is meant is that we have no experience of a completely non-neurotic mind or a mind subjected to its fullest possible development. The hypothesis that neurosis is always abnormal seems to be contradicted by psychoanalytic doctrine itself.[17]

Although it seems to me a model theory in its broad outlines, psychoanalysis is far from general acceptance. Hence I wish to make one final point in defence of the continued relevance of the mental-health concept. Jahoda's milestone survey (1958) of criteria of mental health in current clinical practice reveals a bewildering variety of proposals. This is not surprising, if only because the human mind has a bewildering variety of tasks and abilities. To mention each criterion and assess the likelihood that it objectively describes the human personality design would require lengthy discussion. But it is striking how many of Jahoda's criteria could be subsumed, with some plausibility, under the heading of *maturity*. It is an empirical fact that the usual course of human development shows a growth in knowledge of self and world, informed self-acceptance and sense of identity, unification of life goals, tolerance for stress and frustration, autonomy of thought and action, and various kinds of environmental mastery. At any rate, adults tend to have more of these qualities than children. To whatever extent the increase in these traits can be shown part of a normal developmental sequence, it is correct to call them requirements of health in an adult. Freud is sometimes accused of confusing morals with medicine in taking his 'genital type' to be a health ideal.[18] I have just suggested that this confusion is not unknown among psychoanalysts, but the mere idea of a developmental disease, i.e. arrest or retardation of normal growth, is not a case of it. What is controversial is that Freud's oral, anal, phallic, and genital stages are a genuine series of normal stages of development. It is not controversial that a failure to traverse normal stages is unhealthy.

This point should scarcely be seen as a full vindication of the various criteria just mentioned. Considerable argument would be required to show that the emergence of, say, accurate self-knowledge is objectively a feature of normal human growth in the same way as permanent teeth or secondary sex characteristics. As recent controversy over Piagetian theory illustrates, the notion of a developmental stage is itself in need of detailed analysis. Furthermore, the bare observation that most adults have more self-knowledge than children does not show how much self-knowledge, or of what kind, is a necessary condition of objective maturity. At most, the correlation between existing mental-health criteria and observable maturity provides some evidence that these criteria would remain in a theory free of the methodological deficiencies discussed in section II.

Thus I continue to maintain that the methods used by most theorists of 'mental health' are essentially indefensible. Psychiatrists and psychologists who employ the notion of health must swallow what for some will be a bitter pill. Apart from a theory of the structure and functions of the human mind, virtually all assertions about mental health are either misuses of language or flatly conjectural. It is true that many of the disorders traditionally recognized in clinical theory, e.g. psychoses and serious neuroses, seem likely to be mental diseases in the literal sense. What this means is simply that past confusion about the health concept may not have led clinicians too wide of the mark in practice. But the time has now arrived when the clinical disciplines face a parting of the ways. With Szasz and the behaviourists, they may decide that mental health is not what they are interested in after all and adopt something else, e.g. happiness or social adjustment, as their official aim. Alternatively, they may retain the concepts of health and disease and pursue substantive theories of mental functioning of the psychoanalytic variety.[19] I have tried in this essay to clarify the choice, and to argue that the second option deserves serious inquiry.

Notes

Support from the Delaware Institute for Medical Education and Research and the National Institute of Mental Health (grant RO$_3$ MH 24621) is gratefully acknowledged.

1   Critics of the 'medical model' have some very different interpretations of it (Macklin, 1973). It may or may not be thought to include any of the following assumptions: that individual therapy is the best mode of treatment; that all treatment should be done by physicians; that drugs are better than psychotherapy; that there are classical disease entities in psychology; and that all mental diseases are physical diseases. Interestingly, none of these five theses entails any of the others. In this essay I defend only the basic view that the idea of mental health is coherent and clinically useful.

Apropos of the second of the five listed theses, I should also say that I have longed in vain for a brief term covering all mental-health professionals at once: psychiatrists, clinical psychologists, social workers, counsellors, etc. Specific terms like 'psychiatric' in the text are usually a stylistic convenience with no disciplinary implications.

2   This summary includes the main features of the analysis in my forthcoming essay 'Health as a theoretical concept.' It omits a number of details that also have repercussions for mental health. Further defence of a functional analysis of health in physiology, as well as of the thesis that physiological medicine should be viewed as the paradigm health discipline, can be found in Flew (1973).

3   For the second question, cf. Boorse (1975). The distinction between disease and illness there argued for is one feature that separates my position from that of Flew (1973). I take the term 'disease' to be a technical term belonging to medical theory, and I use it in the textbook sense to cover any and all unhealthy conditions. This broad usage should be kept in mind below in the discussion of mental diseases. In my view 'illness' belongs instead with the institutions of medical practice; hence the analysis just given aims to capture a sort of professionalized ordinary usage.

4   See, for example, Freud (1915), p. 175: 'Our psychical topography has *for the present* nothing to do with anatomy; it has reference not to anatomical localities, but to regions in the mental apparatus, wherever they may be situated in the body' (italics original). Holt (1965) has an illuminating critical discussion of Freud's physiological presuppositions.

5   Putnam (1960) defends the view that mental states are functional states. Davidson (1966) argues for an ontology of event-particulars and applies it to mental events (1970). A connected account of functionalism can also be found in Fodor (1968, ch.3). The term 'functionalism' itself is perhaps uniquely unfortunate for present purposes. It is the mathematical sense of 'function' that seems suggested by Putnam's original discussion; but Fodor's automotive examples allow an alternative interpretation in terms of contributions to goals. Without pursuing this conceptual tangle any further, let me simply state that my claim that mental states have biological functions is entirely independent of the functionalist solution to the mind-body problem.

6   For convenience I ignore the distinction in Smart (1959) between a desire and the having of a desire.

7   Usage of 'mental illness' does not invariably conform to this description. But if physical diseases can have mental symptoms, it is hard to imagine any other basis for distinguishing mental from physical health besides the contrast between mental and physical aetiology. On any account the specialty of psychiatry, as defined by its textbooks, includes some physical diseases, e.g. brain syndromes due to infections, tumours, or alcohol poisoning. It is also worth noting that the scope of 'mental disease' may vary according to one's conception of the mark of the mental.

8   Some endorsements of this view by clinicians and by philosophers are quoted and discussed in Boorse (1975).

9   Concerning the prevalence of the normative route to mental-health criteria, Wootton writes: 'It must, however, be admitted that most of the current definitions of mental health . . . with their visions of 'inner harmonious adjustment,' of 'trustfulness' and of 'socially considerate behavior' – not to mention happy family life, successful sex adjustment, training for citizenship, economic independence and freedom from industrial unrest – most of them are clearly attempts to formulate conceptions of the ideal, under the guise of the healthy, man. They express the personal value-judgments of their authors, rather than scientifically established facts . . .' (1959, 216).

10   Howard and Patry, quoted by Wootton (1959), p. 214.

11   This is a summary by Mowrer (1948) of Alfred Adler's (1939) position. It seems fairly accurate, except for being more specific than any of Adler's own formulations. It is possible that Adler's views should be represented as derived by the second method discussed below, the abstraction route, rather than by pure evaluation.

12   This point is eloquently argued by Szasz (1961); see also Schofield (1964, pp. 22–3).

13   Wootton (1959), p. 218. London (1969) also has a perceptive discussion of the adjustment ideal.

14   Cf. Alexander (1953): 'The function of the ego consists in finding ways and means for the gratification of the subjective needs by adequate behavior.'

15   Hallowell (1965), an evolutionary biologist, gives an interesting treatment of ego and superego functions in the cultural context. It has become commonplace to draw a sharp distinction between biology and culture on the grounds that culture is not genetically inherited. This difference should not obscure the fact that cultural environments play a role in natural selection. Because of this effect, the psychological endowments that allow individuals to succeed within cultures are a biological phenomenon.

16   Hartmann (1964), p. 7. Further discussion of the healthiness of unconscious conflict occurs in the responses to Redlich and Hartmann by Kubie (1954).

17   In connection with these issues, cf. Eidelberg (1968, p. 273): 'From a practical point of view, most analysts agree that an individual who is able to love, to be loved, and to work may be considered normal. While it is true that the presence of repressed infantile wishes interferes with mental health, the decisive factor in determining whether an individual is normal and healthy is the quantitative evaluation of the blocked, repressed mental energy.' What I suggest is that something like this out to be true of theoretical as well as practical health on the psychoanalytic model. Some discussion of more demanding accounts of health than the functional view I defend is contained in my 'Health as a theoretical concept' (forthcoming).

18   Margolis (1966, pp 75 ff); see also Macklin (1972, p. 354).

19   Family therapists often adopt a position that seems to fall between these two options. This position retains the concepts of health and disorder but applies them to the family instead of to the individual. Families are called healthy or disturbed in a sense held not to be reducible to the biological health of their members. It is interesting that from the biological standpoint for which I have argued, there is no difficulty in viewing a family as a functionally organized unit in its own right. The idea is as old as Darwin. But apart from all objections to such a significant alteration in the health concept as application to a group entails, it seems unlikely that family therapists would find the biological approach congenial. It would appear that their use of the family as a unit reflects simply a conviction about therapeutic strategy, together with some distaste for traditional depth psychology. Source material on family therapy may be found in Sager & Kaplan (1972).

References

Adler, A. (1939). *Social Interest: A Challenge to Mankind*. Trans. Linton and Vaughan. New York: G. P. Putnam's Sons.

Alexander, F. (1953). 'The therapeutic applications of psychoanalysis.' In Roy Grinker, ed., *Mid-Century Psychiatry* (Springfield, Ill.: Charles C. Thomas, 1953).

Boorse, C. 'Health as a theoretical concept.' Forthcoming.

Boorse, C. (1975). 'On the distinction between disease and illness.' *Philosophy and Public Affairs*, Fall 1975.

Davidson, D. (1963). 'Actions, reasons, and causes.' *The Journal of Philosophy* **60**, 685–700.

Davidson, D. (1966). 'The logical form of action sentences.' In Nicholas Rescher, ed., *The Logic of Decision and Action* (Pittsburgh: University of Pittsburgh Press).

Davidson, D. (1970). 'Mental events.' In Lawrence Foster and J. W. Swanson, eds., *Experience and Theory* (Amherst: University of Massachusetts Press), pp. 79–101.

Eidelberg, L., ed. (1968). *Encyclopedia of Psychoanalysis*. New York: The Free Press.

Flew, A. (1973). *Crime or Disease?* New York: Barnes and Noble.

Fodor, J. A. (1968). *Psychological Explanation*. New York: Random House.

Freud, S. (1915). 'The Unconscious.' In James Strachey, ed., *The Standard Edition of the Complete Psychological Works of Sigmund Freud*. (London: The Hogarth Press, 1961), vol. **14**, pp. 166–215.

Freud, S. (1927). *The Future of an Illusion*. In Strachey, vol. **21**, pp. 5–56.

Freud, S. (1936). *Analysis Terminable and Interminable*. In Strachey, vol. **23**, pp. 216–53.

Hallowell, A. I. (1965). 'Hominid evolution and culture.' In de Reuck and Porter, eds., *Transcultural Psychiatry* (Boston: Little, Brown, 1965).

Hartmann, H. (1939). 'Psychoanalysis and the concept of health.' In *Essays on Ego Psychology* (New York: International Universities Press, 1964), pp. 1–18.

Hempel, C. G. (1965). *Aspects of Scientific Explanation and Other Essays in the Philosophy of Science*. New York: The Free Press.

Holt, R. R. (1965). 'A review of some of Freud's biological assumptions and their influence on his theories.' In Norman S. Greenfield and William C. Lewis, eds., *Psychoanalysis and Current Biological Thought* (Madison, Wisc.: University of Wisconsin Press, 1965), pp. 93–124.

Jahoda, M. (1958). *Current Concepts of Positive Mental Health*. New York: Basic Books.

Jones, E. (1932). 'The concept of a normal mind.' In Samuel D. Schmalhausen, ed., *Our Neurotic Age* (New York: Farrar and Rinehart, 1932), pp. 65–81.

Kubie, L. (1954). 'The fundamental nature of the distinction between normality and neurosis.' *Psychoanalytic Quarterly* **23**, 167–204, including discussion by Redlich and Hartmann.

London, P. (1969). 'Morals and mental health.' In Stanley C. Plog and Robert B. Edgerton, eds. *Changing Perspectives in Mental Illness* (New York: Holt, Rinehart and Winston, 1969), pp. 32–48.

Macklin, R. (1972). 'Mental health and mental illness: some problems of definition and concept formation.' *Philosophy of Science*, **39**, 341–65.

Macklin, R. (1973). 'The medical model in psychoanalysis and psychotherapy.' *Comprehensive Psychiatry* **14**, 49–69.

Margolis, J. (1966). *Psychotherapy and Morality*. New York: Random House.

Menninger, K. A. (1930). *The Human Mind*. New York: Knopf.

Montagu, M. F. A., ed. (1962). *Culture and the Evolution of Man*. New York: Oxford University Press.

Mowrer, O. H. (1948). 'What is normal behavior?' In L. A. Pennington and Irwin A. Berg, eds., *An Introduction to Clinical Psychology* (New York: Ronald, 1948). Omitted from later editions.

Putnam, H. (1960). 'Minds and machines.' In Sidney Hook, ed., *Dimensions of Mind* (New York: New York University Press, 1960), pp. 138–64.

Redlich, F. C. & Freedman, D. X. (1966). *The Theory and Practice of Psychiatry*. New York: Basic Books.

Roe, A. & Simpson, G. G., eds. (1958). *Behavior and Evolution*. New Haven: Yale University Press.

Sager, C. J. & Kaplan, H. S. (1972). *Progress in Group and Family Therapy*. New York: Brunner-Mazel.

Sarbin, T. (1967). 'On the futility of the proposition that some people be labeled "mentally ill". ' *Journal of Consulting Psychology* **31**, 447–53.

Sarbin, T. (1969). 'The scientific status of the mental illness metaphor.' In Stanley C. Plog and Robert B. Edgerton, eds., *Changing Perspectives in Mental Illness* (New York: Holt, Rinehart and Winston, 1969), pp. 9–31.

Schofield, W. (1964). *Psychotherapy: The Purchase of Friendship*. Englewood Cliffs, N.J.: Prentice-Hall.

Smart, J. J. C. (1959). 'Sensations and brain processes.' *The Philosophical Review* **68**, 141–56.

Stoller, R. J., et al. (1973). 'A symposium: should homosexuality be in the APA nomenclature?' *American Journal of Psychiatry* **130**: 1270–16.

Szasz, T. S. (1961). *The Myth of Mental Illness*. New York: Hoeber-Harper.

Szasz, T. S. (1963). *Law, Liberty, and Psychiatry*. New York: Macmillan.

Szasz, T. S. (1970a). *Ideology and Insanity*. Garden City, N.Y.: Doubleday.

Szasz, T. S. (1970b). *The Manufacture of Madness*. New York: Harper and Row.

Ullmann, L. P. & Krasner, L. (1966). *Case Studies in Behavior Modification*, New York: Holt, Rinehart and Winston.

Wootton, B. (1959). *Social Science and Social Pathology*. London: George Allen and Unwin.

A Symposium: Should Homosexuality be in the APA Nomenclature?*

Robert J. Stoller, Judd Marmor, Irving Bieber, Ronald Gold, Charles W. Socarides, Richard Green and Robert L. Spitzer

Criteria for Psychiatric Diagnosis

Robert J. Stoller

Is homosexuality a diagnosis? A diagnosis is supposed to be a highly compact explanation. To make a proper diagnosis in any branch of medicine there should be: a syndrome – a constellation of signs and symptoms shared by a group of people, visible to an observer; underlying dynamics (pathogenesis) – pathophysiology in the rest of medicine, neuropathophysiology or psychodynamics in psychiatry; and etiology – those factors from which the dynamics originate. When these exist, one can save time by using shorthand, knowing that a word or two – a label, a diagnosis – communicates to others what we know. Unfortunately, the conditions for which our specialty was developed do not usually fulfill these three criteria.

If one uses the above criteria for considering a condition a diagnosis, homosexuality is not a diagnosis because: 1) there is only a sexual preference (noticeable because it frightens many in our society), not a constellation of signs and symptoms; 2) different people with this sexual preference have different psychodynamics underlying their sexual behavior; and 3) quite different life experiences can cause these dynamics and behavior. There *is* homosexual behavior; it is varied. There is no such *thing* as homosexuality. In that sense it should be removed from the nomenclature.

As regards pathogenesis, probably no one these days, not even among those favoring the diagnosis, believes in a unitary cause for homosexual behavior; that would make it a *thing*. The fine reviews of the literature on etiology by Bieber and associates and Socarides, plus their own findings,[1,2] reinforce the impression that many paths lead to one's preferring members of his own sex. This is true even, and especially, with analytic theories of etiology.

Part of a Natural Realm

However, there is something disreputable in using our feeble method of diagnosis and psychiatrists en masse as the whipping boys for the cruel manner in which homosexuals have been and still are treated. These diagnostic issues are not the real source of homosexuals' mistreatment (although they can be borrowed for such use). At our best, we – since Freud's lead – are partly responsible for the fact that homosexuals can begin fighting back against society. Even though we are inaccurate when we call homosexuality a diagnosis, doing so has signified that the homosexual is part of a natural realm and not a member of the species of damned sinners. If homosexuals hate psychiatrists who would oppress them, let them also concede their debts to those who wish them free. If these niceties are bad for strategy, then let homosexuals – and other minorities – continue to flail us; the cause is honorable although the technique may be crude.

In the search for the multiple causes of homosexual behavior, I believe data can be found demonstrating that for many homosexuals the preferences in object choice and some essential, habitual nonerotic behavior (e.g., the effeminacy of some male homosexuals) were developed as the result of trauma and frustration during identity development. Of course, these observations must be understood in the context that I believe they also hold true for most heterosexuals, although the traumas and frustrations are of different sorts and intensities.

Perhaps one can divide humans into two types, heterosexuals and others, as is the custom; if so, we might sort the two in the following idiosyncratic manner (rather as Freud did). I would consider the sexual styles of most humans, including most who prefer homosexual relations, as would-be heterosexual. (Analysts have also shown how heterosexuality may also contain homosexuality.) I believe that the sexual neuroses – the obvious perversions and even most variants of overt heterosexuality, e.g., compulsive promiscuity, use of pornography, preference for prostitutes, adult masturbation – are heterosexual distortions, compromises nonetheless filled with excitement, that allow one to give up certain desires if only others can be salvaged. If it will make the oppressed minorities more comfortable, we can all be given a diagnosis; such pronouncement would certainly not often distort the case. Everyone has his own style and distinctive fantasy content that he daydreams or stages with objects. Everyone is entitled to a category.

But why claim that heterosexuality is mankind's preference? The evidence for this as a biological given is certainly flimsy (although I would guess it is innate in some mild, reversible form). Yet I think that up to the present (not necessarily forever) heterosexuality has been the norm. It is the dominant presence in the ambiance of almost every human in infancy and childhood, because he is created in a family and families are palpably heterosexual (2, pp. 5–6). That sets the standard: heterosexuality is the product of the institution called the family. Then, too, even in childhood we know we are the result of an intimate, highly charged, astonishing, mysterious, unquestionably heterosexual act. So I see perversions (but not all sexual deviations and not all homosexual behaviors) as modifications one must invent in order to preserve some of one's heterosexuality. The form the perversion takes may be far from the extreme of a male preferring a female and vice versa, in which both wholeheartedly enjoy the sexual and loving aspects of their relationship. Yet, while unseen, that ideal may well be buried there in most of us, even if it is manifest in only a few.

A Holding Action

Until the day we know what we are doing, I suggest that – as a holding action – we try the following descriptive syndrome classification system:

A The personality (character) type, habitual since childhood, e.g., obsessive-compulsive, schizophrenic, hysteric, depressive.

 1. The presenting syndrome, e.g., drug dependence, anxiety neurosis, schizophreniform psychosis.

   a. Subsidiary syndromes also present, e.g., alcoholism; nonpsychotic organic brain syndrome with senile brain disease; psychophysiologic respiratory disorder (asthma). Sexual preference, e.g., heterosexual, monogamous, with accompanying fantasies of being raped by a stallion; homosexual, with foreskin fetishism; heterosexual, with preference for cadavers; homosexual, with disembodied penises (tearoom promiscuity); heterosexual, voyeurism; homosexual, expressed only in fantasies during intercourse with wife.

* Stoller, R., Marmor, J., Bieber, I., Gold, R. *et al.*: A symposium: should homosexuality be in the APA nomenclature. *American Journal of Psychiatry* **130**: 1207–1216, 1973.

Only when diagnoses fail to describe succinctly and accurately should they be removed. Since that is the case for homosexuality, it cannot function as a true diagnosis; remove it. And since that is true for most of the rest of the 'diagnoses' of psychiatry, let us scrap the system (although not yet all the labels) and start afresh.

Homosexuality and Cultural Value Systems

Judd Marmor

Proponents of the mental illness label for homosexuality base their arguments on three major themes: 1) that homosexuality is the consequence of 'disordered sexual development,' 2) that it is a deviation from the biological norm, and 3) that psychodynamic studies of homosexuals always reveal them to be deeply disturbed individuals.

The disordered sexual development theme is based on the finding that a certain type of disturbed parent-child relationship is a background factor in most cases. There seems to be an assumption in this theme that if there is a disturbed parent-child relationship in the background of someone with variant sexual behavior this proves that the disturbed relationship is causally responsible and that the individual with such variant behavior must be mentally ill.

There are a number of fallacies in this argument. First, we know that although most homosexuals show the 'typical' family constellation, by no means do all of them. Secondly, not all people who do have such family constellations in their background become homosexual. Third (and most importantly) to call homosexuality the result of disturbed sexual development really says nothing other than that you disapprove of the outcome of that development. *All* personality idiosyncrasies are the result of background developmental differences, and *all* have specific historical antecedents. The concept of illness cannot be extrapolated on the basis of background but must rest on its own merits.

Deviant Behavior not Necessarily Psychopathology

It is my conviction that we do not have the right to label behavior that is deviant from that currently favored by the majority as evidence per se of psychopathology. And, as a matter of fact, we do *not* do so except where we are reflecting our culture's bias toward a particular kind of deviance. In a democratic society we recognize the rights of individuals to hold widely divergent religious or ideational preferences, as long as their holders do not attempt to force their beliefs on others who do not share them. Our attitudes toward divergent sexual preferences, however, are quite different, obviously because moral values – couched in 'medical' and 'scientific' rationalizations – are involved.

There are some psychiatrists who would argue that individuals who adhere to unusual life-styles are indeed neurotic and that they suffer from various developmental fixations or arrests that account for their inability to adhere to the behavioral or ideational standards of the majority. Such labeling tends to define normality in terms of behavioral adjustment to cultural conventions rather than in terms of ego strengths and ego-adaptive capacities, and it puts psychiatry clearly in the role of an agent of cultural control rather than of a branch of the healing arts.

Moreover, the relativity of our contemporary sexual mores should not be ignored in any scientific approach to sexual behavior. In a cross-cultural study of 76 societies other than our own, Ford and Beach[3] found that in nearly two-thirds of them homosexual activities were considered normal and socially acceptable, at least for certain members of the community. Nor were all these societies necessarily 'primitive' ones. In ancient Greece – a society that we admire and feel indebted to culturally, philosophically, and scientifically – overt homosexual relations between older men and youths was not only considered acceptable but was an institutionalized practice cultivated by heterosexual, healthy, honorable, normal men.

Bisexuality – Our Mammalian Inheritance

The second major argument for the illness viewpoint is that homosexuality, in contrast to other forms of behavioral deviance, is biologically unnatural. Dr. Frank Beach, the eminent biologist, has summarized the evidence on this by pointing out that bisexual behavior has been observed in more than a dozen mammalian species and 'undoubtedly occurs in many others not yet studied.' He concluded: 'Human homosexuality reflects the essential bisexual character of our mammalian inheritance. The extreme modifiability of man's sex life makes possible the conversion of this essential bisexuality into a form of unisexuality with the result that a member of the same sex eventually becomes the only acceptable stimulus to arousal'.[4]

Thus, from an objective biological viewpoint there is nothing 'unnatural' about homosexual object choice. To illustrate how specious the argument is concerning the supposed biological unnaturalness of homosexuality let us consider some other conditions that are also outside of the presumably customary biological patterns. What about vegetarians? After all, most human beings are 'naturally' meat-eaters, but we don't automatically label vegetarians as mentally ill. Or what about celibacy? Do we automatically assume that all people who choose a life of sexual abstinence are mentally ill simply because they do not follow the 'natural' biological mating patterns? Obviously, we do not.

The third argument that is often advanced is that any careful study of the personality of homosexuals will show that they are really disturbed individuals. In contrast to Socarides, who holds the view that all homosexuals are practically borderline psychotics, Bieber concedes that many homosexuals can be well-adjusted individuals, but he argues that they still suffer from 'pathology.'

Happy, Constructive, and Realistic Homosexuals

What *does* constitute the intrinsic 'pathology' of a socially well-adjusted homosexual? I submit that in the view of Bieber, Socarides, and others who share their viewpoint, it is primarily that his sexual preference differs from that of the majority of society. I do not deny that there are homosexuals who, just like heterosexuals, suffer from a wide variety of personality disorders and serious mental illnesses, although much of the dis-ease that they suffer from is not intrinsic to their homosexuality but is a consequence of the prejudice and discrimination that they encounter in our society.

But I believe there is now an incontrovertible body of evidence that there are homosexual individuals who, except for their variant object choice, are happy with their lives and have made a constructive and realistic adaptation to being members of a minority group in our society. I consider the kind of evidence that Socarides marshals from his clinical practice as essentially meaningless in this regard. As I have often pointed out, if our judgment about the mental health of heterosexuals were based only on those whom we see in our clinical practices we would have to conclude that all heterosexuals are also mentally ill.

The final absurdity of this is the impossibility of trying to define at what point a person becomes a homosexual who is labeled as having a mental disorder. Some defendants of the illness theory try to justify it by saying that it applies only to obligatory homosexuality. Does this mean that only type 6 homosexuals are mentally ill and all the others are not? Or that types 4, 5, and 6 are ill but not 1, 2, and 3? The whole process of such labeling is unpleasantly reminiscent of the Hitlerian process of trying to determine what fraction of black or Jewish ancestry a person might be permitted to have and still be considered an acceptable member of society with full legal rights.

Surely the time has come for psychiatry to give up the archaic practice of classifying the millions of men and women who accept or prefer homosexual object choices as being, by virtue of that fact alone, mentally ill. The fact that their alternative life-style happens to be out of favor with current cultural conventions must not be a basis in itself for a diagnosis of psychopathology. It is our task as psychiatrists to be healers of the distressed, not watchdogs of our social mores.

Homosexuality – An Adaptive Consequence of Disorder in Psychosexual Development

Irving Bieber

Three Questions seem most relevant to the question of removing the term 'homosexuality' from the *Diagnostic and Statistical Manual of Mental Disorders* or changing the current designation:

1 Is homosexuality a normal variant of sexual development and sexual functioning? The long-term study that my colleagues and I reported in 1962[(1)], further investigations of colleagues, and the extensive clinical experience of myself and others since then leave no doubt that homosexuality is not merely a variation of normal adult sexuality. Observations on olfaction offer supporting evidence that humans born with normal gonads and genitals are biologically programmed for heterosexual development. From early life, olfaction plays a central role in sexual organization and functioning; it steers the infant toward heterosexual objects and works as an important triggering mechanism in sexual arousal.[5,6] Homosexuality does not occur without antecedent heterosexual development; it appears only *after* sexual responsivity to heterosexual objects has been established. Psychoanalytic evidence of heterosexual responses in homosexuals can almost always be demonstrated.

I have repeatedly emphasized that the dislocations in heterosexual organization of biologically normal children occur as a consequence of pathological family contexts – more specifically, pathologic relationships between parents and child. Typically, mothers of homosexuals are inappropriately close, binding, often seductive, and tend to inhibit boyish aggressiveness. The fathers are overtly or covertly hostile; this is expressed in detachment, streaks of cruelty, or frank brutality. The relationship between the parents is generally poor; often the husband is held in contempt by a wife who prefers her son. The prehomosexual child may be exposed to rejection and hostility from other significant males, such as brothers and peer mates. Defective masculine relationships deprive such a boy of needed masculine figures for identification and modeling that are ultimately sought, in part, in homosexuality. It then becomes a substitutive adaptation, replacing the heterosexuality that is made inadequate or unavailable by a network of induced fears about heterosexual behavior. Within a substitutive adaptation, attempts are made to acquire missing sexual and romantic gratification. Through various homosexual maneuvers and activities, reparative attempts are made to strengthen masculine self-esteem and to alleviate profound feelings of rejection from men. Through homosexuality, reassurance and acceptance are sought from other men. Contrary to popular notions, homosexuality is not an adaptation of choice; it is brought about by fears that inhibit satisfactory heterosexual functioning.

Inherent Psychological Pain

The gay activists and their proponents among some psychiatrists claim that many men are neurotic about their homosexuality only because society is prejudiced. Extinct cultures, such as the ancient Greek, are held up as prejudice-free examples, while cultures and present-day societies where there is no homosexuality are disregarded. The animal evidence has rested heavily on statements by Frank Beach. His position on animal homosexuality has changed, however, and in 1971 he wrote, 'I don't know any authenticated instances of males or females in the animal world preferring a homosexual partner, if by homosexuality you mean complete sexual relationships including climax. . . . It's questionable that mounting in itself can be properly called sexual'.[7]

Opponents of my views have accused me and other colleagues with similar ideas of being prejudiced, reactionary, and homophobic. The trouble with such ad hominem attacks is that they do not get to the heart of the matter but serve merely as diversionary methods to discredit without risking an objective engagement with the evidence. As I see it, society at large does not produce a homosexual condition nor can it mitigate the inherent psychological pain. If all discrimination against homosexuals ceased immediately, as indeed it should, I do not think their anxieties, conflicts, loneliness, and frequent depressions would be short-circuited.

2 If homosexuality is not normal, how should it be categorized? In the past century, psychiatry and the allied behavioral sciences have amassed an enormous body of data, although psychiatric diagnostic classification is the weakest part of this extraordinary development. Our present nosology is based on very different categories of criteria. The diagnoses of mania and depression are based on the salient symptom; of schizophrenia, on a constellation or cluster of signs and symptoms; of personality disorders, on psychodynamic formulations; and of sociopathy, on sociologic criteria. Classification of homosexuality has reflected this medley of psychiatric criteria. It is often referred to as 'sexual deviation.' Literally, deviation is a statistical term denoting movement away from a median or statistical norm. Deviation and pathology are not necessarily related; genius is as deviant as is mental deficiency. In my opinion, the term 'sexual deviation' is ambiguous, vague, and not useful as a diagnosis or as a nosologic category.

Homosexuality: Sexual Inadequacy

Masters and Johnson[8] used criteria that qualified as functional and dysfunctional to classify sexual disorders, and they introduced the term 'sexual inadequacy.' Under this rubric, they included frigidity and sexual impotence. The psychodynamic common denominator of frigidity, impotence, premature ejaculation, and homosexuality consists of a network of fears about being, effective in heterosexual activity. I suggest that homosexuality be characterized as a type of sexual inadequacy since most homosexuals (especially those who are exclusively homosexual) cannot function heterosexually.

I think, too, that adaptational concepts are very useful in formulating broader diagnostic contexts. Homosexuality could be classified as an adaptation to inhibited, dislocated heterosexual functioning; this would leave room for an expanded description of the patient's heterosexual difficulties.

3 Does the inclusion of homosexuality in the diagnostic manual make homosexuals 'sick,' as they claim? Discrimination against homosexuals existed long before modern psychiatric and diagnostic manuals. Psychiatry, particularly psychoanalysis, has contributed significantly toward altering archaic, moralistic, and pseudoscientific concepts. Freud[9] was the first to discard the notion that homosexuality was a degenerative disease. He classified it as a disorder of psychosexual development rather than as sinful and antisocial.

There is no reason to believe that if homosexuality were removed from the diagnostic manual there would be a significant alteration in existing social attitudes. Even if it could be shown that improved social attitudes would eventuate, this would not be reason enough to exclude the term if we agree that homosexuality is not normal and is a treatable condition.

Removal of the term from the manual would be tantamount to an official declaration by APA that homosexuality is normal. Undoubtedly it would be interpreted that way. More importantly, dropping the term would be a serious scientific error. Such an action would also interfere with effective prophylaxis. Prehomosexual boys are easily identifiable and should be treated. Further, young men in conflict about their sexual direction may be discouraged from seeking treatment by those who would reassure them that their homosexual proclivities are normal and that it is only 'society,' with its outmoded value system, that makes them reject a homosexual preference.

Stop It, You're Making Me Sick!

Ronald Gold

I have come to an unshakable conclusion: the illness theory of homosexuality is a pack of lies, concocted out of the myths of a patriarchal society for a political purpose. Psychiatry – dedicated to making sick people well – has been the cornerstone of a system of oppression that makes gay people sick.

To be viewed as psychologically disturbed in our society is to be thought of and treated as a second-class citizen; being a second-class citizen is not good for mental health. But that isn't the worst thing about a psychiatric diagnosis. The worst thing is that gay people believe it.

Nothing is more likely to create neurotic anxiety than 'a lack of feeling of wholeness,' and nothing is more likely to alienate you from a major aspect of yourself than to be told incessantly that it's sick.

At 14 years of age I discovered what the 'experts' said about the way I love: 'infantile sex,' 'inevitable emotional bankruptcy,' 'a masquerade of life filled with destruction and self-deceit.' So I went to my older sister and she sent me to a psychiatrist. He shot me full of sodium pentothal and scared me out of my wits. It is amazing how I could have kept on believing this nonsense about homosexuality when so little of it had anything to do with my life. But I went willingly to other psychiatrists and learned from them that a part of me didn't want to give up needed to be excised. I was ready for 'psychic annihilation'; I became a heroin addict. This time I was sent to the Menninger Clinic, and there I was convinced that my 'cure' must include a change in sexual orientation. So when it was agreed that I was through with treatment, it seemed to me I'd done only half a job. But I soon found that all I needed for another person to love me was to like myself better. I met a young man, and we had a good, happy life for 12 years. When we broke up, our conflicts weren't out of the psychiatric literature. They were just like the tales of heterosexual divorce you read about in *Redbook*.

The man I live with now is a warm, loving, open person. For the past two years we've been going through the joyful process of discovering the full repertory of mutuality – easier for two members of the same sex.

Psychological Growth Through Resisting Oppression

There are advantages to being gay. I learned that in the gay movement. And I learned something else: that I was oppressed and must make the choice to do everything I can to cease being an accomplice in my own oppression. I've had an immense sense of psychological growth through this decision. I've fought through to a sense of myself as a whole person – a good, concerned, loving, fighting-mad homosexual. I'm fighting the psychiatric profession now, but I know that a false adversary situation has been drawn between psychiatry and Gay Liberation. We can save you the trouble of treating some people, and we can be a helpful adjunct for many of your patients by pointing them along the road to self-esteem.

After our meeting with your Committee on Nomenclature and Statistics, its chairman said that 'whether a person prefers to have sexual relations with a member of the same or of the opposite sex is in itself not an indicator of mental disorder.' But, he added, 'What are we to do about the homosexual who comes to us and says he's miserable, that he wants to change?' Such people do need help. But is it their homosexuality that's doing them in? Or is it something that psychiatry has helped to create: irrational fear and hatred of homosexuality? Instead of acceding to requests for brainwashing, what you can help these people realize is that there are many successful, well-adjusted people in various professions (including psychiatry) who are homosexual. You can help them to see that successful sexual adjustment of any kind cannot be achieved in a climate of guilt and fear.

When these patients see themselves as people, not sets of stereotypical patterns, I suspect that most of them (about as many as you get with your current techniques) will go on being gay. Only they'll be happy about it. Perhaps the same percentage you have now will wind up predominantly heterosexual. And many of those who had been exclusively homosexual – many more than you now count as treatment 'successes' – will discover a heterosexual component in themselves. We have found that such things happen frequently in the Gay Liberation movement.

I feel better since I've joined Gay Liberation. I work better, I'm happier in love. Would you rather have me the way I am? Or would you suggest another round of therapy? I think you really know that I'm not sick now, that my homosexuality is simply a part of me that in the past I wasn't allowed to accept. And I think you're prepared to agree that my previous

illness was at least in part a direct result of the crimes perpetrated on me by a hostile society. You have been willing accomplices in such crimes. It is now time for you to prevent them. Take the damning label of sickness away from us. Take us out of your nomenclature. Work for repeal of sodomy laws, for civil-rights protections for gay people.

Most important of all, speak out. You've allowed a handful of homophobes to tell the public what you think. It's up to you now to get on the talk shows and write for the weeklies, as they do. You've got to tell the world what you believe – that Gay is Good.

Homosexuality: Findings Derived from 15 Years of Clinical Research

Charles W. Socarides

I've got to get this homosexual monkey off my back. I just frankly can't live with it. I must either extinguish it, if I can, or maybe by religion extinguish all sex. And the other thing is to be dead. To have anonymous sex with other sick men, I can't make a life out of that. The homosexuals I know think I'm copping out, and if it's not hereditary they feel at least that it's impossible to change. They say to me, 'Once homosexuality is established you can't get out or if you do try to get out you'll go nuts.' They tell you that you will be isolated and they keep telling you you're a traitor trying to leave the group, turning against your own kind, that you're trying to do something and be something that you're not. They say you're self-indulgent and selfish, feeding your ego in a very selfish kind of way in that you're enjoying your neurosis in trying to get well.

That quotation from a patient is why some of us treat homosexuals: because people come to us voluntarily and seek our help. They are in agony over their condition.

The Task Force on Homosexuality appointed by the New York County District Branch of the American Psychiatric Association, of which I was the chairman, unanimously agreed in April 1972 that homosexuality arises experientially from a faulty family constellation. (Some few homosexuals come from an institutional background, but in our opinion they present special problems.) It was our finding that homosexuality represents a disorder of sexual development and does not fall within the range of normal sexual behavior. Further, between one-third and one-half of male homosexuals who seek treatment, including those who had formerly been exclusively homosexual, become exclusively heterosexual as a result of psychoanalytically oriented psychotherapy.

The most extensive comparison study oriented to establishing the etiology of male homosexuality was published in 1962.[1] It is a report on 106 male homosexuals and 100 male heterosexuals, distributed in psychoanalytic treatment with 77 members of the Society of Medical Psychoanalysts.

This study established a continuity and severity of pathological parent-child relationships in the background of all the homosexuals studied to an extent not found in the comparison group. The frequency of a parental combination consisting of a close-binding, overintimate mother and a hostile, detached father statistically differentiated the homosexuals from the heterosexual group at the .01 level of confidence.

The majority of mothers of homosexuals interfered with the development of their sons' peer group relationships, heterosexual development, assertiveness, and decision making; the fathers were demasculinizing. One conclusion of this study was that the son who becomes homosexual is the focal point of this intrafamilial pathology.

Preoedipal Theory of Causation

In 1968,[2] after 15 years of clinical research, I introduced the concept that in all homosexuals there has been an inability to make the progression from the mother-child unity of earliest infancy to individuation. This was called the preoedipal theory of causation. This failure in sexual identity, normally achieved by the age of three, is due to a pathological family constellation in which there is a domineering, psychologically crushing mother who will not allow the child to attain autonomy from her and an absent, weak, or rejecting father who is unable to aid the son to overcome the block in maturation. As a result there exists in (obligatory) homosexuals a partial fixation with the concomitant tendency to regression to the earliest mother-child relationship.

It is my conviction that it is necessary for all human beings to complete the separation-individuation of early childhood[10] in order to establish gender identity. Failure to do so results in a deficit in masculinity for boys, with a corresponding intensification and continuation of the primary feminine identification with the mother; thus begins the course toward homosexual development. It may well be clear now why homosexuality is prevalent, has existed since the beginning of recorded history, and spans all sociocultural levels.

While there was total agreement among members of the task force that the parents, consciously or otherwise, are the primary architects of the homosexual psychic organization, some placed major emphasis on the mother's influence in the preoedipal period, while others stressed the inordinate fears of male aggression coupled with a yearning for male acceptance and affection stemming from the deleterious parental attitudes and behavior. Those who subscribe to preoedipal origin emphasize primitive fears of injury by women.

A sound scientific basis for deciding whether the homosexual suffers from a psychosexual disorder has been handicapped by reports of psychological testing that were offered as proof that there are no discernible differences between homosexuals and heterosexuals insofar as such protocols are concerned.[11,12] Having reviewed these data in detail, we strongly recommend that these tests, dating back to 1957 and 1958, be repeated by other investigators with a much more rigorous methodology than was originally used.

Not a 'Sexual Dysfunction'

Scientific knowledge is also damaged when attempts are made to classify homosexuality simply as 'sexual dysfunction,' a term regularly applied to loss of erection, premature ejaculation, retarded ejaculation, or total impotence. These impairments constitute disturbances of the standard male-female pattern. It is characteristic of the standard or normal sex experience that it take place between male and a female. It is also characteristic that orgasm produced by intravaginal penetration is fully within the capability of the male partner, and that this coital activity has the potentiality for reproduction. These criteria are basic to elementary human biology and are not subject to change by social or political movements. Individuals unable to achieve sexual release within this standard pattern, with all its possible variations of foreplay, etc. (of which there are an infinite number), turn to modified patterns for orgastic relief, and these constitute sexual deviations. Thus the immutable distinctions between sexual deviations and sexual dysfunctions cannot be semantically blurred without incurring formidable scientific chaos.

As to the contention that in homosexuality there are no clinical symptoms, no course of development, and no treatment, we strongly disagree. There are symptoms and there is a course and there is a treatment – often a very effective treatment. The limitations of space do not allow me to comment on these here beyond observing that in addition to the uncovering techniques of depth therapy, treatment requires educational and retraining measures, interventions, and modifications in the handling of transference, resistance, and regression.

Let us bear in mind that psychiatrists have been in the forefront in helping homosexuals. It was Freud who opened the gates of freedom and humanity to the homosexual. And it was others after him – investigators who dared, who were not afraid of homosexuals, who had no 'homophobia' of which we are accused – who could therefore treat homosexuals who want to be treated. I urge that all persecutory laws against the homosexual be abolished at once. It is unthinkable that homosexuals be persecuted for something over which they have no choice. Such laws are a direct contradiction to psychiatric as well as humane values.

Should Heterosexuality Be in the APA Nomenclature?

Richard Green

Four major criteria are typically called upon to classify behavior as emotionally disordered. First is gross social dysfunction. Here an individual's behavior is such that to any but the most cynical of observers there is objective evidence that the individual is dysfunctional. The mental functioning of the regressed schizophrenic, the manic, the profoundly depressed, the severely retarded, and the patient with chronic brain syndrome precludes effective social survival.

Second, there exist the less socially obvious emotional limitations. Here inner discord that reduces the efficiency of behavioral functioning is experienced by the individual. Examples include severe anxiety and phobias of various types. Classification of the latter, however, becomes problematic when one considers the relative social consequences of snake phobia, germ phobia, and agoraphobia.

The third criterion of diagnosis is somewhat softer science. This focuses on culturally variant behavior. Using statistical deviance per se as a diagnostic basis evokes problems. Geniuses are deviant. So are the left-handed, vegetarians, pacifists, the celibate, and the esoterically religious. The relationship of idiosyncratic and delusional thinking to cultural accommodation comes into focus when one considers the different view of a religion adhered to by one person, a thousand, or a million. Then too there is the sociopath. His behavior is also deviant and, further, may result in undesirable effects on society. This person may feel no anxiety and not appear grossly dysfunctional. However, his behavior is at odds with external societal values and is labeled as an emotional disorder.

Next, there is a criterion that is scientifically the softest yet. Behavior is judged to be sick or healthy, ordered or disordered, based on a theoretical model of human psychological development. A theory may define specific behavioral phenomena as evidence of disorder. In this regard, classic psychoanalytic theory deems homosexual object choice as psychological immaturity, an arrest of psychosexual development. Castration fear and penis envy are universally posited developmental facts, and resolution of the oedipal crisis is the developmental rite of passage to mature sexuality. The scientific merits of psychoanalytic theory have been debated at length.[13]

Heterosexuality as a Disorder

The title of this paper asks the question whether heterosexuality should be in the APA nomenclature. There are in fact some places where heterosexuality and its derivatives are cited. These include pedophilia (presumably this includes children of the opposite sex), exhibitionism (typically the object is a person of the opposite sex), voyeurism (same as the preceding), sadism and masochism (if it is with a partner of the opposite sex), and transvestism (most transvestites are heterosexual).

One additional diagnostic term in our current nomenclature can refer to heterosexuality. This term is under the heading of psychophysiologic genitourinary disorder. Here psychogenic dyspareunia and impotence can be cited, and presumably also nonorgasmia in the female and premature ejaculation in the male.

Are there other places where heterosexual behavior might be considered worthy of diagnosis and classification? Styles of heterosexual conduct do indeed form much of what is dealt with by psychiatrists. Instability in maintaining a love relationship and neurotic uses of sexuality – in which sexuality is used to control others, as a substitute for other feelings of self-worth, or as a defense against anxiety and depression – constitute a significant bulk of the disorders treated in outpatient psychiatry. Yet there is no specific mention of such ego-dystonic, neurotic uses of heterosexuality in the nomenclature. By contrast, the homosexual is considered to be manifesting a disorder, whether or not he or she is able to maintain a stable interpersonal relationship, feels comfortable about his or her sexuality, and does not utilize it in a self-destructive manner.

Homosexuality as a Disorder

Where in the above gross criteria of mental disorder, other than as a derivative of a theoretical model of personality development, do we place homosexual behavior when it is engaged in by two consenting adults in private? In terms of gross psychologic social functioning the homosexual typically appears no different from his heterosexual counterpart. He or she may hold a responsible occupational and social position. Psychiatrists, other physicians, lawyers, ministers, politicians, authors, etc., may be homosexual. Clearly there is no gross impairment of the kind seen in acute schizophrenia, mania, or organic brain syndromes. With respect to intrapsychic adjustment, the studies that have used comparable samples of nonpatient heterosexual and homosexual subjects typically find no significant differences between the groups on such factors as anxiety and depression.[14] With respect to civil issues, homosexual conduct between consenting adults is not illegal in most western European countries, Canada, and some of the United States.

A Proposed New Classification

Can we attain a compatible coalition between those who consider homosexuality a profound mental disorder and those who view it as an alternate life-style beyond the legitimate purview of the medical profession?

The past few years have witnessed an explosion in the research and treatment of various aspects of sexual behavior. Due to the work of Masters and Johnson, considerable professional attention is now being paid to the problems of sexual dysfunction, particularly impotence and premature ejaculation in the male and nonorgasmia in the female. Sexual dysfunction is externally maladaptive and is accompanied by anxiety, depression, and other inner distress.

The more traditional model of emotional disorder considers sexual relationships as dynamic interpersonal phenomena within the scope of ego functioning. Again, compatibility between the phenomena of the homosexually oriented and the heterosexually oriented can be attained. The classification I am proposing here would include the heterosexual or the homosexual who finds it difficult to maintain desired object relationships, who compulsively uses sexuality to ward off anxiety or depression, or whose sexuality typically leads to depression or anxiety. Within this same general category would also be classed those persons who request reorientation or modification of sexual object preference.

The following classification is proposed:

Sexual dysfunction I. This term is applied when physiological dysfunction of psychogenic origin is the primary presenting symptom.

A) Male impotence: 1) with same-sexed partner, 2) with other-sexed partner; B) male premature ejaculation: 1) with partner of same sex, 2) with partner of opposite sex; C) female nonorgasmia: 1) with partner of same sex, 2) with partner of opposite sex.

Sexual dysfunction II. This term is applied when psychogenic distress is the primary presenting symptom. Physiologic dysfunction may or may not be an accompanying factor.

A) Anxiety, depression, and other neurotic reactions secondary to interpersonal aspects of sexuality, not primarily related to physiologic dysfunction: 1) with partner of same sex, 2) with partner of opposite sex; B) dissatisfaction with sexual orientation: 1) dissatisfaction with exclusive or primary homosexual orientation, 2) dissatisfaction with exclusive or primary heterosexual orientation.

The nomenclature would retain exhibitionism, voyeurism, sadism, masochism, pedophilia (and *add* rapism) when such behavior is of a repetitive nature.

With this new classification, psychiatry would have an objective basis for categorizing sexuality that is free of cultural bias, not based on partially accepted theoretic models, not based on the judgment of an external professional agent, but, rather, is patient-activated. Further, it would not stigmatize the individual and would not reinforce legal, religious, and other forms of social discrimination that are a product of the current classification.

A Proposal About Homosexuality and the APA Nomenclature: Homosexuality as an Irregular Form of Sexual Behavior and Sexual Orientation Disturbance as a Psychiatric Disorder

Robert L. Spitzer

Controversy rages as to whether homosexuality should be regarded as a pathological deviation of normal sexual development or as a normal variant of the human potential for sexual response. Recently this controversy has focused on the American Psychiatric Association's *Diagnostic and Statistical Manual of Mental Disorders*, second edition *(DSM-II)*, in which homosexuality is listed as an official diagnosis in the section on sexual deviations.

The proponents of the view that homosexuality is a normal variant of human sexuality argue for the elimination of any reference to homosexuality in a manual of psychiatric disorders because it is scientifically incorrect, encourages an adversary relationship between psychiatry and the homosexual community, and is misused by some people outside of our profession who wish to deny civil rights to homosexuals. Those who argue that homosexuality is a pathological disturbance in sexual development assert that to remove homosexuality from the nomenclature would be to give official sanction to this form of deviant sexual development, would be a cowardly act of succumbing to the pressure of a small but vocal band of activist homosexuals who defensively attempt to prove that they are not sick, and would tend to discourage homosexuals from seeking much-needed treatment.

When all of the arguments are carefully examined, a few simple statements can be made with which hardly any major psychiatric opinion would disagree.

1 'Homosexuality' refers to an interest in sexual relations or contact with members of the same sex. Some experts in our field believe that predominant or exclusive homosexuality is pathological; other experts believe it is a normal variant.

2 A significant proportion of homosexuals are apparently satisfied with their sexual orientation, show no significant signs of manifest psychopathology (other than their homosexuality, if this is considered by itself psychopathology), and are able to function quite effectively. These individuals may never come for treatment, or they may be seen by a psychiatrist because of external pressure (e.g., court referral, family insistence) or because of other problems requiring psychiatric help (e.g., depression, alcoholism).

3 A significant proportion of homosexuals are quite bothered by, in conflict with, or wish to change their sexual orientation. There is debate within our profession as to why this is so. Some argue that it is an inevitable result of the underlying conflicts that cause homosexual behavior in the first place, while others argue that it is derived from a host of social and cultural pressures that have been internalized. Nonetheless, some of these individuals come voluntarily for treatment, either to be able to accept their sexual feelings toward members of the same sex or to increase their capacity for sexual arousal by members of the opposite sex.

4 Modern methods of treatment enable a significant proportion of homosexuals who wish to change their sexual orientation to do so. The exact percentage is controversial and not at all clear. At the same time, homosexuals who are bothered by or in conflict with their sexual feelings but who are either uninterested in changing or unable to change their sexual orientation can be helped to accept themselves as they are and to rid themselves of self-hatred.

What Is a Manual of Mental Disorders?

Decisions about the labeling problem in *DSM-II* require an understanding of the function of a manual of mental disorders. Its purpose, as its name clearly implies, is to list and define mental (psychiatric) disorders. Its purpose is not to list and describe all of the forms of human psychological functioning that are judged by the profession or some members of the profession as less than optimal, nor is its purpose to imply certainty about the nature of conditions when there is not a consensus in the profession.

For a mental or psychiatric condition to be considered a psychiatric disorder, it must either regularly cause subjective distress or regularly be associated with some generalized impairment in social effectiveness or functioning. With the exception of homosexuality (and perhaps some of the other sexual deviations when they occur in a mild form, such as voyeurism), all of the mental disorders in *DSM-II* fulfill either of these two criteria. (While one may argue that the personality disorders are an exception, on reflection it is clear that it is inappropriate to make a diagnosis of a personality *disorder* merely because of the presence of certain typical personality traits that cause no subjective distress or impairment in social functioning.) Clearly homosexuality per se does not meet the requirements for a psychiatric disorder since, as noted above, many homosexuals are quite satisfied with their sexual orientation and demonstrate no generalized impairment in social effectiveness or functioning.

The only way that homosexuality could therefore be considered a psychiatric disorder would be the criterion of failure to function heterosexually, which is considered optimal in our society and by many members of our profession. However, if failure to function optimally in some important area of life, as judged by either society or the profession, is sufficient to indicate the presence of a psychiatric disorder, then we will have to add to our nomenclature the following conditions: celibacy (failure to function optimally sexually), revolutionary behavior (irrational defiance of social norms), religious fanaticism (dogmatic and rigid adherence to religious doctrine), racism (irrational hatred of certain groups), vegetarianism (unnatural avoidance of carnivorous behavior), and male chauvinism (irrational belief in the inferiority of women).

If homosexuality per se does not meet the criteria for a psychiatric disorder, what is it? Descriptively, it is an irregular form of sexual behavior. Our profession need not now agree on its origin, significance, and value for human happiness when we acknowledge that by itself it does not meet the requirements for a psychiatric disorder.

Sexual Orientation Disturbance

Having suggested that homosexuality per se is not a psychiatric disorder, what about those homosexuals who are troubled by or dissatisfied with their homosexual feelings or behavior? These people have a psychiatric condition by the criterion of subjective distress, whether or not they seek professional help. It is proposed that this condition be given a new diagnostic category, which will replace the current undefined category of homosexuality in subsequent printings of *DSM* defined as follows: 'Sexual orientation disturbance. This is for people whose sexual interests are directed primarily toward people of the same sex and who are bothered by, in conflict with, or wish to change their sexual orientation. This diagnostic category is distinguished from homosexuality, which by itself does not constitute a psychiatric disorder. Homosexuality per se is a form of irregular sexual behavior and, with other forms of irregular sexual behavior that are not by themselves psychiatric disorders, are not listed in this nomenclature.'

What will be the effect of carrying out such a proposal? Homosexual activist groups will no doubt claim that psychiatry has at last recognized that homosexuality is as 'normal' as heterosexuality. They will be wrong. In removing homosexuality per se from the nomenclature we are only recognizing that by itself homosexuality does not meet the criteria for being considered a psychiatric disorder. We will in no way be aligning ourselves with any particular viewpoint regarding the etiology or desirability of homosexual behavior.

By creating a new category, 'sexual orientation disturbance,' we will be applying a label only to those homosexuals who are in some way bothered by their sexual orientation, some of whom may come to us for help. We will no longer insist on a label of sickness for individuals who insist that they are well and who demonstrate no generalized impairment in social effectiveness. We will thus help to answer the charge of some members of our own profession who claim that mental illness is a myth and that by labeling individuals with psychiatric diagnoses we are merely acting as agents of social control. Furthermore, we will be removing one of the justifications for the denial of civil rights to individuals whose only crime is that their sexual orientation is to members of the same sex. In the past, homosexuals have been denied civil, rights in many areas of life on the ground that because they suffer from a 'mental illness' the burden of proof is on them to demonstrate their competence, reliability, or mental stability. (By linking the removal of homosexuality from the diagnostic nomenclature with an affirmation of the civil rights of homosexuals, no implication is intended justifying the irrational denial of civil rights to individuals who do suffer from true psychiatric disorders.)

This revision in the nomenclature provides the possibility of finding a homosexual to be free of psychiatric, disorder, and provides a means to diagnose a mental disorder whose central feature is conflict about homosexual behavior. Therefore, this change should in no way interfere with or embarrass the dedicated psychiatrists and psychoanalysts who have devoted themselves to understanding and treating those homosexuals who have been unhappy with their lot. They, and others in our field, will continue to try to help homosexuals who suffer from what we can now refer to as 'sexual orientation disturbance,' helping the patient accept or live with his current sexual orientation, or, if he desires, helping him to change it.

References

1   Bieber I, Dain HJ, Dince PR, *et al*: *Homosexuality: A Psychoanalytic Study of Male Homosexuals.* New York, Basic Books, 1962.

2   Socarides CW: *The Overt Homosexual.* New York, Grune & Stratton, 1968.

3   Ford CS, Beach FA: *Patterns of Sexual Behavior.* New York, Harper & Bros, 1951, pp 125–143.

4   Beach FA: Sexual Behavior in Animals and Man, in *Harvey Lectures, Series* **43**:1947–48. Springfield, Ill, Charles C Thomas, 1950, p 276.

5   Bieber I: Olfaction in sexual development and adult sexual organization. *Am J Psychother* **13**: 851–859, 1959.

6   Kalogerakis M: The role of olfaction in sexual development. *Psychosom Med* **25**: 420–432, 1963.

7   Karlen A: *Sexuality and Homosexuality.* New York, Norton, 1971, p 309.

8   Masters WH, Johnson VE: *Human Sexual Inadequacy.* Boston, Little, Brown and Co, 1970.

9   Freud S: Three essays on the theory of sexuality (1905), in *Complete Psychological Works*, standard ed, vol 7. Translated and edited by Strachey J. London, Hogarth Press, 1953, pp 125–245.

10   Mahler MS: On human symbiosis and the vicissitudes of individuation. *J Am Psychoanal Assoc* **15**: 740–763, 1967.

11   Hooker E: The adjustment of male homosexuals. *Journal of Projective Techniques* **21**: 17–31, 1957.

12   Hooker E: Male homosexuality in the Rorschach. *Journal of Projective Techniques* **22**: 33–54, 1958.

13   Hook S (ed): Psychoanalysis, *Scientific Method, and Philosophy.* New York. Arone Press, 1959.

14   Siegelman M: Adjustment of male homosexuals and heterosexuals. *Archives of Sexual Behavior* **2**: 9–26, 1972.

On Being Sane in Insane Places*

D. L. Rosenhan

If sanity and insanity exist, how shall we know them?

The question is neither capricious nor itself insane. However much we may be personally convinced that we can tell the normal from the abnormal, the evidence is simply not compelling. It is commonplace, for example, to read about murder trials wherein eminent psychiatrists for the defense are contradicted by equally eminent psychiatrists for the prosecution on the matter of the defendant's sanity. More generally, there are a great deal of conflicting data on the reliability, utility, and meaning of such terms as 'sanity,' 'insanity,' 'mental illness,' and 'schizophrenia'.[1] Finally, as early as 1934, Benedict suggested that normality and abnormality are not universal.[2] What is viewed as normal in one culture may be seen as quite aberrant in another. Thus, notions of normality and abnormality may not be quite as accurate as people believe they are.

To raise questions regarding normality and abnormality is in no way to question the fact that some behaviors' are deviant or odd. Murder is deviant. So, too, are hallucinations. Nor does raising such questions deny the existence of the personal anguish that is often associated with 'mental illness.' Anxiety and depression exist. Psychological suffering exists. But normality and abnormality, sanity and insanity, and the diagnoses that flow from them may be less substantive than many believe them to be.

At its heart, the question of whether the sane can be distinguished from the insane (and whether degrees of insanity can be distinguished from each other) is a simple matter: do the salient characteristics that lead to diagnoses reside in the patients themselves or in the environments and contexts in which observers find them? From Bleuler, through Kretchmer, through the formulators of the recently revised *Diagnostic and Statistical Manual* of the American psychiatric Association, the belief has been strong that patients present symptoms, that those symptoms can be categorized, and, implicitly, that the sane are distinguishable from the insane. More recently, however, this belief has been questioned. Based in part on theoretical and anthropological considerations, but also on philosophical, legal, and therapeutic ones, the view has grown that psychological categorization of mental illness is useless at best and downright harmful, misleading, and pejorative at worst. Psychiatric diagnoses, in this view, are in the minds of the observers and are not valid summaries of characteristics displayed by the observed.[3–5]

Gains can be made in deciding which of these is more nearly accurate by getting normal people (that is, people who do not have, and have never suffered, symptoms of serious psychiatric disorders) admitted to psychiatric hospitals and then determining whether they were discovered to be sane and, if so, how. If the sanity of such pseudopatients were always detected, there would be prima facie evidence that a sane individual can be distinguished from the insane context in which he is found. Normality (and presumably abnormality) is distinct enough that it can be recognized wherever it occurs, for it is carried within the person. If, on the other hand, the sanity of the pseudopatients were never discovered, serious difficulties would arise for those who support traditional modes of psychiatric diagnosis. Given that the hospital staff was not incompetent, that the pseudopatient had been behaving as sanely as he had been outside of the hospital, and that it had never been previously suggested that he belonged in a psychiatric hospital, such an unlikely outcome would support the view that psychiatric diagnosis betrays little about the patient but much about the environment in which an observer finds him.

This article describes such an experiment. Eight sane people gained secret admission to 12 different hospitals.[6] Their diagnostic experiences constitute the data of the first part of this article; the remainder is devoted to a description of their experiences in psychiatric institutions. Too few psychiatrists and psychologists, even those who have worked in such hospitals, know what the experience is like. They rarely talk about it with former patients, perhaps because they distrust information coming from the previously insane. Those who have worked in psychiatric hospitals are likely to have adapted so thoroughly to the settings that they are insensitive to the impact of that experience. And while there have been occasional reports of researchers who submitted themselves to psychiatric hospitalization,[7] these researchers have commonly remained in the hospitals for short periods of time, often with the knowledge of the hospital staff. It is difficult to know the extent to which they were treated like patients or like research colleagues. Nevertheless, their reports about the inside of the psychiatric hospital have been valuable. This article extends those efforts.

Pseudopatients and Their Settings

The eight pseudopatients were a varied group. One was a psychology graduate student in his 20's. The remaining seven were older and 'established.' Among them were three psychologist, a pediatrician, a psychiatrist, a painter, and a housewife. Three pseudopatients were women, five were men. All of them employed pseudonyms, lest their alleged diagnoses embarrass them later. Those who were in mental health professions alleged another occupation in order to avoid the special attentions that might be accorded by staff, as a matter of courtesy or caution, to ailing colleagues.[8] With the exception of myself (I was the first pseudopatient and my presence was known to the hospital administrator and chief psychologist and, so far as I can tell, to them alone), the presence of pseudopatients and the nature of the research program was not known to the hospital staffs.[9]

The settings were similarly varied. In order to generalize the findings, admission into a variety of hospitals was sought. The 12 hospitals in the sample were located in five different states on the East and West coasts. Some were old and shabby, some were quite new. Some were research-oriented, others not. Some had good staff-patient ratios, others were quite understaffed. Only one was a strictly private hospital. All of the others were supported by state or federal funds or, in one instance, by university funds.

After calling the hospital for an appointment, the pseudopatient arrived at the admissions office complaining that he had been hearing voices. Asked what the voices said, he replied that they were often unclear, but as far as he could tell they said 'empty,' 'hollow,' and 'thud.' The voices were unfamiliar and were of the same sex as the pseudopatient. The choice of these symptoms was occasioned by their apparent similarity to existential symptoms. Such symptoms are alleged to arise from painful concerns about the perceived meaninglessness of one's life. It is as if the hallucinating person

* Rosenhan, D.: On being sane in insane places. *Science* **179**: 250–258, 1973.

were saying, 'My life is empty and hollow.' The choice of these symptoms was also determined by the *absence* of a single report of existential psychoses in the literature.

Beyond alleging the symptoms and falsifying name, vocation, and employment, no further alterations of person, history, or circumstances were made. The significant events of the pseudopatient's life history were presented as they had actually occurred. Relationships with parents and siblings, with spouse and children, with people at work and in school, consistent with the aforementioned exceptions, were described as they were or had been. Frustrations and upsets were described along with joys and satisfactions. These facts are important to remember. If anything, they strongly biased the subsequent results in favor of detecting sanity, since none of their histories or current behaviors were seriously pathological in any way.

Immediately upon admission to the psychiatric ward, the pseudopatient ceased simulating *any* symptoms of abnormality. In some cases, there was a brief period of mild nervousness and anxiety, since none of the pseudopatients really believed that they would be admitted so easily. Indeed, their shared fear was that they would be immediately exposed as frauds and greatly embarrassed. Moreover, many of them had never visited a psychiatric ward; even those who had, nevertheless had some genuine fears about what might happen to them. Their nervousness, then, was quite appropriate to the novelty of the hospital setting, and it abated rapidly.

Apart from that short-lived nervousness, the pseudopatient behaved on the ward as he 'normally' behaved. The pseudopatient spoke to patients and staff as he might ordinarily. Because there is uncommonly little to do on a psychiatric ward, he attempted to engage others in conversation. When asked by staff how he was feeling, he indicated that he was fine, that he no longer experienced symptoms. He responded to instructions from attendants, to calls for medication (which was not swallowed), and to dining-hall instructions. Beyond such activities as were available to him on the admissions ward, he spent his time writing down his observations about the ward, its patients, and the staff. Initially these notes were written 'secretly,' but as it soon became clear that no one much cared, they were subsequently written on standard tablets of paper in such public places as the dayroom. No secret was made of these activities.

The pseudopatient, very much as a true psychiatric patient, entered a hospital with no foreknowledge of when he would be discharged. Each was told that he would have to get out by his own devices, essentially by convincing the staff that he was sane. The psychological stresses associated with hospitalization were considerable, and all but one of the pseudopatients desired to be discharged almost immediately after being admitted. They were, therefore, motivated not only to behave sanely, but to be paragons of cooperation. That their behavior was in no way disruptive is confirmed by nursing reports, which have been obtained on most of the patients. These reports uniformly indicate that the patients were 'friendly,' 'cooperative,' and 'exhibited no abnormal indications.'

The Normal Are Not Detectably Sane

Despite their public 'show' of sanity, the pseudopatients were never detected. Admitted, except in one case, with a diagnosis of schizophrenia,[10] each was discharged with a diagnosis of schizophrenia 'in remission.' The label 'in remission' should in no way be dismissed as a formality, for at no time during any hospitalization had any question been raised about any pseudopatient's simulation. Nor are there any indications in the hospital records that the pseudopatient's status was suspect. Rather, the evidence is strong that, once labeled schizophrenic, the pseudopatient was stuck with that label. If the pseudopatient was to be discharged, he must naturally be 'in remission': but he was not sane, nor, in the institution's view, had he ever been sane.

The uniform failure to recognize sanity cannot be attributed to the quality of the hospitals, for, although there were considerable variations among them, several are considered excellent. Nor can it be alleged that there was simply not enough time to observe the pseudopatients. Length of hospitalization ranged from 7 to 52 days, with an average of 19 days. The pseudopatients were not, in fact, carefully observed, but this failure clearly speaks more to traditions within psychiatric hospitals than to lack of opportunity.

Finally, it cannot be said that the failure to recognize the pseudopatients' sanity was due to the fact that they were not behaving sanely. While there was clearly some tension present in all of them, their daily visitors could detect no serious behavioral consequences – nor, indeed, could other patients. It was quite common for the patients to 'detect' the pseudopatients' sanity. During the first three hospitalizations, when accurate counts were kept, 35 of a total of 118 patients on the admissions ward voiced their suspicions, some vigorously. 'You're not crazy. You're a journalist, or a professor [referring to the continual note-taking]. You're checking up on the hospital.' While most of the patients were reassured by the pseudopatient's insistence that he had been sick before he came in but was fine now, some continued to believe that the pseudopatient was sane throughout his hospitalization.[11] The fact that the patients often recognized normality when staff did not raises important questions.

Failure to detect sanity during the course of hospitalization may be due to the fact that physicians operate with a strong bias toward what statisticians call the type 2 error.[5] This is to say that physicians are more inclined to call a healthy person sick (a false positive, type 2) than a sick person healthy (a false negative, type 1). The reasons for this are not hard to find it is clearly more dangerous to misdiagnose illness than health. Better to err on the side of caution, to suspect illness even among the healthy.

But what holds for medicine does not hold equally well for psychiatry. Medical illnesses, while unfortunate, are not commonly pejorative. Psychiatric diagnoses, on the contrary, carry with them personal, legal, and social stigmas.[12] It was therefore important to see whether the tendency toward diagnosing the sane insane could be reversed. The following experiment was arranged at a research and teaching hospital whose staff had heard these findings but doubted that such an error could occur in their hospital. The staff was informed that at some time during the following 3 months, one or more pseudopatients would attempt to be admitted into the psychiatric hospital. Each staff member was asked to rate each patient who presented himself at admissions or on the ward according to the likelihood that the patient was a pseudopatient. A 10-point scale was used, with a 1 and 2 reflecting high confidence that the patient was a pseudopatient.

Judgments were obtained on 193 patients who were admitted for psychiatric treatment. All staff who had had sustained contact with or primary responsibility for the patient – attendants, nurses, psychiatrists, physicians, and psychologists – were asked to make judgments. Forty-one patients were alleged, with high confidence, to be pseudopatients by at least one member of the staff. Twenty-three were considered suspect by at least one psychiatrist. Nineteen were suspected by one psychiatrist *and* one other staff member. Actually, no genuine pseudopatient (at least from my group) presented himself during this period.

The experiment is instructive. It indicates that the tendency to designate sane people as insane can be reversed when the stakes (in this case, prestige and diagnostic acumen) are high. But what can be said of the 19 people who were suspected of being 'sane' by one psychiatrist and another staff member? Were these people truly 'sane,' or was it rather the case that in the course of avoiding the type 2 error the staff tended to make more errors of the first sort – calling the crazy 'sane'? There is no way of knowing. But one thing is certain: any diagnostic process that lends itself so readily to massive errors of this sort cannot be a very reliable one.

The Stickiness of Psychodiagnostic Labels

Beyond the tendency to call the healthy sick – a tendency that accounts better for diagnostic behavior on admission than it does for such behavior after a lengthy period of exposure – the data speak to the massive role of labeling in psychiatric assessment. Having once been labeled schizophrenic, there is nothing the pseudopatient can do to overcome the tag. The tag profoundly colors others' perceptions of him and his behavior.

From one viewpoint, these data are hardly surprising, for it has long been known that elements are given meaning by the context in which they occur. Gestalt psychology made this point vigorously, and Asch[13] demonstrated that there are 'central' personality traits (such as 'warm' versus 'cold') which are so powerful that they markedly color the meaning of other information in forming an impression of a given personality.[14] 'Insane,' 'schizophrenic,' 'manic-depressive,' and 'crazy' are probably among the most powerful of such central traits. Once a person is designated abnormal, all of his other behaviors and characteristics are colored by that label. Indeed, that label is so powerful that many of the pseudopatients' normal behaviors were overlooked entirely or profoundly misinterpreted. Some examples may clarify this issue.

Earlier I indicated that there were no changes in the pseudopatient's personal history and current status beyond those of name, employment, and, where necessary, vocation. Otherwise, a veridical description of personal history and, circumstances was offered. Those circumstances were not psychotic. How were they made consonant with the diagnosis of psychosis? Or were those diagnoses modified in such a way as to bring them into accord with the circumstances of the pseudopatient's life, as described by him?

As far as I can determine, diagnoses were in no way affected by the relative health of the circumstances of a pseudopatient's life. Rather, the reverse occurred: the perception of his circumstances was shaped entirely by the diagnosis. A clear example of such translation is found in the case of a pseudopatient who had had a close relationship with his mother but was rather remote from his father during his early childhool. During adolescence and beyond, however, his father became a close friend, while his relationship with his mother cooled. His present relationship with his wife was characteristically close and warm. Apart from occasional angry exchanges, friction was minimal. The children had rarely been spanked. Surely there is nothing especially pathological about such a history. Indeed, many readers may see a similar pattern in their own experiences, with no markedly deleterious consequences. Observe, however, how such a history was translated in the psychopathological context, this from the case summary prepared after the patient was discharged.

This white 39-year-old male . . . manifests a long history of considerable ambivalence in close relationships, which begins in early childhood. A warm relationship with his mother cools during his adolescence. A distant relationship to his father is described as becoming very intense. Affective stability is absent. His attempts to control emotionality with his wife and children are punctuated by angry outbursts and, in the case of the children, spankings. And while he says that he has several good friends, one senses considerable ambivalence embedded in those relationships also. . . .

The facts of the case were unintentionally distorted by the staff to achieve consistency with a popular theory of the dynamics of a schizophrenic reaction.[15] Nothing of an ambivalent nature had been described in relations with parents, spouse, or friends. To the extent that ambivalence could be inferred, it was probably not greater than is found in all human relationships. It is true the pseudopatient's relationships with his parents changed over time, but in the ordinary context that would hardly be remarkable – indeed, it might very well be expected. Clearly, the meaning ascribed to his verbalizations (that is, ambivalence, affective instability) was determined by the diagnosis: schizophrenia. An entirely different meaning would have been ascribed if it were known that the man was 'normal.'

All pseudopatients took extensive notes publicly. Under ordinary circumstances, such behavior would have raised questions in the minds of observers, as, in fact, it did among patients. Indeed, it seemed so certain that the notes would elicit suspicion that elaborate precautions were taken to remove them from the ward each day. But the precautions proved needless. The closest any staff member came to questioning these notes occurred when one pseudopatient asked his physician what kind of medication he was receiving and began to write down the response. 'You needn't write it,' he was told gently. 'If you have trouble remembering, just ask me again.'

If no questions were asked of the pseudopatients, how was their writing interpreted? Nursing records for three patients indicate that the writing was seen as an aspect of their pathological behavior. 'Patient engages in writing behavior' was the daily nursing comment on one of the pseudopatients who was never questioned about his writing. Given that the patient is in the hospital, he must be psychologically disturbed. And given that he is disturbed, continuous writing must be a behavioral manifestation of that disturbance, perhaps a subset of the compulsive behaviors that are sometimes correlated with schizophrenia.

One tacit characteristic of psychiatric diagnosis is that it locates the sources of aberration within the individual and only rarely within the complex of stimuli that surrounds him. Consequently, behaviors that are stimulated by the environment are commonly misattributed to the patient's disorder. For example, one kindly nurse found a pseudopatient pacing the long hospital corridors. 'Nervous, Mr. X?' she asked. 'No, bored,' he said.

The notes kept by pseudopatients are full of patient behaviors that were misinterpreted by well-intentioned staff. Often enough, a patient would go 'berserk' because he had, wittingly or unwittingly, been mistreated by, say, an attendant. A nurse coming upon the scene would rarely inquire even cursorily into the environmental stimuli of the patient's behavior. Rather, she assumed that his upset derived from his pathology, not from his present interactions with other staff members. Occasionally, the staff might assume that the patient's family (especially when they had recently visited) or other patients had stimulated the outburst. But never were the staff found to assume that one of themselves or the structure of the hospital had anything to do with a patient's behavior. One psychiatrist pointed to a group of patients who were sitting outside the cafeteria entrance half an hour before lunchtime. To a group of young residents he indicated that such behavior was characteristic of the oral-acquisitive nature of the syndrome. It seemed not to occur to him that there were very few things to anticipate in a psychiatric hospital be sides eating.

A psychiatric label has a life and an influence of its own. Once the impression has been formed that the patient is schizophrenic, the expectation is that he will continue to be schizophrenic. When a sufficient amount of time has passed, during which the patient has done nothing bizarre, he is considered to be in remission and available for discharge. But the label endures beyond discharge, with the unconfirmed expectation that he will behave as a schizophrenic again. Such labels, conferred by mental health professionals, are as influential on the patient as they are on his relatives and friends, and it should not surprise anyone that the diagnosis acts on all of them as a self-fulfilling prophecy. Eventually, the patient himself accepts the diagnosis, with all of its surplus meanings and expectations, and behaves accordingly.[5]

The inferences to be made from these matters are quite simple. Much as Zigler and Phillips have demonstrated that there is enormous overlap in the symptoms presented by patients who have been variously diagnosed,[16] so there is enormous overlap in the behaviors of the sane and the insane. The sane are not 'sane' all of the time. We lose our tempers 'for no good reason.' We are occasionally depressed or anxious, again for no good reason. And we may find it difficult to get along with one or another person – again for no reason that we can specify. Similarly, the insane are not always insane. Indeed, it was the impression of the pseudopatients while living with them that they were sane for long periods of time – that the bizarre behaviors upon which their diagnoses were allegedly predicated constituted only a small fraction of their total behavior. If it makes no sense to label ourselves permanently depressed on the basis of an occasional depression, then it takes better evidence than is presently available to label all patients insane or schizophrenic on the basis of bizarre behaviors or cognitions. It seems more useful, as Mischel[17] has pointed out, to limit our discussions to *behaviors*, the stimuli that provoke them, and their correlates.

It is not known why powerful impressions of personality traits, such as 'crazy' or 'insane,' arise. Conceivably, when the origins of and stimuli that give rise to a behavior are remote or unknown, or when the behavior strikes us as immutable, trait labels regarding the *behaver* arise. When, on the other hand, the origins and stimuli are known and available, discourse is limited to the behavior itself. Thus, I may hallucinate because I am sleeping, or I may hallucinate because I have ingested a peculiar drug. These are termed sleep-induced hallucinations, or dreams, and drug-induced hallucinations, respectively. But when the stimuli to my hallucinations are unknown, that is called craziness, or schizophrenia – as if that inference were somehow as illuminating as the others.

The Experience of Psychiatric Hospitalization

The term 'mental illness' is of recent origin. It was coined by people who were humane in their inclinations and who wanted very much to raise the station of (and the public's sympathies toward) the psychologically disturbed from that of witches and 'crazies' to one that was akin to the physically ill. And they were at least partially successful, for the treatment of the mentally ill *has* improved considerably over the years. But while treatment has improved, it is doubtful that people really regard the mentally ill in the same way that they view the physically ill. A broken leg is something one recovers from, but mental illness allegedly endures forever.[18] A broken leg does not threaten the observer, but a crazy schizophrenic? There is by now a host of evidence that attitudes toward the mentally ill are characterized by fear, hostility, aloofness, suspicion, and dread.[19] The mentally ill are society's lepers.

That such attitudes infect the general population is perhaps not surprising, only upsetting. But that they affect the professionals – attendants, nurses, physicians, psychologists, and social workers – who treat and deal with the mentally ill is more disconcerting, both because such attitudes are self-evidently pernicious and because they are unwitting. Most mental health professionals would insist that they are sympathetic toward the mentally ill, that they are neither avoidant nor hostile. But it is more likely that an exquisite ambivalence characterizes their relations with psychiatric patients, such that their avowed impulses are only part of their entire attitude. Negative attitudes are there too and can easily be detected. Such attitudes should not surprise us. They are the natural offspring of the labels patients wear and the places in which they are found.

Consider the structure of the typical psychiatric hospital. Staff and patients are strictly segregated. Staff have their own living space, including their dining facilities, bathrooms, and assembly places. The glassed quarters that contain the professional staff, which the pseudopatients came to call 'the cage,' sit out on every dayroom. The staff emerge primarily for caretaking purposes – to give medication, to conduct a therapy or group meeting, to instruct or reprimand a patient. Otherwise, staff keep to themselves, almost as if the disorder that afflicts their charges is somehow catching.

So much is patient-staff segregation the rule that, for four public hospitals in which an attempt was made to measure the degree to which staff and patients mingle, it was necessary to use 'time out of the staff cage' as the operational measure. While it was not the case that all time spent out of the cage was spent mingling with patients (attendants, for example, would occasionally emerge to watch television in the dayroom), it was the only way in which one could gather reliable data on time for measuring.

The average amount of time spent by attendants outside of the cage was 11.3 percent (range, 3 to 52 percent). This figure does not represent only time spent mingling with patients, but also includes time spent on such chores as folding laundry, supervising patients while they shave, directing ward clean-up, and sending patients to off-ward activities. It was the relatively rare attendant who spent time talking with patients or playing games with them. It proved impossible to obtain a 'percent mingling time' for nurses, since the amount of time they spent out of the cage was too brief. Rather, we counted instances of emergence from the cage. On the average, daytime nurses emerged from the cage 11.5 times per shift, including instances when they left the ward entirely (range, 4 to 39 times). Late afternoon and night nurses were even less available, emerging on the average 9.4 times per shift (range, 4 to 41 times). Data on early morning nurses, who arrived usually after midnight and departed at 8 a.m., are not available because patients were asleep during most of this period.

Physicians, especially psychiatrists, were even less available. They were rarely seen on the wards. Quite commonly, they would be seen only when they arrived and departed, with the remaining time being spent in their offices or in the cage. On the average, physicians emerged on the ward 6.7 times per day (range, 1 to 17 times). It proved difficult to make an accurate estimate in this regard, since physicians often maintained hours that allowed them to come and go at different times.

The hierarchical organization of the psychiatric hospital has been commented on before,[20] but the latent meaning of that kind of organization is worth noting again. Those with the most power have least to do with patients, and those with the least power are most involved with them. Recall, however, that the acquisition of role-appropriate behaviors occurs mainly through the observation of others, with the most powerful having the most influence. Consequently, it is understandable that attendants not only spend more time with patients than do any other members of the staff – that is required by their station in the hierarchy – but also, insofar as they learn from their superiors' behavior, spend as little time with patients as they can. Attendants are seen mainly in the cage, which is where the models, the action, and the power are.

I turn now to a different set of studies, these dealing with staff response to patientinitiated contact. It has long been known that the amount of time a person spends with you can be an index of your significance to him. If he initiates and maintains eye contact, there is reason to believe that he is considering your requests and needs. If he pauses to chat or actually stops and talks, there is added reason to infer that he is individuating you. In four hospitals, the pseudopatient approached the staff member with a request which took the following form: 'Pardon me, Mr. [or Dr. or Mrs.] X, could you tell me when I will be eligible for grounds privileges?' (or '. . . when I will be presented at the staff meeting?' or '. . . when I am likely to be discharged?'). While the content of the question varied according to the appropriateness of the target and the pseudopatient's (apparent) current needs the form was always a courteous and relevant request for information. Care was taken never to approach a particular member of the staff more than once a day, lest the staff member become suspicious or irritated. In examining these data, remember that the behavior of the pseudopatients was neither bizarre nor disruptive. One could indeed engage in good conversation with them.

The data for these experiments are shown in Table 1, separately for physicians (column 1) and for nurses and attendants (column 2). Minor differences between these four institutions were overwhelmed by the degree to which staff avoided continuing contacts that patients had initiated. By far, their most common response consisted of either a brief response to the question, offered while they were 'on the move' and with head averted, or no response at all.

The encounter frequently took the following bizarre form: (pseudopatient) 'Pardon me, Dr. X. Could you tell me when I am eligible for grounds privileges?' (physician) 'Good morning, Dave. How are you today?' (Moves off without waiting for a response.)

It is instructive to compare these data with data recently obtained at Stanford University. It has been alleged that large and eminent universities are characterized by faculty who are so busy that they have no time for students. For this comparison, a young lady approached individual faculty members who seemed to be walking purposefully to some meeting or teaching engagement and asked them the following six questions.

1   'Pardon me, could you direct me to Encina Hall?' (at the medical school: '. . . to the Clinical Research Center?').

2   'Do you know where Fish Annex is?' (there is no Fish Annex at Stanford).

3   'Do you teach here?'

4   'How does one apply for admission to the college?' (at the medical school: '. . . to the medical school?').

5   'Is it difficult to get in?'

6   'Is there financial aid?'

Table 1 Self-initiated contact by pseudopatients with psychiatrists and nurses and attendants, compared to contact with other groups.

| Contact | Psychiatric hospitals | | University campus (nonmedical) | University medical center | | |
| | | | | Physicians | | |
	(1) Psychiatrists	(2) Nurses and attendants	(3) Faculty	(4) 'Looking for a psychiatrist'	(5) 'Looking for an internist'	(6) No additional Comment
Responses						
Moves on, head averted (%)	71	88	0	0	0	0
Makes eye contact (%)	23	10	0	11	0	0
Pauses and chats (%)	2	2	0	11	0	10
Stops and talks (%)	4	0.5	100	78	100	90
Mean number of questions answered (out of 6)	*	*	6	3.8	4.8	4.5
Respondents (No.)	13	47	14	18	15	10
Attempts (No.)	185	1283	14	18	15	10

* Not applicable.

Without exception, as can be seen in Table 1 (column 3), all of the questions were answered. No matter how rushed they were, all respondents not only maintained eye contact, but stopped to talk. Indeed, many of the respondents went out of their way to direct or take the questioner to the office she was seeking, to try to locate 'Fish Annex,' or to discuss with her the possibilities of being admitted to the university.

Similar data, also shown in Table 1 (columns 4, 5, and 6), were obtained in the hospital. Here too, the young lady came prepared with six questions. After the first question, however, she remarked to 18 of her respondents (column 4), 'I'm looking for a psychiatrist,' and to 15 others (column 5), 'I'm looking for an internist.' Ten other respondents received no inserted comment (column 6). The general degree of cooperative responses is considerably higher for these university groups than it was for pseudopatients in psychiatric hospitals. Even so, differences are apparent within the medical school setting. Once having indicated that she was looking for a psychiatrist, the degree of cooperation elicited was less than when she sought an internist.

Powerlessness and Depersonalization

Eye contact and verbal contact reflect concern and individuation; their absence, avoidance and depersonalization. The data I have presented do not do justice to the rich daily encounters that grew up around matters of depersonalization and avoidance. I have records of patients who were beaten by staff for the sin of having initiated verbal contact. During my own experience, for example, one patient was beaten in the presence of other patients for having approached an attendant and told him, 'I like you.' Occasionally, punishment meted out to patients for misdemeanors seemed so excessive that it could not be justified by the most radical interpretations of psychiatric canon. Nevertheless, they appeared to go unquestioned. Tempers were often short. A patient who had not heard a call for medication would be roundly excoriated, and the morning attendants would often wake patients with, 'Come on, you m – f – s, out of bed!'

Neither anecdotal nor 'hard' data can convey the overwhelming sense of powerlessness which invades the individual as he is continually exposed to the depersonalization of the psychiatric hospital. It hardly matters *which* psychiatric hospital – the excellent public ones and the very plush private hospital were better than the rural and shabby ones in this regard, but, again, the features that psychiatric hospitals had in common overwhelmed by far their apparent differences.

Powerlessness was evident everywhere. The patient is deprived of many of his legal rights by dint of his psychiatric commitment.[21] He is shorn of credibility by virtue of his psychiatric label. His freedom of movement is restricted. He cannot initiate contact with the staff, but may only respond to such overtures as they make. Personal privacy is minimal. Patient quarters and possessions can be entered and examined by any staff member, for whatever reason. His personal history and anguish is available to any staff member (often including the 'grey lady' and 'candy striper' volunteer) who chooses to read his folder, regardless of their therapeutic relationship to him. His personal hygiene and waste evacuation are often monitored. The water closets may have no doors.

At times, depersonalization reached such proportions that pseudopatients had the sense that they were invisible, or at least unworthy of account. Upon being admitted, I and other pseudopatients took the initial physical examinations in a semipublic room, where staff members went about their own business as if we were not there.

On the ward, attendants delivered verbal and occasionally serious physical abuse to patients in the presence of other observing patients, some of whom (the pseudopatients) were writing it all down. Abusive behavior, on the other hand, terminated quite abruptly when other staff members were known to be coming. Staff are credible witnesses. Patients are not.

A nurse unbuttoned her uniform to adjust her brassiere in the presence of an entire ward of viewing men. One did not have the sense that she was being seductive. Rather, she didn't notice us. A group of staff persons might point to a patient in the dayroom and discuss him animatedly, as if he were not there.

One illuminating instance of depersonalization and invisibility occurred with regard to medications. All told, the pseudopatients were administered nearly 2100 pills, including Elavil, Stelazine, Compazine, and Thorazine, to name but a few. (That such a variety of medications should have been administered to patients presenting identical symptoms is itself worthy of note.) Only two were swallowed. The rest were either pocketed or deposited in the toilet. The pseudopatients were not alone in this. Although I have no precise records on how many patients rejected their medications, the pseudopatients frequently found the medications of other patients in the toilet before they deposited their own. As long as they were cooperative, their behavior and the pseudopatients' own in this matter, as in other important matters, went unnoticed throughout.

Reactions to such depersonalization among pseudopatients were intense. Although they had come to the hospital as participant observers and were fully aware that they did not 'belong,' they nevertheless found themselves caught up in and fighting the process of depersonalization. Some examples: a graduate student in psychology asked his wife to bring his textbooks to the hospital so he could 'catch up on his homework' – this despite the elaborate precautions taken to conceal his professional association. The same student, who had trained for quite some time to get into the hospital, and who had looked forward to the experience, 'remembered' some drag races that he had wanted to see on the weekend and insisted that he be discharged by that time. Another pseudopatient attempted a romance with a nurse. Subsequently, he informed the staff that he was applying for admission to graduate school in psychology and was very likely to be admitted, since a graduate professor was one of his regular hospital visitors. The same person began to engage in psychotherapy with other patients—all of this as a way of becoming a person in an impersonal environment.

The Sources of Depersonalization

What are the origins of depersonalization? I have already mentioned two. First are attitudes held by all of us toward the mentally ill – including those who treat them – attitudes characterized by fear, distrust, and horrible expectations on the one hand, and benevolent intentions on the other. Our ambivalence leads, in this instance as in others, to avoidance.

Second, and not entirely separate, the hierarchical structure of the psychiatric hospital facilitates depersonalization. Those who are at the top have least to do with patients, and their behavior inspires the rest of the staff. Average daily contact with psychiatrists, psychologists, residents, and physicians combined ranged from 3.9 to 25.1 minutes, with an overall mean of 6.8 (six pseudopatients over a total of 129 days of hospitalization). Included in this average is time spent in the admissions interview, ward meetings in the presence of a senior staff member, group and individual psychotherapy contacts, case presentation conferences, and discharge meetings. Clearly, patients do not spend much time in interpersonal contact with doctoral staff. And doctoral staff serve as models for nurses and attendants.

There are probably other sources. Psychiatric installations are presently in serious financial straits. Staff shortages are pervasive, staff time at a premium. Something has to give, and that something is patient contact. Yet, while financial stresses are realities, too much can be made of them. I have the impression that the psychological forces that result in depersonalization are much stronger than the fiscal ones and that the addition of more staff would not correspondingly improve patient care in this regard. The incidence of staff meetings and the enormous amount of record-keeping on patients, for example, have not been as substantially reduced as has patient contact. Priorities exist, even during hard times. Patient contact is not a significant priority in the traditional psychiatric hospital, and fiscal pressures do not account for this. Avoidance and depersonalization may.

Heavy reliance upon psychotropic medication tacitly, contributes to depersonalization by, convincing staff that treatment is indeed being conducted and that further patient contact may not be necessary. Even here, however, caution needs to be exercised in understanding the role of psychotropic drugs. If patients were powerful rather than powerless, if they were viewed as interesting individuals rather than diagnostic entities, if they were socially significant, rather than social lepers, if their anguish truly and wholly compelled our sympathies and concerns, would we not *seek* contact with them, despite the availability of medications? Perhaps for the pleasure of it all?

The Consequences of Labeling and Depersonalization

Whenever the ratio of what is known to what needs to be known approaches zero, we tend to invent 'knowledge' and assume that we understand more than we actually do. We seem unable to acknowledge that we simply don't know. The needs for diagnosis and remediation of behavioral and emotional problems are enormous. But rather than acknowledge that we are just embarking on understanding, we continue to label patients 'schizophrenic,' 'manic-depressive,' and 'insane,' as if in those words we had captured the essence of understanding. The facts of the matter are that we

have known for a long time that diagnoses are often not useful or reliable, but we have nevertheless continued to use them. We now know that we cannot distinguish insanity from sanity. It is depressing to consider how that information will be used.

Not merely depressing, but frightening. How many people, one wonders, are sane but not recognized as such in our psychiatric institutions? How many have been needlessly stripped of their privileges of citizenship, from the right to vote and drive to that of handling their own accounts? How many have feigned insanity in order to avoid the criminal consequences of their behavior, and, conversely, how many would rather stand trial than live interminably in a psychiatric hospital – but are wrongly thought to be mentally ill? How many have been stigmatized by well-intentioned, but nevertheless erroneous, diagnoses? On the last point, recall again that a 'type 2 error' in psychiatric diagnosis does not have the same consequences it does in medical diagnosis. A diagnosis of cancer that has been found to be in error is cause for celebration. But psychiatric diagnoses are rarely found to be in error. The label sticks, a mark of inadequacy forever.

Finally, how many patients might be 'sane' outside the psychiatric hospital but seem insane in it – not because craziness resides in them, as it were, but because they are responding to a bizarre setting, one that may be unique to institutions which harbor nether people? Goffman (4) calls the process of socialization to such institutions 'mortification' – an apt metaphor that includes the processes of depersonalization that have been described here. And while it is impossible to know whether the pseudopatients' responses to these processes are characteristic of all inmates – they were, after all, not real patients – it is difficult to believe that these processes of socialization to a psychiatric hospital provide useful attitudes or habits of response for living in the 'real world.'

Summary and Conclusions

It is clear that we cannot distinguish the sane from the insane in psychiatric hospitals. The hospital itself imposes a special environment in which the meanings of behavior can easily be misunderstood. The consequences to patients hospitalized in such an environment – the powerlessness, depersonalization, segregation, mortification, and self-labeling – seem undoubtedly counter-therapeutic.

I do not, even now, understand this problem well enough to perceive solutions. But two matters seem to have some promise. The first concerns the proliferation of community mental health facilities, of crisis intervention centers, of the human potential movement, and of behavior therapies that, for all of their own problems, tend to avoid psychiatric labels, to focus on specific problems and behaviors, and to retain the individual in a relatively nonpejorative environment. Clearly, to the extent that we refrain from sending the distressed to insane places, our impressions of them are less likely to be distorted. (The risk of distorted perceptions, it seems to me, is always present, since we are much more sensitive to an individual's behaviors and verbalizations than we are to the subtle contextual stimuli that often promote them. At issue here is a matter of magnitude. And, as I have shown, the magnitude of distortion is exceedingly high in the extreme context that is a psychiatric hospital.)

The second matter that might prove promising speaks to the need to increase the sensitivity of mental health workers and researchers to the *Catch 22* position of psychiatric patients. Simply reading materials in this area will be of help to some such workers and researchers. For others, directly experiencing the impact of psychiatric hospitalization will be of enormous use. Clearly, further research into the social psychology of such total institutions will both facilitate treatment and deepen understanding.

I and the other pseudopatients in the psychiatric setting had distinctly negative reactions. We do not pretend to describe the subjective experiences of true patients. Theirs may be different from ours, particularly with the passage of time and the necessary process of adaptation to one's environment. But we can and do speak to the relatively more objective indices of treatment within the hospital. It could be a mistake, and a very unfortunate one, to consider that what happened to us derived from malice or stupidity on the part of the staff. Quite the contrary, our overwhelming impression of them was of people who really cared, who were committed and who were uncommonly intelligent. Where they failed, as they sometimes did painfully, it would be more accurate to attribute those failures to the environment in which they, too, found themselves than to personal callousness. Their perceptions and behavior were controlled by the situation, rather than being motivated by a malicious disposition. In a more benign environment, one that was less attached to global diagnosis, their behaviors and judgments might have been more benign and effective.

References and Notes

1   **P. Ash**, *J. Abnorm. Soc. Psychol.* 44, 272 (1949); A. T. Beck, *Amer. J. Psychiat.* **119**, 210 (1962); A. T. Boisen, *Psychiatry* **2**, 233 (1938); N. Kreitman, *J. Ment. Sci.* 107, 876 (1961); N. Kreitman, P. Sainsbury, J. Morrisey, J. Towers, J. Scrivener, *ibid.*, p. 887; H. O. Schmitt and C. P. Fonda, *J. Abnorm. Soc. Psychol.* 52, 262 (1956); W. Seeman, *J. Nerv. Ment. Dis.* **118**, 541 (1953). For an analysis of these artifacts and summaries of the disputes, see J. Zubin, *Annu. Rev. Psychol.* **18**, 373 (1967); L. Phillips and J. G. Draguns, *ibid.* **22**, 447 (1971).

2   **R. Benedict**, *J. Gen. Psychol.* **10**, 59 (1934).

3   See in this regard H. Becker, *Outsiders: Studies in the Sociology of Deviance* (Free Press, New York, 1963); B. M. Braginsky, D. D. Braginsky, K. Ring, *Methods of Madness: The Mental Hospital as a Last Resort* (Holt, Rinehart & Winston, New York, 1969); G. M. Crocetti and P. V. Lemkau, *Amer. Social. Rev.* **30**, 577 (1965); E. Goffman, *Behavior in Public Places* (Free Press, New York, 1964); R. D. Laing, *The Divided Self: A Study of Sanity and Madness* (Quadrangle, Chicago, 1960); D. L. Phillips, *Amer. Social. Rev.* 28, 963 (1963); T. R. Sarbin, *Psychol. Today* **6**, 18 (1972); E. Schur, *Amer. J. Sociol.* **75**, 309 (1969); T. Szasz, *Law, Liberty and Psychiatry* (Macmillan. New York, 1963); *The Myth of Mental Illness: Foundations of a Theory of Mental Illness* (Hoeber-Harper, New York, 1963). For a critique of some of these views, see W. R. Gove. *Amer. Social. Rev.* **35**, 873 (1970).

4   **E. Goffman**, *Asylums* (Doubleday, Garden City, N.Y., 1961).

5   **T. J. Scheff**, *Being Mentally Ill: A Sociological Theory* (Aldine, Chicago, 1966).

6   Data from a ninth pseudopatient are not incorporated in this report because, although his sanity went undetected, he falsified aspects of his personal history, including his marital status and parental relationships. His experimental behaviors therefore were not identical to those of the other pseudopatients.

7   A. Barry, Bellevue Is a State of Mind (Harcourt Brace Jovanovich, New York, 1971); I. Belknap, Human Problems of a State Mental Hospital (McGraw-Hill, New York, 1956); W. Caudill, F. C. Redlich, H. R. Gilmore, E. B. Brody, Amer. J. Orthopsychiat. 22, 314 (1952); A. R. Goldman, R. H. Bohr, T. A. Steinberg, Prof. Psychol. 1, 427 (1970); unauthored, Roche Report 1 (No. 13), 8 (1971).

8   Beyond the personal difficulties that the pseudopatient is likely to experience in the hospital, there are legal and social ones that, combined, require considerable attention before entry. For example, once admitted to a psychiatric institution, it is difficult, if not impossible, to be discharged on short notice, state law to the contrary notwithstanding. I was not sensitive to these difficulties at the outset of the project, nor to the personal and situational emergencies that can arise, but later a writ of habeas corpus was prepared for each of the entering pseudopatients and an attorney was kept 'on call' during every hospitalization. I am grateful to John Kaplan and Robert Bartels for legal advice and assistance in these matters.

9   However distasteful such concealment is, it was a necessary first step to examining these questions. Without concealment, there would have been no way to know how valid these experiences were; nor was there any way of knowing whether whatever detections occurred were a tribute to the diagnostic acumen of the staff or to the hospital's rumor network. Obviously, since my concerns are general ones that cut across individual hospitals and staffs, I have respected their anonymity and have eliminated clues that might lead to their identification.

10   Interestingly, of the 12 admissions, 11 were diagnosed as schizophrenic and one, with the identical symptomatology, as manic-depressive psychosis. This diagnosis has a more favorable prognosis, and it was given by the only private hospital in our sample. On the relations between social class and psychiatric diagnosis, see A. deB. Hollingshead and F. C. Redlich. *Social Class and Mental Illness: A Community Study* (Wiley, New York, 1958).

11   It is possible, of course, that patients have quite broad latitudes in diagnosis and therefore are inclined to call many people sane, even those whose behavior is patently aberrant. However, although we have no hard data on this matter, it was our distinct impression that this was not the case. In many instances, patients not only singled us out for attention, but came to imitate our behaviors and styles.

12   **J. Cumming** and **E. Cumming**, *Community Ment. Health* **1**, 135 (1965); A. Farina and K. Ring, *J. Abnorm. Psychol.* **70**. 47 (1965); H. E. Freeman and O. G. Simmons, *The Mental Patient Comes Home* (Wiley, New York, 1963); W. J. Johannsen, *Ment. Hygiene* 53, 218 (1969); A. S. Linsky, *Soc. Psychiat.* **5**, 166 (1970).

13   **S. E. Asch**, *J. Abnorm. Soc. Psychol.* **41**, 258 (1946); *Social Psychology* (Prentice-Hall, New York, 1952).

14   See also **I. N. Mensh** and J. Wishner, *J. Personality* **16**, 188 (1947); J. Wishner, *Psychol. Rev.* **67**, 96 (1960); J. S. Bruner and R. Tagiuri, in *Handbook of Social, Psychology*, G. Lindzey, Ed. (Addison-Wesley, Cambridge, Mass., 1954), vol. 2, pp. 634–654; J. S. Bruner, D. Shapiro, R. Tagiuri, in *Person Perception and Interpersonal Behavior*, R. Tagiuri and L. Petrullo, Eds. (Stanford Univ. Press. Stanford, Calif., 1958), pp. 277–288.

15   For an example of a similar self-fulfilling prophecy, in this instance dealing with the 'central' trait of intelligence, see R. Rosenthal and L. Jacobson, *Pygmalion in the Classroom* (Holt, Rinehart & Winston, New York, 1968).

16   **E. Zigler** and **L. Phillips**, *J. Abnorm. Soc. Psychol.* **63**, 69 (1961). See also R. K. Freudenberg and J. P. Robertson, *A.M.A. Arch. Neurol. Psychiatr.* **76**, 14 (1956).

17   **W. Mischel**, *Personality and Assessment* (Wiley, New York, 1968).

18   The most recent and unfortunate instance of this tenet is that of Senator Thomas Eagleton.

19   **T. R. Sarbin** and **J. C. Mancuso**, *J. Clin. Consult. Psychol.* **35**, 159 (1970); T. R. Sarbin, *ibid.* **31**, 447 (1967); J. C. Nunnally, Jr., *Popular Conceptions of Mental Health* (Holt, Rinehart & Winston, New York, 1961).

20   **A. H. Stanton** and **M. S. Schwartz**, *The Mental Hospital: A Study of Institutional Participation in Psychiatric Illness and Treatment* (Basic, New York, 1954).

21   **D. B. Wexler** and, **S. E. Scoville**, *Ariz. Law Rev.* **13**, 1 (1971).

22   I thank **W. Mischel**, **E. Orne**, and **M. S. Rosenhan** for comments on an earlier draft of this manuscript.

The Concept of Mental Disorder

*On the Boundary Between Biological Facts and Social Values**

Jerome C. Wakefield

This article presents an analysis of the concept of mental disorder. The focus is on *disorder* rather than *mental* because questions about the concept of disorder cause the most heated disputes in the mental health field. I argue that disorder lies on the boundary between the given natural world and the constructed social world; a disorder exists when the failure of a person's internal mechanisms to perform their functions as designed by nature impinges harmfully on the person's well-being as defined by social values and meanings. The order that is disturbed when one has a disorder is thus simultaneously biological and social; neither alone is sufficient to justify the label *disorder*.

There are many reasons why mental health professionals should care about the correct analysis of the concept of disorder. Concerns about the distinction between disorder and nondisorder are omnipresent in the mental health field and range from the sublime (how can one tell the difference between noble self-sacrifice and pathological masochism?) to the ridiculous (is snoring a disorder the treatment of which therefore warrants medical insurance reimbursement?) and on to the tragic (if a person diagnosed with acquired immunodeficiency syndrome expresses suicidal thoughts, is he or she suffering from an adjustment disorder or reacting normally to a life-threatening illness?). In terms of clinical practice, every diagnosis involves the ability to distinguish disorder from normal reactions to stressful environments and from other nonpathological problems, such as the marital, parent-child, and occupational conflicts summarized in the V Code categories of the revised third edition of the *Diagnostic and Statistical Manual of Mental Disorders* (*DSM-III-R*; American Psychiatric Association, 1987). At an institutional level, 'mental disorder' demarcates the special responsibilities of mental health professionals from those of other professionals such as criminal justice lawyers, teachers, and social welfare workers. Thus jurisdictional disputes are often disputes about the application of the term *mental disorder*.

Public concerns about misapplication of the term *disorder* underlie accusations of sexual, racial, and sexual orientational biases in diagnosis (Bayer, 1981; Bayer & Spitzer, 1982; Kaplan, 1983; Spitzer, 1981; Szasz, 1971; Wakefield, 1987, 1988; 1989b; Williams & Spitzer, 1983; Willie, Kramer, & Brown, 1973), as well as more general accusations that psychodiagnosis is often used to control or stigmatize socially undesirable behavior that is not really disordered (Eysenck, J. A. Wakefield, & Friedman, 1983; Foucault, 1964/1965; Goffman, 1963; Gove, 1980; Horwitz, 1982; Laing, 1967; Szasz, 1974). Awareness of past psychodiagnostic errors and abuses, such as diagnoses of 'drapetomania' (the 'disorder' that afflicted slaves who ran away from their masters; Cartwright, 1851/1981; Szasz, 1971), 'childhood mastur-bation disorder' (Englehardt, 1974; Foucault, 1978), and 'lack of vaginal orgasm' (Kaplan, 1983), sets the stage for today's controversies over diagnoses such as 'self-defeating personality disorder' (American Psychiatric Association, 1987; P. J. Caplan, 1984), 'premenstrual syndrome' (American Psychiatric Association, 1987; Ussher, 1989), 'alcoholism' (Fingarette, 1988, 1990; Gorman, 1989a, 1989b; Vaillant, 1990), 'hyperactivity' (Coles, 1987; Cowart, 1988; Kohn, 1989; Pond, 1960; Rutter, Graham, & Yule, 1970),

'homosexuality' (Bayer, 1981; Bayer & Spitzer, 1982; Spitzer, 1981), and many others, all of which controversies would benefit from a clearer understanding of the concept of disorder. Finally, a correct understanding of the concept is essential for constructing 'conceptually valid' (Wakefield, in press) diagnostic criteria that are good discriminators between disorder and nondisorder.

The concept of disorder is not the same as a theory of disorder. Physiological, behavioral, psychoanalytic, and other theories attempt to explain the causes and specify the underlying mechanisms of mental disorder, whereas the concept of disorder is the criterion used to identify the domain that all these theories are trying to explain. The concept is largely shared by professionals and the lay public (Campbell, Scadding, & Roberts, 1979) and is the basis for the attempt in *DSM-III-R* to construct universally acceptable atheoretical diagnostic criteria (Spitzer & Williams, 1983, 1988; Wakefield, in press). The concept is certainly more complex than the simple 'suffering' and 'problems in living' criteria that are sometimes suggested: Grieving a lost spouse involves considerable suffering and being in a bad marriage is a problem in living but neither is a disorder. Despite a vast literature spanning philosophy, psychology, psychiatry, and medicine devoted to the concept of mental disorder, there currently exists no widely accepted analysis that adequately explains even generally agreed upon, uncontroversial judgments about which conditions are disorders. I shall attempt to construct an account that explains such uncontroversial judgments; until such an analysis is available, using a definition of *disorder* as an arbiter of controversies is premature.

Among analyses of the concept of mental disorder, the most basic division is between value and scientific approaches. As Kendell (1986) put it.

> The most fundamental issue, and also the most contentious one, is whether disease and illness are normative concepts based on value judgments, or whether they are value-free scientific terms; in other words, whether they are biomedical terms or sociopolitical ones. (p. 25)

To construct a more adequate analysis and resolve the fact/value debate, I propose a hybrid account of disorder as harmful dysfunction, wherein *dysfunction* is a scientific and factual term based in evolutionary biology that refers to the failure of an internal mechanism to perform a natural function for which it was designed, and *harmful* is a value term referring to the consequences that occur to the person because of the dysfunction and are deemed negative by sociocultural standards.

Because the general concept of disorder, which applies to both mental and physical conditions, is the subject of the present analysis, examples from both the mental and physical realms are equally relevant and are used. I use *internal mechanism* as a general term to refer to both physical structures and organs and mental structures and dispositions, such as motivational, cognitive, affective, and perceptual mechanisms. Also, some writers draw distinctions among *disorder, disease,* and *illness. Disorder* is perhaps the broader term because it covers traumatic injuries as well as disease/ illness. I ignore these differences and use the discussions of related terms as if they refer to *disorder* whenever they contribute useful insights.

First, I review the problems with six standard analyses of the concept of disorder and informally suggest how a harmful dysfunction approach

* Wakefield, J. C.: The concept of mental disorder: on the boundary between biological facts and social values. *American Psychologist* 47:373–388, 1992.

might avoid these problems, if such a view could be precisely and clearly developed. I then analyze the critical concept of natural function so as to have a clear basis for attributing dysfunction (i.e., the loss of a natural function) and thus, in cases in which dysfunction is harmful, disorder.

Problems With Standard Analyses of Mental Disorder

The Myth of the Myth of Mental Disorder

The first question in analyzing the concept of mental disorder is whether the concept exists. Several skeptical writers (e.g., Foucault, 1964/1965, 1978; Sarbin, 1969; Scheff, 1966, 1975; Szasz, 1974) have attempted to cast doubt on the concept's coherence. The skeptics typically claim that 'mental disorder' is merely an evaluative label that justifies the use of medical power (in the broad sense, in which all the professions concerned with pathology, including psychiatry, clinical psychology, and clinical social work, are considered medical) to intervene in socially disapproved behavior. The strength of the skeptical perspective is that it explains the frequency with which the label 'mental disorder' has been misapplied, as in 'drapetomania' and 'childhood masturbation disorder.' However, this strength is bought at a considerable price. According to the skeptical view, all applications of 'mental disorder' are illegitimate, so the ability to distinguish correct from incorrect uses, target criticisms, and improve criteria is lost.

Two arguments are proposed by the skeptics. First. the skeptics present many practical, ethical, and epistemological concerns about psychodiagnosis. They note, for example, that people who are labeled as mentally disordered are often stigmatized, psychodiagnosis is often used for purposes of social control, and it is often difficult to tell whether someone is mentally disordered. Such concerns, legitimate and important though they are, must be separated from questions about the coherence and logic of the concept of disorder (Gorenstein, 1984; Horwitz, 1982). The need for such separation of issues can be illustrated with a physical example: People who are labeled as human immunodeficiency virus (HIV) positive are often socially stigmatized; such labeling is often used for purposes of social control; and, because of imperfections in available tests, it is sometimes hard to establish whether someone is HIV positive. Despite all these problems, the concept of HIV positivity is perfectly coherent and HIV-positive status does truly exist. Thus practical, ethical, and epistemological problems simply do not demonstrate that there is something wrong with the concept of mental disorder. Similar comments apply to attempts to discredit mental disorder through analysis of the historical processes that led up to the adoption of this concept (Foucault, 1964/1965) or of the sociological processes that influence diagnosis (Scheff, 1966, 1975).

The skeptics' second argument is more to the point because it directly addresses the nature of disorder. This argument has been put forward most explicitly by Szasz (1974), but it is implicit in most other skeptical positions as well. Szasz began with the assumption that physical disorder is a legitimate concept based on a clear foundation, namely, that a disorder consists of a physical lesion, with *lesion* referring to a recognizable deviation in anatomical structure. Szasz continued with the observation that mental disorder is an extension of the concept of physical disorder to the mental realm. Therefore, mental disorders exist only if the very same concept of disorder that applies to physical conditions also applies to the mental conditions labeled as disorders. Otherwise, the application of *disorder* to mental conditions is merely an analogy or metaphor. Szasz next maintained that mental disorder is used to label behavior that deviates from social norms and that the psychological functioning that is said to be a mental disorder is typically not accompanied by any identifiable lesion of the brain or of any other part of the body. (Szasz implicitly assumed that no lesions would be found in the future to explain such conditions.) Thus, the lesion concept of disorder that is applicable to physical conditions is not applicable to mental conditions, and mental disorders are not literally disorders. Szasz concluded that 'there is no such thing as "mental illness" ' (1974, p. 1). Sarbin (1969) similarly asserted that

'contemporary users of the mental illness concept are guilty of illicitly shifting from metaphor to myth' (p. 15).

The weakness in Szasz's (1974) argument lies in the inadequacy of the lesion account of physical disorder. The account consists of two theses: (a) that a lesion (or abnormal bodily structure) is simply a statistical deviation from a typical anatomical structure and (b) that a physical disorder is simply a lesion. First, the idea that a lesion can be directly recognized by its deviant anatomical structure is incorrect. Bodily structures normally vary from person to person, and many normal variations are as unusual as any lesion. Moreover, some lesions are statistically nondeviant in a culture, such as atherosclerosis, minor lung irritation, and gum recession in American culture and hookworm and malaria in some others. Therefore recognition of a lesion is not simply a matter of observing anatomical deviance. Second, and more important, it is not the existence of a lesion that defines disorder. There are physical disorders, such as trigeminal neuralgia and senile pruritis (Kendell, 1975), for which there are no known anatomical lesions. Moreover, a lesion can be a harmless abnormality that is nota disorder, such as when the heart is positioned on the right side of the body but retains functional integrity. Kendell compared lesions that are disorders with similar lesions that are not disorders in order to show that the existence of lesions is not what distinguishes disorder from nondisorder in the physical realm:

A child with spina bifida and an oligophrenic imbecile both suffer from congenital diseases – the first by virtue of an anatomical defect acquired early in embryonic development, the second because of the absence of the enzyme needed to convert phenylalanine to tyrosine. But children with fused second and third toes have a similar congenital defect to those with spina bifida, and those with albinism also lack an enzyme involved in tyrosine metabolism, yet despite the presence of these lesions we do not normally wish to regard them as ill. (p. 308)

Thus the lesion account of physical disorder fails, and with it goes the skeptics' case that the concept of disorder cannot literally apply to mental conditions.

How, then, *do* we recognize deviations that are lesions and lesions that are disorders? Roughly, we recognize a variation in anatomical structure as a lesion rather than as a normal variation if the variation impairs the ability of the particular structure to accomplish the functions that it was designed to perform. Such an impairment of a specific mechanism might be referred to as a 'part dysfunction' (Lewis, 1967; see also Klein, 1978). We recognize a part dysfunction/lesion as a disorder only if the deviation in the functioning of the part affects the well-being of the overall organism in a harmful way. For example, the reason that fused toes, albinism, and reversal of heart position are not considered disorders even though they are abnormal anatomical variations is that they do not significantly harm a person. Thus, a harmful dysfunction approach to the concept of disorder would seem to explain what the skeptics' lesion account cannot explain, namely, which anatomical deviations are lesions and which lesions are disorders.

If lesion is essentially a functional concept, then mental conditions and physical conditions can literally be disorders for the very same reason, that is, their functional implications. Considering that mental processes play important species-typical roles in human survival and reproduction, there is no reason to doubt that mental processes were naturally selected and have natural functions, as Darwin himself often emphasized (Boorse, 1976a). Because of our evolutionary heritage, we possess physical mechanisms such as livers and hearts; that same heritage gave us mental mechanisms such as various cognitive, motivational, affective, personological, hedonic, linguistic, and behavioral dispositions and structures. Some mental conditions interfere with the ability of these mental mechanisms to perform the functions that they were designed to perform. In such cases, there is a part dysfunction of the particular mental mechanism. The concept of disorder, whether applied to liver disorders, heart disorders, or mental disorders, refers to part dysfunctions that harm the person. Contrary to Szasz's (1974) and Sarbin's (1967, 1969), claims, the notion of a mental disorder is not a myth based on a bad metaphor but a literal application to the mental realm of the same harmful dysfunction concept of disorder that applies in the physical realm.

Disorder as a Pure Value Concept

The typical response to the skeptics is to argue that mental disorder is an objective scientific concept, like physical disorder (examples of this scientific approach are provided later). However, other thinkers who try to show that mental disorders are genuine disorders accept the skeptics' contention that mental disorder is a value concept and argue that physical disorder is also a value concept.

Quite correctly, the anti-psychiatrists have pointed out that psychopathological categories refer to value-judgments and that mental illness is deviancy. On the other hand, the anti-psychiatric critics themselves are wrong when they imagine physical medicine to be essentially different in its logic from psychiatry. A diagnosis of diabetes, or paresis, includes the recognition of norms or values. (Sedgwick, 1982, p. 38)

The pure value account of disorder asserts that disorder is nothing (or almost nothing) but a value concept, so that social judgments of disorder are nothing but judgments of desirability according to social norms and ideals. The pure value approach is to be distinguished from a mixed or hybrid approach (Boorse, 1975; Klein, 1978), of the kind to be defended later, in which values play some role but in which there are important factual components to the concept of disorder as well.

The value account reflects an important truth: Because disorders are negative conditions that justify social concern, social values are involved. On the other hand, the pure value view has the disadvantage that it makes disorder (both mental and physical) a completely value-and-culture-relative notion with no scientific content whatsoever, thereby leaving the concept open to unconstrained use for purposes of social control. Nonetheless, a considerable number of writers have taken the pure value position or strongly emphasized the evaluative element in their analyses. Ausubel (1971) defined disease as 'any marked deviation, physical, mental, or behavioral, from normally desirable standards of structural or functional integrity' (p. 60). Marmor (1973) stated, 'To call homosexuality the result of disturbed development really says nothing other than that you disapprove of the outcome of that development' (p. 1208). Pichot (1986) asserted, 'The definition of disease in every language is "something bad" ' (p. 56). King (1954/1981) wrote, 'Disease is the aggregate of those conditions which, judged by the prevailing culture, are deemed painful, or disabling, and which, at the same time, deviate from either the statistical norm or from some idealized status' (p. 112). Engelhardt (1974) stated that 'choosing to call a set of phenomena a disease involves . . . judgments closely bound to value judgments' (p. 41). The World Health Organization (1946/1981) defined health as 'a state of complete physical, mental and social well-being' (p. 83). This appears to assume that disorder is any deviation from a completely desirable and ideal state. Sedgwick (1982) was perhaps the most articulate spokesman for the pure value position: 'All sickness is essentially deviancy [from] some alternative state of affairs which is considered more desirable. . . . The attribution of illness always proceeds from the computation of a gap between presented behavior (or feeling) and some social norm' (pp. 32–34).

The fact that all disorders are undesirable and harmful according to social values shows only that values are part of the concept of disorder, not that disorder is composed only of values. Sedgwick (1982) suggested through vivid examples that there is nothing objective or scientific that distinguishes the conditions said to be disorders from other processes in nature, leaving the value element as the only identifying characteristic:

There are no illnesses or diseases in nature. . . . The fracture of a septuagenarian's femur has, within the world of nature, no more significance than the snapping of an autumn leaf from its twig; and the invasion of a human organism by cholera-germs carries with it no more the stamp of 'illness' than does the souring of milk by other forms of bacteria. . . . Out of his anthropocentric self-interest, man has chosen to consider as 'illnesses' or 'diseases' those natural circumstances which precipitate . . . death (or the failure to function according to certain values). (p. 30)

However, completely aside from values, there is a relevant difference between the cracking of a femur and the snapping off of an autumn leaf: The leaf is designed to fall off at a certain stage and the tree is not designed to require the leaf for its continued functioning, whereas the possession of an intact femur is part of the way a person, even an old person, is designed to function. Similarly, once it is extracted from the cow, milk certainly has no natural function, so the bacteria that invade and sour it are not causing a dysfunction, whereas the person who is infected with bacteria is in danger of losing functional integrity. Thus, if natural function is a scientific concept that cannot be reduced to values (as is argued later), then there is a scientifically definable difference between Sedgwick's (1982) examples of natural processes that are disorders and those that are not; that is, the ones that are disorders disrupt a natural function.

The most basic objection to the pure value position is that there are obviously a great many undesirable conditions that are not classifiable as disorders. Recognizing that not all undesirable states are considered disorders, Sedgwick (1982) added to the value account one factual requirement—that the cause of the undesirable condition could not lie entirely in external circumstances but must be inside the individual's body or mind. This would explain why externally caused undesirable conditions such as poverty, bad luck, or being sexually rejected are not disorders. However, it would not explain why other undesirable conditions that are internal, such as ignorance and the pain of teething, are also not considered disorders. A dysfunction account explains why these latter conditions are not disorders: Although they are internal, they do not involve a breakdown in the functioning of an internal mechanism.

Another problem with the pure value position is that it does not explain how people can be mistaken about disorder and how people who share social norms and values can disagree about which conditions are disorders. For example, slaves who ran away from their masters were not in fact suffering from a disorder of 'drapetomania,' even though the dominant social order saw the condition as undesirable, and many incarcerated Soviet dissidents were not in fact mentally disordered despite the fact that they violated social norms. If one embraces the pure value position, one has no grounds for asserting that these diagnoses were incorrect in their context. Moreover, our culture clearly disvalues such conditions as premenstrual syndrome, hyperactivity, and alcoholism, and yet there are ongoing disputes about whether each of these is a disorder. The complex factual arguments presented by both sides in these debates clearly indicate that judgments about disorder depend on much more than values.

To say that a condition is undesirable or socially disvalued does not imply anything about the cause of the condition. Thus, the pure value view fails to account for the fact that attributions of disorder are attempts to partially explain behavior and/or symptoms. For example, the question 'Why is that man talking to himself?' can be coherently answered by explanations in terms of rational action (e.g., 'Because he is trying to memorize a list by repeating it aloud') or the manifestation of a disorder (e.g., 'Because he is suffering from schizophrenia'). Admittedly, an explanation in terms of disorder says very little if nothing more is known about the attributed disorder, but it eliminates enough alternative explanations to be useful. The explanatory content of disorder attributions shows that they involve more than sheer value judgments. We shall see later that the explanatory content of disorder attributions is nicely explained by the functional approach.

Disorder as Whatever Professionals Treat

Frustration with failed attempts to analyze the concept of mental disorder often leads to the practical-sounding suggestion that a disorder is simply any condition that health professionals treat. For example, Taylor (1976) asserted that a disorder consists in part of the 'attribute of therapeutic concern for a person felt by the person himself and/or his social environment' (p. 581), and Kendell (1986) suggested that we stop trying to diagnostically distinguish disorders from 'the problems that psychiatrists are currently consulted about' (pp. 41–42).

However, many concerns that are handled by health professionals clearly are not disorders, but are assigned to health professionals because of their special skills. For example, professionals are regularly called on to provide 'treatment' in cases of childbirth, unwanted pregnancy, circumcision, cosmetic surgery, and distresses due to the normal vicissitudes of life.

DSM-III-R has a special section of V Code diagnostic categories just for conditions that are not disorders but are often treated by mental health professionals, such as marital conflicts, adolescent-parent conflict, and occupational problems. These are conditions in which there is some harm, but not a genuine dysfunction or disorder.

Furthermore, both the patient and the therapist can be wrong about whether a condition is a disorder. For example, Victorian medical books indicate that many people came to physicians seeking treatment of the 'masturbatory disease' from which, under the influence of the writings of the very same physicians, they thought they were suffering, and women sought out treatment—sometimes surgical—for the 'perverse' clitoral orgasms that afflicted them (e.g., Acton, 1871; Barker-Benfield, 1983; Schrenck-Notzing, 1895/1956; Showalter, 1987; Ussher, 1989). Despite what the doctors and patients thought, the patients' masturbatory activities and clitoral orgasms were not in fact disorders, contrary to the whatever-professionals-treat approach. The possibility of error is explained by a functional approach; the diagnostician can simply have an incorrect belief about what a mechanism was naturally designed to do.

Finally, this approach would paradoxically imply that lack of social concern can eliminate disorder. Kendell (1975) himself, in an article in which he criticized the view he later adopted, noted that 'equating illness with "therapeutic concern" implies that no one can be ill until he has been recognized as such, and also gives doctors, and society, free rein to label all deviants as ill' (p. 307).

Disorder as Statistical Deviance

The skeptics claim that physical disorders are lesions and mental disorders are socially deviant behavior and thus the two are not instances of the same concept of disorder. However, if one accepts the skeptics' notion that a lesion is a statistical deviation in anatomical structure, then one might claim that lesions and deviant behavior do have something in common, namely, statistical deviance. If statistical deviance makes either a physical or a mental condition a disorder, then the same concept of disorder can be applied to both domains, and the criterion is purely objective and scientific.

The classical statement of the statistical approach to disorder is Sir Henry Cohen's (1981) definition of disease as 'quantitative deviations from the normal' (p. 218), in which by *normal* he meant the statistical norm. Statistical abnormality is a requirement of many other definitions, including those of Taylor (1971), Scadding (1967), Kendell (1975), King (1954/1981), and even *DSM-III-R* (discussed later). As Claridge (1985) noted, Eysenck's (1986) dimensional system of diagnosis also presupposes a statistical approach to disorder.

One basic problem with this view is that excellence in strength, intelligence, energy, talent, or any other area is just as statistically deviant as its opposite. Moreover, an individual's fingerprint, the precise shape of his or her heart, and endless other neutral features can be deviant and even unique but still normal. An obvious suggestion to avoid this problem is to add the requirement that the deviance must be in a negative direction. (We shall see later that this is essentially the strategy of *DSM-III-R*.) However, there are many behaviors that are statistically deviant and undesirable but are not disorders; for example, such behavior can be criminal, discourteous, ignorant, morally repugnant, or disadvantageous. For a man, being five feet tall is statistically deviant and presumably undesirable but not a disorder; the same goes for men or women being clumsy, having a slow reaction time, and so on.

Another problem with the statistical deviance view of disorder is that many conditions that are statistically normal in their context are still disorders. For example, as noted earlier, minor lung irritation from pollution, atherosclerosis, periodontal disease, and dental caries all seem to be statistically normal in American society, and such disorders as hookworm and malaria are so endemic in other societies as to be statistically normal, but all these conditions are still considered disorders. In fact, there is nothing incoherent about a virtually universal disorder, as might occur as a result of an uncontrolled epidemic or radiation poisoning after a nuclear war. Thus statistical deviance cannot be part of what we mean by disorder.

Although statistical deviance is not the same as disorder, disorder often is statistically deviant. From a functional perspective, this is understandable. In general, mechanisms function as they were naturally designed to function; failures of function are usually deviant. As the preceding examples show, however, functional abnormality and statistical abnormality do not necessarily go together. Dysfunction is judged on the basis of standards set by the design of internal mechanisms rather than by statistical norms.

Disorder as Biological Disadvantage

In order to conceptualize disorder in purely scientific terms, more than sheer statistical deviation is needed. If the definition must equally fit both physical and mental disorders, then a reasonable place to look for an account of disorder is within the biological sciences. The biological sciences are the scientific basis for physical medicine, and the mind is, after all, a part of the organism and has evolved like other parts of the organism. Mental mechanisms like those involved in perception, motivation, emotion, linguistic ability, and cognition play distinctive but coordinated roles in overall mental functioning, much as different organs play distinctive but coordinated roles in physical functioning. Thus, a biological account based on evolutionary theory has seemed to many to be potentially capable of handling the concepts of both mental and physical disorder in a scientific and value-free manner.

Note that although the use of an evolutionary perspective makes an account of the mind biological, it does not necessarily make it physiological or anatomical. The evolutionary approach accepts descriptions of mental and behavioral mechanisms as legitimate biological descriptions of the advantageous mechanisms that were naturally selected (Buss, 1991).

Three different accounts of disorder that involve evolutionary theory are considered in the remainder of this article; confusion might be avoided if they are distinguished here. The first, considered in this section, is the view of Scadding, Kendell, and Boorse, who used the evolution-derived general criterion of lowered survival or lowered reproductive fitness, as a purely scientific means for identifying disorders. The second evolutionary account, suggested in passing in the Disorder as Harmful Dysfunction section, considers an organism disordered when some mental mechanism (e.g., perception or the fear response) does not perform the specific function (e.g., convey information about the environment or help the organism to avoid certain dangers) that it was designed by evolution to perform. This too is a purely scientific criterion. The third evolutionary approach, which is argued in the aforementioned section to be the correct one, combines the second approach (using the specific natural functions of mechanisms) with a value component, so that a person is disordered only when some mechanism fails to perform the specific function it was designed to perform and the failure of the mechanism causes the person real harm.

Scadding (1967, 1990) proposed a purely scientific biological definition of disorder by in effect translating the earlier harmful statistical deviation account into a biologically disadvantageous deviation account:

The name of a disease refers to the sum of the abnormal phenomena displayed by a group of living organisms in association with a specific common characteristic, or set of characteristics, by which they differ from the norm for their species in such a way as to place them at a biological disadvantage. (Scadding, 1990, p. 243)

Kendell (1975) elaborated and extended Scadding's biological disadvantage analysis, and Boorse (1975, 1976a) offered a very similar approach.

Scadding (1967, 1990) never explained what he meant by biological disadvantage, and on the surface it would seem that *disadvantage*, contrary to intent, is a value term. Kendell (1975) and Boorse (1975, 1976a) tried to get around the value implication by using biological theory itself as an objective criterion for what constitutes the relevant type of disadvantage. According to the theory of evolution, the prime advantages to accrue from any internal mechanism or structure are survival and reproductive fitness. (Actually, from an evolutionary perspective, survival also serves the one ultimate goal of reproductive fitness, but so many of the organism's mechanisms are aimed directly at survival in a way that is relatively remote from reproductive activity that it is convenient to use both criteria.) Thus, both

Kendell and Boorse claimed that a disorder is a condition that reduces longevity or fertility. This made the definition value free by in effect equating lowered fertility and longevity with harm (Kendell, 1975).

The equation is faulty, however. A condition can reduce fertility without causing real harm; marginally lowered fertility is serious over the evolutionary time scale, but it may not affect an individual's well-being if the capacity for bearing some children remains intact. And some serious harms, such as chronic pain or loss of pleasure, might not reduce fertility or longevity at all; Kendell (1975) admitted there are many harmful physical conditions, such as postherpetic neuralgia and psoriasis, that are clear cases of disorder but have no effect on mortality or fertility. This is likely to be even more true of mental disorders. It would seem that the harm requirement must be added to, rather than derived from, the evolutionary requirement.

Another problem with Scadding's (1967, 1990) account is that his statistical deviance requirement runs afoul of the counterexamples to the statistical approach presented earlier. As Kendell (1975) noted of both Scadding's and his own position, 'the majority are debarred from being regarded as ill' (p. 309). But this, as we have seen, is not part of our concept of disorder and leads to numerous actual and potential counterexamples. The reason that Scadding and Kendell cannot just scrap the statistical deviation requirement and take biological disadvantage as the whole definition of disorder is that disadvantage is relative. Without the statistical deviation requirement, any disadvantage relative to anyone superior in function could be labeled a disorder, leading to an impossibly demanding criterion. Klein (1978), in an analysis otherwise extremely similar to the one I propose, made this mistake of relativizing disorder to 'optimal' part function: 'Disease is here defined as covert, objective, suboptimal part dysfunction, recognizing that functions are evolved and hierarchically organized' (p. 70). This implies that the existence of even a few people with unusually high functioning would mean that everyone else has a dysfunction. For example, everyone with an IQ lower than 180 has a brain that is functioning less than optimally and so is diseased, according to Klein's proposal. But it is how we are designed to be, not how we might ideally be, that is relevant to judgments of disorder. The same problem, of disorder's including any deviation from optimal functioning, would arise for Scadding if he defined disorder simply as biological disadvantage without specifying that the disadvantage is relative to the statistically normal. If Scadding were to jettison the problematic statistical deviation clause, the validity of the definition in one respect would be increased at the cost of severely decreasing the validity in another respect.

Taken at face value. Scadding's (1967, 1990) account is subject to two additional objections. First, differential fertility rates may exist between populations defined by racial, ethnic, economic, sex, personality, and many other variables. Are all these variables to be considered candidates for pathology? For example, is it a disorder to be a young Black urban male in 1990s America because that 'set of characteristics' corresponds to increased mortality? The problem is that the definition does not distinguish between disadvantage due to dysfunction of internal mechanisms and disadvantage due to harmful environments. Second, the definition implies that a disorder can be 'cured' simply by taking steps to increase the life span and fertility of the people who have the disorder, even if no change is made in their mental condition.

Kendell (1975) recognized these problems and tried to solve them by requiring that the effects of the condition on mortality and fertility be 'innate' or 'intrinsic' rather than due to social factors such as rejection by others: 'The criterion must be, would this individual still be at a disadvantage if his fellows did not recognize his distinguishing features but treated him as they treat one another?' (p. 314). But because humans are social animals, it is impossible to separate the functioning of the organism from all consideration of how others respond. For example, aphasia is certainly a disorder, but language functions as a communication device between individuals, so if the reactions of others to one's attempts to speak are entirely discounted from consideration, then there are no grounds for classifying aphasia as a disorder. Even in the case of schizophrenia, which

Kendell argued is a pathology in part on the grounds that schizophrenic individuals have reduced fertility, it seems likely that the lower fertility is at least in part due to the reactions of potential partners to the schizophrenic person's mental condition, thus putting in question whether schizophrenia is indeed a disorder according to Kendell's account. (Similar questions can be raised about the source of schizophrenic individuals' higher mortality.) Moreover, many conditions, such as being male versus being female, seem to be intrinsically tied to higher mortality and yet are not disorders.

Scadding (1967, 1990), Kendell (1975), and Boorse (1975, 1976a) were right that there must be an evolutionary foundation to our judgments of disorder. The notion that something has gone wrong with the organism's internal functioning, which is critical for distinguishing between disorders and other negative conditions, can be captured only by comparing present functioning with what the organism's mechanisms were designed to do, and this requires a reference to the evolutionary explanation of the mechanism. However, the biological disadvantage approach mistakenly uses decreased longevity and fertility in the present environment as the criterion for mechanism dysfunction. The fact that the organism's mechanisms were originally selected because they increased longevity and fertility in a past environment does not imply that some mechanism is malfunctioning when longevity and fertility decrease in the present environment. Thus, despite its evolutionary roots, the biological disadvantage definition actually fails to require a dysfunction and thus is subject to counterexamples.

By directly relying on reproductive fitness in the present environment as their criterion for health. Scadding (1967, 1990) and Kendell (1975) committed a form of the 'sociobiological fallacy' (Buss, 1991; see also Wakefield, 1989a). This fallacy consists of misinterpreting evolution as conferring on the organism a general tendency to maximize fitness. In fact, evolution confers a multiplicity of specific mechanisms that do not directly aim at fitness but do have fitness as an effect in the environments in which they were selected. For example, sexual attraction is not a mechanism that directly confers maximal reproduction; it confers desire for sexual contact, and that leads to reproduction under the circumstances in which the mechanism evolved. Today, with contraceptive technology available, the sexual attraction mechanism may not ensure reproduction in the same way, but that does not mean that there is something wrong with the mechanism. It is the failure of specific mechanisms to perform their assigned tasks, rather than lowered fitness in itself, that shows that something has gone wrong with the organism. I shall use this insight later to construct a better evolution-based account of the concept of disorder.

Disorder as Unexpectable Distress or Disability

The most influential recent definition of mental disorder is the one developed by Robert Spitzer and his colleagues for *DSM-III-R*. I have presented a detailed analysis and critique of *DSM-III-R*'s definition elsewhere (Wakefield, in press), so the present discussion is limited to a few crucial points. Further support for the claims made here can be found in the aforementioned article.

The definition in *DSM-III-R* is inspired by an overall view of disorder very much like the harmful dysfunction approach I propose. For example, in their discussion of the approach to disorder in the third edition of the *Diagnostic and Statistical Manual of Mental Disorders* (*DSM-III*; American Psychiatric Association, 1980), which is essentially the same as *DSM-III-R*'s, Spitzer and Endicott (1978) listed 'dysfunction' and 'negative consequences' (which can be taken to be equivalent to 'harm') as two of the necessary conditions for disorder. Moreover, *DSM-III-R* explicitly states that a disorder must be 'a manifestation of a behavioral, psychological, or biological dysfunction in the person' (American Psychiatric Association, 1987, p. xxii). It is also required that a disorder must be associated with 'present distress (a painful symptom) or disability (impairment in one or more important areas of functioning) or with a significantly increased risk of suffering death, pain, disability, or an important loss of freedom' (p. xxii), and this list might be considered to be an operationalized approximation to the requirement that there must be harm. So, at least in initial conception, *DSM-III-R's* approach to disorder has much affinity to the harmful dysfunction view.

For two reasons, however, *DSM-III-R* does not actually define disorder as harmful dysfunction. First, as Spitzer and Endicott (1978) noted, one cannot simply define disorder in terms of dysfunction because dysfunction itself is a concept that requires analysis: 'These criteria [for disorder] avoid such terms as 'dysfunction,' 'maladaptive,' or 'abnormal,' terms which themselves beg definition' (p. 17). So, although *DSM-III-R* as well as Spitzer and Endicott indicate in the statement of the definition that a disorder must be a dysfunction, the definition of disorder actually consists of a formula that analyzes dysfunction in clearer terms and in effect replaces dysfunction in the definition. The definition is thus adequate only to the extent that the analysis of dysfunction contained in the definition is adequate.

Second, a central goal of *DSM-III-R* is to present reliable operationalized diagnostic criteria for specific disorders. The definition of disorder is aimed at providing a general framework for constructing such criteria (Spitzer & Endicott, 1978). But dysfunction is not an operational concept, and for *DSM-III-R's* purposes dysfunction must be translated into a more operational and reliable formula that captures the essential idea of dysfunction. The same point applies to harm, which must also be operationalized. Thus, the definition of disorder that actually guides the formulation of specific *DSM-III-R* diagnostic criteria is the operational definition that results after the notions of harm and dysfunction are translated into operational terms. As we shall see, it is in the process of operationalization that the problems with DSM-III-R's definition occur, because the operationalization diverges substantially from the dysfunction requirement that it is meant to capture.

To stand in for the dysfunction requirement (and thus to discriminate those harms that are disorders from all the other harms to which people are subject), *DSM-III-R* specifies that a disorder 'must not be merely an expectable response to a particular event' (American Psychiatric Association, 1987, p. xxii). The basic idea is that normal responses are expectable (e.g., fear is an expectable response to danger, and grief is an expectable response to loss of a loved one), whereas disordered responses are not expectable. *DSM-III-R* translates harm into a list of observable harms such as distress and disability; I shall take the latter two harms as an adequate approximation to *DSM-III-R's* longer list. Thus *DSM-III-R* operationally defines disorder roughly as unexpectable distress or disability. It is this definition that manifests itself in DSM-III-R criteria for specific disorders; the terms dysfunction and harm never appear in those criteria, but statistical unlikelihood and distress/disability do.

However, the unexpectable distress or disability definition fails to capture the notion of a dysfunction, and this results not only in the invalidity of the definition itself, but also in the invalidity of many *DSM-III-R* diagnostic criteria that are patterned on the definition. First, many nondisordered negative reactions (e.g., stress responses and grief) are normally statistically distributed in intensity, so that many of such reactions will be sufficiently above the mean to be 'unexpected' in the sheer statistical sense. The *DSM-III-R* definition allows the incorrect classification of such greater than average normal responses as disorders. For example, *DSM-III-R* classifies a condition as an adjustment disorder if symptoms following a psychosocial stressor 'are in excess of a normal and expectable reaction to the stressors' (American Psychiatric Association, 1987, p. 330). This implies that any reaction to a stressor that is much above the mean in intensity is classifiable as a disorder. Similarly, a child is diagnosed with oppositional defiant disorder when, during a six-month period, he or she displays certain kinds of defiant behavior, such as loss of temper, arguing with adults, refusing to do chores, and swearing, at a rate that is 'considerably more frequent than that of most people of the same age' (p. 57). These criteria confuse normal variation with disorder.

Second, there are many unexpectable conditions, from extreme ignorance to plain misfortune, that can cause distress or disability but are not disorders. Some telling examples are contained in *DSM-III-R's* own V Codes. Although *DSM-III-R* states correctly that these conditions are not disorders, many types and intensities of marital, parent-child, and occupational problems that fall under the V Codes are unexpectable distresses and

disabilities that are classifiable as disorders according to the *DSM-III-R* definition. As another example, consider an adolescent who runs away from home for a second time, breaks into a car, and steals something; these are potentially harmful and unexpectable behaviors. Such an adolescent is disordered according to the criteria for the *DSM-III-R* diagnosis of conduct disorder. Yet this adolescent may just be rebellious, foolish, or desperate rather than disordered.

Third, *DSM-III-R's* diagnostic criteria incorrectly allow normal responses to abusive treatment to be classified as disordered. For example, chronic depressed feelings can be due to a dysfunctional cognitive or affective system, or they can be a normal response to chronically depressing external circumstances such as abuse, neglect, or illness. *DSM-III-R's* criteria for dysthymia do not adequately discriminate these possible sources of depressive symptoms; they merely classify unexpectedly high levels of negative affect as a disorder.

The unexpectability requirement leads to other problems as well. For example, a 'merely expectable response' to an extreme trauma is posttraumatic stress disorder, and an expectable response to lack of contact with a caregiver in infancy is anaclitic depression, but these conditions are disorders nonetheless.

All these problems result from the fact that *DSM-III-R's* operational definition of disorder fails to match the dysfunction requirement that inspired it. For example, a dysfunction requirement would imply that an adjustment disorder would have to involve a breakdown in the way the coping mechanisms were designed to function and not merely a greater than average response to stress. The acts of a desperate teenager may be foolish, but they need not involve a dysfunction. Posttraumatic stress disorder is classifiable as a disorder despite its expectability after trauma if, as appears plausible from the nature of the condition, it involves a breakdown in the functioning of coping mechanisms. What is needed to resolve these problems is a better analysis of dysfunction.

A last point concerns the translation of harm into distress or disability. The list of harms in *DSM-III-R* and various secondary publications is longer than and different from the specific list of harms in *DSM-III*. One suspects that any kind of harm that is due to a dysfunction of some internal mechanism could be called a disorder and therefore the list of possible harms is potentially endless. Although a typology of harms such as that provided by *DSM-III-R* is useful, it should not be forgotten that, as Spitzer and Williams (1982) stated, the underlying reason these effects are relevant to disorder is that they are negative and this evaluative element is fundamental to our judgments about disorder. This value component should be reflected in, rather than obscured by, the definition of disorder.

Disorder as Harmful Dysfunction

Functions as Effects That Explain Their Causes

The preceding critique provides several important lessons. The concept of disorder must include a factual component so that disorders can be distinguished from a myriad of other disvalued conditions. On the other hand, facts alone are not enough; disorder requires harm, which involves values. Thus both values and facts are involved in the concept of disorder. With respect to the factual component of the concept. I suggested earlier that the problems with the lesion, statistical deviation, whatever professionals treat, biological disadvantage, and *DSM-III-R* analyses of disorder could all be avoided, and the facts cited in support of those approaches explained, by a suitable dysfunction analysis. The notions of function and dysfunction are central to the factual-scientific component of disorder.

However, all the preceding points were made informally, without a clear and precise analysis of dysfunction to support them. In a similarly informal way, the view that the concept of disorder somehow involves the concepts of function and dysfunction emerges with remarkable consistency in the remarks of many authors who otherwise differ in their views (e.g., Ausubel, 1971; Boorse, 1975, 1976a; A. L. Caplan, 1981; Flew, 1981; Kendell, 1975, 1986; Klein. 1978; Macklin, 1981; Moore, 1978; Ruse, 1973; Scadding, 1967,

1990; Spitzer & Endicott 1978). Spitzer and Endicott (1978) noted the seeming necessity and virtual universality of using dysfunction to make sense of disorder: 'Our approach makes explicit an underlying assumption that is present in all discussions of disease or disorder, i.e., the concept of organismic dysfunction' (p. 37).

Despite the virtually universal tendency to fall back on dysfunction to explain disorder and the potential explanatory power of the dysfunction approach, *dysfunction* rarely appears in actual definitions of disorder. Because there is no standard account of what dysfunction is, citing dysfunction provides no conclusive insight into disorder. Even the connection I assumed earlier among dysfunction, natural functions, and evolutionary theory is not obvious and needs to be justified. Still, if dysfunction can be analyzed in clearer and more basic terms, then an adequate and generally acceptable criterion for disorder might be constructed using the results.

What, then, is a dysfunction? An obvious place to begin is the supposition that a dysfunction implies an unfulfilled function, that is, a failure of some mechanism in the organism to perform its function. However, not all kinds of functions are relevant. For example, one's nose functions to hold up one's glasses, and the sound of the heart performs a useful function in medical diagnosis. But a person whose nose is shaped in such a way that it does not properly support glasses does not thereby have a nasal disorder, and a person whose heart does not make the usual sounds is not thereby suffering from a cardiac disorder. A disorder is different from a failure to function in a socially preferred manner precisely because a dysfunction exists only when an organ cannot perform as it is naturally (i.e., independently of human intentions) supposed to perform. Presumably, the functions that are relevant are natural functions, about which concept there is a large literature that I draw on shortly (Boorse, 1976b; A. L. Caplan, 1981; Cummins, 1975; Elster, 1983; Hempel, 1965; Klein, 1978; Moore, 1978; Nagel, 1979; Woodfield, 1976; Wright, 1973, 1976). For example, one of the heart's natural functions is to pump the blood, and that is why a cessation of pumping is a dysfunction. A natural function of the perceptual apparatus is to convey roughly accurate information about the immediate environment, and that is why gross hallucinations indicate dysfunctions. Some cognitive mechanisms have the function of providing a person with the capacity for a degree of rationality as expressed in deductive, inductive, and means–end reasoning (I am referring not to ideal rationality as represented by theoretical models, but to simply the degree of rationality that people manifest in everyday inferences), and that is why it is a dysfunction when the capacity for such reasoning breaks down, as in severe psychotic states.

To understand dysfunction, then, we need an analysis of natural function. Hempel (1965) usefully posed the problem of natural function as follows: Each organ has many effects, most of which are not its natural functions. For example, the heart has the effects of pumping the blood and making a sound in the chest, but only pumping the blood is a natural function. An analysis of natural function must specify what distinguishes an organ's natural functions from its other effects.

The concept of function also applies to artifacts, such as automobiles, chairs, and pens. It seems likely that the concept of function was analogically extended from artifacts to organs (Wright, 1973, 1976). Therefore, the use of the term *function* in the case of naturally occurring mechanisms must be a way to refer to properties that such mechanisms share with artifacts. Now, the function of an artifact is just the purpose for which the artifact was designed: for example, the functions of automobiles, chairs, and pens are respectively, to enable us to transport ourselves, to sit, and to write, because those are the benefits the artifacts are designed to provide. But organisms and their organs occur naturally and were not really designed by anyone with a purpose consciously in mind, so design and purpose cannot be the shared property. Of course, evolutionary biologists commonly talk in terms of purpose and design when they talk about natural functions, but that just brings the puzzle back a step: What justifies such talk in the case of naturally occurring mechanisms? The extension of function from artifacts to natural mechanisms must be justified by some other shared property that lies beneath talk of design and purpose and gives that talk its importance.

The function of an artifact is important largely because, via its connection to design and purpose, it has tremendous explanatory value. The function explains why the artifact was made, why it is structured the way it is, why the parts interact as they do, and why one can accomplish certain things with the artifact. For example, we can partially explain why automobiles exist, why automobile engines are structured as they are, and why with suitable learning one can get from place to place with the help of an automobile, all just by referring to the automobile's function of providing transportation.

Functional explanations of artifacts have the odd feature that an effect (e.g., transportation) is claimed to somehow explain the very artifact (e.g., automobiles) that provides the effect. Consequently, it has sometimes been claimed that functional explanations violate the basic principle that a cause must come before its effect. However, a description of the function can legitimately enter into the explanation of the artifact if there is some additional theory that shows that the cited effect plays some role in the events that preceded the artifact's creation. For artifacts, that theory is very simple and well known. The benefit precedes the artifact in the sense that it is represented beforehand in the mind of the person who designs the artifact. Thus, a functional explanation (e.g., 'The function of an automobile is to provide transportation' or, equivalently, 'Automobiles exist in order to provide transportation') is a sketch of a fuller causal explanation: The artifact (e.g., an automobile) exists because someone desired a certain effect (e.g., transportation) and believed that creating that artifact was a way to obtain the effect, and the belief and desire, which preceded the artifact, caused the person to create the artifact.

I have argued that the function of an artifact is important because of its explanatory power and that function explanations of artifacts have a distinctive form—the existence and structure of the artifact are explained by reference to the artifact's effects. It is this form of explanatory implication that statements about artifact functions and natural functions have in common and that justifies extending talk of functions from artifacts to natural mechanisms. Natural mechanisms, like artifacts, can be partially explained by referring to their effects, and natural functions, like artifact functions, are those effects that enter into such explanations. For example, the heart's effect of pumping the blood is also part of the heart's explanation, in that one can legitimately answer a question such as 'Why do we have hearts?' or 'Why do hearts exist?' with 'Because hearts pump the blood.' The effect of pumping the blood also enters into explanations of the detailed structure and activity of the heart. Thus, pumping the blood is a natural function of the heart. Anatomical and physiological research is largely devoted to establishing the natural functions of organs and explaining the features of an organ in terms of their contributions to the organ's natural functions. Talk of design and purpose in the case of naturally occurring mechanisms is just a metaphorical way to refer to this unique explanatory property that the effects of a mechanism explain the mechanism. In sum, the concept of natural function can be analyzed as follows: A natural function of an organ or other mechanism is an effect of the organ or mechanism that enters into an explanation of the existence, structure, or activity of the organ or mechanism.

An important feature of functional explanations is that they can be plausible and very useful even when little is known about the actual nature of a mechanism. With natural mechanisms, as with artifacts, the benefits that they provide are so remarkable and depend on such intricate and harmonious interactions that it is often reasonable to infer that the benefit is not accidental. In such cases, if no alternative explanations exist, it is reasonable to infer that the artifact exists because it has these effects. For example, it cannot be merely a happy accident that the eyes enable us to see, the legs enable us to walk, and the heart pumps the blood any more than it is a happy accident that the automobile provides transportation. The eyes therefore must exist in part because they enable us to see; that is, the fact that the eyes provide sight must somehow enter into the explanation of why we have eyes. This makes seeing a function of the eyes. Obviously, one can go wrong in such explanatory attempts; what seems nonaccidental may turn out to be accidental. But often one is right, and functional explanatory hypotheses communicate complex knowledge that may not be so easily and efficiently communicated in any other way.

The preceding analysis applies equally well to the natural functions of mental mechanisms and thus forms a common basis for the attribution of physical and mental disorder. Like artifacts and organs, mental mechanisms, such as cognitive, linguistic, perceptual, affective, and motivational mechanisms, have such strikingly beneficial effects and depend on such complex and harmonious interactions that the effects cannot be entirely accidental. Thus, functional explanations of mental mechanisms are sometimes justified by what we know about how people manage to survive and reproduce. For example, one function of linguistic mechanisms is to provide a capacity for communication, one function of the fear response is to help a person to avoid danger, and one function of tiredness is to bring about rest and sleep. These functional explanations yield ascriptions of dysfunctions when respective mechanisms fail to perform their functions, as in aphasia, phobia, and insomnia, respectively.

Dysfunction and Evolutionary Theory

We now have an account of natural functions as effects that explain the existence and structure of naturally occurring physical and mental mechanisms. Correspondingly, dysfunction is the failure of a mechanism to perform its natural function. The next step is to provide this abstract analysis with some theoretical substance by linking it to the theory of evolution.

As in the case of artifacts, natural function explanations appear on the surface to violate the principle that a cause comes before its effects. For example, 'Sexual desire exists because it causes people to copulate and reproduce' seems to explain sexual desire in terms of something that normally comes after it. To understand exactly how and in what sense such effects can play a role in causing the respective mechanisms requires an additional theory.

In the case of artifacts, it is a prior mental representation of the effect that explains the existence of the artifact. Coming up with a similar demystifying causal explanation in the case of natural functions has posed an age-old mystery: Why, indeed, should our internal mechanisms be so beneficially designed? Until recently, the mystery could be dealt with only by assuming that there exists a God who purposely created our internal mechanisms with benevolent intentions. According to this theory, our internal mechanisms are artifacts created by a divine entity, so natural functions are reduced to a special case of artifact functions.

Today evolutionary theory provides a better explanation of how a mechanism's effects can explain the mechanism's presence and structure. In brief, those mechanisms that happened to have effects on past organisms that contributed to the organisms' reproductive success over enough generations increased in frequency and hence were 'naturally selected' and exist in today's organisms. Thus, an explanation of a mechanism in terms of its natural function may be considered a roundabout way of referring to a causal explanation in terms of natural selection. Because natural selection is the only known means by which an effect can explain a naturally occurring mechanism that provides it, evolutionary explanations presumably underlie all correct ascriptions of natural functions. Consequently, an evolutionary approach to personality and mental functioning (Buss, 1984, 1991; Wakefield, 1989a) is central to an understanding of psychopathology.

Dysfunction is thus a purely factual scientific concept. However, discovering what in fact is natural or dysfunctional (and thus what is disordered) may be extraordinarily difficult and may be subject to scientific controversy, especially with respect to mental mechanisms, about which we are still in a state of great ignorance. This ignorance is part of the reason for the high degree of confusion and controversy concerning which conditions are really mental disorders. Paradoxically, this ignorance about the detailed nature and causal histories of mental mechanisms also makes it all the more necessary to rely on functional explanations based on inferences about what mental mechanisms are probably designed to do. In this respect, we are now at a stage of understanding that is comparable in some ways to the position of ancient physicians who had to rely on similar inferences in judging physical disorder. For example, although knowing nothing about the mechanisms involved in sight or the natural history of the eye, such physicians still understood on the basis of functional inferences that blindness and other physical conditions are dysfunctions. As we learn more about the naturally selected functions of mental mechanisms, our judgments about dysfunction will become correspondingly more confident.

The Harm Requirement: Why Dysfunction is Not Enough

Given that all disorders must involve failures of naturally selected mechanisms, it is tempting to simply identify disorder with dysfunction as delineated by evolutionary theory. This would realize the long-sought goal of making disorder a purely objective scientific concept. However, as I showed earlier with many examples, a dysfunction is not enough to justify attribution of disorder. To be considered a disorder, the dysfunction must also cause significant harm to the person under present environmental circumstances and according to present cultural standards. For example, a dysfunction in one kidney often has no effect on the overall well-being of a person and so is not considered to be a disorder; physicians will remove a kidney from a live donor for transplant purposes with no sense that they are causing a disorder, even though people are certainly naturally designed to have two kidneys. To take a more speculative example, even if we suppose that people are designed to age and die at roughly a certain rate, someone whose aging mechanism suffered a dysfunction that slowed the aging process and lengthened life would be considered not disordered but lucky, assuming that no harmful side effects occurred as a result. The requirement that there be harm also accounts for why albinism, reversal of heart position, and fused toes are not considered disorders even though each results from a breakdown in the way some mechanism is designed to function. Although every disorder must involve a failure of a naturally selected property, not every such failure is a disorder. The element of harm must also be involved.

There are two reasons for the divergence between harm (in the practical sense that is relevant to diagnostic concerns) and failure of naturally selected effects. First, the natural functions of internal mechanisms were determined by the selective pressures that operated in environments that existed when the human species evolved. In some cases, those selective pressures have changed so that a breakdown in a mechanism now does not have the negative consequences that it would have had then. For example, high levels of male aggression might have been useful under primitive conditions, but in present-day circumstances such aggressive responses might be harmful. Consequently, even if a disposition to highly aggressive responses is the natural function of some mechanism, the loss of that function might not now be considered a disorder.

Second, natural selection of a mechanism occurs when organisms that possess the mechanism have greater reproductive fitness than organisms that do not possess the mechanism. Small decreases in reproductive fitness can be important over the evolutionary time scale, but in the absence of any other negative effects they are not necessarily harmful in the practical sense relevant to disorder. Relative reproductive fitness must be distinguished from possession of some reproductive capacity; the ability to have children is commonly considered a benefit and its deprivation is commonly considered a disorder, although even this has been disputed because of its implications for the classification of homosexuality. The mental health theoretician is interested in the functions that people care about and need within the current social environment, not those that are interesting merely on evolutionary theoretical grounds.

Thus disorder cannot be simply identified with the scientific concept of the inability of an internal mechanism to perform a naturally selected function. Only dysfunctions that are socially disvalued are disorders. Note that in this article I have explored the value element in disorder less thoroughly than the factual element. This is in part because the factual component poses more of a problem for inferences about disorder and in part because the nature of values is such a complex topic in its own right that it requires separate consideration.

The following general concept of disorder results from the preceding analysis: A condition is a disorder if and only if (a) the condition causes some harm or deprivation of benefit to the person as judged by the standards of the person's culture (the value criterion), and (b) the condition results from the inability of some internal mechanism to perform its natural function, wherein a natural function is an effect that is part of the evolutionary explanation of the existence and structure of the mechanism (the explanatory criterion).

This concept of disorder as harmful dysfunction leads directly to a definition of mental disorder as a special case. But first one question must be resolved: Does the 'mental' in 'mental disorder' refer to the nature of the harmful effects (symptoms) or to the nature of the dysfunctional cause of the harm? For example, as already mentioned. *DSM-III-R* asserts that the harm must be 'a manifestation of a behavioral, psychological, or biological dysfunction in the person' (American Psychiatric Association, 1987, p. xxii). The inclusion of biological dysfunctions (by which *DSM-III-R* means physiological as opposed to psychological or behavioral) as causes of mental disorders suggests that what makes a disorder mental is not the kind of dysfunction but the kind of symptom. This interpretation is consistent with Spitzer and Endicott's (1978) statement that 'a mental disorder is a medical disorder whose manifestations are primarily signs or symptoms of a psychological (behavioral) nature, or if physical, can be understood only using psychological concepts' (p. 18). The last clause was added to deal with what would otherwise be the obvious counterexample of psychosomatic illness, in which the symptoms are physical but the disorder is mental. The need for an ad hoc clause to cover psychosomatic disorders already suggests that the definition is incorrect. In fact, it is clearly not the case that mental disorders are disorders with mental symptoms. For example, trigeminal neuralgia has pain as its main symptom, and pain is a mental phenomenon, but trigeminal neuralgia is not a psychological disorder. As the example of psychosomatic illness suggests, it is the nature of the cause of the symptoms, and not the nature of the symptoms themselves, that determines whether a disorder is mental. This is why pain due to a physical dysfunction does not constitute a mental disorder; even extreme pain need not indicate a dysfunction of any mental mechanism. A physiological dysfunction can be the source of mental disorder only if it causes a breakdown in the functioning of some mental mechanism that in turn causes symptoms. So for a disorder to be mental, there must be a mental dysfunction, although the mental dysfunction might be secondary to a physiological dysfunction. This yields the conclusion that a mental disorder is a harmful dysfunction in a mental mechanism or, equivalently, a harmful mental dysfunction. More formally, in parallel to the general concept of disorder, we have the following concept of mental disorder: A condition is a mental disorder if and only if (a) the condition causes some harm or deprivation of benefit to the person as judged by the standards of the person's culture (the value criterion), and (b) the condition results from the inability of some mental mechanism to perform its natural function, wherein a natural function is an effect that is part of the evolutionary explanation of the existence and structure of the mental mechanism (the explanatory criterion). The further question of how to distinguish mental from physical mechanisms in a principled way that goes beyond the sort of list presented earlier (e.g., cognitive, perceptual, emotional, linguistic, and motivational mechanisms) is beyond the scope of this article.

No doubt there is much to be done to clarify, extend, and improve this analysis. But if this analysis does indeed come closer than other analyses to expressing the concept that underlies judgments about mental disorder, then it is this conception that we must scrutinize if we are to understand the strengths and limits of the concept of mental disorder or attempt to improve the conceptual validity of our diagnostic criteria. However, it is worth noting that even the clearest concepts possess areas of ambiguity, indeterminacy, and vagueness, so even a correct analysis of the concept of mental disorder is unlikely to resolve all controversies, although it may illuminate why certain intractable cases are controversial.

The Concept of Disorder and Theories of Disorder

I observed earlier that the concept of disorder has explanatory content; for example, to assert that a person is talking to him- or herself because he or she is suffering from a disorder suggests something about the explanation of the behavior. According to the view developed in the previous section, the explanatory content is as follows: To say that a harm is due to a disorder is to say that the harm is due to the fact that some internal mechanism is not functioning the way it was designed by nature to function. This attribution is inferential and goes beyond either the sheer existence of the manifest symptoms or the value judgment that the symptoms are harmful. However, in itself, a disorder attribution says nothing about the specific nature of the mechanisms that have gone awry. Consequently, judgments of disorder can be based on circumstantial evidence when knowledge of mechanisms is lacking, as when we infer that blindness and hallucinations are disorders without understanding anything about how perception works. Nevertheless, understanding the nature of mental mechanisms is ultimately critical to advancing the mental health field. Specifying the nature and functions of mental mechanisms and why they fail is the task of theories of mental disorder.

Theories of mental disorder are essentially theories of dysfunction. The harm component of the concept of disorder is judged by value standards that transcend the technicalities of any theory. A theory may alert us to hidden processes that have negative implications that we did not know about, but the reason that the processes are negative has to do with pretheoretical values.

The concept of disorder thus places two constraints on any theory of mental disorder. The value criterion implies that any successful theory of disorder must link up in the right way with the commonsense concept of harm. The explanatory criterion implies that any successful theory must offer an account specifically of dysfunctions.

Accounts of disorder in terms of genetic etiology obviously fit well with the approach to disorder I propose. There is a presumption that genetic mechanisms are naturally selected and have natural functions, implying that when something goes wrong there is a dysfunction. Thus, genetic etiology might easily satisfy the explanatory criterion. Moreover, genetic dysfunctions often cause harm, fulfilling the value criterion. However, even dysfunctional genetic mechanisms do not indicate disorder unless there is harm to the organism, as was illustrated in the examples of albinism, fused toes, and reversal of chest organ position.

The harmful dysfunction approach equally fits more psychological theories of disorder. A good example is Freud's repression account of neurotic disorder. It is sometimes mistakenly claimed that repression in itself is neurotic. This position would be bewildering as a theory of mental disorder because it contains no account of the function of repression, of how it comes to be dysfunctional, or of why repression itself is harmful. However. Freud's (1915/1957a, 1915/1957b) theory is much more sophisticated and is quite consistent with the framework imposed by the concept of disorder. Freud maintained that the mechanism of repression is designed to provide the benefit of keeping extremely painful ideas and affects from reaching consciousness and impairing the functioning of the organism. However, according to Freud, repression sometimes fails to perform its function in a satisfactory way, especially under the conditions imposed by modern civilization where so many desires and thoughts must be repressed. Consequently, indirect expressions of the repressed material sometimes reach consciousness in the form of neurotic symptoms. Thus, it is not the repression per se that constitutes the disorder; that would make no sense because neither harm nor dysfunction is necessary in successful repression. Instead the disorder is the failure of repression to do what it was designed to do (which implies a dysfunction) and the fact that harmful symptoms, such as painful anxiety, result from that failure. Note that the link via symptoms to the commonsense concept of harm is essential to the claim that the failure of repression is a disorder.

Similar considerations apply to the opposite end of the therapeutic theory spectrum, behavioral theory. It is sometimes claimed that a behavioral approach to the mind is not compatible with the traditional concept of mental disorder, because behaviorists consider all behavior to be the outcome of the same basic processes of reinforcement and learning, which are normal mechanisms. However, there is no inherent incompatibility between a behavioral approach and the harmful dysfunction concept of disorder. Behavioral theory can link up in a variety of ways with the critical concept of dysfunction (the harm requirement is easily met by many behaviors). One possibility is that learning mechanisms themselves may not operate in the way they were designed to operate. For example, simplifying greatly, Eysenck (1982, 1986) might be interpreted as arguing that certain personological characteristics can cause a person's learning mechanisms to respond to aversive stimuli more sensitively than they are designed to respond, yielding a variety of phobias and other maladaptive behaviors. A second possibility, which is hinted at in Salzinger's (1986) discussion of ethological approaches to behavior, is that there are submechanisms that facilitate the learning of specific classes of behaviors that are essential to survival and reproduction (e.g., ingestive, eliminative, sexual, parental, and agonistic mechanisms) and behavioral disorder results when these innate dispositions are not triggered by learning, as they are designed to be. Third, just as an emotionally normal infant can, in the absence of adequate or 'expectable' caretaking stimuli, develop life-threatening anaclitic depression (Spitz, 1945), and a genetically normal fetus can develop pathological anatomical structures if 'unexpected' chemicals come through the placenta, so a person with normal learning mechanisms can develop pathological behavioral dispositions that are outside the range that the learning mechanism was designed to produce, if the history of reinforcement includes stimuli outside the range that the mechanism was designed to 'expect.' For example, simplifying a bit, suppose that one function of learning mechanisms (i.e., one result of learning that selectively shaped the nature of learning mechanisms) is to associate the response of fear with danger, in such a way that the intensity of fear is roughly proportional to the degree of actual danger. Sometimes a severe trauma or other unusual sequence of stimuli causes the formation of an enduringly exaggerated sense of danger that causes substantial harm to the person. Such a disposition constitutes a disorder, because not only is there a dysfunction (learning is not leading to the kind of adaptive association between fear and danger that partially explains why learning mechanisms exist in the first place), but there is also harm (the exaggerated fear is painful and disabling).

Concluding Comments on the Misapplication of the Concept of 'Disorder'

The requirement that a disorder must involve a dysfunction places severe constraints on which negative conditions can be considered disorders and thus protects against arbitrary labeling of socially disvalued conditions as disorders. Unlike the skeptical view, the harmful dysfunction analysis distinguishes between sound and unsound applications of the term *mental disorder*. Diagnoses such as 'drapetomania' (the 'disorder' of runaway slaves), 'childhood masturbation disorder,' and 'lack of vaginal orgasm' can be seen as unsound applications of a perfectly coherent concept that can be correctly applied to other conditions. Unlike the value view, the harmful dysfunction view allows us to reject these diagnoses on scientific grounds, namely, that the beliefs about natural functioning that underlie them – for example, that slaves are naturally designed to serve, that children are naturally designed to be nonsexual, and that women are naturally designed to have orgasms from vaginal stimulation in intercourse alone – are false.

Because of the complexity of the inferences involved in judgments of dysfunction and our relative ignorance about the evolution of mental functioning, it is easy to arrive at differing judgments about mental dysfunction even on the basis of the same data. For example, according to the eminent Victorian physician and sexologist William Acton (1871), the female sexual organs do not naturally function to produce orgasm during intercourse, and the occurrence of orgasm in a woman is a form of pathology due to an excess of stimulation beyond what her body was designed to tolerate. According

to Masters and Johnson (1966, 1970, 1974), orgasm during intercourse is a natural function of the female sexual organs, and lack of orgasm in a woman is a disorder due to inadequate stimulation of the sort to which her body was designed to respond. Acton and Masters and Johnson knew that there are many women who do have orgasms in intercourse and many women who do not. Acton interpreted these facts to mean that there are a lot of women who are disordered because they suffer from overstimulation, whereas Masters and Johnson interpreted these facts to mean that there are a lot of women who are disordered because they suffer from understimulation. The nonstatistical nature of function and disorder, combined with ignorance of the evolutionary history of female sexual capacities, enabled these opposite beliefs to be consistent with the same set of data and with the same concept of disorder. Only further facts about the nature of the mechanisms involved in female sexual response, and the evolution of those mechanisms, can resolve such debates.

In principle, Acton and Masters and Johnson might have been able to reach agreement on what constitutes female orgasmic dysfunction if they had full knowledge of the evolutionary history of female sexual capacities. However, according to the view presented here, it is possible that agreement on the facts about function and dysfunction might not lead to agreement about which conditions are disorders because of differences in values (e.g., is orgasm in intercourse a desirable goal?). Such value differences, rather than any dispute over facts, may be what makes some diagnostic controversies, such as that over the pathological status of homosexuality, so intractable (Spitzer, 1981). The harmful dysfunction analysis thus provides a framework for identifying both the possibilities and the limits of agreement in such controversies.

References

Acton. W. (1871). *The functions and disorders of the reproductive organs in childhood, youth, adult age, and advanced life, considered in their physiological, social, and moral relations* (5th ed.). London: Churchill.

American Psychiatric Association. (1980). *Diagnostic and statistical manual of mental disorders* (3rd ed.). Washington, DC: Author.

American Psychiatric Association. (1987). *Diagnostic and statistical manual of mental disorders* (3rd ed., rev.). Washington. DC: Author.

Ausubel, D. P. (1971). Personality disorder is disease. *American Psychologist*. **16**, 59–74.

Barker-Benfield. G. J. (1983). The spermatic economy: A nineteenth-century view of sexuality. In T. L. Altherr (Ed.), *Procreation or pleasure? Sexual attitudes in American history* (pp. 47–70). Malabar, FL: Robert E. Krieger.

Bayer, R. (1981). *Homosexuality and American psychiatry: The politics of diagnosis*. New York: Basic Books.

Bayer, R., & Spitzer. R. L. (1982). Edited correspondence on the status of homosexuality in DSM-III. *Journal of the History of the Behavioral Sciences*, **18**, 32–52.

Boorse, C. (1975). On the distinction between disease and illness. *Philosophy and Public Affairs*, **5**, 49–68.

Boorse, C. (1976a). What a theory of mental health should be. *Journal for the Theory of Social Behavior*, **6**, 61–84.

Boorse, C. (1976b). Wright on functions. *Philosophical Review*, **85**, 70–86.

Buss, D. M. (1984). Evolutionary biology and personality psychology: Toward a conception of human nature and individual differences. *American Psychologist*, **39**, 1135–1147.

Buss, D. M. (1991). Evolutionary personality psychology. *Annual Review of Psychology*, **42**, 459–491.

Campbell, E. J. M., Scadding, J. G., & Roberts. R. S. (1979). The concept of disease. *British Medical Journal*, **2**, 757–762.

Caplan, A. L. (1981). The 'unnaturalness' of aging—a sickness unto death? In A. L. Caplan, H. T. Engelhardt. Jr., & J. J. McCartney (Eds.), *Concepts of health and disease: Interdisciplinary perspectives* (pp. 725–738). Reading, MA: Addison-Wesley.

Caplan, P. J. (1984). The myth of women's masochism. *American Psychologist*, **39**, 130–139.

Cartwright, S. A. (1981). Report on the diseases and physical peculiarities of the Negro race. In A. L. Caplan, H. T. Engelhardt, Jr., & J. J. McCartney (Eds.), *Concepts of health and disease: Interdisciplinary perspectives* (pp. 305–326). Reading, MA: Addison-Wesley. (Original work published 1851)

Claridge, G. (1985). *Origins of mental illness*. Oxford, England: Blackwell.

Cohen, H. (1981). The evolution of the concept of disease. In A. L. Caplan, H. T. Engelhardt, Jr., & J. J. McCartney (Eds.), *Concepts of health and disease: Interdisciplinary perspectives* (pp. 209–220). Reading, MA: Addison-Wesley.

Coles, G. (1987). *Learning mystique*. New York: Pantheon.

Cowart, V. (1988). The ritalin controversy: What's made this drug's opponents hyperactive? *Journal of the American Medical Association, 259*, 2521–2523.

Cummins, R. (1975). Functional analysis. *Journal of Philosophy, 72*, 741–765.

Elster, J. (1983). *Explaining technical change*. Cambridge, England: Cambridge University Press.

Engelhardt, H. T., Jr. (1974). The disease of masturbation: Values and the concept of disease. *Bulletin of the History of Medicine, 48*, 234–248.

Eysenck, H. J. (1982). Neobehavioristic (S-R) theory of neurosis. In G. T. Wilson & C. M. Franks (Eds.), *Contemporary behavior therapy* (pp. 205–276). New York: Guilford Press.

Eysenck, H. J. (1986). A critique of contemporary classification and diagnosis. In T. Millon & G. L. Klerman (Eds.), *Contemporary directions in psychopathology: Toward the DSM-IV* (pp. 73–98). New York: Guilford Press.

Eysenck, H. J., Wakefield, J. A., & Friedman, A. F. (1983). Diagnosis and clinical assessment: The DSM-III. *Annual Review of Psychology, 34*, 167–193.

Fingarette, H. (1988). *Heavy drinking: The myth of alcoholism as a disease*. Berkeley: University of California Press.

Fingarette, H. (1990). We should reject the disease concept of alcoholism. *Harvard Medical School Mental Health Letter, 6*(8), 4–6.

Flew. A. (1981). Disease and mental illness. In A. L. Caplan, H. T. Engelhardt. Jr., & J. J. McCartney (Eds.), *Concepts of health and disease: Interdisciplinary perspectives* (pp. 433–442). Reading, MA: Addison-Wesley.

Foucault, M. (1965). *Madness and civilization: A history of insanity in the Age of Reason* (R. Howard, Trans.). New York: Pantheon. (Original work published 1964).

Foucault, M. (1973). *History of sexuality: Vol. 1. An introduction*. New York: Pantheon.

Freud, S. (1957a). Repression. In J. Strachey (Ed. and Trans.), *The standard edition of the complete psychological works of Sigmund Freud* (Vol. 14, pp. 146–158). London: Hogarth Press. (Original work published 1915).

Freud, S. (1957b). The unconscious. In J. Strachey (Ed. and Trans.), *The standard edition of the complete psychological works of Sigmund Freud* (Vol. 14, pp. 166–215). London: Hogarth Press. (Original work published 1915).

Goffman, E. (1963). *Stigma: Notes on the management of spoiled identity*. Englewood Cliffs, NJ: Prentice-Hall.

Gorenstein, E. E. (1984). Debating mental illness: Implications for science, medicine, and social policy. *American Psychologist, 39*, 50–56.

Gorman, D. M. (1989a). Is 'disease model' an appropriate term to describe the alcohol dependence syndrome? *Alcohol and Alcoholism, 24*, 509–512.

Gorman, D. M. (1989b). Is the 'new' problem drinking concept of Heather & Robertson more useful in advancing our scientific knowledge than the 'old' disease concept? *British Journal of Addiction, 84*, 843–845.

Gove, W. R. (1980). Labelling and mental illness: A critique. In W. R. Gove (Ed.), *The labeling of deviance: Evaluating a perspective* (2nd ed., pp. 53–99). Beverly Hills, CA: Sage.

Hempel. C. G. (1965). The logic of functional analysis. In C. G. Hempel (Ed.), *Aspects of scientific explanation and other essays in the philosophy of science* (pp. 297–330). New York: Free Press.

Horwitz, A. V. (1982). *The social control of mental illness*. San Diego. CA: Academic Press.

Kaplan, M. (1983). A woman's view of DSM-III. *American Psychologist, 38*, 786–792.

Kendell, R. E. (1975). The concept of disease and its implications for psychiatry. *British Journal of Psychiatry, 127*, 305–315.

Kendell, R. E. (1986). What are mental disorders? In A. M. Freedman. R. Brotman. I. Silverman, & D. Hutson (Eds.), *Issues in psychiatric classification: Science, practice and social policy* (pp. 23–45). New York: Human Sciences Press.

King, L. (1981). What is disease? In A. L. Caplan, H. T. Engelhardt. Jr., & J. J. McCartney (Eds.), *Concepts of health and disease: Interdisciplinary perspectives* (pp. 107–118). Reading, MA: Addison-Wesley. (Original work published 1954).

Klein, D. F. (1978). A proposed definition of mental illness. In R. L. Spitzer & D. F. Klein (Eds.), *Critical issues in psychiatric diagnosis* (pp. 41–71). New York: Raven Press.

Kohn, A. (1989, November). Suffer the restless children. *Atlantic Monthly*, pp. 90–100.

Laing, R. D. (1967). *The politics of experience*. London: Penguin Books.

Lewis, A. (1967). Health as a social concept. In A. Lewis (Ed.), *The state of psychiatry* (pp. 113–127). New York: Science House.

Macklin, R. (1981). Mental health and mental illness: Some problems of definition and concept formation. In A. L. Caplan, H. T. Engelhardt, Jr., & J. J. McCartney (Eds.), *Concepts of health and disease: Interdisciplinary perspectives* (pp. 391–418). Reading, MA: Addison-Wesley.

Marmor, J. (1973). [Comments]. In A symposium: Should homosexuality be in the APA nomenclature? *American Journal of Psychiatry, 130*, 1270–1316.

Masters, W. H., & Johnson, V. E. (1966). *Human sexual response*. Boston: Little, Brown.

Masters, W. H., & Johnson, V. E. (1970). *Human sexual inadequacy*. Boston: Little, Brown.

Masters, W. H., & Johnson, V. E. (1974). *The pleasure bond: A new look at sexuality and commitment*. Boston: Little, Brown.

Moore, M. S. (1978). Discussion of the Spitzer-Endicott and Klein proposed definitions of mental disorder (illness). In R. L. Spitzer & D. F. Klein (Eds.), *Critical issues in psychiatric diagnosis* (pp. 85–104). New York: Raven Press.

Nagel, E. (1979). *Teleology revisited and other essays in the philosophy and history of science*. New York: Columbia University Press.

Pichot, P. (1986). [Comment in Discussion section]. In A. M. Freedman. R. Brotman, I. Silverman, & D. Hutson (Eds.), *Issues in psychiatric classification: Science, practice and social policy* (p. 56). New York: Human Sciences Press.

Pond, D. (1960). Is there a syndrome of 'brain damage' in children? *Cerebral Paisy Bulletin, 2*, 296.

Ruse, M. (1973). *The philosophy of biology*. London: London University Press.

Rutter, M., Graham, P., & Yule, W. (1970). *A neuropsychiatric study in childhood*. Philadelphia: Lippincott.

Salzinger, K. (1986). Diagnosis: Distinguishing among behaviors. In T. Millon & G. L. Klerman (Eds.), *Contemporary directions in psychopathology: Toward the DSM-IV* (pp. 115–134). New York: Guilford Press.

Sarbin, T. (1967). On the futility of the proposition that some people be labeled 'mentally ill.' *Journal of Consulting Psychology, 31*, 447–453.

Sarbin, T. (1969). The scientific status of the mental illness metaphor. In S. C. Pong & R. B. Edgerton (Eds.), *Changing perspectives in mental illness* (pp. 1–16). New York: Holt, Rinehart & Winston.

Scadding, J. G., (1967). Diagnosis: The clinician and the computer. *Lancet, 2*, 877–882.

Scadding, J. G. (1990). The semantic problem of psychiatry. *Psychological Medicine, 20*, 243–248.

Scheff, T. J. (1966). *Being mentally ill: A sociological theory*. Chicago: Aldine.

Scheff, T. J. (Ed.). (1975). *Labeling madness*. Endlewood Cliffs. NJ: Prentice-Hall.

Schrenck-Notzing, A. (1956). *The use of hypnosis in psychopathia sexualis* (C. D. Chaddock, Trans.). New York: Julian Press. (Original work published 1895).

Sedgwick, P. (1982). *Psycho politics*. New York: Harper & Row.

Showalter, E. (1987). *The female malady: Women, madness, and English culture, 1830–1980*. London: Virago Press.

Spitz, R. (1945). Hospitalism. *The Psychoanalytic Study of the Child, 1*, 53–74.

Spitzer, R. L. (1981). The diagnostic status of homosexuality in DSM-III: A reformulation of the issues. *American Journal of Psychiatry, 138*, 210–215.

Spitzer, R. L., & Endicott. J. (1978). Medical and mental disorder: Proposed definition and criteria. In R. L. Spitzer & D. F. Klein (Eds.), *Critical issues in psychiatric diagnosis* (pp. 15–39). New York: Raven Press.

Spitzer, R. L., & Williams, J. B. W. (1982). The definition and diagnosis of mental disorder. In W. R. Gove (Ed.), *Deviance and mental illness* (pp. 15–31). Beverly Hills, CA: Sage.

Spitzer. R. L., & Williams, J. B. W. (1983). International perspectives: Summary and commentary. In R. L. Spitzer, J. B. W. Williams, & A. E. Skodol (Eds.), *International perspectives on DSM-III* (pp. 339–353). Washington, DC: American Psychiatric Press.

Spitzer, R. L. & Williams, J. B. W. (1988). Basic principles in the development of *DSM-III*. In J. E. Mezzich & M. V. Cranach (Eds.), *International classification in psychiatry: Unity and diversity* (pp. 81–86). Cambridge. England: Cambridge University Press.

Szasz. T. S. (1971). The sane slave. *American Journal of Psychotherapy,* **25**, 228–239.

Szasz, T. S. (1974). *The myth of mental illness: Foundations of a theory of personal conduct* (Rev. ed.). New York: Harper & Row.

Taylor, F. K. (1971). A logical analysis of the medico-psychological concept of disease. *Psychological Medicine,* **1**, 356–364.

Taylor, F. K. (1976). The medical model of the disease concept. *British Journal of Psychiatry,* **128**, 588–594.

Ussher, J. M. (1989). *The psychology of the human body.* New York: Routledge.

Vaillant, G. E. (1990). We should retain the disease concept of alcoholism. *Harvard Medical School Mental Health Letter,* **6**(9), 4–6.

Wakefield, J. C. (1987). Sex bias in the diagnosis of primary orgasmic dysfunction. *American Psychologist,* **42**, 464–471.

Wakefield, J. C. (1988). Female primary orgasmic dysfunction: Masters and Johnson versus DSM-III-R on diagnosis and incidence. *Journal of Sex Research,* **24**, 363–377.

Wakefield, J. C. (1989a). Levels of explanation in personality theory. In D. M. Buss & N. Cantor (Eds.), *Emerging issues in personality psychology* (pp. 333–346). New York: Springer-Verlag.

Wakefield, J. C. (1989b). Manufacturing female dysfunction: A reply to Morokoff. *American Psychologist,* **44**, 75–77.

Wakefield, J. C. (in press). Disorder as harmful dysfunction: A conceptual critique of DSM-III-R's definition of mental disorder. *Psychological Review, 99* (2).

Williams, J. B. W., & Spitzer, R. L. (1983). The issue of sex bias in DSM-III: A critique of 'A woman's view of DSM-III' by Marcie Kaplan. *American Psychologist,* **38**, 793–798.

Willie. C. V., Kramer. B. M., & Brown, B. S. (Eds.). (1973). *Racism and mental health.* Pittsburgh. PA: University of Pittsburgh Press.

Woodfield. A. (1976). *Teleology.* Cambridge, England: Cambridge University Press.

World Health Organization. (1981). Constitution of the World Health Organization. In A. L. Caplan, H. T. Engelhardt, Jr., & J. J. McCartney (Eds.), *Concepts of health and disease: Interdisciplinary perspectives* (pp. 83–84). Reading, MA: Addison-Wesley. (Original work published 1946)

Wright. L. (1973). Functions. *Philosophical Review,* **82**, 139–168.

Wright, L. (1976). *Teleological explanations.* Berkeley: University of California Press.

A Psychiatric Dialogue on the Mind-Body Problem*

Kenneth S. Kendler

Of all the human professions, psychiatry, in its day-to-day work, is most concerned with the relationship of mind and brain. In a typical clinical interaction, psychiatrists are centrally concerned with both subjective, mental, first-person constructs and objective, third-person brain states. In such clinical interventions, the working psychiatrist traverses many times the 'mind-brain' divide. We have tended to view etiologic theories of psychiatric disorders as either brain based (organic or biological) or mind based (functional or psychological). Our therapies are divided into those that impact largely on the mind ('psycho' therapies) and on the brain ('somatic' therapies). The division of the United States government that funds most research in psychiatry is termed the National Institute of 'Mental' Health. The manual of the American Psychiatric Association that is widely used for the diagnosis of psychiatric disorders is called the Diagnostic and Statistical Manual of 'Mental' Disorders.

Therefore, as a discipline, psychiatry should be deeply interested in the mind-body problem. However, although this is an active area of concern within philosophy and some parts of the neuroscientific community, it has been years since a review of these issues has appeared in a major Anglophonic psychiatric journal (although relatively recent articles by Kandel[1, 2] certainly touched on these issues). Almost certainly, part of the problem is terminology. Neither medical nor psychiatric training provides a good background for the conceptual and terminologic approach most frequently taken by those who write on the subject. In fact, training in biomedicine is likely to produce impatience with the philosophical discourse in this area.

The goal of this essay is to provide a selective primer for past and current perspectives on the mind-body problem. No attempt is made to be complete. Indeed, this article reflects several years of reading and musing by an active psychiatric researcher and clinician without formal philosophical training.

Important progress has been recently made in our understanding of the phenomenon of consciousness.[3] Some investigators have proposed general theories (e.g., Edelman and Tononi[4] and Damasio),[5] while others have explored the implications of specific neurologic conditions (e.g., 'blindsight'[6] and 'split-brain').[7] Although this work is of substantial relevance to the mind-body problem, space constraints make it impossible to review all of this material here.

I take a time-honored approach in philosophy and review these issues as a dialogue on rounds between Teacher, a philosophically informed attending psychiatrist, and three residents: Doug, Mary, and Francine. These three have sympathies for the three major theories we will examine: dualism, materialism, and functionalism. Doug has just finished a detailed presentation about a patient, Mr. A, whom he admitted the previous night with major depression.

The Dialogue

TEACHER: That was a nice case presentation, Doug. Can you summarize for us how you understand the causes of Mr. A's depression?

* Kendler, K.: A psychiatric dialogue on the mind–body problem. *American Journal Psychiatry* **158**: 989–1000, 2001.

DOUG: Sure. I think that both psychoanalytic and cognitive theories can be usefully applied. Mr. A has a lot of unresolved anger and competitiveness toward his father and this resulted—

MARY: Doug, come on! That is so old-fashioned. Psychiatry is applied neuroscience now. We shouldn't be talking about parent-child relationships or cognitive schemata but serotonergic dysfunction resulting in deficits in functional transmission at key mood centers in the limbic system.

TEACHER: Mary, I'm glad you raised that point. Let's pursue this discussion further. Could Doug's view and your view of Mr. A's depression both be correct? Could his unresolved anger at his father or his self-derogatory cognitive schemata be expressed through dysfunction in his serotonin system?

DOUG: I am not sure, Teacher. My approach to psychiatry has always been to try to understand how patients feel, to try to make sense of their problems from their own perspectives. People don't feel a dysfunctional serotonin receptor. They have conflicts, wishes, and fears. How can molecules and receptors have wishes or conflicts?

MARY: Wait a minute, Doug! Are you seriously claiming that there are aspects of mental functioning that cannot be due to brain processes? How else do you think we have thoughts or wishes or conflicts? These are all the result of synaptic firings in different parts of our brains.

TEACHER: Let me push you a bit on that, Mary. What precisely do you think is the causal relationship between mind and brain?

MARY: I haven't thought much about this since college! I guess I have always thought that mind and brain were just different words for the same thing, one experienced from the inside—mind—and the other experienced from the outside—brain.

TEACHER: Mary, you are not being very precise with your use of language. A moment ago you said that mind is the result of brain, that is, that synaptic firings are the cause of thoughts and feelings. Just now, you said that mind and brain are the same thing. Which is it?

MARY: I'm not sure. Can you help me understand the distinction?

TEACHER: I can try. It's probably easiest to give examples of what philosophers would call identity relationships. Simply speaking, identity is self-sameness. The most straightforward and, some might say, trivial form of identity occurs when multiple names exist for the same entity. For example, 'Samuel Clemens' is Mark Twain. Of more relevance to the mind-body problem is what have been called theoretical identities, identities revealed by scientists as they discover the way the world works. Theoretical identities take folk concepts and provide for them scientific explanations. Examples include the discoveries that temperature is the mean kinetic energy of molecules, that water is H_2O, and that lightning is a cloud-to-earth electrical discharge.

MARY: I think I get it. It wouldn't make any sense to say that molecular motion causes temperature or that cloud-to-earth electrical discharge causes lightning. Molecular energy just is temperature, and earth-to-cloud discharge of electricity just is lightning.

TEACHER: Exactly! Now, let's get back to the question. Do mind and brain have a causal or an identity relationship? Having looked at identity relationships, let's explore the causal model. Am I correct, Mary, that you said that you think that abnormal serotonin function can cause symptoms of depression? Put more broadly, then, does brain cause mind? Does it only go in that direction?

MARY: Do you mean, can mind cause brain as well as brain cause mind?

TEACHER: Precisely.

DOUG: Wait. I'm lost. I'm still back on the problem of how what we call mind can possibly be the same as brain or even caused by brain. The mind and physical things just seem to be too different.

FRANCINE: Me, too. I can't help but feel that Mary is barking up the wrong tree trying to see mind and brain as the same kind of thing.

TEACHER: I can pick up on both strands of this conversation, as they both lead us back to Descartes (1596–1650), the great scientist and polymath who started modern discourse on the mind-body problem. Descartes agreed with you, Doug. He said that the universe could be divided into two completely different kinds of 'stuff,' material and mental. They differed in three key ways.[8] Material things are spatial; they have a location and dimensions. Mental things do not. Material things have properties, like shape and color, that mental things do not. Finally, material things are public; they can be observed by anyone, whereas mental events are inherently private. They can be directly observed only by the individual in whose mind they occur.

DOUG: Yes. That is exactly what I mean. The physical world has an up and down. Things have mass. But do thoughts have a direction? Can you weigh them?

MARY: Doug, do you realize how antiscientific you are sounding? How can you expect psychiatry to be accepted by the rest of medicine if you talk about psychiatric disorders as due to some ethereal nonphysical thing called mind or spirit?

DOUG: However, maybe that is exactly what psychiatry should do, stand as a bastion of humanism against the overwhelming attacks of biological reductionism. Science is a wonderful and powerful tool, but it is not the answer to everything. Is science going to tell me why I find Mozart's music so lovely or the poetry of Wordsworth so moving?

TEACHER: Hold on, you two. How about if we agree for now to ignore the problem of how psychiatry should relate to the rest of medicine? Let's get back to Descartes. He postulated what we would now call substance dualism, the theory that the universe contains two fundamentally different kinds of stuff: the mental and the material (or physical).

MARY: So, he rejected the idea of an identity relationship?

TEACHER: Absolutely. But he had a big problem, and that is the problem of the apparent bidirectional causal relationship between mind and brain. Even in the 17th century, they knew that damage to the brain could produce changes in mental functioning, so it appeared that brain influences mind. Furthermore, we all know what would happen if a mother were told that her young child had died. One would see trembling, weeping, and agitation – all very physical events. So it would also appear that mind influences brain. Descartes never successfully solved this problem. He came up with the rather unsatisfactory idea that somehow these two fundamentally different kinds of stuff met up in the pineal gland and there influenced each other.

DOUG: But if mind and brain are completely different sorts of things, how could one ever affect the other?

TEACHER: Precisely, Doug. That is one of the main reasons why Descartes's kind of dualism has not been very popular in recent years. It just seems too incredible.

MARY: So, are you saying that the identity relationship makes more sense because causal relationships are hard to imagine between things that are so different as mind and brain?

TEACHER: That is only part of the problem, Mary. There is another that some consider even more serious. It is easy for us to understand what you might call brain-to-brain causation, that is, that different aspects of brain function influence other aspects. We are learning about these all the time, for example, our increasing insights into the biological basis of memory[9]. Many of us can also begin to see how brain events can cause mind events. This is easiest to understand in the perceptual field – let's say vision. We know that applying small electrical currents to the primary and secondary sensory cortices produces the mental experience of perception.

MARY: Those kinds of experiments sure sound like brain-to-mind causation to me.

TEACHER: Yes. I agree that seems like the easiest way to understand them. But I am trying to get at another point. Let's set up a very simple thought experiment. Bill is sitting in a chair eating salty peanuts and reading the newspaper. He has poured himself a beer but is engrossed in an interesting story. In the middle of the story, he feels thirsty, stops reading, and reaches for the glass of beer.

Now, the key question is, what role did the subjective sense of thirst play in this little story? Was it in the causal pathway of events? I am going to have to go to the blackboard here and draw out two versions of this (Figure 1, upper part).

Both versions begin with a set of neurons in Bill's hypothalamus noting that the sodium concentration is rising owing to all those salty peanuts! We will call that brain thirst. The interactionist model assumes that the hypothalamus sends signals to some executive control system (probably involving a network of several structures, including the frontal cortex). Somewhere in that process, brain thirst becomes mind thirst: that is, Bill has the subjective experience of thirst. In his executive control region,

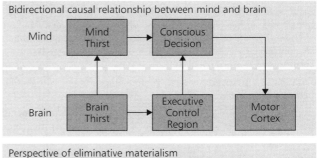
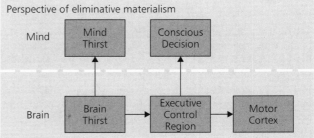

Figure 1 Two Views of the Causal Relationship Between Mind and Brain in the Experience of Thirst and Act of Reaching for a Beer[a]

[a] In the view shown in the top part of the figure, which depicts a bi-directional causal relationship between mind and brain, the critical decision to reach for beer because of thirst is made consciously in the mind; the decision is conveyed to the motor cortex for implementation. From the perspective of eliminative materialism, all causal arrow flow within the brain. The mind is informed of brain processes but has no causal efficacy Conscious decisions apparently made by the mind have, in fact, been previously made by the brain.

then, based on this mind thirst and his memory about the nearby glass of beer, Bill makes the mind-based decision, 'I'm thirsty and that beer would sure taste good.' The decision (in mind) now being made, the executive control region, under the control of mind, sends signals to the motor strip and cerebellum saying, 'Reach for that glass of beer.'

The main advantage of this little story is that it maps well onto our subjective experience. If you asked Bill what happened, he would say, 'I was thirsty and wanted the beer.' He would be clear that it was a volitional act in his mental sphere that made him reach for the beer. But notice in Figure 1 that we are right back into the problem confronted by Descartes. This little story has the causal arrows going from brain to mind and back to brain. A lot of people have trouble with this.

An alternative approach to this problem is offered by the theory of eliminative materialism or, as it is sometimes called, epiphenomenonalism.

DOUG: Ugh. It is these kinds of big words that always turn me off to philosophy.

TEACHER: Bear with me, Doug. It might be worth it. Philosophy certainly does have its terminology, and it can get pretty thick at times. But then again, so do medicine and psychiatry. The concept of eliminative materialism is very simple: that *the sufficient cause for all material events is other material events.* If we were to retell this story from the perspective of eliminative materialism, it would look a lot simpler. All the causal arrows flow between brain states, from the hypothalamus to the frontal cortex to the motor strip (Figure 1, lower part).

DOUG: But what about Bill's subjective experience of thirst and of deciding to reach for the glass of beer?

TEACHER: The theory of eliminative materialism wouldn't deny that Bill experienced that but would maintain that none of those mental states was in the causal loop. The hypothalamic signal might enter consciousness as the feeling of thirst, and the work of the frontal control center might enter consciousness as the sense of having made a decision to reach for the glass, but in fact the mental experiences are all epiphenomenal or, as some say inert. Let me state this clearly. The eliminative materialism theory assumes a one-way casual relation between brain and mind states (brain → mind) and no causal efficacy for mind; that is, there is no mind → brain causality. According to this theory, mind is just froth on the wave or the steam coming out of a steam engine. Mind is a shadow theater that keeps us amused and thinking (incorrectly) that our consciousness really controls things.

DOUG: That is a pretty grim view of the human condition. Why should we believe anything that radical?

TEACHER: Doug, have you ever had the experience of touching something hot like a stove and withdrawing your hand and *then* experiencing the heat and pain?

DOUG: Yes.

TEACHER: If you think about it, that experience is exactly what is predicted by the eliminative materialist theory. Your nervous system sensed the heat, sent a signal to move your hand, and then, by the way, decided to inform your consciousness of what had happened after the fact.

DOUG: OK. I'll accept that. But that is just a reflex arc, probably working in my spinal cord. Are you arguing that that is a general model of brain action?

TEACHER: I'm only suggesting that it needs to be taken seriously as a theory. In famous experiments conducted in the early *1980s*,[10] the neurophysiologist Ben Libet asked students to perform spontaneously a simple motor task: to lift a finger. He found that although the students became aware of the impulse around 200 msec before performing the motor act, EEG recordings showed that the brain was planning the task 500 msec before it occurred. Now, there are a lot of questions about the interpretation of this study, but one way to see it, as predicted by eliminative materialism, is that the brain makes up its mind to do something,

and then the decision enters consciousness. The mind thinks that it really made the decision, but it was actually dictated by the brain 300 msec before. My point with this story and the reference to Libet's work is to raise the question of whether consciousness is as central in brain processes as many of us like to think.

Let me try one more approach to advocating the eliminative materialist perspective. Before the development of modern science, people had many folk conceptions that have since been proven incorrect, such as that thunder is caused by an angry god and that certain diseases are caused by witches. Perhaps the concepts of what has been called folk psychology are the same sort of thing, superstitious beliefs that arose when we didn't know anything about how the brain worked.

DOUG: You mean that believing that our actions are governed by our beliefs and desires is like believing in witches or tribal gods?

MARY: To put it in another way, magnetic resonance imaging (MRI) machines that show the brain basis of perception and cognition are like Ben Franklin's discovery that lightning wasn't caused by Zeus but could be explained as a form of electricity.

TEACHER: Exactly. So, we have now examined some of the problems you get into when you want to try to work out a causal relationship between mind and brain.

MARY: Yeah. That identity theory is looking better and better. After all, it is so simple and elegant that it must be true. Mind is brain and brain is mind.

TEACHER: Not so fast, Mary. There are some problems with this theory too.

FRANCINE: Teacher, isn't one of the biggest problems with identity theories that they assume that the mind is a thing rather than a process?

TEACHER: Yes, Francine. Let's get back to that point in a few minutes. I agree with Mary that identity theories are very appealing in their simplicity and potential power, but, unfortunately, they are not without their problems. Let's review three of them. The first stems from what has been called Leibniz's law, which specifies a critical feature of an identity relationship. This law simply says that if an identity relationship is true between A and B, then A and B must have all the same properties or characteristics. If there is a property possessed by A and not by B, then A and B cannot have an identity relationship.

MARY: That makes sense, and it certainly works for the examples you gave. Whatever is true for water must be true for H_2O, and the same goes for lightning and a cloud-to-earth electrical discharge.

TEACHER: Yes, but what about mind and brain? As Doug said, the brain is physical and has direction, mass, and temperature, whereas the mind has wishes, intentions, and fears. Can two such different things as mind and brain really have an identity relationship?

DOUG: Yes. That is exactly what I have been trying to say. That puts a big hole in your mind-equals-brain and brain-equals-mind ideas, Mary!

MARY: Maybe. But isn't that a pretty narrow view of identity? Perhaps the problem of mind and brain is not like that of lightning and electricity. It might be that mind and brain are one thing, but when you experience it from the inside (as mind) and then from the outside (as brain), it is unrealistic to expect them to appear the same and to have all the same properties.

TEACHER: A good point, Mary. What you have raised is the possibility of another kind of dualism that is less radical than the kind proposed by Descartes. One way to think about it is that there are two levels to what we might call identity. Things can be identical at the level of substance and/or at the level of property. Imagine that brain and mind are the same substance but have two fundamentally different sets of properties.

MARY: Please give me an example. I am having a hard time grasping this.

TEACHER: Sure. If we take any object, it will have several distinct sets of properties: mass, volume, and color, for instance.

MARY: So mind and brain are two distinct properties of the same substance?

TEACHER: Precisely. Not surprisingly, this is called property dualism and is considerably more popular today in philosophical circles than is the substance dualism originally promulgated Descartes.

DOUG: That is quite an appealing theory.

TEACHER: I agree, Doug. Let me get on to the second major problem with the identity theory.

DOUG: Wait, Teacher! At least tell us, is property dualism consistent with identity theories?

TEACHER: A hard question. Most identity theorists suggest that brain and mind have a full theoretical identity just like lightning and cloud-to-earth electrical discharges. But you could argue that property dualism is consistent with an attenuated kind of identity. This might disappoint most identity theorists because it suggests that the relationship of brain to mind is different from that of other aspects of our world in which we are moving from folk knowledge to scientific theories.

DOUG: I think I followed that.

TEACHER: Let's get back to the second major weakness of the classic identity theory. The commonsense or 'strong' form of these identity theories is called a type identity theory. That is, if A and B have an identity relationship, that relationship is fundamental and the same everywhere and always.

MARY: OK. So where does this lead?

TEACHER: Well, let's go back to Mr. A's depression. Let's imagine that in the year 2050 we have a super-duper MRI scanner that can look into Mr. A's brain and completely explain the brain changes that occur with his depression. We can then claim that the brain state for depression and the mind state for depression have identity relationship.

MARY: OK. Makes sense so far.

TEACHER: Now, if Mr. A develops the same kind of depression again in 20 years, would we expect to find the exact same brain state? Or what about if Ms. B comes in with depression. Would her brain state be the same as that seen in Mr. A? Or even worse, imagine an alien race of intelligent sentient beings who might also be prone depression and were able to explain to us how they felt. Is there any credible reason that we would expect the changes in their brains (if they have a brain anything like ours) to be the same as those seen in Mr. A? Philosophers call this the problem of multiple realizability, that is, the probability that many different brain states might all cause the same mind state (e.g., depression).

DOUG: Sounds to me like you are making a pretty strong case against what you call the type identity theory. Is there any other kind?

TEACHER: Yes. It is called a token identity theory, and it postulates a weaker kind of identity relationship.

MARY: Weaker in what way?

TEACHER: It makes no claims for a universal relationship. It only claims that for a given person at a given time there is an identity relationship between the brain state and the mind state.

MARY: That makes clinical sense. I have certainly seen depressed patients who had very similar clinical pictures and got the same treatment, but one got better and the other did not. This might imply that they actually had different brain states underlying their depression.

TEACHER: Precisely. My guess is that if the identity theory is correct, we will find that there is a spectrum extending from primarily type identity to token identity relationships. This will, in part, reflect the plasticity of the central nervous system (CNS) and the level of individual differences. For example, for some subcortical processes, such as stimulation of spinal tracts producing pain, there may be no individual differences, and the type identity theory may apply. It is as if that brain function is hard wired – at least, for all humans. All bets would be off for Martians! On the other hand, for more complex neurobehavioral traits that are controlled by very plastic parts of the human CNS, there may be highly variable interindividual and even intraindividual, across-time differences, so the token identity model may be more appropriate.

FRANCINE: What is the third problem?

TEACHER: The third problem is sometimes referred to as the explanatory gap[11] or the 'hard problem of consciousness'[12]. When most people think about an idenity, they tend to view mind from the outside. For example, recent research with positron emission tomography and functional MRI has produced an increasing number of results supporting identity theories. We can see the effects of vision in the occipital cortex, hearing in the temporal cortex, and the like. We have even been able to see greater metabolic activity in a range of structures, including the temporal association cortex, correlated with the report of auditory hallucinations.

MARY: Yes. My point exactly. This is leading the way to a view of psychiatry as applied neuroscience.

DOUG: I also have to agree that this evidence strongly supports some kind of close relationship between brain and some functions of mind.

TEACHER: Well, the problem of the explanatory gap is that it is easy to establish a correlation or identity between brain activity and a mental function but much harder to get from brain activity to the actual experience. That is, I don't have too much trouble going from the state of looking at a red square to the state of increased blood flow in the visual cortex reflecting increased neuronal firing. Modern neuroscience has been making an increasingly compelling case for viewing this as an identity relationship. However, I have a lot more trouble going from increased blood flow reflecting neuronal firing in the visual cortex to *the actual experience of seeing red*.

In the philosophical literature, this subjective 'feel' of mind is often called 'qualia.' In a famous essay titled 'What Is It Like to Be a Bat?'[13], the philosopher Nagel argued that the qualia problem is fundamental. We will never be able to understand what it feels like to be a bat.

With the qualia problem, we come up against the mind-body divide in a particularly stark and direct way. Even if we got down to the firing of the specific neurons in the cortex that we know are correlated with the perception of color, how does that neuronal firing actually produce the subjective sense of redness with which we are all familiar? Can you have an identity relationship between what seems to be clearly within the material world (neuronal firing) and the raw sensory feel of redness?

I should say that having spoken about this problem with a number of people, I have gotten a wide range of reactions. Some don't see it as a problem at all, and others, like me, feel a sense of existential vertigo when trying to grapple with this question.

DOUG: I think this comes close to describing my concerns. Neuronal firing and the sense of seeing red – they just cannot be the same thing.

MARY: Maybe we have finally gotten to the root of our differences. I have no problem with this. When you stimulate a muscle, it twitches. When you stimulate a liver cell, it makes bile. When you stimulate a cell in the visual cortex, you get the perception of red. What's the difference?

TEACHER: I am glad that the two of you responded so differently to this question. I would only say, Mary, that the major difference is that with stimulating a motor neuron and producing a muscle twitch, you have events that all take place in the material world. On the other hand, stimulation in the visual cortex produces a perception of the color red that is only seen by the person whose brain is being stimulated. In this sense, it is not the same thing at all. It is hard for some of us to see how the nerve cell firing and the experience of seeing red could be the same thing, at least in the way that lightning and an electrical discharge are the same thing.

MARY: It seems to me, Teacher, that you and these philosophers are just getting too precious. That's the way the world is. We humans with our consciousness are not nearly as special as you think. When you poke a paramecium, it moves away. A few hundred million years later you have big-brained primates, but nothing has really changed. It's all biology. I'm losing patience with all this identity-relationship talk. This sounds too much like abstract psychoanalytic theorizing to me.

FRANCINE: I have been patient for a long time, Teacher. Can I have my say now?

TEACHER: Sure, Francine.

FRANCINE: Up until now, all of you have been approaching the mind-body problem the wrong way. Identity theories see the mind as a thing like a rock or a molecule. But the mind isn't a thing; it's a process.

MARY: Help me understand. What is the difference between a thing and a process?

FRANCINE: Sure. There are two ways to answer the question, 'What is it?' If I asked you about a steel girder, you would probably tell me *what it is*, that is, its composition and structure. You would treat it as a thing. However, if I asked you about a clock, you would probably say, 'Something to tell time'; that is, you would tell me *what it does*. In answering what a clock does, you have given a functional (or process) description.

MARY: I think I get it. So how does this explain how brain relates to mind?

FRANCINE: I think that states of mind are functional states of brain.

DOUG: You've lost me! How does a functional state of brain differ from a physical state of brain?

FRANCINE: Think about a computer. You can change its physical state by adding more random-access memory or getting a bigger hard drive, or you can change its functional state by loading different software programs.

TEACHER: Let me interrupt for a moment. Francine is advocating what has been called functionalism, which is almost certainly the most popular current philosophical approach to the mind-body problem. Functionalism has strong historical roots in computer science, artificial intelligence, and the cognitive neurosciences.

MARY: Why has it been so popular?

TEACHER: Well, maybe we can let Francine explain. But its advocates say that it avoids the worst problems of dualism and the identity theories.

FRANCINE: Let me start with how this approach is superior to the type identity theories. When we think about mental states from a functional perspective, the problems of multiple realizabilty go away.

MARY: How?

FRANCINE: A functional theory would say depression is a functional state defined by responses to certain inputs with specific outputs.

DOUG: Such as crying when you took at a picture of an old boyfriend or having a very sad facial expression when waking up in the morning?

FRANCINE: Correct. Functionalism doesn't try to say that depression is a particular physiological brain state. It defines it at a more abstract level as any brain state that plays this particular functional role of causing someone to cry, to look sad, etc.

MARY: So functionalism would not be so concerned about whether the basic biology of depression in different humans or humans and aliens was the same as long as the state of depression in these organisms played the same functional role?

FRANCINE: Yes. I find this especially attractive.

MARY: So functionally equivalent need not say anything about biologically equivalent?

FRANCINE: Right. You can see how well functionalism lends itself to cognitive science and artificial intelligence. If brain states are functions connecting certain inputs with certain outputs (stub your toe → experience pain → swear, get red in the face, and dance around holding your toe and cursing), then this kind of state could be realized in a variety of different physical systems, including neurons or silicon chips.

MARY: I think I understand. But are functionalists materialists?

FRANCINE: Can I try to answer this?

TEACHER: Sure.

FRANCINE: I think the answer is mostly yes but a little bit no. Functional states are realized in material systems, but they are not essentially material states.

MARY: Can you translate that into plain English?

FRANCINE: OK. Let's go back to clocks. Their functional role is to tell time. But we could design a machine to tell time that used springs, pendulums, batteries, or even water. In each case, the clock is a material thing, but very different kinds of material things that were nonidentical on a physical level could all have the same function – of telling time.

TEACHER: Let me try to clarify. I think Francine is right that functionalism avoids the unattractive feature of dualism, which postulates a nonmaterial mental substance. But it resembles dualism in that it postulates two levels of reality. That is, there is the physical apparatus – I like to think of a huge series of switches – and then there is the functional state of those switches. Let's imagine a computer program that controls the railroad. You have thousands of switches in the form of transistors. Depending on whether one of those thousands of switches is on or off, you send a train to New York or Chicago. Recall that the fundamental physical nature of a transistor or any switch is not changed as a function of which position it is in. What is important are the rules of your program, that is, the functional significance of what that switch means.

MARY: I think I see more clearly. The switch is physical, but the significance of its on-ness or off-ness is really a function of the rules of the system – the program, in this case.

TEACHER: Yes. Philosophers would say that the functional status of the switch is *realized* in some physical structure.

DOUG: I think that I only dimly see the difference between functionalism and identity theories.

TEACHER: Doug, let me try one more approach, and this, for me, is perhaps the most important insight that functionalism has given me. Identity theorists want to equate a specific physiological aspect of brain function with specific mental events. A problem with this is that at a basic level, a lot of what goes on in the brain (ions crossing through membranes, second messenger systems being activated, neurotransmitters binding receptors) is nonspecific. If you looked at the biophysics of cell firing, it would probably look similar whether the neuron was involved in a pain pathway, the visual system, or a motor pathway. So, on one level, I would wager that the functionalists are right: that the specific mental consequences of a brain event cannot be fully specified at a purely physical level (e.g., as ions crossing membranes) but must also be a consequence of the functional organization of the brain. The same action potential could initiate the activity of neuronal arrays associated with a perception of pain, the color red, or the pitch of middle C, depending on where that neuron is located, that is, its functional position in the various brain pathways.

DOUG: That helps a lot. Thanks.

MARY: If we accept functionalism, aren't we at risk of sliding back into the whole functional-versus-organic mess? Am I not correct that functionalism might predict that some psychiatric illness is in the software, hence, functional, whereas others might be in the hardware? That has been a pretty sterile approach, hasn't it? I still want to stick up for the identity theories.

TEACHER: That is quite insightful, Mary. Maybe we will have time to look quickly at the implications of these theories for psychiatry. Let me briefly outline how the philosophical community has responded to functionalism. I will focus on two main objections. The first, and probably most profound, addresses the question of whether a software program is really a good model of the mind. This approach, known as the 'Chinese room problem,' was developed by the Berkeley philosopher John Searle[14]. It goes like this. Assume that you are part of a program designed to simulate naturally spoken Chinese, about which you know absolutely nothing. You have an input function, a window in your room through which you receive Chinese characters. You then have a complex manual in which you look up instructions. You go to the piles of Chinese characters in this room and, carefully following the instruction manual, you assemble a response that you produce as the output function of your room. If the manual is good enough, it is possible that to someone outside the room it might appear that you know Chinese – but, of course, you do not.

MARY: So, what is the point?

TEACHER: The point that Searle is making is that software is a bad model of the mind because it is only rules with no understanding (or, more technically, 'syntax without semantics'). An aspect of mind that has to be taken into account in any model of the mind-body problem is that minds understand things. You know what the words 'box,' 'love,' and 'sky' mean. Meaning is a key, basic aspect of some critical dimensions of mental functioning.

FRANCINE: But there have been a number of strong rebuttals to this argument!

TEACHER: I know, Francine, but if we are going to get done with these rounds, let me outline the second main problem with the functionalist approach: it defines mind-brain operations solely in terms of their functional status.

DOUG: Yes. So, where is the problem?

TEACHER: Well, for example, say I am faced with a color-discrimination task: having to learn which kind of fruit is bitter and poisonous (let's say green) and which is sweet and nutritions (let's say red). The state of my perception of color in this context is only meaningful to a functionalist because it enables me to predict taste and nutritional status.

In what is called the 'inverted-spectrum problem,' if the wiring from your eye to your brain for color were somehow reversed so that you saw green where I saw red and vice versa, from a functional perspective, we would never know. You would learn just as quickly as I would that green fruit is bitter and to be avoided and red fruit is good and can be eaten safely. However, our subjective experiences would be exactly the opposite. You would have learned to associate the subjective sense of redness (which you would have learned to call greenness because that it what everyone else would call it) with fruit to be avoided and greenness with fruit to be eaten.

MARY: I think I see.

TEACHER: We need to move on to another of the most puzzling aspects of the mind-body problem.

MARY: How many more are there? My head is starting to swim.

TEACHER: Hold on, Mary. Just a few more minutes, and we'll be done. The first issue we need to talk about has a bunch of names, which I will call the problem of intentionality. If we reject dualistic models and accept one of the family of identity theories or functionalism, how do we explain that when I want to scratch my nose, amazingly, my arm and hand move and my fingers scratch?

DOUG: Isn't your big term 'intentionality' another word for, free will?

TEACHER: Sort of, Doug, but I don't want to get into all the ethical and religious implications of free will. I would argue that it is an absolutely compelling subjective impression of every human being I have spoken to that we have a will. We can wish to do things, and then our body executes those wishes. This phenomenon, which in the old dualistic theory might be called mind-brain causality, is pretty hard to explain using identity and functionalist theories.

MARY: The eliminative materialists have a solution: that the perception of having a will is false.

DOUG: Isn't there any philosophically defensible alternative to this rather grim view?

MARY: I'd be more interested in a scientifically defensible alternative. But I'm a little confused. If we accept the identity theory, aren't we then saying that brain and mind are the same thing? So, if the brain wishes something – has intention, to use your words – then so does the mind.

TEACHER: Technically you're right, Mary. But here is the problem. How do carbon atoms, sodium ions, and cAMP have intentions or wishes?

MARY: Hmm. I'll have to think about that.

TEACHER: Although there are several different approaches to this problem, I want to focus here on only one: that of emergent properties and the closely associated issues of bottom-up versus top-down causation.

FRANCINE: Can you define emergent properties for us?

TEACHER: Sure. But first we have to review issues about levels of causation. Most of us accept that there are certain laws of subatomic particles that govern how atoms work and function. The rules for how atoms work can then explain chemical reactions, the rules that explain biochemical systems like DNA replication, and these in turn can explain the biology of life. I could keep going, but I think that you get the basic idea.

MARY: Yes. So what does this have to do with the mind-body problem?

TEACHER: The concept of emergent properties is that at higher levels of complexity, new features of systems emerge that could not be predicted from the more basic levels. With these new features come new capabilities.

FRANCINE: Can you give us some examples?

TEACHER: Sure. One example that is often used is water and wetness. It makes no sense to say that one water molecular is wet. Wetness is an emergent property of water in its liquid form. Probably a better analogy is life itself. Imagine two test tubes full of all the constituents of life: oxygen, carbon, nitrogen, etc. In one of them, there are only chemicals – no living forms – and in the other, there are single-celled organisms. You would be hard pressed to deny that although the physical constituents of the two tubes are the same, there are not some new properties that arise in the tube with life.

DOUG: Couldn't you say the same things about family or social systems, that they have emergent properties that were not predictable from the behavior of single individuals?

TEACHER: Yes, Doug. Many would argue that. One critical concept of emergent properties is that all the laws of the lower level operate at the higher level, but new ones come online. So, the question this all leads to is whether we can view many aspects of mind, such as intentionality, consciousness, or qualia, as emergent properties of brain.

The theory of emergent properties can challenge traditional scientific ideas about the direction or causality. Traditional reductionist models of science see causation flowing unidirectionally through these hierarchical systems, from the bottom up. Changes in subatomic particles might influence atomic structure, which in turn would affect molecular structure, etc. But no change in a biological system would affect the laws of quantum mechanics. However, if we adopt this perspective on the mind-body problem, it is very difficult to see how volition could ever work.

DOUG: I think I need an example here to understand what you're driving at.

TEACHER: Let's look at evolution. Most of us accept that life is explicable on the basis of understood principles of chemistry. However, life is a classic emergent property. Evolution does not work directly on atoms, molecules, or cells. The unit of selection by which evolution works is the whole organism, which will or will not succeed in passing on its genes to the next generation. So your and my DNA are in fact influenced by natural selection acting on the whole organisms of our ancestors. Thus, in addition to the traditional bottom-up causality we usually think about – DNA produces RNA, which makes protein – DNA itself is shaped over evolutionary time by the self-organizing emergent properties of the whole organism that it creates. That is an example of top-down causality. But, critically, this hypothesis is nothing like dualism. Organisms are entirely material beings that operate by the rules of physics and chemistry.

MARY: So you see this as a possible model for the mind/brain?

TEACHER: This is one of the main ways that people try to accommodate two seemingly contradictory positions, that dualism is not acceptable and is probably false and that the mind/brain truly has causal powers, so that human volition is not a fantasy as proposed by the eliminative materialists.

I need to see a patient in a few minutes. But before we end, we have to touch on two more issues. The first returns us to where we started, with dualism. As I said before, few working scientists today give much credence to classical Cartesian substance dualism, although property dualism does have some current adherents. However, there is a third form of dualism that may be highly relevant to modern neuroscience, especially psychiatry.

FRANCINE: What is that, Teacher?

TEACHER: It is called explanatory dualism and might be defined as follows: to have a complete understanding of humans, two different kinds of explanations are required. Lots of different names have been applied to these two kinds of explanations. The first can be called mental, psychological, or first person. The second can be called material biological, or third person.

DOUG: Aren't those just different names for Descartes' mental and material spheres?

TEACHER: Yes. But with one critical difference. Descartes spoke of the existence of two fundamentally different kinds of 'stuff.' Technically, he was talking about ontology, the discipline in philosophy that examines the fundamental basis of reality. Explanatory dualism, by contrast, deals with two different ways of knowing or understanding. This is a concern of the discipline of epistemology, or the problem of the nature of knowledge.

MARY: Can you explain that without all the big words?

TEACHER: A fair question! Explanatory dualism makes no assumptions about the nature of the relationship between mind and brain. It just says that there are two different and complementary ways of explaining events in the mind/brain.

DOUG: To accept explanatory dualism, do you have to accept Descartes' substance dualism?

TEACHER: No. In fact, explanatory dualism is consistent with identity theories or functionalism. Let's assume that the token identity theory about Mr. A's depression is true; that is, the serotonergic dysfunction in certain critical limbic regions in his brain is his depression. Explanatory dualism suggests that even if these brain and mind states have an identity relationship, to understand these states completely requires explanations both from the perspective of mind (perhaps the psychological issues that Doug first raised at the beginning of our discussion) and the perspective of brain. Neither approach provides a complete explanation.

DOUG: That is very attractive. This makes it possible to believe that mind and brain are the same thing and yet not deny the unique status of mental experiences.

TEACHER: Yes, if you accept explanatory dualism.

MARY: Isn't this theory a bit unusual in that most events in the material world have only one explanation? We wouldn't think that you would have one explanation for lightning and another for earth-to-cloud electrical discharges. Why should events in the brain be different?

TEACHER: I agree, Mary. Explanatory dualism suggests that there is something unique about mind-brain events that does not apply to material events that do not occur in brains, that they can be validly explained from two perspectives, not just one.

DOUG: What is appealing about explanatory dualism is that it seems to describe what we do every day when we see psychiatric patients, despite all these discussions, and it may be that mind really is brain. I am still impressed with the basic fact that we have fundamentally different ways in which we can know brains versus minds. One is public and the other private. Getting back to Mr. A, the optimal treatment for him requires me to be able to view Mr. A's depression from both the perspectives of brain and mind. We need to be able to view the depression as a product of Mr. A's brain to consider whether his disorder might be due to a neurologic and endocrine disease and to evaluate the efficacy and understand the mode of action of antidepressant medications. But to provide good quality humanistic clinical care, and especially psychotherapy, I need to be able to use and develop my natural intuitive and empathic powers to understand his depression from the perspective of mind, thinking about his wishes, conflicts, anger, sadness, and the impact of life events in addition to autoreceptors; uptake pumps, and down-regulation.

TEACHER: There is a lot that is very sensible in what you say, Doug. I would add that it is critically important for us to understand both the strengths and limitations of and the important differences between knowing our patients from the perspective of brain versus from the perspective of mind.

DOUG: I agree.

TEACHER: One last issue, and then I really have to go. When we look at major theories in psychiatry, like the dopamine hypothesis of schizophrenia or trying to tie Mr. A's depression to dysfunction in the serotonin system, what assumptions are we making about the relationship between mind and brain?

MARY: It is pretty clearly materialistic at least in the sense that changes in brain explain the mental symptoms of these syndromes.

TEACHER: So these theories embody the assumption of brain-to-mind causality?

DOUG: I am not clear on this. Do these biological theories of psychiatric illness assume a causal or an identity relationship between mind and brain?

TEACHER: Good question, Doug. If you listen to biological researchers closely, they actually use causal language quite commonly. They might say, 'An excess of dopamine transmission in key limbic forebrain structures causes schizophrenia.'

FRANCINE: Do they mean that, or do they actually mean that an excess of dopamine transmission is schizophrenia?

TEACHER: I am not sure. My bet is that most biological psychiatrists prefer some kind of identity theory. I wonder if they use causal language because Cartesian assumptions about the separation of material and mental spheres are so deeply rooted in the way we think.

MARY: So they may not be very precise about the philosophical assumptions they are making?

TEACHER: That's my impression.

MARY: What about the multiple-realizability problem? Are they likely to assume type identity theories that imply that a single mental state (e.g., auditory hallucinations) has an identity relationship with a single brain state or token identity states that suggest that multiple brain states might produce the same mental state, such as hearing voices?

TEACHER: My guess is that most researchers suggest that token identity models are most realistic. They would be more likely to call it 'etiologic heterogeneity,' but I think it is the same concept in different garb.

DOUG: After all, we know that hearing voices can arise from drugs of abuse, schizophrenia, affective illness, and dementia.

MARY: What about eliminative materialism? That would have pretty radical implications for the practice of psychiatry!

TEACHER: Yes, it would, Mary. If you took that theory literally – that mental processes are without causal efficacy, like froth on the wave – then any psychiatric interventions that are purely mental in nature, like psychotherapy, could not possibly work.

DOUG: We have a lot of evidence that psychological interventions work and can produce changes in biology. That would be strong evidence against eliminative materialism, wouldn't it?

TEACHER: That's how I see it, Doug.

FRANCINE: What about functionalism? Certainly theories of schizophrenia and affective illness have pointed toward defective information processing and mood control modules, respectively.

TEACHER: This gets to a pretty basic point. Etiologic heterogeneity aside, are specific forms of mental illness "things" that have a defined material basis or abnormalities at a functional level, like an error in a module of software?

FRANCINE: This gets at what you said before. Functionalism is different from identity theories in that it implies abnormalities are possible in psychiatric illness at two levels: the functional 'software' level that affects mind or the material 'hardware' level that affects brain.

TEACHER: Yes. I am ambivalent about that implication. It suggests two different pathways to psychiatric illness. Is it helpful to ask whether Mr. A developed depression with a normal brain that was 'misprogrammed' perhaps through faulty rearing or because there is a structural abnormality in his brain? I'm not sure. I continue to feel that functionalism makes sense if you think about computers and artificial intelligence, but when you deal with brains like we do, I have my doubts. But as I said, this is still the most popular theory about the mind-body problem among philosophers. I have to go. I look forward to seeing you on rounds tomorrow. This was fun.

DOUG, FRANCINE, AND MARY: Good bye, Teacher.

Conclusions

The goal of this introductory dialogue was to provide a helpful, user-friendly introduction to some of the current thinking on the mind-body problem, as seen from a psychiatric perspective. Many interesting topics were not considered (including, for example, philosophical behaviorism and the details of theories propounded by leading workers in the field, such as Searle and Dennett), and others were discussed only superficially. Those interested in pursuing this fascinating area might wish to consult the list of references and web sites below.

Recommendations

Web Sites

The *Stanford Encyclopedia of Philosophy*[15] has a number of entries relevant to the mind-body problem. For example, see 'Epiphenomenalism,' 'Identity Theory of Mind,' and 'Multiple Realizability.' See, also, the *Dictionary of Philosophy of Mind*[16].

David Chalmers has compiled a very useful list of 'Online Papers on Consciousness' as part of a larger web site titled 'Contemporary Philosophy of Mind: An Annotated Bibliography'[17].

Further Reading

Bechtel's *Philosophy of Mind: An Overview for Cognitive Science*[18] is a good overview from the perspective of psychology, although rather technical in places.

A Companion to the Philosophy of Mind[19] is a helpful but somewhat difficult introductory essay followed by short entries on nearly all topics of importance in the mind-body problem. Very useful.

Gennaro's *Mind and Brain: A Dialogue on the Mind-Body Problem*[20] is a brief, easily understood introduction to the mind-body problem, also in the form of a dialogue.

Churchland's *Matter and Consciousness: A Contemporary Introduction to the Philosophy of Mind*[21] is a good introduction to the mind-body problem. Although a strong advocate for eliminative materialism, Churchland fairly presents the other main perspectives. The chapter on neuroscience is dated.

Brook and Stainton's *Knowledge and Mind: A Physical Introduction*[22] is a charming, accessible, and up-to-date introduction that includes sections on epistemology and the problem of free will.

Priest's *Theories of the Mind*[23] is a quite useful, albeit somewhat more advanced, treatment of the mind-body problem. Priest takes a different approach from the other books listed here, summarizing the views of this problem by 17 major philosophers, from Plato to Wittgenstein.

Heil's *Philosophy of Mind: A Contemporary Introduction*[24] is a recent introductory book, with an emphasis on the metaphysical aspects of the mind-body problem. A bit hard to follow in the later chapters.

Searle's *The Rediscovery of the Mind*[25] is probably the most important book by this influential philosopher who has been very critical of functionalism. He writes clearly and with a minimum of philosophical jargon.

Nagel's *The View From Nowhere*[26] is a brilliant book-length treatment of the key epistemic issue raised by the mind-body problem: that we see the world from a third-person perspective but ourselves from a first-person perspective.

Hannan's *Subjectivity and Reduction: An Introduction to the Mind-Body Problem*[27] is a short and relatively clear introduction. The author makes no attempt to hide her views about the problem.

The Nature of Consciousness: Philosophical Debates[28] is probably the most up-to-date of the several available collections of key articles in this area, with an emphasis on problems related to consciousness.

Cunningham's *What Is a Mind? An Integrative Introduction to the Philosophy of Mind*[29] is a particularly clear and up-to-date summary of the mind/body and related philosophical topics. It is one of the best available introductions.

Audiotapes

If you want to probe the mind-body problem on your way to work, you might want to try Searle's *The Philosophy of Mind*[30] audiotapes. Searle has his own specific 'take' on this problem, but he is down-to-earth and rather accessible for the beginner.

References

1   **Kandel ER**: A new intellectual framework for psychiatry. *Am J Psychiatry* 1998; **155**:457–469.

2   **Kandel ER**: Biology and the future of psychoanalysis: a new intellectual framework for psychiatry revisited. *Am J Psychiatry* 1999; **156**:505–524.

3   **Seager W**: *Theories of Consciousness: An Introduction and Assessment*, 1st ed. London, Routledge, 1999.

4   **Edelman GM, Tononi G**: *A Universe of Consciousness*. New York, Basic Books, 2000.

5   **Damasio A**: *The Feeling of What Happens: Body and Emotion in the Making of Consciousness*. San Diego, Harcourt Brace, 1999.

6   **Guzeldere G, Flanagan O, Hardcastle VG**: The nature and function of consciousness: lessons from blindsight, in *The New Cognitive Neurosciences*, 2nd ed. Edited by Gazzaniga MS. Cambridge, Mass, MIT Press, 2000. pp 1277–1284.

7   **Baynes K., Gazzaniga MS**: Consciousness: introspection, and the split-brain: the two minds/one body problem. Ibid, pp 1355–1364.

8   **Descartes R**: *Meditations on First Philosophy*. Translated by **Lafleur LJ**. New York. Macmillan, 1985.

9   **Squire LR, Kandel ER**: *Memory: From Mind to Molecules*. New York, Scientific American Library, 1999.

10 **Libet B**: Unconscious cerebral initiative and the role of conscious will in voluntary action. *Behav Brain Sci* 1985; **8**:529–566.

11 **Levine J**: Materialism and qualia: the explanatory gap. *Pacific Philosophical Quarterly* 1983: **64**:354–361.

12 **Chalmers D**: Facing up to the problem of consciousness. *J Consciousness Studies* 1995; **2**:200–219.

13 **Nagel T**: What is it like to be a bat, in *Mortal Questions*. New York, Cambridge University Press, 1979, pp 165–180.

14 **Searle JR**: Minds, brains, and programs. *Behav Brain Sci* 1980; **3**:417–424.

15 Stanford University, Metaphysics Research Lab, Center for the Study of Language and Information: *Stanford Encyclopedia of Philosophy.* http://plato.stantord.edu.

16 **Eliasmith C** (ed): *Dictionary of Philosophy of Mind.* http://www.artsci.wustl.edu/ ~philos/MindDict/index.html

17 **Chalmers D**: *Online Papers on Consciousness.* http://www.u.arizona.edu/ ~chalmers/online.html

18 **Bechtel W**: *Philosophy of Mind: An Overview for Cognitive Science.* **Hillsdale, NJ.** Lawrence Erlbaum Associates, 1988.

19 **Guttenplan S** (ed): *A Companion to the Philosophy of Mind.* Cambridge, Mass. Blackwell, 1994.

20 **Gennaro RJ**: *Mind and Brain: A Dialogue on the Mind-Body Problem.* Indianapolis, Hackett, 1996.

21 **Churchland PM**: *Matter and Consciousness: A Contemporary Introduction to the Philosophy of Mind*, revised ed. Cambridge, Mass, MIT Press, 1988.

22 **Brook A, Stainton RJ**: *Knowledge and Mind: A Physical Introduction.* Cambridge, Mass, MIT Press, 2000.

23 **Priest S**: *Theories of the Mind.* New York, Houghton Mifflin, 1991.

24 **Heil J**: *Philosophy of Mind: A Contemporary Introduction.* London. Routledge, 1998.

25 **Searle JR**: *The Rediscovery of the Mind.* Cambridge, Mass, MIT Press, 1992.

26 **Nagel T**: *The View From Nowhere.* New York, Oxford University Press, 1986.

27 **Hannan B**: *Subjectivity and Reduction: An Introduction to the Mind-Body Problem.* Boulder, Colo, Westview Press, 1994.

28 **Block N. Flanagan O, Guzeldere G** (eds): *The Nature of Consciousness: Philosophical Debates.* Cambridge, Mass, MIT Press, 1997.

29 **Cunningham S**: *What Is a Mind? An Integrative Introduction to the Philosophy of Mind.* Indianapolis. Hackett, 2000.

30 **Searle JR**: *The Philosophy of Mind.* Springfield, Va, Teaching Company, 1996 (audiotapes).

4 Confidentiality

Preserving the secrets of patients has its provenance in Ancient Greece. The Oath of Hippocrates makes this duty explicit

What I may see or hear in the course of the treatment or even outside of the treatment in regard to the life of men which on no account one must spread abroad, I will keep to myself holding such things shameful to be spoken about[1]

In modern times, the psychiatrist's assurance to his patients that whatever transpires between them will remain confidential, is a hallmark of the therapeutic relationship. However, many forces, including the changing nature of clinical practice and the society in which that practice is embedded, have limited the capacity of psychiatrists to guarantee absolute confidentiality, and have even raised questions about the moral basis of such assurance.

The chapters and articles we have selected and referred to in this section cover the place of confidentiality in contemporary clinical psychiatry and highlight the ethical dilemmas that arise and potential responses to them (see also Chapter 9).

What is confidentiality?

Confidentiality is a key facet of the concept of privacy whereby we deem it a value to insist that all people have the right to control access to themselves or not be intruded upon. Stated more positively, every person has the right to be left alone.

Privilege, a related concept, refers to the right of a person to determine what information will be divulged in a judicial or administrative context and prevails when legal statute specifies its function. The clearest illustration of its role in psychiatry is articulated in Jaffee v. Redmond (1995), where the US Supreme Court ruled that communication between therapist and patient is privileged and '. . . rooted in the imperative need for confidence and trust' in the therapeutic encounter. Mary Redmond, a policewoman, shot and killed a man while on duty. She soon started to receive psychotherapy from a social worker. The deceased's relatives then sued Ms Redmond and asked to access the therapist's notes. This was refused on the grounds of the privileged status of the material. In the majority decision (7:2) psychotherapist-patient privilege was upheld although it could be waived by the patient and be put aside to avert serious harm to the patient or to others.[2]

As can be seen in this example, confidentiality pertaining to the clinical sphere has special relevance in psychiatry. The nature of the patient's disclosures to the therapist are frequently personal in the extreme. Patients may share their innermost secrets with psychiatrists who commonly serve as the first recipients of these disclosures. An account of sexual or physical abuse or a shameful act or a guilt-laden experience are but a few instances which testify to the salience of the therapist-patient relationship as a forum for sharing the most intensely personal details about oneself.

Sissela Bok, in her splendid book, *Secrets*,[3] from which we have selected Chapter 9 for our anthology, outlines four premises for justifying confidentiality, although certain caveats obtrude. Central for Bok is respect for individual autonomy – a person is entitled to have secrets. However, this entitlement is not complete. For example, bearing a contagious disease calls for respecting the interests of others. The second premise relates to the notion of shared secrets as exemplified in an intimate marriage. Again, circumstances may arise which warrant disclosing a marital secret to other parties. A third premise deals with keeping a confidence if this has been promised, although questions arise as to potential situations that could override that obligation. The last premise focuses on professional confidentiality in that various professionals including priests, lawyers and doctors, commit themselves to keeping the secrets divulged to them. Here, the value of confidentiality is made explicit. As Bok puts it: 'People benefit from confidentiality because it allows them to seek help they might otherwise fear to ask for.' The fact that such profession-based confidentiality cannot be absolute raises genuine ethical dilemmas which we tackle below.

The recurrent theme in Bok's chapter – preserving confidentiality – is the focus in a chapter by Douglas Black[4] suitably entitled 'Absolute confidentiality?' in Gillon's monumental volume, *Principles of health care ethics*. Black's argument rests on three propositions: an ethical position can be valid and useful but not necessarily apply to all situations; legitimate exceptions are likely; and two or more accepted ethical principles may clash and prove incompatible. All three propositions may apply to the obligation to safeguard confidences in medical practice. The example of a train driver suffering a myocardial infarction is used to stress the possible need for his doctor to inform the employer about the risks of the person returning to his former job. In releasing that information, however, two cogent issues arise: who needs to know and how much do they need to know? Black invokes the hallowed process of informed consent as a valuable means to expedite disclosure of information to another party and also reminds us of the range of statutory and legal requirements for the doctor to inform.

The centrality of confidentiality in clinical psychiatry

Mark Siegler's[5] description of confidentiality in medicine as a 'decrepit concept' has resonated for over two decades and is often quoted. He was certainly not exaggerating when pointing out that at least six dozen people have legitimate access to the hospital medical record but a corollary that the principle of medical confidentiality therefore '. . . no longer exists' does not follow. On the contrary, it means that clinicians have to work that much harder to safeguard patients' confidences. David Joseph and Joseph Onek have pointed this out impressively in their comprehensive chapter in our sister volume *Psychiatric Ethics*.[6] They cover a vast range of pertinent topics (only some of which we can tackle below): the interface between confidentiality and the law, clinical records (this is especially problematic in an era of information technology when much personal clinical data are computerized, transferred between information systems including medical databases, and accessible to the patient), the requirements of, and pressures from, third parties (eg. insurers, employers, statutory authorities), the Tarasoff situation, sexual abuse, AIDS, psychiatric genetics, group, family and couple therapy, multiple clinicians, teaching and medical writing.

We could not possibly select papers and chapters from the published literature on every one of these subjects; it would assume the dimensions of an anthology unto itself. We have therefore opted to focus on some key topics which challenge the psychiatrist particularly and have, consequently, attracted ethical attention, namely the potential breach of confidentiality when a patient threatens to harm others, the question of sharing information with the caregiver of the psychotic patient and the tension between the psychotherapy patient's need for complete privacy and the professional's need to advance the field (the latter topic is covered in lively fashion by a team of psychoanalysts who presented at an international conference in Montreal in 2000.[7]

The Tarasoff judgment

Informed consent makes a doctor's potential breach of confidentiality considerably easier to handle since the action stems from a partnership. By contrast, when the patient prohibits the doctor from divulging any information about himself or is not mentally competent to arrive at a sound judgment, ethical complications arise.

The landmark case in this context is the Tarasoff judgment delivered in the Californian Supreme Court, initially in 1974 and with a follow-up two years later. In brief, a student, Prosenjit Poddar, murdered Tatiana Tarasoff, whom he was eager to befriend, having divulged his intention to do so to his psychologist-therapist two months earlier. Concerned by the prospect of harm befalling Ms Tarasoff, the therapist consulted his seniors and, on their advice, the police. The latter questioned Mr Poddar and concluded that he did not pose a threat to Ms Tarasoff but obtained a promise that he would not contact her.

The 1976[8] judgment can be summarized as follows: in the event of a patient intending to harm an identified person, 'protective privilege ends when the public peril begins'. In other words, the therapist is duty-bound to protect an intended victim if that person can be identified. The 1974 decision referred only to a 'duty to warn'.

The judgment has endured for over a quarter of a century and been taken up in various ways by several other jurisdictions (about half the States in the US, for example, have passed legislation), so testifying to its coherence. However, we should note arguments mounted against the judgment, including a dissenting opinion in the original decision. Virtually all criticism revolves around the threat Tarasoff poses to the integrity of the therapeutic relationship. As Stone[9] proclaimed at the time of the 1976 judgment, using a utilitarian argument (also the basis of the dissenting opinion in the Californian Supreme Court decision), imposing a duty to protect would undermine a patient's expectation of confidentiality and so jeopardize treatment. This in turn would reduce public safety. (Stone changed his mind about this matter later.)

Gurevitz[10] argued that a Tarasoff duty leads to clinical practice that makes the psychotherapist more concerned with protecting society than with treating patients. Put another way, Tarasoff elevates psychiatry's social control function.

A clinically-oriented position has been advocated by Wulson et al.[11] who assert that the duty of care to both intended victim and patient can lead to an optimal outcome. How can this be so? Conceding that breaches of confidentiality are inevitable, the treatment alliance need not suffer. Informing the patient honestly and directly, exploiting the customary ambivalence towards the victim and demonstrating that the clinician is taking responsibility to protect both parties combine to reinforce the integrity of the alliance.

Ironically, a professor of law has argued trenchantly for a shift in how clinicians should deal with the patient threatening to cause harm and the intended victim. The law, David Wexler[12] avers, has played itself out but paved the way for a 'post-Tarasoff scenario' whose principal feature is abandonment of an intrapsychic model of interpersonal violence in favour of an interactionist framework; his sights are on both patient and intended victim. The latter, empirical research reveals, is typically a family member or other known person who is aware of the patient's participation in treatment, and of his hostility. The therapist, accordingly, strives to obtain the patient's consent to establish contact with the potential victim. The advantage of a meeting between therapist and the person at risk is acquisition of valuable knowledge about the patient's motives as well as the intended victim's possible contributions to the problematic interaction. This additional body of information is, in Wexler's thesis, likely to enhance treatment. There is a snag, however, with this ostensibly reasonable interactionist position – the possible, if not likely, lack of psychological insight in the patient to consent to the contact deemed so vital by Wexler. If consent is forthcoming, it is likely that the risk of actual violence is considerably reduced. Notwithstanding, the proposition to exploit the patient's trust in therapist and treatment is designed to prevent a breach of confidentiality with all the ethical and legal repercussions that ensue.

The Wexler account is appealing when we consider that although Tarasoff has become a legislative feature of many American jurisdictions, it has been applied inconsistently. Anfang and Appelbaum[13] have usefully examined how a duty to protect has been handled in the US over the first two decades post-Tarasoff. As they put it, the precedent 'continues to confuse and confound'. No wonder when so many variations have evolved. The authors paint a rich canvas, showing how complex Tarasoff has become. For instance, in a Nebraskan case, the court finds a duty to protect even in the absence of a specifically identifiable victim while in a Delaware ruling the question of duration of the prediction of violence is raised. Can a psychiatrist realistically know that his patient may be violently disposed several months following his discharge from hospital treatment? In Iowa, a patient held her own psychiatrist negligent in not preventing her from murdering her first husband. Farcically, her current husband got into the act by suing the same psychiatrist for the loss of the marital relationship. This is taking Tarasoff to an absurd level. Fortunately, the authors recommend an appropriate response to the duty to protect which brings reason to a messy picture.

Possibly anticipating the uniqueness of each Tarasoff situation, jurisdictions outside of the US, among them the UK, Canada and Australia,[14] have shied away from legislating or setting a precedent. In the UK, the Royal College of Psychiatrists produced a series of guidelines designed to assist the clinician to make the best possible judgement.[15] The decision may be 'finely balanced' but takes into account a range of factors including the duty to maintain confidences, an interest in a health service preserving such confidences, the scope of an actual disclosure, the risk of not disclosing (e.g. death or serious harm), the ability to identify an intended victim and dual obligation in the psychiatrist's workplace. When breaching confidentiality is regarded as essential, the College offers recommendations on how to carry out the process.

Notwithstanding the adoption by many States in the US of legal measures, a tendency may have began to dilute the potency of the law by limiting the scope of the duty to protect.[16] *Parri passu*, clinicians are regarded as less liable than in the past. The legal situation in Australia shows an absence of statutory law and no legal precedent, with emphasis on the centrality of the doctor-patient relationship. On the other hand, empirical research demonstrates that most psychiatrists are familiar with the Tarasoff duty and have given it much thought.[17]

The pervasiveness of Tarasoff is also exemplified by the threat of law being raised in psychiatric research.[18] Argued hypothetically because an act of violence has not been recorded in research, the authors list the issues that investigators should consider were such a situation to arise. The paramount question is grounded in whether a 'special relationship' akin to a therapeutic relationship can be said to exist in the research setting. The answer will probably differ according to the nature of the study. Thus, the more similar the researcher-subject relationship is to the therapeutic one, the more likely a Tarasoff duty warrants consideration. The idea of the investigator raising the possibility of a duty to protect as part of informed consent is not regarded as useful since it is likely to discourage people from participating in research.

If we return to the clinical arena, psychiatrists as part of the medical profession face other quandaries when a threat of, or actual, harm to an identified person is discovered. A classical example is child abuse, for which jurisdictions in many enlightened societies have legislated that it is mandatory to report this to relevant authorities. Forewarning the limits of confidentiality becomes a challenging ethical issue in these circumstances.

The dilemma is highlighted in a symposium revolving around the sexual abuse of a 13-year-old girl by her stepfather.[19] The case involves the disclosure by a mother and her daughter to their general practitioner of continuing sexual abuse by the stepfather (also a patient of the practitioner), and the mother's insistence upon absolute confidentiality. The doctor agrees to counsel mother and daughter under this condition and does so for 18 months. At the end of this time the girl indicates that the abuse has not occurred for a substantial period. The counselling programme is ended by agreement of the three protagonists. Five months later, the girl is sexually assaulted and strangled by the stepfather. Should the general practitioner have shared the information regarding sexual abuse with other authorities at the outset even if it meant doing so without the patient and the mother's (as proxy) consent?

In the discussion that follows, a consistent attitude emerges. A general practitioner argues that it was incumbent upon the doctor to seek expert advice from a paediatrician who could, as an impartial third party, adjudicate between the needs of the child and the welfare of the family. A paediatric panellist is forthright about the overriding obligation to the patient, in this case the girl. In colluding with the mother, the general practitioner failed to keep the patient's interests paramount.

The child psychiatrist sees the matter similarly: '. . . the safety of the child must in all circumstances be of paramount importance and must override all considerations'. The contribution from a medical ethicist points to the same conclusion but one derived from an interesting analysis. The two arguments in favour of confidentiality – that it is an absolute principle or can only be trumped where extreme harm will result – are outweighed by three counter-arguments: that preserving confidentiality does not respect the girl's autonomy, does not serve the common good and is against the child's interests. Although child sexual abuse may present unique features, the case discussion illuminates well the complex aspects of confidentiality.

Pamela Budai[20] examines the arguments for legally mandated reporting, illuminating how different jurisdictions, even in a small country like Australia, can adopt a diverse array of policies – from no legislation at all through voluntary reporting to mandatory reporting of abuse. She also deals clearly with the arguments for and against the latter, raising the possibility of professionally derived standards to guide reporting.

HIV infection and AIDS, like child sexual abuse, have generated hugely challenging ethical dilemmas for the clinician, including the psychiatrist. In his overview on the subject, Kelly[21] argues for the respect of confidentiality except in a few limited circumstances: a past sexual partner of a virus carrier should be notified of his exposure in order to prevent the spread of the virus; a potential sexual partner or spouse of a virus carrier should be advised about the potentiality of becoming infected; and medical staff who are in contact with infected body fluids have a right to know this in order to take protective measures. Otherwise, Kelly asserts, the principle of confidentiality applies, not only in respect of the patient's diagnosis but also concerning his or her lifestyle, i.e. sexual and drug habits. Although Kelly implicitly refers to respect for the patient's autonomy and the desirability of maximizing the common good, the guidelines he offers do not stem from any obvious process of ethical reasoning.

The American Psychiatric Association (APA) began to tackle the issues covered by Kelly in the early 1980s, establishing its first AIDs work group in 1984, its charge to make psychiatrists aware of the psychosocial dimension. It soon emerged that ethical aspects were prominent, particularly the conflict between patient confidentiality and the clinician's 'duty to protect'. A policy crystallized in 1987, subsequently subject to revision. In essence, the APA's official position on confidentiality, disclosure and the protection of others, encompassed the following guidelines: there are specified limits of confidentiality concerning HIV/AIDS; the law may require reporting names of HIV positive patients; patients placing others at risk of infection should be counselled to cease that behaviour or inform the person/s concerned; it is ethically justifiable in the case of a non-cooperative patient to notify identified people at risk or to request a statutory health authority to do so; it is equally justifiable to contact an authority when the risk is to unidentifiable persons; hospital commitment is permissible when hazardous behaviour is the result of a mental illness; psychiatrists should counsel HIV patients to inform past contacts or ask a relevant health authority to do so; and if the patient refuses or is unable to do this (eg. a demented patient), the psychiatrist is ethically justified to notify the authority.[22]

In the UK, a working party of the independent Institute of Medical Ethics launched its consideration of the confidentiality/HIV-AIDS interface in the wake of the General Medical Council's 1988 guidelines. Examining those aspects also tackled by the APA, they arrived at broadly similar guidelines concerning the need to breach patient confidentiality; interestingly no psychiatrists served on the UK working party.[23]

The family and confidentiality

With the growth of community psychiatry has come an examination of the role of the family as informal carer for patients with enduring or recurring mental illnesses such as schizophrenia, bipolar disorder, recurrent depression and schizoaffective disorder. The question of how family members should be involved in the care of their relative-patient has been much influenced by ethical factors. Szmukler and Bloch[24] argue for a methodical approach to collaborating with the family in these circumstances in order that ethical challenges, such as whether to breach confidentiality, can be addressed rationally. Their focus is on patients with a psychotic condition, since it is in this type of situation that ethical problems arise.

With considerable research pointing to the benefits of enlisting help of relatives to treat patients with psychosis though psychoeducation, counseling and the opportunity to obtain pertinent information, it would appear counterproductive to be thwarted by a patient's insightless refusal to provide consent. Yet to act against the patient's wishes places the relationship in jeopardy.

Szmukler and Bloch's line of argument rests on the premise that a morally neutral encounter with patient and family is fanciful. Values are central, particularly their influence on how to balance the interests and needs of all members. Informed consent is the cornerstone upon which ethically sound care of patients and their families may occur, a process involving a continuing dialogue between clinician and family (including the patient). It is when informed consent is inoperative that ethical dilemmas multiply. Through a series of sequential contentions the authors conclude that justification for disclosing information to (and also obtaining from) the family, contrary to the patient's wishes, is most robust when the harms to be avoided are serious and likely, acceptable alternatives are unavailable, the capacity of the patient to judge his or her interests is obviously impaired, the family's values embrace mutual concern and care and non-involvement of the family will lead inevitably to even greater restrictions on liberty.

Health authorities have come to appreciate this sort of reasoning. For instance, the Victoria (Australia) Mental Health Act was amended in 1996 to enable provision of information about the patient to family members serving in a caregiver role on the assumption that their interests and needs are as cogent as those of the patient.[25]

The above ideas are echoed in the work of Furlong and Leggatt[26] (also working in the Victoria context) and Petrila and Sadoff.[27] The latter present two vivid, tragic clinical stories to illustrate the point that 'Families should not be kept at arm's length because of a notion of confidentiality that far exceeds in application what is necessary to protect the values that is serves.' Disclosing patient's private communications to caregiving families is consistent with good risk management and relevant ethical principles.

Individual case material and confidentiality

Psychoanalysis grew out of the individual case report as we well know from the classical studies of Freud in the 1890s and early part of the twentieth century. Dora, Little Hans, the Rat Man, the Wolf Man and Anna O ushered in a novel way to understand the underlying dynamics of neurotic symptoms. In the Dora case, Freud himself pronounced that it was a doctor's duty to publish material about his patients '. . . as long as he can avoid causing personal injury to the patient concerned'.[28]

A century later, the humble case report may have been eclipsed by the bandwagon of evidence-based medicine but it remains a respected means to share ideas in many journals, especially those of a psychotherapy type. A threat to its continuing role is, however, the issue of preserving confidences. For many years, the author's discretion determined how they went about disseminating relevant details of a patient in a publication. In the late 1990s, a movement on the part of certain journal editors began to work out an ethically based policy. For instance, the *British Journal of Psychiatry* (BJP) launched a requirement in 1994[29] that informed consent should be obtained from the patient or, if that was impossible, from an 'authorized person'. In addition, sufficient concealment of the patient's identity through alteration of personal details was called for. Panellists invited to debate the topic differed predictably in response to these instructions. On the one hand, the need for informed consent, it was asserted, would probably discourage preparation of case reports while on the other hand instructions were vital to promote ethical standards. Interestingly, BJP policy was later amended to include the situation in which a patient refuses to consent. The case study in these circumstances could be considered for publication if details which might identify the person were omitted, so preventing a possible breach of confidentiality. Glen Gabbard,[30] co-editor of the *International Journal of Psychoanalysis*, depicted the issue as a conflict of interest – safeguarding privacy versus scientific progress. A further dimension was the case report serving the writer's own professional advancement. Gabbard resisted a single remedy (like the original BJP policy), proposing five options: thick disguise; informed consent from the patient; composites, that is, features of several patients combined into a single case study; a colleague writing up the report in order to protect the original clinician's anonymity; and focusing on the process of treatment rather than on the patient. Whatever strategy or combination of strategies selected, protecting privacy remained paramount.

This matter came dramatically to the fore in the Anne Sexton case. A celebrated American poet, her sessions with a distinguished psychiatrist, Martin Orne, were taped so that the patient could make better use of the therapeutic process. Years later, (following her suicidal death), when Sexton's biographer sought, with the support of the patient's daughter/ literary executor, the tapes for her research, Dr Orne, after considerable wavering, permitted the material to be thus used.

The ensuing heated debated revolved around confidentiality with the inevitable contrary positions. Release of the material on utilitarian grounds was justified in an argument offered by Paul Chodoff[31] inasmuch as the use of clinical material '. . . augment(s) knowledge of the causes and treatment of mental and emotional disorders, and thus benefit(s) present and future patients and the society as a whole'.

Prohibition of disclosure rests on the premise, as advanced by Edmund Pellegrino,[32] that people have a right to privacy that leads to a corresponding duty not to invade it. Trust lies at the heart of both these aspects. Pellegrino uses other arguments too – beneficence or promoting a person's best interests, keeping promises (assuming that the therapist does this) and respecting autonomy (really an umbrella under which sits respect for privacy). The author ends his paper with a *cri de couer*:

The Sexton biography should serve to sensitise all of us – therapists, patients and biographers – to the serious and complex nature of the moral covenant that entrusts us with the private life of our fellow human beings – living or dead

A laudable statement and one that permeates our selected material. However, and unfortunately, we cannot end without reiterating the caveat that confidentiality can never be absolute, and therein lies its ethical intricacy.

References

1   **Edelstein, L.**: The Hippocratic Oath, text, translation and interpretation, in *Ancient Medicine*, ed. O. Temkin and C.L. Temkin. Baltimore, Maryland, Johns Hopkins University Press, 1967, pp. 17–18.

2   **Jaffee *v.* Redmond**, 116 S. Ct. 1923, 1996.

*3   **Bok, S.**: *Secrets*. Oxford, Oxford University Press, 1996, pp. 116–135.

*4   **Black, D.**: Absolute confidentiality, in *Principles of health care ethics*, ed. R. Gillon. Chichester, Wiley, 1994, pp. 479–488.

5   **Siegler, M.**: Confidentiality in medicine. *New England Journal of Medicine* **307**:1518–1521, 1982.

6   **Joseph, D. and Onek, J.**: Confidentiality in psychiatry, in *Psychiatric Ethics*, 3rd edn. S. Bloch, P. Chodoff and S. Green. Oxford, Oxford University Press, 1999, pp. 105–140.

7   **Levin, C., Furlong, A. and O'Neil, M.**: (eds) *Confidentiality: Ethical perspectives and clinical dilemmas*. Hillsdale, NJ., Analytic Press, 2003.

*8   ***Tarasoff v. Regents of the University of California***. 131 Cal Rptr 14, 17 Cal. 3d 425, 551P. 2d 334, 1976.

9   **Stone, A.**: The Tarasoff case and some of its progeny: suing psychotherapists to safeguard society, in *Law, psychiatry and society*. Washington D.C., American Psychiatric Press, pp. 161–190, 1984.

10   **Gurewitz, H.**: Tarasoff: protective privilege versus public peril. *American Journal of Psychiatry* **134**:289–292, 1977.

11   **Wulsin, L., Bursztajn, H. and Gutheil, T.**: Unexpected clincial features of the Tarasoff decision: the therapeutic alliance and the 'duty to warn'. *American Journal of Psychiatry* **140**:601–603, 1983.

12   **Wexler, D.**: Patients, therapist, and third parties: The victimological virtues of Tarasoff. *International Journal of Law and Psychiatry* **2**:1–28, 1979.

13   **Anfang, S. and Appelbaum, P.**: Twenty years after Tarasoff: reviewing duty to protect. *Harvard Review of Psychiatry* **4**:67–76, 1996.

14   **Mendelson, D. and Mendelson, G.**: Tarasoff down under: the psychiatrist's duty to warn in Australia. *Journal of Psychiatry and Law* Spring–Summer, 33–61, 1991.

15   *Good psychiatric practices: confidentiality*. London, Royal College of Psychiatrists, 2000.

16   **Walcott, D., Cerundolo, P. and Beck, J.**: Current analysis of the Tarasoff duty: an evolution towards the limitations of duty to protect. *Behavioural Sciences and the Law* **19**:325–343, 2001.

17   **Beck, J.**: Violent patients and the Tarasoff duty in private psychiatric practice. *Journal of Psychiatry and the Law*. Fall–Winter: 361–376, 1985.

18   **Appelbaum, P. and Rosenbaum, A.**: Tarasoff and the researcher. does the duty to protect apply in the research setting? *American Psychologist* **44**:885–894, 1989.

19   **Williams, R., Singh, T., Naish, J.** *et al*. Medical confidentiality and multidisciplinary work: child sexual abuse and mental handicap registers. *British Medical Journal* **295**:1315–1319, 1987.

20   **Budai, P.**: Mandatory reporting of child abuse: is it in the best interest of the child? *Australian and New Zealand Journal of Psychiatry* **30**:794–804, 1996.

21   **Kelly K.** AIDS and ethics: an overview. *General Hospital Psychiatry* **9**:331–340, 1987.

22   **AIDS policy: Position statement on confidentiality disclosure and protection of others. *American Journal of Psychiatry* 150:852, 1993.**

23   **Boyd, K.** HIV infection and AIDS: The ethics of medical confidentiality. *Journal of Medical Ethics* **18**:173–179, 1992.

*24   **Szmukler, G. and Bloch, S.**: Family involvement in the care of people with psychoses. *British Journal of Psychiatry* **171**:401–405, 1997.

25 *Mental Health Act, 1986*, amended 19/6/97, Melbourne, State of Victoria, pp. 133–137, 1997.

26 **Furlong, M.** and **Leggatt, M.**: Reconciling the patient's right to confidentiality and the family's need to know. *Australian and New Zealand Journal of Psychiatry* **30**:614–622, 1996.

27 **Petrila, J.** and **Sadoff, R.**: Confidentiality and the family as caregiver. *Hospital and Community Psychiatry* **43**:136–139, 1992.

28 **Freud, S.** Fragment of an analysis of a case of hysteria, in *Standard edition*, vol **7**. London, Hogarth Press, 1953, pp. 7–122.

29 **Wilkinson, G., Fahy, T., Russell, G., Healy, D., Marks, I., Tantam, D** and **Dimond, B.**: Case reports and confidentiality. *British Journal of Psychiatry* **166**:555–558, 1995.

30 **Gabbard, G.**: Disguise or consent. *International Journal of Psychoanalysis* **81**: 1071–1086, 2000.

31 **Chodoff, P.**: The Anne Sexton biography: the limits of confidentiality. *Journal of the American Academy of Psychoanalysis* **20**:639–643, 1992.

*32 **Pellegrino, E.**: Secrets of the couch and the grave: the Anne Sexton case. *Cambridge Quarterly of Healthcare Ethics* **5**: 189–203, 1996.

The Limits of Confidentiality*

Sissela Bok

The Professional Secret

Fiercely defended, yet under ever greater stress, the duty of professional confidentiality spans all the issues of control over secrecy and openness discussed in earlier chapters. Individual and collective secrecy combine in its defense. And it is invoked with respect to increasing amounts and kinds of information that are, in turn, due to new forms of record-keeping and collaboration, ever more difficult to keep secret.

Doctors, lawyers, and priests have traditionally recognized the duty of professional secrecy regarding what individuals confide to them: personal matters such as alcoholism or depression, marital difficulties, corporate or political problems, and indeed most concerns that patients or clients want to share with someone, yet keep from all others.[1] Accountants, bankers, social workers, and growing numbers of professionals now invoke a similar duty to guard confidences. As codes of ethics take form in old and new professions, the duty of confidentiality serves in part to reinforce their claim to professional status, and in part to strengthen their capacity to offer help to clients.

Confidential information may be more or less intimate, more or less discrediting, more or less accurate and complete. No matter how false or trivial the substance of what clients or patients convey, they may ask that it be kept confidential, or assume that it will be even in the absence of such a request, taking it for granted that professionals owe them secrecy. Professionals, in turn, must not only receive and respect such confidences; the very nature of the help they can give may depend on their searching for even the most deeply buried knowledge.

All the pressures for and against secrecy noted in earlier chapters are present in such relationships. But the duty of confidentiality is no longer what it was when lawyers or doctors simply kept to themselves the confidences of those who sought their help. How can it be, when office personnel and collaborators and team members must have access to the information as well, and when clients and patients with numerous interdependent needs consult different professionals who must in turn communicate with one another? And how can it be, given the vast increase in information collected, stored, and retrievable that has expanded the opportunities for access by outsiders? How can it be, finally, when employers, school officials, law enforcement agencies, insurance companies, tax inspectors, and credit bureaus all press to see some of this confidential information?

So much confidential information is now being gathered and recorded and requested by so many about so many that confidentiality, though as strenuously invoked as in the past, is turning out to be a weaker reed than ever. Employers, schools, government agencies, and mental health and social service organizations are among the many groups now delving into personal affairs as never before. Those with fewest defenses find their affairs most closely picked over. Schools, for instance, are looking into the home conditions of students with problems, sometimes even requesting psychiatric evaluations of entire families, regardless of objections from health professionals on grounds of confidentiality. And access to public welfare assistance, work training programs, and many forms of employment may depend on the degree to which someone is willing to answer highly personal questions.

At the same time, paradoxically, a growing number of discreditable, often unlawful secrets never even entered into computer banks or medical records have come to burden lawyers, financial advisers, journalists, and many others who take themselves to be professionally bound to silence. Faced with growing demands for both revelation and secrecy, those who have to make decisions about whether or not to uphold confidentiality face numerous difficult moral quandaries. Legislation can sometimes dictate their choice. But the law differs from state to state and from nation to nation, and does not necessarily prescribe what is right from a moral point of view. Even if it did, it could never entirely resolve many of the quandaries that arise, since they often present strong moral arguments on both sides. Consider, for example, the following case:

A forty-seven-year-old engineer has polycystic kidney disease, in his case a genetic disorder, and must have his blood purified by hemodialysis with an artificial kidney machine. Victims of the disease [at the time of his diagnosis] usually die a few years after symptoms appear, often in their forties, though dialysis and transplants can stave off death for as much as ten years.

The patient has two children: a son, eighteen, just starting college, and a daughter, sixteen. Though the parents know that the disease is genetic – that their children may carry it and might transmit it to their own offspring – the son and daughter are kept in the dark. The parents insist the children should not be told because it would frighten them unnecessarily, would inhibit their social life, and would make them feel hopeless about the future. They are firm in saying that the hospital staff should not tell the children; the knowledge, they believe, is privileged and must be kept secret. Yet the hospital staff worries about the children innocently involving their future spouses and victimizing their own children.[2]

It is not difficult to see the conflicting and, in themselves, quite legitimate claims on each side in this case: the parents' insistence on privacy and on the right to decide when to speak to their children about a matter of such importance to the family; and the staff members' concern for the welfare of the children. But the question of whether the parents are wrong to keep the information from the children must be separated from that of what the staff members should do about what they see as harmful secrecy. Should they reject their obligation of confidentiality in this case?

Even those who arrive at clear answers concerning the parents' responsibility may recognize that their views could change if the facts were somewhat different. If they conclude, for example, that the children have a right to be told, they might decide differently if the disease were less severe, if a cure seemed likely to be found shortly, if the chances of the illness striking the children were low, or if the children were much younger. And those who decide that the parents are right to insist on secrecy might similarly come to a different conclusion if the illness were more certain to strike the children, or to afflict them sooner. A few might hold rigidly to one choice or the other no matter what the circumstances, but many would discern cases where the conflicting claims are so nearly equal that choice is difficult. At such times, the additional weight to be placed on confidentiality becomes crucial. Should it matter at all? If so, why? And in what sorts of conflicts should it be rejected?

These questions require us to look more closely at the nature of confidentiality and its powerful hold and to ask what it is that makes so many professionals regard it as the first and most binding of their duties.

Confidentiality refers to the boundaries surrounding shared secrets and to the process of guarding these boundaries. While confidentiality protects much that is not in fact secret, personal secrets lie at its core. The innermost, the vulnerable, often the shameful: these aspects of self-disclosure

* Bok, S.: *Secrets*. Oxford, Oxford University Press, 1996, pp. 116–135.

help explain why one name for professional confidentiality has been 'the professional secret.' Such secrecy is sometimes mistakenly confused with privacy; yet it can concern many matters in no way private, but that someone wishes to keep from the knowledge of third parties.

Confidentiality must also be distinguished from the testimonial privilege that protects information possessed by spouses or members of the clergy or lawyers against coerced revelations in court. While a great many professional groups invoke confidentiality, the law recognizes the privilege only in limited cases. In some states, only lawyers can invoke it; in others, physicians and clergy can as well; more recently, psychiatrists and other professionals have been added to their number. Who ought and who ought not to be able to guarantee such a privilege is under ceaseless debate. Every newly established professional group seeks the privileges of existing ones. Established ones, on the other hand, work to exclude those whom they take to be encroaching on their territory.

The principle of confidentiality postulates a duty to protect confidences against third parties under certain circumstances. Professionals appeal to such a principle in keeping secrets from all outsiders, and seek to protect even what they would otherwise feel bound to reveal. While few regard the principle as absolute, most see the burden of proof as resting squarely on anyone who claims a reason for overriding it. Why should confidentiality bind thus? And why should it constrain professionals to silence more than, say, close friends?

Justification and Rationale

The justification for confidentiality rests on four premises, three supporting confidentiality in general and the fourth, professional secrecy in particular. They concern human autonomy regarding personal information, respect for relationships, respect for the bonds and promises that protect shared information, and the benefits of confidentiality to those in need of advice, sanctuary, and aid, and in turn to society. The first and fundamental premise is that of individual autonomy over personal information. It asks that we respect individuals as capable of having secrets. Without some control over secrecy and openness about themselves, their thoughts and plans, their actions, and in part their property, people could neither maintain privacy nor guard against danger. But of course this control should be only partial. Matters such as contagious disease place individual autonomy in conflict with the rights of others. And a variety of matters cannot easily be concealed. No one can maintain control, for example, over others' seeing that they have a broken leg or a perennially vile temper.[3]

The second premise is closely linked to the first. It presupposes the legitimacy not only of having personal secrets but of sharing them, and assumes respect for relationships among human beings and for intimacy. It is rooted in loyalties that precede the formulation of moral justification and that preserve collective survival for one's tribe, one's kin, one's clan. Building on such a sense of loyalty, the premise holds that it is not only natural but often also right to respect the secrets of intimates and associates, and that human relationships could not survive without such respect.

This premise is fundamental to the marital privilege upheld in American law, according to which one spouse cannot be forced to testify against the other; and to the ancient Chinese legal tradition, so strongly attacked in the Maoist period, that forbade relatives to report on one another's misdeeds and penalized such revelations severely.[4] No more than the first premise, however, does this second one suffice to justify all confidentiality. It can conflict with other duties, so that individuals have to choose, say, between betraying country or friend, parents or children; and it can be undercut by the nature of the secret one is asked to keep.

The third premise holds that a pledge of silence creates an obligation beyond the respect due to persons and to existing relationships. Once we promise someone secrecy, we no longer start from scratch in weighing the moral factors of a situation. They matter differently, once the promise is given, so that full impartiality is no longer called for.

In promising one alienates, as Grotius said, either a thing or some portion of one's freedom of action: 'To the former category belong promises to give; to the latter, promises to perform.'[5] Promises of secrecy

are unusual in both respects. What they promise to give is allegiance; what they promise to perform is some action that will guard the secret – to keep silent, at least, and perhaps to do more. Just what performance is promised, and at what cost it will be carried out, are questions that go to the heart of conflicts over confidentiality.[6] To invoke a promise, therefore, while it is surely to point to a *prima facie* ground of obligation, is not to close the debate over pledges of secrecy. Rather, one must go on to ask whether it was right to make the pledge in the first place, and right to accept it; whether the promise is a binding one, and even if it is, what circumstances might nevertheless justify overriding it.[7]

Individuals vary with respect to the seriousness with which they make a promise and the consequent weight of the reasons they see as sufficient to override it. Consider the CIA agent who takes an oath of secrecy before gaining access to classified information; the White House butler who pledges never to publish confidential memoirs; the relatives who give their word to a dying author never to publish her diaries; the religious initiate who swears on all he holds sacred not to divulge the mysteries he is about to share; the engineer who signs a pledge not to give away company trade secrets as a condition of employment. Some of these individuals take the pledge casually, others in utter seriousness. If the latter still break their pledge, they may argue that they were coerced into making their promise, or that they did not understand how it bound them. Or else they may claim that something is important enough to override their promise – as when the relatives publish the author's diaries after her death for a sum of money they cannot resist, or in the belief that the reading public would be deprived without such documents.

For many, a promise involves their integrity and can create a bond that is closer than kinship, as the ceremonies by which people become blood brothers indicate. The strength of promising is conveyed in such early practices as those in which promisors might offer as a pledge their wife, their child, or a part of their body.[8] And promises of *secrecy* have been invested with special meaning, in part because of the respect for persons and for relationships called for by the first two premises.

Taken together, the three premises give strong prima facie reasons to support confidentiality. With certain limitations, I accept each one as binding on those who have accepted information in confidence. But of course there are reasons sufficient to override the force of all these premises, as when secrecy would allow violence to be done to innocent persons, or turn someone into an unwitting accomplice in crime. At such times, autonomy and relationship no longer provide sufficient legitimacy. And the promise of silence should never be given, or if given, can be breached.

It is here that the fourth premise enters in to add strength to the particular pledges of silence given by professionals.[9] This premise assigns weight beyond ordinary loyalty to professional confidentiality, because of its utility to persons and to society. As a result, professionals grant their clients secrecy even when they would otherwise have reason to speak out: thus lawyers feel justified in concealing past crimes of their clients, bankers the suspect provenance of investors' funds, and priests the sins they hear in confession.

According to this premise, individuals benefit from such confidentiality because it allows them to seek help they might otherwise fear to ask for; those most vulnerable or at risk might otherwise not go for help to doctors or lawyers or others trained to provide it. In this way, innocent persons might end up convicted of crimes for lack of competent legal defense, and disease could take a greater toll among those ashamed of the nature of their ailment. Society therefore gains in turn from allowing such professional refuge, the argument holds, in spite of the undoubted risks of not learning about certain dangers to the community; and everyone is better off when professionals can probe for the secrets that will make them more capable of providing the needed help.

The nature of the helpfulness thought to override the importance of revealing some confidences differs from one profession to another. The social worker can offer support, counsel, sometimes therapy; physicians provide means of relieving suffering and of curing disease; lawyers give assistance in self-protection against the state or other individuals. These efforts may conflict, as for army psychiatrists whenever their mission is both to receive the confidences of troubled military personnel and to serve as agents of the state, obligated to report on the condition of their patients. And the help held to justify confidentiality about informants by police and journalists is not directed to individuals in need of relief at all, but rather to society by encouraging disclosures of abuses and crime.

Such claims to individual and social utility touch on the *raison d'être* of the professions themselves; but they are also potentially treacherous. For if it were found that a professional group or subspecialty not only did not help but actually hurt individuals, and increased the social burden of, say, illness or crime, then there would be a strong case for not allowing it to promise professional confidentiality. To question its special reason for being able to promise confidentiality of unusual strength is therefore seen as an attack on its special purposes, and on the power it acquires in being able to give assurances beyond those which nonprofessionals can offer.

A purely strategic reason for stressing professional confidentiality is that, while needed by clients, it is so easily breached and under such strong pressures to begin with. In schools and in offices, at hospitals and in social gatherings, confidential information may be casually passed around. Other items are conveyed 'off the record' or leaked in secret. The prohibition against breaching confidentiality must be especially strong in order to combat the pressures on insiders to do so, especially in view of the ease and frequency with which it is done.

Together with the first three premises for confidentiality, the defense of the fourth helps explain the ritualistic tone in which the duty of preserving secrets is repeatedly set forth in professional oaths and codes of ethics. Still more is needed, however, to explain the sacrosanct nature often ascribed to this duty. The ritualistic nature of confidentiality in certain religious traditions has surely had an effect on its role in law and medicine. A powerful esoteric rationale for secrecy linked the earliest practices of medicine and religion. Thus Henry Sigerist points out that in Mesopotamia medicine, like other sacred knowledge, was kept secret and not divulged to the profane; conversely, many religious texts ended with a warning that 'he who does not keep the secret will not remain in health. His days will be shortened.'[10]

However strong, these historical links between faith and professional practice give *no* added justification to professional confidentiality. The sacramental nature of religious confession is a matter of faith for believers. It may be respected even in secular law on grounds of religious freedom; but it adds no legitimacy to that of the four premises when it comes to what professionals conceal for clients.[11]

The four premises are not usually separated and evaluated in the context of individual cases or practices. Rather, they blend with the ritualistic nature attributed to confidentiality to support a rigid stance that I shall call the rationale of confidentiality. Not only does this rationale point to links with the most fundamental grounds of autonomy and relationship and trust and help; it also serves as a rationalization that helps deflect ethical inquiry. The very self-evidence that it claims can then expand beyond its legitimate applications. Confidentiality, like all secrecy, can then cover up for and in turn lead to a great deal of error, injury, pathology, and abuse.

When professionals advance confidentiality as a shield, their action is, to be sure, in part intentional and manipulative, but in part it also results from a failure to examine the roots of confidentiality and to spell out the limits of its application. It can lead then to sweeping claims such as that made by the World Medical Association in its 1949 International Code of Medical Ethics: 'A doctor shall preserve absolute secrecy on all he knows about his patient because of the confidence entrusted in him.'[12]

If such claims go too far, where and how should the lines be drawn? Granting the *prima facie* importance of the principle of confidentiality in the light of the premises which support it, when and for what reasons must it be set aside? I shall consider such limits with respect to the secrets of individual clients, of professionals themselves, and of institutional or corporate clients.

Individual Clients and Their Secrets

Among the most difficult choices for physicians and others are those which arise with respect to confidences by children, mentally incompetent persons, and those who are temporarily not fully capable of guiding their affairs.

While some such confidences – as about fears or hopes – can be kept secret without difficulty, others are more troubling. Consider the following case:

Janet M., a thirteen-year-old girl in the seventh grade of a small-town junior high school, comes to the office of a family physician. She has known him from childhood, and he has cared for all the members of her family. She tells him that she is pregnant, and that she has had a lab test performed at an out-of-town clinic. She wants to have an abortion. She is afraid that her family, already burdened by unemployment and illness, would be thrown into a crisis by the news. Her boyfriend, fifteen, would probably be opposed to the abortion. She asks the doctor for help in securing the abortion, and for assurance that he will not reveal her condition to anyone.

Cases such as Janet's are no longer rare. In small towns as in large cities, teen-age pregnancy is on the rise, teen-age abortion commonplace. Many families do provide the guidance and understanding so desperately needed at such times; but when girls request confidentiality, it is often out of fear of their families' reaction. Health professionals should clearly make every effort to help these girls communicate with their families. But sometimes there is no functioning family. Or else family members may have been so brutal or so unable to cope with crisis in the past that it is legitimate to be concerned about the risks in informing them. At times, it is even the case that a member of the girl's own family has abused her sexually.[13]

Health professionals are then caught in a conflict between their traditional obligation of confidentiality and the normal procedure of consulting with a child's parents before an irreversible step is taken. In this conflict, the premises supporting confidentiality are themselves in doubt. Just how autonomous should thirteen-year-olds be with respect to decisions about pregnancy? They are children still, but with an adult's choice to make. And what about even younger girls? In what relation does a physician stand to them, and to their parents, regarding such secrets?

Because the premises of autonomy and of relationship do not necessarily mandate secrecy at such times, deciding whether or not to pledge silence is much harder. Even the professional help that confidentiality allows is then in doubt. Pregnant young girls are in need of advice and assistance more than most others; confidentiality too routinely extended may lock them into an attitude of frightened concealment that can do permanent damage. Health professionals owe it to these patients, therefore, to encourage and help them to communicate with their families or others responsible for their support. But to *mandate*, as some seek to do, consultation with family members, no matter how brutal or psychologically abusive, would be to take a shortsighted view. Not only would it injure those pregnant girls forced into family confrontations; many others would end by not seeking professional help at all, at a time when they need it most.

Childhood and adolescent pregnancies are far from the only conditions that present professionals with conflicts over confidentiality. Venereal disease, drug and alcohol addiction among the young, as well as a great many problems of incompetent and disturbed individuals past childhood, render confidentiality similarly problematic.

Even where there is no question about maturity or competence, professionals worry about the secrecy asked of them when someone confides to them plans that seem self-injurious: to enter into a clearly disastrous business arrangement, or to give all his possessions to an exploitative 'guru,' or to abandon life-prolonging medical treatment. He may have no intention of hurting anyone else (though relatives and others may in fact be profoundly affected by his choice) and may be fully within his rights in acting as he does. But his judgment may itself be in doubt, depending on how self-destructive the plans are that he is confiding.

Here again, an absolute insistence on confidentiality would be unreasonable. No one would hesitate to reveal the secret of a temporarily deranged person about to do himself irreversible harm. Patients and clients do not have the requisite balance at such a time to justify silence – and thus complicity – regarding their self-destructive acts, the less so as the very revelation of such plans to a professional is often correctly interpreted as a call for help.

If, on the other hand, the act has been carefully thought through, breaches of confidentiality are much less justified, no matter how irrational the project might at first seem to outsiders. Say the person planning to give his money away wants to live the rest of his life as a contemplative, or that the patient planning to abandon medical treatment has decided to cease delaying death in view of his progressively debilitating and painful disease; it is harder to see the basis for a breach of professional confidentiality in such cases,* since it is more difficult to prove that the person's act is necessarily self-destructive from his point of view. Professionals are constantly at risk of assuming too readily that the purposes they take to be overriding and to which they have dedicated their careers – financial prudence, for instance – are necessarily more rational for all others than conflicting aims. This professional bias has to be taken into account in any decision to override confidentiality on grounds of irrationality and self-harm.

Sometimes, however, a patient's insistence on confidentiality can bring quite unintended risks. Because people live longer, and often suffer from multiple chronic diseases, their records have to be accessible to many different health professionals. Their reluctance to have certain facts on their medical records may then be dangerous. One physician has pointed to some of the possible consequences of such concealment:

The man who insists that no record be made of a psychiatric history, or the drugs that would suggest that there is one, and wants no record of his syphilis and penicillin injections and subsequent recovery, is the same man who must face squarely the risk of future syphilitic disease of the nervous system or even lethal penicillin reactions because future medical personnel never followed through in the right manner. They do not even know that the problem existed; they and the patient stumbled blindly into trouble.[14]

At times, the insistence on secrecy can become obsessive, so that confidentiality may come to surround the most trivial matters, even when less secrecy could be useful not only to oneself but to others. Thus many refuse to release information about their blood types or past illnesses, even at the cost of slowing down research that might help other sufferers. Here as always, secrecy can shut out many forms of feedback and assistance and consequently encourage poor judgment.

Do patients have the same claims to confidentiality about personal information when persons from whom it is kept run serious risks? Consider again the family mentioned earlier in which the father wishes to conceal from his children that he suffers from polycystic kidney disease. It is now two years later. The father, much closer to death, has told his two children about the genetic nature of his disease. He was prompted to do so, in part, by his daughter's plans to marry. She, however, fears disclosing to her future husband that the same disease may strike her and affect their children. Now it is her turn to insist on confidentiality, not only from her father but from all others who know the facts, including the health professionals involved.

The dilemma they face is in one sense very old, in another quite new. It resembles all the choices through the ages about whether or not to reveal to intimates and future spouses that someone suffers from incurable venereal disease, sexual problems, a recurring psychiatric condition, or a degenerative disease as yet in its early stages. But it has taken on a new frequency because there is now so much more information, especially of a genetic nature, than even a hundred years ago. The category of problematic and troubling predictions has expanded, raising new conflicts of secrecy for parents, prospective spouses, and many others, and of confidentiality for health professionals. Lacking the genetic information, this family would not have faced the same choice in an earlier period. With increased knowledge of risks, therefore, the collective burden of confidentiality has grown as well.

Does a professional owe confidentiality to clients who reveal plans or acts that endanger others directly? Such a question arises for the lawyer whose client lets slip that he plans a bank robbery, or that he has committed an assault for which an innocent man is standing trial; for the pediatrician who suspects that a mother drugs her children to keep them quiet; and for the psychiatrist whose patient discloses that he is obsessed by jealousy and thoughts of violence to his wife.

---

* A number of questions having to do with paternalism arise in these cases. It is important to note, however, that breaching confidence for paternalistic reasons does not necessarily involve interfering with the persons whose confidences are revealed, nor coercing them.

The conflicts that psychotherapists face in this respect were brought to public attention by the murder in 1969 of a young woman, Tatiana Tarasoff. The young man who killed her had earlier told his psychotherapist that he wanted to do so. The psychotherapist had alerted the police, who detained the student briefly, then released him after determining that he seemed 'rational' and asking him to promise to leave Miss Tarasoff alone. When the police reported the matter back to the director of psychiatry, he asked that the matter be dropped and that the correspondence with the police be destroyed. The student did not return for further treatment, and no effort was made to get in touch with him. Two months later, he went to Miss Tarasoff's home and shot and stabbed her to death. Her parents then brought suit against the university, the campus police, and the therapists for negligence in failing to warn either their daughter or themselves.

The California Supreme Court concluded that the psychotherapists had breached a duty overriding that of confidentiality: the duty to use reasonable care when they determine that a patient presents a serious danger of violence to another, to protect the intended victim against such danger.[15] 'The privilege ends,' the court held, 'when the public peril begins.'

The Tarasoff decision troubled psychiatrists. They argued, first, that one cannot know whether a threat uttered by a patient will be put into effect: that it usually is not, and that as a group psychiatrists often overpredict violence, being more often wrong than right. But such an argument does not stand up under scrutiny. Obviously, if a threat of violence is a vain boast only, or a fantasy never to be put into effect, no one is at risk; a psychiatrist who can be sure of the harmlessness of such a threat has no reason to breach confidentiality. But if there is a reasonable chance that it might be put into effect, the psychiatrist's inability to predict accurately is no reason not to consider the danger to the potential victim. It is no consolation to survivors to learn that the victim's risk had been, say, merely one in five, once the threat has been carried out. The potential victims or their family members have every interest in knowing about even such dangers. And they might legitimately argue that speculations about the degree of risk, once it is known to exist at all, should not be left up to the psychotherapist alone.

Psychiatrists have argued, moreover, that the duty to warn potential victims threatens the trust between patient and therapist. They might concede that the first premise supporting confidentiality – the claim to patient autonomy with respect to personal information – no longer holds when that information concerns serious harm to others. Just as no one is granted autonomy when it comes to *doing* violence to others, so there is no reason to concede such autonomy and control for *plans* to do so, once divulged. Having conceded the first premise, however, psychiatrists who oppose the Tarasoff decision stress the remaining three, all the more. They argue that the therapeutic relationship and its implicit promise must be inviolate if therapy is to stand a chance.[16] This is especially the case in psychiatry, where probing secrets serves special purposes. If pain and fear and hatred can be brought into the open, healing may take place, so that the patient will have better control over the relations between inner and shared experience. The promise of secrecy, impicit or explicit, allows this process to take place. Many patients have already felt betrayed in ways that left them vulnerable, and the assurance of full loyalty is therefore indispensable. A duty to warn potential clients prevents doctors from offering such assurance. Such a duty, Alan Stone has argued, 'will deter both patients and therapists from undertaking treatment, thereby further increasing the risk of violence to which society is exposed.'[17]

Two objections arise to this line of argument. The first is empirical. No evidence suggests that therapy will be imperiled if patients know that therapists have the duty to reveal their plans of violence. Even if therapy were thus imperiled, it is not clear that more violence would result. Not only have such contentions not been proved; many doubt that they are even probable. Patients rarely place much trust in confidentiality regarding their most extreme statements anyway, and may even hope that their threats *will* lead to some preventive action.[18]

The second objection is independent of such a weighing of benefit and harm. Even if we were to concede, for the sake of argument, that patients will fare better and society be less burdened by violence if psychotherapists have no duty to reveal threats to potential victims, such a duty might nevertheless still be owed to those who risk their lives without knowing it. It is not right, according to such an objection, to risk one person's life in order to help patients and reduce the violence in society. Tatiana Tarasoff should not have had to run that risk without having consented thereto.

I agree with these objections. Once psychiatrists undertake to receive and even probe for information threatening to others, they can no longer ignore those others, out of concern either for their patients or for society. The prima facie premises supporting confidentiality are overridden at such times.

The autonomy we grant individuals over personal secrets, first of all, cannot reasonably be thought to extend to plans of violence against *innocent persons*; at such times, on the contrary, someone who knows of plans that endanger others owes it to them to counteract those plans, and, if he is not sure he can forestall them, to warn the potential victims. Nor, in the second place, can patients who voice serious threats against innocent persons invoke confidentiality on the basis of their relationship with therapists or anyone else without asking them to be partially complicitous. The third premise, basing confidentiality in part on a promise, is likewise overridden, since in the absence of legitimacy for the first two, it ought to be clearly understood that no one, whether professionally trained or not, should give such a pledge. The benefits invoked in the fourth premise, finally, are not only not demonstrated in these cases; even if they were, they could not override the injustice done to those unwittingly placed at risk.*

Long before psychiatrists worried about these problems, Catholic theologians had studied them with a thoroughness often lacking in contemporary discussions. The distinctions they worked out over the centuries concerning different types of secrets and the obligations of professionals were detailed and well reasoned. Most theologians agreed that certain types of secrets were not binding on professional recipients, foremost among them grave threats against the public good or against innocent third persons.[19]

An example they often described is the following: What should a doctor do if he has a patient who suffers from an incurable and highly contagious venereal disease and who plans to marry without disclosing this fact to his fiancée? According to many theologians, the doctor's obligation of secrecy would then cease: the young man forfeits such consideration through his intent to act in a way that might gravely injure his fiancée. The doctor is therefore free to speak, but with certain limitations: he must reveal only so much of the secret as is necessary to avert the harm, and only to the person threatened, who has a right to this information, rather than to family members, neighbors, or the curious or gossip-hungry at large.

These commentators also discussed a subject that still divides the contemporary debate: should the breach of secrecy to avert grave harm be obligatory, or merely permitted? Should the professional feel free to choose whether or not to warn the endangered person, or acknowledge a duty to do so? It is one thing to say that he no longer owes the client confidentiality; but does he also owe the endangered person the information? Do lawyers, for example, owe any information to persons who may be injured by their clients' unlawful tax schemes, plans for extortion, or threats of violence? And if they do recognize some such obligation, how does it weigh against that of confidentiality?

The duty of confidentiality clearly has some weight; as a result, the obligation to warn potential victims is not as great for professionals as it might be for others who happen to hear of the danger. Yet it is a strong one nevertheless, especially where serious harm is likely to occur. In such cases, the duty to warn ought to be overriding. Professionals should not then be free to promise confidentiality, nor should a client expect to be able to entrust them with such projects, any more than with stolen goods or lethal weapons.[20]

The same is true for confidences regarding past crimes. Here, too, confidentiality counts; but it must be weighed against other aims – of social

justice and restitution. It is therefore hard to agree with those lawyers who argue as a matter of course that they owe clients silence about past, unsolved murders; it is equally hard to agree with Swiss bankers claiming that confidentiality suffices to legitimate the secret bank accounts that attract so many depositors enriched through crime, conspiracy, and political exploitation.

Secrecy as a Shield

The greatest burden of secrecy imposed by confidentiality, however, is that of the secrets professionals keep to protect themselves rather than patients and clients. Confidentiality can be used, here as elsewhere, as a shield for activities that could ill afford to see the light of day. An example of how dangerous such shielding can be is afforded by the story of the death in 1976 of Anneliese Michel, a young German student, after ten months of exorcism.[21]

Anneliese Michel had been under periodic medical care since she was sixteen years old. She had been diagnosed as suffering both from recurrent epileptic seizures and from anorexia nervosa. When she was twenty-two, her parents persuaded her to withdraw from university studies. Ernst Alt, the local parish priest, suspected that she might be possessed by devils and that exorcism might cure her. He saw the seizures as evidence of such possession rather than of epilepsy, and decided to consult Germany's leading 'satanologist,' the eighty-three-year-old Adolf Rodewyk, S.J. Father Rodewyk concluded that the convulsions were trancelike states of possession in which, among other manifestations, a devil calling himself Judas made no secret of his identity.

Father Rodewyk recommended exorcism. The *Rituale Romanum* of 1614, still followed in cases of exorcism, prescribes that a bishop must agree to the procedure before it can be undertaken, and that the person thus treated must be beyond medical help. Father Rodewyk assured Bishop Joseph Stangl of Wurzburg that Anneliese's case was one for exorcists, not for doctors; and the bishop authorized the rites, ordering 'strictest secrecy and total discretion.'

For ten months, the young woman took part in lengthy sessions with the parish priest and Father Wilhelm Renz, an expert called in for the exorcism. The two prayed with her and tried, by means of holy water, adjurations, and commands, to drive out the devils – by then thought to number at least six and calling themselves, in addition to Judas, by such names as Lucifer, Nero, and Hitler. Anneliese was convinced that she was thus possessed and that the powers of good and of evil were fighting over her soul. She wrote in her diary that the Savior had told her she was a great saint. Fearing that doctors might diagnose her voices and seizures as psychiatric symptoms and send her to a mental hospital, she avoided health professionals. As the months wore on, she grew weaker, eating and drinking next to nothing. During one particularly stormy session of exorcism, she rushed head first against the wall facing her bed, then lay back exhausted. The devils were finally declared to have left. The next morning, she was found dead in her bed.

In April 1978, her parents and the two priests who had conducted the exorcism were brought to trial. They were convicted of negligent homicide for having failed to seek medical help up to the very end. Physicians testified that, even as late as a few days before Anneliese died, her life could have been saved had she had medical attention. The four accused were sentenced to six months imprisonment.

The priests sincerely believed that they were doing their best to save Anneliese Michel. Insofar as they believed Father Rodewyk's attesting to the presence of devils, they could hardly think medical treatment appropriate. But they knew their belief that Anneliese was possessed by devils would be shared by few, and so they conspired with her parents to keep the sessions of exorcism secret to the very end. Two kinds of confidentiality come together here: that between priest and penitent, and that between caretaker and patient. But neither one should have been honored in this case, for while they protect much that is spoken by penitents and by patients, they were never intended to protect all that is done by priests or caretakers in response, least of all when it constitutes treatment of very sick persons by dangerous methods without medical assistance.

---

* Such a conclusion carries with it line-drawing problems: how likely the danger should be before one assumes serious risk; how sure one should be about the identity of the potential victim; how much this individual already knows about the risk; the degree of precautions already in place, etc. But line-drawing problems would occur no matter what the conclusion unless one postulated either no duty to breach confidentiality under any conditions whatsoever, or, on the contrary, no obligation of confidentiality at all.

The case is an extreme one. Strict adherence to the stipulation in the *Rituale Romanum* of 1614 that someone must be beyond medical help would have required much more careful consultation with physicians before leaping to the conclusion that exorcism was called for. When publicity about the case arose, Catholics and non-Catholics alike were distressed at how the young woman had been treated. What is worth noting, however, is that her need for medical help went unnoticed because of the secrecy in which the exorcism was conducted. The case illustrates, therefore, what can happen in almost any system of advising and helping those in need whenever secrecy shrouds what is done to them. And it raises broader questions about confidentiality: Exactly whose secret should it protect? The patient's or client's alone? Or the professional's? Or all that transpires between them?

In principle, confidentiality should protect only the first. But in practice, it can expand, like all other practices of secrecy, to cover much more. It may even be stretched so far as to include what professionals hide *from* patients, clients, and the public at large.

The sick, the poor, the mentally ill, the aged, and the very young are in a paradoxical situation in this respect. While their right to confidentiality is often breached and their most intimate problems openly bandied about, the poor care they may receive is just as often covered up under the same name of confidentiality. That is the shield held forth to prevent outsiders from finding out about negligence, overcharging, unnecessary surgery, or institutionalization. And far more than individual mistakes and misdeeds are thus covered up, for confidentiality is also the shield that professionals invoke to protect incompetent colleagues and negligence and unexpected accidents in, for instance, hospitals, factories, or entire industries.

The word 'confidentiality' has by now become a means of covering up a multitude of questionable and often dangerous practices. When lawyers use it to justify keeping secret their client's plans to construct housing so shoddy as to be life-threatening, or when government officials invoke it in concealing the risks of nuclear weapons, confidentiality no longer serves the purpose for which it was intended; it has become, rather, a means for deflecting legitimate public attention.

Such invocations of confidentiality are facilitated by the ease with which many transpose the confidentiality owed to individuals to the collective level. Consider, for example, the prolonged collaboration between asbestos manufacturers and company physicians to conceal the risks from exposure to asbestos dust. These risks were kept secret from the public, from workers in plants manufacturing asbestos insulation, and even from those workers found in medical checkups to be in the early stages of asbestos-induced disease. When a reporter approached a physician associated with the concealment as consultant for a large manufacturer, the physician turned down his request for an interview on grounds of confidentiality owed as a matter of 'the patient's rights,' and explained, when the astonished reporter inquired who the 'patient' was, that it was the *company*.[22]

Government agencies sometimes request confidentiality, not so much to deflect inquiry as to be able to conduct it in the manner most likely to resolve difficult problems. Thus the United States Center for Disease Control argued, in 1980, that it needed to be able to promise confidentiality to hospitals seeking its help for nosocomial, or hospital-induced, infections. Such infection is a major health risk, conservatively estimated as killing 20,000 persons a year in the United States alone, and contributing to the deaths of over 40,000 others in a substantial manner. When a hospital experiences an outbreak of nosocomial infection, it can call on the expert advice of the Center for Disease Control in order to find the cause of the infection and to reverse its course; but to do so under conditions of publicity is to invite rumor, lawsuits, and patient anxiety, according to those who argued in favor of extending confidentiality to the hospitals.[23] The center saw a need to promise such confidentiality to a hospital in order to help it combat infection, much as a doctor might promise silence to an individual patient with a similar affliction.

The center's request for an exemption from the Freedom of Information Act on such grounds was turned down. No proof had been advanced that the dangers the hospitals feared were realistic. Patients did not appear to be staying away from hospitals that had experienced outbreaks of nosocomial infection; and no suit had been won on the basis of information provided by the center.

The step from patient confidentiality to hospital confidentiality is a large one, but it is often lightly taken in arguments that ignore the differences between the two. The first two premises underlying confidentiality, of autonomy regarding personal information and the respect for intimacy and human bonds, are obviously applicable, if at all, in a different manner when it comes to institutions. And the fourth premise, concerning the benefit to individuals from having somewhere to turn when vulnerable and in need of help, and the indirect benefit to society from allowing professionals to give counsel in strict confidence, must be scrutinized with care whenever the claim is made that it applies to government agencies, law firms, or corporations. We ask of them a much higher degree of accountability.

To be sure, these institutions should be able to invoke confidentiality for legitimate activities such as internal memoranda and personnel files; but it is a different matter altogether to claim confidentiality for plans that endanger others. Such protection attracts all who seek surreptitious assistance with bribery, tax evasion, and similar schemes. And because corporate or consulting law is so lucrative, the power to exercise confidentiality for such secrets then shields not merely the company and the client but the lawyer's own links to, and rewards from, highly questionable practices.

The premises supporting confidentiality are strong, but they cannot support practices of secrecy – whether by individual clients, institutions, or professionals themselves – that undermine and contradict the very respect for persons and for human bonds that confidentiality was meant to protect.

References

1. See Robert E. Regan, *Professional Secrecy in the light of Moral Principles* (Washington, D. C.: Augustinian Press, 1943); Alan H. Goldman, *The Moral foundations of Professional Ethics* (Totowa, N.J.: Rowman & Littleffield, 1980); LeRoy Walters, 'Ethical Aspects of Medical Confidentiality,' in Tom L. Beauchamp and LeRoy Walters, eds., *Contemporary Issues in Bioethics* (Encino, Calif.: Dickenson Publishing Co., 1978), pp. 169–75; Susanna J. Wilson, *Confidentiality in Social Work* (New York: Free Press, 1978); William Harold Tiemann, *The Right to Silence: Privileged Communication and the Pastor* (Richmond, Va.: John Knox Press, 1964); William W. Meissner, 'Threats to Confidentiality,' *Psychiatric Annals* 2 (1979): 54–71.

2. From the newsletter *Hard Choices*, of the Office for Radio and Television for Learning (Boston, 1980), p. 9.

3. For a discussion of whether this partial autonomy over personal information should be defended in terms of property, see Arthur R. Miller, *The Assault on Privacy* (Ann Arbor: University of Michigan Press, 1971), pp. 211–16.

4. For the marital privilege, see Sanford Levinson, *The State and Structures of Intimacy* (New York: Basic Books, forthcoming). For the Chinese tradition, see Derk Bodde and Clarence Morris, *Law in Imperial China* (Cambridge, Mass.: Harvard University Press, 1967), p. 40.

5. **Hugo Grotius**, *The Law of War and Peace*, trans. Francis Kelsey (Indianapolis: Bobbs-Merrill Co., 1925), bk. 2, chap. 11, p. 331.

6. I discussed the question of lying to protect confidences in *Lying*, chap. 11.

7. For different views on the binding force of promises, see William Godwin, *Enquiry Concerning Political Justice* (1793; 3rd ed. 1798), bk. 3, chap. 3; Richard Price, *A Review of the Principal Questions in Morals* (1758; 3rd ed. 1787), chap. 7 (both in D. H. Munro, ed., *A Guide to the British Moralists* [London: William Collins, Sons & Co., 1972], pp. 187–97, 180–86). For more general treatments of promising, see Grotius, *Law of War and Peace*, bk. 2, chap. 11, pp. 328–42; John Searle, *Speech Acts* (Cambridge: Cambridge University Press, 1969); Charles Fried, *Contract as Promise* (Cambridge, Mass.: Harvard University Press, 1981).

8. Nietzsche, in *Ecce Homo*, trans. Kaufmann, p. 64, relates such pledges to the bond between debtor and creditor; he argues that the memory necessary for people to keep promises only developed through such painful, often cruel experiences.

9. For discussions of whether some or all of these premises should be accepted, and whether they are grounded on utilitarian or deontological considerations, see Goldman, *Moral Foundations of Professional Ethics*; Leo J. Cass and William J. Curran, 'Rights of Privacy in Medical Practice,' partially reprinted in Samuel Gorovitz et al., *Moral Problems in Medicine* (Englewood Cliffs, N.J.: Prentice-Hall, 1976), pp. 82–85; Benjamin Freedman, 'A Meta-Ethics for

Professional Morality,' *Ethics* 89 (1978): 1–79; Benjamin Freedman, 'What Really Makes Professional Morality Different: Response to Martin,' *Ethics* 91 (1981):626–30; Mike W. Martin, "Rights and the Meta-Ethics of Professional Morality," *Ethics* **91** (1981):619–25.

10. **Henry E. Sigerist**, *A History of Medicine*, vol. 1, *Primitive and Archaic Medicine* (New York: Oxford University Press, 1951), p. 433.

11. **Jeremy Bentham**, otherwise opposed to testimonial privileges for professionals, argues in favor of 'excluding the evidence of a Catholic priest respecting the confessions intrusted to him,' holding that freedom of religion outweighs the social costs of such practices. See *Works of Jeremy Bentham*, **7**:366–68.

12. Code of Ethics, 1949 World Medical Association, in *Encyclopedia of Bioethics* (New York: Free Press, 1978), pp. 1749–50.

13. I have discussed abortion in 'Ethical Problems of Abortion,' *Hastings Center Studies* 2 (1974):33–52.

14. **Lawrence Weed**, *Your Health Care and How to Manage it* (Arlington, Vt.: Essex Publishing Co., 1978), p. 79.

15. See Judge Tobriner, *Tarasoff* v. *Regents of the University of California*, Opinion #551, 1. 2d 334, 131 Cal. Rptr. 14 (1976).

16. See, for example, Harvey L. Ruben and Diana D. Ruben, 'Confidentiality and Privileged Communication: The Psychotherapeutic Relationship Revisited,' *Medical Annals of the District of Columbia* 41 (1972):365: 'The patient in analysis must learn to free associate and to break down resistances to deal with unconscious threatening thoughts and feelings. To revoke secrecy after encouraging such risk-taking is to threaten all further interaction.'

17. **Alan A. Stone**, 'The Tarasoff Decisions: Suing Psychotherapists to Safeguard Society,' *Harvard Law Review* **90** (1976):358–78.

18. **David Wechsler**, in "Patients, Therapists, and Third Parties: The Victimological Virtues of Tarasoff," *International Journal of Law and Psychiatry* 2 (1979):1–28, argues that, as a practical matter, most threats by patients concern family members or close associates, who usually know about the hostility aimed at them. Requiring psychotherapists to disclose such dangers, Wechsler argues, may force them to give up their counterproductive focus on the patient alone and to consider much more carefully, as well, his relationship with others.

19. See Regan, *Professional Secrecy*, pp 104–13.

20. For diverging views of the lawyer's responsibility of confidentiality, see American Bar Association, Proposed Final Draft, Model Rules of Professional Conduct, 1981, pp 37–47; and the Roscoe Pound-American Trial Lawyers Foundation, Discussion Draft, The American Lawyer's Code of Conduct, June 1980, pp. 101–10.

21. For accounts of the story of Anneliese Michel and of the trial after her death, I have relied on *Die Zeit*, July 30, 1976, and April 7, 1978; *Der Spiegel*, July 2, 1976, and April 3, 1978; and *Süddeutsche Zeitung*, which had stories almost daily during the period of the trial, March 30–April 24, 1978.

22. See Paul Brodeur, *Expendable Americans* (New York: Viking Press, 1973).

23. Ethics Advisory Board, Department of Health and Human Services, The Request of the Center for Disease Control for a Limited Exemption from the Freedom of Information Act. 1980.

Absolute Confidentiality?*

Sir Douglas Black

Since I have been allotted, and been glad to accept, the ostensibly negative role of denying that confidentiality in the doctor–patient relationship is absolute, I must pre-empt possible misunderstanding by emphasizing my adherence to two important positive positions, which may be summarily expressed thus:

1. The doctor–patient relationship is both so important and so potentially fragile as to require the support of a clear ethical framework, understood and accepted implicitly or even explicitly by both doctor and patient.

2. I accept both the general value of stated ethical principles, and in particular the validity of the principles indicated by the terms 'autonomy, beneficence, non-maleficence, and justice'.

What then can be my grounds for questioning the absolute character of what is undoubtedly a major ethical requirement in the relationships between doctors and patients? The detailed arguments and instances which I see as supporting these grounds should, of course, form the content of this chapter, but it may make the nature of my argument clearer if even at this early stage I indicate its general course in the form of three summary propositions:

1. The statement of an ethical position can be valid, valuable, and generally acceptable, without its having the qualities of universality in acceptance and application which would justify its designation as 'absolute'.

2. There are likely to be 'legitimate exceptions' in the practical application of ethical principles, even those which are soundly based and generally accepted.

3. There are practical situations, both in clinical medicine and in public health medicine, where two or even more agreed ethical principles would appear to be in conflict, in the sense that action dictated by one of them would be incompatible with courses of action dictated by the other or others.

Can ethical propositions be 'absolute'?

Warned by the fate of the anti-hero who maddened himself by the quest of the absolute in Balzac's novel, it is not my ambition to define the absolute as a 'thing-in-itself'; but more modestly to raise the question whether the propositions of medical ethics are of such a nature that they can properly be described as 'absolute', in the sense in which that adjective is generally used – 'Die Bedeutung eines Wortes ist sein Gebrauch in der Sprache'. The first definition of absolute given in *Chambers 20th–century dictionary* (1983) is 'free from limits, restrictions, or conditions', which I take to be the common usage. Later on there is another definition, qualified by '(*philos*)', which reads 'existing in and by itself without necessary relation to anything else' – a usage which certainly could not be relevant to practical medical ethics. But could even the first, less 'free-standing', definition be sensibly applied to the type of proposition commonly made in medical ethics?

* Black, D.: Absolute confidentiality, in *Principles of health care ethics*, ed. R. Gillon. Chichester, Wiley, 1994, pp. 479–488.

At the (commonly accepted) risk of putting words into the mouths of hypothetical others, I suppose a deontologist might argue that some such propositions might rank as 'categorical imperatives', in the sense that they would be willed by all intelligences; and might give 'Thou shalt not kill' as an example. But even in relation to that precept, and among those intelligences to which we can obtain limited access by observing their behaviour and actions, there is a disturbing lack of unanimity, with deviance all too overtly expressed by terrorists, by other murderers, and more legitimately perhaps by agents of the state – and of course the different ethical standards of different countries and societies indicate that there is no escape from individual aberration by resort to organized collectivity.

There have, of course, been attempts, still within a deontological framework, and without rushing to naked utilitarianism, to escape from the difficulty imposed by the extreme variability of observed human behaviour, often accompanied by bizarre attempts at justification, such as the Nazi defence of slaying the mentally handicapped, even before they embarked on wholesale murder on racial grounds. For example, a distinction has been made between *prima facie ethical principles* (which should prevail in the absence of conflicting obligations); and *absolute duty* (which presumably must govern conduct without exception, and which seems difficult to exemplify)[1]. Another approach recognizes the general validity of moral principles, but would resolve such conflicts as may arise between them by having set them in a hierarchical or *lexical ordering*, such that the 'higher' principles be satisfied before observing those 'lower' in the imposed order[2].

In the later, more pragmatic, sections of this chapter I shall be illustrating what I believe to be justifiable transgressions of the general principle of confidentiality of information given in the context of health care by patients to doctors, and indeed to other 'health care professionals', to use the accepted if somewhat cumbrous phrase used to denote the many groups other than doctors who give a professional service related to health. If confidentiality in these situations were indeed 'absolute', all such transgressions would be illegitimate and immoral; and it would obviously be wrong even to discuss them without having attained a prior conviction that confidentiality is not in fact 'absolute'. That is certainly my own belief; it may be an intuitive one, though I have laboured in preceding paragraphs to give it some groundwork in theory.

Those who, like myself, have a mistrust of absolutes, or to put it more simply are chary of the words 'always' and 'never' in our ethical discourse, are quite likely to be considered as ethical reprobates by those who take the opposite view. Let me therefore lay it on the line that I believe in the formulation and study of ethical principles and of the practical precepts which may flow from them; and that they represent a norm of proper conduct, deviations from which require to be justified. To go further in the specific matter of confidentiality, it has both historical acceptance going back to the ancient world; and a very strong ethical base, involving at least two of the four *prima facie* principles which inform this whole volume – those of autonomy and non-maleficence. To elaborate on the ethical base, release of personal health information supplied by patients is a breach of their *autonomy*, unless of course they have given specific informed consent. The dissemination of health information, whether by careless leakage or deliberate malice, offends against the principle of *non-maleficence*. Further, confidentiality of health information is compatible in almost all circumstances with the principles of beneficence and of justice; although later I shall hope to produce instances in which the need for beneficence or for justice may override the obligation to maintain the confidentiality of personal health information.

Thus far the argument has been largely theoretical, hoping to establish that ethical principles in general are not 'absolute', in the accepted sense of the word; but they constitute valuable guides to attitudes, which will then conduce to ethically acceptable behaviour. Within this framework a duty to maintain the confidentiality of personal health information is clearly in accord with ethical standards, and to do so represents the norm of proper action. But, like other guides to ethical conduct, it does not stand detached from the situations which adorn or perplex our daily lives. Questions which remain to be considered are, What constitutes a breach of confidentiality? Are there legitimate exceptions to confidentiality in the ordinary run of clinical practice? What are the special problems of confidentiality of health records in public health medicine and in society?

What constitutes a breach of confidentiality?

Not every disclosure of personal health information represents a breach of confidentiality. With one important proviso, any disclosure of information can be legitimated by the patient's consent to the disclosure. The proviso is, of course, that of *adequately informed consent*. This means that, for any disclosure of importance, the patient must know what is to be disclosed, the purpose of the disclosure, the person or persons to whom the disclosure is to be made, and that his consent is 'specific', i.e. he is sanctioning, unless otherwise agreed, *one* disclosure of a *specified part* of his record. These are the strict requirements, perhaps more easily stated than fulfilled, and of such gravamen that they may be strictly appropriate to areas in which possible damage or hurt to the patient may be foreseen. But in any matter of possible moment the necessary rigour of consent should be judged by the patient, whose trust or ignorance is not something to be abused.

Legitimation by adequately informed consent is the most valid guarantee that a disclosure does not constitute a breach of confidentiality. But of course it is now the rule rather than the exception that health care is provided not by an isolated doctor, but by a team of health professionals, and also in many cases social workers. Transfers of information are a necessary part of the care of any major episode of illness; and it would be unrealistic to subject each such transfer to the formal sanctions of informed consent. In actual practice the assumption is made that the patient in his own interests would agree to transfer of information relevant to his care and hopefully cure; this assumption of what may be called *implied consent* is pragmatically useful, if not even necessary in the interests of reasonable efficiency. It is, however, ethically and perhaps even legally frail, in that it could be construed as a derogation from the patient's autonomy. There is one safeguard which should certainly be applied to pragmatic transfers of personal health information, that they should be made only to those who require the information to enable them to serve the patient's own interests – it is this which constitutes the criterion known as the *right to know*.

It is transfer of personal health information without the consent of the patient to those who do not need to know such information for purposes of legitimate health or social care, which constitutes a breach of confidentiality. A deliberate breach of this kind, with malicious intent, is a serious ethical offence, and may also be a criminal act. Consideration of the numbers of people who may, quite legitimately, become possessed of health information about a patient, must arouse some concern about leakage of information, not through malice, but through inattention to proper reticence, or to carelessness in the handling of records. The important safeguard here lies in professional adherence to codes of confidentiality, and to similar obligations laid on other employees as part of their terms and conditions of service.

Confidentiality in a Clinical Setting

'All happy families are more or less like one another; every unhappy family is unhappy in its own particular way.' Without suggesting that clinicians are either unhappy or, like Tolstoy's Oblonsky family, in 'a complete state of confusion', it is important to recognize that the welcome recognition that 'all patients are different' might in justice be extended to their doctors, and not least in their ethical attitudes and behaviour. At the level of ethical principle, doctors in general would assent to the sentence in the Hippocratic oath which says, 'Whatever I see or hear, professionally or privately, which ought not to be divulged, I will keep secret and tell no one.' But it should be noted that this obligation comes well short of the absolute secrecy attributed to the clergy in the confessional; the phrase 'which ought not to be divulged' leaves room for the exercise of professionally informed ethical judgement. Freedom commonly opens the way to error, and the particular temptation here is to act according to our own ethical preconceptions, rather than to discover the patient's own judgement of what should or should not be told. Of course, common sense has to enter, in the recognition that in the majority of clinical settings no particular problems are likely to arise, particularly if for sound pragmatic reasons we assume that if a patient agrees, at our suggestion, to see a colleague for a further opinion, he will not simply agree, but will positively expect that we will pass on information about his state of health. Such an assumption comes naturally to me, as a doctor who practised in a hospital setting, and dealt with general medical problems in which the help of a colleague was often needed, and in relation to which 'stigmatization' was not a likely issue. Even so, from time to time things would come to light with a bearing on life insurance, on fitness for employment, on disease communicable in various ways, or even on accident associated with previous treatment. As a rest from the theory, let me recall two specific examples of the kind of thing which can arise even in the humdrum practice of a general physician.

A train-driver, appropriately from Crewe, was referred to me with central chest pain of a few days' duration, made worse by exertion, but still present at rest, and associated with shortness of breath on quite slight effort. His clinically suspected 'heart attack' was confirmed on investigation. I explained the situation to him, and pointed out that if he continued his present occupation he might be endangering others as well as himself; and I asked his permission to notify the railway's own doctor, so that after he had recovered from his immediate illness alternative safer employment could be arranged for him, as is usually possible in a large organization. Fortunately, he accepted this advice. Had he not done so, I believe it would have been my duty to notify the occupational physician of the railway in any case, rather than risk both harm to the man himself, and a distinct risk to public safety.

A patient came with a story of cough and chest pain of several months' duration, of sudden onset after previous good health. He fortunately mentioned that he had had a tooth out shortly before his trouble began; but the true state of affairs would have come out in any case, as the chest X-ray showed collapse of the right lower lobe, and a large molar tooth in the corresponding bronchus. This was removed by bronchoscopy, but again I saw no alternative to explaining the nature of the illness, and the dentist involved became the subject of a successful claim, which he did not contest.

Perhaps these two experiences are in some sort of balance, since in one I could be considered to have 'shopped' a patient, had the need arisen; and in the other I 'shopped' a dental colleague. In relation to the thesis of this chapter, 'absolute confidentiality' would have prevented me from notifying the railway doctor, but would have allowed me presumably, in the patient's interest, to do the second; while in each case another doctor might well have acted differently.

As I hinted, perhaps somewhat obliquely, at the beginning of this section, the attitudes and consequent behaviour of doctors in relation to confidentiality are likely to be affected by the type of practice in which they are engaged. My own perspective as a general physician may well be different from that of an occupational physician, who has a degree of responsibility to an employer as well as to a patient; and even more different from that of a venereologist, whose access to patients is critically dependent on perception by the prospective patient that confidentiality will be absolute. This emphasis on absolute confidentiality has largely dictated the conventional wisdom on the ethical dilemmas posed by AIDS; but I personally share the view expressed in a statement made in relation to AIDS by the General Medical Council in 1988, that 'most doctors are now prepared to regard these conditions as similar in principle to other infections and life-threatening conditions, and are willing to apply established principles in approaching their diagnosis and management, rather than treating them as medical conditions quite distinct from all others'. Thankfully, the public health aspects of AIDS are to be considered in a later chapter; but at the clinical level I would be prepared, in the face of absolute refusal by the patient, to divulge to a spouse, with the promise of appropriate counselling, that her partner had AIDS; and I support the action of surgeons in testing patients for HIV, when there is a risk that they might pass on the virus to other patients – just as I would see it as the surgeon's duty to notify an infection which he had acquired. I think I am consistent at any rate with the thrust of this chapter in considering the principle of autonomy not as absolute, but capable in the right circumstances of having to yield place to the principle of non-maleficence.

Confidentiality and society

Although considerations of confidentiality are of the utmost importance in clinical settings, such settings are so much a relationship between individuals, some of them idiosyncratic by nature or as a result of illness, that the general principles by which they are undoubtedly informed are not easily extracted from the complex scene for demonstration purposes. However, society, or rather the agents acting on its behalf, quite rightly ask for a more formal definition of principles and of practical safeguards. From my background of clinical practice (which I can only hope to have been ethical in the manner of Molière's M. Jourdain's prose, i.e. adequate in practice without prior conscious study of the rules), I was called to the chair of a committee set up at the initiative of the British Medical Association (BMA), and with the support of the Department of Health, to consider matters of confidentiality as they affected personal health information. The immediate context of this was the prospect of legislation designed to protect from improper access any information held generally in computerized systems; but our own remit was 'limited' to health information. Because of the variety of professions concerned in the provision of health care, and because of the interface between health and social care, the committee was both large and multidisciplinary; it became known as the Interprofessional Working Group (IPWG). The large size and the number of different interests in the IPWG, and changes in representation over a number of years, did not make for rapid decisions; on the other hand, we were greatly benefited by the drive and enthusiasm of Dr John Dawson of the Science Board of the BMA, and by the legal expertise and clarity of mind of Paul Sieghart. The group held well over 50 meetings, spread over so many years that the Bill which stimulated its formation has long overtaken it, and has indeed been the Data Protection Act since 1984. I mention my long-standing involvement with the IPWG not either to commend my patience as a chairman or to expose my ineptitude; but to explain the stimulus and the background to my own thinking on these matters, and perhaps also to persuade you that the problems, even if they lack the infinite personal variety of clinical transactions, are not without a complexity of their own. The general shape of the problems, and the principles underlying them, had become clear at least five years ago, and we had produced guidelines and an explanatory handbook which satisfied almost everyone – but in ethical matters as in many others, the desire to please everyone without exception is an *ignis fatuus*, offering its followers a choice of morasses, in one or other of which the consultation processes of government have now submerged our efforts. However, we did owe largely to representatives from the Department of Health a wise and clarifying decision – that although the Data Protection Act itself was limited in scope to mechanically processed information, in the health field the same principles of confidentiality should equally apply to the much greater amount of personal health information held on ordinary paper – the so-called 'manual record'. So in what follows I shall be speaking of personal health information in general, irrespective of the manner in which it is recorded.

In these matters the general principle, and also the public expectation, is that when an individual provides or a doctor elicits information on that individual's state of health, such information will not be divulged. To do so would breach the *prima facie* principle of *autonomy*. I suggested at the beginning of this chapter that departures from conduct apparently dictated by *prima facie* ethical principles could be justified either by the recognition of *legitimate exceptions*, or by *conflict between principles*.

Legitimate Exceptions

The most obvious of these is when a patient voluntarily abrogates his own autonomy, by giving free informed consent to the release of health information contained in his record. When information is to be used for other than clinical purposes – e.g. for insurance, welfare or housing – the patient's consent should have been preceded by explanation of the possible consequences of release of his personal health information to the authority concerned. A less important gloss, at least in most cases, on the release of information legitimated by consent is that a patient can abrogate his own autonomy but not, without the other's consent, someone else's. For example, if the record includes a family history attributing to relatives a condition which they might not wish generally known, their consent should formally be obtained to disclosure of that part of the record. Common sense might suggest, however, that sensitive matter of this kind is not frequent, and that when it does occur it may be less cumbrous to delete that part of the record than to go through a formal consent procedure with a distant relative.

It was suggested earlier that, in a clinical context, those looking after the patient in various ways could have legitimate access to his record either in whole or in necessary part; and more debatably perhaps, that such transfers might be legitimated by the consent implied in having had recourse to health care. But when we go outside the clinical field the possibility of release on a 'right to know' basis is limited in two particular ways, which can be expressed in the form of questions which should be answered before the information is released:

> Who needs to know?
> How much of the record is needed?

On the first of these questions, it is the *need* to know, and not just the *wish* to know, which confers the *right*. When the disclosure is made in the interests of the patient, his consent should still be sought. Even so, the transfer of information should still be made to a responsible individual, not broadcast to an institution. On the second question, it is often preferable to make a specific disclosure, appropriate to the particular need, than to adopt the inherently sloppy course of sending unedited material. To go back for an illustration to the clinical field, I have on occasion seen patients referred from other hospitals bringing with them their entire notes and X-rays, but no summary of the specific problem at issue. I felt sad for the patient sitting there while I ploughed through this material; but I fell short of my duty of *agape* to the referring registrar.

These are but examples of possible legitimate exceptions to the principle of confidentiality of health information. In any material case their legitimacy should rest on a considered decision, taken in the interests of the patient. But there are also cases of conflict between the interests of individuals, between individuals and society, and even conflict between principles themselves.

Conflict Between Principles

It is a matter of common observation that one man's autonomy may be at another's expense; banal examples in the health field are in the 'freedom' to transmit colds, or to smoke in public. Some such conflicts of interest reflect discordance not simply in the application of a principle, but between principles themselves. As examples, I will discuss first the conflict between 'autonomy' and 'benevolence', using as illustration the possible constraints on research; and then the conflict between 'autonomy' and 'non-maleficence', illustrating it by legal pressures to use health information in the detection or prevention of crime.

Research

In order to avoid an argument tangential to the main theme, let me join the good company of Thomas Jefferson, and say that 'I hold it to be a self-evident truth' that it is desirable to increase knowledge by carrying out research; and it is further beneficial if the results of such research can be applied to the prevention and cure of illness. Clinical research has its ethical problems, soluble in the main by truly informed consent; but they are not particularly those arising from disclosing information, rather perhaps arising from withholding it. But one very important branch of research is based on the use of records, with as a rule no direct interview between researcher and subject in which explanation can be given and consent sought. The academic and practical values of epidemiological studies are not in question; argument focuses on how the patient's right of confidentiality can be secured. One extreme position, strongly held by nursing organizations, is that any access to records must be preceded by explicit informed consent given by the patient; in other words, complete preservation of autonomy, at whatever cost to research or its possible fruits. There are not, of course, any advocates of the theoretical other extreme, which would be research without consent and without safeguards. The middle position, taken by the majority of the IPWG, is that any proposal for epidemiological study of records should be submitted to a research ethics committee; and that the results should be published in such a way that no individual patient could be identified – 'anonymized publication', in the jargon. Much valuable epidemiological research is based in part on death certificates, for example the effect of smoking on heart disease and lung cancer; a rigid stipulation of 'consent' would prevent such research.

Law Enforcement

The principle of 'non-maleficence' would seem to favour the arrest of criminals and the detection of crime; but the criminal himself might see things rather differently, especially if health information volunteered by him for another purpose was made instrumental in his pursuit. Absolute 'autonomy' would preclude the use of such information – would indeed preclude either arrest or prevention. On the other hand – and not fancifully – rigid devotees of law and order have happily suggested that the immigration officer or the tax inspector might get some useful information from clinical records. But I think most people might see this as a matter of degree, giving the preference to autonomy for trivial offences, but becoming skewed to non-maleficence in case of terrorism or other serious crime. But in the practical world two specific problems arise, how to define 'serious crime'; and who is to make the disclosure.

On the first of these, the Police and Criminal Evidence Act (1985) gives some help, which wisely falls short of the catgorical, but instances the 'security of the state', the processes of criminal investigation and trial, and the life and health of individuals as things worthy of protection, even at some cost to autonomy. Representative crimes include homicide, rape, treason and kidnapping.

Formal disclosures to the police of health information are not a daily occurrence, but authorities must have a mechanism for deciding on them. In family practice the onus is presumably on the individual doctor; and in hospital the doctor in charge of the patient is the first choice; but he or she may not always be available in an emergency, and it may then be necessary to fall back on an administrative arrangement – which should not, however, be the first choice, as administrators, however strong their personal integrity, are under no professional constraint, and have not got the traditions of confidentiality which medical training and practice should inculcate.

Where a doctor finds himself possessed of information which may be relevant to the detection or prevention of serious crime, he can as a rule make his decision as a free agent. But there are quite a number of statutory provisions which may variously require, permit, or prevent disclosure; and in some of these contexts the requirement is on the health authority, with or in some cases without the necessary awareness of the doctor. A doctor may also be ordered by a court of law to disclose health information on his patient, and he is then under a legal obligation to do so. It is unlikely, but not impossible, that a legal requirement would be in flagrant conflict with personal or professional ethics; but if it were, the damage to personal integrity would have to be balanced against the penalty likely to be imposed by the court.

Recapitulation

Doctors and other health workers should not divulge personal health information given them by patients. This is a norm of conduct, not a categorical ethical imperative. Disclosures can be legitimated by the informed consent of the patient, and by the 'need to know' of other health professionals directly involved in the care of that patient. For information to go outside the health care field and into society generally, stringent safeguards are needed; but even so, other ethical principles in particular contexts may take precedence over the principle of confidentiality based on autonomy. There are also statutory and legal constraints to be taken into account.

References

1   **Ross, W. D.**. *The right and the good*. Oxford University Press, Oxford.
2   **Rawls, J.** 1976. *A theory of justice*. Oxford University Press, Oxford.

Tarasoff v. Regents of the University of California*

Tobriner, Justice.

On October 27, 1969, Prosenjit Poddar killed Tatiana Tarasoff. Plaintiffs, Tatiana's parents, allege that two months earlier Poddar confided his intention to kill Tatiana to Dr. Lawrence Moore, a psychologist employed by the Cowell Memorial Hospital at the University of California at Berkeley. They allege that on Moore's request, the campus police briefly detained Poddar, but released him when he appeared rational. They further claim that Dr. Harvey Powelson, Moore's superior, then directed that no further action be taken to detain Poddar. No one warned plaintiffs of Tatiana's peril.

. . .

We shall explain that defendant therapists cannot escape liability merely because Tatiana herself was not their patient. When a therapist determines, or pursuant to the standards of his profession should determine, that his patient presents a serious danger of violence to another, he incurs an obligation to use reasonable care to protect the intended victim against such danger. The discharge of this duty may require the therapist to take one or more of various steps, depending upon the nature of the case. Thus it may call for him to warn the intended victim or others likely to apprise the victim of the danger, to notify the police, or to take whatever other steps are reasonably necessary under the circumstances.

. . .

1. Plaintiffs' complaints

Plaintiffs, Tatiana's mother and father, filed separate but virtually identical second amended complaints. The issue before us on this appeal is whether those complaints now state, or can be amended to state, causes of action against defendants. We therefore begin by setting forth the pertinent allegations of the complaints.

Plaintiffs' first cause of action, entitled 'Failure to Detain a Dangerous Patient,' alleges that on August 20, 1969, Poddar was a voluntary outpatient receiving therapy at Cowell Memorial Hospital. Poddar informed Moore, his therapist, that he was going to kill an unnamed girl, readily identifiable as Tatiana, when she returned home from spending the summer in Brazil. Moore, with the concurrence of Dr. Gold, who had initially examined Poddar, and Dr. Yandell, assistant to the director of the department of psychiatry, decided that Poddar should be committed for observation in a mental hospital. Moore orally notified Officers Atkinson and Teel of the campus police that he would request commitment. He then sent a letter to Police Chief William Beall requesting the assistance of the police department in securing Poddar's confinement.

Officers Atkinson, Brownrigg, and Halleran took Poddar into custody, but, satisfied that Poddar was rational, released him on his promise to stay

* Tarasoff v. *Regents of the University of California*. 131 Cal Rptr 14, 17 Cal. 3d 425, 551P. 2d 334, 1976.

away from Tatiana. Powelson, director of the department of psychiatry at Cowell Memorial Hospital, then asked the police to return Moore's letter, directed that all copies of the letter and notes that Moore had taken as therapist be destroyed, and 'ordered no action to place Prosenjit Poddar in 72-hour treatment and evaluation facility.'

Plaintiffs' second cause of action, entitled 'Failure to Warn On a Dangerous Patient,' incorporates the allegations of the first cause of action, but adds the assertion that defendants negligently permitted Poddar to be released from police custody without 'notifying the parents of Tatiana Tarasoff that their daughter was in grave danger from Prosenjit Poddar.' Pod persuaded Tatiana's brother to share an apartment with him near Tatiana's residence; shortly after her return from Brazil, Poddar went to her residence and killed her.

. . .

Plaintiffs can state a cause of action against defendant therapists for negligent failure to protect Tatiana

The second cause of action can be amended to allege that Tatiana's death proximately resulted from defendants' negligent failure to warn Tatiana or others likely to apprise her of her danger. Plaintiffs contend that as amended, such allegations of negligence and proximate causation, with resulting damages, establish a cause of action. Defendants, however, contend that in the circumstances of the present case they owed no duty of care to Tatiana or her parents and that, in the absence of such duty, they were free to act in careless disregard of Tatiana's life and safety.

In analyzing this issue, we bear in mind that legal duties are not discoverable facts of nature, but merely conclusory expressions that, in cases of a particular type, liability should be imposed for damage done. As stated in *Dillion v. Legg* (1968): 'The assertion that liability must . . . be denied because defendant bears no 'duty' to plaintiff 'begs the essential question – whether the plaintiff's interests are entitled to legal protection against the defendant's conduct . . . [Duty] is not sacrosanct itself, but only an expression of the sum total of those considerations of policy which lead the law to say that the particular plaintiff is entitled to protection.' (Prosser, Law of Torts [3d ed. 1964] at pp. 332–333.)'

In the landmark case of *Rowland v. Christian* (1968), Justice Peters recognized that liability should be imposed 'for an injury occasioned to another by his want of ordinary care or skill' as expressed in section 1714 of the Civil Code. Thus, Justice Peters, quoting from *Heaven v. Pender* (1883) stated: ' "whenever one person is by circumstances placed in such a position with regard to another . . . that if he did not use ordinary care and skill in his own conduct . . . he would cause danger of injury to the person or property of the other, a duty arises to use ordinary care and skill to avoid such danger." '

We depart from 'this fundamental principle' only upon the 'balancing of a number of considerations'; major ones 'are the foreseeability of harm to the plaintiff, the degree of certainty that the plaintiff suffered injury, the closeness of the connection between the defendant's conduct and the injury suffered, the moral blame attached to the defendant's conduct, the policy of preventing future harm, the extent of the burden to the defendant and consequences to the community of imposing a duty to exercise care with resulting liability for breach, and the availability, cost and prevalence of insurance for the risk involved.'

The most important of these considerations in establishing duty is foreseeability. As a general principle, a 'defendant owes a duty of care to all persons who are foreseeably endangered by his conduct, with respect to all risks which make the conduct unreasonably dangerous.'

As we shall explain, however, when the avoidance of foreseeable harm requires a defendant to control the conduct of another person, or to warn of such conduct, the common law has traditionally imposed liability only if the defendant bears some special relationship to the dangerous person or to the potential victim. Since the relationship between a therapist and his patient satisfies this requirement, we need not here decide whether foreseeability alone is sufficient to create a duty to exercise reasonable care to protect a potential victim of another's conduct.

Although, as we have stated above, under the common law, as a general rule, one person owed no duty to control the conduct of another, . . . nor to warn those endangered by such conduct, the courts have carved out an exception to this rule in cases in which the defendant stands in some special relationship to either the person whose conduct needs to be controlled or in a relationship to the foreseeable victim of that conduct. Applying this exception to the present case, we note that a relationship of defendant therapists to either Tatiana or Poddar will suffice to establish a duty of care; as explained in section 315 of the Restatement Second of Torts, a duty of care may arise from either '(a) a special relation . . . between the actor and the third person which imposes a duty upon the actor to control the third person's conduct, or (b) a special relation . . . between the actor and the other which gives to the other a right of protection.'

Although plaintiffs' pleadings assert no special relation between Tatiana and defendant therapists, they establish as between Poddar and defendant therapists the special relation that arises between a patient and his doctor or psychotherapist. Such a relationship may support affirmative duties for the benefit of third persons. Thus, for example, a hospital must exercise reasonable care to control the behavior of a patient which may endanger other persons. A doctor must also warn a patient if the patient's condition or medication renders certain conduct, such as driving a car, dangerous to others.

Although the California decisions that recognize this duty have involved cases in which the defendant stood in a special relationship *both* to the victim and to the person whose conduct created the danger, we do not think that the duty should logically be constricted to such situations. Decisions of other jurisdictions hold that the single relationship of a doctor to his patient is sufficient to support the duty to exercise reasonable care to protect others against dangers emanating from the patient's illness. The courts hold that a doctor is liable to persons infected by his patient if he negligently fails to diagnose a contagious disease, or, having diagnosed the illness, fails to warn members of the patient's family.

Since it involved a dangerous mental patient, the decision in *Merchants Nat. Bank & Trust Co. of Fargo v. United States* (1967) comes closer to the issue. The Veterans Administration arranged for the patient to work on a local farm, but did not inform the farmer of the man's background. The farmer consequently permitted the patient to come and go freely during nonworking hours; the patient borrowed a car, drove to his wife's residence and killed her. Notwithstanding the lack of any 'special relationship' between the Veterans Administration and the wife, the court found the Veterans Administration liable for the wrongful death of the wife.

In their summary of the relevant rulings Fleming and Maximov conclude that the 'case law should dispel any notion that to impose on the therapists a duty to take precautions for the safety of persons threatened by a patient, where due care so requires, is in any way opposed to contemporary ground rules on the duty relationship. On the contrary, there now seems to be sufficient authority to support the conclusion that by entering into a doctor-patient relationship the therapist becomes sufficiently involved to assume some responsibility for the safety, not only of the patient himself, but also of any third person whom the doctor knows to be threatened by the patient.' (Fleming & Maximov, *The Patient or His Victim: The Therapist's Dilemma* [1974] 62 Cal.L.Rev. 1025, 1030.)

Defendants contend, however, that imposition of a duty to exercise reasonable care to protect third persons is unworkable because therapists cannot accurately predict whether or not a patient will resort to violence. In support of this argument amicus representing the American Psychiatric Association and other professional societies cites numerous articles which indicate that therapists, in the present state of the art, are unable reliably to predict violent acts; their forecasts, amicus claims, tend consistently to over-predict violence, and indeed are more often wrong than right. Since predictions of violence are often erroneous, amicus concludes, the courts should not render rulings that predicate the liability of therapists upon the validity of such predictions.

The role of the psychiatrist, who is indeed a practitioner of medicine, and that of the psychologist who performs an allied function, are like that of the physician who must conform to the standards of the profession and who must often make diagnoses and predictions based upon such evaluations. Thus the judgment of the therapist in diagnosing emotional disorders and in predicting whether a patient presents a serious danger of violence is comparable to the judgment which doctors and professionals must regularly render under accepted rules of responsibility.

We recognize the difficulty that a therapist encounters in attempting to forecast whether a patient presents a serious danger of violence. Obviously we do not require that the therapist, in making that determination, render a perfect performance; the therapist need only exercise 'that reasonable degree of skill, knowledge, and care ordinarily possessed and exercised by members of [that professional specialty] under similar circumstances.' Within the broad range of reasonable practice and treatment in which professional opinion and judgment may differ, the therapist is free to exercise his or her own best judgment without liability; proof, aided by hindsight, that he or she judged wrongly is insufficient to establish negligence.

In the instant case, however, the pleadings do not raise any question as to failure of defendant therapists to predict that Poddar presented a serious danger of violence. On the contrary, the present complaints allege that defendant therapists did in fact predict that Poddar would kill, but were negligent in failing to warn.

Amicus contends, however, that even when a therapist does in fact predict that a patient poses a serious danger of violence to others, the therapist should be absolved of any responsibility for failing to act to protect the potential victim. In our view, however, once a therapist does in fact determine, or under applicable professional standards reasonably should have determined, that a patient poses a serious danger of violence to others, he bears a duty to exercise reasonable care to protect the foreseeable victim of that danger. While the discharge of this duty of due care will necessarily vary with the facts of each case, in each instance the adequacy of the therapist's conduct must be measured against the traditional negligence standard of the rendition of reasonable care under the circumstances. As explained in Fleming and Maximov, *The Patient or His Victim: The Therapist's Dilemma* (1974) 62 Cal.L.Rev. 1025, 1967: '. . . the ultimate question of resolving the tension between the conflicting interests of patient and potential victim is one of social policy, not professional expertise. . . . In sum, the therapist owes a legal duty not only to his patient, but also to his patient's would-be victim and is subject in both respects to scrutiny by judge and jury.'

Contrary to the assertion of amicus, this conclusion is not inconsistent with our recent decision in *People v. Burnick* (1975). Taking note of the uncertain character of therapeutic prediction, we held in *Burnick* that a person cannot be committed as a mentally disordered sex offender unless found to be such by proof beyond a reasonable doubt. The issue in the present context, however, is not whether the patient should be incarcerated, but whether the therapist should take any steps at all to protect the threatened victim; some of the alternatives open to the therapist, such as warning the victim, will not result in the drastic consequences of depriving the patient of his liberty. Weighing the uncertain and conjectural character of the alleged damage done the patient by such a warning against the peril to the victim's life, we conclude that professional inaccuracy in predicting violence cannot negate the therapist's duty to protect the threatened victim.

The risk that unnecessary warnings may be given is a reasonable price to pay for the lives of possible victims that may be saved. We would hesitate to hold that the therapist who is aware that his patient expects to attempt to assassinate the President of the United States would not be obligated to warn the authorities because the therapist cannot predict with accuracy that his patient will commit the crime.

Defendants further argue that free and open communication is essential to psychotherapy, that 'Unless a patient . . . is assured that . . . information [revealed to him] can and will be held in utmost confidence, he will be reluctant to make the full disclosure upon which diagnosis and treatment . . . depends.' The giving of a warning, defendants contend, constitutes a breach of trust which entails the revelation of confidential communications.

We recognize the public interest in supporting effective treatment of mental illness and in protecting the rights of patients to privacy, and the consequent public importance of safeguarding the confidential character of psychotherapeutic communication. Against this interest, however, we must weigh the public interest in safety from violent assault. The Legislature has undertaken the difficult task of balancing the countervailing concerns. In Evidence Code section 1014, it established a broad rule of privilege to protect confidential communications between patient and psychotherapist. In Evidence Code section 1024, the Legislature created a specific and limited exception to the psychotherapist-patient privilege: 'There is no privilege . . . if the psychotherapist has reasonable cause to believe that the patient is in such mental or emotional condition as to be dangerous to himself or to the person or property of another and that disclosure of the communication is necessary to prevent the threatened danger.'

We realize that the open and confidential character of psychotherapeutic dialogue encourages patients to express threats of violence, few of which are ever executed. Certainly a therapist should not be encouraged routinely to reveal such threats; such disclosures could seriously disrupt the patient's relationship with his therapist and with the persons threatened. To the contrary, the therapist's obligations to his patient require that he not disclose a confidence unless such disclosure is necessary to avert danger to others, and even then that he do so discreetly, and in a fashion that would preserve the privacy of his patient to the fullest extent compatible with the prevention of the threatened danger.

The revelation of a communication under the above circumstances is not a breach of trust or a violation of professional ethics; as stated in the Principles of Medical Ethics of the American Medical Association (1957), section 9: 'A physician may not reveal the confidence entrusted to him in the course of medical attendance . . . *unless he is required to do so by law or unless it becomes necessary in order to protect the welfare of the individual or of the community*.' (Emphasis added.) We conclude that the public policy favoring protection of the confidential character of patient-psychotherapist communications must yield to the extent to which disclosure is essential to avert danger to others. The protective privilege ends where the public peril begins.

Our current crowded and computerized society compels the interdependence of its members. In this risk-infested society we can hardly tolerate the further exposure to danger that would result from a concealed knowledge of the therapist that his patient was lethal. If the exercise of reasonable care to protect the threatened victim requires the therapist to warn the endangered party or those who can reasonably be expected to notify him, we see no sufficient societal interest that would protect and justify concealment. The containment of such risks lies in the public interest. For the foregoing reasons, we find that plaintiffs' complaints can be amended to state a cause of action against defendants Moore, Powelson, Gold, and Yandell and against the Regents as their employer, for breach of a duty to exercise reasonable care to protect Tatiana.

. . .

Clark, Justice (dissenting).

Until today's majority opinion, both legal and medical authorities have agreed that confidentiality is essential to effectively treat the mentally ill, and that imposing a duty on doctors to disclose patient threats to potential victims would greatly impair treatment. Further, recognizing that effective treatment and society's safety are necessarily intertwined, the Legislature has already decided effective and confidential treatment is preferred over imposition of a duty to warn.

The issue of whether effective treatment for the mentally ill should be sacrificed to a system of warnings is, in my opinion, properly one for the Legislature, and we are bound by its judgment. Moreover, even in the absence of clear legislative direction, we must reach the same conclusion because imposing the majority's new duty is certain to result in a net increase in violence.

. . .

Common Law Analysis

Entirely apart from the statutory provisions, the same result must be reached upon considering both general tort principles and the public policies favoring effective treatment, reduction of violence, and justified commitment.

Generally, a person owes no duty to control the conduct of another. Exceptions are recognized only in limited situations where (1) a special relationship exists between the defendant and injured party, or (2) a special relationship exists between defendant and the active wrongdoer, imposing a duty on defendant to control the wrongdoer's conduct. The majority does not contend the first exception is appropriate to this case.

Policy generally determines duty. Principal policy considerations include foreseeability of harm, certainty of the plaintiff's injury, proximity of the defendant's conduct to the plaintiff's injury, moral blame attributable to defendant's conduct, prevention of future harm, burden on the defendant, and consequences to the community.

Overwhelming policy considerations weigh against imposing a duty on psychotherapists to warn a potential victim against harm. While offering virtually no benefit to society, such a duty will frustrate psychiatric treatment, invade fundamental patient rights and increase violence.

The importance of psychiatric treatment and its need for confidentiality have been recognized by this court. 'It is clearly recognized that the very practice of psychiatry vitally depends upon the reputation in the community that the psychiatrist will not tell.' (Slovenko, *Psychiatry and a Second Look at the Medical Privilege* (1960) 6 Wayne L.Rev. 175, 188.)

Assurance of confidentiality is important for three reasons.

Deterrence from Treatment

First, without substantial assurance of confidentiality, those requiring treatment will be deterred from seeking assistance. It remains an unfortunate fact in our society that people seeking psychiatric guidance tend to become stigmatized. Apprehension of such stigma – apparently increased by the propensity of people considering treatment to see themselves in the worst possible light – creates a well-recognized reluctance to seek aid. This reluctance is alleviated by the psychiatrist's assurance of confidentiality.

Full Disclosure

Second, the guarantee of confidentiality is essential in eliciting the full disclosure necessary for effective treatment. The psychiatric patient approaches treatment with conscious and unconscious inhibitions against revealing his innermost thoughts. 'Every person, however well-motivated, has to overcome resistances to therapeutic exploration. These resistances seek support from every possible source and the possibility of disclosure would easily be employed in the service of resistance.' (Goldstein & Katz, 36 Conn. Bar J. 175, 179.) Until a patient can trust his psychiatrist not to violate their confidential relationship, 'the unconscious psychological control mechanism of repression will prevent the recall of past experiences.' (Butler, *Psychotherapy and Griswold: Is Confidentiality a Privilege or a Right?* (1971) 3 Conn.L.Rev. 599, 604.)

Successful Treatment

Third, even if the patient fully discloses his thoughts, assurance that the confidential relationship will not be breached is necessary to maintain his trust in his psychiatrist – the very means by which treatment is effected. '[T]he essence of much psychotherapy is the contribution of trust in the external world and ultimately in the self, modelled upon the trusting relationship established during therapy.' (Dawidoff, *The Malpractice of Psychiatrists*, 1966 Duke L.J. 696, 704.) Patients will be helped only if they can form a trusting relationship with the psychiatrist. All authorities appear to agree that if the trust relationship cannot be developed because of collusive communication between the psychiatrist and others, treatment will be frustrated.

Given the importance of confidentiality to the practice of psychiatry, it becomes clear the duty to warn imposed by the majority will cripple the use and effectiveness of psychiatry. Many people, potentially violent – yet susceptible to treatment – will be deterred from seeking it; those seeking it will be inhibited from making revelations necessary to effective treatment; and, forcing the psychiatrist to violate the patient's trust will destroy the interpersonal relationship by which treatment is effected.

Violence and Civil Commitment

By imposing a duty to warn, the majority contributes to the danger to society of violence by the mentally ill and greatly increases the risk of civil commitment – the total deprivation of liberty – of those who should not be confined. The impairment of treatment and risk of improper commitment resulting from the new duty to warn will not be limited to a few patients but will extend to a large number of the mentally ill. Although under existing psychiatric procedures only a relatively few receiving treatment will ever present a risk of violence, the number making threats is huge, and it is the latter group – not just the former – whose treatment will be impaired and whose risk of commitment will be increased.

Both the legal and psychiatric communities recognize that the process of determining potential violence in a patient is far from exact, being fraught with complexity and uncertainty. In fact precision has not even been attained in predicting who of those having already committed violent acts will again become violent, a task recognized to be of much simpler proportions.

This predictive uncertainty means that the number of disclosures will necessarily be large. As noted above, psychiatric patients are encouraged to discuss all thoughts of violence, and they often express such thoughts. However, unlike this court, the psychiatrist does not enjoy the benefit of overwhelming hindsight in seeing which few, if any, of his patients will ultimately become violent. Now, confronted by the majority's new duty, the psychiatrist must instantaneously calculate potential violence from each patient on each visit. The difficulties researchers have encountered in accurately predicting violence will be heightened for the practicing psychiatrist dealing for brief periods in his office with heretofore nonviolent patients. And, given the decision not to warn or commit must always be made at the psychiatrist's civil peril, one can expect most doubts will be resolved in favor of the psychiatrist protecting himself.

Neither alternative open to the psychiatrist seeking to protect himself is in the public interest. The warning itself is an impairment of the psychiatrist's ability to treat, depriving many patients of adequate treatment. It is to be expected that after disclosing their threats, a significant number of patients, who would not become violent if treated according to existing practices, will engage in violent conduct as a result of unsuccessful treatment. In short, the majority's duty to warn will not only impair treatment of many who would never become violent but worse, will result in a net increase in violence.

The second alternative open to the psychiatrist is to commit his patient rather than to warn. Even in the absence of threat of civil liability, the doubts of psychiatrists as to the seriousness of patient threats have led psychiatrists to overcommit to mental institutions. This overcommitment has been authoritatively documented in both legal and psychiatric studies. This practice is so prevalent that it has been estimated that 'as many as twenty harmless persons are incarcerated for every one who will commit a violent act.' (Steadman & Cocozza, *Stimulus/Response: We Can't Predict Who Is Dangerous* (Jan. 1975) 8 Psych. Today 32, 35.)

Given the incentive to commit created by the majority's duty, this already serious situation will be worsened, contrary to Chief Justice Wright's admonition 'that liberty is no less precious because forfeited in a civil proceeding than when taken as a consequence of a criminal conviction.'

Family Involvement in the Care of People with Psychoses

An ethical argument*

George I. Szmukler and Sidney Bloch

Growing evidence points to the benefits of involving relatives (or other informal carers) in treating people suffering from a psychosis. Psychoeducational approaches, for instance, are associated with a reduced relapse rate in schizophrenia and offer potential for better family coping and a diminution in their distress (Falloon & Pederson, 1985; Lam, 1991; Bloch *et al*, 1994). Furthermore, the family commonly provides useful information about the patient and their illness; this facilitates a treatment plan in which the family can play a prominent role in helping to supervise medication, encouraging participation in rehabilitation programmes, and generally providing an environment conducive to promoting recovery or reducing disability. However, achieving optimal collaboration with the family is often beset with difficulties of an ethical nature, especially revolving around confidentiality, and its potential breach. A specially taxing problem concerns the circumstances when the involvement of the family is justified despite a patient's refusal to provide consent.

We focus on patients with psychotic disorders because the benefits of family involvement are established and because the validity of their refusal is sometimes unclear in that their illness may affect their capacity to judge what is in their best interests. Furthermore, the crucial role of carers in making 'community care' possible is increasingly recognised, carrying with it a right to respect their needs.

The purposes of this paper are twofold. The first is to outline an approach to family collaboration sensitive to the issues of confidentiality and the potentially competing interests of patient and family. We hope that such an approach will establish from the outset a treatment relationship with both patient and family in which later ethical dilemmas are mostly avoided. The second is to offer guidelines where a patient refuses family involvement even though the interests of one or both are likely to be served. We hope our suggestions will provoke discussion of a neglected area, and so lead to agreed principles of good practice.

Before proceeding further we enter a major caveat concerning cultural differences in value systems, both inside and outside the family. Our discussion is geared to psychiatry in Western countries, but even here value differences between ethnic groups, or even generations within families, may create difficulties. A consultation with a patient in an Indian family may encounter different expectations of family involvement – for example, who should be present, who is entitled to know what, and who should make decisions – to an English one. Such differences cannot be addressed in this paper, but we ask the reader to bear in mind their possible influences.

Confidentiality

Confidentiality, a core ethical principle in medicine as part of respect for a person's privacy, is supported by other values which enhance the doctor-patient relationship (Beauchamp & Childress, 1988). These include respect for autonomy and a community interest in encouraging patients to feel secure in being open with their doctors, thus facilitating accurate diagnosis and treatment. However, confidentiality cannot be absolute and may be justifiably breached as a result of competing interests. For example, in many jurisdictions notifying authorities of specified diseases is mandatory, and information about patients may be revealed where failure to do so could expose them or others to risk of serious harm. Here patient consent is not essential, although it should be sought whenever possible as part of good practice.

Frequently in the course of a psychosis, confidentiality is necessarily breached in the patient's interests or to protect others. A clear example is in the instigation of compulsory treatment under mental health law where others (relatives, other doctors, social workers, police, ambulance officers) become involved even if this is contrary to the patient's wishes. Other situations commonly arise, short of those warranting compulsory treatment, in which the interests of patient or others, especially family, appear to necessitate disclosure of confidential information. But uncertainty prevails about when such action is justified. Psychiatrists' concerns may hinder both effective treatment of the seriously ill and the addressing of their carers' needs.

Before offering our ideas on dealing with these challenging circumstances, we provide an ethical framework for engaging families in treatment, which seeks to clarify key aspects of their participation.

An Ethically Sensitive Approach to Family Involvement

An ethical framework for all psychiatric interventions with the family entails the role of values, the question of how to balance the interests of its members, informed consent, and confidentiality.

Values and family intervention

Whatever the form of family engagement, the psychiatrist enters a moral arena. The concept of a morally neutral clinical encounter is fanciful despite the determination to maintain an objective ethical stance. A value system is crucial to a family's welfare; if undetermined its stability could well be jeopardised. These risks are magnified in the clinical context since values held by family members may be linked to the patient's difficulties or to related systemic problems. Helpful guidelines have been elaborated by Aponte (1985) and Bloch *et al* (1994) for dealing with this issue:

(a) The family's role in trying to understand its difficulties and seeking to work out solutions is respected, and kept to the forefront throughout treatment.

(b) The clinician offers professional knowledge and skills as required, but not at the expense of depriving the family of the opportunity to use their own strengths.

(c) The clinician takes care to withhold his or her values, especially avoiding the imposition of what he or she regards as 'right' for the family.

(d) The clinician does, however, convey when appropriate the desirability for the family to explore their values so that related changes in functioning can be considered.

* Szmukler, G. and Bloch, S.: Family involvement in the care of people with psychoses. *British Journal of Psychiatry* 171:401–405, 1997.

(e) The clinician is active in highlighting any conflicting values in the family in the expectation that differences can be explored and dealt with.

The relative interests of family members

How does the psychiatrist respond to the interests of family members, especially if they clash with one another? Three basic positions have been proposed:

(a) The patient's interests always take priority, with the rest of the family regarded as ancillary. Although their potential contribution is sought, this is construed as assistance to the patient.

(b) While the interests of family members are taken into account, the particular features of the therapeutic situation guide the clinician's responses. Thus, he or she may attend to the patient at one point but switch to other members, for example, the patient's principal carer at another time. The patient is not always the chief priority; indeed, satisfactory functioning may sometimes be at the expense of others. Moreover, given that family members' well-being may change during treatment, the clinician monitors the welfare of each and adjusts interventions accordingly.

(c) The interests of all family members are relevant without exception, on the premise that their dynamics as a social group and the patient's difficulties are inextricably linked. The psychiatrist is correspondingly obliged to consider carefully and take into account as far as possible the interests of each.

The third position is least applicable to the psychoses since systemic explanations of their origins are weak. One could argue pragmatically that any of the three positions could prevail according to specific clinical circumstances. We think otherwise and suggest that the second option best suits the majority of interventions with the family. By adopting a broad-based approach, we commit ourselves to a stance which gives due place to the contribution of the family in understanding the causes, outcome and treatment of mental illness. We convey that all may need to participate if the treatment is to be well implemented. It follows that clinicians have a responsibility to ensure that all family members' interests are respected. Thus, whatever their status (especially as patient or otherwise) or values, all are given appropriate attention. Given the nature of psychosis, it is likely that the patient will require more of the psychiatrist's expertise, but still not at the expense of the rest of the family.

A key point here is that this potentially disproportionate therapeutic allocation must be clarified with patient and family when the latter are recruited. The procedure of informed consent served well to engage the family according to our preferred position. We turn to this subject now to note its central role in working with the family.

Informed consent

Informed consent is the foundation upon which ethically sound care of patients and their families occurs. A common sequence in the case of the psychotic patient entails psychiatric assessment followed by interviews with one or more family members, then possible meetings as a group. The ingredients of the consent process are that the psychiatrist: (a) explains the purposes, benefits and risks of the family's involvement; (b) ensures that all participants including the patient comprehend this information; (c) ensures that the family consents freely – without coercion – although they may harbour concerns; and (d) stipulates that although consent is being sought at this juncture, it is subject to re-negotiation if family members should wish it.

Informed consent is thus a dynamic process – a continuing dialogue between psychiatrist and family. Psychiatrist, patient and family unite in determining what is therapeutically advantageous. The clinician accepts that some members may refuse to participate. In the event, he or she adheres to the principle of respect for autonomy in recognising the family's varied preferences. Neither family members declining nor remaining are discriminated against by,

for instance, veiled threats that further help will not be offered unless all cooperate.

Confidentiality in working with the family

Preserving confidences where the family is involved is unquestionably problematic (Fieldsteel, 1982; Lakin, 1988; Doherty & Boss, 1991; Goldenberg & Goldenberg, 1991). The process may entail sharing sensitive information about not only the patient but also the family: The patient or family member may request, even insist, the specified material should not be divulged. Yet the information may be necessary for the optimal conduct of treatment (examples are a history of sexual or physical abuse, domestic violence or an extra-marital affair). The psychiatrist the faces a dilemma. The material may be central to the family's welfare, or to an understanding of the patient's problems. But insistence on breaching confidentiality may well jeopardise the alliance with patient or family. Similar difficulties may arise when clinically relevant secrets are shared by some family members, excluding others.

Solutions for these dilemmas are elusive; they both rest and legitimise 'professionalism'. However, three options can be proposed (Margolin, 1982):

(a) Confidences are sacrosanct and family members are not pressed to divulge them.

(b) The psychiatrist discourages family members from confiding in him alone. He contracts with the family not to be shackled by secrets, perhaps by not meeting with any member separately, thus pre-empting any collusion.

(c) The psychiatrist is flexible inasmuch as information is generally shared among family members but on the understanding they have the right to keep intensely personal information private.

Arguments can be advanced for each but the degree of difference between them points to the question resisting a straightforward remedy. However, one issue is none the less clear: the clinician is obliged to share his or her preferred option with the family, together with its rationale, advantages and risks (although flexibility is retained with the possibility of re-negotiation later if circumstances change).

Situations Where Patients Refuse Family Involvement

We anticipate that the approach we have outlined will reduce dilemmas concerning family involvement in the treatment of psychotic patients. However, complicated instances remain when the psychiatrist will consider contacting relatives despite the patient's refusal to give consent. We start with the premise that confidentiality is presumed. When it is breached, the onus falls on the psychiatrist for justification. We divide our discussion as follows: we first consider further attempts to obtain the patient's consent; we then discuss the grounds for acting without consent, firstly in the patient's interests, and secondly in the family's interests.

An initial response

The clinician can persevere in seeking the patient's consent. Two aspects are relevant. The first is a detailed explanation of the reasons for seeking family involvement. If our advice, above, concerning family recruitment is accepted, it is emphasised that this is routine. The benefits can be high lighted – the patient's problems can be better understood, the family can provide support, the clinician needs the family's help with treatment, the outcome will probably be enhanced, and family members may well have their own need to understand the nature of the illness and the treatment proposed. The second aspect is an attempt to understand the reasons behind the patient's refusal. Does it arise out of set patterns of family communication, or the family's value system, or previous unhappy incidents? Exploring the patient's predictions about how family members might react to receiving certain information about his or her condition may yield fears in a non-confronting way. Family involvement might also significantly alter the patient's relationship with the clinician as well as others, like peers or a partner. An undertaking to address the patient's anxieties can be made explicit in these circumstances. Further more, the psychiatrist weighs up the advantages of asking the patient to be present when the relatives are seen.

If approval for family contact is still unobtainable, the psychiatrist can negotiate restricted conditions. For example, only agreed questions will be posed or agreed items of information disclosed (e.g. medication and side-effects, self-help organisations for carers). If this strategy fails, the patient might agree to contact by correspondence, including reading the letter.

When might a patient's refusal be overridden?

If this initial response fails, the complex matter of overriding the patient's refusal comes into play. Grounds for such drastic action are either clearly established or more ambiguous. The former correspond in general with the grounds for considering compulsory admission to hospital. Central to these is a serious risk to the patient's safety or health or to the safety of others. For example, under section 3 of the Mental Health Act 1983 for England and Wales, the approved social worker is obliged to discuss the patient's plight with the nearest relative and to obtain his or her agreement.

Our discussion will now focus on less clearly established grounds. These involve risks, short of dangers to physical safety, (a) to the health or well-being of the patient or (b) to the well-being of the family. Different 'ends' apply to these two sets of circumstances, requiring consideration of separate principles.

Risks to the patient's health or well-being

The risk falls short of that warranting compulsory admission. The patient is often in the process of relapse with a likelihood that compulsion will become necessary later. Preventing further deterioration may be an immediate goal. Common risks include severe self-neglect, loss of accommodation, job, money or friends, intense distress, exploitation by others, predictable worsening of symptoms, or deterioration to a point which jeopardises future rehabilitation. The psychiatrist may judge that the patient's family may be able to help by, for example, providing information, offering support, supervising medication or ensuring a safe environment.

The dilemma concerning confidentiality posed by a patient who refuses contact with the family turns on the balance between the competing values of respect for autonomy versus paternalism. A further consideration is the future doctor–patient relationship if confidentiality is breached. Many psychiatrists hold that without grounds for compulsory admission, respect for autonomy is paramount. This may be a considered position, but may well arise out of a fear of departing from a hallowed principle.

If respect for autonomy is not an absolute determinant, what factors should be weighed in the balance in deciding to act against the patient's wishes? We propose the following:

(a) The nature and magnitude of the harms to be avoided, and the probability of their occurrence.

(b) The availability of alternatives which might reduce the likelihood of harm. Other people or helping agencies which the patient may be happy to deal with may be able to alleviate the harms.

(c) The patient's capacity to make choices. In assessing the patient's capacity to make decisions about treatment, we consider the ability to comprehend the nature and purpose of the proposed treatment, the likely outcome if treatment is not given, and possible adverse effects. Furthermore, the patient should be able to make a 'true choice', that is, one unaffected by distorted ideas such as delusions. If such a test were to be applied, would the patient be deemed to have capacity to decide on the value of family involvement?

(d) The values of patient and family might suggest how family contact will be received. A family typified by good relationships and mutual support, but which the patient, as a result of the psychosis, sees as rejecting, might be regarded differently to a long-standing dysfunctional one. Cultural norms concerning the role of the family of an ill person in general may also be relevant. Following recovery, would the patient be likely to see family involvement as having been desirable? Has previous discussion with patient or family revealed that contact would be acceptable, given the current circumstances?

(e) The principle of 'the least restrictive' option could apply when family involvement will reduce the likelihood of a greater restriction on the patient's freedom, especially involuntary hospitalisation. This principle is explicit in some mental health statutes, for example in Victoria, Australia, but not in others. But even in the latter case, it is implicit in certain circumstances, as in the requirement to consult the nearest relative before compelling admission under section 3 of the Mental Health Act 1983 for England and Wales.

In summary, justification for involving the family contrary to the patient's wishes would be strongest when: the harms to be avoided are serious and highly probable; no acceptable alternatives are available; the patient's capacity to make a genuine choice is impaired; the family's values embody mutual concern and assistance; and not recruiting the family may lead to even greater restrictions on the patient's liberty. Also to be kept in mind is the potential effect on the future doctor–patient relationship were confidentiality to be breached, and whether harms avoided in the short term will be outweighed by those in the long term arising from a breakdown in the therapeutic alliance. The clinical context may be important here. The psychiatrist may act differently depending on how long he or she has known the patient and the quality of their relationship.

Risks to the well-being of the family

At present it is unlikely that many psychiatrists would involve the family without the patient's consent out of concern about their well-being (short of serious, physical danger). Yet we are all familiar with families who experience bafflement, anguish, burdensome behaviours, and even intimidation as a result of their relative's illness. Some may approach the clinician for help; others may wish to do so but feel too frightened. It comes as a harsh blow if they are told that information cannot be given because of 'patient confidentiality'.

Does the psychiatrist have a duty of care towards such carers, over and above that to the patient? The question has been largely ignored and we recognise we are moving into largely uncharted waters. However, with increased family participation in treatment, ambiguities abound which do need sorting out. Consider the following developments.

The 1995 Mental Health (Patients in the Community) Act for England and Wales introduced 'supervised discharge' for certain categories of patient who pose risks of serious harm to themselves or others in the absence of after-care services. It is noteworthy that an informal carer must be consulted when making an application, as well as later if changes to the care plan prove necessary, including stopping the order. The patient cannot object to this consultation, but can object to the 'nearest relative' being informed if this person is not the 'carer'.

Guidance from the Department of Health (1996) in England and Wales – *The Protection and Use of Patient Information* – shows inconsistency concerning carers. In one section (2.6) which deals with information being divulged to others without the patient's consent, a recipient who 'needs the information because he or she is or may be concerned with the patient's care and treatment' has this right on a 'need to know basis'. A footnote states that 'carers are often regarded as members of the care team' and are thus presumably covered. However, we read elsewhere (section 5.1): 'With the patient's consent, the significant role of carers may need to be recognised in the type of information provided: for example, on discharge from hospital and to make arrangements for continuing care'.

The Australian Medical Association's (1996) revised *Code of Ethics* states: 'Keep in confidence information derived from your patient, and divulge it only with the patient's permission. Exceptions may arise where the *health of others is at risk* or you are required by order of a court to breach patient confidentiality' (emphasis added).

An explicit provision for carers to be informed is contained in recent changes to the Victoria (Australia) Mental Health Act, in which Section 120A (3) allows:

the giving of information relating to a person who is, or has been, receiving services from a relevant psychiatric service by a member of the medical staff, or a member of a prescribed class of staff, to a guardian, family member or primary carer of the person to whom the information relates if – (i) the information is reasonably required for the ongoing care of the person to whom it relates: and (ii) the guardian, family member or primary carer will be involved in providing the care.

Thus, a trend towards the recognition of carers' interests has emerged recently, and this is likely to grow in parallel with the expanding role of informal carers as members of the care team in the community.

Several arguments can be marshalled for involving relatives, primarily for their own benefit, but against the patient's wishes. The first is to view the family as the unit of treatment. The best care of the patient requires the family's support. Moreover, the impact on the family of a member with a severe mental illness is so major that the psychiatrist has a duty of care to them. This case is strengthened by the philosophy of community care, which aims to preserve the patient's social links and to avoid institutional treatment. Further, it could be argued that often the treatment team alone has the requisite knowledge about the patient's illness to be able to help the family effectively. A more limited assistance might be obtainable by relatives seeking help elsewhere, for example from a self-help organisation or the general practitioner (GP). Presumably the GP would be just as constrained by the patient's objections as the psychiatrist. Indeed, if the GP serves both patient and family, a conflict of loyalty may prove even more troublesome. In any event, the 'unit of treatment' argument probably represents too radical a departure from traditional practice to gain widespread acceptance at present; for example, current General Medical Council (1995) guidance on confidentiality in the UK is unlikely to sanction it.

A further, more robust argument invokes the principle of justice or fairness. This has usually been applied to resolve competing claims for allocation of resources, but is also relevant in judging entitlements to other 'goods'. Such adjudication entails the identification of 'material principles' on which allocation should be determined, for example, 'needs' or 'equity'. In our context, should the needs of the family merit distinctive attention? If these can be met by someone outside the treatment team (for example, a self-help organisation) then the clinician's quandary is possibly alleviated. Alternatively, if resources capable of meeting the family's needs reside in major part within the treatment team, a set of duties to the family would seem to follow.

Probably the most compelling argument is to re-frame relatives' relationships to the patient as not only familial but also as 'carer'. As such they enjoy rights intrinsically attached to all carers, whether relatives or not. These cover at least an account of the illness and guidance about how to deal with the ill person's problems insofar as they impinge on the carer's life (Bloch *et al*, 1995). This might include details about other agencies that offer assistance. Provision of information is best governed by the 'need to know' principle. This would bring the family's position into alignment, for example, with that of a hostel support worker. A counter-argument might be that the patient has agreed to reside in a hostel and accepted that the terms include disclosure of relevant information. An ill relative may not 'choose' to live with the family in the same way. Against this, it could be asserted that obligations exist between family members so that if one is expected to care for another, he or she also has a claim to a necessary minimum of professional assistance. This type of thinking is consistent with the trend in legislation illustrated earlier which views 'carers' as having special status vis-à-vis the patient.

In summary, we contend that justifications can be advanced for providing family carers with material information aimed at meeting their interests. Several factors should be weighed up in judging when this is appropriate, some resembling those considered earlier: the seriousness of risk to the family's well-being, available alternatives, the patient's capacity to recognise actual and potential harms, and pre-existing family values. If information is to be disclosed non-consensually, it should be confined to a 'need to know' level, that is the minimum necessary for the carer to cope with the situation.

Conclusions

Radical changes in clinical practice require us to think differently about the interests of patients' families. In the era of community care we expect much from them, but this has not been balanced by mapping out our duties towards them. The time has arrived for mental health professionals to develop ethically sound practice guidelines facilitating family intervention. To this end we have offered our ideas on ways of engaging families which take account of confidentiality and competing interests. We have also considered grounds for involving families despite a patient's refusal. A central difficulty is that medical ethics in a traditional Western sense is concerned with the individual. Hence the struggle in attempting to marry it to a family-orientated model of clinical practice. We hope our contribution will stimulate debate and pave the way for a consensus about what is ethically sound as well as clinically beneficial.

Acknowledgements

We thank Edwin Harari, Helen Herrman and James Barrett for their helpful comments on earlier drafts.

References

Aponte, H. J. (1985) The negotiation of values in therapy. *Family Process*. **24**. 323–338.

Australian Medical Association (1996) *Code of Ethics* Australian Capital Territory: AMA.

Beauchamp, T. L. & Childress, J. F. (1983) *Principles of Biomedical Ethics*, 2nd edn. New York: Oxford University Press.

Bloch, S., Hafner, J., Harari, E., et al (1993) *The Family in Clinical Psychiatry*. Oxford: Oxford University Press.

——, Szmukler, G., Herrman, H., et al (1995) Counseling caregivers of relatives with schizophrenia: Themes. interventions, and caveats. *Family Process*. **34**. 413–425.

Department of Health (1996) *The Protection and Use of Patient Information*. London: HMSO.

Doherty, W. & Boss, P. (1991) Values and ethics in family therapy. In *Handbook of Family Therapy*. vol. 2 (eds A. S. Gurman & D. P. Kniskern), pp. 606–637. New York: Brunner/Mazel.

Falloon, I. R. & Pederson, J. (1985) Family management in the prevention of morbidity of schizophrenia: the adjustment of the family unit. *British Journal of Psychiatry*. **147**. 156–163.

Fieldsteel, N. D. (1982) Ethical issues in family therapy. In *Ethics and Values in Psychotherapy: A Guidebook* (ed. M. Rosenbaum). New York: Free Press.

General Medical Council (1995) *Confidentiality: Duties of a Doctor*. London: GMC.

Goldenberg, I. & Goldenberg, H. (1991) *Family Therapy: An Overview*, 3rd edn. Pacific Grave. CA: Brookes/Coles.

Lakin, M. (1988) *Ethical Issues in the Psychotherapies*. New York: Oxford University Press.

Lam, D. H. (1991) Psychological family intervention in schizophrenia: A review of empirical studies. *Psychological Medicine*. **21**. 788–801.

Margolin, G. (1982) Ethical and legal considerations in martial and family therapy. *American Psychologist*. **37**. 788–801.

Secrets of the Couch and the Grave:

*The Anne Sexton Case**

Edmund D. Pellegrino

The dead have no right of redress. The biographer, for better or worse, has the last word.

Ronald Steel

Introduction

In 1991, Diane Wood Middlebrook,[1] a professor of English at Stanford University, published a biography of the poet Anne Sexton in which, among other things, she used as source material some 300 tapes of Sexton's psychotherapeutic sessions with her psychiatrist, Dr. Martin Orne. After some years of reluctance and with the concurrence of Sexton's daughter and literary executor, Linda Gray Sexton, Orne released the tapes to Professor Middlebrook. Middlebrook's picture of Sexton drew heavily on the tapes, supplemented by scrapbooks, letters, photos, clippings, unpublished poems, and hospital records.

The book was met by a storm of immediate controversy and an extra-ordinary spate of reviews and commentaries in the popular press.[2–8] The book was praised for carrying out the presumed wishes of the poet to share her sufferings for the benefit of those similarly afflicted, for providing insight into the connections between psychosis and creativity, for destigmatizing emotional illness, for its witness against paternalism, and for underscoring the need for psychiatric treatment. The critics, on the other hand, were severe in their condemnation of Dr. Orne's violation of the ethics of confidentiality, of the adverse impact of the revelations on members of Sexton's family who did not share the enthusiasm of other members for opening the tapes to public scrutiny, and of the dubiety about claims that others might possibly gain benefit from revelations of Sexton's sexual aberrations, constant emotional turmoil, and eventual suicide. One detailed legal analysis found that Dr. Orne and, to a lesser extent, Linda Sexton committed infractions of the laws of torts, contract, and fiduciary relationships.[9] Others deem the whole controversy a teapot tempest inspired by fear of frank discussions of sex, by anti-feminist bias, and outmoded notions of the rights of the dead. In any case, they argued, this appeared to be a 'victimless' crime.

Given the ubiquity and seeming insatiability of the public for salacious details of the biographies of artists and celebrities, one would have thought such revelations would occasion scant commentary: the plethora of comments and book reviews was, therefore, surprising.[10] What was unusual was the question of violation of confidentiality by the psychotherapist. A similar ethical issue was raised by recent revelations about the life of Chairman Mao by his personal physician.[11] The legal issues aside, a number of serious questions of professional ethics are raised by the book. The central issue is the ethical propriety of release of the tapes and their use by the biographer. But there were also questions about the ethical infraction of Sexton's second psychiatrist, who had sexual relations with her, the associated question of the responsibility of the first psychiatrist to report that fact, and the possible responsibility of the third psychiatrist for Sexton's suicide and its possible relationship to her terminating Sexton's treatment because of frustration with Sexton's behavior as a patient.[12]

* Pellegrino, E.: Secrets of the couch and the grave: the Anne Sexton case. *Cambridge Quarterly of Healthcare Ethics* 5: 189–203, 1996.

This essay focuses only on the central issue of confidentiality. The second psychiatrist's conduct in having sexual relations with his patient during therapy – and charging for those sessions! – is beyond ethical defense. As to the first psychiatrist's obligation to report his knowledge of the second psychiatrist's sexual misbehavior, there is some evidence that he tried to do so, although perhaps tardily. The details of the third psychiatrist's treatment of Ms. Sexton and its relationship to her suicide are far too problematic for consideration without more information than is available at this writing.

I will examine the confidentiality issue in a series of questions: What is the nature of confidentiality in general? How does it differ in psychotherapeutic relationships? When, if ever, may confidentiality be breached? Does it belong solely to the patient, or is it shared by family, friends, and others who might be hurt by revelations of secrets? Does the public have a right to know all the details of the lives of public personages? Do psychiatric patients have a special claim on knowledge of the psychotherapy of other persons similarly afflicted? Does the moral right of confidentiality extend beyond the couch to the grave? Do dead persons have a claim on their psychiatrist, and, if so, for how long?

On the way to examining these questions, I will examine the ethical propriety of the conduct of Anne Sexton's psychiatrist, her daughter and executor, Linda, and her biographer, Professor Middlebrook. My purpose is not so much to pass judgment as to provide an ethical framework against which such judgments might be made. I will use the details in the biography, but only parenthetically, to illustrate the ways in which Sexton's biographer, literary executor, and therapist justified their release of the tapes.

Some Facts About the Biography

There is little real question about the sincerity of the motivations of Anne Sexton's psychiatrist, daughter, and biographer to act in her interests, to do so in an ethically justifiable way that might help others, and to fulfill Anne Sexton's wishes. The question is whether, in fact, they achieved these ends and by what ethical criteria we might judge their actions.

At the outset, it should be clear that Professor Middlebrook's biography is not a piece of sensationalizing semifiction like so many psychobiographies of famous people these days. Middlebrook attempts a somber, factual, and sympathetic narrative adhering to the facts available to her. Her subject was an unusually complex, disturbed, suicidal, and remarkably gifted woman. Middlebrook quite accurately characterizes Sexton as, among other things: '. . . a suburban housewife, . . . a New England WASP, . . . half-cracked, . . . intimate, confessional, . . . insistently female, [and] . . . a serious, disciplined artist whose work had been admired from the beginning by distinguished peers.'[13]

If there is sensation in the biography, it is because the subject was a source of sensation. The revelations of adultery, alcohol and drug abuse, probable incest and sexual abuse, the torments of feelings of inadequacy, the acting and posturing, the conscious attempt to fashion a public persona – all of this belonged to Sexton's life and was accurately portrayed. In the face of all her emotional sufferings, Sexton produced a highly regarded body of poetry, won a Pulitzer Prize, and became a professor at Boston University. Her success notwithstanding, her emotional distress was not allayed, and she committed suicide at age 45 after many years of inpatient and outpatient psychotherapy.

It is against the background reality of this complicated life narrative that I shall consider some of the ethical aspects of confidentiality in psychotherapy and psychobiography.

Moral Basis for Keeping Confidences

What Is the Nature of the Obligation?

The moral right to protection of secrets and the corresponding duty of others not to reveal them is fundamental in human relationships. Both are rooted in the respect owed other persons and in the trust essential to interpersonal transactions. Without these, we would lose the benefits of intimacy, counseling, and advice on matters of personal interest that we may wish to share with selected persons. We would also be vulnerable to harm from information broadcast about us that others chance upon.

Violations of confidence are violations of our person inasmuch as our innermost thoughts, personal experiences, promises, foibles, or vices are parts of our person. We may yield them voluntarily to some and withhold them from others as we choose. Confidences are possessions entrusted to others over which those who receive them have stewardship but not ownership. This applies to confidences one person tells us about her/himself or about someone else. To voluntarily accept such confidences is to enter a trust covenant. If we are not willing to keep the promise of confidentiality, we must not accept the information in the first place.

Sometimes we stumble fortuitously upon secrets about other persons without the opportunity to refuse the information. Even then, there is an implicit obligation not to reveal what we learn even though we did not voluntarily promise to keep what we learned secret. This is true also of confidences others confide in us before we know what we are being told is a secret. Under these circumstances, there is the additional problem of deciding what should or should not be revealed. The obligation to protect secrets is indirect, but is binding regardless of whether the intermediary informer has failed to swear us to confidentiality. No matter how we come into possession of secrets, we are bound to treat them with circumspection and safeguard them from revelation to others. The gravity of this obligation is in direct proportion to the harm to the person or her/his reputation that would accrue if the confidence were violated.

The obligation to protect confidences is related to, but not identical with, the protection of a person's privacy. Privacy centers on the moral right to be free of the invasion of our physical or emotional lives by those who have no permission to do so. Privacy derives from our nature as rational creatures capable of fashioning our own identity, and making choices about how much of ourselves to conceal or reveal to others. We violate privacy when we search out information about others by reading their mail, eavesdropping, wiretapping a phone, etc. In violations of privacy, we do not ask or invite the sharing of a secret. We steal the secret and, thus, take a part of a person's identity from him/her. This is an act of moral theft because privacy invasions involve the acquisition of secrets to which we have not been given privileged access in the first place.

What Is Special About Confidentiality in Psychotherapy?

The duty to protect confidences takes on special urgency and special stricture in therapeutic relationships among physicians, psychotherapists, and all who have privileged access to the patient or to the patient's records. This access is a necessity if the patient is to be helped. She/he must reveal details of her/his innermost private life that would ordinarily be closed to family members and intimate friends. The patient must disclose this information in a state of vulnerability at a time when the capacity and the resolve to make judicious decisions is compromised.

The patient is dependent upon the therapist, who, in turn, elicits the patient's confidence and trust as intrinsic to fulfillment of the therapeutic role. It is this trust that motivates the patient to reveal confidences. Receiving confidences, the physician implicitly promises to safeguard what is revealed and to use it only for the purposes for which it was revealed. Through this covenant of trust, the patient's expectation is that he/she will retain control over the release of what has been disclosed. To release the

physician from the promise, the patient must give morally valid consent, that is, consent that is informed, competent, and made without coercion.

These realities pertain to every kind of therapeutic relationship, but they are especially true in psychiatry. Here the innermost details of a patient's most personal and intimate life are, of necessity, laid bare. The vulnerability of the patient is heightened many times by the volatile and unpredictable chemistry of transference and countertransference.[14, 15] The chemistry of transference is unique for each relationship. It determines what is explored and what will be revealed. That chemistry makes the probability of truly informed consent problematic at best. What is revealed in a psychotherapeutic session may be highly detrimental to the patient's job and social and familial relationships. In the case of the forensic psychiatrist, what is disclosed can contribute to conviction of a crime or even the death penalty. Here, the serious question arises of whether it is ever possible to separate the psychiatrist as therapist from the psychiatrist as technical legal expert.[16]

Psychiatrists and other physicians are familiar with the obligation to preserve confidences found in the Oath of Hippocrates, and in the statements on Medical Ethics of the American Medical Association and the American Psychiatric Association.[17] It is the probable infraction of these traditional injunctions against disclosing confidences that has generated much of the debate over the release of the tapes of Anne Sexton's therapeutic sessions. Few would quarrel with the validity of the *prima facie* obligation to protect what is revealed in a therapeutic session.[18] What is at issue is when, if ever, such confidences can be revealed and under what conditions.

When Confidences May Be Disclosed

In the matter of confidentiality, the language of the Hippocratic Oath is open to at least two interpretations. It says '. . . whatever in connection with my professional practice, or not in connection with it, I see or hear in the life of men which ought not to be spoken abroad, I will not divulge as reckoning that all such should be kept secret.'[19] Some take this to mean that whatever is observed or heard must be kept secret always; others take it to mean that what must be kept secret is what *ought not* be told, implying that some things ought to be told. This latter interpretation grants the physician discretion in judging what ought to be revealed. No further elaboration of what might constitute the limits of the duty of confidence is provided, however.

The same ambiguity persists in the treatment of confidences in modern codes. Thus, the International Code of Medical Ethics (1949) speaks of 'absolute secrecy.' The Declaration of Geneva (1968) goes further: 'I will respect the secrets which are confided in me even after the person has died.' The British Medical Association, likewise, holds that the patient's death does not absolve the doctor from the obligation of secrecy. The AMA Principles of 1980 call for preservation of confidences '. . . within the constraints of law,' thus opening the way for conflict between what is morally a *prima facie* obligation and what law may dictate.

It is increasingly difficult to protect confidentiality in the complicated, fragmented, and team-oriented healthcare system of today. Confidential information is no longer confined to the physician. Patient care today makes it necessary to share information about the patient with many others who need to speak to the patient or read his/her chart if they are to fulfill their professional responsibilities. Many of these persons have only brief, intermittent, and superficial personal contact with the patient. Others, like pathologists, radiologists, or imaging specialists, may never enter personally into the patient–physician relationship at all. This is especially true of third party payers, utilization reviewers, medical students, or social workers. Usually, the patient has little suspicion about the number or identity of these persons, many of whom, in small communities, will easily be able to identify the patient.[20] No patient could give anything more than implicit or tacit consent to the vast array of persons who, for a variety of reasons, may become party to the most intimate details of that patient's life.

Yet the complexity of modern medicine and the multiplication of persons who may have access to privileged information (and who may not handle it with discretion) do not make the concept of confidentiality a 'deception' as Siegler suggests.[21] In psychiatric practice, for example, separate charts can be prepared, and kept under lock and key, for the more sensitive material. To be sure, the way modern medicine is practiced compounds the difficulties. But, the difficulties cannot eradicate so fundamental an obligation. It is dangerous to patient welfare to minimize the obligation of maintaining confidentiality. Rather, it is essential to reaffirm its moral significance despite the difficulties and to take the measures required to protect professional secrets as much as possible. The burden of proof certainly must be borne by any psychiatrist who chooses to breach confidentiality.

To reveal a confidence is a violation of the *prima facie* principles of beneficence, respect for persons, promise keeping, and trust. However, justice is also a *prima facie* obligation. Justice may require that we override one obligation to satisfy another. Justice is an underdeveloped concept in the Hippocratic ethic which is so strongly focused on the patient–physician dyad.[22] This deficiency also characterizes most of the codes that have been patterned upon the Hippocratic ethic for 2,500 years.

The contemporary predominance of the principle of self-determination in medical ethics strongly affirms the patient as the central factor in medical ethics. But, like confidentiality, self-determination itself is a *prima facie*, not an absolute, principle. Freedom and autonomy are to be limited if they result in compromise of the freedom of other persons. This is the first principle of Mill's *On Liberty*,[23] which is at the conceptual heart of the idea of personal freedom. Mill's second principle allows individuals to be subject to social coercion if respecting their freedom results in violation of some socially definable obligation to another, or to fulfill rightful expectations others may have of us.

Under both of Mill's stipulations, confidentiality – which can be interpreted as a means of self-governance and, therefore, of personal liberty – is itself subject to limitation. There are circumstances under which promises to safeguard confidentiality would not be valid and under which there would be a positive obligation in the interests of justice to violate the patient's normal claim to confidentiality. This is true of the obligation to preserve confidentiality in general, and in the medical relationship in particular. What are these conditions, and did they exist in the Sexton case?

Conditions for Ethical Disclosure of Confidences

Disclosure of confidences may be voluntary or involuntary. When they are voluntary, the patient releases the physician, hospital, or other persons from obligation by giving morally valid consent. He/she may still withhold certain aspects of his/her record, particularly in psychiatric illnesses. But even with voluntary consent, patients must be made aware of the uses to which the confidential information is to be put. They must be warned of any dangers in granting consent of the harmful uses to which knowledge of their personal lives may be subject. The physician must release only what is essential for the purpose – informing a consultant, a family member, or supplying data for insurance purposes or a court proceeding.

A morally valid consent to release confidential information should be explicit and demonstrable by some form of concrete evidence, like a signed and witnessed statement. To assure the proper handling of case histories, some have suggested a living will to protect psychiatric case files specifically. The stringency of those conditions is in direct proportion to the gravity and potential dangers in release of the information in question. When the patient is not competent to give consent, a morally valid surrogate takes his/her place – one who knows the patient's values, and has no conflicts of interest in release of the information. The surrogate is under moral compulsion to act as the patient would have desired.

Under certain circumstances, confidences must be breached, nonvoluntarily or involuntarily, over the objections of patients or their valid surrogates. Some clear examples are the reporting of child abuse, gunshot wounds, tuberculosis, or venereal diseases. These actions are required by both law and morality on the principle of protection of the public good.

More debatable are instances of involuntary release of confidential information for the benefit of the patient. A physician may find his patient depressed, suicidal, or alcohol addicted. The patient may refuse to be treated and want the information kept confidential, yet the physician might ask a psychiatrist colleague to see the patient over the patient's objection. A psychiatrist might be informed by a spouse of her husband's drinking, abuse of medication, dangerous driving, etc., on the condition that the information be kept secret.[24] To withhold this information from the patient is deceptive and undermines trust. But to reveal it may disrupt relationships with a well-intentioned spouse or friend. The uncertainties are compounded when we realize that the information we are told in secret, even when well intentioned, may be erroneous or unrelated to the patient's problem.

An argument can be made that most secrets of this type should be told to the patient and the information should be disclosed. Informants should be told their information is likely to be revealed. Occasionally, secrecy may be justified.[25] But if this is the case, a heavy burden of proof rests with the physician to show that, on balance, omission of disclosure is a beneficent act.

Violations of confidence are justified when there is foreseeable harm that is serious, probable, and definable to an identifiable third party or parties. The Tarasoff case[26] is a well-known example involving a patient who confided to his psychologist his intention to kill his girlfriend. The psychologist failed to warn the victim or the police. He was sued by the family when the patient killed the woman.

The majority opinion of the California Supreme Court held that the therapist had an obligation to protect the victim. A minority of the justices, however, assessed the harm differently, arguing against disclosure on grounds that confidence in psychotherapists would be undermined. As a result, patients would not seek to be treated or would withhold knowledge about their violent tendencies, thus reducing the chance for treatment and increasing the likelihood of violence.

The difficulties of ascertaining the seriousness of threats to harm others, their frequency, and the lack of quantifying measures are concerns for conscientious therapists. But the arguments of the judicial minority and therapists notwithstanding, it is difficult to see how a therapist in possession of knowledge that might prevent serious harm or death to others could be excused from an obligation of disclosure. Obviously, there needs to be a reasonable probability that harm would occur. Also, a due proportionality must exist between the harm done by breaking confidence and the harm of not doing so. Clearly, there will be gradations in the obligation to disclose information based on the amount of harm, the number of people at risk, the practical exigencies of identifying them, the patient's therapeutic needs, and the patient's right to confidentiality. Some balance must be struck among these factors.

Some of the difficulties of finding a balance are illustrated in cases of known seropositivity to the HIV virus. The patient's spouse or identified sexual partner(s) should be told after the patient has been given a chance to do so, but refuses or fails to do so. When there are multiple partners whose identity would be difficult to ascertain, the obligation of disclosure is mitigated. On the other hand, disclosure is mandatory when a health professional suffers a needle prick in fulfillment of her/his duties to patients. The health worker is entitled to the chance for early treatment if the patient whose blood was involved was HIV positive, and relief of anxiety if the patient was negative. Indeed, this is an instance in which, out of justice for the health worker, mandatory testing would be morally defensible if a patient did not know his/her HIV serology or refused to reveal it.[27]

In short, there is no justification to conceal knowledge of the possibility of exposure to a uniformly fatal disease like AIDS in the name of either autonomy or confidentiality if harm to an identifiable other person is a possibility. This is likewise the case when a patient's job entails responsibility for the welfare and lives of others. The therapist who is aware of substance abuse, psychological disorder, epilepsy, etc., in a truck driver, airline pilot, or locomotive engineer is under obligation to reveal that knowledge to appropriate persons.

Obviously, no simple formula will resolve the tensions between the *prima facie* obligations to preserve confidences on the one hand, and to serve justice and beneficence on the other. The difficulties do not excuse therapists from a serious effort to engage in some form of a moral calculus involving degree and probability of harm to the patient from disclosure or to others from concealment, the number of people involved, and the reliability of the data in question. Such an analysis will certainly not guarantee moral certitude. But it will set some limits on the *prima facie* obligation to guard confidences and the conditions that might warrant violation of this serious moral proscription.

Confidentiality and the Sexton Tapes

Anne Sexton's psychiatrist, Dr. Martin Orne, initiated the taping sessions as an aid to therapy because Sexton often could not remember from one session to the next.[28] With the taping sessions Orne felt he could maintain continuity across sessions and sustain therapeutic progress. He also felt the tapes helped Sexton's poetic efforts, which he had suggested and encouraged as part of her therapy early in their association.

Anne Sexton made no mention of these tapes in her otherwise detailed will. Only four tapes were found in her papers at her death. Sexton's biographer, Diane Middlebrook, seems sure from what she learned about Sexton that she would not have held back the tapes that were then in the possession of Dr. Orne. Middlebrook bases her presumption of permission on her appraisal that Sexton did not have a strong sense of privacy and was considered exhibitionistic and lacking in reserve. From this, she concludes that Sexton would have found meaning in her suffering only by communicating it with others.[29]

Similarly, Dr. Orne, after several years of reluctance, agreed to release the tapes to Middlebrook because he felt they could help others afflicted like Anne Sexton. He did not have explicit permission to do so, but inferred from his intimate knowledge of Sexton's personality that she would want them released if they could relieve the suffering of others. Thus, he became Middlebrook's willing collaborator in her use of the tapes he had recorded.

The reasons for release of the tapes and material therein asserted by Martin Orne, Linda Sexton, and Diane Middlebrook do not square very well with the reasons outlined earlier in this essay for breaching confidences ethically. No identifiable third parties would have been harmed in a definable way by keeping the confidence. However, there was potential harm to others in making the revelations, that is, members of the family who did not entirely share Linda Sexton's confidence that Anne Sexton would have wanted the material released. Other patients under psychotherapy with Orne or other psychiatrists could identify with Sexton and be depressed by her suicide. Furthermore, it is not known how many patients or potential patients had their trust in psychotherapy undermined by knowing their analyses might one day be revealed.

The two major reasons given for release of the tapes were that Anne, herself, would have wanted the tapes made public (a right of disclosure) and that if the tapes were released, some good might come to other patients in psychotherapy or, more distantly, that a better understanding of literary creativity might be obtained.

There is insufficient evidence that Sexton did give, or would have given, permission for the use of the information contained in her taped therapy sessions. The evidence to which Dr. Orne and Linda Sexton appeal in their argument that permission would have been granted is entirely presumptive. It is based in the facts that Sexton was a 'confessional' poet (and, by this simple fact, would have wanted to confess all), that she was exhibitionistic, and that her therapy appeared in her poetry anyway.

It must be pointed out that Sexton was ambiguous even about her exhibitionism. She took great pains to present herself as she wanted to be perceived by her public. She admitted, 'I can be deeply personal, but I'm not being personal about myself.'[30] Further, it is not at all clear how much of Dr. Orne's assumption of consent is the result of the transference-counter transference dynamic. Some have suggested he was motivated by a desire to share in his patient's limelight.[31,32] They ask why he did not destroy the tapes at Anne's death, a practice some psychiatrists regard as mandatory with highly sensitive material. It is unfair to attribute selfish motives to Dr. Orne, but it is also unfair to assume they were not possible in a relationship as complicated as any relationship with Anne Sexton seems destined to have been.

Similar allegations of self-interest have been leveled against Linda Sexton. It has been suggested that she may have been sexually abused by her mother and may have suffered emotional trauma from her mother's psychological aberrancies. The urge to recount traumatic childhood experiences of this kind and to work out feelings of victimization are realities that cannot be totally ignored. Again, it would be unfair to impute such motives to Linda, but equally unfair to her mother not to consider them at all.

The upshot of the matter is that the evidence for Anne Sexton's consent is based primarily on assumptions and inferences. This kind of evidence is indirect and open to alternative explanations. There does not appear to be enough solid evidence to justify breaching confidences of such sensitive material as the tapes contained. Certainly, the conditions outlined earlier in this paper for a morally justifiable release from the obligation of confidentiality do not seem to be present.

But what about the putative good for others that Orne, Middlebrook, Linda Sexton, and Maxine Kumin, Anne's poet friend, all put forth as justification for release? What might some of those presumptive goods be?

There is little or no evidence that intimate knowledge of another person's psychosocial and sexual torments are, in themselves, therapeutic or prophylactic for others similarly afflicted. Because the outcome in this case was suicide, harm might just as arguably occur. One could reasonably argue that some benefit could accrue to students of psychiatry from a study of Martin Orne's method of therapy or the intricacies of Ms. Sexton's case. If Sexton had, in fact, intended the tapes for such use, there could be little quarrel with their release. They would be used by a limited audience with some social claim on knowledge of psychoanalytic procedure. The identity of the patient would be concealed. In any case, justification for use of the tapes for residents in psychiatry does not translate easily into their release to a biographer or to the general public.

Some might argue that any insight we might gather into the connections between the creative poetic life and the interstices of Anne Sexton's psychosexual life would tell us something about the mysteries of artistic creativity. Erica Jong argues that we must understand all we can about the artist's surrender to her subject matter.[33] But Freud, himself, warned us against this kind of psychologism. In his own analysis of the creative life of Leonardo daVinci, he said, 'We have to admit that the nature of artistic attainment is psychoanalytically inaccessible to us.'[34] The perilousness of such analyses is further illustrated in Peter Gay's compendious biography of Freud.[35] Gay points out that Freud attributed all of Leonardo's artistic attainments and presumed homosexuality to a childhood fantasy involving a vulture. Freud, himself, was the victim of the German mistranslation of the Italian word for 'kite' or 'hawk.' The kite has a very different symbolic significance from that constructed by Freud for the 'vulture.' In any case, as Barzun points out, psychobiographical constructs are notoriously deceptive, especially about sexual matters.[36]

Equally precarious as an argument for releasing the tapes is the claim that, as a literary figure, Anne Sexton was 'in the public domain.' There is no justifiable moral claim to confidential information on the part of the general public to intimate details of a celebrity's life unless the public has some very good reason to be informed. Knowledge of the serious psychiatric pathology of a public official could be in the public interest. The First Amendment right to free flow of information, however, is not an automatic right of access to intimate details of the lives of public figures that would serve no purpose beyond feeding salacious interests. Anne Sexton's poetry is in the public domain, not her psychiatric case file. To grant any sort of moral claim to so nebulous an entity as the public domain is to give sanction to the all too common temptation of the media and the public for psychological voyeurism.

Moreover, we hardly need to encourage the current obsessive fixation on the sex lives of public figures. It helps little to understand writing, sculpting, painting, or composing to know about every convolution in the emotional life of the artist. Freud, himself, is more prudent in these matters than some of his disciples: 'It behooves us,' he said, 'to be very careful not to forget that, after all, we are dealing with analogies and that it is dangerous to drag them out of the region where they have originated and have matured.'[37] Would it change the artistic achievements of Dante, Shakespeare, or T.S. Eliot, or help us to understand their genius better to have access to their therapeutic sessions if these were available? Would it help anyone to write poetry like theirs?

To Whom Does the Right of Confidentiality Belong?

Even in the absence of the possibility of informed consent, the obligation of confidentiality could be abrogated legitimately by a morally valid surrogate under certain circumstances, that is, if a previously competent patient becomes incompetent, or, as in the case of Anne Sexton, the patient dies. (We will examine postmortem confidentiality a little later.) To be a morally valid surrogate requires that the surrogate him/herself be competent, be charged with stewardship of the confidential information, and have no obvious conflict of interest in its release.

We have already dealt with the problematic nature of delegated authority by Anne Sexton to her psychiatrist and/or her daughter during her life. Whether either would qualify as a 'morally valid' surrogate must remain an open question. Certainly the possibility of real conflicts of interest cannot be ruled out by people so intimately involved as Sexton's psychiatrist, daughter, and biographer.

Two problems arise when we examine the question of surrogacy. First of all, in the foreword to Middlebrook's book, Dr. Orne makes quite a point of how much his audiotaping contributed to Sexton's therapy, to his discovery of her poetic talent, and to his suggestion that her progress was undercut by her subsequent psychotherapists. He refers to the undermining of Anne's relationship with her husband, who was necessary to her mental health. He complains that he was not allowed to see Sexton intermittently, as was his wont, and he even suggests that all of this contributed to her suicide. The final paragraph of his foreword is especially revealing[38]:

... although I felt obliged not to interfere with the guidelines that had been established for Anne's treatment in the last years of her life. Anne called to say that she would be in Philadelphia and that she hoped she could see me. I expected to see her, but she never made it. Sadly, in therapy, had Anne been encouraged to hold onto the vital supports that had helped her build the innovative career that meant so much to her and others, it is my view that Anne Sexton would be alive today.

This is, no doubt, a heartfelt but a very grave indictment of Orne's colleagues. Without indulging in psychoanalysis at a distance, one cannot help but wonder what role his own emotional state played in Dr. Orne's decision to release the tapes.

From the Couch to the Grave

One might argue that the death of Anne Sexton relieved her surrogates of all obligations, because the dead cannot be harmed. This ignores the real harm that can be done to the memory of a dead person. A person does not lose all identity or dignity after death. Death does not eradicate covenants and promises made in good faith during life. If this were so, wills would be meaningless. In fact, we do show respect for the body of the dead person. We respect their wishes about distribution of their material possessions or bodily parts. Is not the person's intimate life worthy of at least equal respect?

Some have called the allegations of breach of confidentiality a 'victimless crime,' because the dead cannot be harmed physically or emotionally. On this view, there seems to be no substance to the requirement of codes of medical ethics that hold the physician to confidentiality after the patient's death. Jefferson held this view when he said, 'The dead have no rights. They are nothing and nothing cannot own something.' Ecclesiastes puts it this way: 'For the living know that they shall die but the dead know not anything, neither have they anymore a reward; for the memory of them is forgotten' (Ecclesiastes 9:15). Erica Jong, commenting on the Sexton case, takes the same view.[39]

Yet this flies in the face of the fact that, in most cultures, the dead are respected and revered; their memory is a sacred heritage, meaningful to families, friends, and nations. Memory of the dead is something not to be dishonored. Indeed, many families struggle to refurbish the reputation of deceased members whom they deem to have been unjustly judged during life, sometimes centuries after they died. Moreover, few would say that they are totally indifferent to what posterity thinks of them. Indeed, those who deny an afterlife are often most insistent that their genuine immortality lies in the way future generations will judge them. Cicero puts it well: 'The life of the dead consists in being present in the minds of the living.'

Perhaps the wisest attitude to the rights of the dead is captured by Confucius: 'If we treat the dead as if they were wholly dead, it shows want of affection; if we treat them as wholly alive, it shows want of sense.' This is

a little more practical than the ancient adage 'De mortuis nil nisi bonum.' Sometimes truth, justice, and history require that we set the record straight and reveal the evil that humans do as well as the good.

This does not mean that confidentiality cannot be overridden after death; rather, despite death, it remains a prima facie obligation. We must judge when to override the confidentiality of the dead by the same ethical criteria we use to make judgments about release of confidences about living people. Revealing confidences about the dead when doing so would restore justice to them or to another person, refurbish their or another person's reputation, straighten out claims on estates or authorship, or verify important points of history is a mandatory breach of confidentiality. None of these justifications, however, seems to have been present in the release of the Anne Sexton tapes.

Who Owns Secrets?

Throughout this discussion, I have emphasized the moral claim of confidentiality during life and even after death of a patient undergoing psychotherapy. But, a further question is the degree to which others who are mentioned or affected by the release of confidences also have a claim on confidentiality. All members of Sexton's family did not agree that release of the tapes was a good thing.[40] There is information about the lives of Sexton's father and mother that could be damaging to their memories. Other family members could be offended by what was made public about Anne.

Generally speaking, the right of confidentiality extends to those about whom a secret is told, as well as those who reveal the secret. Whatever secrets we chance upon concerning intimate parts of other people's lives imposes the obligation of stewardship, even if we did not seek out that stewardship. The same ethical criteria apply to safeguarding and releasing secrets about others as apply to the secrets we tell others in confidence.

Finally, what about the rights to disclosure? To whom does the right of disclosure belong in psychotherapeutic relationships? Certainly, the patient has the primary right to disclose what he/she deems fit for disclosure. But is this right absolute? As mentioned earlier, this right is abrogated if grave harm to others occurs as a result of secrecy. What happens when the patient wishes to disclose, but the therapist does not? Some have argued that the therapist must maintain such absolute hold on confidentiality that neither the patient nor the family can request him/her to reveal confidences; only the patient can reveal those confidences.[41] Here we confront the recurrent conflict between absolute patient autonomy and absolute physician authority. As I have tried to show elsewhere,[42] this calls for a judicious balancing of benevolence and autonomy that cannot be detailed here.

A Few Words About Psychobiography

This discussion has centered primarily on the ethics of the psychiatric relationship. Little has been said of the obligations of biographers. It can be argued that, by definition, biography involves some invasion of a living or dead person's privacy. Biographers, therefore, cannot be accused ipso facto and en masse of unethical invasion of privacy. Yet the precise limit of the invasion they are permitted is an ethical question that has not yet been carefully examined. Suffice it to say that the use of tapes of psychotherapeutic sessions is sufficiently usual to permit raising privacy as well as confidentiality questions. One can easily imagine future cases of this type, that, given the ubiquity and technical ingenuity of modern audio and visual recording devices, are certain to occur. What will the information highway do to even the confidentiality of a psychotherapeutic session?

Often those with literary interests and capabilities are understandably impatient with the difficult and not always definitive methodology of ethical analysis. There is even a suggestion that literature and ethics are examples of the 'right-brain/left-brain polarity' that irrevocably divides art and reason. But the imaginative and the rational dimensions of human existence cannot be so neatly separated. Good ethics should not, and cannot, destroy genuine art; nor can or should art, however great, obliterate ethics or substitute for it. Gauguin's conduct toward his family remains despicable. The beauty of his paintings does not redeem the kind of life he led.

Certainly, biography is an important and often socially useful enterprise. Society and our culture would lose much if we did not have critical studies of the lives of other persons in our own time and in times past. But a question remains about the degree to which physicians, and psychotherapists in particular, should provide material for the biographer. In the Sexton case, Willard Gaylin is firm in his insistence that Dr. Orne should not have been Middlebrook's 'research assistant.' He goes further and claims that physicians have no 'obligation to history.'[43] Clearly, the ethics of biography, the way confidential material is discovered and revealed, and the part physicians might play in either deserves study.

Conclusion

Anne Sexton's case is important in itself, but also for the precedent it establishes. To be sure, there are, and have been, numerous postmortem revelations of the intimacies of artists' lives. Indeed, this is almost the rule of late 20th century biography, particularly when it comes to the sexual persona. These revelations seem not to have had the ethical scrutiny they deserve. Once the criteria for maintaining confidentiality are loosened, especially in a widely publicized case like Sexton's, a logical gradient is established in the direction of further loosening of the traditional bonds of confidentiality. Gradually, the concept of confidentiality can become so diluted as to be meaningless. The ethically defensible boundaries that should protect confidentiality can become so flexible that they lose their restraining influence. As a result, one of the pediments upon which the covenant of trust, central to any therapeutic relationship, is based, can be irreparably damaged, to the peril of the patient and the profession.

What I have tried to show is that, far from being a 'decrepit' concept, confidentiality remains a vital element in all human relationships, especially those of a psychotherapeutic nature. The obligation to protect confidences has a strong moral foundation in the ethics of liberty, autonomy, and privacy. It is a *prima facie* obligation, but not an absolute obligation. It may be overridden in certain specific circumstances. These circumstances are applicable to the living as to the dead, and they bind surrogates as well as therapists. The whole subject of confidentiality, especially in pursuit of the art of biography, deserves closer empirical and ethical examination. The tendency to see confidentiality as outmoded is seriously in error. Rather, its complexities should stimulate us to a more careful analysis of its limits in unusual cases like Anne Sexton's.

The Sexton biography should serve to sensitize all of us – therapists, patients, and biographers – to the serious and complex nature of the moral covenant that entrusts us with the private life of our fellow human beings – living or dead.

> The doctors should fear arrogance
> more than cardiac arrest.
> If they are too proud,
> and some are,
> then they leave home on horseback.
> But God returns them on foot.
>
> – Anne Sexton, Doctors

Notes

1   Middlebrook DW. *Anne Sexton, A Biography*. Boston, Massachusetts: Houghton Mifflin, 1991.

2   Ablow KR. Whose life is it, anyway? Keeping confidences shared in psychotherapy. *Washington Post Health* 1991;7:9, 24.

3   Burnam JF. Secrets about patients. *New England Journal of Medicine* 1991;24:1130–3.

4   Chaffin DS, Goldstein RL. The Anne Sexton case: protecting confidentiality? [Letter and Reply]. *Psychiatric Annals* 1992;22:586–7.

5   Eisenberg C. Confidentiality in psychotherapy – the case of Anne Sexton [Review of Middlebrook biography]. *New England Journal of Medicine* 1991;325:1451.

6   Goldstein RL. Psychiatric poetic license? Post-mortem disclosure of confidential information in the Anne Sexton case. *Psychiatric Annals* 1992;22:341–8.

7   Kibel HB, Bloom V. Sexton's psychiatrist violated ethics. *New York Times* 1991;Sept 8:A26 (col. 1).

8   Stone AA. Confidentiality in psychotherapy the case of Anne Sexton. *New England Journal of Medicine* 1991;325;1450–1.

9   Carton S. The poet, the bibliographer, and the shrink: psychiatrist–patient confidentiality and the Anne Sexton biography. *University of Miami Entertainment and Sports Law Review* 1993;10:117–64.

10 At this writing, there are 36 published book reviews. Surprisingly, little or nothing has been said by ethicists on this case.

11 Zhisui L. *The Private Life of Chairman Mao* [Trans H-C Tai]. New York: Random House, 1994.

12 See note 8. Stone. 1991;325:1450.

13 See note 1. Middlebrook. 1991:xix.

14 Langs R. *The Bi-Personal Field*. New York: Jason Aronson, 1976.

15 Tiefer L. Personal perspective: the neurotic need of psychotherapists to exploit their patient's problems. *Los Angeles Times* 1991;June 21:M1.

16 Pellegrino ED. Societal duty and moral complicity: the physician's dilemma of divided loyalty. *International Journal of Law and Psychiatry* 1993;16:371–91.

17 American Psychiatric Association. *The Principles of Medical Ethics With Annotations Especially Applicable to Psychiatry*. Washington, DC: American Psychiatric Association, 1989; Section IV.

18 Beauchamp TL, Childress JF. *Principles of Bioethics*, 3rd ed. New York: Oxford University Press, 1989:335–41.

19 Hippocrates. *Hippocrates*, Vol. I [Trans WHS Jones]. Boston: Loeb Classical Library, Harvard University Press, 1972:289–302.

20 Weiss BD. Confidentiality expectations of patients, physicians, and medical students. *Journal of the American Medical Association* 1982;247:2695–7.

21 Siegler M. Confidentiality in medicine – a decrepit concept. *New England Journal of Medicine* 1982;307:1518–21.

22 Pellegrino ED. Toward an expanded medical ethics: the Hippocratic ethic revisited. In: Bulger RJ, Ed. *Hippocrates Revisited*. New York: MEDCOM Press, 1973:133–47.

23 Mills JS. *On Liberty* [Edited with an introduction by E Rappaport]. Indianapolis, Indiana: Hackett Publishing Company, 1978:73–91.

24 See note 3. Burnam. 1991;24:1130–3.

25 See note 3. Burnam. 1991;24:1130–3.

26 *Tarasoff v. Regents of the University of California*. California Supreme Court 17, California Reports 3rd Series, 425, July 1, 1976.

27 Pellegrino ED. HIV infection and the ethics of clinical care. *The Journal of Legal Medicine* 1989;10:29–46.

28 Orne M. Sexton tapes. *New York Times* 1991;July 23:A21.

29 See note 1. Middlebrook. 1991:xxii-iii.

30 See note 1. Middlebrook. 1991:158.

31 See note 8. Stone. 1991;325:1451.

32 See note 15. Tiefer. 1991;June 21:M1.

33 Jong E. Anne Sexton's river of words. *New York Times* 1991;Aug 17:A21, A17.

34 Freud S. *Leonardo da Vinci: A Study in Psychosexuality* [Trans AA Brill]. New York: Random House, 1947:130.

35 Gay P. *Freud: A Life for Our Time*. New York: W.W. Norton, 1988:273.

36 Barzun J. *Clio and the Doctors*. Chicago University Press, 1974:42–5.

37 Freud S. *Civilization and Its Discontents* [Trans J Riviere]. Michigan: Anchor Books, 1958:103–4.

38 See note 1. Middlebrook. 1991:xviii.

39 See note 33. Jong. 1991;Aug 17:A21, A17.

40 Stocker C. The late poet's sister and nieces are battling to tell their slice of the family's story. *Boston Globe* 1991;Aug 13:A20 (col 1.).

41 Weissberg JA. The poet's art mined, the patient's anguish. *New York Times* 1991;July 26:A26.

42 Pellegrino ED. Patient and physician autonomy: conflicting rights and obligations in the physician–patient relationship. *The Journal of Contemporary Health, Law, and Policy* 1994;10:47–68.

43 As quoted in Stanley A. Poet told all; therapist provides the record. *New York Times* 1991;July 15:C13.

5 Psychiatric Treatment and Services

Assessing and treating patients, the cardinal interrelated tasks of the clinical psychiatrist, depend on establishing a working alliance and obtaining informed consent. We have dealt with the ethical aspects of the alliance in Chapter 2 on the psychiatrist-patient relationship. We have also examined informed consent as it applies to research in psychiatry in chapter 9 on research ethics. We now turn to the place of informed consent and its ramifications in the clinical sphere.

A conundrum immediately arises. Given that the organ of rational decision-making is the same one that is impaired in its function in many psychiatric conditions, profound ethical complications ensue. On the other hand, we also know confidently that a sizeable proportion of those seeking psychiatric care are in a position to understand and appreciate what they are letting themselves in for. Thus, they are able to decide on a particular treatment once all pertinent treatments have been clearly laid out before them. In this regard, psychiatry is like the rest of medical practice. Provided the process of informed consent is diligently and responsibly handled by the clinician, particularly with reference to the relative benefits and risks of pertinent therapeutic options, patients undergoing psychiatric treatment are in a comparable position to their counterparts facing, say, chemotherapy or surgery.

We can summarize this comparability in the words – competence and voluntarism. Competence covers the required criterion that the person facing choices in medical treatment enjoys the 'critical faculties' to comprehend and appreciate the implications for himself of each course of therapeutic action. Voluntarism refers to a condition whereby he is free to make a choice. Thus, the process of consent is devoid of such buffeting forces as coercion, suggestion and advice. Laura Roberts'[1] fluent account has dissected out the features of voluntarism.

Since informed consent has been comprehensively considered in the general bioethics literature,[2,3] we shall not discuss the subject further here, but refer you instead to key texts. A splendid book in this regard is *The silent world of doctor and patient* by Jay Katz[4] which has achieved the status of a classic. Chapter 5 on respecting autonomy is particularly noteworthy in its exploration of conscious and unconscious, and rational and irrational forces in the doctor-patient encounter and their effects on patient self-determination.

We now turn to aspects of providing care and treatment to psychiatric patients that are ethically challenging and complex, namely involuntary hospitalization and treatment and the interrelated rights to receive treatment, to refuse treatment and to receive the correct treatment. We will also cover specific ethical facets of the major treatments in psychiatry – medication, psychotherapy and electroconvulsive therapy (ECT).

Involuntary treatment

A consensus has prevailed for generations (Thomas Szasz is a notable but, perhaps, iconoclastic exception) that a proportion of psychiatric patients lose their capacity for self-determination, (i.e. lose their critical faculties to discern what is in their best interests.) They become vulnerable to harming themselves and/or others, acting in ways they will later regret, e.g. a manic patient's sexual indiscretions or squandering of financial resources; and suffer from self-neglect (e.g. chronic schizophrenic patients who are homeless, exposed to the elements, malnourished and physically ill). What is not universally agreed, within psychiatry and beyond, is how best to deal with such exceedingly vulnerable people. Society has, generally, assigned the law to serve as the vehicle to deal with the thorny issue of when and how to protect this group. However, substantial variations in resultant legislation and its application are legion, reflecting, in part, the ethical underpinnings of the process. It is in this regard that psychiatrists and the society they serve need robust, coherent arguments as to the moral principles we should heed. A good start is J. S. Mill,[5] the originator of the libertarian tradition, in his essay, *On Liberty*:

The only purpose for which power can be rightfully exercised over any member of a civilised community, against his will, is to prevent harm to others. His own good, either physical or moral, is not a sufficient warrant. He cannot rightfully be compelled to do or forebear because it will be better for him to do so, because it will make him happier, because, in the opinion of others, to do so would be wise, or even right. (p. 15)

We hasten to supplement this position with Mill's own caveats – that an exception must be made in the case of children and in people who are mentally disturbed. Mill thus opines that a person who is 'delirious' or in a 'state of excitement or absorption incompatible with the full use of the reflecting faculty' can legitimately be assisted. Mill's rationale is clear and succinct – such a person is not actually aware of the risks to which he subjects himself and is therefore not experiencing true liberty.

Paul Chodoff[6] has written eloquently on the awesome question of depriving a person of his liberty on the grounds of mental illness and applied the libertarian thesis espoused by Mill. In a notably humanistic spirit, Chodoff observes that since values pervade the issue, and values inevitably differ, consensus is elusive.

Then, citing utilitarian and deontological theories, he finds both of them wanting. Instead, Chodoff proposes a paternalism which is typically 'chastened and self-critical', one 'willing to commit to strong safeguards against abuse'. He is certainly aware of that potential outcome, since he played a prominent role in the campaign to eliminate the misuse of psychiatry for political purposes in the former Soviet Union in the late 1970s and 1980s.

His humanism is epitomized in the concluding sentiment of his argument: involuntary hospitalization of the mentally ill is not a conflict of right against wrong but rather a conflict over the right to remain at liberty against the right 'to be free from dehumanizing disease'. The notion of being imprisoned by one's illness certainly resonates with any psychiatrist who has treated psychotic patients.

This emphasis on humanism is not simply an example of 'motherhood is good' piety. Procedural justice has come into its own since the 1990s with regard to compulsory admission to hospital. The argument is explicit – the need to detain a proportion of people with disordered minds who are not competent to safeguard their own interests (and may also harm the welfare of others) is an unfortunate but inescapable duty of the psychiatrist. But it should be accompanied by particular respect for people's dignity, concerns and anxieties. Charles Lidz[7] and his colleagues have demonstrated that psychiatric patients admitted into hospital, whether voluntary or involuntary, harbour feelings about the process according to the way they perceive the degree of coercion applied by clinicians. There are also implications for the patient's subsequent willingness to cooperate with treatment.

Our account hitherto refers to patients as a homogeneous group. Loss of critical faculties as discussed in the context of Mill (or incompetence in more familiar clinical discourse) may be a unifying feature but the argument can be marshalled that ethical factors will vary according to the particulars of the patient's clinical state. The obvious example is suicidal behaviour.

Thomas Szasz[8] sees suicide as an act of a moral agent who is ultimately responsible for that act. In essence, he avers that we are dealing with an 'ethic of self-responsibility'. Therefore, the State through psychiatrists and relevant authorities such as the police (as well as other mental health professionals) should not assume power to prevent self-killing, although they may opt to advise for or against it in a given situation. In effect, the argument is libertarian in nature, with the corollary that everyone should have the right to end their life as they wish. However, concession to professional intervention (albeit informal and brief) is permitted by Szasz in a case where abundant, objective evidence points to 'brain malfunctioning', and in the situation where a person has prepared a 'psychiatric will' (see later) which states unambiguously that they wish, under specific circumstances, to submit to involuntary intervention. Otherwise the pairing of liberty and responsibility should prevail.

Szasz has obviously neglected to incorporate into his thesis the caveat by Mill about respecting a person's right to liberty – the loss of critical faculties. The distinction between brain malfunctioning and other clinical circumstances in which suicidality is a prominent feature are, for the critics of Szasz, spurious and unworkable. This is not to negate, we rush to add, that all suicidal behaviour is a function of a disordered mind. The suicide of the author Arthur Koestler, in the wake of his leukaemia and Parkinson's Disease and a long-standing commitment to euthanasia, seemed to be based on rational and coherent grounds. His suicide note leaves us in little doubt that he arrived at his decision to kill himself authentically and with all his critical faculties intact.

This account of the ethics of suicide has been covered by Heyd and Bloch[9], and we will not pursue it further here. Suffice to say, the suicidal patient epitomizes the psychiatrist's dilemma in having no choice but to foist assessment and treatment in various clinical circumstances and having to declare a person's incapacity, by dint of mental illness, to make rational judgments about what is in their best interests.

A succinct contribution by two South African psychiatrists, Van Staden and Kruger,[10] covers this topic of incapacity by highlighting its dimensions: failure to understand relevant information provided by the psychiatrist, choose decisively between options, communicate consent or accept that the need for treatment exists. In this selection, the authors refer to the utility of a 'functional approach' in determining capacity, especially concerning time, namely that a patient may be incapable of deciding at one point but become capable at another.

The philosopher Loretta Kopelman[11] focuses on another feature of competence, an evaluative one, in arguing that professional assessment is influenced by internal and external values, and that these extend well beyond legalistic constraints. But external values are more clear cut in that most clinicians would agree on the primacy of certain values in assessing capacity: say truthfulness and fairness. Internal values relate to task – specific matters such as whether the person is capable of reaching an explicit goal and the threshold required.

We have discussed the inevitable resort to compulsory treatment in the aforementioned account of suicide. The picture becomes all the more challenging since the introduction in the 1990s, in several jurisdictions, of compulsory treatment in the community. The ethical arguments brought into play to justify detention in a hospital can legitimately be extrapolated into the community setting. After all, similar restrictions on liberty lie at the heart of the moral dilemma and the psychiatrist again has to consider patients' degree of competence.

Munetz and his colleagues[12] have tackled the ethics of mandatory community treatment coherently, their paper warranting inclusion in the anthology. They turn to three ethical arguments in considering such a drastic step – utilitarian, communitarian and beneficence – concluding that all three support the application of compulsory community treatment.

In brief, utilitarianism looks to the outcome of such an intervention. If it can be demonstrated that compulsory community treatment can reduce the rate of a patient's readmission to hospital, prolong his living in the community and promote compliance with treatment, then such a procedure is ethically justified. Here, we have to draw on the results of empirical research. The accumulated evidence does in fact suggest that worthwhile benefits accrue.

The communitarian position revolves around the benefits that compulsory treatment may generate for society. Munetz et al. emphasize the social gains of promoting the values of humanity, safety and promotion of health. The corollary, however, is that the community responds to the needs of the mentally ill, whose rights are necessarily infringed (but not violated), by formulating sound plans of treatment for them and committing adequate resources to the task.

Beneficence relates most directly to incapacity in that the State is obliged 'to make decisions on behalf of individuals who are unable to make informed decisions for themselves'. Through such a process, patients who need specific treatment are assured of obtaining it. The contribution by Munetz and his colleagues is valuable on several accounts: the skilful marshalling of relevant ethical theories so reinforcing justification for compulsory community treatment, applying the product of empirical research to support the theoretical argument and, by paying heed to potential risks, alerting us to cogent caveats.

We have mentioned the authors' emphasis on society responding to the needs of patients by providing adequate treatment. This brings us conveniently to our next topic – the right to treatment in circumstances where patient liberty is restricted.

The right to treatment

The era of the asylum for the most part was (and still is in many parts of the world) marked by tragic neglect of the needs and interests of patients.[13] Ultimately, the overcrowded institution became little more than a custodial warehouse. We could possibly reconcile ourselves to the inevitability of such a development if we accept that the asylum became a repository for increasing numbers of the incurably mentally ill for which little could be done. However, the custodial character persisted into the modern era, which saw the advent of psychotropic medication and the evolution of psychosocial forms of therapy. As is so often the case, it took a plaintiff, Kenneth Donaldson,[14] to determine that a person involuntarily committed to a mental hospital did have the 'right to receive such individual treatment as will give him a reasonable opportunity to be cured or to improved his mental condition'. The Donaldson case, which eventually reached the US Supreme Court in 1975, had its origin in his compulsory admission to the Florida State Hospital in January 1957. Diagnosed with paranoid schizophrenia there for the next decade and a half, he received minimal treatment. The situation was not quite so straightforward. As a Christian Scientist, Donaldson refused at times to take prescribed medication. Nonetheless, the court in a unanimous judgment concluded that a patient who does not pose a danger to himself or to others or who is not a recipient of treatment has a constitutional right to be released from hospital if he is able to live safely in the community. The 14th Amendment of the American Constitution states that no person shall be deprived of life, liberty or property without due process of law.

We need to bear in mind that Donaldson won this right in the context of a decade of civil rights campaigning in the US, which included respect for the rights of the mentally ill. Indeed, a few years before, in 1971, a class action in the State of Alabama had led Judge Johnson, in the case of *Wyatt v Stickney*[15] to declare that due process had been violated in circumstances where a citizen was confined ostensibly for humane purposes but then not given adequate treatment. The judge subsequently set explicit, detailed standards of care for all psychiatric patients in Alabama.

The right to effective treatment

Alan Stone[16] has discussed the Alabama and Florida cases (as well as other relevant judgments), albeit mainly in legal terms. The right to treatment issue has been revisited on a number of occasions in other court judgments, predominantly American. What the right has never encompassed is a guarantee that a patient will receive optimal or effective treatment. These two desiderata both open up a Pandora's box. The right to effective treatment has indeed been examined, although only by a tribunal, therefore not setting a legal precedent. We include two notable contributions on the subject by two seasoned protagonists on the US academic psychiatric scene – Alan Stone and Gerald Klerman.

In *Osheroff v Chestnut Lodge*, the plaintiff sued a private psychiatric hospital for failure to provide antidepressant medication in the face of his severe, deteriorating depression. The hospital's continuing application of psychoanalytic psychotherapy as the single treatment of his mood disorder constituted malpractice. Dr Osheroff, the claimant, ultimately agreed to an out of court settlement.

The contradictory points of view of Klerman and Stone vividly illuminate the question of whether psychiatrists can guarantee the most effective treatment for their patients. Klerman[17] argues that this is possible in the light of accumulated scientific evidence on efficacy. The clinician therefore is duty-bound to use only 'those treatments for which there is substantial evidence' and also a plan of treatment or seek a second opinion if a patient does not respond. Put another way, the psychiatrist should not rely on a single therapeutic approach, (e.g., medication or psychotherapy, alone).

Klerman is clearly an advocate of evidence-based medicine and randomized controlled trials. Not so Alan Stone,[18] who contends that Klerman's position is tantamount to '. . . promulgating more uniformed scientific standards of treatment in psychiatry, based on . . . opinion about science and clinical practice'. Moreover, legal standards of care cannot be established by one psychiatric school for the profession as a whole, even if enveloped in science. Instead, we should depend on 'the collective sense of the profession', as well as apply the 'respectable minority rule'. Stone thus supports diversity and pluralism and eschews 'authoritarian control'.

Revealingly, both protagonists are aware that the process of informed consent remains central to all treatments – much along the lines discussed above.

The right to refuse treatment

As a voluntary patient, Osheroff could obviously have refused any treatment as part of the process of informed consent. His lawsuit revolved around the institution's failure to offer him an alternative treatment in the face of his clinical worsening with the sole treatment offered. We could talk here about coercion, but if the principles of informed consent had been applied properly, his freedom to choose one treatment above others and to withdraw consent at any stage thereafter should have prevailed.

The situation differs radically when the patient is involuntarily committed to hospital or to community treatment. The right to refuse treatment in this context looms large as an ethical question.[19] A key event in this story is another legal judgement in the United States. In 1979, a district court in Boston ruled that detained patients had a constitutional right to refuse treatment.[20] This coincided with the changing face of commitment laws in many American jurisdictions, from criteria linked to need for treatment to an emphasis on the level of danger posed to self and/or others. Ultimately,

in 1983, the Massachussetts Supreme Court delivered its decision in the case of *Rogers v Okin*.[20] All psychiatric in-patients, whether competent or not, had a right to refuse antipsychotics except in an emergency. In the case of their refusal, substituted legal judgment was mandated.

The ethical repercussions are profound. If psychiatrists are legally empowered to detain patients against their will, is it not a contradiction in terms if they are then unable to offer them treatment in the face of refusal? The argument rests on the premise that a person sufficiently disturbed to warrant involuntary admission is axiomatically entitled to treatment, and the consulting psychiatrist suitably placed to provide it. Without this arrangement, the psychiatrist's functions are reduced to custodial.

A countervailing argument is grounded on fundamental constitutional rights. Merely because people are committed does not mean that they are incapable of participating in the process of informed consent. In the event they cannot understand or appreciate the rationale for a therapeutic course of action, the argument follows, a form of substituted judgment is cause for so ensuring that rights remain in the foreground.

Given the inherent ethical quandary in the above tussle, an assortment of legal remedies has evolved, ranging from a full adversarial process to reliance on a guardian's decision.

Paul Appelbaum[21] has offered us a lucid account of the range of available options and shared his predilection for a treatment-driven model whereby patients are committed on the grounds that their capacity to decide about treatment is lacking as part of their disturbed mental state. He is, no doubt, influenced in coming to this determination by his own research done with Tom Gutheil, a decade earlier, that most legal arguments supporting the right to refuse medication were not in accord with clinical reality, most refusing patients voluntarily accepting treatment within 24 hours.[22]

On the other hand, the question remains as to whether a single psychiatrist should be given 'unbridled discretion' or some form of independent review to safeguard rights of patients as a preferable alternative. With respect to the latter, Gutheil and his colleagues[23] have usefully examined the place of various types of legal guardianship and pointed out their relative strengths and limitations. Together with Schouten,[24] Gutheil has also addressed pragmatic considerations of the court's involvement in 'right to refuse' situations, highlighting economic realities of taking every refusal of treatment case to court.

In another pragmatically oriented account, Stone[25] proposes that 'presumption of competency is dealt with *before* hospitalisation in a legally acceptable manner'. Dealing with the issues of commitment and patient competence to decide about treatment, he asserts, would obviate the problem of compulsory hospitalization without treatment. The difficulty here is the fluidity of the mental state. What patients think about treatment during the maelstrom of a process of detention may well change once they are admitted to a ward and suitably cared for.

The role of advanced directives

An ingenious idea evolved in the 1980s to deal with many of the aforementioned ethical quandaries – variously named advanced directive, a Ulysses contract, self-binding contract and advanced treatment authorization. In summary, psychiatric patients prone to recurrence of their illness during which they may be too disturbed to provide informed consent reach an agreement with their psychiatrist about what constitutes the best course of action should they suffer a future episode and be unable to decide appropriately what treatment is in their best interest.

In this way patients can determine specific treatment preferences in the event they become incompetent when ill in the future. Given that several major mental illnesses recur and are associated with incapacity, advanced directives would appear, on the face of it, to have a useful role.

Alongside the plethora of labels for this situation is a range of methods whereby the process may be expedited. Srebnik and La Fond[26] have mapped out the terrain for us and identified two general types: instructional and proxy. In the former, patients specify when competent a set of instructions concerning, *inter alia*, use of drugs, electroconvulsive therapy and other treatments, methods such as seclusion to deal with an emergency, people that need to be contacted, location of treatment and any financial aspects.

An inherent limitation of this instructional approach is the considerable difficulty of anticipating all contingencies. This hurdle is overcome, to a degree, by the proxy method. Here, patients assign the task of consent to a designated person who then uses what is usually referred to as substituted judgment. Thus, a decision about treatment is made in accord with what the patient would probably have preferred were they able to express it. The alternative is the best interest approach in which the proxy judges what he or she believes is in the patient's best interest.

A combination of instructional and proxy is a third option.

Theorizing about the merits of different approaches to advanced directives to satisfy the goals of empowering the patient and enabling appropriate treatment is one strategy to examine their relevant advantages and disadvantages. Another option is to go up an empirical track and actually test out the strengths and limitations of specific alternatives. Henderson et al.[27] have done just this in carrying out a single-blind randomized controlled trial in the south of England. One hundred and sixty people diagnosed with a psychotic disorder or non-psychotic bipolar illness who had been psychiatric inpatients in the previous two years were randomly allocated to either an intervention or control condition. In the former, a joint plan was devised with specification of the patient's treatment preferences as paramount. Over a 15 month follow-up the rate of compulsory admission and treatment was substantially less in the intervention group compared to the controls. The study is clearly pertinent since it demonstrates that an advanced agreement can reduce the rate of legal compulsion in treating the severely mentally ill.

However, as the authors concede, two-thirds of those eligible to participate declined to do so. The team had presumably anticipated this possibility by examining the feasibility of introducing a 'joint crisis plan' into their service in a pilot study.[28] They were sufficiently encouraged then to proceed with the main trial by the 40 per cent take-up by patients with a psychosis of the offer to formulate a plan.

This extensive reluctance would undoubtedly disappoint psychiatrists who find coercive treatment disdainful and seek to establish a viable alternative. On the other hand, this type of research is crucial to validate the concept of the advance directive.[29]

Widdershoven and Berghmans[30] are, similarly, aware of the need for sound empirical research to examine the practical limitations of advance directives as well as related ethical questions. They tackle their task within what they refer to as a 'narrative' perspective. They stress the potential misuse of the process, particularly by the mental health professional assuming, unjustifiably, leverage to exert control over patients. 'Shared power', their slogan to prevent abuse, is linked to a perspective in which the patient's illness is viewed in the context of his or her life history, and the advanced directive as a genuine expression of core values. In this way, what the patient truly desires is the outcome of a collaborative endeavour.

Thomas and Cahill[29] also tackle the 'story' in order to understand the ambivalence patients may show to advance directives. The mental health profession, they assert, has to be sensitive to possible feelings of demoralization and disempowerment. Their own experience in Bradford in the UK is sobering. Despite two years of systematic preparation, only 1 out of 70 eligible patients opted to negotiate an advanced directive.

Legal aspects of advanced directives are covered by a Canadian team.[31] Specifically, they advocate a role for legal provisions to ensure that the goals of advanced directives are achieved, namely that patients are treated in the light of their declared preferences and that the dialogue between patient and doctor becomes more transparent. At the time of reaching an agreement, patients should stipulate whether they are prepared to have their status overridden in the future should the doctor judge this to be necessary; doctors should formally state whether the patient is competent or not; in the event of a dispute regarding competence and what is in the patient's best interests, an independent tribunal should adjudicate (this recommendation is put rather vaguely); and patients should indicate whether they agree to possible involuntary treatment should they be unable to provide informed consent.

This legalistic perspective appears to offer the treating doctor a degree of leverage to deal with the unexpected but also reduces the inherent advantage of an advance directive to have an articulated preference respected in the face of future illness typified by incompetence.

Suvalescu and Dickenson[32] adopt a contrary view by placing considerable weight on the present 'dispositional' preferences of the patient. They posit that 'advance directives are only relevant in that they provide some evidence for what a person's present dispositional preferences might be'. Moreover, they espouse a libertarian view inasmuch as the State 'should not interfere in a person's life for his or her own good'; this applies equally to the mentally ill who may formulate rational preferences for their own lives and treatment. The difficulty with their argument concerns patients who are quite unable to decide about their treatment and may be unable to identify and/or communicate their preferences. It would seem inconceivable to us to dispense with mental health law in circumstances where treatment is critical to save a life, alleviate acute suffering or prevent major deterioration.

Ethical aspects in using medication

In dealing with informed consent and the three related rights to receive treatment, to refuse treatment and to obtain the correct treatment, we have covered much that pertains to the ethical dimension of treatment with psychotropic drugs. However, we need to tackle a topic that has provoked much ethical debate, namely the inappropriate use of medication. Those that clamour for special attention are the role of antidepressants in children and adolescents and prescribing stimulants for ADHD. The potential use of psychotropics to enhance specific psychological states – 'cosmetic psychopharmacology' – is another ethically challenging situation we shall address.

The concept of the 'therapeutic orphan'[33] captures the dilemma of research data being generally unavailable to determine the effectiveness and safety of drugs in children; the psychotropics are no exception. Whereas we have built up a reasonably accurate picture of the proper place of antipsychotics and antidepressants in adult patients (albeit less so in the elderly), the situation in younger people is unclear.[34] The cause is obvious – drug companies commonly test out their products in adults only since the procedure to obtain consent in children and young adolescents is much more complex.

The clinician is between a rock and a hard place. For instance, what should she do when facing a young person presenting with moderate to severe depression whose adult counterpart would be prescribed an SSRI without much hesitation? Responses include: a ban on prescribing until solid data become available; the use of the psychotherapies in place of medications on the grounds of safety, even though medication could potentially be beneficial; combining medication and psychotherapy;[35] the requirement that pharmaceutical companies are legally forced to conduct trials in all age groups and prescribing in the absence of robust research findings on the assumption that potential benefits outweigh possible harms.

Clinicians have been left to find their own remedy for many years. The possibility of an increased rate of suicidal thinking and self-harm behaviour in children and teenagers on antidepressants has altered the situation substantially.[36,37] In the United Kingdom, the Committee on Safety of Medicines (CSM) examined published and unpublished material and, as a result, introduced a warning to the effect that SSRIs, with one exception, were contraindicated in children.[38]

In the US, the Food and Drug Administration has not gone to such extreme lengths but instructed pharmaceutical companies to include a strong warning on information sheets of antidepressants for patients and doctors to the effect that they can lead to suicidality in young people.[39] Moreover, the warning incorporates a statement that few antidepressants have been demonstrated to be of value in this age group.

We could infer that these policies are reasonable. After all, suicide is irreversible. On the other hand, as the American Psychiatric Association[39] has stated, patients with serious depression may be at grave risk without medication. The Australian authorities have adopted yet another position. Its relevant advisory body, the Adverse Reactions Advisory Committee, recommends careful monitoring of suicidality when using the SSRIs for major depression in children and adolescents (in the context of national clinical practice guidelines) and doctors keeping abreast of new research knowledge and product information issued by the drug companies.[40]

This is more or less the position adopted by Peter Jensen[41] of the child and adolescent research division of the American National Institute of Mental Health. In a well-balanced and pragmatic overview of the role of psychotropics in young children, which we have selected for the anthology, he calls for

... caution and an in-depth evaluation of the possible alternatives for each child .... Anything that compromises that process ... should be regarded as unethical .... Appropriate and judicious use, even in the absence of safety and efficacy data, may be warranted.

This is particularly the case in a patient with what he refers to as substantial ongoing impairment. On the other hand, psychotherapy is the most sensible first step.

Fisher and Fisher[42] are of a different view in arguing that where scientific data on effectiveness are lacking or stem from poor methodology as is the case, in their view, of antidepressants in children and adolescents, the question of how much freedom should be accorded to individual practitioners to use their own clinical judgment is crucial. The related matter of what constitutes informed consent in these circumstances is also raised by these authors but left unanswered.

Stimulants and Attention Deficit Hyperactivity Disorder (ADHD)

Although ADHD (and its previous incarnations, e.g. minimal brain dysfunction, hyperkinetic syndrome) has been recognized by child psychiatrists as a clinical entity for decades, it is still shrouded in intense controversy. This is principally because of the stimulant drugs used to treat it. As long ago as 1971, the distinguished psychiatrist Leon Eisenberg[43] coherently addressed four key dimensions, all of which continue to be contentious: limited research knowledge; the risks of adverse effects in the long term; the issue of whether it is the child that is being treated or another party such as parents, teachers or the courts; and the social costs inasmuch as medication use may lead to a relative neglect of counselling parents, instituting remedial educational programs, encouraging creativity and so forth.

Since the 1990s, the debate concerning ADHD and its treatment has become even more heated in the wake of the massive escalation in the number of children diagnosed and medicated. Consider developments in the US as illustrative. These have been thoroughly documented by Laurence Diller, academic and clinical paediatrician.[44,45] Although survey data are not entirely national it is estimated that stimulant use soared in the US during the 1990s by several hundred percent, with over four million children, mostly boys aged between 6 and 13, on methylphenidate, a synthetic stimulant, or amphetamines. This vast increase in prescriptions has also occurred in Canada and in parts of Australia.

Whether medication is over-used depends on the rate of ADHD in these countries. A snag immediately arises. The diagnosis may be valid but objective biological or psychological tests to confirm its presence in a particular case are unavailable. Considerable variation in diagnostic decision-making leads to over and under-diagnosis. One repercussion is the application of stimulant drugs when these are inappropriate. George Halasz[46] has highlighted the need for a 'comprehensive assessment of the child in a family context, with additional information obtained, if needed, from the school and related settings'. In its absence, he suggests, the question of whether the child has the diagnosis or is exhibiting a variation of normal temperament or is struggling with the effects of a noxious environment, is not readily sorted out.

The Great Smoky Mountain Study[47] shows how the aforementioned blurred boundaries have therapeutic implications. Having identified that 5 percent of the community of over 4000 children could be diagnosed with ADHD (in keeping with rates commonly found in scientific studies), the investigating team then ascertained that 7 percent of the children were receiving stimulants. However, over half of the children on medication did *not* satisfy ADHD criteria, and were evidently being treated for a range of behavioural and learning difficulties.

This brings us conveniently to Eisenberg's aforementioned point of *who is being treated*? If attaching the ADHD label so 'easily' to problems of behaviour and learning occurs, is there not the potential for its misuse? Given that the child lacks the power to determine whether to be treated or not with stimulants, we need to examine the roles of parents, teachers, doctors, statutory health agencies and the pharmaceutical industry. Each group may be motivated to reach out for the tablet solution. For parents and teachers, medicalization may exonerate them from any possible blame for their 'failing' child and student, respectively, serve as a means to quell unruly behaviour and lack of discipline and attract special 'disability' benefits.

Recourse to the prescription pad by doctors spares them a time-consuming biopsychosocial assessment and possible psychological and social interventions. For State health and educational authorities, economic factors may prevail. A tablet is considerably cheaper than complex family therapy or remedial educational programs. The drug company will want a good return on its investment; the more children who take their brand of stimulant, the greater their profit margin.

Eisenberg's[43] point about long-term effects remains problematic over three decades later. While research during this period has confirmed the effectiveness of stimulants in accurately diagnosed ADHD, its mechanism of action continues to elude the investigator. The effects of long-term use also remains relatively understudied, including the risk of substance abuse in adult life.

Cosmetic psychopharmacology

The final drug therapy scenario with profound ethical indications that we tackle is reflected in the title of a brief paper by Gerald Klerman[48] from the early 1970s – *Psychotropic hedonism vs. pharmacological Calvinism*. He raises a pivotal question for any society – should psychotropics be used in people who experience such psychological states as tension, melancholy and insomnia, which are customarily construed as reasonable responses to the vicissitudes of daily life? At one extreme of the prescribing continuum, the Calvinistic, is a view that drugs should only be used when stringently indicated, that is for states of mind that have been scientifically determined to constitute psychiatric diagnoses (e.g., schizophrenia, bipolar disorder and postnatal depression.) Abstinence is viewed as ideal since the individual is then truly self-reliant. At the other pole, protagonists argue that psychotropics may play a valuable role in promoting a sense of calm, boosting self-confidence or facilitating social relationships.

The psychiatrist may well be caught in the tussle between the two positions, becoming uncertain as to where to draw the line between legitimate clinical need and drugs as a form of palliation.[49] Pharmaceutical companies will be tempted to broaden the indications for their products. An obvious example is extending psychotropic use from marked generalized anxiety and panic attacks to social anxiety, even shyness.

Ordinary citizens who lack full knowledge of the potential role of psychotropics are presumably puzzled about the proper place of these drugs in dealing with everyday stress. When does the feeling of grief, sadness or tension become that severe and/or enduring to warrant their relief through medication? Whom should they trust – the drug companies, the family doctor, the specialist psychiatrist, a relative or friend who encourages them to seek relief through drugs or to deal with stress head-on? All these parties will necessarily be influenced, overtly or covertly, by ethical considerations in arriving at their particular judgment.

For instance, if they had consulted the late George Carstairs,[50] a leading British psychiatrist, they would have heard him offer the following opinion:

A particular aberration has entered into public thinking. Everyone nowadays expects to be happy. What is more, if anyone feels unhappy, he immediately thinks that something must be wrong either with him or with the state of the world, if not both.

They would also have heard him declaim: 'I do not mean to imply that I approve of unnecessary suffering, but rather that suffering, like pain, is a part of human experience which is not entirely negative'. In summary, Carstairs espouses a view that society, including its psychiatrists, should reject the 'tranquillising anodyne'.

The argument for and against this position has continued unabated, and without resolution, for decades. The publication of *Listening to Prozac* by Peter Kramer[51] in the 1990s certainly provoked a fulsome debate. In that bestseller, we are confronted by a new way of articulating Klerman's 'Psychotropic hedonism' but one which bears a similar value-based quality – cosmetic psychopharmacology. Kramer[52] presents his central thesis in a later philosophically oriented paper entitled 'The valorization of sadness' (a selection). We are invited to entertain the possibility of employing a medication that has the potential to shift one normal psychological state into another normal psychological state but where the latter has more sought-after qualities.

For Kramer antidepressants are an example of such a medication, and the shift is from a melancholic temperament characterized by such personal features as pessimism and self-doubt to a non-melancholic temperament. As a clinical practitioner, Kramer is no doubt aware that psychotherapy has played that role for years, but he now poses a challenge as to why cosmetic psychopharmacology should be seen as any less valuable and any less morally acceptable if the aim of both approaches – to reduce melancholy – is similar.

Kramer's further contentions are in response to criticisms that have been levelled against him by the ethicist, Carl Elliott.[53] Echoing Carstair's repudiation of a tranquillizing solution, Elliot casts his net even wider with a proposition that psychiatry, with its heavy reliance on medication, fails to perceive that what people are really grappling with is a sense of alienation. He identifies three overlapping forms: personal, cultural and existential. Examples of the first are problematic questions about where to live, whom to marry, what job to do and the like. Cultural alienation is best illustrated by the destruction of an indigenous people's traditional ways of living their lives. The existential form revolves around a person questioning their own values and not knowing what to do with their life. Whatever the type of alienation, Elliott suggests, drugs cannot possibly alter it. Any associated depression may lift but the predicament in which a person is stuck will persist. They need help to consider how to live their life and to locate a sense of meaning. We have returned, it would appear, to the psychotherapies that Kramer acknowledges but is possibly ambivalent about. We are also challenged through Elliott's position to ascertain what role psychiatrists should assume in the face of adverse social circumstances such as the harrowing plight of many indigenous cultural groups, worldwide.

Kwame McKenzie, in a debate in the *British Journal of Psychiatry*,[49] clearly supports Elliott in his opposition to cosmetic psychopharmacology but asserts that any 'science of wellness', as he quaintly puts it, has not got off the ground. Producing such wellness may not be a function of medicine at all since we do not actually know what that aim represents. Instead, governments may be the responsible agencies, especially if lack of wellness is linked to such social forces as economic inequality, crime and occupational stress.

We have alluded to the potential role of the 'talking' treatments to wield changes in perspective on how one is living one's life. This is a crucial dimension of our account of the ethical aspects of the psychotherapies that we address later in this essay.

Ethical aspects of electroconvulsive treatment

As Max Fink,[54] a leading figure in research on electroconvulsive treatment (ECT) reminds us, the treatment seems unable to shake off its controversial status. Notwithstanding its long-standing demonstrated utility in melancholia and psychotic depression, two of the most severe psychiatric disorders, ECT remains tainted.

The controversy revolves mainly around the fact that ECT is a form of physical manipulation of the brain whose rationale is not yet determined. Instead of dealing with identified pathology like the removal of a brain tumour, the intervention is applied to normal brain tissue. The emotional tumult – commonly manifesting as abhorrence of an electrically based treatment causing a seizure – often precludes rational appraisal of the potential role of ECT to treat specific psychiatric conditions. Multiple myths abound.[55] Fink together with another prominent ECT researcher, Jan-Otto Ottosson, hit the nail on the head when entitling the opening chapter of their book on ethics in ECT, 'The stigmatisation of ECT'.[56] Even in the face of well conducted, systematic research since the 1980s, stigma prevails. The history of the application of ECT no doubt contributes to this. The treatment was introduced during an era of 'great and desperate cures', when therapeutic nihilism was rampant and any potentially useful intervention was greeted enthusiastically but unfortunately, applied uncritically.

Six decades after its discovery, ECT warrants more erudite deliberation, both scientific and ethical. What follows is our attempt to clarify the ethical dimension. Indubitably, the principal issue revolves around informed consent.[57–59] The typical clinical scenario readily illustrates this. A patient's morbid state of melancholia coupled with loss of contact with reality because the mood change has a distinct psychotic quality, can well lead to an incapacity to (a) comprehend information about ECT and (b) to appreciate the implications of agreeing or refusing to have the treatment. This is not to suggest that in every case of depression in which ECT is scientifically indicated, a patient is axiomatically incompetent to decide about treatment. On the contrary, as suggested by Culver and his colleagues,[60] depressed patients can, and do, consent freely to receiving ECT. The problem facing the psychiatrist is how to deal with the minority in which ECT is either life-saving or the treatment of choice, and competence is compromised. A further complicating feature is the competent patient who refuses treatment, ostensibly for irrational reasons, i.e. declines ECT when sound scientific evidence points to the likelihood that it is the treatment of choice and the probability high that benefits will follow its use.

Culver *et al.* carefully differentiate between these two ethical situations with the aid of prototypical clinical illustrations. Thus, in the patient incompetent to decide about treatment by virtue of disordered mental functioning, the clinician is powerless to convey pertinent information which can then be appraised by the patient. Proxy consent by relatives or guardians is recommended in these circumstances, in tandem with the consideration of any views that have been previously expressed by the patient. Given the recurrent pattern of severe depression, evidence is commonly available of a patient's attitude to ECT ranging from immense gratitude that it was prescribed in a past episode to consistent refusal on the grounds that its long term safety is unproven.

In the latter situation, the patient is deemed competent but refuses ECT despite the psychiatrist's objective view that the treatment is soundly indicated. Here, competence refers to the patient's capacity to understand the information provided by the psychiatrist. The irrationality is grounded in the profound depressed mood which leads the patient to believe that they deserve a terrible fate like death. Then, the decision to refuse ECT, or any other treatment, according to Culver *et al.*, constitutes a justifiable basis for forcible treatment, but only after strenuous efforts have been made to obtain consent.

The third clinical scenario concerns a patient who, worried about the side-effects of memory impairment, cannot be reassured that a conventional course of ECT has been shown objectively to be associated with temporary impairment only, and that this level of impairment can be minimized with the use of unilateral electrode placement. The process of informed consent comes into its own in this context as myths and misconceptions are diligently dealt with by the treating psychiatrist.

Martin and Bean[61] grapple systematically with the issue of what constitutes competence to consent to ECT. After considering the components of the process in general, they recommend a series of specific questions to guide the clinician: is the patient aware that they have been asked to make a decision about receiving ECT; are they troubled arriving at a decision, do they want to make their decision independently; are they willing to rely on a third party? A further group of questions are listed to ascertain whether the patient can (a) understand information relevant to the decision regarding ECT (b) 'manipulate' the information rationally, particularly with reference to evincing a wish to recover from the illness and a concern for his own well-being and (c) appreciate pertinent clinical factors, namely that they have an illness, that it requires treatment and that their condition is likely to worsen in the absence of treatment.

Setting these questions appears, on the face of it, to be useful pragmatically. The authors, however, stress a caveat that competence in the context of ECT remains 'an elusive concept'. On the other hand they are hopeful that their line of enquiry constitutes a paving stone towards a legal definition.

Legally mandated criteria to assess competence are not likely given the considerable variation in clinical presentation. Other contributors to the literature do not pursue this option. The law, on the contrary, can vitiate what should be a clinically based encounter, governed by ethical principles. For example, the decision in a public referendum in Berkeley, California in 1982 to proscribe the use of ECT in the city was ill-conceived in the light of the treatment regularly saving the lives of severely melancholic patients. The anti-psychiatry movement, in this context, is irresponsible in campaigning for a total ban of ECT.[54]

The potentially destructive effects of legal forces is obvious in a poignant account of a 23 year-old woman with intractable mania, a feature of her stormy course of bipolar disorder, who failed to respond to maximum doses of mood stabilizers and antipsychotics.[62] Given this dire situation, the grossly psychotic patient was considered unable to consent to ECT. The treating psychiatrist reports on his futile efforts, over several months, to obtain court approval. The difficulty revolved primarily around the patient's incapacity to consent. The tragic outcome was her cardiac arrest and death, possibly as part of a malignant neuroleptic syndrome.

What a pity that the legal authorities in this tragic case did not consult Richard Sherlock,[63] an American bioethicist who, in a symposium on consent, competency and ECT, argues convincingly that when benefit from ECT is likely but that from alternative treatments non-existent or 'very doubtful', the doctor may, in fact, be morally obligated to use ECT, even without consent. Sherlock posits the justification of such paternalism in cases where the complete irrationality of a patient's decision-making indicates incompetence to act in his own interests.

Another contributor to this symposium, the English philosopher Harry Lesser,[64] is not as confident as Sherlock in the clinician's ability to determine that a patient's decision is 'really' irrational, that ECT 'really' will be beneficial (he does exclude situations of a life in danger and refusal of nutrition), and that alternative treatments are unavailable. Lesser adds other confounders such as a doctor's legal obligations and the availability of clinical resources but these appear quite marginal. He concludes that the patient should be considered 'rational until proved irrational'. No doubt every treating psychiatrist would espouse this position but also feel obligated to wrestle with the possibility of patient irrationality. The limitation in Lesser's argument is his requirement for proof. If only this were so! Lack of an objective yardstick in determining incompetence and irrationality is what makes application of ECT in certain clinical circumstances so much of an ethical dilemma.

Finally, we turn to Jan-Otto Ottosson,[65] the doyen of ECT research in Europe. In a lecture delivered to the Association of Convulsive Therapy in 1985 he chose the ethical dimension of ECT as his theme. Given his pre-eminent role in the development of ECT as a mainstream treatment, and his pioneering research contribution, we have included this address as a selection. Ottosson deals with a range of ethical issues within the framework of principlism. Thus, in terms of beneficence and non-maleficence, he draws on research data which show that ECT has a 'very favourable' risk-benefit ratio. In conditions such as severe depression and acute catatonia, he avers that ECT has distinct benefits. The only risk, and then a small one at that, is long-term difficulty with memory which, he argues, is of minimal importance compared to the pain of persistent melancholia.

In the context of the principle of justice, Ottosson laments the patchy availability of ECT around the world, citing considerable disparities in its deployment, even in the same country.

Respect for autonomy, as applied to ECT, brings us back to the issue of rational capacity. Conceding that this can resist accurate assessment with depressed patients, Ottosson nonetheless asserts that compulsory treatment is legitimate in specific circumstances where autonomous functioning is lacking eg. in many deluded patients. In borderline cases, respect for autonomy is preferable to imposing ECT but psychiatrists may have no choice but to make a judgement to trump it on the basis of the principle of beneficence, even in the face of resistance from patient and/or family.

The final section of his lecture is devoted to the ethical obligation to pursue research in ECT in the quest to relieve suffering in patients with some of the most severe mental illnesses who fail to respond to alternative treatments.

Ethical aspects of psychosurgery

Psychosurgery is rarely used in contemporary psychiatry, having been supplanted by treatments which are equally effective and far less invasive. However, we can learn many lessons from the history of its deployment over more than half a century which bears on ethical aspects of psychiatric treatment in general.

Mersky[66] addresses many of these issues in his chapter in *Psychiatric ethics* on physical manipulation of the brain. Having described the procedures that have been used for affective disorders, pain and aggression, he highlights the problems which arise when informed consent is not forthcoming because of a patient's disordered mental state. Unlike the case of ECT (which Mersky also covers), psychosurgery should never be performed on patients 'who decline explicitly or are implicitly unwilling' for three main reasons: treatment involves permanent brain change, it is ethically impermissible to impose potentially permanent alterations in mental functioning and psychosurgery may lead to a change in personality and the source of all future judgments.

For an account of psychosurgery in all its ramifications, one can do no better than turn to Eliot Valenstein's[67] *Great and desperate cures: The rise and the decline of psychosurgery and other radical treatments for mental illness.* One of the author's motives is clearly articulated – to offer a cautionary tale. By carefully examining factors that lay behind the uncritical acceptance of psychosurgery, we may avoid doing the same with respect to other potentially hazardous treatments in the future. Another volume on this subject, *Ethical issues in psychosurgery* by John Kleinig[68] and published contemporaneously, also alerts us to the ethical perils inherent in embracing a treatment which alters brain structure permanently. He considers several pertinent issues such as the right to treatment, the right to refuse treatment, proxy consent in the face of the incompetent patient and essential characteristics of valid consent. Like Valenstein, Kleinig sees psychosurgery as a splendid advantage point for a broader consideration of key aspects of medical ethics.

Finally, we can recommend an essay by Stagno and his colleagues[69] on informed consent in psychosurgery, with associated commentary by Edward Hundert.[70]

Ethical aspects of psychotherapy

The practice of psychotherapy requires many decisions which involve an ethical dimension. The following are merely illustrative. The definition of psychotherapy is elusive: is it an art, a branch of science, a blend of both, or comparable to a trusting friendship? Psychotherapists do not belong to a unitary profession: they may be, *inter alia*, psychiatrists, psychologists, social workers, chaplains, lay-analysts, psychiatric nurses, or counselors of all forms; and each of these disciplines practices with a certain set of assumptions and premises. The goals they strive for are frequently ill-defined, ranging from symptom relief to ambitious personality change. The multiplicity of objectives is matched by the number of 'schools', each with its own theory of what constitutes normal and abnormal mental health. Finally, the effectiveness of various modes of treatment is subject to much debate.

Who should be offered psychotherapy?

It may seem surprising that the issue of selecting patients for psychotherapy should involve an ethical dimension. Although psychotherapy has a place in psychiatry the question still arises whether a substantial proportion of people receiving it are, as Szasz[71] puts it, wrestling with 'problems of living' rather than psychiatrically ill. A fundamental question follows: should psychotherapy be 'prescribed' only for those who have a clearly defined psychiatric disorder? An explicit form of therapy would then be selected from an established range of treatments and outcome measured in terms of specific, objective criteria. Thus, a satisfactory outcome for a person with depressive symptoms would be elevation of mood, for a bulimic patient cessation of bingeing and vomiting, and for a socially phobic student the ability to dine in the college canteen and participate in social events. This scientific approach owes much to Freud,[72] who developed a mode of treatment to deal with specific neurotic symptoms such as hysterical conversion, obsessions and anxiety. Psychoanalysts, including Freud himself, soon loosened themselves from those moorings and explored uncharted waters. The result has been acceptance of a remit to address the need of a much expanded group of people.

The medical model in this view is constraining and ill-suited to the psychotherapeutic pursuit; first, because legitimate goals may encompass much more than symptomatic relief and second, because pinpointing a diagnosis and plan of treatment is contrary to the notion of psychotherapy as a journey of personal exploration. An opportunity is thus offered to acquire greater self-knowledge or self-awareness and self-actualization or self-realization. This conception also embraces the notion of personal growth, in such spheres as the interpersonal, the spiritual, the sexual, and so on. The quest for self-awareness and self-fulfillment assumes priority.

This broadening of psychotherapy is not without ethical difficulty. Freud[73] captures the dilemma in *Analysis terminable and interminable* when arguing that the aim of psychoanalysis is:

. . . not to rub off every peculiarity of human character for the sake of a schematic 'normality', nor yet to demand that the person who has been 'thoroughly analyzed' shall feel no passions and develop no internal conflicts. The business of the analysis is to secure the best possible psychological conditions for the functions of the ego; with that it has discharged its tasks. (p 250)

Existentially oriented psychotherapy emphasizes self-confrontation and making choices. As Sartre[74] puts it: '[Existential psychoanalysis] is a method destined to bring to light, in a strictly objective form, the subjective choice by which each living person makes himself a person; that is, makes known to himself what he is.'

Yet another position is Jung's[75] concept of 'individuation', whereby a patient becomes a 'separate, indivisible unity or "whole" through a union of conscious and unconscious experience. New creative potential emerges, amounting to the "rounding out" of the personality into a whole'.

It will be evident from these three illustrations that they eschew a focus on symptoms but rather stress personal maturity.

Ethical issues in the therapeutic process

No matter who is selected for psychotherapy and what goals are set, new ethical issues arise as therapist and patient embark on the process; these are best considered in the context of the relationship that evolves between them. The nature of this tie makes the ethical dimension of therapy so salient. The protagonists are virtually polarized with respect to their initial positions. The patient is inevitably bewildered and distressed. The route taken to reach the therapist is likely to have been tortuous and protracted: consultation with family or friend, assessment by a GP, referral to a specialist, further referral to psychotherapy itself. At long last, the encounter with *the*

expert! The inequality is striking – the dependent, vulnerable patient and the ostensibly omniscient therapist. The dependency increases the power and authority already vested in the therapist, and may be reinforced by his opting to divulge little about himself or the nature of treatment on the premise that disclosure would undermine transference (the irrational feelings and attitudes the patient develops towards the therapist), regarded by dynamically oriented schools as central to the therapeutic process. Obfuscation may be the product of the encounter.

Informed consent[76] is one means to dispel this air of mystery. An admirably clear model, provided by Carl Goldberg,[77] invokes the concept of 'therapeutic partnership', its cornerstone a 'mutually agreed upon and explicitly articulated working plan'. This becomes subject to regular review throughout therapy. Among its elements are: identifying goals and methods to reach them, monitoring efficacy and permitting either partner to voice any dissatisfaction with the plan. Moreover, respective roles, tasks and responsibilities are outlined and examined as necessary.

The partnership does not imply an equal share of power, rather an agreement about how the power inherent in the relationship will be allocated at various times. Thus, total autonomy in the patient whereby he enjoys the capacity to reflect, to decide and to act freely on the basis of reflection, may not always be apt. A patient in the throes of an intense crisis, for instance, may lack the wherewithal to appreciate what is in his best interests and, in collaboration with the therapist, agree to a redistribution of responsibility; the therapist is then assigned a more paternalistic role. As the crisis wanes so is there restoration of the patient's autonomy state. The key feature of such shifts is his recognition and determination by both protagonists.

Dyer and Bloch,[78] in reviewing models pertinent to informed consent in the therapeutic relationship, propose that a fiduciary approach is most apt by dint of its emphasis on trust and time. Thus, the therapist works to earn the patient's trust. The process occurs over time and is not a one-off negotiation at the outset of treatment. The fiduciary-based relationship also enhances a sense of responsibility in the therapist, who seeks to respond to particular needs in the patient. Although patient autonomy is always a pre-eminent goal, it is not the therapist's sole preoccupation. They may need to act paternalistically on occasion, comparable to the concern manifest by responsible parents for their child.

Values and psychotherapy

A therapeutic, fiduciary-based partnership obviates many ethical pitfalls intrinsic to psychotherapy. The partnership is a necessary but *not* sufficient condition for sound clinical practice. Permeation of treatment by values of many types is another complication which must be addressed. Given that the problems for which patients seek help are inextricably bound up with the question of how they should live their lives, the therapist inevitably is at risk of imposing their values, intentionally or unwittingly.[79]

The ethicist, Tristram Engelhardt,[80] deals with this issue by positing that psychotherapy is not about ethics but about *meta-ethics*, that is, it paves the way for ethical decision-making by patients. The aim is not for them to adopt a particular set of values as a result of treatment. Indeed, the therapist takes care to avoid offering specific recommendations about how patients shall live their lives. Instead, they are helped to reach a point where they can make their own choices *freely*, unhindered by internal psychological conflict or unconscious influences. But in affirming the therapist's role to help patients become autonomous and therefore able to map out their own values, Engelhardt is necessarily accepting an inescapable feature of psychotherapy, that it is value-bound. To think otherwise is, as Strupp[81] stresses, a fallacy.

Freud[82] was also intent on promoting value-free treatment. Indeed, he argued that: 'The [therapist] should be opaque to his patients and, like a mirror, should show them nothing but what is shown to him' (p. 118) and he insisted that the task of therapy was limited to the 'freeing of someone from his neurotic symptoms, inhibitions and abnormalities of character'[73] through making the unconscious conscious. Freud was stressing the essential character of the task as he saw it: for the patient to reach certain goals, uninfluenced by the therapist's beliefs and attitudes. On the other hand, he also pointed out an educative role for the therapist.[83] As he put it '[the analyst] must possess some kind of superiority, so that in certain analytic situations he can act as a model for his patient and in others as a teacher' (p. 248).

It is difficult to conceive this hybrid role of mirror, model and teacher as being value-free, even if the ultimate goal in analysis is to promote an autonomy free of the influence of unconscious, irrational forces.

An appraisal by leading figures in psychotherapy suggests that therapists inevitably embrace values in their work. Thus, Strupp[81] asserts that moral values are always 'in the picture', the therapist unable to espouse a 'value-free' position. Whether they are aware of it or not, the therapist influences the values of the patient.

Sidney Crown[84] reminds us that the therapist's influence occurs at both verbal and non-verbal levels. While they may be aware of their utterances and attempt to control these, 'his non-verbal communication through gesture, facial expression, nods of approval or disapproval, can be almost unconscious'. Erik Erikson[85] echoes and extends these views when proposing that psychotherapy is essentially an ethical intervention. In a thoughtful paper he concludes: 'What the healing professionals advocate . . . is always part of the value struggle of the times and, whether 'avowed' or not, will be – therefore had better be – ethical intervention.'

If therapy must, to a degree, amount to ethical intervention, the question of how the therapist should handle this follows. They could make every effort to minimize the ethical role, but the likelihood of success is slim since their 'unavowed' values will manifest through non-verbal signs. It is inconceivable that a therapist could maintain an ethically neutral stance without a crippling level of self-consciousness.

Another option is to accept the inevitability of 'ethical interventionism' but recognize this as a 'problem' for the therapist, not the patient. The latter is not burdened by a dilemma that does not belong to them. The therapist by contrast has the responsibility to remain aware of this potential role as moral agent and to regard their values as a factor in the therapeutic encounter, remaining sensitive to his own values and monitors any unconsciously derived impulses to influence the patient. A process of value-testing occurs constantly to ensure that intrusion of values is never neglected and to preclude their imposition unwittingly.

A third radical option is for the therapist to declare their own value system as a value in itself. The argument runs as follows: psychotherapy is a means of social influence; the therapist is more powerfully placed to influence patients than vice versa; the therapist acknowledges this state of affairs; and is entirely 'transparent' regarding the values they espouse.

The psychoanalyst, Robert Jay Lifton,[86] is an eloquent spokesman for this position. Illustrative is his work with US veterans of the Vietnam War. He elaborated a view in which the professional avoids the 'trap of pseudo-neutrality'; instead, he combines attitudes of advocacy and detachment. The process entails voicing 'moral advocacies' in tandem with 'maintaining sufficient detachment to apply the technical and scientific principles of one's discipline'. In helping the veterans, Lifton articulated his anti-war position explicitly to former soldiers who had shared the experience of fighting an allegedly unjust war and who wished to make sense of it.

Other examples of such 'affinity' have evolved in psychotherapy, all typified by the therapist assuming the role of moral advocate. Certain homosexual therapists, for example, have aligned themselves with the 'gay movement' when treating homosexual patients. A distinguished psychotherapist and committed Christian, Alan Bergin,[87] has evolved a school of 'theistic realism' in which the therapist shares specific values derived from a Judeo-Christian tradition, including forgiveness, reconciliation, spiritual belief, supremacy of God, marital fidelity and primacy of love. Some therapists who functioned in the context of apartheid in South Africa declared their rejection of racism and demonstrated their support of traumatized Blacks, especially those who had been victims of detention and torture.[88]

Particular constituencies are being served in all these illustrations. A therapist's explicit avowal of personal values can be applied more generally. A therapist may adopt an approach with *all* patients in which they will be

transparent about their ethical attitudes in various clinical circumstances. This is done on the premise that values are central in assessing a problem, formulating goals and selecting therapeutic options.[89] The corollary is unambiguous: 'Therapists do not have a choice about whether they need to deal with their values in therapy, only how well.'

Another valuable contribution on this theme is by Jeremy Holmes.[79] As a long-standing scholar of the ethics of psychotherapy and a practitioner of psychodynamic therapy, he is well placed to consider the interface between values and psychological treatment – historically, philosophically and practically. Accepting that psychotherapy cannot be value-free, Holmes offers therapists a way of examining their 'ethical countertransference'. In using this notion, he points to the need for therapists to be aware of unconscious influences which may be the opposite of what they overtly espouse.

References

1 Roberts, L.: Informed consent and the capacity for voluntarism. *American Journal of Psychiatry* **159**:705–712, 2002.

2 Lidz, CW., Meisel, A., Zerubavel, E., Carter, M., Sestak, R. and Roth, L.: *Informed consent: A study of decision making in psychiatry.* New York, Guilford, 1984.

3 Faden, R. and Beauchamp, T.: *A history and theory of informed consent.* New York, Oxford University Press, 1986.

4 Katz, J.: *The silent world of doctor and patient.* New York, Free Press, 1984.

5 Mill, J.: On liberty, in *Three essays.* Oxford University Press, 1976, pp. 15.

*6 Chodoff, P.: Involuntary hospitalization of the mentally ill as a moral issue. *American Journal of Psychiatry* **141**:384–389, 1984.

7 Lidz, C., Hoge, S., Gardner, W., Bennett, N., Monahan, J., Mulvey, E. and Roth, L.: Perceived coercion in mental hospital admission. *Archives of General Psychiatry* **52**:1034–1039, 1995.

*8 Szasz, T.: The case against suicide prevention. *American Psychologist* **41**:806–812, 1986.

9 Heyd, D. and Bloch, S.: The ethics of suicide, in *Psychiatric ethics*, 3rd edn, ed. S. Bloch, P. Chodoff, and S. Green. Oxford University Press, 1999, pp. 441–460.

*10 Van Staden, C.W. and Kruger, C. Incapacity to give informed consent owing to mental disorder. *Journal of Medical Ethics* **29**:41–43, 2003.

11 Kopelman, L.: On the evaluative nature of competency and capacity judgements. *International Journal of Law and Psychiatry* **13**:309–329, 1990.

*12 Munetz, M.R., Galon, P.A. and Frese, F.J.: The ethics of mandatory community treatment. *Journal of the American Academy of Psychiatry and the Law* **31**:173–183, 2003.

13 Pargiter, R. and Bloch, S. A history of psychiatric ethics. *Psychiatric Clinics of North America* **25**:509–524, 2002.

*14 Donaldson v O'Connor, F.2d 5th Cir, decided April 26, 1974, *O'Connor v Donaldson* 422US. 563, 1975.

15 Wyatt v Stickney 325F Supp 781 (1971); *Wyatt v Stickney* 344 F Supp 373, 376, 379–385 (1972)

16 Stone, A.: Overview: the right to treatment – comments on the law and its impact. *American Journal of Psychiatry* **132**:1125–1134, 1975.

*17 Klerman, G.: The psychiatric patient's right to effective treatment: Implications of *Osheroff v Chestnut Lodge. American Journal of Psychiatry* **147**:419–427, 1990.

*18 Stone, A.: Law, science, and psychiatric malpractice: A response to Klerman's indictment on psychoanalytic psychiatry. *American Journal of Psychiatry* **147**:419–427, 1990.

19 Radden, J.: Forced medication, patients' rights and values conflicts. *Psychiatry, Psychology and Law* **10**: 1–11, 2003.

20 Rogers v Okin, 478 F Supp 1342 (D Mass, 1979); *Rogers v Commissioner of the Department of Mental Health*, 458NE 2d 308 (Mass Sup Jud Ct, 1983)

21 Appelbaum, P.: The right to refuse treatment with antipsychotic medications: retrospect and prospect. *American Journal of Psychiatry* **145**:413–419, 1988.

22 Appelbaum, P. and Gutheil, T.: 'Rotting with their rights on': Constitutional theory and clinical reality in drug refusal by psychiatric patients. *Bulletin of the American Academy of Psychiatry and the Law* 7:308–317, 1979.

23 Gutheil, T., Shapiro, R. and St. Clair, L.: Legal guardianship in drug refusal: An illusory solution. *American Journal of Psychiatry* 137: 347–352, 1980.

24 Schouten, R. and Gutheil, T.: Aftermath of the Rogers decision: Assessing the costs. *American Journal of Psychiatry* 147:1348–1352, 1990.

25 Stone, A.: The right to refuse treatment: Why psychiatrists should and can make it work. *Archives of General Psychiatry* 38:358–362, 1981.

26 Srebnik, D. and La Fond, J. Advanced directives for mental health treatment. *Psychiatric Services* 50:919–925, 1999.

*27 Henderson, C., Flood, C., Leese, M., Thornicroft, G., Sutherby, K. and Szmukler, G.: Effect of joint crisis plans on the use of compulsory treatment in psychiatry: single blind randomised controlled trial. *British Medical Journal* 329:136–138, 2004.

28 Sutherby, K., Szmukler, G., Halpern, A., Alexander, M., Thornicroft, G., Johnson, G. and Wright, S.: A study of 'crisis cards' in a community psychiatric service. *Acta Psychiatrica Scandinavica* 100:56–61, 1999.

29 Thomas, P. and Cahill, A.: Compulsion and psychiatry: the role of advanced statements (editorial). *British Medical Journal* 329:122–123, 2004.

30 Widdershoven, G. and Berghmans, R.: Advanced directives in psychiatric care: a narrative approach. *Journal of Medical Ethics* 27:92–97, 2001.

31 Ritchie, J., Sklar, R. and Steiner, W.: Advanced directives in psychiatry. *International Journal of Law and Psychiatry* 21:245–260, 1998.

32 Savulescu, J. and Dickenson, D.: The time frame of preferences, dispositions, and the validity of advanced directives for the mentally ill. *Psychiatry, Psychology and Philosophy* 5:225–266, 1998.

33 Cote, C., Kaufmann, R., Troendle, G. and Lambert, G.: Is the therapeutic orphan about to be adopted? *Paediatrics* 98:115–123, 1996.

34 Coffey, B.: Ethical issues in child and adolescent psychopharmacology. *Child and Adolescent Psychiatric Clinics of North America* 4:793–807, 1995.

35 Treatment for adolescents with depression study (TADS) team.: Fluoxetine, cognitive-behavioural therapy, and their combination for adolescents with depression. *JAMA* 292:807–20, 2004.

36 Martinez, C., Rietbrock, S., Wise, L. *et al.*: Antidepressant treatment and the risk of fatal and non-fatal self-harm in first-episode depression: nest case controlled study. *BMJ* 330:389–393, 2005.

37 Cipriani, A., Barbui, C. and Geddes, J.: Suicide, depression and antidepressants (editorial). *BMJ* 330:373–374, 2005.

38 Whittington, C.J., Kendall, T., Fonagy, P., Cottrell, D., Cotgrove, A. and Boddington, E.: Selective serotonin reuptake inhibitors in childhood depression: systematic review of published versus unpublished data. *Lancet* 363:1341–1345, 2004.

39 *New York Times*, 16 October 2004. FDA toughens warning on antidepressant drugs.

40 Adverse Drug Reactions Advisory Committee, 17 June 2004. Use of SSRI antidepressants in children and adolescents. See: www.tga.gov.au/adr/adrac_ssri.htm

*41 Jensen, P.: Ethical and pragmatic issues in the use of psychotropic agents in young children. *Canadian Journal of Psychiatry* 43: 585–588, 1998.

*42 Fisher, R. L. and Fisher, S.: Antidepressants for children. Is scientific support necessary? *Journal of Nervous and Mental Disease* 184:99–102, 1996.

43 Eisenberg, L.: Principles of drug therapy in child psychiatry with special reference to stimulant drugs. *American Journal of Orthopsychiatry* 41:371–379, 1971.

44 Diller, L.: The run on Ritalin. Attention deficit disorder and stimulant treatment in the 1990s. *Hastings Center Report* 26:12–18, 1996.

45 Diller, L.: Prescription stimulant use in America: Ethical issues. *President's Council on Bioethics*, 24 January 2003. See www.bioethicsprint.bioethics.gov.

46 Halasz, G.: Symposium on Attention Deficit Hyperactivity Disorder (ADHD): An ethical perspective. *Australian and New Zealand Journal of Psychiatry* 36:472–487, 2002.

47 Angold, A., Erkanli, A., Egger, H. and Costello, J.: Stimulant treatment for children: a community perspective. *Journal of the American Academy of Child and Adolescent Psychiatry* 39:975–984, 2000.

48 Klerman, G.: Psychotropic hedonism vs. pharmacological Calvinism. *Hastings Center Report* 2: 1–3, 1972.

49 Charlton, B. and McKenzie, K.: Treating unhappiness – society needs palliative psychopharmacology. *British Journal of Psychiatry* 185:194–195, 2004.

50 Carstairs, G.: A land of lotus eaters? *American Journal of Psychiatry* 125:1576–1580, 1969.

51 Kramer, P.: *Listening to Prozac*. London, Fourth Estate, 1994.

*52 Kramer, P.: The valorization of sadness. *Hastings Center Report* 30:13–18, 2000.

*53 Elliott, C.: Pursued by happiness and beaten senseless. *Hastings Center Report* 30:7–12, 2000.

54 Fink, M.: Impact of the antipsychiatry movement on the revival of electroconvulsive therapy in the United States. *Psychiatric Clinics of North America* 14:793–801, 1991.

55 Fink, M.: Myths of 'shock therapy'. *American Journal of Psychiatry* 134:991–996, 1977.

56 Fink, M. and Ottosson, J-O.: *Ethics in convulsive therapy*. New York, Brunner-Routledge, 2004.

57 Salzman, C.: ECT and ethical psychiatry. *American Journal of Psychiatry* 134:1006–1009, 1977.

58 Reiter-Theil, S.: Autonomy and beneficence: Ethical issues in electroconvulsive therapy. *Convulsive Therapy* 8:237–244, 1992.

59 Leong, G.B. and Eth, S.: Legal and ethical issues in electroconvulsive therapy. *Psychiatric Clinics of North America* 14:1007–1019, 1991.

60 Culver, C.M., Ferrell, R.B. and Green, R.M.: ECT and special problems of informed consent. *American Journal of Psychiatry* 137:586–591, 1980.

61 Martin, B.A. and Bean, G.J.: Competence to consent to electroconvulsive therapy. *Convulsive Therapy* 8:92–102, 1992.

62 Parry, B.: The tragedy of legal impediments involved in obtaining ECT for patients unable to give informed consent (letter). *American Journal of Psychiatry* 138:1128–1129, 1981.

63 Sherlock, R.: Consent, competency and ECT: some critical suggestions. *Journal of Medical Ethics* 9:141–143, 1983.

64 Lesser, H.: Consent, competency and ECT: a philosopher's comment. *Journal of Medical Ethics* 9:144–145, 1983.

*65 Ottosson, J.-O.: Ethical aspects of research and practice of ECT. *Convulsive Therapy* 11:288–299, 1995.

66 Merskey, H.: Ethical aspects of the physical manipulation of the brain, in *Psychiatric ethics*, 3rd edn, ed. S. Bloch, P. Chodoff and S. Green. Oxford, Oxford University Press, 1999.

67 Valenstein, E.: *Great and desperate cures: The rise and decline of psychosurgery and other radical treatments for mental illness*. New York, Basic Books, 1986, and *The psychosurgery debate*, ed. E. Valenstein. San Francisco, Freeman, 1980.

68 Kleinig, J.: *Ethical issues in psychosurgery*. London, Allen and Unwin, 1985.

69 Stagno, S., Smith, M. and Hassenbusch, S.: Reconsidering psychosurgery: Issues of informed consent and physician responsibility. *Journal of Clinical Ethics* 5:217–223, 1994.

70 Hundert, E.: Autonomy, informed consent and psychosurgery. *Journal of Clinical Ethics* 5:264–266, 1994.

71 Szasz, T.: *The myth of mental illness*. Harper and Row, New York, 1974.

72 Freud, S.: The psychotherapy of hysteria. In *Studies on hysteria* by J. Breuer and S. Freud, Standard edition 2, Hogarth Press, London. pp. 255–305, 1895.

73 Freud, S.: *Analysis terminable and interminable*. Standard edition, 23, Hogarth Press, London. pp. 211–53, 1937.

74 Sartre, J.P.: (no year stated) *Existentialism and human emotions*. Castle, New York. p. 81.

75 Jung, C. G.: Conscious, unconscious and individuation. In *The essential Jung*, ed. A. Storr, Princeton University Press, Princeton, pp. 212–226, 1983.

76 Beahrs, J. and Gutheil, T.: Informed consent in psychotherapy. *American Journal of Psychiatry* 158:4–10, 2001.

77 Goldberg, C.: *Therapeutic partnership: ethical concerns in psychotherapy*. New York, Springer, 1977.

78   Dyer, A. and Bloch, S.: Informed consent and the psychiatric patient. *Journal of Medical Ethics* **13**:12–16, 1987.

*79   Holmes, J.: Values in psychotherapy. *American Journal of Psychotherapy* **50**:259–273, 1996.

80   Engelhardt, H.T.: Psychotherapy as meta-ethics. *Psychiatry* **36**:440–445, 1973.

81   Strupp, H.: Observation on the fallacy of value-free psychotherapy and the empty organism. *Journal of Abnormal Psychology* **20**:11–15, 1990.

82   Freud, S.: *Recommendations to physicians practising psychoanalysis.* Standard edition 12, Hogarth Press London, pp.111–120, 1924.

83   Freud, S.: *An outline of psychoanalysis.* Standard edition 23, Hogarth Press, London, p. 144, 1940.

84   Crown, S.: Psychotherapy. In *Dictionary of medical ethics*, eds A. S. Duncan, G. R. Dunstan, and R. B. Wellbourn. London, Darton, Longman and Todd; pp. 264–268, 1977.

*85   Erikson, E.H.: Psychoanalysis and ethics-avowed and unavowed. *International Review of Psychoanalysis* **3**:409–415, 1976.

*86   Lifton, R. J.: Advocacy and corruption in the healing professions. *International Review of Psychoanalysis* **3**: 385–398, 1976.

*87   Bergin, A. E.: Psychotherapy and religious values. *Journal of Consulting and Clinical Psychology* **48**:95–105, 1980.

88   Steere, J. and Dowdall, T.: On being ethical in unethical places. The dilemma of South African clinical psychologists. *Hastings Center Report* **20**:11–15, 1990.

*89   Aponte, H. J.: The negotiation of values in therapy. *Family Process* **24**:323–338, 1985.

Involuntary Hospitalization of the Mentally Ill as a Moral Issue*

Paul Chodoff

Some years ago I was invited to debate Dr. Thomas Szasz on the legitimacy of involuntary hospitalization for mental illness. I undertook the assignment, and my views on the matter were published in 1976 under the title 'The Case for Involuntary Hospitalization of the Mentally Ill'.[1] Since that time I have maintained an active interest in this controversial issue. I have tried to keep abreast of changes and developments and have been involved in many discussions about it in both formal and informal settings. Although it is clear that I have a particular point of view, I believe I have maintained sufficient objectivity to have noted that (as happens whenever differing opinions are held with emotional intensity) a complex matter has become polarized into blacks and whites.

On one side are those who regret the necessity for involuntary hospitalization but regard it as an essential last resort enabling the care and treatment of a small proportion of patients whose severe mental illnesses substantially interfere with their capacity to accept such treatment voluntarily. This is the medical model approach, and I count myself among its adherents along with, I believe, a majority of psychiatrists and some lawyers as well. The contrary position is maintained in varying degrees by a smaller but very articulate segment of the psychiatric profession and by a number of lawyers who have banded together under the designation of the 'mental health bar.' This is the civil liberties approach. Those who hold it have in common the conviction that the psychiatric hospitalization of a person against his or her will is a dangerous assault on individual freedom. The members of this group, however, are by no means monolithic in the intensity with which they oppose involuntary hospitalization. Some of them support Szaszian absolutism. They regard the forced hospitalization of anyone for the sake of his mental health as anathema; there are no circumstances under which it can be justified.[2]

Another and currently more influential civil liberties position is to accept forced hospitalization under certain circumstances but only in the most gingerly fashion and when hedged about with rigid restrictions. Rejecting medical necessity as a proper criterion, these civil libertarians would permit the state to act only under the sanction of the police power when behavior that is physically dangerous to the self or others has been demonstrated unequivocally and immediately. In addition to the police power, the medical model psychiatrist would also like to be able to invoke the doctrine of *parens patriae*, under which the state takes protective action toward a citizen, sometimes without his permission, as a parent may do with a child.

As a consequence of this fundamental disagreement, the two sides interpret the considerable amount of data that has accumulated about involuntary hospitalization in very different fashions. They disagree about the nature and effects of mental illness and even about its very existence; about whether the mentally ill can accurately be differentiated from the idiosyncratic normal and, if so, whether the behavioral deviance of the former is sufficient cause to justify depriving them of their liberty. Can mentally ill persons be adequately treated even if they are committed? Are enough properly equipped facilities and sufficient funds available? Is hospitalization really necessary, or will less restrictive alternatives not involving deprivation of liberty be just as effective?

Each side hurls its thunderbolts of horrible examples at the other. The civil libertarians attack with their Donaldsons incarcerated for years without treatment in a gulag of warehouses or 'treated' by powerful drugs with irremediable side effects. They point to such atrocities as the Alabama state hospital system before Judge Johnson. They bring forward instances of 'putting away' relatives for vindictive or economic reasons with the collusion or indifference of doctors and hospital authorities. The psychiatrists fire back with the multiple dislocations and the misery caused by the fiasco of deinstitutionalization. They decry what they call the criminalization of the mental health system. They are scornful of lawyers sitting comfortably in their offices who are willing to sacrifice the real, desperate needs of individuals for the sake of an abstract principle. They deplore the legal roadblocks preventing them from providing proper and helpful treatment for sick and suffering people not 'dangerous' enough to be hospitalized.

Can this conflict be resolved fully by the continued careful amassing and analysis of data, which will demonstrate the extent to which the opposing views are correct or incorrect? I do not think so.

We are dealing primarily here not with questions of fact but with questions of value or at least with a situation in which differing values influence perceptions and thus make it very difficult to arrive at a consensual interpretation of whatever data are accumulated. Through the ages moral philosophers have been grappling with the question of whether values can be derived from facts, and no definitive answer has emerged.

Is it morally right or wrong to hospitalize someone against his will for mental health reasons? This is the value issue underlying the debate. If we grant, as I think we should, the basic good will of both the medical model and the civil liberties groups, their differing attitudes toward this issue are determined to a significant degree by the differing moral stances from which they approach it. In the remainder of this paper I shall discuss some aspects of the moral philosophies that inform and motivate contrary judgments about involuntary hospitalization for mental illness. Although I have acknowledged where my sympathies lie, I will attempt to be evenhanded in my discussion and will make it clear when I am becoming partisan.

For at least as long as we have had records of man as a self-conscious entity facing the ambiguities of the world, there have been disagreements about how to determine the rightness or wrongness of ideas and actions. I do not intend, nor am I qualified, to give an account of this infinitely subtle debate. However, in order to clarify my discussion, it is necessary to undertake some preliminary definitions.[3]

Utilitarian versus Deontological Approaches

One of the main divisions in moral philosophy is whether the right is always a function of the good (however the good is defined). One position is held by the utilitarians, who believe that the morality of an act is determined by the extent

* Chodoff, P.: Involuntary hospitalization of the mentally ill as a moral issue. *American Journal of Psychiatry* 141:384–389, 1984.

to which that act serves the good of the individual or the society. The main opponent of utilitarianism in the philosophical arena is the deontological school. The deontologists maintain that whether an act has good consequences should not be the only factor determining its rightness or wrongness. Certain fundamentally intuited principles such as liberty, fairness, and justice must also enter into the judgment and, on occasion, may be important enough to override or, to use Dworkin's term,[4] 'trump' the good as the sole criterion of right action. It is obvious that neither of these approaches to morality (or any other approach) has triumphed. The literature and folklore of ethics abound in examples of the ambiguity confronting those who attempt to use either utilitarian or deontological principles to resolve specific moral dilemmas. Is it right to throw into the water one or more occupants of an overcrowded lifeboat to save the other occupants? At least theoretically, the utilitarian answer would be in the affirmative; that of the deontologists would be negative.

How does this somewhat abstruse distinction apply to the moral legitimacy of involuntary hospitalization for mental illness? I suggest that these labels are useful ways of describing the attitudes of the two sides in the debate we are discussing. The doctors who embrace the medical approach are following a utilitarian ideal. For them the removal or diminishing of the barriers that mental illness imposes on the healthy functioning of their patients is the right thing to do. It justifies temporary deprivation of physical liberty. These physicians take as their moral guideline that involuntary hospitalization serves the good of their patients and of the society within which the patients reside.

For the civil libertarians, however, the fact that the patient may benefit from being forcibly hospitalized is not the only consideration determining the morality of such an act. They are more concerned with its coercive aspects and with the loss of liberty that it entails. Like John Stuart Mill (cited in reference 3), they conceive liberty to be so important a value to society that it transcends other values. For its sake, they are even willing, if necessary, to sacrifice the immediate good of certain mentally ill individuals.[5] I suggest that the fervor with which they pursue this end has a deontological rather than a utilitarian flavor. It is more concerned with threats to liberty than with the welfare of individuals.

The unequivocality of this civil liberties passion for liberty has certain advantages at a time when personal liberty is under assault in so many places in the world. Witness the perversion of psychiatry in the Soviet Union, where people are being cast into prison hospitals for their dissident opinions and behavior rather than for mental illness.[6] A cautionary restraint is needed for those psychiatrists who take too lightly the seriousness of the decision to undertake involuntary commitment in the absence of absolutely clear-cut indications. I believe from my own years of experience in the field that this attitude was present among some psychiatrists in the not-too-distant past; it seems less likely to be a danger today.

However, it can also be argued that too absolute an emphasis on liberty can itself result in serious abuses. Defining liberty only in terms of freedom from coercive hospitalization fails to take into account that such liberty may be meaningless in the presence of the debilitating effects of untreated disease. Even in a setting of involuntary hospitalization, proper treatment can offer the promise of psychological and physiological freedom to the hospitalized patient and can increase his or her options. It is worth pointing out that even John Stuart Mill exempted from his libertarian principles those whose behavior was 'incompatible with the full use of the reflecting faculty'.[3] (It seems somewhat ironic that the liberty which the great utilitarians identified as the supreme good in general is being used in a nonutilitarian fashion to justify depriving the mentally ill of other, very important, goods.) A corollary of the emphasis on liberty as the supreme value is that the only moral justification for deprivation of freedom is bad (violent) behavior. Therefore, for the mentally ill to be confined, they must be proven to be dangerous and thus bad.

This need to justify abridgment of liberty only on the grounds of antisocial behavior is a powerful if covert motive in the growing tendency to prescribe involuntary hospitalization for actions dangerous to the self or others and for no other reason. One effect is to redefine the mental health system as a subset of the criminal justice system, a triumph of principle perhaps, but one of doubtful advantage to either society or the suffering patient.[7]

In my opinion (and here I am departing from my 'objective' role), such criteria of dangerousness are no more objective or reliable than the medical criteria, which are under legal attack as fuzzy and subjective. The need to demonstrate dangerousness makes psychiatrists into policeman enforcing preventive detention. It also promotes a galling kind of hypocrisy when, in order to effect a necessary commitment, dangerousness must be invented or exaggerated. Total reliance on such standards is inimical to treatment considerations, since within the ranks of seriously disturbed mental patients the most dangerous are often not treatable and the most treatable may not be particularly dangerous. If carried to its ultimate, total replacement of the criteria of medical necessity by those of dangerousness may end involuntary hospitalization altogether. The consequences to mentally disordered persons and to society of an even greater degree of deinstitutionalization than is already taking place are cause for real concern.

Rights versus Obligations

To return to my theme that presuppositions rather than interpretations of facts are largely responsible for generating attitudes about involuntary hospitalization, the utilitarian-deontological dichotomy is not the only way of trying to understand the differences in value judgments between civil liberties and medical model points of view. Another distinction is the relative weight the two sides give to the importance of rights on the one hand and obligations on the other. Civil libertarians are particularly concerned with the rights of patients, obviously their right not to be hospitalized if they do not wish to be, and incidentally and more recently, their right to refuse treatment even if hospitalized. This position is an instance of the emphasis on individual human rights that is one of the strongest currents sweeping the Western world today. It is the heir and direct outgrowth of that ideal of egalitarianism which developed during the period of the Enlightenment and reached its climax in the French Revolution. In its light, hierarchal arrangements between superiors and inferiors have increasingly been replaced by a legal model emphasizing contractual agreement between equals. This egalitarian ideal leaves little room for the exercise of an unregulated benevolence from the powerful to the needy. Witness the burgeoning of informed consent procedures in biomedical settings. The traditional attitudes of physicians toward patients are less likely today to be accepted uncritically and gratefully as a form of benevolence. Rather, these attitudes are likely to be considered as paternalistic, and paternalism in our society has become an almost stigmatic term.[8] Adherence to egalitarian principles leaves little moral justification for the deprivation of rights that occurs in the forced hospitalization of someone for his or her own good.

Are the Mentally Ill Autonomous?

However, diverse and eminent figures of philosophy have held that morality requires autonomous persons. Can severely mentally ill persons with gross defects in their reasoning processes be autonomous in the sense required for their inclusion within a vision of morality that regards human beings as equals? I take it as given that neither medical model nor civil liberties adherents would condone involuntary hospitalization for any reason (dangerousness or medical necessity) without the existence of reason-damaging mental illness. Therefore, differences of opinion on the legitimacy of the practice will be determined largely by attitudes to the question just posed. The radical civil libertarians such as Szasz[2] dispose of the problem easily. For them mental illness is a myth, and a myth cannot interfere with the responsible autonomy that claims freedom as its natural right. A large body of literature disputes this assertion. Among other objections, it appears that by equating mental illness exclusively with organicity, Szasz's definition is inordinately narrow. A more general contrary view has been expressed by Moore:[9] 'The problem is that mental illness is not a myth. It is not some palpable falsehood propagated among the populace by power mad psychiatrists, but a cruel and bitter reality that has been with the human race since antiquity.'

Other civil libertarians, such as Stephen J. Morse,[5] accept the legitimacy of mental disease. They claim, however, that the effects of such illness on autonomy, in the sense of decision-making ability, do not differentiate mental patients from the idiosyncratic normal with sufficient exactness to warrant disregarding the wishes of either group concerning hospitalization. This is an argument from the facts that has a certain degree of cogency. The ability of psychiatrists to make regular and reliable distinctions between peculiar and psychotic people certainly can be challenged.

However, in accordance with my thesis that underlying processes which are not entirely in awareness determine attitudes about the 'facts' of involuntary hospitalization, I believe that there are elements of rationalization in this contention. Through the denial of significant differences between the normal and the mentally ill with regard to autonomy, the latter can be considered capable of moral responsibility for dangerous (i.e., bad) behavior. Thus, the moral conviction that all people have an equal right to liberty unless they are criminals can be reinforced.

Those espousing the medical model side would deny that the severely mentally ill are truly autonomous persons, that is, capable of self-governance and of exercising independent judgment. Their deficit in rationality prevents them from being able to respond positively to the bracing winds of equality; to such shorn lambs these winds must be tempered by some measure of benevolence. The psychiatrists who take this position are harking back to a much earlier tradition than the egalitarianism of the civil liberties advocates. They are clinging to that priestly role which since the dawn of history has been so important a component of the identity of the physician.

However, like the civil libertarians on the other side of the question, the psychiatric arguments that the mentally ill lack autonomy and therefore cannot be held to standards of moral responsibility may not be free of bias. Medical model reasoning, too, may be distorted by the need of its proponents to assert their utilitarian desire to enhance the good of mentally ill patients and to downplay the cost of depriving them temporarily of their liberty. This need is, of course, a very natural outgrowth and concomitant of the clinical situation in which medicine, including psychiatry, is practiced. There is an inevitable disparity between the role of physician and of patient that requires an attitude of benevolence and caring on the part of the physician. The atmosphere in which the doctor-patient relationship is conducted, incidentally, is very different from that of legal practice. Although lawyers act on behalf of their clients, their daily contact is predominantly with other lawyers, who are their adversarial equals.

Can Paternalism be Justified?

But can a physician who deprives a person of his liberty for the sake of his mental health be regarded as acting benevolently? Or are such actions intrusive and even malevolent? To the extent, then, that the utilitarian role of the psychiatrist encompasses paternalism, it is necessary to discuss and if possible to justify that concept.

A useful distinction can be made between strong and weak forms of paternalism.[3] If the choice to be overridden is voluntary and informed, we are dealing with a strong paternalism that is clearly coercive and, in a medical context, ignores the patient's right not to be interfered with if he does not wish such interference. An example would be the refusal of a rational victim of irreversible kidney failure to undergo further dialysis. But the decision of a psychiatrist to override the refusal of lifesaving antidepressant treatment by a suicidal depressed patient is not paternalism of this sort. Rather, it is an exercise of a weak paternalism because the mental illness prevents the patient's choice from being truly voluntary. The psychiatrist in such a case is acting to restore that control over the self which is the essence of autonomy and which has been lost through the mental disorder. However, it needs to be pointed out that paternalism requires more than nonvoluntarism to be morally justified. Some other assurance of beneficent interest is needed. As John Rawls[10] has stipulated, 'Paternalistic intervention must also be guided by the principles of justice and what is known about the subject's more permanent aims and preferences.'

Reducing the argument to a simple conflict between autonomy and paternalistic beneficence can be done only by accepting that autonomy is

consistent with severe mental illness. For those who do not believe in a meaningful autonomy for patients with such illnesses, a certain degree of paternalism is unavoidable. It should be emphasized that not all patients who in the psychiatrist's judgment would benefit from hospital treatment should have it imposed on them against their will. What, then, are the particular characteristics of some mentally disabled patients that legitimate paternalistic intervention?

An example of a narrow defense of the paternalistic principle is contained in an article by Culver and Gert.[11] They hold that a moral violation (deprivation of liberty) can be justified only by demonstrated irrationality and an overwhelming preponderance of good done and harm prevented by the intervener's action as opposed to his failure to act. For practical purposes they confine such instances to the strong likelihood that the irrational patient will suffer physical harm in the absence of such intervention. As an example of a case not meeting this criterion and in which, therefore (although reluctantly), they could not condone involuntary hospitalization, they cite a writer who after a previous manic episode had been working productively and had been supplied by his publisher with a sum of money that was all he had to live on. At this point, manic behavior recurred. One of its manifestations was that the writer began burning the money he had just received. Culver and Gert[11] justify their decision not to intervene on the grounds that money burning by itself cannot be taken as a general rule compelling hospitalization of the burner. I find this a weak argument, since it would never, of course, be the single reason why anyone would advocate commitment of such a person but might constitute one symptom among others pointing to a serious, diagnosable, and treatable mental illness interfering with rational judgment. In addition, since in most jurisdictions physical dangerousness to the self is included within police power rather than *parens patriae* commitments, there is some question whether such cases afford a fair test of the morality of paternalistic commitments.

Can the forced hospitalization of mentally ill patients who are not dangerous to either themselves or others but who meet medical model criteria be justified on moral grounds? I have already given my reasons for rejecting dangerousness as the sole criterion. A case in point is Culver and Gert's manic patient,[11] who, while not dangerous, appears to me eminently suitable for paternalistic commitment. One possible but limited reassurance for those inclined to the negative decision would be to take into account the prior expressed wishes of individuals who have been subject to discrete psychotic episodes that they be hospitalized if they become ill again[11-14] — a kind of living will. Theoretically, such a principle might be implied in a broader way in some variety of social contract theory. As expressed by Rawls,[10] this would require agreement by representatives of society, acting behind a veil of ignorance that keeps them from awareness of the consequences of their decisions to themselves, on the steps that society should take for the good of mentally ill patients.

However, although such considerations are interesting and provocative, they will likely have little direct effect on the debate over the moral validity of involuntary hospitalization. Stephen Toulmin[15] has referred to Rawls's work as 'an ethic for strangers,' and the emotionally heated real-life situations in which psychiatrists must make decisions about mentally ill patients are hardly the encounters of strangers. Toulmin, incidentally, decries the 'tyranny of principles' that underlie our concepts of justice through laws. He seeks to leave at least a little room for an alternative to the justice of laws and rules through the intermediation of the ancient concept of equity, which is defined as 'the resort to general principles of justice to correct or supplement the provisions of the law' (*Oxford English Dictionary*). Thus, equity permits clemency to the individual on the basis of a kind of justice that exists behind and without a system of codified laws. In a way, psychiatrists may unknowingly be using equity considerations when they seek clemency for their patients rather than strict legal justice. Toulmin[15] quotes Tolstoy that an ethics modeled on law rather than equity is no ethics at all. In a similar vein, it has been said that medical ethics, to the extent that it becomes codified in a set of principles, has had an ambiguous effect and has contributed to the dehumanization of medicine by 'abstracting ethics from the arena of clinical decision making'.[16]

Conclusions

At this point I will return to the personal note on which I began this discussion. I doubt if any intellectual calculus, no matter how well informed and subtle, will ever fully resolve the antinomian moral issues that lie behind the dispute over involuntary hospitalization. Ethics is 'inescapably controversial';[17] the summum bonum of the philosophers is yet to be achieved. In the final analysis no set of rules – utilitarian, deontologic, or whatever – can fully determine moral attitudes; there will always be a substantial subjective element, the product of the complex series of antecedents that form each individual outlook. With regard to the questions I have raised, my own view is in favor, as an ideal, of a wise and benevolent paternalism that accepts the obligation to help suffering patients who through no fault of their own are incapable of voluntarily accepting help. This statement is in accord with a utilitarian ethic at a logical level; however, the feeling from which it stems is not logical but is intuitive, generated in the heat of clinical action demanding decision. And, as the Oxford philosopher R.M. Hare[18] has pointed out, this is the way most people make moral judgments.

However, I am aware that my call for a 'wise and benevolent paternalism' may be pounced upon as a pious fraud by those who take the fallibility of psychiatrists and their frequent inability to function in such a lofty empyrean as reasons why paternalism must inevitably be corrupt. These opponents of paternalism, too, are convinced at a feeling level of the moral rightness of the judgments that underlie their arguments. Although I believe that these arguments are basically flawed, certainly they have had an impact on those who follow the medical model. It cannot be denied that there may be an ugly side to the utilitarian ethic when it maintains a coarse concentration on ends over means (although I feel impelled also to point out the opposite peril of restricting the achievement of worthwhile ends only to those for which the means have been immaculate). The civil liberties objections have at least moderated the hubris that can contaminate the paternalistic approach. Therefore, the paternalism I espouse should not be assumed to be wise and benevolent; rather, chastened and self-critical, it should be willing to submit to strong safeguards against abuse.

To the extent that the question of involuntary hospitalization for mentally ill patients is a moral problem, it is not an easy but a very difficult one. In a theatrical analogy, we are confronted not with melodrama, a contest of right against wrong, but rather with tragedy, a conflict of one right – to be at physical liberty – against another right – to be free from dehumanizing disease.

References

1. Chodoff P: The case for involuntary hospitalization of the mentally ill. *Am J Psychiatry* **133**:496–501, 1976.
2. Szasz T: *Psychiatric Slavery*. New York, Free Press, 1977.
3. Beauchamp TL, Childers JF: *Principles of Biomedical Ethics*. New York, Oxford University Press, 1979.
4. Dworkin R: *Taking Rights Seriously*. Cambridge, Mass, Harvard University Press, 1977.
5. Morse SJ: A preference for liberty: the case against involuntary commitment of the mentally disordered. *California Law Review* **70**:54–106, 1982.
6. Bloch S: The political misuse of psychiatry in the Soviet Union, in *Psychiatric Ethics*. Edited by Bloch S, Chodoff P. New York, Oxford University Press, 1981.
7. Stone AA: *Mental Health and Law: A System in Transition*. Rockville, Md, NIMH Center for Studies of Crime and Delinquency, 1975.
8. Chodoff P: Paternalism versus autonomy in medicine and psychiatry. *Psychiatric Annals* **13**:318–320, 1983.
9. Moore MS: Some myths about mental illness. *Arch Gen Psychiatry* **32**:1483–1497, 1975.
10. Rawls J: *A Theory of Justice*. Cambridge, Mass, Harvard University Press, 1971.
11. Culver CM, Gert, B: The morality of involuntary hospitalization, in *The Law-Medicine Relation: A Philosophical Critique*. Edited by Englehardt HT, Spicker SF. Boston, Reidel, 1979.
12. Reinert RE: A living will for a commitment hearing. *Hosp Community Psychiatry* **31**:857–858, 1980.
13. Szasz TS: The psychiatric will: a new mechanism for protecting persons against 'psychosis' and psychiatry. *Am Psychol* **37**:762–770, 1982.
14. Chodoff P, Peele R: The psychiatric will of Dr Szasz. *Hastings Cent Rep* **13**:11–13, 1983.
15. Toulmin S: The tyranny of principles. *Hastings Cent Rep* **11**:31–39, 1981.
16. Dyer A: The problem of the moral inversion in medical ethics, in *Ethical Dimensions of Clinical Medicine*. Edited by Robbins DA, Dyer AR. Springfield, Ill, Charles C Thomas, 1981.
17. Fletcher J: How do we go about making moral decisions? Ibid.
18. Hare R: The philosophical basis of psychiatric ethics, in *Psychiatric Ethics*. Edited by Bloch S, Chodoff P. New York, Oxford University Press, 1981.

The Case Against Suicide Prevention*

Thomas Szasz

Failure to prevent suicide is now one of the leading reasons for successful malpractice suits against mental health professionals and institutions. Although such a suit brought against a Protestant church and its ministers was, in the middle of the trial, dismissed by the judge on the grounds that it violated the freedom of religion clause of the First Amendment, an appellate court in California had earlier considered the case to be appropriate for jury trial, and after the trial ended, a member of the jury told the press, 'I feel strongly the church would have lost. I'd say at least 80 percent [of the jury] felt that' ('$1M Lawsuit,' 1985). Although psychiatrists and psychiatric hospitals now bear the brunt of such litigation, all mental health practitioners run the risk of being accused of professional negligence for failing to prevent a client's or patient's suicide. As I shall show, this situation is an inexorable consequence of the way suicide is now viewed by mental health professionals, lawyers, judges, and other educated persons.

Suicide: From Sin to Sickness

Insofar as suicide is perceived as immoral or undesirable, it is inevitable that people will hold someone or something responsible for it. In the history of Western civilization, the end of the Enlightenment – roughly the year 1800 – marks a dramatic change in the perception of suicide. Before that time, suicide was considered to be both a sin and a crime for which the actor was responsible; since then, suicide has increasingly been regarded as a manifestation of madness for which the actor is not responsible (Fedden, 1938; Sprott, 1961). Exemplifying both views, and the transformation of the former into the latter, are the following records of two suicides in the Louisiana colony in the 18th century. A man named Jean Baptiste, who killed himself in 1765, was punished by having his corpse tied to the back of a cart and dragged to the public square, where it was hung upside down from the scaffold for 24 hours. Another man, named André Sauvinien, who killed himself in 1752, was sentenced to similar degradations as well as to the seizure of all of his property. Probably because of the latter penalty, Sauvinien's family succeeded in having the superior council of the colony overturn the sentence on the ground that Sauvinien was insane when he killed himself ('Convicted,' 1982). In short, long before suicide was decriminalized, the responsibility of self-murderers for their deeds was annulled by declaring them, posthumously, *non compos mentis*.

Not surprisingly, many people immediately saw through this ruse. The famed English jurist William Blackstone (1755/1962) sounded this warning against such a 'reform':

But this excuse [of lunacy] ought not to be strained to the length to which our coroner's juries are apt to carry it, viz., that every act of suicide is an evidence of insanity; as if every man who acts contrary to reason had no reason at all; for the same argument would prove every other criminal *non compos*, as well as the self-murderer.

(p. 212)

Although Blackstone foresaw and forewarned against such use of the idea of insanity, it is precisely the elastic and strategic character of the concept that makes mental illness so attractive to the modern mind (Szasz, 1983).

Because the history of suicide is not germane to our present concerns, suffice it here to note that the definition of suicide as self-murder originates from a specifically Judeo-Christian cosmology in which God is viewed as both 'giving' and 'taking' each human being's life: Hence, taking one's own life is a most grievous offense against God. The modern 'scientific' view of suicide represents a secularized version of the same belief concerning the impermissibility of the act. 'We are now . . . in agreement,' declared Stanley Yolles in 1967, then the director of the National Institute of Mental Health, 'that this [suicide] is a public health matter and that the state should combat the disease of suicide' (pp. 16–17). The idea that anyone who kills himself or herself is crazy reinforces the negative valuation of the act, exonerates the suicide from wrongdoing, and excuses the survivors from punishing the deed.

The dominant image of suicide today – as a mental abnormality or illness (or as a symptom of such a condition) – explains why mental health professionals, philosophers, and ethicists, as well as laypersons, are all so skittish about suicide that it is virtually impossible to engage in a reasoned examination of this subject. If suicide is 'bad' because it injures society, then why is it not a crime (as it used to be) and punished accordingly by the state? If suicide is 'bad' because it injures the soul or spirit of the 'victim,' then why is it not a sin (as it used to be) and punished accordingly by the church? (Individuals who die by suicide are no longer denied a Christian burial.) Finally, if suicide is 'bad' because it injures both the suicide and others, like a disease (as people now seem to believe), then why is it not treated as such? Other potentially life-threatening diseases are treated by professionals who claim competence to treat such conditions and are formally accorded the privilege of doing so. Instead of seriously pondering such questions, people now prefer to explain away the problem of suicide by claiming to view it 'scientifically,' creating an image of it that combines the features not only of sin, sickness, and crime, but also of irrationality, incompetence, and insanity. The result is a stubborn unwillingness to view suicide as we view other morally freighted acts – like abortion or divorce – as good or bad, desirable or undesirable, depending on the circumstances in which they occur and the criteria by which they are judged.

Professional Liability for Suicide

If clients suffer harm that they attribute to their relationship with a professional, it does not automatically follow that the professional is guilty of negligence ('malpractice'). To successfully prosecute a suit for professional negligence, the plaintiff must show that the professional had a specific duty to perform (typically, because he or she voluntarily assumed said duty); that this duty was performed negligently or not at all; that the plaintiff suffered injuries as a result; and that the injury is directly attributable to the malperformance or nonperformance of the professional's duty (Warren, 1978, Vol. 2C, pp. 729–752).[1]

The main reason mental health professionals and mental institutions are found liable for a patient's or client's suicide is because they assume the duty (responsibility) of preventing suicide. It is important to emphasize

* Szasz, T.: The case against suicide prevention. *American Psychologist* **41**:806–812, 1986.

that, in our free society, people can (as a rule) choose to seek or not seek professional help and that professionals can (as a rule) choose to assume or not assume a particular duty. For example, a Catholic gynecologist, who wishes to obey the strictures of his or her faith, is free to refuse to perform an abortion; a neurosurgeon, burdened by astronomical malpractice insurance premiums, is free to refuse to perform surgery (and to limit his or her practice to neurology); and a mental health professional is free, if he or she so chooses, to refrain from assuming the duty of trying to prevent a patient's or client's suicide. It must, of course, be clear and explicit what duties one assumes or does not assume. An ophthalmologist cannot be successfully sued for not administering a Rorschach test, nor can a clinical psychologist for not performing an appendectomy. Similarly, mental health professionals and institutions could not be successfully sued for failing to prevent suicide if they explicitly eschewed assuming the duty of suicide prevention as a professional service. In short, as long as mental health professionals insist on imposing their services on unwilling recipients by claiming that the clients or patients are 'dangerous to themselves,' they should not be surprised that when clients or patients commit suicide (or otherwise injure themselves while under professional care), the clients or their families insist on holding the mental health professionals responsible for failing to fulfill their promises, and courts find them guilty of professional negligence. The fact that suicide prevention – with or without the cooperation of patients or clients – is one of the duties and services now specifically attributed to, accepted by, and expected from mental health professionals and institutions constitutes the context for my following remarks.

If troubled individuals confide their 'suicidal ideation' to a priest, the priest is not expected to intervene coercively to prevent their suicide. Neither is the lawyer who, especially if engaged in matrimonial disputes, often hears clients say such things as, 'If my wife (or husband) leaves me, I will kill myself', or 'If my child is taken from me, I will kill myself.' Mental health professionals, however, are expected to prevent suicide: If they are psychiatrists, they have the duty to commit the 'patient'; if they are psychologists, social workers, nurse practitioners, or lay therapists – who are not (or not yet) licensed, or even required, by the state to commit – then they are expected to make an appropriate referral to a physician (who may or may not be a psychiatrist) to forcibly prevent the patient's suicide. Although mental health professionals sometimes complain about the burden this duty entails, in the main they clearly enjoy the power and prestige that go along with it. After all, if psychiatrists did not want to engage in coercive suicide prevention, they could say so and could refuse to participate in such work. Similarly, if psychologists viewed coercive suicide prevention negatively, they too could say so, instead of seeking (as many do) the professional privilege and legal authority to involuntarily confine persons deemed to be dangerous to themselves.

I should like to add that, strictly speaking, I am opposed only to coercive methods of preventing, or trying to prevent, suicide. It would be hypocritical, however, to deny that in practice suicide prevention rests on the actual or potential use of force to restrain the would-be suicide: The term *prevention* itself, especially when coupled with *suicide*, implies coercion. Preventive medical measures, exemplified by vaccinating children against contagious diseases, are typically (although not necessarily) backed by the force of the law. Psychological counseling in connection with conflicts about pregnancy or marriage are thus properly called abortion and divorce *counseling*. It would be wrong – indeed, it would be absurd – to refer to such counseling as abortion or divorce prevention.

It is sobering to keep in mind in this connection that no one, not even the politically or professionally most powerful person, can serve all masters or good ends simultaneously. Each of us, like Jesus, must render unto God what is God's and unto Caesar what is Caesar's. To be sure, Jesus did not say what belongs to the one and what to the other. That is for us to decide, and we constantly make that decision, individually as moral agents and collectively as members of a profession and as citizens. Mental health professionals bear an especially heavy burden with respect to the moral and social dilemmas posed by suicide; hence, they must be especially thoughtful and forthright in coming down on one side or the other on the issue of (coercive) suicide prevention. Mental health professionals could do this together, combining their forces in a united front, or separately as differing factions, each clearly identified to the public by the professional duties they assume and decline. Psychiatrists, psychologists, social workers, family therapists, nurse practitioners, clinical sociologists – everyone who identifies himself or herself as a 'therapist' or member of a 'helping profession' – could thus choose to embrace coercive suicide prevention, as psychiatrists (qua physicians) typically do, or eschew such coercion, as the clergy (qua priests or ministers) typically do. Opting for either course would be defensible and moral. Trying to go both ways and claiming to serve the 'best interests' of both the individual and society, despite the dilemma that suicide poses, is impossible to achieve and immoral to attempt.

On Preventing Suicide

Why do we now give mental health professionals (especially psychiatrists) and judges special privileges and powers to intervene vis-à-vis suicidal persons? The reason is that in the modern 'scientifically enlightened' view, the person who threatens to commit suicide or actually does so is considered to be irrational or mentally ill (Szasz, 1971). However, there is neither philosophical nor empirical support for viewing suicide as different, in principle, from other acts, such as getting married.

The phrase 'suicide prevention' is itself a misleading slogan characteristic of our therapeutic age. Insofar as suicide is a physical possibility, there can be no suicide prevention; insofar as suicide is a fundamental right, there ought to be no such thing. If one person is to prevent another person from killing himself or herself, the former clearly cannot, and should not be expected to, accomplish that task unless he or she can exercise complete control over the suicidal person. But it is either impossible to do this, or would require reducing the so-called patient to a social state beneath that of a slave. The slave is compelled only to labor against his or her will, whereas the suicidal person would thus be compelled to live against his or her will. Such a life is not the life of a person or human being, but only that of a human organism or 'living human thing.'

This does not mean that individuals troubled by suicidal ideas or impulses should not be able to secure the assistance they seek, provided they can find others willing to render such assistance. It only means that expressions of so-called suicidal behavior – in any of their now-familiar psychopathological forms or shapes, such as 'suicidal ideation,' 'suicidal impulse,' 'suicide attempt,' and so forth – would no longer qualify as a justification for coercing the subject. Were such a policy adopted, people would have to make do with noncoercive methods of preventing suicide, just as they must now make do with noncoercive methods of preventing other forms of 'self-harming' actions – such as warnings from the Surgeon General on packages of cigarettes or diet soda.

No one can deny that policies aimed at preventing suicide by means of legal and psychiatric coercion imply a paternalistic attitude toward the 'client' or 'patient' and require giving certain privileges and powers to a special class of 'protectors' vis-à-vis a special class of 'victims.' Clearly, all such 'solutions' to human or social problems are purchased at the cost of creating the classic problem of 'Who shall guard the guardians?' The demonstrable harms generated by the mistakes and misuses of the powers of mental health professionals and judges (delegated to them on the grounds that they are 'protecting' suicidal persons from themselves) must be balanced against the alleged or ostensible benefits generated by coercive policies of suicide prevention. Inasmuch as we have no generally agreed upon criteria for adjudicating controversies concerning such a trade-off, our acceptance or rejection of coercive suicide prevention is perhaps best viewed as a manifestation of our moral and political (existential, religious) beliefs in certain ideas and their practical implications – such as free will and personal responsibility on the one hand and 'mental illness' and therapeutic paternalism on the other hand.

It is worth noting in this connection that psychiatrists now stigmatize and 'punish' suicide much as priests did before them, but with one important difference: The theory and practice of coercive suicide prevention also stigmatizes the psychiatrists. By assuming control over persons who want to kill themselves, psychiatrists patronize their patients and promise more than they can deliver, doubly compromising their integrity. By trying to prevent suicide, psychiatrists ally themselves with the police powers of the state and resort to coercion, thus defining themselves as foes rather than friends of individual liberty and responsibility. It is no wonder that policies of coercive suicide prevention are at once an indispensable source of prestige and power for psychiatrists and an embarrassing emblem of the fateful antagonism lurking in their relationship to 'mental patients.' That such policies should now also constitute a vast reservoir of complex legal problems for psychiatrists should not surprise us. Psychologists and social workers aspiring to share the privileges and powers of psychiatrists could do well to heed these considerations.

Assigning and Assuming Responsibility for Suicide

We are ready now to consider the question of the mental health professional's responsibility for the suicide of a client or patient. However, before examining the specific question of the mental health professional's responsibility for the so-called suicidal patient, let us clarify what we mean, more generally, when we speak of one person's responsibility for another, especially of a professional person's responsibility for a client or patient. We use the term *responsible* to describe a person's accountability for the conduct or welfare of others or himself or herself. For example, parents are responsible for their children (especially when the children are young), whereas competent adults are responsible for themselves.

The idea of responsibility is intertwined with two other concepts: liberty and control. Liberty and responsibility are, in fact, two sides of the same coin. Ordinarily, we assume that adults are moral agents endowed with free will; that is, they choose their behavior from among a range of options, large or small. We also assume that they are responsible for their actions; that is, they are praised or blamed, rewarded or punished, depending on whether their conduct is judged to be good or bad.

Where there is no freedom, there is no responsibility: We do not hold infants responsible for their behavior; duress is a complete excuse in the criminal law; and so forth. And where there is no control, there can be no responsibility: A person cannot be held responsible for something he or she does not control. Asserting that 'X is responsible for Y' (for Y's welfare, health, not committing suicide, and so on) is tantamount to asserting that X can, and indeed must, have enough control over Y to bring about the desired condition of Y. This is why persons who want to assume control over others typically claim to be responsible for them (called 'paternalism') and why persons who want to reject responsibility for their own conduct typically claim to have no control over their actions (called 'mental illness').

These principles are recognized in countless contractual arrangements, as, for example, when a bank trustee is empowered to manage someone else's money or an anesthesiologist to put someone else to sleep. Such experts undertake to exercise a specific responsibility, for the proper discharge of which they are granted control over specific objects or functions (money, respiration, and so forth). In every such situation, the controllers become responsible for what they control, and only for what they control. It follows, then, that anyone who assumes the task of preventing another person from committing suicide must assume the most far-reaching control over that person's capacity to act. Because, in fact, it is virtually impossible to prevent the suicide of a person determined on killing himself or herself, and because forcibly imposed interventions to prevent suicide deprive the patient of liberty and dignity, the use of psychiatric coercion to prevent suicide is at once impractical and immoral. It should, of course, be noted that because children have neither the rights nor responsibilities of adults, and because, unlike adults, children are typically treated coercively by the medical system (as well as in other situations), we must always clearly distinguish between policies aimed at children and policies aimed at adults. The

principle of coercive paternalism obliterates this basic distinction. In this discussion, I shall be concerned only with *adult* suicidal persons and moreover only with those subjected to *involuntary* interventions. (Interventions by mental health professionals provided noncoercively for voluntary clients or patients pose no special conceptual or moral problems.)

Suicide and the Mental Health Professional

What, then, *is* the mental health professional's responsibility insofar as he or she deals with (counsels, ministers to, treats) suicidal clients or patients? What *should be* the clinician's responsibility in that situation? These are different questions, requiring different answers. To the first question, I would answer that the clinician's responsibility for his or her patient's suicide is whatever the law and social custom say it is. To the second I would answer that the clinician's responsibility vis-à-vis the suicidal patient should be the same as any other physician's or psychologist's vis-à-vis his or her competent adult patient or client. If the patient or client wants or is willing to accept help for 'being suicidal,' the mental health professional has a moral obligation – and, depending on the circumstances, perhaps also a legal obligation – to provide some sort of help for that person. However, if the patient or client does not want such help and actively rejects it, then the mental health professional's duty ought to be to leave him or her alone (or, perhaps, to try to persuade him or her to accept help).

In short, my position on *coercive suicide prevention* is similar to the abolitionist position on the death penalty. If people say, as many now do, that they are morally opposed to the judicial system's killing anyone, then it would be inconsistent for them to inquire into a defendant's criminal deeds to ascertain whether he or she should be executed. It would also be pointless for an interlocutor to try to change the speaker's mind by emphasizing the depravity of any particular criminal. I am similarly opposed, as a matter of principle, to coercive interventions – legally formalized and psychiatrically administered – vis-à-vis suicidal persons. The contention that the 'patient' or 'client' is 'psychotic' or 'treatable' is thus irrelevant to my argument.

A brief clarification of my views concerning the management of what are now considered to be especially difficult cases – such as the delirious or acutely psychotic person or the so-called impulsive suicide – may be in order here. Clearly, there are many situations, exemplified by that of the semiconscious postoperative patient, where restraining the person is an integral part of caring for him or her. Such restraint seems to me to be appropriate and justified because it is informal, of brief duration, and strictly limited to situations where there is strong objective evidence that the person's unusual behavior is caused by a demonstrable malfunctioning of his or her brain. It is important to bear in mind, however, that there is a vast difference between the informal restraint of a patient in a medical setting and the formal restraint of a patient under psychiatric auspices. No applicant for a driver's license, admission to college, or a job is asked 'Have you ever been restrained after general anesthesia?' but every such applicant is asked 'Have you ever been a patient in a mental hospital?' The personal and social consequences of legally formalized psychiatric 'protection' are too obvious and too complex for further discussion here. Concerning so-called impulsive suicide, suffice it to say that impulsiveness is a basic human trait, characteristic of childhood, which we are enjoined and expected to outgrow. Coercion is neither necessary nor particularly effective for moderating a person's impulsive desire, whether for suicide, marriage, or some other important enterprise. (Indeed, coercion is likely, in the long run, to make the person even more impulsive.) To be sure, it is easier and quicker to coerce than to truly care, because caring entails lavishing personal attention on the object of our affection and requires much effort and patience.

Inasmuch as my views on suicide prevention are contrary to the presently accepted views on it, I want to further clarify the issues by comparing my position on suicide to Justice Hugo Black's position on pornography. Before deciding whether to permit or prohibit the distribution of a particular item deemed by lower courts to be pornographic, it was the custom of the justices of the Supreme Court to view the evidence. Hugo Black refused to participate in such collective acts of judicial voyeurism. Why? Because he believed that it did not matter whether a particular book or film was or was not 'pornographic'; all that mattered was whether the Constitution, as he understood and interpreted it, authorized the government to prohibit the sale of such materials because, in the opinion of the law enforcement authorities, they were 'prurient.' Having concluded that the First Amendment protects the sale of pornographic and non-pornographic materials alike, Justice Black felt that there was no point in his viewing an allegedly pornographic film before deciding whether the Supreme Court should make its distribution illegal (Dunne, 1977, p. 356).

In other words, there is a fundamental difference between deciding what sort of social policy vis-à-vis pornography we approve or disapprove and deciding whether a particular film is pornographic. Similarly, there is a difference between deciding what sort of social policy vis-à-vis suicide we approve or disapprove and deciding whether a particular suicidal person is 'psychotic.' Accordingly, if on moral and political grounds we decide that we oppose a social policy authorizing coercive mental health interventions vis-à-vis so-called suicidal persons, then the mental state of any particular suicidal person becomes irrelevant to judging whether, in that specific case, such a policy should or should not be implemented. This does not mean that a suicidal person's mental state is irrelevant for other purposes; on the contrary, it is highly relevant for an intelligent pursuit of certain other tasks, for example, determining how best to help such a person noncoercively, what such help might entail or require, and whether we (as particular moral agents in a universe of many such agents) want to participate in such efforts.

I object to our present policies of suicide prevention because they downgrade the responsibility of the individual (who is typically called a 'patient' or 'client' even if he or she rejects such a role) for the conduct of his or her own life and death. Because I value individual liberty highly and am convinced that liberty and responsibility are indivisible, I want to enlarge the scope of liberty and responsibility. In the present instance, this means opposing policies of suicide prevention that minimize the responsibility of individuals for killing themselves and supporting policies that maximize their responsibility for doing so. In other words, we should make it more difficult for suicidal persons to reject responsibility for deliberately taking their own lives and for mental health professionals to assume responsibility for keeping such persons alive. To achieve this goal, we would have to hold every adult responsible for his or her behavior and, temporarily perhaps, make use of a 'psychiatric will' (a legal–psychiatric instrument that I have described elsewhere; Szasz. 1982). The adoption of such a will would symbolize the presumption that adults are responsible (when sane) for deciding how they want to be treated should they be deemed (because of mental illness, however diagnosed) to require coercive methods of suicide prevention. Such a mechanism would protect individuals from being coercively paternalized by mental health professionals, unless they themselves wanted to submit to specific involuntary interventions; it would also protect mental health professionals from being held responsible for the self-destructive actions of suicidal persons, unless they chose to assume such an obligation. Adopting such a mechanism would shift our policies of suicide prevention from coercive to contractual methods, restoring self-responsibility to all of the parties involved in the drama of suicide and its 'prevention.'

The Right to Suicide

In a free society a person is not only presumed to be innocent until proven guilty but also sane until proven insane.[2] This presumption has far-reaching implications, especially insofar as a person's right to his or her own body is concerned. Consider, for example, our contemporary attitude toward procreation. Whether a person creates another human life is now almost completely separated from 'nature.' Contraception and abortion are legal and widely accepted, and we possess biologically and morally complex tech-

niques of artificial fertilization and surrogate motherhood. The decision of creating or not creating new life has thus been rendered independent of many biological constraints and from most social constraints (such as marriage or the ability or willingness to support a child). The result is that having a child is now treated as if it were an inalienable right.

I submit that there is an instructive symmetry between procreation and suicide: One consists of multiplying one's life, the other of nullifying it, with both decisions and acts having a profound impact, for good or ill, on the actors, their families, and the society of which they form a part. In the case of procreation, we recognize the moral complexity; namely, that a newborn baby's life is infinitely precious, but that irresponsible procreation is dangerous, destructive of the welfare of both the individuals responsible for it and society. Nevertheless, we in the West, impose no coercive measures on anyone (not even on minors) to prevent procreation, as if procreation were never undesirable enough to warrant coercive measures to prevent it.

In contrast to procreation, when it comes to suicide we deny the moral complexity; namely, that although life is precious, disease, disability, and dishonor may render a person's life not worth living and thus may make suicide a blessing for himself or herself as well as for others and society. Nevertheless, we, in the West, impose coercive measures on every would-be suicide (even the hopelessly sick and very aged), as if suicide were never desirable enough to justify it.

The similarities between choosing procreation or contraception and choosing life or death – and the differences between our unwillingness to use coercion in the one case and our eagerness to use it in the other – become even more striking if we keep in mind that a man's impregnating a willing woman, a woman's allowing herself to become pregnant, and a person's committing suicide are all acts that lend themselves very poorly (if at all) to prevention by coercive sanctions. (As noted earlier, in order to be effective the sanctions must be so savage that those subject to them would rightly be regarded as less than fully human.)

All this points toward the desirability of according suicide the status of a basic human right (in its strict, political–philosophical sense). I do not mean that killing oneself is always good or praiseworthy; I mean only that the power of the state should not be legitimately invoked or deployed to prohibit or prevent persons from killing themselves.[3]

This distinction between the illegal and the immoral is, in fact, deeply ingrained in Anglo-American law. Some acts are thus regarded not only as crimes but also as violations of widely shared moral values. For example, the unprovoked killing of another person is a *malum in se*, a wrong in itself. Other acts are regarded as crimes because they violate existing laws without being immoral, for example, exceeding the speed limit by 10 miles per hour on the open road or harboring an illegal alien. Such an act is *malum prohibitum*, a wrong because it is prohibited. Finally, there are acts that only some people may consider wrongs, for example, the use of artificial methods of birth control or eating pork. In a secular society, such acts are not illegal but are, of course, against the precepts of one or another religion. In my opinion, some suicidal behavior – for example, causing a public disturbance by threatening to jump from a high building in the middle of the day – ought to be treated as wrongs in themselves. Other types of suicidal behavior, such as killing oneself with an illegally obtained drug or gun, ought to be treated as prohibited wrongs, and still others – for example, killing oneself to avoid great pain or suffering, without creating dependents who would be public charges – ought not to be treated as legal wrongs at all. (Mental health professionals, could, of course, repudiate all suicide, just as Catholic priests can repudiate all artificial birth control.) Further consideration of the subject of suicidal 'dangers' and 'threats' must await another occasion.

Thus, treating suicide as a right does not mean that we must accept committing suicide as a morally legitimate option; it means only that we must abstain from empowering agents of the state to coercively prevent it. Mental health professionals could then treat suicide as they treat, say, abortion – in other words, as an act they may approve or disapprove in general and may choose to counsel for or against in any particular case.

Suicide or Death Control?

The effort to seriously ponder the issue of suicide probes some of our most passionately held, but not universally shared, beliefs about ending our own lives. Is such an act like homicide and accordingly properly called 'suicide?' Or is it more like birth control and accordingly better termed 'death control'? The behavior of countless successful and prominent persons shows us unmistakably that most Americans view suicide ambivalently, as a dreaded enemy as well as a trusted friend.

The belief that it is the legitimate function of the state to coerce persons because they might kill themselves is a characteristically modern, quasi-therapeutic idea, catering at once to our craving for dependency and omnipotence. The result is an intricate web of interventions and institutions that have themselves become powerful engines of hypocrisy and seemingly indispensable mechanisms for satisfying human needs now buried in hidden agendas.

It has taken a long time to get mental health professionals deeply enmeshed in the suicide business, and it will take a long time to get them out of it. In the meantime, mental health professionals and their clients and patients are doomed to wander aimlessly in the existential–legal labyrinth generated by treating suicide as if it constituted a mental health problem. However, if we refuse to play a part in the drama of coercive suicide prevention, then we shall be sorely tempted to conclude that mental health professionals and their partners in suicide richly deserve each other and the torment each is so ready and eager to inflict on the other.

Notes

1   *Black's Law Dictionary* states that, 'As a technical term of the law, 'duty' signifies . . . that which is due from another person; that which a person owes to another. An obligation to do a thing' (Black, 1968, p. 595). How does a person or party incur such an obligation? In one or both of two ways: *explicitly*, by contracting for it, as airline companies do, for example, when they promise, in exchange for a sum of money, to transport a passenger from place A to place B; and *implicitly*, by promising to do so without causing injuries to the passengers during the flight.

2   This fundamental principle is now being eroded, due in no small part to the ideology of mental illness and the activities of mental health professionals. The far-advanced state of this erosion is exemplified by the fact that competent (sane), adult Americans now claim that they are not responsible for smoking cigarettes, that mental health professionals eagerly support this claim with 'expert' opinions and testimony, and that judges legitimize this claim by allowing smokers to sue tobacco companies for causing 'tobacco addiction' (Bean, 1985; Margolick, 1985). The belief that we can have liberty without responsibility is, of course, an illusion people are often unwilling to relinquish until it is too late to do so.

3   Asserting that X is a right does not mean that doing X is (always or sometimes or ever) good or praiseworthy, it means only that the power of the state cannot be legitimately invoked or deployed to prevent or prohibit doing X. For example, treating freedom of religion as a right does not compel us to accept abortion as a morally legitimate act; it compels us only to abstain from using the power of the state to impose that judgment on those who fail to impose it on themselves.

References

Bean, E. (1985, May 1). Cigarettes and cancer. Lawyers in U.S. gird to battle tobacco firms on liability. *The Wall Street Journal*, p. 1.

Black, H. C. (1968). *Black's law dictionary*. St. Paul, MN: West.

Blackstone, W. (1962). *Commentaries on the laws of England: Of public wrongs*. Boston: Beacon Press. (Original work published 1755–1765.)

Convicted of killing themselves. (1982, September 19). *Parade*, p. 23.

Dunne, G. T. (1977). *Hugo Black and the judicial revolution*. New York: Simon & Schuster.

Fedden, H. R. (1938). *Suicide: A social and historical study*. London: Peter Davies.

Margolick, D. (1985, March 15). Antismoking is encouraging suits against the tobacco industry. *The New York Times*, p. 15.

$1M lawsuit against clergy dismissed. (1985, May 18). *Syracuse Herald Journal*, p. A–11.

Sprott, S. E. (1961). *The English debate on suicide: From Donne to Hume*. Lasalle, IL: Open Court.

Szasz, T. S. (1971). The ethics of suicide. *The Antioch Review*, **31**, 7–17.

Szasz, T. S. (1982). The psychiatric will: A new mechanism for protecting persons against 'psychosis' and psychiatry. *American Psychologist*, **37**, 762–770.

Szasz, T. S. (1983). Mental illness as strategy. In P. Bean (Ed.), *Mental illness: Changes and trends* (pp. 93–113). Chichester, England: Wiley.

Warren, O. L. (1978). *Negligence in New York courts*. New York: Matthew Bender.

Yolles, S. F. (1967). The tragedy of suicide in the United States. In L. Yochelson (Ed.), *Symposium on suicide* (pp. 15–26). Washington, DC: George Washington University.

Incapacity to give informed consent owing to mental disorder*

C. W. Van Staden, C. Krüger

What renders some mentally disordered patients incapable of informed consent? It may be claimed, for example, that someone who is psychotic cannot give informed consent. This claim is over-inclusive, however, since it is based on the general clinical features implied by a diagnosis.[1,2] It is not based on the assessment of a particular patient's capacity to give consent, neither specifically for each intervention nor at the time when the consent has to be given. Such assessment may be guided by considering specific conditions necessary for informed consent, especially those that cannot be met owing to a mental disorder.

It is important to define with clarity these necessary conditions, for decisions have to be made routinely about a mentally disordered patient's capacity to give informed consent if clinical practice in psychiatry is to be ethically acceptable. We shall illustrate how clarity about conditions necessary for informed consent may be decisive clinically in the assessment of a patient's capacity to give informed consent.

We take it that a patient's consent is required for any medical intervention unless s/he is incapable of consenting, or unless the law requires a doctor to intervene even if against a patient's wishes.[3] But even when a doctor's intervention is required by law, it remains good ethical and clinical practice to obtain a patient's consent if at all possible.[4] For present purposes, the medical interventions for which informed consent is considered to be necessary are treatment interventions, participation in clinical research as well as, rarely addressed in the literature, mental and physical clinical examinations.

Necessary Conditions for Informed Consent

Notwithstanding standard conditions such as information,[5] trust,[6] and lack of coercion,[7] we shall confine the consideration of the conditions necessary for informed consent to those that typically cannot be met owing to mental disorder. Thus, they are presented not as sufficient conditions, but each of them being necessary. They are:

i) a mental disorder should not prevent a patient from *understanding* what s/he consents to;

ii) a mental disorder should not prevent a patient from *choosing* decisively for/against the intervention;

iii) a mental disorder should not prevent a patient from *communicating* his/her consent (presuming that at least reasonable steps have been taken to understand the patient's communication if present at all), and

iv) a mental disorder should not prevent a patient from *accepting* the need for a medical intervention.

The inability of some mentally disordered patients to meet the first three conditions is commonly cited.[8–14] For some disorders, these conditions are indeed appropriately identified as those which at times cannot be met owing to the mental disorder. Some mental disorders prevent patients from understanding the nature and purposes of a medical intervention, or

prevent patients from choosing decisively, or prevent patients from communicating their consent. Examples are dementia and learning disability of sufficient severity.[12] A manic episode or a major depressive episode, for example, may entail marked indifference, ambivalence, or indecisiveness, any of which may prevent a patient from choosing decisively. Psychotic illnesses may also cause patients significant difficulty in understanding the nature and purposes of a medical intervention, or in choosing, or communicating their consent, as found in – for example, hebephrenic schizophrenia with markedly disorganised thoughts.

The Mental Health Act Code of Practice, reflecting the law in England and Wales, emphasises a patient's *understanding* of the information about the proposed treatment, potential risks and benefits of treatment, and the consequences of not taking the treatment.[4] It also requires a patient to have the capacity to make a *choice*. The Law Commission, in its consultation paper on mental incapacity, and the British government also consider 'incapacity' in terms of 'understanding' and 'communication'.[8–10] They say a mentally disordered person should be considered unable to take a decision on medical treatment in question if s/he is 'unable to *understand* or retain the information relevant to the decision, unable to make a decision based on that information, or unable to communicate a decision'. Medical defence societies[15,16] and various papers[17–19] also take a patient's *understanding* of information about treatment as the main determinant of his/her capacity to give informed consent.

The main problem that renders some mentally disordered patients incapable of informed consent does not, however, involve these conditions. The problem is that mental disorder prevents some patients from accepting that they need a medical intervention. We see this particularly in patients suffering from psychotic illnesses such as schizophrenia. They may understand the treatment proposed but still decline or refuse it because, in their judgment, they are not ill or do not need treatment for their difficulties. For example, a patient suffering from psychotic illness may assert adamantly: 'I understand that you think I am ill, I understand your proposed treatment and potential consequences of my taking or my not taking the treatment, but I am *not* ill', or: 'I know I am ill, I understand the proposed nature and purposes of the treatment, but I don't need treatment for it, because my illness will disappear in the near future when I will be God'. Such impaired judgment in patients suffering from psychotic illnesses is inherent to their illness. We clinicians commonly refer to this kind of judgment about their state of health as a 'lack of insight' into their condition.

That the patient's *acceptance* of the need for a medical intervention should *not* be prevented by his/her mental disorder, is a condition *necessary* for informed consent. If any patient, even if not mentally disordered, were to agree to treatment when s/he did not accept that treatment was warranted or necessary, it would cast serious doubt, to say the least, on whether such a patient actually gave informed consent for this intervention. Of course, there may be many reasons, valid or invalid, for not accepting that treatment is required. Clinical practice has it that a patient's lack of acceptance that treatment is necessary is dealt with by honouring the patient's choice irrespective of the reasons given.[20] Patient refusals are presumed to be valid exercises of autonomy. Congruently, the Law Commission has recommended a 'presumption against lack of capacity' and that the resulting

* Van Staden, C.W. and Kruger, C. Incapacity to give informed consent owing to mental disorder. *Journal of Medical Ethics* **29**:41–43, 2003.

decision should not be regarded as invalid just because it would not be made by a person with ordinary prudence'.[8]

However, in the case of a patient who cannot accept that an intervention is warranted or necessary, *owing to a mental disorder*, such a patient's choice is not autonomous because it is determined by the mental disorder. This also means that even if such a patient were to agree to an intervention, it would be farfetched to attest that s/he actually gave informed consent.

That a patient should *believe* the information about a proposed intervention, as suggested in case law,[21,22] is also not always the appropriate necessary condition to determine capacity to give informed consent. For example, a deluded patient may state: 'I believe the information you have given me about the proposed treatment, I believe the treatment may be beneficial for some and even for me, but I shall not take it because it does not befit me, being royalty from outer space, to take the medicine from common humans'.

Of course, mental disorder does not necessarily prevent a patient from accepting his/her illness and the need for a medical intervention. Many patients, including those suffering from psychotic illnesses, do accept their illness and the need for medical intervention. And, while some may not realise the full extent of their illness, they can none the less give informed consent.

The clinician may find it helpful to have the above list of four necessary conditions at hand when questions arise about a patient's capacity to give consent. It may be helpful in decisions about specific treatments. For example, say consent is sought to proceed with electro-convulsive treatment (ECT) for a severely depressed patient who suffers from the Cotard's delusion that he is dead already and who therefore considers treatment to be futile. Say the patient *understands* what he consents to – that is ECT, he *communicates* his decision to go ahead with the ECT, and he has *chosen to* follow the recommended advice. He thus meets the first three conditions necessary for informed consent. He will still not be capable of giving informed consent to the ECT, however, because his mental illness prevents him from accepting that he requires treatment.

The list of four necessary conditions may also be helpful in decisions about a patient's capacity to consent to participation in research. For example, a patient who does not accept, owing to his/her mental disorder, that s/he requires treatment is also incapable of consenting to participation in research on medication for his/her illness. This is the case even though s/he understands the nature and potential consequences of the research, s/he chooses to participate, and communicates his/her willingness to participate. The reason is that his/her mental illness causes him/her to refute the need for efficacious (non-placebo) treatment. S/he might even think that his/her participating in the research serves to prove that treatment is not really necessary. An argument against this stance might claim that it is not necessary that this patient accept the need for treatment, because a healthy person may consent to the use of research medication even though s/he does not need it. In fact, it is common practice to use healthy volunteers as controls in medication research. The difference, however, is that a healthy volunteer's acceptance of *not* requiring the treatment, is not affected by mental illness.

The capacity of a mentally ill patient to give informed consent for a mental and physical clinical examination is a difficult issue practically, rarely addressed in the literature. The problem is that it is hardly possible for a clinician to assess a mentally ill patient's capacity to give informed consent for a clinical examination until s/he has examined the mental state of the patient. Practically, this dilemma is eased in most civilised countries by provisions of law – for example, a mental health act, which may order or require a doctor to examine a patient even without a patient's consent. When informed consent for a mental and physical examination is required, though, the same conditions are necessary as for informed consent to treatment and participation in research. A mental disorder should not prevent a patient from understanding the nature and purpose of the examination, from choosing decisively whether to have it done or not to have it done, from communicating his/her consent, and from accepting that the examination is needed or warranted.

The Extent of Incapacity to Give Informed Consent

The Law Commission recommended, and the British government accepted, a 'functional approach' in determining whether a person has the capacity to make a particular decision.[8–10] This approach focuses on whether the individual is able to make a decision at the time when it has to be made. It allows for an individual to be incapable of making a particular decision at one point in time, but indeed capable to make it at another time – for example, after recovery. It also allows for situations where the individual is capable of making some decisions, but incapable of making others.

The conditions necessary to give informed consent, as they have been identified above, are concordant with this 'functional approach' to making decisions. Capacity to make decisions is not to be confused, however, with the capacity to give informed consent. Capacity to make decisions is required for someone to give informed consent, but informed consent requires more than capacity to make decisions. It requires – for example, trust and lack of coercion.[6,7] Moreover, informed consent requires more than mere capacity. As seen above, it requires that a mental disorder does not prevent 'actual' understanding of what is being consented to (rather than a mere capacity to understand).

Furthermore, incapacity to give informed consent extends to incapacity to give informed consent to medical interventions for mental as well as physical conditions. For example, say a patient were to agree to a medical intervention for his gangrenous leg, but his mental disorder prevented him from understanding the nature and purpose of the intervention, or prevented him from communicating his consent despite all practical steps to understand him, or prevented him from choosing decisively whether to have it done owing to severe ambivalence, or prevented him from accepting the need for the intervention. Then, it would plainly be mistaken to claim that this patient's assent to the intervention would constitute informed consent, for he fails, owing to mental disorder, to meet the conditions necessary for informed consent.

The same would apply in the following vignette. The patient suffered from paranoid schizophrenia with multiple delusions of persecutory, somatic, and grandiose types. He presented with a peptic ulcer that had ruptured into the abdominal cavity – a condition that required immediate life saving surgery. He understood the nature and the purpose of the proposed surgery, but he clearly communicated his choice not to have the surgery. On further inquiry, he revealed his delusions that he had magical spirits in his abdomen, which were the sources of his super human powers. He was certain that opening his abdomen by laparotomy would allow the magical spirits to escape, and without these sources of power he would die. He took it that the magical spirits would, in fact, heal the ruptured ulcer. Hence, his decision not to have had the surgery. Clearly, this patient's mental illness prevented his acceptance of the need for surgery. He could not give informed consent for the procedure. Even if he had chosen to have the surgery despite having these delusions, thus believing his cure would come from the magical spirits rather than surgery, he would still not be capable of giving informed consent. His illness would still prevent his acceptance of the real need for the surgery.

Similarly, say a patient were to agree to participate in research on the treatment of an acute myocardial infarction, but his/her mental disorder prevented him/her from understanding the nature and purpose of the research, or from communicating his/her consent to participate in the research, or from choosing to participate in the research, or prevented him/her from accepting that s/he did *not* have to participate in the research. Certainly, such a patient's assent would not constitute informed consent.

Incapacity to give informed consent to be examined is also not confined to examinations for mental disorders. For example, when a patient who suffers from advanced dementia does not understand the nature and purpose of, say, a genital examination, he/she cannot give informed consent for this (physical) examination.

A patient's incapacity to give informed consent to one intervention should not be assumed to imply incapacity to give consent to *all* medical interventions. It is well established in ethics and law that a patient may be incapable of giving consent to one intervention but capable of giving consent to another.[21] For example, a patient suffering from schizophrenia may be capable of giving informed consent to the treatment of his/her diabetes but not to the treatment for his/her schizophrenia (or vice versa). Simply, a patient may meet the conditions necessary to give informed consent to the one intervention but not to the other. Thus, each proposed intervention would require an assessment of the particular patient's capacity to give informed consent for that specific intervention.

The same is true of capacity in other respects, and particularly regarding performing actions. For example, a patient may be incapable of giving informed consent owing to his/her mental disorder, yet be capable of another action, say, making a cup of tea.

By acknowledging that incapacity to give informed consent does not necessarily imply incapacity to perform other actions, however, another clinical and ethical problem is laid bare: even if a patient is incapable of giving informed consent owing to a mental disorder, the question remains whether this patient is also incapable of the actions of *declining* or even *refusing* a medical intervention.

For practical purposes, the case may usually be that if a patient is incapable of giving informed consent, this patient would also be incapable of declining or refusing intervention. Nonetheless, the conditions necessary for someone to be capable of declining or refusing a medical intervention are not quite the same as the conditions necessary for giving informed consent. Consider the role of understanding: one might be capable of refusing an intervention without understanding the intervention. For example, one could refuse the hawker who approaches you even before you know what he actually wants (to sell). It could therefore be worth while teasing out, similarly to the present paper, the conditions necessary to decline or refuse a medical intervention, especially those conditions that cannot be met owing to a mental disorder.

In conclusion, the clinical assessment of a particular patient's capacity to give informed consent in a case of mental disorder is better informed by the consideration of conditions necessary to give informed consent than by making inferences from the general features implied by a specific diagnosis. An assessment of a particular patient's capacity to give informed consent by the consideration of conditions necessary to give informed consent may remain difficult clinically, yet such an assessment may strengthen ethically a clinical decision about a mentally disordered patient's capacity to give informed consent.

References

1 **Royal College of Psychiatrists.** Guidelines for research ethics committees an psychiatric research involving human subjects. *Psychiatric Bulletin* 1990; **14**:48–6.

2 **Davies T.** Informed consent in psychiatric research. *British Journal of Psychiatry* 2001; **178**:379–98.

3 **Gendreau C.** The rights of psychiatric patients in the light of the principles announced by the United Nations: a recognition of the right to consent to treatment. *International Journal of law and Psychiatry* 1997; **20**:259–78.

4 **Department of Health and Welsh Office.** *Code of practice: Mental Health Act,* 1983. London: HMSO, 1993.

5 **Osborn DPJ.** Research and ethics: leaving exclusion behind. *Current Opinion in Psychiatry* 1999; **12**:601–4.

6 **Davies T.** Consent to treatment: trust matters as much as information. *Psychiatric Bulletin* 1997; **21**:200–1.

7 **Wing J.** Ethics in psychiatric research. In: Bloch 5, Chodoff P, Green SA, eds. *Psychiatric ethics* [3rd ed]. Oxford: Oxford University Press, **1999**:461–77.

8 **Law Commission.** *Mental incapacity.* London: HMSO, 1995. (Consultation paper no 231.)

9 **Lord Chancellor's Department.** *Who decides? Making decisions on behalf of mentally incapacitated adults: a consultation paper.* London: HMSO, 1997.

10 **Lord High Chancellor.** *Making decisions: the government's proposals for making decisions on behalf of mentally incapacitated adults.* London: The Stationery Office, 1999. (Cmnd 4465.)

11 **Brabbins C, Butler J, Bentall R.** Consent to neuroleptic medication for schizophrenia: clinical, ethical and legal issues. *British Journal of Psychiatry* 1996; **168**:540–4.

12 **Arscott K, Dagnan D, Kroese BS.** Assessing the ability of people with a learning disability to give informed consent to treatment. *Psychological Medicine* 1999; **29**:1367–75.

13 **Fulford KWM, Howse K.** Ethics of research with psychiatric patients: principles, problems and the primary responsibility of researchers. *Journal of Medical Ethics* 1993; **19**:85–91.

14 **Appelbaum PS, Grisso T.** Assessing patients' capacities to consent to treatment *New England Journal of Medicine* 1988; **319**:1635–9.

15 **Medical Protection Society.** *Consent and confidentiality.* London: Medical Protection Society, 1991.

16 **Medical Defence Union.** *Consent to treatment.* London: Medical Defence Union, 1992.

17 **Carpenter WT, Gold JM, Lahti AC,** *et al.* Decisional capacity for informed consent in schizophrenia research. *Archives of General Psychiatry* 2000; **57**:533–8.

18 **Appelbaum BC, Appelbaum PS, Grisso T.** Competence to consent to voluntary psychiatric hospitalization: a test of standard proposed by the American Psychiatric Association. *Psychiatric Services* 1998; **49**:1193–6.

19 **Appelbaum PS.** Missing the boat: competence and consent in psychiatric research. *American Journal of Psychiatry* 1998; **155**:1486–8.

20 **Beauchamp TL, Childress JF.** *Principles of biomedical ethics.* [5th ed] Oxford: Oxford University Press, 2001:160–2.

21 In Re C (adult: refusal of treatment) [1994] 1 WLR 290.

22 In Re MB (medical treatment) [1997] 2 FLR, CA.

The Ethics of Mandatory Community Treatment*

Mark R. Munetz, Patricia A. Galon and Frederick J. Frese III

The appropriate role of coercion in psychiatric treatment remains controversial. In recent years, the locus and focus of the controversy has shifted from hospitals to the community. Involuntary hospital confinement through civil commitment statutes is available in all states in the *United States*. By the 1970s, most states modified their commitment statutes to emphasize dangerousness as a major criterion for involuntary hospitalization. With such revisions, inpatient civil commitment is generally accepted as a necessary intervention for acutely ill individuals who present an imminent risk of harm to themselves or others because of mental illness. Patients confined as a result of the civil commitment process generally retain the right to refuse treatment in the hospital absent an emergency. Non-emergency treatment of a committed patient generally can be given only after the patient has been found, through an appropriate judicial or administrative process, to lack decision making capacity and therefore to be unable to give informed consent to treatment.

As patients with serious mental illness have largely moved from institutions to community settings during the past four decades, so too has most of the controversy about mandatory interventions with this population. There are at least three groups of people with serious mental illness who may be confronted with mandates to accept treatment: forensic psychiatric patients, mentally ill offenders, and patients being treated within the community mental health system who have no criminal justice system involvement (i.e., *civil patients*).

This article confines its consideration to the last group, focusing on patients with serious mental disorders (i.e., *schizophrenia* spectrum and *bipolar* and *major depressive* disorders) who are not necessarily involved with the criminal justice system but who do not voluntarily adhere to treatment and who appear to be unable to live successfully in the community without coercive interventions. Such patients are often referred to as revolving-door patients. For such patients, mandatory community treatment has been proposed as an alternative to repeated inpatient hospitalizations in which involuntary treatment with medication is often required. It has been argued that there are patients with serious mental disorders who do not believe they are ill or need treatment, who when ill deteriorate to the point of meeting involuntary commitment criteria, who respond well to treatment when treated in the hospital, bur who repeatedly discontinue treatment after discharge and repeat the cycle, again and again. For such patients, mandatory outpatient treatment has been proposed as a less restrictive alternative to repeated inpatient hospitalization. Mandatory outpatient treatment, which depending on the jurisdiction, may be provided under a commitment statute [outpatient commitment (OPC)], through conservatorship or limited guardianship, or through conditional release from a hospital, is a preventive intervention aimed at maintaining stability in a person who otherwise would predictably, based on a well-established history, become ill and commitable.[1]

According to the recent American Psychiatric Association (APA) Resource Document on Mandatory Outpatient Treatment,[1] such *treatment is permitted* by *statute in 40 states* and the District of Columbia. While mandatory outpatient treatment is not implemented systematically in many states where it is permitted, a number of states are *actively looking* at enacting or amending statutes to implement mandatory outpatient treatment. The recent passage of *Kendra's Law* in New York and the ongoing advocacy of OPC by groups like the Treatment Advocacy Center have brought the debate about OPC to prominence. Position statements representing two sides of the debate nicely highlight the controversy. The National Alliance for the Mentally Ill *(NAMI)*,[2] in its policy statement on OPC states: 'Court ordered outpatient treatment should be considered as a less restrictive, more beneficial, and less costly alternative to involuntary inpatient treatment.' The Bazelon Center[3] in counterpoint states:

Outpatient commitment laws – statutes authorizing courts to require an individual to accept outpatient mental health treatment – are being proposed as a solution to the problem of people with mental illness in jails, homeless on the streets or engaging in violence. In addition to an unacceptable infringement of individuals' constitutional rights, such laws are a simplistic response that cannot compensate for the lack of appropriate and effective services in the community.[3]

While consumer advocates have been characterized historically as opposing coercive treatment, it is increasingly apparent that individuals with serious mental disorders themselves have a spectrum of opinions similar to those of the community at large.[4] Increasingly, there are vocal consumer advocates in support of mandatory community treatment, along with those who oppose such interventions.

Whether mandatory community treatment can be an ethical intervention for some individuals with a serious mental disorder is the focus of the remainder of this article, along with some specific matters related to the ethics of such treatment.

The authors believe that, when used judiciously, mandatory community treatment is both ethically and clinically sound; but if used casually, coercive interventions can be clinically inappropriate and unethical. There are a variety of ethical approaches to the question of mandatory community treatment. Herein, three arguments will be reviewed in turn.

Rights-Based Versus Beneficence

Liberal individualism is one of the most powerful ethics arguments raised against coercive treatment. This rights-based theory provided the impetus in the 1970s to change civil commitment laws from a need-for-treatment standard to a standard of imminent dangerousness. Proponents of this theory declare that (the) right is before the good.[5] Liberalism occupies a near sacred position within Western democracies, and many believe 'that no part of the moral vocabulary has done more to protect the legitimate interests of citizens in political states' (Ref. 6, p 77). In this context liberalism does not refer to the current political philosophy but instead refers to a tradition of thought that emphasizes tolerance and respect for individual rights that spans the philosophical tradition from John Locke (17th century England) to John Rawls, a living American rights-based political and social

* Munetz, M.R., Galon, P.A. and Frese, F.J.: The ethics of mandatory community treatment. *Journal of the American Academy of Psychiatry and the Law* 31:173–183, 2003.

philosopher. Within the framework of liberalism, rights are justified claims that individuals and groups can make on others and the state.

Rights are divided into two categories: positive and negative. Positive rights are best described as entitlements, such as a free public education. Negative rights entail the right of individuals to be left alone. Negative rights, or freedom from interference, are viewed as more powerful claims than positive rights. Rights have been described as 'trumps' by the legal philosopher Ronald Dworkin.[7] The powerful position of rights in the Anglo-American tradition has been bolstered within the past 30 years by the predominance of liberal individualism theories in the fields of ethics, law, and political philosophy.

Two other essential features of the liberal theory of ethics are neutrality and equality. Neutrality describes the condition in which the state must tolerate differing conceptions of the good life or what gives value to life. Liberal neutrality is probably the most challenged aspect of liberalism when considering the ethics of involuntary treatment overall and involuntary outpatient treatment in particular. Equality, the final tenet of liberalism, implies equal access to rights and benefits in a society, as well as the provision that enforcing the law will not unduly burden any particular segment of society.

Clearly, our society greatly values individual freedom. Individuals have the right to make lawful decisions about all aspects of their life without undue intrusion from the state or others. The courts have emphasized the principle that 'every human being of adult years and sound mind has a right to determine what shall be done with his own body . . .' (Ref. 8, p 1). The legal doctrine of informed consent essentially elaborates the principle that, with certain exceptions, nothing can be done to one's body without explicit agreement after a careful review of the risks, benefits, and alternatives, including the alternative of doing nothing. Informed consent must be voluntary, knowing, and competent.[9]

Competence to make decisions (or the clinical term decisionmaking capacity) may be problematic among persons with serious mental disorders. Grisso and Appelbaum[10] in their MacArthur Foundation competency studies looked most systematically at this matter. They describe four tests of competence: evidencing a choice, understanding, reasoning, and appreciation. They found about a quarter of acutely ill, hospitalized patients with schizophrenia failed any one of these three tests: understanding, reasoning, and appreciation. When a compound standard was used requiring adequate performance in all three tests, results showed that over half had impaired decisionmaking capacity. Presumably, after treatment, a portion of these patients will regain decisionmaking capacity by the time of discharge from the hospital. This has not been well studied, but it is apparent that, despite treatment, a portion of patients have a more persistent lack of capacity. In a research context, Carpenter and associates[11] have shown that an educational intervention can be a remedy for impaired capacity to give informed consent to research in subjects with schizophrenia.

It is likely that a substantial portion of patients with a persistent lack of capacity are the people commonly referred to as lacking insight into their illnesses. Studies have demonstrated that response to treatment for psychosis is independent of insight; in other words, psychotic patients who do not appreciate that they are ill may, with treatment, have substantial improvement in psychotic symptoms such as delusions and hallucinations, but continue to believe that they are not ill.[12,13] Lack of insight into illness appears to overlap substantially with one of the tests for competency developed by Grisso and Appelbaum,[10] the appreciation test. This tests the ability 'to appreciate the significance for one's own situation of the information disclosed about the illness and possible treatments.' It appears that a patient who does not believe he/she is ill (i.e., who lacks insight) would fail the appreciation test and, on that basis, could be found to lack decision-making capacity. Recent evidence suggests that this unawareness of illness has a neurobiologic basis inherent in schizophrenia and is therefore more than defensive denial.[14–18] Accordingly, a strong argument can be made that there are patients with schizophrenia who meet the description of the revolving-door patient who cannot make an autonomous refusal. Their brain disorders prevent them from making an informed decision. In such cases, rights-based arguments appear to give way to the notion of beneficence, using the *parens patriae* powers of the state to *make decisions on* behalf of individuals who are unable to make informed decisions for themselves. A beneficence argument holds that in these circumstances the ethical solution is to develop a mechanism to assure that such patients get the treatment that they need. Without such imposed treatment, a patient is allowed to be a victim of his or her illness. More than two decades ago, in an essay, 'The Myth of Advocacy,' Alan Stone argued persuasively that advocating on behalf of such patient's right to refuse treatment is misguided advocacy at best.[19] Actions based on *parens patriae* are appropriate responses for persons who are unable to make decisions in their own best interest.

Critics who do not believe in the reality of schizophrenia are quick to point out the apparent circularity of clinician's reasoning in support of mandatory intervention. Critics argue that saying that a patient who denies he or she is ill does not have decision making capacity is tantamount to saying that if a patient does not agree with the doctor, then the patient is incompetent. If schizophrenia were not to have a biologic basis and if there were an acceptable alternative explanation (e.g., mislabeled social deviance or an appropriate response to an insane society) then such an argument might carry weight. However, today the evidence that schizophrenia (or the group of schizophrenias) is a brain-based disorder greatly weaken the critics' arguments. The argument is further weakened by the growing evidence that the lack of awareness of schizophrenia itself has a biologic basis, similar to the anosognosia in stroke patients.[18]

A beneficence approach supports the appropriateness of intervention for an individual who lacks decisionmaking capacity. In creating a process for an alternate decision maker, the question remains as to what standard should be used to make decisions on the impaired individual's behalf. Two approaches are possible: a substituted-judgment approach and a best-interest approach. A substituted-judgment approach requires that the assigned decision maker consent to the decision that the incapacitated individual would have made if he or she were competent. A best-interest approach requires only consideration of what the decision maker deems to be in the incapacitated person's best interest. The substituted-judgment approach appears to provide the possibility of maintaining greater autonomy. In cases in which the individual's values and opinions about his or her illness and treatment options were known during a time that the person clearly was a capable decision-maker, the use of a substituted judgment comes closest to a rights-based approach. Unfortunately for the patients who are most often candidates for mandatory outpatient treatment, their lack of decision making capacity is commonly long-standing. Therefore, it is extremely difficult to know what they would have wanted if competent. In such cases a best-interest standard appears to be the preferable option.

Utilitarianism

Utilitarianism, a consequentialist theory of ethics, has one basic principle, that of utility. It is most often defined as the greatest good for the greatest number. The effective use of a utilitarian argument in the instance of outpatient commitment requires appreciation that it is not used as a common sense, expedient approach to what some see as a social ill. Such an approach, sometimes termed hedonistic utilitarianism, does not appropriately inform the practice of mental health professionals in general or in a case-specific context. For example, the use of outpatient commitment solely for convenience or resource management at the cost of individual freedom is not acceptable. Nevertheless, the type of direct utilitarian approach that seeks to produce agent-neutral or intrinsic good, the type of good that rational people value, can legitimately inform public health policy positions. The utilitarian requirement of an objective assessment of overall interest and reasoned, fair choice to optimize good results for all involved parties is an acceptable alternative to a totally rights-based versus beneficent position.

There is evidence that delay of treatment of persons with severe mental illness may negatively affect recovery.[20,21] In addition, reports of the lifetime suicide rate, among those with major mental illnesses, range from 10 to 17 percent, compared with 1 percent in the general population.[22] Persons with chronic mental disorders are also more likely to neglect medical treatment for co-occurring illnesses, significantly reducing the length and quality of their lives.

Recently, there has been much discussion concerning the frequency of violence in the mentally ill and there have been several high profile cases that have intensified the interest in the use of outpatient commitment in the prevention of violence. The relationship of violence to mental illness is complex, but recent studies support the argument that the two are at least somewhat positively correlated. Torrey[22] notes three risk factors that increase the likelihood of violence in the mentally ill: a history of violence, substance abuse, and noncompliance with medication. To the extent that outpatient commitment could decrease the likelihood of noncompliance with medication and substance abuse, it might decrease the risk of violent behavior in committed individuals with such histories. It is likely that more mentally ill persons are victims of violence rather than perpetrators. The literature chronicles frequent reports of the homeless mentally ill being robbed, beaten, and sexually assaulted. Cognitive disorganization can leave such individuals particularly unable to defend themselves. Using a utilitarian framework of balancing goods would appear to favor the beneficent/paternalistic course. Because of the seriousness of the possible harms, the utilitarian is likely to believe that avoidance of those harms is preferable to preserving autonomy. When the risk of harm is slight, then it is likely the utilitarian would opt to preserve autonomy, because in most situations, self-determination promotes the greatest good. It is important to remember, in this instance, that the utilitarian is likely to favor the more intrusive beneficent option only if the results of the use of outpatient commitment indeed significantly reduce the risk of harm. That implies that outpatient commitment must demonstrate, on average, more positive outcomes to continue to be considered an appropriate utilitarian option. The APA Resource Document reports that a growing body of research demonstrates that the 'Use of mandatory outpatient treatment is strongly and consistently associated with reduced rates of rehospitalization, longer stays in the community, and increased treatment compliance among patients with severe and persistent mental illness' (Ref. 1, p 23). However, a recent Rand review of the empirical literature and the experience of eight states on the effectiveness of involuntary outpatient treatment conducted for the California legislature was more circumspect. The Rand researchers acknowledged that there 'is some evidence that the combination of court orders and intensive treatment' may reduce rates of hospitalization, violent behavior, and arrests but considering the complexity of an underfunded California mental health system they did not believe there were enough data to determine whether 'the development of an involuntary outpatient treatment system in California is worth the additional cost to mental health treatment systems, the courts, and law enforcement' (Ref. 22, p xx).

Communitarianism

A serious challenge to a rights-based argument against outpatient commitment can be derived from communitarian ethics. Communitarian ideals are rooted in the philosophical and political traditions of the 18th century Scottish philosopher David Hume, through the writings of Thomas Jefferson, to the present day in the works of Michael Sandel and Michael Walzer. Communitarians oppose the fundamental positions of liberalism, especially neutrality, as well as the current societal network of structures that support those ideals. Briefly, communitarians propose that ethical decision making should be based on promoting communal good, traditional practices, and cooperation. Another common thread among communitarians is the necessity of involvement in public life signified by increased participation in micro- and macrocommunities.

As noted earlier, part of the liberal objection to all types of involuntary treatment is based on the preservation of negative rights through noninterference. However, it is also based on the liberal notion of neutrality, described as the presumption that government or institutions must not presuppose any conception of the good life. The embodiment of policies, based on the liberal notion of neutrality, has ill served revolving-door patients. The affront that episodic, crisis-oriented treatment has caused the

community of families, treating professionals, and society at large forces communitarians to point to this situation as another example of how unrestrained liberalism has promoted moral harms. In challenging the exercise of the negative right to refuse treatment, the communitarian would be likely to note that an infringement (not a violation) of that right would be justified to promote the communal values of humanity, safety, and health promotion. Without question, the communitarian would require the community to develop an adequate treatment plan and resources as a response to those same values.

Communitarians continue their skepticism of liberalism, particularly neutrality, by questioning the impossible liberal ideal of the unencumbered self. This term refers to the position that ethics decisions must be made with a conscious effort to assure freedom from the influence of values that often inform such decisions, notably cultural, religious, social, or even professional values. Michael Sandel, a prominent communitarian, criticizes this idea noting: 'Despite its powerful appeal, the image is flawed. It cannot make sense of our experience nor account for commonly recognized obligations such as solidarity, family ties etc. . . . Such loyalties are not as some liberals contend, matters of sentiment rather than morality' (Ref. 24, p 13). Sandel also correctly notes that liberal notions of neutrality are also based on values. They are based on the values that liberals hold dear such as tolerance, freedom, and fairness. It is an equal violation of the principle of neutrality to promote liberal values in preference to communitarian values.[24] Descriptions abound in the literature describing the dire circumstances into which revolving-door patients sink between episodes of intensive involuntary treatment. They are often accompanied by incredulous accounts of lawyers defending the individual's rights to remain in such situations.[25] Sandel criticizes the liberal position on neutrality and equality noting: 'We have seen how problems in theory show up in practice . . . . Treating persons as freely choosing independent selves may fail to respect persons encumbered by convictions or life circumstances that do not permit the independence the liberal self image requires' (Ref. 24, p 116).

Communitarians, based on their convictions regarding traditional roles, are also likely to criticize mental health professionals for their reluctance to involve themselves in the care of persons requiring more legally intrusive interventions. They would be likely to view a reluctance to pursue individual treatment options that include the additional burdens of involuntary outpatient treatment as not fulfilling one's obligation as helper and healer. Based on the value of community participation, mental health professionals would be expected to pursue policies to facilitate the availability of effective treatment options that might include involuntary outpatient treatment. Finally, communitarians believe the route to true liberty does not begin with the defense of rights but in civil engagement in one's political and social community. Engagement in recovery, described later in this article, is one sphere of common interest in which persons with mental illness may choose to participate if afforded opportunities.

Having considered three ethical arguments about the appropriateness of mandatory community treatment we now turn to several specific issues when implementation of such interventions is considered.

How Long Should Mandatory Community Treatment Be Maintained?

In a recent large scale, methodologically sound study of outpatient commitment, the investigators found that for outpatient commitment to be effective, the commitment order must be maintained for more than 180 days, a longer duration than that required simply to stabilize the person.[26] However, based on a traditional interpretation of the concept of least restrictive alternative, a well-established value within rights-based theories, such lengthy interventions could not be supported. Some ethicists would challenge that such an interpretation of rights-based theory is superficial and not totally accurate.

Waithe[27] challenges the notion quite effectively in examining the writings of John Stuart Mill, a 19th century philosopher and an exemplar of rights-based theorists. She examines his consideration of the conditions that justify paternalism within his classic work, *On Liberty*, originally published in 1859.[28] Waithe's use of Mill's ideas in justifying a beneficence-based approach is particularly relevant because his work is often quoted by liberal individualists seeking to limit coercive forms of treatment. For example, Mill is cited in the *Lessard* decision, one of the most prominent cases in the change of commitment criteria from need for treatment to dangerousness.[29]

Briefly, Waithe[27] presents Mill's position as follows: The potentially paternalized must be morally nonresponsible for actions in the specific circumstances in which paternalism is contemplated. Mill references the mentally ill in the category of the morally nonresponsible. The second condition of morally defensible paternalism is that such individuals are about to cause harm to their own interests, notably those involving their ability to exercise their rights fully. The third condition is that the potentially paternalized will experience an enhancement in his or her capacity to self-govern or that further deterioration is prevented. The final condition is that the potential paternalization takes place in the least restrictive manner. Waithe believes that, based on the sum of the conditions outlined by Mill, he (Mill) would champion the form of treatment that, while the least restrictive, would be most conducive to the restoration of the paternalized person to the fullest capacity for self-government. In light of the research noted earlier, Mill's conditions, considered together, seem to permit the use of more restrictive but restorative treatment (i.e., longer term outpatient commitment) even if the less restrictive treatment regimen would be sufficient to stabilize the person. Waithe also believes that Mill's third condition clearly supports legal decisions concerning the right to treatment and wider latitude in choice of treatments. If there is good evidence that repeated but insufficient treatment episodes are not as effective as a prolonged period of outpatient commitment following stabilization, Mill would be likely to deem such repeated brief interventions as unjustified paternalism. Considering this, the current practice of repeated, brief, intense treatment for stabilization of revolving-door patients would appear less morally defensible than maintaining a more lengthy outpatient commitment.

What Are Appropriate Criteria for Mandatory Community Treatment?

The use of dangerousness as the primary criterion for mandatory community treatment is *problematic*.[30,31] While dangerousness criteria are appropriate when considering the need for involuntary confinement, their appropriateness is much less clear when considering outpatient treatment. If a person is imminently dangerous, a strong argument can be made for involuntary confinement. However, such a person, unless determined also to lack decision making capacity, can still refuse treatment. Confinement without treatment, for the protection of self or others, appears ethically justifiable only for short periods. For community treatment, in which treatment rather than confinement is the fundamental goal, there are three critical problems with a dangerousness approach: it contributes to stigma, it is an unsustainable argument over time, and it fails to permit mandatory treatment.

Requiring dangerousness in order for someone in need to receive mandatory outpatient treatment is at odds with efforts to reduce the stigma associated with serious mental illness. The dangerousness argument with outpatients, what might be called the 'but for treatment' argument, is hard to sustain for the length of time that a person needs mandatory treatment. The following is a typical scenario:

A patient with a well established history of repeated decompensations resulting eventually in dangerous behavior and inpatient commitment has been treated, stabilized, and discharged into the community under an outpatient commitment order. The treating psychiatrist believes the patient's continued success in the community is contingent on maintaining an outpatient commitment order. A request for continued commitment is filed with the court, and during the hearing the psychiatrist testifies that while the patient is not imminently dangerous, he would predictably become dangerous again 'but for treatment.'

While this argument may be appropriate shortly after an acute episode, as time passes it becomes increasingly difficult to sustain the argument that such a person remains dangerous.

With dangerousness as a criterion for commitment, whether inpatient or outpatient, there is not generally a finding of decisionmaking incapacity and, accordingly, mandatory treatment (e.g., with medication) is not included in the court order. This results in paradoxical and potentially deceitful court orders in which a patient is ordered for outpatient treatment that can be refused. The court and clinicians may imply, for example, that the patient must take medication, but that is not actually part of the commitment. An outpatient commitment order that is essentially a bluff, while often effective, is ethically suspect.[31–33] In such cases, no actual harm is done, but in light of the clinician's role obligation to be truthful, moral harm is perpetrated by such a bluff. Such actions create a sense of moral regret for the clinician acting in good faith. Demarco[34] notes that moral regret in such circumstances may be interpreted as a sign of a need for reform within the circumstances, obligations, or social/professional roles creating the dissonance.

For these reasons, capacity-based criteria for mandatory outpatient treatment appears to be a better alternative than dangerousness. Capacity-based approaches seem to be less stigmatizing, are sustainable over whatever period of time the individual is determined to lack decisionmaking capacity, and directly result in a substitute decisionmaking process to obtain consent for needed treatment. A capacity-based approach also appears to address another important concern that critics of mandatory community treatment raise – what is referred to as the 'problem of the slippery slope.'

The Problem of the Slippery Slope

There is great concern of how widely mandatory approaches to treatment will be used for individuals with serious mental disorders and how the concept of mandatory outpatient treatment might be expanded to other populations. Regarding individuals with serious mental disorders, the question of what proportion of the population is appropriate for mandatory treatment is a serious public policy issue for which there is not yet a clear answer. A mainstream view of ethics appears to be that it is that portion of the population with a serious mental disorder who persistently lack decisionmaking capacity beyond an acute episode of illness and who, without coercion, refuse needed treatment. The size of that population is unknown but is certainly open to empirical investigation. Studies to date, most prominently the MacArthur Foundation competency studies, provide data on the lack of capacity during an acute episode. Studies extending the methodology over time in the community, to our knowledge, have yet to be done.

When in the course of a patient's illness should mandatory interventions be tried? If mandatory treatment becomes readily available, might it be tried prematurely, before a person has had an opportunity to enter recovery on a voluntary basis? This appears to be a valid concern and requires that careful clinical consideration be given to criteria for mandatory community treatment. While elsewhere we have argued that mandatory treatment is not incompatible with a recovery paradigm, such interventions may complicate the therapeutic relationship and the recovery effort early in the course of a person's illness.[35] Geller[36] promulgated clinical guidelines that suggested mandatory outpatient interventions should be considered only when a person has demonstrated repeatedly an inability to live independently in the community. According to such guidelines, a person would not be a likely candidate for a court-ordered intervention following a first or second psychotic episode. Such determinations almost certainly must be made on a case-by-case basis, using clinical criteria with some flexibility. Lack of decisionmaking capacity may be necessary but not sufficient as a criterion for an involuntary community intervention.

A major criticism of mandatory community treatment is that it may be promoted as an alternative to a community's provision of adequate voluntary community services. It is clear that before mandatory community treatment can be considered, the community has to offer adequate mental health services to meet the needs of the population of patients with serious mental disorders. Mandatory treatment can in no way serve to fix an underfunded service system in which appropriate services are not available. Before a program of mandatory community treatment is put into place in a community, that community must have an appropriately functional mental health system. An ethical society must fulfill its obligation to provide sufficient support, both financial and political, to assure that an adequate and accessible system of services is available to meet the needs of its citizens with serious mental illness. Too often this obligation remains unfulfilled. On the other hand, since an ideal mental health system remains a largely unattained goal, it could be concluded that a system will rarely be ready to offer mandatory community treatment. A decision to keep the very sickest individuals in that community stuck in the revolving door would be ethically suspect.

If our society becomes comfortable with mandating treatment of people with serious and persistent mental illness, will this lead to expansion of mandated treatment into other populations? The concern that we will slide down such a slippery slope is widespread, especially if we are not careful with the criteria used for such interventions. If dangerousness, especially over the long term, and refusal of treatment are the primary criteria for mandatory treatment, can we not argue for inclusion of alcohol and other substance abusers, for which there may be effective interventions,[37] and sex-offenders, for whom the effective intervention may essentially be quarantine.[38] Taken to the extreme, it has been facetiously suggested that it is only a matter of time before mandatory treatment is required for nicotine addiction, obesity, diabetes, or any number of chronic medical conditions. While many non-mentally ill people with chronic conditions fail to comply with recommended interventions, often for no good reason, thereby putting themselves at long term health risk, few could be considered to lack the capacity to make an informed decision about such interventions. Careful use of decisionmaking incapacity as a primary criterion for mandated intervention appears to reduce the basis for concern about sliding into overuse of mandatory interventions.

The Importance of Consumer Participation: Nothing About Us Without Us

The recovery approach to treatment of persons with serious mental illness has become increasingly influential during the past decade.[39–42] Indeed, states such as Wisconsin and Ohio have started to redesign their mental health systems so as to incorporate recovery values.[41] While there are various facets to the recovery model, one of the more salient features is that of empowerment of the consumer. Empowerment has been described as having many aspects. Some have suggested that, consonant with empowerment precepts, 'Consumers should play a key role in the development, implementation, and evaluation of all services' (Ref. 40, p 10).

As the mental health field increasingly embraces the recovery paradigm, consideration should be given to affording consumers a role in the decision making procedures of the involuntary treatment process (as well as other aspects of the mental health delivery system). Such consumer involvement would have the effect of increasing the collective experiential base of those participating in the process, helping to insure that decisionmakers remain sensitive to the various possible consequences of their actions for those most affected by their mandates.

However, in that consumer views on involuntary treatment are not monolithic,[42] care must be taken to ensure consumer input is representative and responsible. Frese[43] has reviewed the evolution of consumer advocacy activities during the past few decades. He points out that consumer advocates who have been primarily interested in increased consumer rights and liberties have tended to focus their advocacy efforts on opposing the use of forced treatment. In developing this stance, they have forged relationships with consumer rights attorneys and others who place a particularly high value on these considerations.

On the other hand, consumer advocates who place high value on the need for psychiatrically disabled persons to receive effective treatment, tend to be supportive of delivering such treatment, even in those circumstances in which such persons' disability interferes with their ability to appreciate that they have the disability.

Because the libertarian consumer advocates and their attorney allies have been so successful, the no-forced-treatment stance has been perceived as that of consumers as a whole. This is an unfortunate circumstance, one that fails to reflect the view and opinions of the growing number of consumer advocates who feel strongly that such a rights-oriented perspective tends to do serious injustice to those with the most severe psychiatric disabilities.

Consumer advocates in this latter category often find themselves comfortable working with the consumer/family advocacy organization NAMI. NAMI has many thousands of consumer members. Currently, such members make up fully one-fourth of the members of the NAMI Board of Directors.

Recently, consumers with these more treatment oriented views have become active as both board and staff members of the Treatment Advocacy Center (TAC). The TAC is a legal advocacy organization that has recently been established for the purpose of ensuring that effective treatment can be made available to those who are most seriously disabled with psychiatric conditions.

However, even consumer advocates who recognize the value of selected use of mandated treatment seldom argue that decisions concerning the employment of such an approach to treatment should be left entirely in the hands of mental health professionals or attorneys who have not themselves personally experienced these conditions.

Increasingly, the often-repeated refrain of the more treatment-focused consumer advocates has been, 'Nothing about us without us.' More recently, leaders of the rights-oriented consumer advocates have also begun to recognize the value of this position,[44] which demands consumer representation at all levels of the decisionmaking process, including those decisions concerning the use of forced treatment.

Mechanisms for possible consumer involvement in the mandatory treatment decision making process have been described.[31,35] Such mechanisms include the establishment of a consumer review panel and the possibility of employing persons who are in recovery from mental illness as guardians for those with similar but more severe disabilities.

Briefly described, a capacity review panel could be established that might, for example, consist of three members from the mental health community, with at least one member being a person who has personally experienced serious mental illness. The primary duty of such a panel would be to review decisions concerning mandatory treatment, perhaps before the issue of decisionmaking incapacity is presented at a formal hearing. Such inclusion of a recovered person ensures that these decisions are not made without the involvement of members of the class of persons who are, or have been, the recipients of treatments similar to those that could be mandated.

Likewise, involving a recovered consumer as the appointed guardian of an impaired person would serve a similar purpose. In this case, however, recovered persons could have even more direct and ongoing influence concerning mandated care. In such a role, a consumer guardian may help disabled persons accept treatment that they might otherwise refuse.

In any event, either of these two approaches serves a critical function by ensuring that decisions concerning mandated treatment are not left entirely in the hands of persons who have no direct personal experience as recipients of such treatments.

Conclusions

The authors have presented three ethics arguments that support the use of mandatory community treatment in appropriate circumstances for individuals with serious mental disorders. Mandatory outpatient treatment can never serve in place of a comprehensive, quality mental health service system and is not an effective solution for inadequately funded or structured systems. With an adequate system in place, however, we believe a program of mandatory community treatment may play an important role. In considering mandatory outpatient treatment, the authors argue that a capacity-based approach to determining the appropriateness of mandatory community treatment is preferable to a dangerousness-based approach; that clinical criteria with some flexibility should be developed so that mandatory community treatment is only used when less intrusive alternatives have failed; that mandatory community treatment should be implemented long enough to be effective; and that consumers must be involved in the ongoing development and implementation of mandatory outpatient treatment programs.

References

1   Gerbasi JB, Bonnie RJ, Binder RL: Resource document on mandatory outpatient treatment. *J Am Acad Psychiatry Law* 28:127–44, 2000.

2   National Alliance for the Mentally Ill: *Policy on involuntary commitment and court-ordered treatment*. Arlington. VA: Author, October, 1995.

3   Judge David A. Bazelon Center for Mental Health Law: *Position Statement on Involuntary Commitment*. Washington, DC: Author, 1999 (available at http://www.bazelon.org/involcom.html).

4   Frese FJ: The mental health consumer's perspective on mandatory treatment, in *Can Mandatory Treatment be Therapeutic? New Directions for Mental Health Services*. Number 75, Edited by Munetz MR. San Francisco: Jossey-Bass, 1997, pp 17–26.

5   Rawls J: *A Theory of Justice*. New York: Oxford University Press, 1971.

6   Beauchamp TL, Childress JF: *Principles of Biomedical Ethics*. New York: Oxford University Press, 1994.

7   Dworkin R: *Taking Rights Seriously* (ed 4). Cambridge, MA: Harvard University Press, 1977.

8   Schloendorff v. Society of N.Y. Hosp., 105 N.E. 92 (N.Y. 1914), overruled, *Bing v. Thunig*, 143 N.E.2d 3 (N.Y. 1957).

9   Appelbaum PS, Lidz CW, Meisel A: *Informed Consent: Legal Theory and Clinical Practice*. New York: Oxford University Press, 1987.

10 Grisso T, Appelbaum PS: Comparison of standards for assessing patients' capacities to make treatment decisions. *Am J Psychiatry* 152: 1033–7, 1995.

11 Carpenter WT, Gold JM, Lahti AC, *et al*: Decisional capacity for informed consent in schizophrenia research. *Arch Gen Psychiatry* 57:533–8, 2000.

12 McEvoy JP, Apperson LJ, Appelbaum PS. *et al*: Insight in schizophrenia: its relationship to acute psychopathology. *J Nerv Ment Dis* 177:43–7, 1989.

13 McEvoy JP: The relationship between insight in psychosis and compliance with medications, in *Insight and Psychosis*. Edited by Amador XF, David AS. New York: Oxford University Press, 1998, pp 289–306.

14 Lysaker PH, Bell MD, Bryson G, *et al*: Neurocognitive function and insight in schizophrenia: support for an association with impairments in executive function but not with impairments in global function. *Acta Psychiatry Scand* 97:297–301, 1997.

15 Flashman LA. McAllister T, Andreasen NC, *et al*: Smaller brain size associated with unawareness of illness in patients with schizophrenia. *Am J Psychiatry* 157:1167–9, 2000.

16 Young DA, Zakzanis KK Bailey C, *et al*: Further parameters of insight and neuropsychological deficit in schizophrenia and other chronic mental disease. *J Nerv Ment Dis* 186:44–50, 1998.

17 Mohamed S, Fleming S, Penn DL, *et al*: Insight in schizophrenia: its relationship to measures of executive functions. *J Nerv Ment Dis* 187: 525–31, 1999.

18 Keefe RSE: The neurobiology of disturbances of the self: autonoetic agnosia in schizophrenia, in *Insight and Psychosis*. Edited by Amador XF, David AS. New York: Oxford University Press, 1998, pp 142–73.

19 Stone AA: The myth of advocacy. *Hosp Community Psychiatry* 30:819–22, 1979.

20 Edwards J, Maude D, McGorry PD, *et al*: Prolonged recovery in first-episode psychosis. *Br J Psychiatry* (suppl) 172:107–16, 1998.

21 Harrow M, Sands JR, Silverstein ML, *et al*: Course and outcome for schizophrenia versus other psychotic patients: a longitudinal study. *Schizophr Bull* 23:287–303, 1997.

22 Torrey EF: *Out of the Shadows: Confronting America's Mental Illness Crisis*. New York: John Wiley & Sons, 1997.

23 Ridgely MS, Borum R, Petrila J: *The Effectiveness of Involuntary Outpatient Treatment: Empirical Evidence and Experience of Eight States*. Santa Monica, CA: RAND Health, RAND Institute of Civil Justice, 2001.

24 Sandel MJ: *Democracy's Discontent: America in Search of a Public Philosophy*. Cambridge, MA: The Belknap Press of Harvard University Press, 1996.

25 Isaac RJ, Armat VC: *Madness in the Streets: How Psychiatry and the Law Abandoned the Mentally Ill*. New York: The Free Press, 1990.

26 Swartz MS, Swanson JW, Wagner HR, *et al*: Can involuntary outpatient commitment reduce hospital recidivism? – findings from a randomized trial of severely mentally ill individuals. *Am J Psychiatry* 156:1968–75, 1999.

27 Waithe ME: Why Mill was for paternalism. *Int J Law Psychiatry* 6:101–11, 1983.

28 Mill JS: On liberty, in On Liberty (original work published in 1859). *Norton critical edition: annotated text sources and background criticism*. Edited by Spitz D. New York: Norton Co., 1975.

29 Lessard v. Schmidt, 349 F-Supp. 1078 (E.D. Wis. 1972).

30 Goldman HH: Book review of Coercion and Aggressive Community Treatment: A New Frontier in Mental Health Law (edited by Dennis DL, Monahan J). *Psychiatr Serv* 47:1270–1, 1996.

31 Munetz MR, Geller JL, Frese FJ: Commentary: capacity-based involuntary outpatient treatment. *J Am Acad Psychiatry Law* 28: 145–8, 2000.

32 Geller JL: The quandaries of enforced community treatment and unenforceable outpatient commitment statutes. *J Psychiatry Law* 14:149–58, 1986.

33 Borum R, Swartz M, Riley S, *et al*: Consumer perceptions of involuntary outpatient commitment statutes. *J Psychiatr Serv* 50:1489–91, 1999.

34 Demarco J: *Moral Theory: A Contemporary View*. Boston: Jones and Bartlert, 1996.

35 Munetz MR, Frese FJ: Getting ready for recovery: reconciling mandatory treatment with the recovery vision. *Psychiatr Rehabil J* 25:35–42, 2001.

36 Geller JL: Clinical guidelines for the use of involuntary outpatient treatment. *Hosp Community Psychiatry* 41:749–55, 1990.

37 Maynard C, Cox GB, Krupski A, *et al*: Utilization of services by persons discharged from involuntary chemical dependency treatment. *J Addict Dis* 19:83–93, 2000.

38 LaFond JQ: The future of involuntary civil commitment in the U.S.A. after *Kansas v. Hendricks. Behav Sci Law* 18:153–67, 2000.

39 Anthony W: Recovery from mental illness: the guiding vision of the mental health system in the 1990's. *Psychosoc Rehabil J* 16:11–23, 1992.

40 Beale V, Lambric T: The recovery concept: implementation in the mental health system, in *A Report by the Community Support Service Advisory Committee*. Columbus. OH: Ohio Department of Mental health, August 1995, pp 1–20.

41 Jacobson N, Greenley D: What is recovery? – a conceptual model and explication, *Psychiatr Serv* 52:482–5, 2001.

42 Frese FJ, Stanley J, Kress K, *et al*: Integrating evidence-based practices and the recovery model. *Psychiatr Serv* 52:1462–8, 2002.

43 Frese FJ: Advocacy, recovery, and the challenges of consumerism for schizophrenia. *Psychiatr Clin North Am* 21:233–49, 1998.

44 Pelka F: Shrink *rap. Mainstream*. June/July, 1998, pp 22–7.

Donaldson v. O'Connor*

F.2d – (5th Cir., decided April 26, 1974)

Before RIVES, WISDOM and MORGAN, Circuit Judges

WISDOM, Circuit Judge: This case requires us to decide for the first time the far-reaching question whether the Fourteenth Amendment guarantees a right to treatment to persons involuntarily civilly committed to state mental hospitals. The plaintiff-appellee, Kenneth Donaldson, was civilly committed to the Florida State Hospital at Chattahootchee in January 1957, diagnosed as a 'paranoid schizophrenic.' He remained in that hospital for the next fourteen and a half years. During that time he received little or no psychiatric care or treatment.

Donaldson contends that he had a constitutional right to receive treatment or to be released from the state hospital. In this action, filed February 24, 1971, he seeks damages under 42 U.S.C. § 1983[1] against five hospital and state mental health officials who allegedly deprived him of this constitutional right.[2] A jury returned a verdict of $28,500 in compensatory damages, and $10,000 in punitive damages against the two defendants-appellants, Dr. J. B. O'Connor and Dr. John Gumanis. Dr. O'Connor, as Acting Clinical Director of the Hospital, was Donaldson's attending physician from the time of his admission until mid-1959. He was Clinical Director of the Hospital from mid-1959 until late 1963, and Superintendent thereafter until his retirement February 1, 1971. Dr. John Gumanis was Donaldson's attending physician from the fall of 1959 until the spring of 1967. He was added as a defendant by an amended complaint filed April 20, 1972. The jury returned a verdict in favor of the other three defendants.

Gumanis and O'Connor bring separate appeals to this Court. They challenge the sufficiency of the evidence to support the jury verdict[3] and they contend that the Constitution does not guarantee a right to treatment to mental patients involuntarily civilly committed. Both argue, therefore, that the trial judge erred in denying a motion to dismiss for failure to state a claim and in instructing the jury that civilly committed mental patients have a constitutional right to treatment. In addition, Gumanis raises a number of lesser issues. We hold that the Fourteenth Amendment guarantees involuntarily civilly committed mental patients a right to treatment, and that the evidence was sufficient to support the verdict. We also reject the numerous lesser contentions advanced by Gumanis. Accordingly, we affirm the judgment in Donaldson's favor.

I

To put the legal issues in proper context as well as to discuss the defendants' challenge to the sufficiency of the evidence, it is essential to review the facts in unusual detail.

Donaldson was committed January 3, 1957, on the petition of his father and after a brief hearing before a county judge of Pinellas County, Florida. He was admitted to the Florida State Hospital twelve days later, and soon thereafter was diagnosed as a 'paranoid schizophrenic.' The committing judge told Donaldson that he was being sent to the hospital for 'a few weeks' to 'take some of this new medication,' after which the judge said that he was certain that Donaldson would be 'all right' and would 'come back here.' Donaldson was not released until July 31, 1971, after he had instituted this suit.

There is little dispute about the general nature of the conditions under which Donaldson was confined for almost fifteen years. Donaldson received no commonly accepted psychiatric treatment. Shortly after his first mental examination, Donaldson, a Christian Scientist, refused to take any medication or to submit to electroshock treatments, and he consistently refused to submit to either of these forms of therapy. No other therapy was offered. At trial, Gumanis mentioned 'recreational' and 'religious' therapy as forms of therapy given Donaldson; but this amounted to allowing Donaldson to attend church and to engage in recreational activities, privileges he probably would have been allowed in a prison. In the oral argument on appeal the appellants' counsel made much of what they called 'milieu therapy,' which they said was given Donaldson. This was nothing more than keeping Donaldson in a sheltered hospital 'milieu' with other mental patients; the defendants did not refer to anything specific about the 'milieu' that was in any special way therapeutic.[4] Donaldson was usually confined in a locked room, where, according to his testimony, there were about sixty beds, with little more room between beds than was necessary for a chair; his possessions were kept under the bed.

At night he was often wakened by some who had fits and by some 'who would torment other patients, screaming and hollering.' Then there was 'the fear, always the fear you have in your heart, I suppose, when you go to sleep that maybe somebody would jump on you during the night.' A third of the patients in the ward were criminals. Indeed, Donaldson testified, 'The entire operation of the ward was geared to criminal patients.'[5]

During his first ten years at the hospital, progress reports on his condition were irregularly entered at intervals averaging about one every two and a half months. During those first ten years, he requested grounds privileges and occupational therapy; his requests were denied. In short, he received only the kind of subsistence level custodial care he would have received in a prison, and perhaps less psychiatric treatment than a criminally committed inmate would have received.

At the time Donaldson was admitted to the hospital in 1957, O'Connor was Assistant Clinical Director of the hospital. As Assistant Clinical Director, he was in charge of the hospital's Department A, then the white male ward, where Donaldson was assigned upon his admission to the hospital. In that position, O'Connor was Donaldson's attending physician. At that time, Gumanis was a staff physician in Department A. On July 1, 1959, O'Connor became Clinical Director of the hospital, and in the fall of 1959, Gumanis was placed in charge of Department A, and became Donaldson's attending physician. O'Connor was promoted from the position of Clinical Director to the position of Superintendent July 30, 1963, and served as Superintendent until he retired February 1, 1971. Gumanis served as Donaldson's attending physician until April 18, 1967, when Donaldson was transferred to Department C, until that time the Negro male ward. After the transfer, Donaldson's attending physician was Dr. Israel Hanenson, the head of

Department C until Dr. Hanenson's death in the fall of 1970. After that, until his release, Donaldson's attending physician was Dr. Jesus Rodriguez.

Donaldson brought this suit while he was still a patient at the hospital. In his original complaint, Donaldson sought to bring this suit as a class action on behalf of all patients in the hospital's Department C. In addition to damages, to the plaintiff and to the class, the complaint sought habeas corpus relief directing the release of Donaldson and of the entire class, and sought broad declaratory and injunctive relief requiring the hospital to provide adequate psychiatric treatment.

After Donaldson's release, and after the district court dismissed the action as a class suit, Donaldson, on August 30, 1971, filed his First Amended Complaint. This complaint sought individual damages and renewed Donaldson's prayers for declaratory and injunctive relief to restrain the enforcement of Florida's civil commitment statutes unless Florida provided adequate treatment to its civilly committed mental patients. The complaint asked the district court to convene a three-judge district court to consider the plaintiff's attack on the constitutionality of the civil commitment statutes as they then operated. On November 30 however, the plaintiff in a memorandum brief abandoned the prayer that a three-judge court be convened. The prayers for injunctive and declaratory relief therefore were effectively eliminated from the case.

The key allegation in the amended complaint charged that the defendants O'Connor and Walls had 'acted in bad faith toward plaintiff and with intentional, malicious, and reckless disregard of his constitutional rights.' The complaint alleged examples of such actions, including the denial to Donaldson of grounds privileges; the refusal of the psychiatrists to speak with him, even at his own request; refusal or obstruction of his opportunities for out-of-state discharge, despite a recommendation by a staff conference that he be given such a discharge, and despite the presentation of a signed parental consent to such a discharge. The core of the charge, however, was that Walls and O'Connor acted intentionally and maliciously in 'confining Donaldson against his will, knowing that [he] was not physically dangerous to himself or others'; in confining him 'knowing that [he] was not receiving adequate treatment, and knowing that absent such treatment the period of his hospitalization would be prolonged'; and that they 'intentionally limit[ed] [his] "treatment" program to "custodial care" for the greater part of his hospitalization.' Corresponding to these allegations, the complaint sought $100,000 damages against Walls and O'Connor.

The trial began November 21, 1972, and continued for four days. The jury returned a verdict awarding Donaldson $17,000 in compensatory damages and $5,000 in punitive damages against O'Connor, and $11,500 in compensatory damages and $5,000 in punitive damages against Gumanis. The jury returned verdicts in favor of the other three defendants. From the judgment entered on this verdict, Gumanis and O'Connor appeal.

The trial centered, of course, upon the conditions of Donaldson's confinement and upon the defendants' behavior toward Donaldson. On the record as a whole, there was ample evidence to support the jury's reaching any or all of the conclusions set forth in the following subsections in Part I of this opinion.

A. The defendants unjustifiably withheld from Donaldson specific forms of treatment

The evidence establishes that there were at least three forms of treatment the defendants withheld from Donaldson.

First, he was denied grounds privileges. Since the purpose of hospitalization is to restore the capacity for independent community living, one of the most basic modes of treatment is giving a patient an increasing degree of independence and personal responsibility. One of the plaintiff's expert witnesses was Dr. Walter Fox, Director of the Arizona Mental Health Department and former president of the Association of Medical Superintendents of Mental Hospitals. He had interviewed Donaldson and examined his hospital record. Fox testified that confining Donaldson to a locked building, with no opportunity for grounds privileges was not 'consistent' with a treatment plan for a patient with Donaldson's history.

Gumanis denied Donaldson a privilege card, even after Donaldson had asked him for one. Fox testified that it would have been 'standard psychiatric practice' to extend grounds privileges to a patient of Donaldson's background, condition, and history. Gumanis, in his testimony at trial, could not give a convincing explanation for his refusal of grounds privileges to Donaldson.[6] At one point he sought to shift the responsibility for the refusal to O'Connor's shoulders, saying that he recalled having denied privileges after consultation with O'Connor. Later, he testified that at the time in question Donaldson had appeared to him to be 'really upset,' and that he had 'probably' made the decision to deny Donaldson a privilege card on his own.

Donaldson testified that soon after his transfer to Department C, Dr. Hanenson, the physician in charge of that department, gave him a privilege card.

The second form of treatment denied Donaldson was occupational therapy. Donaldson testified that Gumanis consistently refused to allow him to enter occupational therapy. This testimony was borne out by a progress note entered in Donaldson's hospital record January 17, 1964. Again, Fox testified that given what he called Donaldson's 'social history,' Donaldson would have been ideally suited to benefit from occupational therapy. According to Donaldson, Gumanis did not want him to go into occupational therapy, because Gumanis feared that he would learn touch-typing and would use this skill, in Donaldson's words, to 'write writs,' that is, to prepare habeas corpus petitions. Gumanis gave no reason why he denied Donaldson occupational therapy, although in the course of his testimony he did allude to the fact that he had done so. Not until Donaldson was transferred to Dr. Hanenson's care was he allowed to enter occupational therapy.

Third, the simplest and most routine form of psychiatric treatment is to have a patient talk with a psychiatrist. Donaldson testified that in the eighteen months O'Connor was in direct charge of his case, he spoke with O'Connor 'not more than six times,' and that the total time he spent talking to O'Connor did not consume more than one hour. He testified that in the eight and one-half years he spent under Gumanis' care, he did not speak with Gumanis more than a total of two hours – an average of about fourteen minutes a year. He testified that neither Gumanis nor O'Connor ever heeded his requests to discuss his case. On one occasion Gumanis said that he 'talked only to patients that he wanted to.' Gumanis did not recall that conversation. Once again, there was evidence to show that the situation improved when Donaldson was transferred to Dr. Hanenson's care. Donaldson testified that Hanenson managed to speak with him once a week, even though, according to Donaldson, patients were more numerous, psychiatrists fewer, and conditions worse in Hanenson's Department C than they had been in Gumanis' Department A.

B. The defendants recklessly failed to attend to and treat Donaldson at precisely those junctures when treatment could have most helped Donaldson recover and therefore be released

The jury could have concluded that Donaldson should have been marked, at his entrance to the hospital, as a prime candidate for an early release, and that the defendants acted recklessly in failing to treat or attend to him during the early stage of his confinement. Fox testified that, given Donaldson's history,[7] he should have been 'pegged' for an 'early discharge.' Moreover, a progress note entered by Gumanis after his first diagnostic interview with Donaldson, March 25, 1957, recorded that Donaldson 'appeared' to be 'in remission.' Gumanis defined 'remission' for the jury as a state 'when the patient does not express delusions or paranoid ideas,' and told the jury that it was hospital practice to release patients who were in remission. He testified that Donaldson was not released because he wanted to 'observe [Donaldson] further.' But after that interview the first progress note entered in Donaldson's hospital record is dated four months later; and the next report five months after that. Asked about this, Gumanis first replied, 'When you have 900 patients you do that'; later, he insisted that he had seen Donaldson frequently, but had not recorded progress notes after each observation. The jury, however, could have discounted this testimony and concluded that Gumanis acted wantonly in giving a patient who had appeared to be 'in remission' the same treatment he gave his 900 other patients.

C. The defendants wantonly, maliciously, or oppressively blocked efforts by responsible and interested friends and organizations to have Donaldson released to their custody

At issue here are two efforts made to secure Donaldson's release, one by Helping Hands, Inc., a Minneapolis organization which runs halfway houses for mental patients and John H. Lembcke, a college friend of Donaldson.

1. *The Helping Hands' attempt to obtain Donaldson's release.* Helping Hands made an inquiry to the hospital concerning the possibility of releasing Donaldson to its custody by a letter dated June 6, 1963:

We are interested in the possibility of signing out your patient, Kenneth Donaldson, and taking him as a resident at our halfway house at 3800 Columbus Avenue, Minneapolis. A maximum of six people live here, including our house mother, and myself, as president. At this time we have a room for Kenneth, who has interested us very much through his letters.

Enclosed with the letter was a brochure describing Helping Hands and a letter from the Minneapolis Clinic of Psychiatry and Neurology, stating that 'it would be impossible in any of our State Hospitals for a patient to receive the type of attention and care' provided at Helping Hands. The author of this letter pointed out that the woman identified by the letterhead as the founder and director of Helping Hands had 'rehabilitated well over a thousand over the years.' The letter requested information concerning Donaldson's age, health, and 'qualifications for work.'

The hospital responded June 17, 1973, in a letter signed by O'Connor, then Clinical Director of the hospital. It gave Donaldson's age, and answered inquiries concerning his health and qualifications for work with the bare statement that Donaldson was 'mentally incompetent at the present time.' The crisp concluding paragraph read:

Should he [Donaldson] be released from this Hospital, he will require very strict supervision, which he would not tolerate. Such a release would be to the parents. We see no prospects of his release to any third party at any time in the near future.

The jury could have decided that Gumanis and O'Connor acted wantonly and maliciously in issuing this response, and that this conduct foreclosed an opportunity for Donaldson to win back at least a part of his freedom, and to gain access to a level of psychiatric treatment unavailable to him at the Florida Hospital. Each of the defendants sought to shift the responsibility for sending this curt reply to the other's shoulders. They discussed the question in terms of whether hospital rules, in general, fixed responsibility for deciding whether a patient could be furloughed by the attending physician, or the Superintendent or Clinical Director; they did not discuss it in terms of their recollections of the particular event. The jury would have been justified in finding the two jointly responsible for the incident.

2. *The Lembcke attempt to obtain Donaldson's release.* John H. Lembcke, a certified public accountant, in Binghamton, New York, who is married and has three children, had been a classmate of Donaldson's at Syracuse University in the 1920's. On four occasions, Lembcke sought to have Donaldson released to his custody. The first was on July 3, 1964, when Lembcke informed the hospital that Donaldson was a friend of his, and inquired whether there were 'any conditions under which he would be released so that I could bring him back to New York State.' The same day the hospital received the letter, O'Connor pencilled a note to Gumanis that is attached to the letter in Donaldson's hospital record. The note said:

This man must not be well himself to want to get involved with someone like this patient, who even the recent visiting psychologist considered *dangerous* – Recommend turn it down.

Rich, the new Clinical Director, wrote Lembcke saying that Donaldson had 'shown no particular changes mentally,' and that if released he would 'require complete supervision.'

The second inquiry came by letter of November 27, 1964. Again O'Connor appended a note to Gumanis that is in the hospital records. This note gave three reasons for denying Lembcke's request to have Donaldson released to him: parental consent would be required; the patient 'would not stay with party mentioned'; and 'we don't know anything about party.' Gumanis prepared a letter, dated November 27 and again signed by Dr. Rich, 'advis[ing]' Lembcke that Donaldson would 'require further hospitalization.' The reply did not mention the three reasons for the denial set out in O'Connor's note, and did not request any further information from Lembcke, even though Lembcke in his November 23 letter had offered to provide any information the hospital should request.

The third attempt by Lembcke began with another letter to the hospital, dated December 21, 1965. According to Lembcke's testimony, the hospital responded by saying Donaldson could be released on two conditions: (1) that Lembcke would give Donaldson 'adequate supervision' so that the release would not be detrimental to his mental health; and (2) that Lembcke would secure parental permission for Donaldson to go to New York with Lembcke. In May 1966, Lembcke went to Florida, and met with Gumanis and O'Connor. While in Florida he saw Donaldson and obtained from Donaldson's parents a letter dated May 14, 1966, giving their consent to Donaldson's being released to him. Nothing happened. In his testimony Lembcke did not explain how or why he came to abandon this 1966 effort to secure his friend's release.

Lembcke's final and most important effort to secure Donaldson's release began in March 1968. On March 21, the General Staff, at a meeting attended by Gumanis and Hanenson but not by O'Connor, recommended Donaldson's release on a trial visit or out-of-state discharge. On March 24, Lembcke wrote the hospital renewing his offer to take Donaldson. On March 28, the hospital responded, imposing three conditions on Donaldson's release: (1) that Lembcke be willing to come for Donaldson; (2) that he be willing to supervise Donaldson; and (3) that he be willing to take Donaldson to a psychiatrist if Donaldson needed treatment. By letter of March 31, Lembcke acceded to these conditions. On April 4, the hospital replied with a letter imposing two additional conditions: (1) a detailed statement concerning the home supervision Donaldson would be given; and (2) written authorization for the release from Donaldson's parents. Lembcke wrote back giving the hospital the information about home supervision it requested. The hospital replied by again saying it would be necessary to obtain the written consent of Donaldson's parents.

On September 18, 1968, Lembcke wrote the hospital, enclosing a photocopy of the notarized written permission Donaldson's parents had signed May 14, 1966. The hospital responded in a letter dated September 24, signed by Dr. Rich. The letter informed Lembcke that Donaldson had been mentally ill for many years, that he 'still express[ed] delusional thinking' and that 'it would not be fair to you or to him to release him from the hospital at this time without adequate planning.' The letter added, in its final paragraph, that it would be necessary for the hospital to have more recent authorization from Donaldson's nearest relative than the one Lembcke had proffered. At that point, Lembcke gave up; whenever he met the conditions imposed by the hospital officials, new conditions were imposed. As he put it, 'after requirements were met, requirements were increased.'

One other facet of Lembcke's last attempt to secure Donaldson's release bears mention. As noted, O'Connor did not attend the Staff Conference which had recommended Donaldson's release March 21. O'Connor first learned of the hospital's recommendation in June, when Donaldson wrote to the Division Director of the hospital concerning the effort being made to release him. The division director forwarded the letter to O'Connor, who in turn forwarded it to Hanenson, asking for information concerning the proposed release. Hanenson responded with a memorandum dated June 17. Across the bottom of this memorandum, O'Connor pencilled in the remark, 'the record will show, I believe, we have been through this before and decided Mr. Lembcke would not properly supervise the patient.' It was not clear when O'Connor supposed this 'decision' to have been made, and in his deposition O'Connor was unable to locate any record of it in the hospital record. Moreover, there were suggestions in the record that Dr. O'Connor's conduct, in this and other respects, was influenced by his knowledge of Donaldson's history of writing letters to the press and to outside officials. From all of this evidence, the jury would have been justified in concluding that the frustration of Lembcke's effort to secure Donaldson's release in 1968 was entirely or primarily the result of O'Connor's bad faith intervention or, at the least, that the intervention was in reckless disregard of Donaldson's rights.

D. The defendants continued to confine Donaldson knowing he was not dangerous, or with reckless disregard for whether he was dangerous

Three of the plaintiff's expert witnesses – Fox, Raymond D. Flowler, Jr., Chairman of the Psychology Department at the University of Alabama and former President of both the Alabama and Southern Psychological Associations, and Julian Davis, Director of the Psychology Department at the Florida State Hospital – testified that they did not believe Donaldson was dangerous. Fox's and Flowler's opinions were based upon readings of the hospital records, Donaldson's psychological reports, Donaldson's past history, and raw data from his psychological examination. Lembcke testified that in his half century of having known Donaldson, he had never known Donaldson to be 'violent,' 'aggressive,' or 'belligerent'; that, on the contrary, he knew Donaldson to be a 'gentle' man. Dr. Walls testified that he did not believe Donaldson was physically dangerous; Gumanis himself conceded that he did not think Donaldson dangerous while Donaldson was in the hospital, although he said he could not predict what Donaldson would be like outside the hospital. There was no evidence in the record of Donaldson's ever having been violent in any way.

On the basis of this testimony the jury would have been justified in finding that Donaldson was not dangerous, and in inferring that the defendants knew him to be so.

E. The defendants did not do the best they could with available resources

As they did in the district court, the defendants on appeal pitch their defense in substantial part on their contention that they did the best they could with limited resources available to the state psychiatric hospital. Donaldson rebuts this contention, first, by pointing out the contrast between the treatment he received from the defendants and that he received from Hanenson. Hanenson allowed him grounds privileges and occupational therapy, spoke with him frequently, and within a year of taking charge of his case arranged a staff conference that recommended his release. Second, he relies on the testimony of Fox and the other experts to the effect that Gumanis and O'Connor failed to take steps that would have been open to them to take, even given the admittedly stark limitations on the resources available to them. We agree that these two considerations were a sufficient basis for the jury to reject the defendants' defense that they did the best they could with available resources.

We turn now to the novel and important question whether civilly committed mental patients have a constitutional right to treatment.

II

The theory of Donaldson's cause of action under section 1983 was set forth in three of the instructions given by the trial judge. The first, instruction number 34, was, a variation of a standard form 'boiler plate' instruction found in 2 Dewitt & Blackmer's Federal Jury Practice & Instructions, 1970, §87.05 (2d ed.) This instruction stated that there were four basic elements Donaldson had to prove to make out a claim under §1983: (1) that the defendants 'confined plaintiff against his will, knowing that he was not

mentally ill or dangerous, and knowing that if mentally ill he was not receiving treatment for his mental illness'; (2) that defendants 'then and there acted under the color of state law'; (3) that defendants' 'acts and conduct deprived the plaintiff of his federal constitutional right not to be denied his liberty without due process of law as that phrase is defined and explained in these instructions'; and (4) that the defendants' 'acts and conduct were the proximate cause of injury and consequent damage to the plaintiff.' The other two instructions, 37 and 38, were the relevant instructions 'defin[ing] and explain[ing]' the 'phrase,' 'federal constitutional right not to be denied or deprived of his liberty without due process of law,' within the meaning of instruction 34. These instructions told the jury:

37 You are instructed that a person who is involuntarily civilly committed to a mental hospital does have a constitutional right to receive such individual treatment as will give him a realistic opportunity to be cured or to improve his mental condition.

38 The purpose of involuntary hospitalization is treatment and not mere custodial care or punishment if a patient is not dangerous to himself or others. Without such treatment there is no justification, from a constitutional standpoint, for continued confinement.'

The propriety of these two instructions is the heart of the question raised by both O'Connor and Gumanis in their appeals.[8]

The question for decision, whether patients involuntarily civilly committed in state mental hospitals have a constitutional right to treatment, has never been addressed by any of the federal courts of appeals. Three district courts, however, have decided the question within the last three years, two of which held that there is a constitutional right to treatment.[9] The Court of Appeals for the District of Columbia Circuit, in a case decided eight years ago, took note in dictum of the existence and seriousness of the question, although in the same case the court held that the Hospitalization of the Mentally Ill Act of 1964[10] creates a *statutory* right to treatment on the part of mental patients in the District of Columbia.[11] The idea of a constitutional right to treatment has received an unusual amount of scholarly discussion and support,[12] and there is now an enormous range of precedent relevant to, although not squarely in point with, the issue.[13] The idea has been current at least since 1960, since the publication in the May 1960 issue of the American Bar Association Journal of an article by Dr. Morton Birnbaum, a forensic medical doctor now generally credited with being the father of the idea of a right to treatment.[14] The A.B.A. Journal editorially endorsed the idea shortly after the publication of Dr. Birnbaum's article.[15]

We hold that a person involuntarily civilly committed to a state mental hospital has a constitutional right to receive such individual treatment as will give him a reasonable opportunity to be cured or to improve his mental condition.

In reaching this result, we begin by noting the indisputable fact that civil commitment entails a 'massive curtailment of liberty' in the constitutional sense. Humphrey v. Cady, 1972, 405 U.S. 504, 509, 92 S. Ct. 1048, 31 L. Ed. 2d 394. The destruction of an individual's personal freedoms effected by civil commitment is scarcely less total than that effected by confinement in a penitentiary. Indeed, civil commitment, because it is for an indefinite term, may in some ways involve a more serious abridgement of personal freedom than imprisonment for commission of a crime usually does. Civil commitment involves stigmatizing the affected individuals, and the stigma attached, though in theory less severe than the stigma attached to criminal conviction, may in reality be as severe, or more so.[16] Since civil commitment involves deprivations of liberty of the kind with which the due process clause is frequently concerned, that clause has the major role in regulating government actions in this area.

Beyond this, the conclusion that the due process clause guarantees a right to treatment rests upon a two-part theory. The first part begins with the fundamental, and all but universally accepted, proposition that 'any non-trivial governmental abridgement of [any] freedom [which is part of the "liberty" the Fourteenth Amendment says shall be denied without due process of law] must be justified in terms of some "permissible governmental goal." ' Tribe, Foreword – Toward a Model of Roles in the Due

Process of Life and Law, 86 Harv. L. Rev. 1, 17 (1973). Once this 'fairly sweeping concept of substantive due process' is assumed, id. at 5 n. 26,[17] the next step is to ask precisely what government interests justify the massive abridgement of liberty civil commitment entails. Typically, three distinct grounds for civil commitment are recognized by state statutes: danger to self; danger to others; and need for treatment, or for 'care,' 'custody,' or 'supervision.' Jackson v. Indiana, 1972, 406 U.S. 715, 737, 92 S. Ct. 1845, 32 L. Ed. 2d 435; see Note, Civil Commitment of the Mentally Ill: Theories and Procedures, 1966, 79 Harv. L. Rev. 1288, 1289–97; Note, 1967, The Nascent Right to Treatment, 53 Va. L. Rev. 1134, 1138–39.[18] It is analytically useful to conceive of these grounds as falling into two categories; one a 'police power' rationale for confinement, the other a 'parens patriae' rationale.[19] Danger to others is a 'police power' rationale; need for care or treatment a 'parens patriae' rationale. Danger to self combines elements of both.

The key point of the first part of the theory of a due process right to treatment is that where, as in Donaldson's case, the rationale for confinement is the 'parens patriae' rationale that the patient is in need of treatment, the due process clause requires that minimally adequate treatment be in fact provided. This in turn requires that, at least for the nondangerous patient, constitutionally minimum standards of treatment be established and enforced. As Judge Johnson expressed in the Wyatt case: 'To deprive any citizen of his or her liberty upon the altruistic theory that the confinement is for humane therapeutic reasons and then fail to provide adequate treatment violates the very fundamentals of due process.' Wyatt v. Stickney, supra, 325 F. Supp. at 785. Or as Justice Cutter, speaking for the Supreme Judicial Court of Massachusetts, put it: 'Confinement of mentally ill persons, not found guilty of crime, without affording them reasonable treatment also raises serious questions of deprivation of liberty without due process of law. As we said in the Page case [citation omitted], of a statute permitting comparable confinement, "to be sustained as a nonpenal statute . . . it is necessary that the remedial aspect of confinement . . . have foundation in fact." ' Nason v. Superintendent, Bridgewater Hospital, 1968, 353 Mass: 604, 612, 233 N.E.2d 908, 913. This key step in the theory also draws considerable support from, if indeed it is not compelled by, the Supreme Court's recent decision in Jackson v. Indiana, 1972, 406 U.S. 715, 92 S. Ct. 1845, 32 L. Ed. 2d 435. In Jackson, the Supreme Court established the rule that '[a]t the least, due process requires that the nature and duration of commitment bear some reasonable relation to the purposes for which the individual is committed.' 406 U.S. at 738.[20] If the 'purpose' of commitment is treatment, and treatment is not provided, then the 'nature' of the commitment bears no 'reasonable relation' to its 'purpose,' and the constitutional rule of Jackson is violated.

This much represents the first part of the theory of a due process right to treatment; persons committed under what we have termed a parens patriae ground for commitment must be given treatment lest the involuntary commitment amount to an arbitrary exercise of government power proscribed by the due process clause. The second part of the theory draws no distinctions between persons committed under 'parens patriae' rationales and those committed under 'police power' rationales. This part begins with the recognition that, under our system of justice, long-term detention is, as a matter of due process, generally permitted only when an individual is (1) proved, in a proceeding subject to the rigorous constitutional limitations of the due process clause of the fourteenth amendment and the Bill of Rights, (2) to have committed a *specific act* defined as an offense against the state. See Powell v. Texas, 1968, 392 U.S. 514, 533, 542–543, 88 S. Ct. 2145, 20 L. Ed. 2d 1254 (Black, J., concurring). Moreover, detention, under the criminal process, is usually allowed only for a period of time explicitly fixed by the prisoner's sentence. The second part of the theory of a due process right to treatment is based on the principle that when the three central limitations on the government's power to detain – that detention be in retribution for a specific offense; that it be limited to a fixed term; and that it be permitted after a proceeding where fundamental procedural safeguards are observed – are absent, there must be a quid pro quo extended by the government to justify confinement.[21] And the quid pro quo most commonly recognized is the provision of rehabilitative treatment, or, where rehabilitation is impossible, minimally adequate

habilitation and care, beyond the subsistence level custodial care that would be provided in a penitentiary.[22]

This second part of the theory draws a wide range of support from a variety of precedents. The relevant cases have arisen in five major procedural contexts.

The earliest group of relevant cases consists of cases decided on habeas corpus petitions brought by citizens held under provisions for various kinds of 'nonpenal' confinement, who were being held in correctional facilities for prisoners convicted of crimes. These cases uniformly held that, where detention is 'nonpenal' in theory, the very least that is required is that the persons be confined in a facility other than a prison.[23]

Later cases expand the view of these cases by holding not only that persons held under provisions for 'nonpenal' confinement be held elsewhere than in a prison, but that they must be held in places where the conditions are *actually* therapeutic.[24]

The third line of relevant cases are those where the constitutionality of various modern 'nonpenal' statutes – notably sex-offender and defective-delinquent statutes – provide for the confinement of habitual criminal offenders to protect society and to provide rehabilitative care. The decisions have upheld such statutes, but the courts have usually added the proviso that the constitutionality of the statute is conditioned upon the *realization* of the statutory promise of rehabilitative treatment.[25]

The fourth set of cases, highlighted by Rouse v. Cameron[26] and Nason v. Superintendent of Bridgewater State Hospital,[27] consists of cases where individuals under confinement have brought habeas corpus petitions challenging their confinement on the ground that they were not receiving treatment. This is a diverse group of cases; in most of them, the challenge to confinement for lack of treatment has been combined with challenges brought on other grounds, and often the other grounds are the subject of the decisions. Among these cases, however, we have found none where any court has declared that no right to treatment exists, and we have found none explicitly recognizing a *constitutional* right to treatment. When they hold that there is a right to treatment, the cases usually either rest on statutory grounds, or are ambiguous as to whether they are resting upon statutory or constitutional grounds.[28] But in all cases, the courts have at least sustained the right of a petitioner to a hearing to develop the facts supporting his claim that he is not receiving treatment.[29]

Fifth, and last, among the groups of cases is the spate of recent cases brought as class actions in federal court, seeking broad forms of injunctive and declaratory relief requiring that adequate treatment be provided in state-run facilities. The cases have included attacks on conditions in many types of facilities – including facilities for the mentally ill,[30] the mentally retarded,[31] juvenile delinquents[32] or nondelinquent juveniles held as being 'persons in need of supervision.'[33]

Taken together, these five sets of cases constitute a near unanimous recognition that governments must afford a quid pro quo when they confine citizens in circumstances where the conventional limitations of the criminal process are inapplicable. These five groups include cases decided by all levels of courts – the Supreme Court,[34] the courts of appeals,[35] the federal district courts,[36] and the state courts.[37] One or another of them concerns each of the major forms of 'nonpenal confinement': from those with a heavy police power emphasis, such as confinement of sex offenders[38] or defective delinquents,[39] of persons acquitted by reason of insanity,[40] or of persons held incompetent to stand trial;[41] those with a heavy parens patriae emphasis, such as confinement of the mentally retarded,[42] or of juveniles;[43] and those – such as civil commitment of the mentally ill[44] – with elements of both rationales behind them.

The appellants argue strenuously that a right to constitutionally adequate treatment should not be recognized, because such a right cannot be governed by judicially manageable or ascertainable standards. In making the argument, they rely heavily upon the Northern District of Georgia's decision in Burnham v. Department of Public Health, 1972, 349 F. Supp. 1335, 1341–1343. In Burnham, the district judge held that a class action seeking declaratory and injunctive relief requiring the Georgia Department of Public Health to provide treatment at Georgia mental hospitals presented a nonjusticiable controversy. He quoted Baker v. Carr, 1962, 369 U.S. 186, 198, 82 S. Ct. 691, 700, 7 L. Ed. 2d 663, for the proposition that determining whether a suit was justiciable requires determining whether 'the duty asserted can be judicially identified and its breach judicially determined, and whether protection for the right asserted can be judicially molded.' 349 F. Supp. at 1341, quoting 369 U.S. at 198. He then cited the ambiguity of the dictionary definition of treatment, a passage from a law review article noting the fact that there are as many as forty different methods of psychotherapy,[45] and a passage from the Supreme Court's decision in Greenwood v. United States, 1956, 350 U.S. 366, 76 S. Ct. 410, 100 L. Ed. 412, concerning the 'tentativeness' and 'uncertainty' of 'professional judgment' in the mental health field.[46] He concluded: '[T]he claimed duty (i.e., to "adequately" or "constitutionally treat") defies judicial identity and therefore prohibits its breach from being judicially defined.' 349 F. Supp. at 1342.

The defendants' argument can be answered on two levels. First, we doubt whether, even if we were to concede that courts are incapable of formulating standards of adequate treatment in the abstract, that we could or should for that reason alone hold that no right to treatment can be recognized or enforced. There will be cases – and the case at bar is one – where it will be possible to make determination whether a given individual has been denied his right to treatment without formulating in the abstract what constitutes 'adequate' treatment. In this case, the jury properly could have concluded that Donaldson had been denied his rights simply by comparing the treatment he received while he was under Gumanis's and O'Connor's care with that he received while under Hanenson's care; or it could have concluded that Donaldson's rights had been violated on the basis of the evidence that the defendants obstructed his release even though they knew he was receiving no treatment. Neither judgment required any a priori determination of what constitutes or would have constituted adequate treatment, and of course no such determination was made.

We do not, however, concede that determining what constitutes adequate treatment is beyond the competence of the judiciary. In deciding in individual cases whether treatment is adequate, there are a number of devices open to the courts, as Judge Bazelon noted in discussing the implementation of the statutory right to treatment in the landmark case of Rouse v. Cameron:

But lack of finality [of professional judgment] cannot relieve the court of its duty to render an informed decision. Counsel for the patient and the government can be helpful in presenting pertinent data concerning standards for mental care, and, particularly when the patient is indigent and cannot present experts of his own, the court may appoint independent experts. Assistance might be obtained from such sources as the American Psychiatric Association, which has published standards and is continually engaged in studying the problems of mental care. The court could also consider inviting the psychiatric and legal communities to establish procedures by which expert assistance can be best provided. [Footnotes omitted].

373 F.2d at 457. There are by now many cases where courts have undertaken to determine whether treatment in an individual case is adequate or have ordered that determination to be made by a trial court.[47] Even in cases like Wyatt and Burnham, when courts are asked to undertake the more difficult task of fashioning institution-wide standards of adequacy, the task should not be beyond them. The experience of the Wyatt case bears this out. In Wyatt, agreement was reached among the parties on almost all of the minimum standards for adequate treatment ordered by the district court, and the defendants joined in submitting the standards to the district court. These stipulated standards were supported and supplemented by testimony from numerous expert witnesses. Moreover, there was a striking degree of consensus among the experts, including the experts presented by the defendants, as to the minimum standards for adequate treatment. The standards developed have not been challenged by the defendants in the appeal now pending before this Court. See Wyatt v. Stickney, M.D. Ala. 1972, 344 F. Supp. 373, 375–376.

In summary, we hold that where a nondangerous patient is involuntarily civilly committed to a state mental hospital, the only constitutionally permissible purpose of confinement is to provide treatment, and that such a patient has a constitutional right to such treatment as will help him in be

cured or to improve his mental condition. We hold that the district court did not err in so instructing the jury.

[In the balance of the opinion the court decided, inter alia: (1) that the evidence supported the jury's finding that the defendants did not act in good faith; (2) that Donaldson's claim was not barred by the statute of limitations; (3) that the district court did not err in refusing to instruct the jury that the defendants were entitled to a defense of quasi-judicial immunity under the Civil Rights Act; and, finally, (4) that the trial judge did not err in allowing the jury to award punitive damages.

Useful background facts concerning the Donaldson case are to be found in B. Ennis, Prisoners of Psychiatry: Mental Patients, Psychiatrists and the Law 83–108 (1972).]

Notes

1   42 U.S.C. §1983 provides: 'Every person who, under color of any statute, ordinance, regulation, custom, or usage, of any State or Territory, subjects, or causes to be subjected, any citizen of the United States or other person within the jurisdiction thereof to the deprivation of any rights, privileges, or immunities secured by the Constitution and laws, shall be liable to the party injured in an action at law, suit in equity, or other proper proceeding for redress.'

2   Except when the text clearly indicates otherwise, we use the term 'defendants' in this opinion to refer to Dr. Gumanis and Dr. O'Connor, against whom judgments were rendered. The other three who were sued were: Dr. Francis G. Walls, who became Acting Superintendent of the Hospital when O'Connor retired from that position in February 1971, and who held that position for about four months; Dr. Milton J. Hirschberg, who became permanent Superintendent, succeeding O'Connor, in June 1971: and Emmett S. Roberts, Secretary of the Department of Health and Rehabilitative Services in Florida at the time Donaldson filed his First Amended Complaint August 30, 1971.

3   The defendants raised the question of the sufficiency of the evidence on a motion for directed verdict made at the close of the plaintiff's evidence, and renewed at the close of all evidence. The defendants apparently did not move for judgment notwithstanding the verdict after the verdict was returned, but they did move for a new trial. The first ground they asserted in their motion for new trial was that '[t]he verdict is contrary to the clear weight of the evidence, which evidence showed that Defendants reasonably believed in good faith that due to his mental illness and need of treatment Plaintiff was properly confined'.

4   'Milieu therapy' is a frequent response by doctors and hospitals to claims by patients that they are receiving inadequate treatment. See Halpern, A Practicing Lawyer Views the Right to Treatment, 1969, 57 Geo. L.J. 782, 786–87, n. 19. Halpern discusses 'milieu therapy' in discussing Rouse v. Cameron, 1966, 125 U.S. App. D.C. 366, 373 F.2d 451, in which the District of Columbia Court of Appeals held that there was a statutory right to treatment. He notes that 'milieu therapy' is an 'amorphous and intangible' concept, 'the easiest therapeutic claim for an institution to assert and the most difficult for a patient to refute', Halpern, supra, at 787 n. 19.

5   Some of Donaldson's testimony relating the conditions under which he lived is worth quoting:
  'Q. Now, in the buildings you lived in Department A, were those buildings locked?
  A. Yes, sir.
  Q. Were the wards you lived on locked?
  A. Yes.
  Q. Were there metal enclosures on the windows?
  A. Yes, padlocks on each window.
  Q. Approximately how many beds were there in the rooms where you slept?
  A. Sixty some beds.
  Q. How close together were they?
  A. Some of the beds were touching, the sides touched, and others there was room enough to put a straight chair if we had had a chair.
  Q. Did you have chairs in the room you were in?

A. There wasn't a chair in the room I was in.

Q. All right, was there an outside exercise yard for your department?

A. Yes, there was one period in particular when nobody went out for two years.

Q. Now, Mr. Donaldson, you were civilly committed. You had not been charged with any crime, is that right?

A. That is right.

Q. Were there criminal patients on your ward?

A. There were criminal patients on the ward.

Q. Approximately what percent of the population on your ward were criminals?

A. Looking back, roughly, I would say a third. I do not know the figures for the whole department.

Q. Let's just talk about your ward.

A. Okay, I would say about a third in the wards I was in.

Q. Now, did you sleep in the same rooms as the criminal patients?

A. Yes.

Q. Did you get up at the same time?

A. Yes.

Q. Did you eat the same food?

A. Yes.

Q. In the same dining room?

A. Yes.

Q. Did you wear the same clothes?

A. Yes. The entire operation of the wards I was on was geared to the criminal patients.

Q. Let me ask you, were you treated any differently from the criminal patients?

A. I was treated worse than the criminal patients.

Q. In what sense were you treated worse?

A. The criminal patients got the attention of the doctors. Generally a doctor makes a report to the court every month.

Q. For the criminal?

A. On the criminal patients, and that would be a pretty heavy case load. It didn't give them time to see the ones who weren't criminal patients.

Q. Was there a place on the ward you had access to for keeping personal possessions?

A. No, not at that time.

Q. What did you do with your personal possessions?

A. I kept mine in a cedar box under the mattress of my bed.

Q. Was there a place in the wards where you could get some privacy?

A. No, not anytime in all of the years I was locked up.

Q. Were you able to get a good nights sleep?

A. No.

Q. Why not?

A. On all of the wards there was the same mixture of patients. There were some patients who had fits during the night. There were some patients who would torment other patients, screaming and hollering, and the fear, always the fear you have in your mind, I suppose, when you go to sleep that maybe somebody will jump on you during the night.

      They never did, but you think about those things. It was a lunatic asylum.'

6   Donaldson testified that he had once escaped from the hospital. This occurred around Christmastime 1957, shortly before the end of the first year Donaldson had spent at Florida State. The hospital records, however, did not show that a fear Donaldson would attempt to escape again motivated the denial of grounds privileges; nor have Gumanis and O'Connor asserted before this Court that such a fear was their reason for denying Donaldson a card.

7   Fourteen years before he was hospitalized in Florida, Donaldson had been hospitalized at the Marcy State Hospital in New York, with the same diagnosis as that made by the Florida doctors – 'paranoid schizophrenic'. On that occasion, Donaldson was released after three months.

8   As a threshold matter, Donaldson suggests that the objections to these instructions are not properly before this Court. He notes that the defendants did not object to that instruction either when the proposed instructions were discussed in chambers, or after the charge was read to the jury. The defendants did, however, object to what were then the plaintiff's proposed instructions 37 and 38 in a pretrial brief filed before the Court. There they asked that those instructions be replaced with an instruction that '[y]ou are instructed that a person who is committed to a mental hospital has a right to be released through judicial process when through no fault of his own treatment is not afforded and he is not dangerous to society or to himself'. The trial judge refused this request, and gave the two instructions as the plaintiffs had proposed them. It is settled that 'a failure to object may be disregarded if a party's position has previously been made clear to the court and it is plain that a further objection would be unavailing'. 9 C. Wright & A. Miller, Federal Practice & Procedure §2553 at 639–40; see, e.g., Mays v. Dealers Transit, 7 Cir. 1971, 441 F.2d 1344; Steinhauser v. Hertz Corp., 2 Cir. 1970, 421 F.2d 1169. We find that was the case here, and therefore we consider that the objections are properly before the Court.

9   Two cases hold that there is a right to treatment for civilly committed mentally ill patients. Wyatt v. Stickney, M.D. Ala. 1971, 325 F. Supp. 781, on submission of proposed standards by defendants, 334 F. Supp. 1341, enforced, 1972, 344 F. Supp. 373, 387, appeal docketed sub nom., Wyatt v. Aderholt, No. 72-2634, 5 Cir. Aug. 1, 1972; Stachulak v. Coughlin, N.D. Ill., 1973, 364 F. Supp. 686. One has held civilly committed mentally ill patients enjoy no right to treatment. Burnham v. Department of Public Health, N.D. Ga. 1972, 349 F. Supp. 1335, appeal docketed, No. 72-3110, 5 Cir., Oct. 4, 1972.

      A fourth case has recently held that civilly committed mentally retarded patients have a right to treatment. Welsch v. Likins, No. 4-72-Civ. 451, D. Minn. Feb. 15, 1974, – F. Supp. –.

10   D.C. Code Ann. §21–501.

11   Rouse v. Cameron, 1966, 125 U.S. App. D.C. 366, 373 F.2d 451. Chief Judge Bazelon wrote for the Court: 'Absence of treatment "might draw into question 'the constitutionality of [this] mandatory commitment section' as applied." (1) Lack of improvement raises a question of procedural due process where the commitment is under D.C. Code §24-301 rather than under the civil commitment statute, for under §24-301 commitment is summary, in contrast with civil commitment safeguards. It does not rest on any finding of present insanity and dangerousness but, on the contrary, on a jury's reasonable doubt that the defendant was sane when he committed the act charged. Commitment on this basis is permissible because of its humane therapeutic goals. (2) Had appellant been found criminally responsible, he could have been confined a year, at most, however dangerous he might have been. He has been confined four years and the end is not in sight. Since this difference rests only on need for treatment, a failure to supply treatment may raise a question of due process of law. It has also been suggested that a failure to supply treatment may violate the equal protection clause. (3) Indefinite commitment without treatment of one who has been found not criminally responsible may be so inhumane as to be "cruel and unusual punishment." [Footnotes and citations omitted.]' Id. at 453.

12   The landmark article in the field is Birnbaum, The Right to Treatment, 1960, 46 A.B.A. Journal 499. Much of the commentary in the area was stimulated by the Rouse decision. E.g., Symposium – The Right to Treatment, 1969, 57 Geo. L.J. 673 (11 articles, 218 pages); Bazelon, Implementing the Right to Treatment, 1969, 36 U. Chi. L. Rev. 742; Birnbaum, Some Remarks on 'The Right to Treatment,' 1971, 23 Ala. L. Rev. 623; Chambers, Alternatives to Civil Commitment of the Mentally Ill: Practical Guides and Constitutional Imperatives, 1969, 70 Mich. L. Rev. 1108; Katz, The Right to Treatment – An Enchanting Legal Fiction? 1969, U. Chi. L. Rev. 755; Drake, Enforcing the Right to Treatment: Wyatt v. Stickney. 1972, 10 Am. Crim. L. Rev. 587; Morris, 'Criminality' and the Right to Treatment, 1969, U. Chi. L. Rev. 784; Note, The Nascent Right to Treatment, 1967, 53 Va. L. Rev. 1134; Note, Civil Restraint, Mental Illness, and the Right to Treatment, 1967, 77 Yale L.J. 87; 80 Harv. L. Rev. 898 (1967).

13   See cases cited at nn. 23–44 infra.

14 Birnbaum, The Right to Treatment, 1960, 46 A.B.A.J. 499.

15 Editorial, A New Right, 1960, 46 A.B.A.J. 516.

16 On the recognition that stigmatization constitutes a deprivation of liberty in the constitutional sense, see Board of Regents v. Roth, 1972, 408 U.S. 564, 573, 92 S. Ct. 2701, 33 L. Ed. 2d 548, 558–559.

17 See also Ely, The Wages of Crying Wolf: A Comment on Roe v. Wade, 1973, 82 Yale L.J. 920, 935 & n. 91; Roe v. Wade, 1973, 410 U.S. 113, 172–173, 93 S. Ct. 705, 35 L. Ed. 2d 147 (Rehnquist, J., dissenting); Doe v. Bolton, 1973, 410 U.S. 179, 223, 93 S. Ct. 739, 35 L. Ed. 2d 201 (White, J., dissenting).

18 In Jackson, the Supreme Court, relying upon an American Bar Foundation study, found that in nine states the sole criterion for involuntary commitment was the danger to self or others; that in 18 other states the patient's need for care or treatment was an alternative basis; that the need for care or treatment was the sole basis in six other states; and a few states had no statutory criteria at all and 'presumably le[ft] the determination to judicial discretion'. 406 U.S. at 737 n. 19, citing American Bar Foundation, The Mentally Disabled and the Law (rev. ed. 1971) at 36–49.

19 See Note, The Nascent Right to Treatment, 1967, 53 Va. L. Rev. 1134, 1138–39.

20 Jackson involved a mentally defective deaf mute who was committed after the court determined that he was incompetent to stand trial. Since the mental and physical defects which were the cause of his inability were not susceptible to treatment and not likely to improve during his confinement, it was unlikely that he would ever become competent to stand trial. In the circumstances, the Supreme Court held that its rule that 'the nature and duration of commitment bear some reasonable relation to the purpose for which the individual is committed' permitted the state to confine Jackson under the provisions for the commitment of those found incompetent to stand trial only for 'the reasonable period of time necessary to determine whether there is a substantial probability that he will attain that capacity [to stand trial] in the foreseeable future'. It held further that even if it were determined that he was likely to become able to stand trial, 'his continued commitment [would have to be] justified by progress toward that goal'. 406 U.S. at 738.

21 'One theory is that commitment pursuant to civil statutes generally lacks the procedural safeguards afforded those charged with criminal offense. The constitutional justification for this abridgment of *procedural rights* is that the purpose of commitment is treatment.' (Emphasis supplied). Welsch v. Likins, No. 4-72-Civ. 451, D. Minn., Feb. 15, 1974, – F. Supp. – at –. See also Inmates of Boys' Training School v. Affleck, D.R.I. 1972, 346 F. Supp. 1354, 1368; Rouse v. Cameron, 1966, 125 U.S. App. D.C. 366, 373 F.2d 451, 453 (Bazelon, C.J.); Note, Civil Restraint, Mental Illness, and the Right to Treatment, 1967, 77 Yale L.J. 87, 90–91, 102–03 & nn. 62–63.

22 'Adequate and effective treatment is constitutionally required because, absent treatment, the hospital is transformed "into a penitentiary where one could be held indefinitely for no convicted offense." ' Wyatt v. Stickney, M.D. Ala. 1971, 325 F. Supp. 781, 784, quoting Ragsdale v. Overholser, 1960, 108 U.S. App. D.C. 308, 281 F.2d 943, 950 (Fahy, J., concurring). See also cases cited in nn. 23–24 infra.

Of the various formulations of this 'quid pro quo' theory we have found, perhaps the most successful is that made by Professor Nicholas Kittrie, writing specifically about confinement of juveniles, but articulating a theory equally applicable to civil commitment of mentally ill persons: 'Our society has increasingly divested certain groups from the traditional criminal justice court and, acting under its asserted role of parens patriae, substituted new therapeutic controls . . . A new concept of substantive due process is evolving in [this] therapeutic realm. This concept is founded upon a recognition of the concurrency between the state's exercise of sanctioning powers and its assumption of the duties of social responsibility. Its implication is that effective treatment must be the quid pro quo for society's right to exercise its parens patriae controls. Whether specifically recognized by statutory enactment or implicitly derived from the constitutional requirements of due process, the right to treatment exists.' Kittrie, Can the Right to Treatment Remedy the Ills of the Juvenile Process? 1969, 57 Geo. L.J. 851–52, 870.

23 Benton v. Reid, 1956, 98 U.S. App. D.C. 27, 231 F.2d 780; Commonwealth v. Page, 1958, 339 Mass. 313, 159 N.E.2d 82; In re Maddox, 1958, 351 Mich. 358, 88 N.W.2d 470; cf. Miller v. Overholser, 1953, 92 U.S. App. D.C. 110, 206 F.2d 415.

24 'But this mandatory commitment provision rests upon a supposition, namely, the necessity for treatment of the mental condition which led to the acquittal by reason of insanity. And this necessity for treatment presupposes in turn that treatment will be accorded.' Ragsdale v. Overholser, 1960, 108 U.S. App. D.C. 308, 281 F.2d 943, 950 (Fahy, J., concurring), quoted with approval, Darnell v. Cameron, 1965, 121 U.S. App. D.C. 58, 348 F.2d 64, 67–68, (Bazelon, C.J.); Sas v. Maryland, 4 Cir. 1964, 334 F.2d 506, 517, cert. dismissed as improvidently granted sub nom. Murel V. Baltimore City Crim. Ct., 1972, 407 U.S. 355, 92 S. Ct. 2091, 32 L. Ed. 2d 791; Commonwealth v. Page, 1959, 339 Mass. 313, 317, 159 N.E.2d 82, 85.

25 'For those in the category [of defective delinquents] it [the defective delinquents statute] would substitute psychiatric treatment for punishment in the conventional sense and would free them from confinement, not when they have "paid their debt to society," but when they have been sufficiently cured to make it reasonably safe to release them. With this humanitarian and progressive approach to the problem no person who has deplored the inadequacies of conventional penological practices can complain. But a statute though "fair on its face and impartial in appearance" may be fraught with the possibility of abuse in that if not administered in the spirit in which it is conceived it can become a mere device for warehousing the obnoxious and antisocial elements of society. . . . *Deficiencies in staff, facilities, and finances would undermine the efficacy of the institution and the justification for the law, and ultimately the constitutionality of its application.* [Footnotes omitted]' Sas v. Maryland, 4 Cir. 1964, 334 F.2d 506, 517, cert. dismissed as improvidently granted sub nom. Murel v. Baltimore City Crim. Ct., 1972. 407 U.S. 355, 92 S. Ct. 2091, 32 L. Ed. 2d 791 (emphasis supplied). See also Davy v. Sullivan, M.D. Ala. 1973, 354 F. Supp. 1320, (sex offender statute) (three-judge court).

26 1966, 125 U.S. App. D.C. 366, 373 F.2d 451 (Bazelon, C.J.). The District of Columbia Circuit has reaffirmed its Rouse holding on numerous occasions. See, e.g., In re Curry, 1971, 147 U.S. App. D.C. 28, 452 F.2d 1360; Covington v. Harris, 1969. 136 U.S. App. D.C. 35, 419 F.2d 617; Tribby v. Cameron, 1967, 126 U.S. App. D.C. 327, 379 F.2d 104; Dobson v. Cameron, 127 U.S. App. D.C. 324, 383 F.2d 519; Millard v. Cameron, 1966, 125 U.S. App. D.C. 383, 373 F.2d 468.

27 353 Mass. 604, 233 N.E.2d 908 (1968) (Cutter, J.).

28 But see Stachulak v. Coughlin, N.D. Ill. 1973, 364 F. Supp. 686, a case of this kind, citing Wyatt and holding there is a constitutional right to treatment.

29 E.g., Humphrey v. Cady, 1972, 405 U.S. 504, 92 S. Ct. 1048, 31 L. Ed. 2d 394 (characterizing committed sex offender's claim that he was not receiving treatment a 'substantial constitutional claim', and remanding for a hearing on, inter alia, that issue).

30 See cases cited in note 9 supra.

31 Wyatt v. Stickney, M.D. Ala. 1972, 344 F. Supp. 387; Welsch v. Likins, No. 4-72-Civ. 451, D. Minn. Feb. 15, 1974, – F. Supp. –. Contra, New York State Ass'n for Retarded Children, Inc. v. Rockefeller, E.D.N.Y. 1973, 357 F. Supp. 752.

32 Nelson v. Heyne, 7 Cir. 1974, 491 F.2d 352, aff'g N.D. Ind. 1972, 355 F. Supp. 451; Inmates of Boys' Training School v. Affleck, D.R.I. 1972, 346 F. Supp. 1354; Morales v. Turman, E.D. Tex. 1973, 364 F. Supp. 166.

33 Martarella v. Kelley, S.D.N.Y. 1972, 349 F. Supp. 575, enforced, 359 F. Supp. 478.

The closest the Supreme Court has come to speaking directly on the second, more important part of the due process right to treatment theory we articulate, came in In re Gault, 1967, 387 U.S. 1, 22 n. 30, 87 S. Ct. 1428, 18 L. Ed. 2d 527, in which the Court, discussing the context of juvenile confinement, wrote: 'While we are concerned only with procedure before the juvenile court in this case, it should be noted that to the extent that the special procedures for juveniles are thought to be justified by the special consideration and treatment afforded them, there is reason to doubt that juveniles always receive the benefits of such a quid pro quo. . . . The high rate of juvenile recidivism casts some doubt upon the adequacy of treatment afforded juveniles . . . .

'In fact some courts have recently indicated that appropriate treatment is essential to the validity of juvenile custody, and therefore that a juvenile may challenge the validity of his custody on the ground that he is not in fact receiving any special treatment.'

34 Jackson v. Indiana, 1972, 406 U.S. 715, 92 S. Ct. 1845, 32 L. Ed. 2d 435; Humphrey v. Cady, 1972, 405 U.S. 504, 92 S. Ct. 1048, 31 L. Ed. 2d 394; McNeil v. Director, Patuxent Institution, 1972, 407 U.S. 245, 92 S. Ct. 2083, 32 L. Ed. 2d 719.

35 E.g., Nelson v. Heyne, supra note 39; Sas v. Maryland, 4 Cir. 1964, 334 F.2d 506, cert. dismissed as improvidently granted sub nom. Murel v. Baltimore City Crim. Ct., 1972, 407 U.S. 355, 92 S. Ct. 2091, 32 L. Ed. 2d 791; Rouse v. Cameron, 1966, 125 U.S. App. D.C. 366, 373 F.2d 541.

36 E.g., cases cited in nn. 9, 31–33, supra.

37 E.g., Nason v. Superintendent, Bridgewater Hospital, 1968, 353 Muss. 604, 233 N.E.2d 908; Commonwealth v. Page, 1959, 339 Mass. 313, 159 N.E.2d 82; In re Maddox, 1958, 351 Mich. 358, 88 N.W.2d 470.

38 E.g., Humphrey v. Cady, 1972, 405 U.S. 504, 92 S. Ct. 1048, 31 L. Ed. 2d 394; Davy v. Sullivan, M.D. Ala. 1973, 354 F. Supp. 1320 (three-judge court); Commonwealth v. Page, 1959, 339 Mass. 313, 159 N.E.2d 82.

39 E.g., Sas v. Maryland, 4 Cir. 1964, 334 F.2d 506, cert. dismissed as improvidently granted sub nom. Murel v. Balitmore City Crim. Ct., 407 U.S. 355, 92 S. Ct. 2091, 32 L. Ed. 2d 791.

40 E.g., Rouse v. Cameron, 1966, 125 U.S. App. D.C. 366, 373 F.2d 451 (Bazelon, C.J.); Darnell v. Cameron, 1965, 121 U.S. App. D.C. 58, 348 F.2d 64 (Bazelon, C.J.); Ragsdale v. Overholser, 1960, 108 U.S. App. D.C. 308, 281 F.2d 943 (Burger, J.).

41 Jackson v. Indiana, 1972, 406 U.S. 715, 92 S. Ct. 1845, 32 L. Ed. 2d 435. See also Greenwood v. United States, 1956, 350 U.S. 366, 76 S. Ct. 410, 100 L. Ed. 412; United States v. Pardue, D. Conn. 1973, 354 F. Supp. 1377; United States v. Jackson, N.D. Cal. 1969, 306 F. Supp. 4.

42 E.g., Wyatt v. Stickney, M.D. Ala. 1972, 344 F. Supp. 387; Welsch v. Likins, No. 4-72-Civ. 451, D. Minn. Feb. 15, 1974, noted, 42 U.S.L.W. 1141–42.

43 Cases cited in notes 32–33.

44 Cases cited in note 9 supra.

45 'Levine [M. Levine, Psychotherapy in Medical Practice] lists 40 methods of psychotherapy. Among these, he includes physical treatment, medicinal treatment, reassurance, authoritative firmness, hospitalization, ignoring of certain symptoms and attitudes, satisfaction of neurotic needs and bibliotherapy. In addition, there are physical methods of psychiatric therapy, such as the prescription of sedatives and tranquilizers, the induction of convulsions by drugs and electricity, and brain surgery. *Obviously, the term 'psychiatric treatment' covers everything that may be done under medical auspices – and more.*

'If mental treatment is all the things Levine and others tell us it is, how are we to determine whether or not patients in mental hospitals receive adequate amounts of it?' Szasz, The Right to Psychiatric Treatment: Rhetoric and Reality, 1969, 57 Geo. L.J. 740, 741.

46 '. . . [T]heir [two court-appointed psychiatrists] testimony illustrates the uncertainty of diagnosis in this field and the tentativeness of professional judgment. The only certain thing that can be said about the present state of knowledge and therapy regarding mental disease is that science has not reached finality of judgment.' Greenwood v. United States, 1956, 350 U.S. 366, 375, 76 S. Ct. 410, 415, 100 L. Ed. 412.

47 See, e.g., Humphrey v. Cady, 1972, 405 U.S. 504, 92 S. Ct. 1048, 31 L. Ed. 2d 394; In re Curry, 1971, 147 U.S. App. D.C. 28, 452 F.2d 1360; United States v. Waters, 1970, 141 U.S. App. D.C. 289, 437 F.2d 722; Dobson v. Cameron, 1967, 127 U.S. App. D.C. 324, 383 F.2d 519; Tribby v. Cameron, 126 U.S. App. D.C. 327, 379 F.2d 104; Millard v. Cameron, 1966, 125 U.S. App. D.C. 383, 373 F.2d 468; Sas v. Maryland, 4 Cir. 1964, 334 F.2d 506, remanding, D. Md., 1969, 295 F. Supp. 389, aff'd sub nom. Tippett v. Maryland, 1971, 436 F.2d 1153, cert. dismissed as improvidently granted sub nom. Murel v. Baltimore City Crim. Ct., 1972, 407 U.S. 355, 92 S. Ct. 2091, 32 L. Ed. 2d 791; Dixon v. Atty. Gen'l of Pennsylvania, M.D. Pa. 1971, 325 F. Supp. 966 (three-judge); In re Jones, D.D.C. 1972, 338 F. Supp. 428; Clatterbuck v. Harris, D.D.C. 1968, 295 F. Supp. 84; Nason v. Supt. of Bridgewater State Hospital, 1968, 353 Mass. 604, 233 N.E.2d 908.

The Psychiatric Patient's Right to Effective Treatment:

Implications of Osheroff v. Chestnut Lodge*

Gerald L. Klerman

In recent decades, the courts have played a growing role in setting standards for psychiatric treatment. Important court decisions have established the patient's right to treatment, the patient's right to refuse treatment, and the patient's right to the least restrictive environment. Most of these court decisions have concerned patients in public institutions, many of whom have been hospitalized involuntarily under civil commitment statutes. With regard to nongovernmental institutions and the private practice of psychiatry, the courts have mainly been involved in cases of negligence, many of which involved adverse consequences of biological treatments, such as drugs and convulsive therapy, or issues related to suicide (unpublished 1985 paper by K. Livingston).

Recently, the lawsuit of *Osheroff v. Chestnut Lodge* was settled out of court. The plaintiff claimed negligence because the institution failed to institute drug treatment and persisted in the use of individual psychotherapy as the sole treatment for his severe depression. This lawsuit is considered a landmark case dealing with a number of important issues confronting psychiatry – particularly the need for standards for psychiatric treatment and the ethical and legal consequences of the absence of such standards. The case has been widely discussed in legal journals,[1] in the lay press,[2] and in psychiatric circles;[3–5] it was also discussed by Alan Stone in a paper given at the 1988 meeting of the American College of Psychiatrists.

The standards for psychiatric treatment include the safety, efficacy, and appropriateness of psychiatric treatment. These have long been subjects of controversy among the medical profession, psychiatry, and the public in general. The controversies have increased in recent years due to the introduction of new psychotropic drugs, new forms of psychotherapy and behavior therapy, increases in the types and numbers of mental health professionals, and the growing utilization of mental health services.[6]

The lawsuit of *Osheroff v. Chestnut Lodge* raises a number of important clinical, scientific, public policy, and legal issues. The clinical issues have to do with the validity of psychiatric diagnoses and the criteria used in making treatment decisions. The scientific issues pertain to the nature of evidence for the safety and efficacy of psychiatric treatments. The public policy issues pertain to the respective roles and responsibilities of federal and state governments, the courts, and professional organizations in the protection of the welfare of patients with psychiatric conditions and the provision of careful, valid diagnoses and effective, humane treatment and care. The legal issues have to do with the definition of standards of care in the criteria for malpractice and negligence.

I will summarize the salient clinical and legal developments in Dr. Osheroff's case, reviewing issues that have clinical, scientific, public policy, and legal implications. I will conclude with recommendations for clinical practitioners and for the profession.

* Klerman, G.: The psychiatric patient's right to effective treatment: Implications of *Osheroff v Chestnut Lodge*. *American Journal of Psychiatry* 147:419–427, 1990.

The Case of Dr. Osheroff

Permission has been obtained from the patient to use his name and to report details of his history and treatment. Under usual circumstances, the patient's identity and that of the institutions where he was treated would not be given. However, since this case has already been discussed in the lay press[2] and in professional journals where the patient and the institutions have been frequently identified, further attempts at anonymity would be unjustified.

The patient, Dr. Rafael Osheroff a 42-year-old, white male physician, was admitted to Chestnut Lodge in Maryland (in the Washington, D.C., metropolitan area) on Jan. 2, 1979. His history included brief periods of depressive and anxious symptoms as an adult; these had been treated on an outpatient basis. He had completed medical school and residency training, was certified as an internist, and became a subspecialist in nephrology. He was married and had three children – one with his current wife and two with his ex-wife.

Before his 1979 hospitalization, Dr. Osheroff had been suffering from anxious and depressive symptoms for approximately 2 years and had been treated as an outpatient with individual psychotherapy and tricyclic antidepressant medications. Dr. Nathan Kline, a prominent psychopharmacologist in New York, had initiated outpatient treatment with tricyclic medication, which, according to Dr. Kline's notes, produced moderate improvement. The patient, however, did not maintain the recommended dose, his clinical condition gradually worsened, and hospitalization was recommended.

The patient was hospitalized at Chestnut Lodge for approximately 7 months. During this time he was treated with individual psychotherapy four times a week. He lost 40 pounds, experienced severe insomnia, and had marked psychomotor agitation. His agitation, manifested by incessant pacing, was so extreme that his feet became swollen and blistered, requiring medical attention.

The patient's family became distressed by the length of the hospitalization and by his lack of improvement. They consulted a psychiatrist in the Washington, D.C., area, who spoke to the hospital leadership on the patient's behalf. In response, the staff at Chestnut Lodge held a clinical case conference to review the patient's treatment. They decided not to make any major changes – specifically, not to institute any medication regimen but to continue the intensive individual psychotherapy. Dr. Osheroff's clinical condition continued to worsen. At the end of 7 months, his family had him discharged from Chestnut Lodge and admitted to Silver Hill Foundation in Connecticut.

On admission to Silver Hill Foundation, Dr. Osheroff was diagnosed as having a psychotic depressive reaction. His treating physician began treatment with a combination of phenothiazines and tricyclic antidepressants. Dr. Osheroff showed improvement within 3 weeks and was discharged from Silver Hill Foundation within 3 months. His final diagnosis was manic-depressive illness, depressed type.

Although the patient's final diagnosis on discharge from Silver Hill was manic-depressive illness, depressed type, testimony of the treating physician at Silver Hill revealed that, of the two *DSM-II* diagnoses that would subsume a depressive illness as severe as Dr. Osheroff's (manic-depressive illness, depressed type, and psychotic depressive reaction), the diagnosis of manic-depressive illness, depressed type, was selected because of the potential future complications regarding child custody that could arise from a diagnostic label including the term 'psychotic.' The Silver Hill physician further testified that she did not find evidence of a narcissistic personality disorder in Dr. Osheroff and that the correct diagnosis according to DSM-III terminology would be major depressive episode with psychotic features.

Following his discharge from Silver Hill Foundation in the summer of 1979, the patient resumed his medical practice. He has been in outpatient treatment, receiving psychotherapy and medication. He has not been hospitalized and has not experienced any episodes of depressive symptoms severe enough to interfere with his professional or social functioning. He has resumed contact with his children and has also become active socially.

The Legal Actions

In 1982, Dr. Osheroff initiated a lawsuit against Chestnut Lodge. He claimed that as a result of the negligence of Chestnut Lodge in not administering drug treatment, which would have quickly returned him to normal functioning, in the course of a year he lost a lucrative medical practice, his standing in the medical community, and custody of two of his children.

When Dr. Osheroff's suit came before the Maryland Health Care Arbitration Panel it was marked, among other things, by the large number of expert witnesses for the plaintiff, including Drs. Donald Klein, Bernard Carroll, Frank Ayd, and myself. The Arbitration Panel found for the plaintiff and awarded him financial damages.[7] This was not a majority decision, however, and the director of the Arbitration Panel sent the panel back for an amended decision, which reduced the award. Under Maryland statute, once an arbitration process is concluded, any party to the proceedings may reject the panel's arbitration and call for court review. Both sides appealed. The claimant, Dr. Osheroff, requested a jury trial, which was to have taken place in October 1987. However, before any action was taken by the court, a settlement was agreed on by both parties.

Clinical and Scientific Issues

This case raises a number of clinical and scientific issues. The clinical issues have to do with the validity of the diagnosis and the process of decision making with regard to treatment. The scientific issues have to do with the nature of evidence for safety and efficacy of psychiatric treatments.

Divisions Within Psychiatry in the United States

Resolution of both the clinical and scientific issues is made difficult by the divisions within psychiatry in the United States, where psychiatry is divided theoretically and clinically into different schools – biological, psychoanalytic, and behavioral.[7] This aspect of the sociology of psychiatry and other mental health professions and its effect on training and practice have been documented for a number of years.[8-11] Various terms have been used to describe these divisions and splits – schools, movements, ideologies, and paradigms, for example.[10, 12, 13] Whatever term is used, there is agreement that the differences in theory and practice involve controversies over the nature of mental illness, the appropriateness of different forms of treatment, and the nature of the evidence for the safety and efficacy of such treatments.

Chestnut Lodge has played an important role in the modern history of psychiatry in the United States. For more than 40 years, Chestnut Lodge has been one of the major centers of theory and clinical practice in intensive

individual psychotherapy based on psychoanalytic and interpersonal paradigms.[14] Harry Stack Sullivan[15], who formulated the interpersonal theory of psychiatry, was a consultant to the institution. Many of his lectures and seminars at Chestnut Lodge have been published posthumously. Frieda Fromm-Reichmann was also on the staff at the same time. She had immigrated to the United States from Germany along with a large number of other leading psychoanalysts driven out of Europe by the Nazi regime. Fromm-Reichmann wrote a number of influential papers and books about the psychotherapeutic treatment of schizophrenia and manic-depressive illness.[16, 17]

Several prominent U.S. psychiatrists were trained at Chestnut Lodge; many subsequently became leaders in clinical psychiatry. Alfred Stanton, who became psychiatrist-in-chief at McLean Hospital in Massachusetts, and Otto Will, who became medical director of the Austin Riggs Center in Massachusetts, are two notable examples. The writings of Sullivan[15], Fromm-Reichmann[16], Will[18], and others were influential in many psychiatric residency training programs from 1950 through the 1970s.

In the 1950s and 1960s, new psychopharmacological agents and the findings of neuroscientific research began to influence psychiatric teaching, practice, and research. New forms of psychotherapy based on approaches other than psychoanalytic were applied. Professional controversies increased, particularly over the comparison of the therapeutic efficacy of the different forms of psychotherapy (psychoanalytic, behavioral, family, group) and over the relative efficacy and safety of the psychotherapies, used either alone or in combination with psychopharmacological agents[19].

Diagnostic Issues in Dr. Osheroff's Hospitalization

At both Chestnut Lodge and Silver Hill Foundation there was agreement that Dr. Osheroff suffered from a severe depressive condition. There was disagreement, however, as to the diagnosis of narcissistic personality disorder. In a discussion of this case, Dr. Stone[3] described a 'dispute' over the appropriate diagnosis: 'The patient's psychiatric experts, in depositions that reflected their biological orientation, diagnosed him as having an obvious case of biological depression, emphasizing his vegetative disturbances. The private psychiatric hospital contended that the patient was properly diagnosed as having a narcissistic personality disorder.'

It is to be noted that Dr. Osheroff's diagnoses at both Chestnut Lodge and Silver Hill Foundation were made in 1979 in accordance with *DSM-II*, APA's official nomenclature at the time of his hospitalization. *DSM-III*, which is the current diagnostic nomenclature for clinical psychiatric practice in the United States, did not come into use until 1980. DSM-II does not include a diagnostic category of narcissistic personality disorder, although that diagnostic category is included in DSM-I and in DSM-III.

DSM-II includes diagnostic categories of psychotic depressive reaction and manic-depressive illness, depressed type. Both refer to severe forms of depression. There is no evidence of clinical features of hypomania or mania in Dr. Osheroff's history or in the case records from either institution. The patient would not meet *DSM-III* criteria for bipolar disorder or *DSM-II*, criteria for manic-depressive illness, manic or circular types.

The *DSM-II* diagnostic category of psychotic depressive reaction was replaced in *DSM-III* by major depressive episode with melancholia and/or major depressive episode with psychotic features. Melancholia is a term from the past denoting a particularly severe form of depression uniquely responsive to somatic drugs and/or ECT therapies. It is of note that the term 'biological depression' does not appear in *DSM-II*, *DSM-III*, or *ICD-9*.

According to Chestnut Lodge records, there were differences in medical opinion as to the relative importance to be given to the patient's personality conflicts and his depressive diagnosis as they influenced treatment decisions, not over the depressive diagnosis itself. As was the practice at that institution, the patient had two physicians, psychiatrist-administrator and a psychotherapist.[20] The hospital records suggest there may have been disagreement between these two physicians: the psychotherapist emphasized the need to treat the patient's personality problems as the major condition, and the administrator expressed concern over the continued severity of the patient's depressive symptoms and distressed behavior.

This aspect of the clinical process illustrates the tendency for many psychoanalytically oriented psychotherapists, both in institutional and in community practice, to focus treatment on a patient's personality conflict and character pathology rather than on symptoms. In *DSM-III* terms, there tends to be an emphasis on the axis II diagnosis and relatively less attention given to the axis I diagnosis. The axis I diagnosis, a severe depression in the case of Dr. Osheroff, is often missed, or, even if it is formulated, the personality disorder is chosen as the major target for treatment planning.

The Disputed Diagnosis of Personality Disorder

An important clinical consideration at issue in Osheroff is whether the patient suffered from a personality disorder as well as from depression and whether the presence of the narcissistic personality disorder militated against the use of medication for the depression. Long-term psychoanalytically oriented psychotherapy is often justified by the theory that some states of clinical depression derive from unresolved personality conflicts whose origins lie in developmental problems related to childhood intrafamilial psychopathology.[17, 21] This theory of etiology and pathogenesis of depression is the subject of scientific research and professional discussion.[22] Expert witnesses testified on this issue at the Osheroff hearings.

It should be noted that the psychiatric experts who testified in this case did not agree on the validity of the diagnosis of narcissistic personality disorder for the patient. One expert, a trained psychoanalyst who is currently responsible for Dr. Osheroff's treatment and who had treated him when the patient was 29 years old and at the time of his divorce (when he was 34 years old), did not accept the diagnosis of narcissistic personality disorder and testified to this effect at the court hearing. He noted the patient's successful life achievements before the onset of the illness episode that led to hospitalization at Chestnut Lodge, including his professional success as a nephrologist, his ability to sustain a high income, and his loving, empathic, and sensitive relationship with his children.

The admitting psychiatrist at Silver Hill Foundation did not make the diagnosis of any personality disorder. An expert witness called by Chestnut Lodge to testify at the court hearing also did not think that the patient had a narcissistic personality disorder. In contrast to the near-unanimity of expert opinion as to the patient's severe depressive condition, disagreement existed as to whether the patient met any criteria for narcissistic personality disorder.

Scientific Evidence for Evaluating Psychiatric Treatment

With regard to all kinds of therapeutics – pharmacotherapy, surgery, radiation, psychotherapy – the most scientifically valid evidence as to the safety and efficacy of a treatment comes from randomized controlled trials when these are available. Although there may be other methods of generating evidence, such as naturalistic and follow-up studies, the most convincing evidence comes from randomized controlled trials.

There have been many controlled clinical trials of psychiatric treatments; most have been conducted to evaluate psychopharmacological agents. These trials were initiated in the 1950s and 1960s in response to the controversy that followed the introduction of chlorpromazine, reserpine, and the other 'tranquilizers.' The application of controlled trials in psychopharmacology expanded after the passage in 1962 of the Kefauver-Harris Amendments to the Food, Drug, and Cosmetic Act, which mandated evidence of efficacy before a pharmaceutical compound could be approved by the Food and Drug Administration and marketed.

Research on the efficacy of psychotherapy has lagged behind that of psychopharmacology but has, nevertheless, been extensive. Smith et al.[23] analyzed more than 400 reports of psychotherapy research. Specific reviews of the evidence have appeared with regard to psychotherapy of neurosis[24], schizophrenia[25], depression[26], and obsessive-compulsive disorders[27].

In view of these developments, a review of the state of evidence regarding the treatments of the two psychiatric conditions diagnosed for Dr. Osheroff at the time of his hospitalization is in order.

With regard to the treatment of the patient's diagnosis of narcissistic personality disorder, there were no of reports of controlled trials of any pharmacological or psychotherapeutic treatment for this condition at the time of his hospitalization[28]. The doctors at Chestnut Lodge decided to treat Dr. Osheroff's personality disorder with intensive individual psychotherapy based on psychodynamic theory.

With regard to the treatment of the patient's DSM-II diagnosis of psychotic depressive reaction, there was very good evidence at the time of his hospitalization for the efficacy of two biological treatments – ECT and the combination of phenothiazines and tricyclic antidepressants. The combination pharmacotherapy was the treatment later prescribed at Silver Hill Foundation.

There are no reports of controlled trials supporting the claims for efficacy of psychoanalytically oriented intensive individual psychotherapy of the type advocated and practiced at Chestnut Lodge and administered to Dr. Osheroff. The closest approximation to a controlled clinical trial of this form of intensive individual psychotherapy has been reported with hospitalized schizophrenic patients at two institutions in the Boston area[30]. Contrary to the expectations of the investigators, one of whom was Dr. Alfred Stanton (who had held a senior position at Chestnut Lodge and was one of the authors of The Mental Hospital[20], which describes the Chestnut Lodge institution), the results indicated that intensive individual psychotherapy offered no advantage over standard-treatment (hospitalization, medication, and supportive psychotherapy) for these patients.

McGlashan and Dingman[30, 31] have reported results from follow-up studies of groups of patients treated at Chestnut Lodge. The findings from this naturalistic study do not support the efficacy of long-term psychotherapy and hospitalization for severely depressed patients such as Dr. Osheroff.

It should not be concluded there is no evidence for the value of any psychotherapy in the treatment of depressive states. Depressive states are heterogeneous, and there are many forms of psychotherapy. There is very good evidence from controlled clinical trials for the value of a number of brief psychotherapies for nonpsychotic and nonbipolar forms of depression in ambulatory patients[26]. The psychotherapies for which there is evidence include cognitive-behavioral therapy[32], interpersonal psychotherapy[14], and behavioral therapy[33]. However, no clinical trials have been reported that support the claims for efficacy of psychoanalysis or intensive individual psychotherapy based on psychoanalytic theory for any form of depression.

Personality Disorder and Depressed Patients' Response to Pharmacotherapy

An important clinical issue raised by Osheroff has to do with the possible influence of a patient's diagnosis of personality disorder on the decision to use medication and on the expected response to medication of depressed patients treated either with medication alone or with medication in conjunction with psychotherapy.

Even if we assume that the personality disorder was correctly diagnosed in Dr. Osheroff's case, there is no evidence to support the premise that the presence of a narcissistic personality disorder militates against the use of antidepressant medication. Patients with a personality disorder in addition to depressive illness may be relatively less responsive to medication than those without an associated personality disorder[34]. However, the presence of a personality disorder by itself does not contraindicate the prescription of appropriate medication or predict complete failure to respond.

A related therapeutic issue raised by the case has to do with the possible negative interactions between psychotherapy and pharmacotherapy for depression. Many psychoanalytically oriented psychotherapists have argued against the use of medication in patients receiving psychotherapy because of the possible adverse effects of the pharmacotherapy on the conduct of the psychotherapy[35], although there is evidence that the combination of drugs and psychotherapy does not interfere with the psychotherapy of depression[36]. Moreover, findings from controlled trials suggest that the combination of drugs and psychotherapy may have beneficial additive effects in the treatment of depression[37].

Decision Making in Psychiatry

Given this state of evidence, it is difficult to justify the rationale used by the Chestnut Lodge staff in forming their treatment plan and in making specific decisions. On the one hand, there was a body of scientific evidence from controlled trials attesting to the value of medication and/or ECT for the type of severe depression that the institution diagnosed this patient as having. On the other hand, there was no scientific evidence for the value of psychodynamically oriented intensive individual psychotherapy for either the patient's depressive condition or his diagnosis of personality disorder. Nevertheless, the patient was treated only with intensive psychotherapy.

It might have been reasonable to have undertaken a period of psychotherapy, particularly in view of the tendency of many depressive states to remit spontaneously. However, several clinical studies[38, 39] have concluded that, in the absence of intervention with somatic treatments, severe health impairment and greater mortality are associated with deep depressions.

The hospital continued its treatment plan for many months in the face of continued worsening of the patient's clinical state. Meanwhile, the prolonged hospitalization was having adverse effects on the patient's medical practice, financial resources, and marital and family relations.

Public Policy Issues

In addition to clinical and scientific issues regarding diagnosis and treatment, this case raises some important issues regarding public policy. The policy issues have to do with the locus of responsibility for the protection and welfare of psychiatric patients and the activities of the government, the courts, and professional groups in establishing criteria for diagnosis and treatment.

The Roles of the Federal and State Governments

There is a federal agency, the Food and Drug Administration, that has statutory authority to review the evidence for the efficacy and safety of pharmacological treatments. Because of the Kefauver-Harris Amendments, a pharmaceutical firm that makes promotional claims for the efficacy of a drug is expected to present evidence from controlled trials in support of its assertions.

Consider, however, the situation with regard to psychotherapy. There are no statutory constraints on claims made for psychotherapy. No government body is authorized to review the evidence for psychotherapy or comment on its status. In the late 1970s, the Senate considered the creation of a National Commission on Mental Health Treatments, but the proposal was opposed by the mental health professions and was not enacted into law[40].

The National institutes of Health (NIH) conduct consensus development conferences to review the evidence about specific procedures relevant to health and medicine, including the efficacy of treatments. An NIH consensus development conference was held on long-term drug treatments of affective disorders in 1984[41], and a conference on electroconvulsive therapies was held in June 1985. However, the efficacy of psychotherapies has not been addressed by NIH.

It might be expected that two other federal government agencies concerned with health financing and disability – the Health Care Financing Administration and the Social Security Administration – would be involved in judgments as to the appropriateness of treatment, inasmuch as they are involved in the disbursement of large amounts of funds. The Health Care Financing Administration provides reimbursement under both Medicare and Medicaid, and the Social Security Administration determines the disability status of individuals with psychiatric illness. However, only limited efforts have been undertaken by these agencies to establish criteria for the safety and efficacy of treatments for which reimbursement will be provided. In this respect it is of note that the legislation establishing Medicaid and Medicare did not include criteria of safety or efficacy but, rather, discussed the criteria of reasonable and medical necessities. These criteria have not been explicated in specific regulations or procedures.

Although the federal government has no direct regulatory role with regard to psychotherapy, as it does with regard to drugs, it has a major role in supporting scientific research on mental illnesses and their treatment. The current imbalance in available evidence for efficacy of psychotherapy in relation to psychopharmacology has many sources; one is the social and economic structure of treatment research. In the case of pharmacological agents, the pharmaceutical industry is organized into large corporate bodies with considerable resources and incentives for research on the efficacy and safety of their products. In contrast, the psychotherapy 'industry' is made up of many small firms and practitioners whose resources are less extensive and who are less capable of concerted action. It might be expected that the institutes of the Alcohol, Drug Abuse, and Mental Health Administration, particularly the National Institute of Mental Health (NIMH), would devote leadership and resources to treatment research, but here again, for complex reasons, NIMH's record on funding psychotherapy research is inadequate in total grants and not reflective of clinical practice or professional judgment. Efforts to correct this imbalance require greater cooperation between officials of the Alcohol, Drug Abuse, and Mental Health Administration and the professional leadership than has been achieved to date.

State governments have an important potential role with respect to these issues because licensure and certification of health professionals are the responsibility of state governments, as is the licensing of hospitals and clinics. Almost all state governments have established standards for professional licensing of physicians. An increasing number of state governments have established criteria for licensing and/or certification of psychotherapists, particularly psychologists and social workers. Similarly, almost all hospitals, including private psychiatric hospitals such as Chestnut Lodge and Silver Hill Foundation, require licensing in their respective states. However, no state has attempted to establish guidelines for the selection of treatments based on efficacy as part of licensing or certification requirements.

The Role of the Psychiatric Profession

In the absence of a government body similar to the Food and Drug Administration, patients and the public might expect that professional associations such as APA, the American Psychological Association, or the National Association of Social Workers would undertake to provide this service to the public. No guidelines for treatment have emerged, however, although peer review criteria have been established. APA issued a report on the status of ECT in 1978[42]. The Royal Australian and New Zealand College of Physicians has contracted with the Australian Ministry of Social Security to undertake a quality assurance program, which has issued a series of reports reviewing the state of scientific evidence for selected diagnoses, including depression[43].

As of the late 1970s, when Dr. Osheroff was hospitalized, APA had published a manual for peer review of hospital utilization[44]. With regard to the DSM-II diagnosis of psychotic depressive reaction, this manual recommended the use of drugs or ECT. It did not recommend individual psychotherapy. Furthermore, this manual recommended that if hospitalization has continued beyond 1 or 2 months, the case should be reviewed and the use of ECT or drug treatments considered. Therefore, although there were no government bodies offering legal guidelines, APA had established peer review criteria for the hospital treatment of psychotic depressive reaction[44].

APA is currently completing a project on psychiatric treatments under the leadership of T. Byram Karasu[45]. Preliminary reports from this project have been published[46].

The Role of the Courts

Given that there are no government bodies judging the efficacy of claims for psychotherapy, and given the limited efforts undertaken by professional associations, it is understandable that individual patients use the courts to seek redress for their grievances.

Governmental and professional bodies have been urged to issue judgments recommending treatments so that these criteria could be used by reimbursement agencies. In response, the Senate considered possible legislation to establish a National Commission on Mental Health Treatments in the late 1970s and, more recently, APA established the Commission on Psychiatric Therapies, led by Dr. Karasu. Some have advocated that the profession not make such recommendations in regard to treatment, assuming that if the profession did not take such actions the courts would ignore the issue or not take a position. The opposite seems to be the case. In the absence of professional criteria for standards of care, the courts are increasingly becoming the arena in which these disputes are adjudicated. Thus, case law and individual precedents may become the criteria for adequacy of diagnosis and treatment.

Biological Versus Psychodynamic Psychiatry

Dr. Stone[3] raised the possibility that patients who have not improved after prolonged psychotherapeutic treatment may have found a way around their frustrations – a way provided by 'biological psychiatrists. Dr. Stone noted that biological psychiatry appears to be on the scientific ascendancy over psychodynamic psychiatry due to the prestige of the neurosciences and the evidence for efficacy of biological treatments.

My conclusion, however, is that the issue is not psychotherapy versus biological therapy but, rather, opinion versus evidence. The efficacy of drugs and other biological treatments is supported by a large body of controlled clinical trials. This body of evidence is all the more relevant to public policy in view of the paucity of studies indicating efficacy for individual psychotherapy.

It is regrettable that psychoanalysts and psychodynamic psychotherapists have not developed evidence in support of their claims for therapeutic efficacy. Twenty years ago, psychodynamic psychotherapy was the dominant paradigm of psychiatry in the United States, particularly in academic centers. A number of European psychiatrists, mostly psychoanalysts, contributed intellectual leadership and imaginative ideas to psychiatry here. Currently, however, psychoanalysis is on the scientific and professional defensive. This situation is, in part, a consequence of the failure of psychoanalysis to provide evidence for the efficacy of psychoanalysis and psychodynamic treatments for psychiatric disorders[47, 48].

In the period between World War I and World War II, biological psychiatry was in poor repute. Numerous treatments, often of a heroic nature, were advocated: colonic resection, adrenalectomy, excision of teeth, lobotomy. These interventions were based on biological laboratory research of dubious quality and without any systematic studies of safety and efficacy. The situation changed after World War II, with evidence for the value of ECT for depression and insulin coma therapy for schizophrenia and, later, with the introduction of chlorpromazine and other drugs.

The Respectable Minority Doctrine

The case of *Osheroff v. Chestnut Lodge* prompts a reevaluation of the doctrine of the respectable minority. Until recently, this doctrine held that if a minority of respected and qualified practitioners maintained a standard of care, this was an adequate defense against malpractice. I propose that this doctrine no longer holds if there is a body of evidence supporting the efficacy of a particular treatment and if there is agreement within the profession that this is the proper treatment of a given condition. Moreover, the respectable minority have a duty to inform the patient of the alternative treatments. In an unpublished 1985 paper discussing *Osheroff v. Chestnut Lodge*, K. Livingston wrote,

Under this view, the respectable minority view would still constitute a defense to a malpractice action where even 10% of practitioners would adhere to the treatment in question. However, the shield of the respectable minority rule would not be available unless the patient had been given informed consent after a disclosure of risk/benefits and alternatives to the therapy.

How Do We Proceed in the Absence of Consensus?

When there is consensus in the profession as to the appropriate treatment for a given condition (in the case of *Osheroff*, the essential nature of biological treatment for severe depression), then a standard of care can be agreed on and can provide the basis for malpractice action.

However, how are we to evaluate claims for the efficacy of treatments for clinical conditions about which there is no consensus? What are the standards to be applied in diagnostic and clinical situations where there is no consensus within the field with regard to the treatment of the particular disorder? This is a serious policy question that, in the future, may become a legal question. In my opinion, there are three aspects to this issue: 1) What constitutes evidence for efficacy? 2) Who is responsible for generating the evidence? and 3) Who is to make the appropriate evaluation of treatments?

What constitutes evidence of treatment? In my view, the best available evidence as to efficacy comes from controlled trials. I am not taking the position that the only source of evidence for efficacy comes from such trials. Clinical experience, naturalistic studies, and follow-up studies are also sources of relevant evidence. However, when results from controlled clinical trials are available, they should be given priority in any discussion of scientific evidence.

Who should be responsible for generating the evidence? What should be society's policy in regard to treatments for which there is no positive or negative evidence? This issue has not reached resolution, and I feel it merits further discussion within the profession.

My opinion is that the responsibility for generating evidence for efficacy rests with the individual, group, or organization that makes the claim for the safety and efficacy of a particular treatment. In the case of drugs, this responsibility is established by statute. If a pharmaceutical firm makes a claim for the efficacy of one of its products, it must generate enough evidence to satisfy the Food and Drug Administration before it can market the drug for prescription use.

No such mandate of responsibility exists for psychotherapy. Anyone can make a claim for the value of a form of psychotherapy – psychoanalysis, Gestalt, est, primal scream, etc. – with no evidence as to its efficacy.

What should be our position toward the claims of the efficacy in certain conditions of multiple treatments for which the evidence varies in quality and quantity? In my view, those treatments which make claims but have not generated evidence are in a weak position.

The efficacy of psychoanalysis and psychoanalytic treatments is in question for conditions for which there is evidence of efficacy with other treatments. For example, how many psychiatrists would justify long-term psychoanalytic treatment of panic disorder and/or agoraphobia when there is no evidence that this treatment works for these disorders but reasonably good evidence for the efficacy of certain drugs and/or forms of behavioral psychotherapy?

Who is to evaluate the evidence? A major problem arises as to the process by which the evidence regarding psychiatric treatments is to be evaluated. I believe there are serious deficiencies in our current professional and governmental arrangements for evaluating psychiatric treatments. In the case of drugs, we have the Food and Drug Administration, which makes such judgments according to established legal statutes and regulatory processes. There is no comparable statutory mandate for assessing the efficacy and safety of nonpharmacological treatments such as radiation, surgery, and psychotherapy.

In this situation, I believe the public has the right to expect that the medical profession will provide appropriate judgments as to the state of the evidence for treatments and establish criteria for standards of care. I maintain that the psychiatric profession has been lax in this responsibility and that the absence of professional consensus statements in our field leaves it open for the courts to be used by individuals, such as Dr. Osheroff, who feel they have been poorly treated and who believe they are entitled to redress of their grievances.

The fact that evidence changes is to my mind irrelevant to any policy or clinical discussion. The judgment on treatment of individual patients should be made according to the state of knowledge and professional practice at the time the individual patient is treated. In the case of *Osheroff*, this was 1979.

My strong preference would be for the profession to be more vigorous and more responsible in accepting this responsibility. I have stated these views on a number of occasions.

Recommendations for the Practicing Clinician

What lessons can be learned from the case of Osheroff v. Chestnut Lodge that can be used by the practicing clinician, whether in institutional or community settings? As Dr. Stone pointed out in a paper given at the 1988 meeting of the American College of Psychiatrists, this case has no formal legal status because it was settled out of court. However, it has been widely discussed and will likely provide the basis for possible further legal actions in similar cases. In my opinion, this case goes a long way toward establishing the patient's right to effective treatment. The following recommendations are not intended to be legal standards for negligence or malpractice but, rather, to clarify professional responsibility.

1 The psychiatrist has a responsibility to make a comprehensive assessment, including determination of the proper diagnosis. The patient should be evaluated as to social and personal background, symptoms, and medical history, including personality, need for hospitalization, and possible suicidal risk. As part of this assessment, a diagnostic formulation should be made and, wherever possible, the formulation should be in accord with *DSM-III-R*. Of course, investigators and clinicians can and do depart from *DSM-III-R* categories and criteria whenever they have good scientific or professional reasons to do so (unpublished 1988 paper of Alan Stone). However, in my opinion, when this departure is done for an individual patient, in teaching, or in research, the psychiatrist should make explicit the departure from *DSM-III-R* and name the alternative diagnostic system used.

2 The psychiatrist has a responsibility to communicate to the patient the conclusions of the assessment, including a proper diagnosis. The patient has a right to be informed as to his or her diagnosis. Wherever possible, this should be communicated in a manner consistent with *DSM-III-R* terminology and criteria. I recognize that there is a legal as well as a professional dispute as to the nature of informed consent that is expected in different jurisdictions, but the fullest possible transmission of information will facilitate trust and integrity in the doctor-patient relationship (unpublished 1988 paper of Alan Stone).

3 The psychiatrist has a responsibility to provide information as to alternative treatments. The patient has the right to be informed as to the alternative treatments available, their relative efficacy and safety, and the likely outcomes of these treatments. This is a special requirement on the respectable minority of physicians, since they should inform the patient that their treatment is not the one most widely held within the profession. In communicating these alternatives to the patient, the clinician should not make pejorative statements about former types of treatment. Statements such as 'Drug treatment is only a crutch,' 'I don't believe in drug treatment,' 'ECT will cause brain damage,' and 'I don't believe in psychotherapy' are ill-advised and may be used by the patient against the clinician in subsequent complaints, including legal action.

4 The psychiatrist has a responsibility to use effective treatment. The patient has the right to the proper treatment. Proper treatment involves those treatments for which there is substantial evidence.

5 The psychiatrist has a responsibility to modify treatment plans or seek consultation if the patient does not improve. To quote K. Livingston (unpublished 1985 manuscript):

While psychiatry is not obliged to guarantee a cure, the courts may consider sympathetically arguments based upon the disparity between lengthy and costly treatment and the patient's failure to improve. Commentators note that when a patient fails to improve or deteriorates during treatment, there may be a duty upon the psychiatrist to abandon the treatment or to seek consultation.

Applied to the treatment of depression, the available evidence indicates that patients should begin to show improvement with medication within 4–8 weeks or with psychotherapy within 12–16 weeks. Failure of the patient to improve on a given treatment program within 3–4 months should prompt a reevaluation of the treatment plan, including consultation and consideration of alternative treatment.

Conclusions

Dr. Stone[3] stated, 'When it deals with psychiatry, the law must deal with a world of complexity, dubiety, and increasing conflict about efficacy.' The availability of scientific evidence will increasingly be considered by the courts as relevant to such decisions. In large part this is because of the major advances in psychiatric therapeutic research. The availability of this growing body of evidence prompts new criteria for judging standards of care and treatment. In the presence of such evidence, practitioners and institutions who continue to rely on forms of treatment with limited efficacy will be on the defensive and at possible jeopardy for legal action.

Resolution of professional issues through the courts is far from ideal and has substantial social costs. Ideally, the profession is the best judge of the available evidence. The courts are a poor tribunal in which to resolve scientific and professional issues. However, in the case of *Osheroff v. Chestnut Lodge*, there had been some professional agreement, as reflected in the APA peer review manual (44). The courts may be an appropriate arena for litigation when a small minority of the profession persist in practices that scientific evidence and professional judgment have deemed obsolete.

The problem of differences of opinion within a professional group has its analogy in issues of civil liberties – when should the majority insist that the minority accept its views? In the case of professional issues in psychiatry and medicine, however, the persistence of a minority dissent has implications beyond those of the profession because certain professional practices may involve harm to individual patients.

In the current situation in psychiatric practice, where there are large areas of ignorance, it behooves individual practitioners and institutions to avoid relying on single treatment approaches or theoretical paradigms. Thus, in modern psychiatry, treatment programs based only on psychotherapy or only on drugs are subject to criticism. Professionalism requires balancing available knowledge against clinical experience and promoting the advancement of scientific knowledge. In the case of treatment practices, such knowledge best comes from controlled trials.

References

1 **Malcolm JG:** Treatment choices and informed consent in psychiatry: implications of the Osheroff case for the profession. *J Psychiatry Law* 1986; **14**:9–107.

2 **Sifford D:** An improper diagnosis case that changed psychiatry. *Philadelphia Inquirer*, March 24, 1988, p 4E.

3 **Stone AA:** The new paradox of psychiatric malpractice. *N Engl J Med* 1984; **311**:384–1387.

4 **Fink PJ:** Response to the presidential address: is 'biopsychosocial' the psychiatric shibboleth? *Am J Psychiatry* 1988; **145**:1061–1067.

5 **Campbell RJ III:** Psychiatrists take law into own hands. *Psychiatr News*, April 1, 1988, p 4.

6 **Klerman GL:** Trends in utilization of mental health services: perspectives for health services research. *Med Care* 1985; **23**: 584–587.

7   State of Maryland Health Claims Arbitration Board Amended Arbitration Panel Determination 82–262, Jan 18, 1984. Baltimore, Health Claims Arbitration Board, 1984.

8   Hollingshead A, Redlich F: *Social Class and Mental Illness*. New York, John Wiley & Sons, 1958.

9   Armor DJ, Klerman GL: Psychiatric treatment orientations and professional ideology. *J Health Soc Behav*, 1968: **9**:243–255.

10 Strauss A, Schatzman L, Bucher R, *et al* (eds): *Psychiatric Ideologies and Institutions*, New York, Free Press, 1964.

11 Havens L: *Approaches to the Mind*. Boston, Little, Brown, 1973.

12 Kuhn TS: *The Structure of Scientific Revolutions*, 2nd ed: International Encyclopedia of Unified Science, vol 2, number 2. Chicago, University of Chicago Press, 1970.

13 Klerman GL: The scope of depression, in *The Origins of Depression: Current Concepts and Approaches*. Edited by Angst J. New York, Springer-Verlag, 1983.

14 Klerman GL, Weissman MM, Rounsaville BJ, *et al*: *Interpersonal Psychotherapy of Depression*. New York, Basic Books, 1984.

15 Sullivan HS: *The Interpersonal Theory of Psychiatry*. New York, WW Norton, 1953.

16 Fromm-Reichmann F: *Principles of Intensive Psychotherapy*. Chicago, Phoenix Books, 1960.

17 Cohen MB, Baker G, Cohen R, *et al*: An intensive study of twelve cases of manic-depressive psychosis. *Psychiatry* 1954; **17**:103–137.

18 Will O: Schizophrenia: psychological treatment, in *Comprehensive Textbook of Psychiatry*, 3rd ed. vol 2. Edited by Kaplan HI, Freedman AM, Sadock BJ. Baltimore, Williams & Wilkins, 1980.

19 Klerman GL: Drugs and psychotherapy, in *Handbook of Psychotherapy and Behavior Change: An Empirical Analysis*, 3rd ed. Edited by Garfield SL, Bergin AE. New York, John Wiley & Sons, 1986.

20 Stanton AH, Schwartz MS: *The Mental Hospital*. New York, Basic Books, 1954.

21 Arieti S, Bemporad J: *Severe and Mild Depression: The Psychotherapeutic Approach*. New York, Basic Books. 1978.

22 Hirschfeld RMA, Klerman GL, Clayton PJ, *et al*: Assessing personality: effects of the depressive state on trait measurement. *Am I Psychiatry*, 1983: **140**:695–699.

23 Smith ML, Glass GV. Miller TI: *The Benefits of Psychotherapy*. Baltimore. John, Hopkins University Press. 1980.

24 Andrews G, Harvey R: Does psychotherapy benefit neurotic patients: *Arch Gen Psychiatry* 1981; **38**:1203–1208.

25 Stanton AH. Gunderson JG, Knapp PH, *et al*: Effects of psychotherapy in schizophrenia, I: design and implementation of a controlled study. *Schizophr Bull*. 1984; **10**:520–563.

26 Weissman MM, Jarrett RB, Rush AJ: Psychotherapy and its relevance to the pharmacotherapy of major depression, in *Psychopharmacology: The Third Generation of Progress*, Edited by Meltzer HY. New York, Raven Press, 1987.

27 Marks I: Review of behavioral psychotherapy, I: obsessive-compulsive disorders. *Am J Psychiatry* 1981; **138**:584–592.

28 Griest JH, Jefferson JW, Spitzer RL: *Treatment of Mental Disorders*. New York, Oxford University Press, 1982.

29 Klerman GL: Ideology and science in the individual psychotherapy of schizophrenia. *Schizophr Bull* 1984; **10**:608–612.

30 McGlashan TH: The Chestnut Lodge follow-up study, III: long-term outcome of borderline personalities. *Arch Gen Psychiatry* 1986; **43**:20–30.

31 Dingman CW, McGlashan TH: Discriminating characteristics of suicides: Chesnut Lodge follow-up sample including patients with affective disorder, schizophrenia and schizoaffective disorder. *Acta Psychiatr Scand* 1986; **74**:91–97.

32 Beck AT, Rush AJ. Shaw BF, *et al*: *Cognitive Therapy of Depression*. New York, Guilford Press, 1979.

33 Lewinsohn PM: A behavioral approach to depression, in *The Psychology of Depression: Contemporary Theory and Research*. Edited by Friedman RJ, Katz MM. Washington, DC, VH Winston & Sons, 1974.

34 Shea T, Glass DR, Pilkonis PA, *et al*: Frequency and implications of personality disorders in a sample of depressed out-patients. *J Personality Disorders* 1987: **1**:27–42.

35 Klerman GL: Psychotherapies and somatic therapies in affective disorders. *Psyhiatr Clin North Am*. 1983; **6**:85–103.

36 Rounsaville BJ, Klerman GL, Weissman MM: Do psychotherapy and pharmacotherapy for depression conflict? *Arch Gen Psychiatry* 1981; **38**:24–29.

37 Beitman BD, Klerman GL (eds): *Combining Psychotherapy and Drug Therapy in Clinical Practice*. Jamaica, NY, SP Medical & Scientific Books, 1984.

38 Gottlieb JS, Huston PE: Treatment of schizophrenia: a comparison of three methods–brief psychotherapy, insulin coma, and electric shock. *J Nerv Ment Dis* 1951; **113**:211–235.

39 Avery D, Winokur G: Mortality in depressed patients treated with electroconvulsive therapy and antidepressant. *Arch Gen Psychiatry* 1976; **33**:1029–1037.

40 Klerman GL: The efficacy of psychotherapy as the basis for public policy. *Am Psychol* 1983; **38**:929–934.

41 Consensus Development Panel: NIMH/NIH Consensus Development Conference Statement: mood disorders: pharmacological prevention of recurrences. *Am J Psychiatry* 1985; **142**:469–476.

42 American Psychiatric Association Task Force Report 14: *Electroconvulsive Therapy*. Washington, DC, APA, 1978.

43 Andrews G: A treatment outline for depressive disorders. *Aust. NZ J Psychiatry* 1983; **17**:129–146.

44 American Psychiatric Association Peer Review Committee: *Manual of Psychiatric Peer Review*. Washington, DC, APA, 1982.

45 American Psychiatric Association Commission on Psychotherapies: *Psychotherapy Research: Methodological and Efficacy Issues*. Washington, DC, APA, 1982.

46 American Psychiatric Association Commission on Psychiatric Therapies: *The Psychiatric Therapies*. Washington, DC, APA, 1984.

47 Grunbaum A: *The Foundations of Psychoanalysis: A Philosophical Critique*. Berkeley, University of California Press, 1984.

48 Klerman GL: The scientific tasks confronting psychoanalysis: a review of Grunbaum's *Foundations of Psychoanalysis*. *Behavioral and Brain Sciences* 1986; **9**:245.

Law, Science, and Psychiatric Malpractice

A Response to Klerman's Indictment of Psychoanalytic Psychiatry*

Alan A. Stone

It is the potential legal implications of Klerman's conclusions that will be most noteworthy to his colleagues, insurance companies, and the lawyers for whom these matters are relevant. It is therefore necessary for me to set out here what I think is the potential legal import of Klerman's paper, recognizing that he can claim I have misunderstood what he intended merely as clinical recommendations. The problem is that clinical recommendations made by one of the leading authorities in psychiatry carry legal weight in court as standards of care. This point will be amplified in what follows. I also assume that what Klerman says in his paper he is prepared to say in court or in depositions, just as he did in the Osheroff litigation. The principal inquiry to be considered here, therefore, is how Klerman's paper would be understood by a lawyer contemplating a malpractice suit against a psychoanalytically oriented psychiatrist.

As Klerman et al.[1] have written elsewhere, this is the age of depression; the treatment of depression, therefore, is the principal task of clinical psychiatry. The significance of Klerman's recommendations, implicit in his paper, is that it is clinically improper and therefore negligent to provide exclusively psychoanalytic treatment or psychoanalytically based psychotherapy for any patient with any depressive disorder. It is also reasonable to conclude that Klerman recommends that the provision of such exclusive treatments should be deemed improper for any other DSM-III-R disorder for which there is an alternative treatment, that has any demonstrated efficacy in a clinical trial.

The reader might suppose that such exclusive treatments are not negligent, in Klerman's view, if the patients have been appropriately informed of the more efficacious treatment alternatives and have been told that the kind of treatment being proposed has no 'scientifically' proven efficacy. Patients could choose exclusive psychoanalytic treatment in this scenario, despite being appropriately informed about the 'scientific' evidence. The law of informed consent might then insulate the psychiatrist from liability. However, Klerman's paradigm of professional responsibility is aimed at regulating the exclusive practice of personal psychiatry. It includes as its fourth responsibility that of providing treatments for which there is substantial evidence, regardless of the patient's consent. He chastises psychiatry for its failure 'to provide evidence for the efficacy of psychoanalysis and psychodynamic psychotherapies as treatments for psychiatric disorders.' Although he acknowledges other kinds of evidence for efficacy, controlled clinical trials provide the key evidence. He writes, 'Those treatments which make claims but have not generated evidence are in a weak position.' Certainly, nothing in his paper indicates that he thinks there is substantial evidence for treatments in this weak position.

It is by no means certain that a psychiatric patient's informed consent would in fact insulate a psychiatrist. Malpractice is always a retrospective determination after an adverse outcome. Therefore. I believe the import of Klerman's recommendations can be understood by a reasonable lawyer as

stating that, in the absence of new efficacy studies, exclusive use of psychoanalysis, psychodynamic psychotherapy, or, perhaps, other humanistic psychotherapies that are not scientifically substantiated is improper, in a weak position. and subject to serious, if not dispositive, challenge in any malpractice litigation. Those are the legal inferences I have drawn from Klerman's presentation. What follows, therefore, is based on that interpretation and will further demonstrate the basis for it. Hereafter, I will refer to psychoanalysis and psychoanalytic therapy as traditional psychiatry, recognizing, as does Klerman, that the psychoanalytic approach has been a dominant force in psychiatry in the United States since World War II.

The Law

Klerman's title, 'The Psychiatric Patient's Right to Effective Treatment,' will suggest to most psychiatrists that the law has announced some new Constitutional right and that it has something to do with Osheroff v. Chestnut Lodge. However, as Klerman recognizes, this litigation was settled out of court. No Constitutional claim was made, and no judge formulated any legal theory about the so-called right to effective treatment. There is no clear legal precedent for anything Klerman states in his paper.

I have therefore carefully eschewed the phrase the 'Osheroff case' to emphasize that there is no decided case establishing any relevant legal precedent about rights or about negligence in the law of Maryland or any other jurisdiction. (There was an arbitration report and a published decision on a narrow procedural question.) Furthermore, when Dr. Osheroff agreed to settle his legal claims, he undoubtedly signed documents indicating that Chestnut Lodge was not to be deemed negligent on any ground. Therefore, the legal precedent of the Osheroff litigation is unknown and unknowable. It does not exist.

Klerman also asserts that 'the case has been widely discussed in legal journals.' He then cites an article that began as required written work by Malcolm as a Harvard law student.[2] This work has since been expanded into a book.[3] Malcolm's article and an unpublished paper by Livingston are the only citations Klerman relies on for the legal implications he draws from Osheroff. It is totally without legal precedent and without any other legal authority or evidence that Klerman writes, 'In my opinion, this case goes a long way toward establishing the patient's right to effective treatment.' Particularly troubling is Klerman's use of the phrase 'the right to effective treatment.' Patients' rights usually refer to Constitutional or statutory rights. For instance, the familiar right to treatment is based on the Bill of Rights or on legislation. Klerman describes no such basis for this new right. Furthermore, Dr. Osheroff's litigation involved allegations of malpractice. With the exception of the so-called right to informed consent,[4] malpractice law is not ordinarily conceptualized in terms of a patient's rights but about a physician's negligence.[5] Legal scholars would certainly argue that even in negligence law and malpractice one can speak of every duty in terms of a countervailing right. Klerman, however, provides no legal basis for either a

* Stone, A.: Law, science, and psychiatric malpractice: A response to Klerman's indictment on psychoanalytic psychiatry. American Journal of Psychiatry 147:419–427, 1990.

duty or a right. Klerman's concluding recommendations suggest that the right to effective treatment is somehow derived from the right to informed consent. That would be a radical legal departure from existing law. Although the courts have broadened the legal requirements of disclosure in informed consent, their goal has always been to increase the patient's autonomy and not to regulate or restrict methods of treatment. Furthermore, empirical research suggests that the law of informed consent is already out of touch with clinical reality.[6] Nonetheless, Klerman's recommendations would further expand and rigidly specify this legal obligation. In any event, the right to effective treatment is never clarified; its legal basis is never documented; its use is confused and confusing; and Klerman acknowledges that he has not confronted the legal complexities or consequences involved in informed consent, which vary from state to state according to statutes and case law.[7]

Malpractice law quintessentially concerns duties translated into standards of care. The standard of care depends on the facts of the situation. Familiarity with a malpractice treatise would make it clear that it is difficult, if not impossible, to generalize about the standard of care in all of psychiatric practice based on one actual situation.[5] Yet that is exactly what Klerman seems to be doing in making conclusions about the legal implications of *Osheroff*.

Once it becomes clear that there is neither legal precedent nor established legal authority for what Klerman writes here, it becomes possible to discern more clearly the nature of his paper. It is not about law; rather, it is an attempt to promulgate more uniform scientific standards of treatment in psychiatry, based on his own opinions about science and clinical practice. Klerman notes the large number of expert witnesses for Dr. Osheroff, including Drs. Donald Klein, Bernard Carroll, Frank Ayd, and himself. Their number is less impressive than their professional qualifications and their shared 'scientific' perspective. This panel of experts certainly rivals in eminence any group that was ever assembled to testify on the patient's side of a malpractice case in psychiatry. None of them, however, is by reputation an authority on informed consent. They were all willing to testify on other grounds that Chestnut Lodge was negligent in its diagnosis and/or treatment. I take it that Klerman defends that testimony in his paper and suggests that his basic rationale should be accepted by like-minded colleagues who might testify in future malpractice litigation. Klerman's recommendations may have considerable legal consequences, even if his ideas have no basis in law and are intended only as clinical recommendations. The basic practical consideration for a contingency-fee lawyer in malpractice litigation is whether one or more expert witnesses can be found with sufficient professional authority who are willing to testify convincingly that their colleagues are guilty of negligence.[5] Whatever claim a lawyer makes against a traditional psychiatrist can only be helped by any expert witness who accepts Klerman's opinions. For example, any traditional psychiatrist whose patient commits suicide might face expert testimony stating that the treatment provided was not proper and lacked substantial evidence of efficacy, which could lead to liability. Thus, Klerman's paper has potentially serious legal consequences for all practitioners of traditional psychiatry.

The Standard of Care in *Osheroff*

Klerman clearly recognizes, and it must he emphasized, that the alleged malpractice in *Osheroff* took place in 1979. Therefore, the legal standard of care to be applied is the accepted practice of the psychiatric profession more than a decade ago. Much has happened in psychiatry in the past decade, both in our diagnostic approaches and in our treatment armamentaria. Those developments cannot be the basis for an expert witness's opinion about the standard of care in 1979. In his chapter on affective disorders in *The Harvard Guide to Modern Psychiatry*, published in 1978,[8] Klerman suggested the accepted practices of the time. Two things should be noted about this chapter. First, he recognized that many respectable clinicians held to a unitary (psychoanalytic) theory of mental illness in general and of depression in particular but that he had himself accepted the concept of 'multiple symptom complexes' as the more enlightened approach to nosology.

Second, although he clearly favored combined chemotherapy and psychotherapy and a pluralistic approach to etiology and treatment, Klerman wrote, 'Individual psychotherapy based on psychodynamic principles remains the most widely used form of psychotherapy. Although systematic, controlled clinical studies do not exist, clinical observations strongly support the value of this form of psychotherapy during both acute and long-term treatments.' He even suggested that traditional psychoanalysis might be 'indicated for neurotic depressions in individuals with long-standing personality disorders.' Thus, Klerman's own 1978 publication summarizing what was known then about affective disorders would by itself go a long way as a legal defense of Chestnut Lodge. Ironically, except for the word 'strongly,' his revised chapter in the 1988 *New Harvard-Guide to Psychiatry*,[9] quoted at the end of this paper, contains almost identical language.

It is essential that the reader distinguish between the narrow legal question of what was negligent in 1979 and the much broader arguments about scientific evidence and policy advanced by Klerman. He attempts to link together the *Osheroff* litigation, the legal standard of care in malpractice, efficacy research, and public policy based on efficacy research. It is possible to argue that he presents each of these issues and their supposed connections in a one-sided and partisan fashion. Therefore, I shall here present the other side. First, if there was malpractice in *Osheroff*, the strongest argument is that under the facts of that case, as described by Klerman, negligence arose from the persistence in a course of exclusive psychodynamic treatment despite obvious psychotic deterioration. This argument does not depend on the latest scientific research on efficacy or the scientific status of psychoanalysis or psychodynamic psychotherapy. Second, the legal standard of care in malpractice is not and should not be a universal rule set by one school of psychiatry for the others, even if it wraps itself in the mantle of modern science. Rather, the legal standard of care should reflect the 'collective sense of the profession',[10] not the partisan opinions or one particular group and certainly not the latest unreplicated and evolving scientific evidence.[5] Third, efficacy research, including controlled clinical trials, is of varying quality, Much of it is far from being based on solid methodological grounds,[11] and the leap from controlled trials to clinical practice often produces unexpected results. Public policy based on such a limited scientific foundation and enforced by malpractice litigation is unlikely to benefit our patients or our profession. If the kind of efficacy research now available to psychiatry led to decisively beneficial treatment for most patients with minimal side effects and long-term improvement, there would be no professional debate. However, it should be obvious that all of Klerman's arguments about law, science, efficacy, and policy stand or fall without regard to the *Osheroff* litigation.

A Restatement of the Case History

Klerman's brief description of Dr. Osheroff s history makes the diagnosis of narcissistic personality disorder seem ridiculous. The details of Dr. Osheroff's case history, including excerpts from his own autobiographical account, have been published by Malcolm[3] and are the basis for what follows here. I have no professional relationship with Dr. Osheroff or the litigation. Furthermore, I would emphasize that everything reported here is available to the general public in Malcolm's book. There are still reasons to have qualms about republishing the personal details of an identified patient's case history. On the other hand, Klerman has made this case the centerpiece of his paper and Dr. Osheroff himself participated in a session at the 1989 APA annual meeting.

Malcolm's book reports that Dr. Osheroff was married three times before his hospitalization. His first marital relationship began while he was in college and ended in divorce after 21 months because his wife had allegedly been unfaithful. He thought of leaving medical school but saw a psychiatrist who convinced him to return. During his internship he met and married a nurse. That second marriage lasted much longer but deteriorated after the birth of two children. Dr. Osheroff saw a psychiatrist again during these years while he was establishing his practice. According to Malcolm,[3] he wrote about this period of time in his autobiography, which he entitled *A Symbolic Death:*

All during the early years of my (second) marriage, I had been rather immature and insensitive and my energies seemed to be so devoted to and focused on my career, that I perhaps was not listening and if I was listening, perhaps I wasn't hearing. I was seemingly oblivious to the stresses that were developing in my marriage at the time.

Psychotherapy for Dr. Osheroff and marital therapy for the couple did not save the marriage. His second wife eventually left the children with him and went off with another man. Dr. Osheroff lost 40 pounds during this time, living 'a life that was almost devoid of the usual types of satisfaction.' His nephrology practice, nonetheless, grew and prospered as he opened his own dialysis center. He then met his third wife, a medical student on her clinical clerkship, and married her after a 'whirlwind romance.' This was at first a happy and successful marriage, and symptoms of depression apparently disappeared. He and his wife were, in his words, 'one of the most celebrated and sought after medical couples in the . . . area.'

There were continuing conflicts, however, with his second wife, who now wanted custody of their two children. Conflicts also began with his third wife. They were precipitated, according to her, by his seemingly inconsiderate behavior during the birth of their first child (his third) and his lack of attention to the baby and her.

Dr. Osheroff also began to have serious disagreements with his professional associates in practice. With these conflicts and the deterioration of his third marriage, he saw at least three different psychiatrists, two of whom prescribed antidepressive medication, which was not successful – perhaps because of lack of compliance. It is well recognized that 'drug manipulation and drug compliance are anticipated problems' in patients whose affective symptoms are complicated by personality disorders.[12] No doubt, such problems can be even greater when the patient is himself a physician and may have his own opinions about treatment.

I do not mean to suggest that Klerman intentionally selected from the history only those features which support his diagnosis and the basic thesis of his paper. Perhaps the kinds of subjective experiences revealed in Dr. Osheroff's autobiographical account and the interpersonal difficulties he experienced with the important people in his life, which suggest problems in the sphere of object relations and character, have become less relevant to psychiatrists who tend to overemphasize *DSM-III's* axis I in comparison with axis II. Perhaps these two quite different histories indicate that there is an incorrigible diagnostic and conceptual difference between Klerman's school and traditional psychiatrists. The 'scientific' psychiatrist now looks for the symptoms. The traditional psychiatrist still looks for the person. Each school can criticize the blindness of the other on the basis of its own criteria.

In any event, when Dr. Osheroff entered Chestnut Lodge he was not a neophyte as to psychiatry or its various therapeutic approaches, nor was he professionally or personally ignorant about depression. He was a physician who, I have no doubt, had already several times in his life been diagnosed, fully informed about his diagnosis, and treated exactly in the manner recommended by Klerman in his paper. Those treatment methods had failed. All of this seems relevant to any judgment about Chestnut Lodge's alleged negligence and the lessons Klerman claims are to be learned from this litigation.

The Diagnosis

Klerman relies on a strict construction of *DSM-II, DSM-III,* and *DSM-III-R* in his discussion of the standard of care for diagnosis. He points out that there was no narcissistic personality disorder in *DSM-III.* Therefore, Chestnut Lodge used a diagnosis not listed in psychiatry's official nomenclature.

DSM-II, however, was certainly not regarded with the same authority the profession has given its successors. Psychodynamic etiological diagnoses were commonly used whether or not they were in *DSM-III* and narcissistic

personality was perhaps the most frequently used. Indeed, it became the diagnosis of an entire culture.[13] Given my restatement of the case history, I believe that the vast majority of psychiatrists would agree that a diagnosis of narcissistic or some other personality disorder at the time of admission was not evidence of negligence, particularly since a diagnosis of affective disorder was also made. Most psychiatrists in 1979 would not have considered it a breach of professional standards merely to depart from official nomenclature in this way.

Dr. Osheroff's own autobiographical account of his illness would substantiate many, if not all, of the typical features of narcissistic personality disorder described by Kernberg.[14] Certainly, the restated case history presents relevant evidence omitted by Klerman.

The Treatment

The breakdown of Dr. Osheroff's third marriage and his professional conflicts, which precipitated his hospitalization, could reasonably have been understood at the time as classic examples of the kind of psychosocial crises that destroy the precarious balance of the narcissistic personality. Even if Klerman believes that this kind of psychodynamic formulation and approach to treatment is no longer 'scientifically' acceptable, there can be little doubt that it was well within the collective sense of the profession in 1979. Thus, I suggest that the initial treatment program for Dr. Osheroff was acceptable, particularly in the light of a history of previous unsuccessful drug treatment provided by a leading psychopharmacologist and implemented by his traditional psychotherapist.

With only this psychodynamically oriented psychotherapy, however, the patient's condition obviously deteriorated. Whatever the original diagnosis and treatment plan were, reevaluation and consultation are required at some point when a treatment regimen has such obviously negative consequences. I have no doubt that during the 1950s, 1960s, and 1970s at Chestnut Lodge and other similarly oriented hospitals, traditional therapists did persist in exclusive psychoanalytic psychotherapy, despite similar situations of obvious symptomatic deterioration. My own clinical experience at McLean Hospital during these years certainly confirms this impression.

If Klerman had stayed with this narrow fact of the situation and stated that exclusively psychoanalytic treatment of a hospitalized patient in the face of obvious psychotic deterioration is no longer clinically acceptable, I believe he could have claimed to speak for the collective sense of the profession, including the vast majority of traditional psychiatrists.

It is important to recognize that this marks an important historical moment of transition in modern psychiatry. Many new considerations as well as efficacy studies have led to this change. The biological dimensions of serious mental disorders and their treatment have been better understood, and this understanding has been more widely accepted. The consequences of long periods of psychotic decompensation have been more fully recognized. The distinction between social recovery with improvement of symptoms and the cure of serious mental illnesses has been better appreciated and psychiatric hospitalization has increasingly focused on the former. The negative implications of long-term hospitalization of patients with psychotic disorders have been well documented. Psychiatrists have recognized the importance of improvement in symptoms for the therapeutic alliance and, therefore, as a necessary part of treatment with seriously disturbed patients. The limitations of traditional therapy with psychotic patients are widely accepted, and successful treatment is more often attributed to the unique qualities of the therapist or the relationship rather than to the method of the psychotherapy. All of these factors and not just the available efficacy studies have led to the changes in the collective sense of the profession.

At Chestnut Lodge, Dr. Osheroff apparently developed a negative therapeutic reaction and a negative transference to both the therapist and the hospital. The person suffering from these serious symptoms of depression was in revolt against his treatment. The recommendation to change hospitals seems to me eminently sound on psychodynamic grounds. Klerman suggests that Dr. Osheroff's remarkable cure at the Silver Hill Foundation was a function of his finally being provided the efficacious combination of tricyclics and phenothiazines. If all patients like Dr. Osheroff had such remarkable cures with these drugs, psychiatry would be a different profession. But Dr. Osheroff's psychological response to Silver Hill Foundation, as described in his autobiography, suggests that other, equally important, psychodynamic factors were involved. He had escaped, if not narcissistically triumphed over, Chestnut Lodge and his therapist. His negative transference had been vindicated. Such psychodynamic conceptions still seem as relevant to our clinical understanding of such remarkable cures as does psychopharmacology.

Biological Versus Psychodynamic Psychiatry

Klerman and Klein have both objected to my characterization of the *Osheroff* dispute as one between biological and psychodynamic psychiatry.[15] Klerman here states that it is, rather, a matter of opinion versus evidence. Klein[16] has made the same point in stronger and more colorful language. Both of them contend that they are speaking as scientists and that the issue is one of scientific evidence versus dogmatic opinion. Klerman makes this a thesis of his current paper, applying it as a standard to all psychiatric treatments. I believe that both men ignore the very real problem of differing opinions about scientific evidence and the canons of science within the psychiatric profession. Klerman and Klein surely recognize that the quality of the evidence, even in their own impressive research, leaves room for other scientists to make interpretations and raise questions. The basic assumptions on which clinical research on depression and panic states proceeds are subject to fundamental questions by serious scientists.[17] Klerman is no doubt correct that at a meeting of scientists, the person with evidence should take precedence over the person without evidence. Even a small amount of evidence is better than opinion when the question is what can science say about a subject. But that does not mean the science is good enough to create a uniform policy or to dictate to clinicians the clinical standards of care.

Klerman also objects to the 'biological' designation because of his longstanding pluralistic approach to etiology and treatment. My intention, however, was not to suggest that he was a biological psychiatrist but that he brought a biological perspective, as opposed to the psychodynamic perspective of Chestnut Lodge, to the *Osheroff* dispute. My objective was to explain what I understood to be the basis of the dispute. Certainly, if I had been responsible for Dr. Osheroff's care I would have insisted on 'biological treatment' in the face of obvious psychotic deterioration. It has been my long-standing contention that in similar actual situations, judges upholding the right to refuse treatment were forcing psychiatrists to commit malpractice[18]. Unfortunately, Klerman's paper goes well beyond the facts of *Osheroff*. His standards are meant to apply to the treatment of any *DSM-III-R* disorder, and the onus he places on traditional psychiatry is unmistakable.

Efficacy Research and Public Policy Concerns

There is an apocryphal story told about male lawyers. One asks the other, 'How is your spouse?' The other replies, 'Compared to what?' 'Compared to what' is the appropriate perspective to bring to Klerman's discussion of efficacy research and policy. He compares psychotherapy and drugs. In that comparison he criticizes the failure of various government agencies at the federal and state levels. He also criticizes his colleagues in research and in professional associations. When compared to Food and Drug Administration safety and efficacy standards for drugs, the regulation of psychotherapy seems to stand out as a public policy disaster. But virtually everything Klerman says about psychotherapy applies with equal force to

surgery and almost everything else that physicians do which does not come under the Food and Drug Administration's authority. Much of what all physicians do has no demonstrated effectiveness – even the prescription of supposedly efficacious medication. Thus, if psychotherapy is compared to surgery, for example, one might get a totally different impression about the nature and significance of the public policy problem posed by traditional psychotherapy. It turns out that the Food and Drug Administration is quite unique, holding the massive pharmaceutical industry hostage and able to require it to invest vast resources in research into efficacy and safety. Thus, Klerman's use of the Food and Drug Administration as a model is less relevant and less meaningful than it seems.

All health policy experts are concerned about efficacy. Indeed, efficacy research has become the central requirement of what Relman[19] called the third revolution in medical care, requiring increased attention to assessment and accountability. In order to meet the pressing objectives of quality and cost control, however, Relman wrote, 'We will also need to know much more about the relative costs, safety, and effectiveness of all the things physicians do or employ in the diagnosis, treatment and prevention of disease'.[19] Relman was commenting on an article by Roper *et al.*[20] of the Health Care Financing Administration, who described new 'effectiveness initiatives.' These will increasingly involve the federal government in the collection and distribution of efficacy and outcome data concerning many branches of medicine. Roper *et al.*, along with Relman, stated that more comprehensive assessment of medical effectiveness will eventually improve the quality of care and eventually help curtail costs. Unlike Klerman, they suggested that the science of efficacy research currently available in the rest of medicine is inadequate to the task. The focus of the Health Care Financing Administration was on surgery. For example, they cited carotid endarterectomy and the implantation of cardiac pacemakers as examples of surgical practices often used inappropriately because of the lack of adequate efficacy studies. More money is certainly spent on these procedures than on all of the traditional psychotherapy provided in the United States – and the immediate risks of their use or misuse are much greater. Roper et al.[20] clearly recognized what Klerman has not: that the 'science of health care evaluation, still in its formative stages, requires certain resources: money, data, and people trained in the evaluative sciences' and that 'methods of gathering and synthesizing data on health outcomes and effectiveness are correspondingly underdeveloped.'

Roper *et al.* made it clear that a whole new infrastructure for gathering data is necessary before sensible public policy can be developed to control clinical practice. They did not blame the medical profession for this gap in our scientific knowledge. Klerman's paper, in contrast, seems to be a rush to judgment, with the first stop at the courthouse. Klerman does not even acknowledge that there is any legitimate opposition to his views. He is prepared to argue that 'the absence of professional consensus statements in our field leaves it open for the courts to be used by individuals, such as Dr. Osheroff, who feel they have been poorly treated and who believe they are entitled to redress of their grievances.' This is to suggest that the psychiatric profession is now being punished for its own sins of laxity, which opened the door to the courtroom. This is simply nonsense. Every legal scholar writing on the subject of psychiatric malpractice has pointed to the lack of professional consensus in psychiatry as a major cause for the remarkable dearth of such litigation compared to other specialties over the past century.[5, 21] In fact, any experienced lawyer would say that Dr. Osheroff was able to litigate because he was able to obtain expert witnesses like Klerman and his distinguished colleagues, who were willing to testify that there is a consensus about efficacious treatment. Indeed, Klerman's paper is an attempt to assert and establish this thesis.

The use of the courtroom and malpractice litigation to enforce a consensus policy on efficacy would have serious consequences for biological psychiatry as well as for the field as a whole. The history of neuroleptic medication for schizophrenic disorders presents a striking example. Psychiatry's understanding of efficacious doses and deleterious side effects has changed dramatically over the past two decades. We have gone from smaller doses to megadoses back to smaller doses. We have gone from routine maintenance to selective maintenance. We went through a brief phase of rapid intramuscular 'neurolepticization' for acute psychotic disorders and abandoned it.[22] All of these changing standards of care were based on clinical experience, available scientific evidence, and a genuine concern for providing effective treatment. If, at any early point in this history, biological psychiatrists had gone to court or to any other official authority to impose efficacious dose standards on all their colleagues, it would have been a disaster for our patients and for biological psychiatry. If it is Klerman's idea that psychiatry should be ruled by the courts applying the prevailing scientific evidence of the day, he has a recipe for disaster.

Klerman's Specific Recommendations

Responsibility to Make a Diagnosis According to DSM-III-R

DSM-III and DSM-III-R constitute officially recognized diagnostic nomenclature. Furthermore, the use of this nomenclature is now widely accepted in the profession. Thus, Klerman's first recommendation is not obviously controversial. Looking back to the Osheroff litigation, Klerman strongly objected to the diagnosis of narcissistic personality disorder based on psychodynamic considerations. Presumably, this requirement is intended to prevent similar lapses. Traditional psychiatrists writing in modern psychiatric textbooks continue to emphasize psychodynamic formulations and criticize DSM-III and DSM-III-R. Nemiah,[23] for example, wrote, 'The new nomenclature and diagnostic grouping are a mixed blessing, particularly if one wishes to go beyond purely phenomenological description to a consideration of the psychodynamic mechanisms involved in the formation of symptoms – an activity that the framers of DSM-III would like to discourage.' Klerman would not only discourage such activity but also delegitimize the psychodynamic diagnostic formulations of traditional psychiatry. The essence of the first responsibility is that it locks the traditional psychiatrist into the scientific paradigm urged by Klerman.

Responsibility to Inform the Patient

Having made a diagnosis, the psychiatrist would be required to communicate it to the patient in a manner consistent with DSM-III-R. Ironically, Klerman cites me as supporting this requirement. I value DSM-III-R as a basis for more reliable communication within the psychiatric profession. I do not believe that all of its diagnostic categories have scientific validity or that they all have value in helping patients to understand their human problems or their mental disorders. Some DSM-III-R diagnoses seem quite helpful in this respect, and others do not. For some patients a psychodynamic diagnostic formation may be more helpful. Even when the diagnosis is helpful to the patient, there is the matter of timing, which Klerman fails to emphasize.

It is certainly my belief that psychiatrists should view helping patients understand their problems as one of their professional responsibilities. In that sense, informed consent is an essential goal and principle of psychiatry and of all psychiatric treatments. It is a predicate for a therapeutic alliance. But informed consent is a process, not an immediate one-time recitation of a formula regardless of the actual situation. DSM-III-R may or may not be helpful in that enterprise and therefore ought not to be forced on all patients by a blanket rule that places the clinician in a pseudoscientific ideological straightjacket. We should not confuse the valuable function DSM-III-R serves in clarifying communication among psychiatrists with its value in communication with our patients. Whatever the law of informed consent may be, it does not require uniform behavior in every actual situation. The law requires a reasonably prudent physician,[5] not a scientific automaton. Klerman's criteria suggest an emphasis on controlling his colleagues rather than on promoting a therapeutic relationship.

Responsibility to Describe Alternative Treatments

The psychiatrist, having made a DSM-III-R diagnosis and revealed it to the patient, is next required by Klerman to discuss with the patient the efficacious treatment alternatives. The burden here is heaviest on traditional psychiatrists, whom Klerman now relegates to a respectable minority. ('This is a special requirement on the respectable minority of physicians, since they should inform the patient that their treatment is not the one most widely held within the profession.') Klerman is prepared to abolish the legal concept of the respectable minority on scientific grounds. He seems not to recognize that this legal concept is intended, among other things, to protect scientific innovation against rigid orthodoxy in standards of care. Thus, the concept has no specific numerical definition.[5] Relying on Livingston's unpublished student paper. Klerman selects 10% as a numerical definition of the legal concept. He suggests that traditional psychiatrists comprising such a respectable minority (although he provides no empirical evidence about their actual numbers) have a special burden. The burden seems to be to familiarize themselves with the claims of scientific efficacy put forward by all other therapies, present them to the patient, and inform the patient that their own traditional psychotherapy has no demonstrated efficacy.

I first injected the idea of the respectable minority into the Osheroff controversy from quite a different perspective.[15] The question I had addressed was whether a hospital could hold itself out as providing exclusively psychoanalytic and psychosocial treatments for patients who had serious mental disorders under the respectable minority rule. The rule, despite its legal ambiguity, seemed to recognize that the practice of medicine was characterized by different schools of thought, not by uniform orthodox criteria.[5] I assumed that such a hospital would accept only patients who chose not to have drug treatment or ECT. Klerman's deposition in the Osheroff litigation[3] seemed to indicate that in his expert opinion such a hospital would be negligent per se. This is by no means an entirely obsolete question, since advertisements apparently describing such a hospital have regularly appeared in the American Journal of Psychiatry (for instance, in the January 1989 issue, page A 14).

If the respectable minority rule in law and other legal doctrine relevant to the necessary qualifications of experts have any role at all, it is to protect the diversity of reasonably prudent professional opinion and different approaches to the practice of the healing arts[5] against the rigid orthodoxy proposed by Klerman. Similarly, organized psychiatry, when it accepted DSM-III, specifically indicated that this was not intended as an endorsement of any etiological theory or therapy of mental disorder. Rather, it was agnostic, recognizing the diversity of professional views and opinions. Klerman's criteria for professional responsibility would repudiate the traditional commitment of both the law and psychiatry to diversity. It would further narrow the practice of psychiatry and the choices available to patients. In his quest for efficacious standards, Klerman endorses an authoritarian control of psychiatric practice. The lessons of the history of science suggest that this would be detrimental, even to the aspirations of 'scientific psychiatry.'

Responsibility to Provide Proper Treatment

Klerman's definition of a responsibility to provide effective treatment drives home the nails on the coffin he has devised for traditional psychiatry. He says, 'The patient has the right to the proper treatment. Proper treatment involves those treatments for which there is substantial evidence.' His paper makes clear that he believes there is no such substantial evidence for traditional psychotherapy in the treatment of any DSM-III-R disorder. Thus, psychiatrists who apply traditional psychotherapy cannot claim to provide effective treatment or to fulfill the patient's 'right' to proper treatment. This criterion alone, given his arguments, might well raise the specter of malpractice, not for a respectable minority but for the majority of psychiatrists in the United States who at least in some of their practice provide such treatments to patients with DSM-III-R diagnoses. I again emphasize the point that if anything should go wrong during such treatment the claim could be made under Klerman's criteria that the therapist had failed to provide proper treatment.

The special burden placed on traditional psychiatrists by Klerman cannot be fully appreciated if one does not consider the quite different impact of these criteria on psychiatrists specializing in psychopharmacology. They can take Klerman's paper as authority for the proposition that they need never discuss or refer a patient for traditional therapy, since such treatments have no demonstrated efficacy compared to their own. Thus, they need to do nothing further to familiarize themselves with these unscientific theories and therapies. Furthermore, they need have no concern about their own responsibility to provide proper therapy. Klerman seems to accept Food and Drug Administration approval of efficacy as a sufficient minimum guarantee of proper treatment to appropriate patients. Thus, all standard psychopharmacology is by definition proper. Ironically, it is not at all uncommon in the treatment of panic disorder, the example given by Klerman, for different psychopharmacologists to reach contradictory conclusions about the relevant scientific literature on the basis of their judgment and professional opinion. Klerman has no intention of preventing these colleagues from telling patients that despite demonstrated efficacy, Food and Drug Administration approval, and widespread use a particular drug is worthless and even dangerous in their opinion. It is only traditional psychiatrists who are not permitted to have such professional opinions about scientific evidence.

Responsibility to Consult and Refer

There is a great deal of law as well as ethical principles in psychiatry that establish a responsibility to seek expert consultation when a patient's condition obviously deteriorates on a given regimen of treatment.[5,24] Psychiatrists have not always respected this legal and ethical requirement, perhaps because, as Klerman suggests, they have failed to recognize the safety and efficacy of alternative treatments. If Klerman had made this the central feature of his discussion of the facts of the *Osheroff* litigation and its implications for psychiatry and for legal policy, there would have been no need for a response.

Conclusions

If it is correct that Klerman's arguments and recommendations are not required by law or by any legal precedent of *Osheroff*, then it would appear that Klerman is invoking the threat of malpractice liability to further his own 'scientific' approach and his own vision of what clinical psychiatry is and should be. This strategy of seeking legal empowerment is an unfortunate and increasing tendency in the psychiatric profession. Advocates of various partisan positions in psychiatry have gone to the courtroom and to the law to advance their own schools and ideologies. It is striking to me how often legal decisions that offend the psychiatric profession as a whole are based on the expert opinions of psychiatrists advocating their own partisan positions. The psychiatric profession has often complained about the constraints the law was placing on us and our patients.[25] What we have failed to recognize is how often what the law did was based on the partisan and adversarial testimony of our colleagues. We have less reason to fear our litigious patients and their lawyers than our partisan colleagues in this new era of psychiatric malpractice. Unfortunately, Klerman has chosen to attack traditional psychiatry in the context of a legal dispute and in a manner that may have consequences he did not intend. Law is a blunt instrument; it can be used to beat down the opposition, but no one should think that the law can chart the path of scientific progress in clinical psychiatry.

Klerman has often been able to speak for the collective wisdom of the psychiatric profession. His own words, in *The New Harvard Guide to Psychiatry*,[9] are the best answer in the courtroom to the partisan position he has asserted here: 'Individual psychotherapy based on psychodynamic principles remains the most widely used form of psychotherapy. Although systematic, controlled clinical studies do not exist, clinical experience supports the value of this form of treatment.'

References

1. **Klerman GL, Weissman MM, Rounsaville BJ**, *et al*: *Interpersonal Psychotherapy of Depression*. New York, Basic Books, 1984.

2. **Malcolm JG**: Treatment choices and informed consent in psychiatry: implications of the Osheroff case for the profession. *J Psychiatry Law* 1986: **14**:9–107.

3. **Malcolm JG**: *Treatment Chokes and Informed Consent: Current Controversies in Psychiatric Malpractice Litigation*. Spring field, III, Charles C Thomas, 1988. pp 22–37.

4. Canterbury v Spence. 464 F 2d 772 (DC Or 1972).

5. **Louisell DW, Williams H**: *Medical Malpractice*, rev ed. New York, Matthew Bender, 1983.

6. President's Commission (or the Study of Ethical Problems in Medicine and Biomedical Research: *Making Health Care Decisions*, vol 2: Appendices. Washington, DC, US Government Printing Office, Oct 1982.

7. President's Commission for the Study of Ethical Problems in Medicine and Biomedical Research: *Making Health Care Decisions*, vol 3: Report. Washington, DC, US Government Priming Office. Oct 1982.

8. **Klerman GL**: Affective disorders, in *The Harvard Guide to Modern Psychiatry*. Edited by Nicholi AM Jr. Cambridge, Mass, Belknap Press (Harvard University Press), 1978.

9. **Klerman GL**: Depression and related disorders of mood (affective disorders), in *The New Harvard Guide to Psychiatry*. Edited by Nicholi AM Jr. Cambridge, Mass, Belknap Press (Harvard University Press), 1988.

10. **King JH**: *The Law of Medical Malpractice*. St Paul. West. 1986. P 51.

11. **Elkin I, Pilkonis PA, Docherty JP**, *et al*: Conceptual ad methodological issues in comparative studies of psychotherapy and pharmacotherapy. II: nature and timing of treatment effects. *Am J Psychiatry* 1988; **145**: 1070–1076.

12. **Cole JO, Sunderland PS 111**: The drug treatment of borderline patients, in *Psychiatry 1982: The American Psychiatric Association Annual Review*. Edited by Grinspoon L. Washington, DC, American Psychiatric Press, 1982.

13. **Lasch C**: *The Culture of Narcissism: American Life in an Age of Diminishing Expectations*. New York. Warner Books, 1979.

14. **Kernberg OF**: An ego psychology and object relations approach to the narcissistic personality, in *Psychiatry 1982: The American Psychiatric Association Annual Review*. Edited by Grinspoon L. Washington, DC, American Psychiatric Press, 1982.

15. **Stone AA**: The new paradox of psychiatric malpractice. *N Engl J Med* 1984; **311**:1384–1387.

16. **Klein DF**: The *Osheroff case*: a rebuttal. *Psychiatr News*, April 7, 1989, p 26.

17. **Baldessarini RJ**: Update on recent advances in antidepressant pharmacology and pharmacotherapy, in *Psychobiology and Psychopharmacology*. Edited by Flach F. New York, WW Norton. 1988.

18. **Stone AA**: *Law. Psychiatry, and Morality: Essays and Analysis*. Washington, DC, American Psychiatric Press, 1984.

19. **Relman AS**: Assessment and accountability: the third revolution in medical care (editorial). *N Engl J Med* 1988; **319**:1220–1222.

20. **Roper WL, Winkenwerder W, Hackbarth GM**, *et al*: Effectiveness in health care: an initiative to evaluate and improve medical practice. *N Engl J Med* 1988: **319**:1197–1202.

21. **Furrow BR**: *Malpractice in Psychotherapy*. Lexington, Mass, Lexington Books, 1980.

22. **Kane JM**: Somatic therapy, in *Psychiatry Update: American Psychiatric Association Annual Review*. vol 5. Edited by Frances AJ, Hales RE. Washington, DC. American Psychiatric Press. 1986.

23. **Nemiah JC**: Psychoneurotic disorders, in *The New Harvard Guide to Psychiatry*. Edited by Nicholi AM Jr. Cambridge, Mass, Belknap Press (Harvard University Press), 1988.

24. American Psychiatric Association: *The Principles of Medical Ethics With Annotations Especially Applicable to Psychiatry*, rev ed. Washington, DC, APA, 1981.

25. **Stone AA**: The myth of advocacy. *Hosp Community Psychiatry* 1979; **30**:319–322.

Effect of Joint Crisis Plans on use of Compulsory Treatment in Psychiatry

Single blind randomised controlled trial*

Claire Henderson, Chris Flood, Morven Leese, Graham Thornicroft, Kim Sutherby and George Szmukler

Introduction

For patients receiving psychiatric treatment a joint crisis plan aims to empower the holder and to facilitate detection and treatment of relapse.[1] It is developed by a patient together with mental health staff. Held by the patient, it contains his or her choice of information, which can include an advance agreement for treatment preferences for any future emergency, when he or she might be too unwell to express coherent views.

The format was developed after consultation with national user groups, interviews with organisations and individuals using crisis cards,[2] and detailed development work with service users in south London.

Use of the Mental Health Act has increased in English mental health services. Data returned to the Department of Health[3] show a 57% increase in civil cases of compulsory detention under the Mental Health Act 1983 between 1988 and 1998.[3] Legal detention can have serious negative consequences for patients, including restricted access to travel visas and financial services. Current policy in England is towards greater involvement of patients as partners in care.[4,5] In the review of the Mental Health Act 1983, the Legislation Scoping Study Committee referred to the desirability of reducing compulsory treatment through the use of advance agreements; in the context of new mental health legislation to be introduced 'the creation and recognition of advance agreements about care would greatly assist in the promotion of informal and consensual care.'[6]

We evaluated the effectiveness of joint crisis plans at reducing use of inpatient services and objective coercion at and during admission.

Methods

Setting and participants

We recruited patients in 2000 and 2001 from seven community mental health teams in south London and one in Kent.

To be eligible, patients had to be in contact with their local team; have been admitted to a psychiatric inpatient service at least once in the previous two years; and have a diagnosis of psychotic illness or bipolar affective disorder without psychotic symptoms. We excluded those unable to give informed consent because of mental incapacity or insufficient command of English. Current inpatients were not recruited to avoid any coercion to participate.

* Henderson, C., Flood, C., Leese, M., Thornicroft, G., Sutherby, K. and Szmukler, G.: Effect of joint crisis plans on the use of compulsory treatment in psychiatry: single blind randomised controlled trial. *British Medical Journal* **329**:136–138, 2004.

Study procedures

We used minimisation to allocate patients to the intervention or the control group (see bmj.com). The nature of the interventions meant that neither participants nor staff could be blinded to allocation. The outcome assessor, however, was blinded to the intervention.

Intervention group – At the first meeting the project worker (CF) explained the procedure to the patient and, if possible, the care coordinator. To finalise each plan, the patient was encouraged to bring a carer, friend, or advocate to a second meeting. This meeting was to discuss the views of patients and professionals on what to do in a crisis and to negotiate agreed solutions. The selection of information to include and the exact wording were the patient's choice alone. Full details of how plans were produced are given in reports of our pilot study.[1,2]

Control group – Patients in the control group received information leaflets about local services, mental illness and treatments, the Mental Health Act, local provider organisations, and relevant policies. In accordance with standard practice in England, all patients received written copies of their care plan, within the care programme approach.[7]

Baseline and outcome measures – We collected data on sociodemographic variables, clinical details, history of adverse events – for instance, self harm and harm to others, and compliance with mental health treatment, rated by the care coordinator on a 7 point rating scale.[8] Our primary outcomes were admission to hospital and length of time spent in hospital. Our secondary outcome was objective coercion – that is, compulsory treatment under the Mental Health Act 1983. Follow up was conducted 15 months after randomisation.

Results

Participants

We assessed 466 sets of case notes for eligibility. Twenty three people did not meet the inclusion criteria and 282 were either not contacted or declined to take part; we therefore randomised 160. During follow up there were fewer adverse outcomes in the intervention group; we shall be addressing this fully in a future paper (table 1). Baseline sociodemographic and clinical features were similar (table 2).

Hospital admissions

A smaller proportion of the intervention group were admitted (risk ratio 0.69, 95% confidence interval 0.45 to 1.04) (table 3). There was no significant difference in mean bed days (difference 4, −18 to 26, P = 0.15, for the whole sample; difference −24, −72 to 24, P = 0.39, for those admitted). Overall about a quarter of patients were admitted for more than one month (23% in the intervention group and 29% in the control group).

Table 1 Adverse events in psychiatric patients randomised to receive joint crisis plan (intervention) or standard treatment (control). Figures are numbers (percentages) of patients

	Intervention group (n = 80)	Control group (n = 80)	P value*
Declined further participation	5 (6)	4 (5)	1.0
Self harm:			
None	73 (99)	69 (91)	0.09
Not resulting in admission of close observations	1 (1)	5 (6)	
Resulting in admission or close observations	0 (0)	2 (3)	
Violence:			
None	71 (96)	65 (85)	0.03
Not major†	1 (1)	9 (12)	
Major†	2 (3)	2 (3)	

* Fisher's exact test.

† Incidents requiring attendance of police or seclusion on ward or special civil law admissions to place of safety.

‡ Homicide, sex attacks, demoted or actual serious assault.

Table 2 Baseline demographic and clinical characteristics of participant groups. Figures are numbers (percentages) unless stated otherwise

	Intervention group (n = 80)	Control group (n = 80)
Mean (SD) age (years)	39.5 (12.1)	38.6 (10.6)
Men	47 (59)	47 (59)
Country of birth:		
UK	48 (60)	43 (54)
Outside UK	30 (37)	25 (31)
Missing	2 (2)	12 (15)
Ethnic group:		
White	29 (36)	34 (42)
Black	44 (55)	40 (50)
Other	7 (9)	6 (7)
Household composition:		
Alone	36 (45)	33 (41)
With family member(s)	20 (25)	28 (35)
Others	19 (24)	17 (21)
Missing	5 (6)	2 (2)
Median (range) years of education	11 (8–18)	11 (9–20)
Median No of previous psychiatric admissions	5 (n = 75)	5 (n = 69)
Days in psychiatric hospital in 6 months before recruitment (median)	29	42
Ever admitted on section:		
Yes	70 (67)	73 (91)
Ever had police involved in admission:		
Yes	48 (60)	37 (46)
No	17 (21)	23 (29)
Not known	15 (19)	20 (25)
History of self harm:		
None	53 (66)	45 (56)
Yes, not resulting in admission or observations	5 (5)	6 (7)
Yes, resulting in admission or observations	20 (25)	19 (24)
Missing	2 (2)	10 (12)

Table 2 (*Continued*)

	Intervention group (n = 80)	Control group (n = 80)
History of violence:		
None	48 (60)	44 (55)
Not major	13 (19)	15 (19)
Major†	17 (21)	12 (15)
Missing	2 (2)	9 (11)
High current care programme approach†	71 (89)	70 (88)
Mean (SD) compliance rating	4.8 (1.3)	4.9 (1.3)

* Incidents requiring attendance of police or seclusion on ward or special civil law admissions to place of safety.

† Homicide, sex attacks, attempted or actual serious assault.

‡ Defined as having more than one member of the community mental health team involved in providing care as per the treatment plan.

Table 3 Hospital admission and use of the Mental Health Act 1983

	Intervention group (n = 80)	Control group (n = 80)	Test statistic*	P value
Missing data	0	1	–	–
No (%) patient admitted at least once	24 (30)	35 (44)	3.25	0.07
Mean (median) No of bed days†:				
Whole sample	32 (0)	36 (0)	1.52	0.15
Those admitted	107 (75)	83 (48)	0.74	0.39
No (%) of patients with at least one compulsory admission	10 (12.5)	21 (26.5)	4.84	0.03
Mean (median) time on section (days):				
Whole sample	14 (0)	31 (0)	4.13	0.04
For those on section	114 (104)	117 (99)	0.00	0.98

* x2 values from Mann-Whitney tests, except proportions admitted or on section, which were from Pearson's x2 tests.

† For 34 participants in control group because of missing data.

Use of the Mental Health Act

Compulsory admission and treatment were significantly less common in the intervention group (risk ratio 0.48, 0.24 to 0.95, $\chi2 = 4.84$, P = 0.03, table 3). The mean number of days of detention for the intervention group was 14 compared with 31 for the control group (difference 17, 0 to 36, P = 0.04). For those admitted on a section, the mean number of days on a section was similar in the two groups (difference 3, −61 to 67, P = 0.98).

Discussion

We have shown that a type of advance agreement significantly reduces use of the Mental Health Act both at and during hospital admission. Evidence that it can also reduce number of admissions was weaker, and there was no significant difference for number of bed days used.

Methodological considerations

This study has several important limitations. The rate of hospital admission among the control group was lower than expected from our pilot study, which reduced the power of the study to detect a difference in this outcome and resulted in wide confidence intervals for the mean differences in bed days, consistent with either an increase or a decrease in length of hospital stay. Only 36% of eligible patients agreed to participate, so the results may not be widely generalisable. Those who declined to participate when interviewed reported that the plan would not help them, they were unlikely to become ill again, that a plan was already in place, or that no one would take any notice of it. On the other hand, generalisability was strengthened by the various settings for recruitment (inner city, suburban, small town) and the broad ethnic representation of patients. The follow up rate for the outcomes reported was high.

Implications for services

The reduction in use of the Mental Health Act has important implications for mental health services. Although the provision of a written care plan, signed by the patient, is now required in England, the joint crisis plan is substantially different. Making a joint crisis plan is voluntary, while the standard care plan is a statutory requirement. Thus, joint crisis plans can be used only when staff and patients want to formulate and use them. Furthermore, a third party, with knowledge of severe mental health problems and who is not a team member, mediates between the parties in producing each joint crisis plan. Such facilitation requires extra resources.

The joint crisis plan is therefore different from a self completed advance directive[9] because it is fully agreed with staff, increasing the likelihood that it will be implemented.

Finally, the process of writing a joint crisis plan is deliberately one of negotiation. We intend to undertake further investigation in future to understand what such negotiation means for staff and patients, to explore the power relationships between staff and patients, and to investigate more fully other contextual factors which may impact on such a complex intervention.[9-14] We can find no other evidence in the literature that a structured clinical intervention can significantly reduce compulsory psychiatric admission and treatment. This study suggests that the committee reviewing the Mental Health Act 1983 was correct in its assertion that advance agreements can promote more consensual and less coercive care.[6]

We thank all participants, their informal carers, and care staff for their help in conducting the study.

Contributors: See bmj.com

Funding: CH was supported by a Medical Research Council health service research training fellowship, and CF was supported by a South London and Maudsley Trust health services research committee grant.

Competing interests: None declared.

Ethical approval: Ethics Committees of the South London and Maudsley NHS Trust, Lewisham University Hospital, South West London and St George's NHS Trust, and Thames Gateway NHS Trust.

References

1 Sutherby K, Szmukler GI, Halpern A, Alexander M, Thornicroft G. Johnson C, et al. A study of 'crisis cards' in a community psychiatric service. *Acta Psychiatr Scand* 1999; **100**: 56–61.

2 Sutherby K, Szmukler GI. Crisis cards and self-help crisis initiatives. *Psychiatric Bulletin* 1998; **22**:4–7.

3 Department of Health. *Inpatients formally detained in hospitals under the Mental Health Act 1983 and other legislation, England: 1988–89 to 1998–99.* London: Government Statistical Service, 1999.

4 Department of Health. *The national service framework for mental health. Modern standards and service models.* London: Department of Health, 1999.

5 Department of Health. *The NHS plan.* London: Department of Health, 2000.

6 Department of Health. *Report of the expert committee. Review of the Mental Health Act 1983.* London: Stationery Office, 1999.

7 Department of Health. *Effective care co-ordination in mental health services. Modernising the care programme approach. A policy booklet.* London: Department of Health, 2000.

8 Kemp RA, Lambert TJ. Insight in schizophrenia and its relationship to psychopathology. *Schizophr Res* 1995; **18**:21–8.

9 Papageorgiou A, King M. Janmohamed A, Davidson O. Dawson J. Advance directives for patients compulsorily admitted to hospital with serious mental illness: randomised controlled trial. *Br J Psychiatry* 2002: **181**:513–9.

10 Campbell M, Fitzpatrick R, Haines A, Kinmonth AL, Sandercock P, Spiegelhalter D, et al. Framework for design and evaluation of complex interventions to improve health. *BMJ* 2000: **321**:694–7.

11 Medical Research Council. *A framework for development and evaluation of RCTs for complex interventions to improve health.* London: Medical Research Council, Health Services and Public Health Research Board, 2000.

12 Pawson R, Tilley N. *Realistic evaluation.* London: Sage Publications, 1997.

13 Thomas P. How should advance statements be implemented? (letter). *Br J Psychiatry* 2003; **182**:548–9.

14 Bracken P, Thomas P. Postpsychiatry: a new direction for mental health. *BMJ* 2001; **322**:724–7.

Ethical and Pragmatic Issues in the Use of Psychotropic Agents in Young Children*

Peter S Jensen

In the last 2 decades, we have become increasingly aware that mental, behavioural, and emotional disorders that afflict adults and adolescents also can strike and devastate the lives of prepubertal children and their families. While severe developmental disorders such as autism and mental retardation have been well established, only recently has more information emerged about the diagnosis of other emotional and behavioural disorders in this young age-group. Thus, we now know that attention-deficit hyperactivity disorder (ADHD) and oppositional defiant disorder (ODD) can be described and reliably diagnosed in young children. Much of this knowledge has become part of 'mainstream thinking' among child psychiatrists, psychologists, and others who treat the mental health problems of very young children. Disorders reported for preschool and early school-age children now include early-onset schizophrenia, major depressive disorder, and even bipolar disorder.[1–3] While many child psychiatrists and other mental health professionals may have begun their work with children on the premise that intervening at a young age offered the opportunity to make a greater difference with more malleable conditions, it also has become increasingly apparent that mental disorders afflicting children at young ages may have a more severe and pernicious course, possibly with the highest genetic loading and/or a combination of other environmental factors, all of which have merged to result in early expression of a disorder.

Not surprisingly, given the increasing use and apparent effectiveness of *psychotropic agents* for behavioural and emotional disorders among adults and adolescents, these same agents are being applied increasingly in the treatments of preschool and early school-age children. In part, these patterns of increased use result from their apparent efficacy and relative ease of use, as well as from fiscal pressures from managed care companies interested in the 'bottom line.' The potential benefits of medications, if they can be shown to be safe and to yield long-term gains that consolidate as the child ages, seem clear.

Unfortunately, however, in the United States (US), very few psychotropic agents approved by the Food and Drug Administration (FDA) for use in adults have been tested and approved for use in younger children. Thus, of all of the psychotropic agents used in preschool children, only some antipsychotic agents (for example, haloperidol) have received testing sufficient for the FDA to allow labeling their use for child mental and behavioural disorders.[4] The lack of childhood safety and efficacy data for medications developed and tested principally in adults is actually a very widespread problem that applies to 80% of all medications (including antibiotics and anesthetics) currently available in the US formulary.[5] Children have often been termed 'therapeutic orphans' because the kind of research needed to demonstrate the safety and efficacy of various therapeutics in children has been left largely undetermined.[6] Consequently, parents and clinicians have had to make difficult treatment decisions, relying principally on sporadic case reports, small pilot studies, or downward

extrapolations of adult data to make assumptions about apparent benefits, safety, and efficacy of these agents in children.[4]

The central nervous system and the neurotransmitters and receptors on which psychotropic agents act are in a period of substantial growth, development, and refinement through childhood and adolescence.[7] Because some animal data suggest the possibility of permanent up-or down regulation of receptor systems as a function of exposure to psychotropic agents in the developing mammalian brain, great caution is warranted when using such agents in children, particularly for those agents with which we have not had extensive experience or for which no safety and efficacy data exist. Another reason for caution in the use of psychotropic agents is the evidence that a number of psychotherapeutic interventions have been shown to be effective for young children with certain types of behavioural problems. Thus, early behavioural interventions with children with autism can reduce stereotypies and self-injurious behaviour and increase prosocial behaviour. Similarly, well-delivered contingency management programs, either through direct behavioural reinforcement of the children by mental health professionals or through parent training programs, have been shown to reduce oppositional and aggressive behaviours in young children. (Hibbs and Jensen[8] provide an extensive review of research-based psychosocial treatments.)

While the possibility of side effects, lack of efficacy data, and availability of alternative therapies do not comprise a universal proscription against the use of medication in young children, they do suggest the need for caution and an in-depth evaluation of the possible alternatives for each child. This is the core component of ethical clinical practice, namely, ensuring a process that allows the clinician to provide the best therapeutic strategy for each child based on the particular needs of that child and family. Anything that compromises that process, whether it be a shortened assessment period that curtails the evaluation or fiscal pressures to use a less effective or less safe form of treatment over another, should be regarded as unethical.

Unfortunately, the evidence is not always clear as to which alternative is preferable, particularly with young children, for whom little formal data exist. Nonetheless, because a core principle of ethical practice is to do no harm, therapeutic uncertainty should be shared with the parents and family.[9] Just because no firm data exist to support the clinical use of psychotropic agents in young children, medication may be required and may be the most ethical alternative for a given child. Likewise, even though the FDA may have allowed the labeling of a given psychotropic agent for a specific indication (for example, haloperidol for severely aggressive behaviour in children with autism), it does not automatically follow that the prescribing of that agent is the most appropriate or ethical alternative for all cases involving children.

Under what conditions should behavioural alternatives be considered or given top priority? Given the potential for lifelong neurologic effects (such as tardive dyskinesia), a behavioural intervention may seem to be the most appropriate (ethical) choice, but the condition's degree of severity, clinical response, and other contextual factors are also important factors in the clinician's and family's decision-making process. Hence, no single, uniform prescriptive or proscriptive process can replace the clinician's

* Jensen, P.: Ethical and pragmatic issues in the use of psychotropic agents in young children. *Canadian Journal of Psychiatry* **43**: 585–588, 1998.

case-by-case decision-making based on a thorough assessment of the child's needs.[10]

Obviously, given the overall lack of data concerning safety and efficacy of psychotropic agents in young children (and the lack of similar data concerning psychosocial interventions), a vigorous research effort is needed to determine what works for whom under what circumstances, as is a careful examination of potential short- and long-term behavioural toxicities of all forms of treatment, pharmacologic and psychotherapeutic.

So what is known about the current level of use of psychotropic medications in young children? Many databases are available that could help address this question. Unfortunately, these data sources are limited by their relatively small samples of young children, making it difficult to reliably determine the rate of prescriptions of psychotropic agents in this age-group. For example, information from the National Ambulatory Medical Care Evaluation Survey (NAMCES) indicates that psychotropic prescriptions for young children (aged 5 years and under) are being delivered at appreciable levels during physician visits throughout the US. Reliable information concerning the exact level of prescribing of specific psychotropic agents is not available. Nonetheless, preliminary evidence suggests the likelihood that prescriptions for these agents are in the tens of thousands.[13]

While we should be concerned about prescribing practices in the absence of solid safety and efficacy information. We should also be concerned about being overly cautious or pessimistic. It is quite possible that many of the agents that are increasingly available on the market may be both safe and effective for target conditions for young children. Difficulty stems from the fact that, whether or not we should use such agents, We really do not know if they are safe and effective. Although there are probably risks on both sides of the to-use-or-not-to-use question, we must obtain evidence concerning safety and efficacy for parents and clinicians to make appropriate decisions regarding the children that present for our evaluation and treatment.

To increase this program of research, a number of activities will be essential. First, we require better studies of diagnosis to ensure the reliability, validity, and predictive validity in terms of longer term outcomes. For the child with early, persistent, and severe behavioural or emotional difficulties that have been unresponsive to environmental manipulations, what is the risk of this condition in and of itself in terms of the child's long-term development? What are the risks versus benefits of treatment? How well do these early behavioural problems predict later problems, with or without treatment? The ethical issues of such research considerations, including whether or not to use placebo, can be thorny. However, when safety and efficacy data are lacking, placebos can and should be used. Their use is well justified in the absence of certainty regarding whether a medication is an appropriate alternative.[14]

Because of these difficulties, the NIMH has developed and recently funded 7 research units for pediatric psychopharmacology. Under the guidance of Ben Vitiello, MD, these research units are conducting multisite investigations to determine the safety and efficacy of those medications more commonly used for mental disorders.

As another strategy to increase pediatric research in general, the National Institutes of Health are now revising policy guidelines such that all studies will presume the inclusion of children and adolescents, so that children are not systematically excluded from research. Thus, whenever an investigator would study an adult disorder also found in children, to obtain federal funding he or she would also have to shoulder the responsibility (and seize the opportunity!) to study the particular condition across the life span, unless ethical factors would preclude the inclusion of children in such studies.

In addition, over the last several years the FDA has been in the process of implementing its pediatric initiative. The FDA, encouraged by the White House to work with the pharmaceutical industry to identify those agents commonly used in children for which research data are lacking, is urging drug companies to mount trials of safety and efficacy in children

Clinical Implications

- Few medications have been adequately tested for safety and efficacy in young children.

- Behavioural and psychotherapeutic strategies are often the wisest first therapeutic intervention for this age group.

- Psychotropic medications may be required but should be used cautiously in young children.

Limitations

- More studies of psychotropic agents in young children are needed.

- Clinicians need to fully acquaint themselves with available data concerning the safety and efficacy of psychoactive medications in young children.

- More training on the use of psychotropic agents is needed for primary care and specialty care physicians.

and adolescents as part of their ongoing new drug applications, either immediately prior to or shortly after receiving the approval for an indication in adults.[15] These are hopeful signs that the next decade will provide substantial new knowledge concerning the appropriate, judicious, effective, and safe use of these agents in children.

What should clinicians do in the interim? The answer to this question is complex. First and foremost, we must understand that medications are not a panacea, neither are they the bane of pediatric psychiatric practice. Appropriate and judicious use, even in the absence of safety and efficacy data, may be warranted. Clinicians should be thoroughly versed in all literature concerning the use of psychotropic agents in adults, including their safety and efficacy, and aware of any case reports or studies in progress concerning these agents. Whenever possible, consultation with more experienced colleagues is advisable. Consideration of all available therapeutic alternatives in terms of the benefits, safety, and efficacy is always appropriate, and succumbing to the clinical or pecuniary pressures of the easiest alternative appearing in the pharmacopeia or managed care menu should be avoided.

Most clinicians, myself included, often begin with environmental and behavioural manipulations to address behavioural and emotional disorders in young children, but for substantial ongoing impairment, judicious use of psychotropic agents can and should be considered in view of the severe prognosis for many of the conditions affecting children and preschoolers.

References

1 Lahey B, Applegate B, McBumett K, Biederman J, Greenhill L, Hynd G, and others. DSM-IV field trials for attention deficit/hyperactivity disorder in children and adolescents. *Am J Psychiatry* 1994; **151**:1673–85.

2 Nottelmann ED, Jensen PS. Special section: bipolar disorder and ADHD. *J Affect, Disord.* Forthcoming.

3 Narrow, W. National Institute of Mental Health (NIMH). Personal communication.

4 Jensen PS, Vitiello B, Leonard H, Laughren T. Child and adolescent psychopharmacology: expanding the research base. *Psychopharmacol Bull* 1994; **30**:3–8.

5 Committee on Drugs. Unapproved uses of approved drugs: the physician, the package insert, and the Food and Drug Administration: subject review. *Pediatrics* 1996; **98**:143–5.

6 Coté CJ, Kauffman RE, Troendle GJ, Lambert GH. Is the 'therapeutic orphan' about to be adopted? *Pediatrics* 1996; **98**:118–23.

7   Vitiello B, Jensen PS. Developmental perspectives in pediatric psychopharmacology. *Psychopharmacol Bull* 1995; **31**:75–81.

8   Hibbs E, Jensen PS, editors. *Psychosocial treatments for children and adolescents: empirically-based approaches.* Washington (DC): American Psychological Association; 1996.

9   Jensen PS, Josephson AM, Frey J. Informed consent: legal content versus therapeutic process. *Am J Psychother* 1989; **43**:378–86.

10 Coffey B J. Ethical issues in child and adolescent psychopharmacology. *Child and Adolescent Psychiatric Clinics of North America* 1995; **4**:793–807.

11 Jensen P, Vitiello B, Bhatara V, Hoagwood K, Fell M. Current trends in psychotropic prescribing practices. Clinical and policy implications. *J Am Acad Child Adolesc Psychiatry*. In review.

12 Jensen PS, Fisher CB, Hoagwood H. Special issues in mental health/disorder research with children and adolescents. In: Pincus H, Zarin D, editors. *Ethical issues.* Washington (DC): American Psychiatric Press. Forthcoming.

13 Food and Drug Administration. Specific requirements on content and format of labeling for human prescription drugs; revision of pediatric use subsection in the labeling. *Federal Register* 1994; **59**:64240–50.

Antidepressants for Children

*Is Scientific Support Necessary?**

Rhoda L. Fisher and Seymour Fisher

Our intention is to clarify certain issues concerning the role of scientific data in therapeutic decisions. Although it is generally accepted that there should be a scientific rationale for treatment, the application of this concept is complex and overlaid with ambiguity and even (as we will illustrate) defensive rationalization.

We will present our observations in the context of the widespread practice of treating depressed children with antidepressants. Literally millions of depressed children are being treated with agents like imipramine and fluoxetine. Goleman (1993) reports that 4 to 6 million prescriptions for desipramine and related medications were issued for children 18 and under in 1992. Prescribing antidepressants for children is occurring with increasing frequency and in many locales is accepted as a standard practice (Popper, 1992). Some textbooks (Green, 1991) recommend such use of antidepressants and offer detailed procedural advice.

However, after reviewing the pertinent scientific literature, we cannot find a body of data demonstrating that antidepressants are more therapeutic for childhood depression than are placebos. We located 13 double-blind placebo-controlled studies (e.g., Boulos et al., 1991; Geller et al., 1990, 1992; Hughes et al., 1990; Kashani et al., 1994; Kramer and Feiguine, 1981; Kutcher et al., 1994; Lucas et al., 1965; Petti and Law, 1982; Prieskorn et al., 1987; Puig-Antich et al., 1979, 1987; Simeon et al., 1990) that have tested the efficacy of antidepressants for children and adolescents.

Except for two possible borderline instances of the drug exceeding placebo in efficacy, there has been a consistent failure to demonstrate any advantage over placebo. A few studies (e.g., Geller et al., 1990; Puig-Antich et al., 1979) suggested that placebo was more successful than the active drug. Various other observers, after reviewing the pertinent literature, have arrived at a similar negative appraisal. Gadow (1991) stated: 'To date, none of the placebo-controlled, double-blind studies of tricyclics in depressed prepubertal children have found drug therapy to be superior to placebo . . . Equally discouraging are the findings from drug studies of depressed adolescents' (pp. 843–844).

Green (1991) notes: 'A literature review of the use of tricyclic antidepressants in children and adolescents with major depression found them to be clinically effective in several open studies, but no double-blind placebo-controlled study reported that tricyclics were superior to placebo' (p. 115).

Ambrosini et al. (1993) concluded: 'The empirical data reviewed does not support antidepressant efficacy in child and adolescent major depressive disorder, neither when results are collated nor when the few double-blind placebo-controlled studies are reviewed individually' (p. 3)

Conners (1992) remarked:

Widespread use of tricyclic antidepressant (TCA) drug treatment for depressed adolescents reflects a momentum continuing from early uncontrolled trials in adolescents and children, as well as the apparent success of controlled trials of TCA therapy among adults. The results of more recent controlled trials in youths, however, are uniformly negative.

(p. 11)

* Fisher, R. L. and Fisher, S.: Antidepressants for children. Is scientific support necessary? *Journal of Nervous and Mental Disease* 184:99–102, 1996.

Elliot (1992) stated:

It is sobering . . . to recall that the best-designed existing studies do not confirm the efficacy of antidepressants in relieving depression in either children or adolescents. To date, no study has shown that any antidepressant is unequivocally superior to placebo. Results from clinical studies of adolescents with depression have been especially problematic. A few investigators have failed to find even a suggestion of a drug response, in fact, in some studies, antidepressants actually appear to be less effective than placebo.

(p. 7)

The evidence is unanimous that antidepressants are no more effective than placebos in treating children with symptoms of depression. These negative findings have been described in various journals. However, as earlier indicated, the prescribing of antidepressants for children continues to be widely practiced. This has aroused uneasiness in some child psychiatrists who have sought to conjure up a rationale for a practice that has no documented scientific justification. Incidentally, the entire matter has been further complicated by the fact that several children taking antidepressants have suddenly and unexpectedly died (e.g., Riddle et al., 1993). By 1992, an official editorial written by Charles Popper (1992) in the *Journal of Child and Adolescent Psychopharmacology* addressed the dilemma. The editorial noted: 'But there is no escaping the fact that research studies certainly have not supported the efficacy of tricyclic antidepressants in treating depressed adolescents. There are critical questions about this treatment which, simply put, appears to have been demonstrated to be ineffective. Yet clinicians have come to use antidepressants to treat adolescent depression on such a wide scale that it has become essentially a standard of practice in many locales. Even many of the researchers who have found negative findings in their studies continue to use tricyclic antidepressants in treating adolescents in their clinical practice.

'What is going on here? What has become of the tradition of research in laying the groundwork and leading the way to improved clinical care?' (p. 1).

The editorial then proceeds to enumerate various reasons why clinicians may actually 'know better' than the published research whether antidepressants are effective with children. For example, the editorial argues that clinical treatment is more flexible; that the individual outcomes are evaluated in a more complex and detailed fashion than is true of research protocols; that the clinician's definition of depression may be more realistic than the DSM-III-R criteria used by researchers; and so forth. Finally, it is recommended: 'At present, clinicians must again use their professional judgment when making treatment recommendations, bearing in mind the uncertainties. Among the uncertainties regarding antidepressant treatment of adolescents, we have to ask whether the clinicians are ahead of the researchers, or whether the handwriting on the wall is just hard to believe' (Popper, 1992, p. 3).

In essence, the editorial tells practicing clinicians that although the published double-blind, placebo-controlled studies unanimously demonstrate that antidepressants are no better than placebo, they should feel free to judge whether to continue to use them therapeutically. The rationale is that the research studies are not perfect and may be flawed in various ways (which would, of course, be true of all research studies).

A recently published *Handbook of Depression in Children and Adolescents* (Johnston and Fruehling, 1994) adopts an analogous strategy. In this volume, Johnston and Fruehling, after reviewing the series of double-blind studies indicating that antidepressants do not exceed placebos in efficacy, concluded that still it was premature to conclude that antidepressants are not a valid form of treatment for children. To justify this position they state: 'Perhaps the most persuasive reason is the widespread clinical use of these medications in depressed children. *It, seems unlikely that clinicians would continue to prescribe these medications if no clinical benefit were being realized.* Second, the studies completed thus far are all methodologically compromised, yet many of them show trends toward efficacy that are not statistically significant' (p. 388). The authors' position is that if the scientific data do not come out as expected, one can appeal to a different set of justifying criteria.

Other observers (*e.g.*, Pellegrino and Thomasma, 1981) have similarly leaned toward the right of clinicians to bypass the research findings if their individual judgments so dictate. One is immediately prompted to ask why such a permissive orientation would not justify any clinician selectively ignoring the existing scientific data pertinent to his or her treatment specialty?

While the results of studies of therapeutic efficacy are stated in terms of probabilities of success in groups or samples of patients, clinicians deal with the individual patient. They have to decide how applicable the group findings are to the circumstances of a particular individual. They have to integrate multiple facts applicable to the individual case with the modal data harvested from scientific studies. This was pointed out by Wulff (1986) in an issue of the *Journal of Medicine and Philosophy* entirely devoted to the nature of rational decision making in medicine. He indicated that this meant there was typically a significant area of ambiguity in arriving at therapeutic (also diagnostic) decisions about individual cases. It is in this ambiguous region that practitioners find some permission whether to go beyond the pertinent scientific information available to them. The prerogative of physician-practitioners to retain final authority with respect to choice of treatment has been a powerful theme in physician identity. There has been continued resistance to adopting a definition of physician activity that is synonymous with taking a scientific orientation. Note what Pellegrino and Thomasma (1981) have to say about this point:

A large part of the physician's specific activity . . . depends upon skills outside of the traditional scientific paradigm. Whenever the physician resorts to experience or empirical data, he or she must use the scientific canon, but once the data are in, the physician's internal dialogue conforms more closely to the canons of the liberal arts. This does not mean that these canons are not susceptible to explicit analysis, but only that any unitary theory of medicine which identifies it exclusively with science is doomed to failure.

(p. 147)

They highlight a 'tension between the scientific-actuarial and the artist-intuitionist models of clinical judgment' (p. 120).

Other medical ethicists take an opposed position. Thus, Lynoe (1992) declares: 'For a physician with an academic medical education it would be unethical and irreconcilable with the tenets of science and proven experience to provide a treatment, the effect of which is indistinguishable from the placebo effect' (p. 221).

Relatedly, Roy (1986) suggested: 'When there is uncertainty or definite doubt about the safety or efficacy of an innovative or established treatment, there *is*, not simply *may* be, a higher moral obligation to test it critically than to prescribe it year-in, year-out with the support of custom or wishful thinking' (p. 286).

Whatever the explicit theoretical positions taken, there is no doubt that many clinicians do make therapeutic decisions that are not anchored in existing scientific data. The prescribing of antidepressants for children clearly illustrates how a significant group of practitioners (child psychiatrists and pediatricians) can persist in using a procedure that is actually contradicted by research data and at the same time muster justifications for doing so. There is obviously a need to define more precisely how far individual practitioners are at liberty to deviate from modal scientific findings.

A number of articles (*e.g.*, Banta and Thacker, 1990; *Evidence-Based Working Group*, 1992; Grimes, 1993) have examined the issue of how responsible physicians should be for basing their decisions on the most up-to-date and reliable scientific data. These articles have commented on the fact that the medical school curiculum often does not encourage skepticism or an interest in independently appraising the evidence pertinent to specific treatment alternatives. Strong recommendations have been made by Bishop (1984), Grimes (1993), and others to the effect that medical students be taught the essentials of experimental design, statistical significance, and meta-analysis so that they can, with some autonomy, question new procedures, drugs, and technologies that are recommended to them. The apparent inability of child psychiatrists to grasp the significance of the literature concerning the efficacy of antidepressants for children has been duplicated in other areas of medicine in relation to such diverse procedures as fetal monitoring, episiotomy, and electroencephalography (*e.g.*, Banta and Thacker, 1990).

In this context, one can see that various troublesome questions need to be resolved. For example, how can adequate access to the most current scientific findings concerning specific treatments be guaranteed to the average practitioner? Should practitioners feel justified in applying treatments that have been anecdotally recommended in letters to journals? Should practitioners clearly communicate to patients whether given therapies have or have not been scientifically validated? However, the most basic issue is whether physicians as a community will explicitly accept the idea that what they do must be supported by the most up-to-date scientific findings. At the least, is there a willingness to agree that no therapeutic procedure should be applied that has been empirically shown not to be effective?

References

Ambrosini PJ, Bianchi MD, Rabinovish H, Ella J (1993) Antidepressant treatments in children and adolescents. I. Affective disorders. *J Am Acad Child Adolesc Psychiatry* **32**:1–5.

Banta HD, Thacker SB (1990) The case for reassessment of health care technology: Once is not enough. *JAMA* **264**:235–246.

Bishop JM (1984) Infuriating tensions: Science and the medical student. *J Med Educ* **59**:91–102.

Boulos C, Kutcher S, Marton P, Simeon J, Ferguson B, Roberts N (1991) Response to desimpramine treatment in adolescent major depression. *Psychopharmacol Bull* **27**:59–65.

Conners CK (1992) Methodology of antidepressant drug trials for treating depression in adolescents. *J Child Adolesc Psychopharmacol* **2**:11–22.

Elliott GR (1992) Dilemmas for clinicians and researchers using antidepressants to treat adolescents with depression. *J Child Adolesc Psychopharmacol* **2**:7–9.

Evidence-Based Medicine Working Group (1992) Evidence-based medicine: A new aproach to teaching the practice of medicine. *JAMA* **268**:2420–2425.

Gadow KD (1991) Clinical issues in child and adolescent psychopharmacology. *J Consult Clin Psychol* **59**:842–852.

Geller B, Cooper TB, Graham DL, Fetner HH, Marsfeller FA, Wells J (1992) Pharmacokinetically designed double-blind placebo-controlled study of nortriptyline in 6 to 12 year olds with major depressive disorder. *J Am Acad Child Adolesc Psychiatry* **31**:34–44.

Geller B, Cooper TB, Graham DL, Marsfeller FA, Bryant DM (1990) Double-blind placebo-controlled study of nortriptyline in depressed adolescents using a 'fixed plasma level' design. *Psychopharmacol Bull* **26**:85–90.

Goleman D (1993, December 15) Use of antidepressants in children at issue. *The New York Times*, p. 17.

Green WH (1991) *Child and adolescent clinical psychopharmacology.* Baltimore: Williams & Wilkins.

Grimes DA (1993) Technology follies: The uncritical acceptance of medical innovation. *JAMA* **269**:3030–3033.

Hughes CW, Preskorn SH, Woller E, Woller R, Hassamein R, Tucker S (1990) The effect of concomitant disorders in childhood depression on predicting treatment response. *Psychopharmacol Bull* **26**:235–238.

Johnston HF, Fruehling JJ (1994) Pharmacological therapy for depression in children and adolescents. In WM Reynolds, HF Johnston (Eds) *Handbook of Depression in Children and Adolescents*. New York, Plenum.

Kashani JH, Shekim WO, Reid JC (1994) Amitriptyline in children with major depressive disorder: A double-blind crossover pilot study. *J Am Acad Child Adolesc Psychiatry* **23**:348–351.

Kramer A, Feiguine R (1981) Clinical effects of amitriptyline in adolescent depression: A double-blind crossover pilot study. *J Am Acad Child Adolesc Psychiatry* **20**:36–44.

Kutcher S, Boulos C, Ward B, Marton P (1994) Response to desipramine treatment in adolescent depression: A fixed-dose placebo controlled trial. *J Am Acad Child Adolesc Psychiatry* **33**:686–694.

Lucas A, Lockett H, Grimm F (1965) Amitriptyline in childhood depressions. *Dis Nerv Syst* **26**:105–110.

Lynoe N (1992) Ethical and professional aspects of practice of alternative medicine. *Scand J Soc Med* **4**:217–225.

Pellegrino ED, Thomasma DC (1981) *A Philosophical Basis of Medical Practice*. New York: Oxford University Press.

Petti T, Law W (1982) Imipramine treatment of depressed children: A double-blind pilot study. *J Clin Psychopharmacol* **2**: 107–110.

Popper CW (1992) Are clinicians ahead of researchers in finding a treatment for adolescent depression? [Editorial] *J Child Adolesc Psychopharmacol* **2**:1–3.

Preiskorn SH, Weller EB, Hughes C, Weller RA, Bolte K (1987) Depression in prepubertal children: Dexamethasone nonsuppression predicts differential response to imipramine vs. placebo. *Psychopharmacol Bull* **23**: 265–268.

Puig-Antich J, Perel JM, Lupatkin W, Chambers W, Shea C, Tabrize MA, Stiller R (1979) Plasma levels of imipramine and desmethylimipramine (DMI) and clinical response in prepubertal major depressive disorders. *J Am Acad Child Adolesc Psychiatry* **18**:616–627.

Puig-Antich J, Perel JM, Lupatkin W, Chambers WJ, Tabrizi MA, King J, Goetz R, Davies M, Stiller RL (1987) Imipramine in prepubertal major depressive disorders. *Arch Gen Psychiatry* **44**:81–89.

Riddle MA, Geller B, Ryan N (1993) Another sudden death in a child treated with desipramine. *J Am Acad Child Adolesc Psychiatry* **9**:283–289.

Roy DJ (1986) Ethics in clinical research and clinical practice. *Clin Invest Med* **9**:283–289.

Simeon J, DiNicola V, Phil M, Ferguson H, Copping W (1990) Adolescent depression: A placebo-controlled fluoxetine treatment study and follow-up. *Prog Neuropsychopharmacol Biol Psychiatry* **14**:791–795.

Wulff HR (1986) Rational diagnoses and treatment. *J Med Philos* **11**:123–134.

The Valorization of Sadness

Alienation and the Melancholic Temperament*

Peter D. Kramer

At the heart of *Listening to Prozac* is a thought experiment: Imagine that we have to hand a medication that can move a person from a normal psychological state to another normal psychological state that is more desired or better socially rewarded.1 What are the moral consequences of that potential, the one I called 'cosmetic psychopharmacology'?

The question would be overgeneral except that it occurs in the context of a discussion of psychic consequences of technologies. People now experience the self in the light of psychotherapeutic medications as lately they experienced it through psychoanalysis. In the thought experiment, the medication we are to imagine is rather like Prozac, and the less desired state is something like melancholy, when that term refers to a personality style rather than an illness. Melancholics are well described in literature that stretches back for centuries. They are pessimistic, self-doubting, moralistic, and obsessive. They have low energy but use that energy productively. They are creative in the arts. They are prone to depression, especially in response to social disappointments.

Listening to Prozac argues that the important action of new medications may be on the melancholic temperament as much as on depression, although the two are presumed to be related. The book's assessment of cosmetic psychopharmacology begins with the observation that for decades, psychotherapy has been the technology applied to melancholy. In this account, psychotherapy includes approaches, such as supportive or strategic therapies, in which self-understanding is not the means or end of cure – where the goal is change in affective state merely. Asking why cosmetic psychopharmacology makes us so uneasy, I did not neglect to consider the targets of treatment – in particular, claims that suffering is an indicator of the human condition; that psychic pain serves an adaptive function; and that melancholy is an element of authentic self. But since the premise of 'cosmesis' is movement from normal to normal, the post-treatment state as much as the pretreatment should meet the criteria of Darwinian fitness and human completeness. And those who hope psychotherapy succeeds must be comfortable with the diminution of melancholy. For these reasons, I came to believe that a critical element in a principled objection to cosmetic psychopharmacology must involve the method of change, namely, medication, more than the goals of intervention.

To my delight, moral philosophers have taken up this thought experiment, particularly the medical ethicist Carl Elliott, in a series of essays distinguished by their literary appeal. These discussions are a continuation of *Listening to Prozac*, but they are also a form of backtracking, because the element that interests Elliott is cosmesis's goal. Elliott is worried about the diminution of alienation.

I hope here to use Elliott's essays to ask, as rule-keeper for a certain sort of game, whether the concept of alienation successfully identifies grounds on which cosmetic psychopharmacology might be morally suspect. At the same time, I will want to reopen the issue of the legitimate goals of treatment. To preview my conclusion – my impression is that the concern over Prozac, and with imagined medications extrapolated from

experience with Prozac, turns almost entirely on an aesthetic valuation of melancholy.

. . .

Elliott's central claim is that addressing alienation as a psychiatric issue is like treating holy communion as a dietary issue – a category mistake. Included in this claim is the understanding that alienation has a particular moral worth. Neither of these assertions strikes me as obvious. In particular, I want to say that both are thrown into doubt by a premise of our discussion, namely that medication can lessen alienation. The nature of the technology may cause us to reassess the category, and the significance, of the target.

To begin with the question of category: Clearly *some* alienation is an aspect of mental illness, indeed alienation is an element in schizophrenia. It is not absurd to imagine that alienation might be 'psychiatric.' Often Elliott equates alienation with depression, as when he paraphrases Walker Percy to this effect: 'Take a look around you; it would take a moron not to be depressed.'2 The arguments Elliott makes regarding depression and alienation, as worrisome targets for pharmacology, are identical. It is not always clear whether the depression referred to is a stance or a syndrome.

As regards category, then, the question is, alienation of what sort? Elliott recognizes 'that alienation comes in many forms, and he describes personal, cultural, and existential alienation. But from a psychiatric point of view, the people Elliott suggests as candidates for antidepressant use are homogeneous. They are not primarily mistrustful, in a way that might make us think of a paranoid alienation; nor are they socially unaware and distanced from their fellows in way that might suggest an autistic alienation. Elliott's subjects are sad, obsessive, and questing. They worry. Their alienation is of a single sort, the sort that is an element of the melancholic personality.

When I say that the premise 'medication diminishes alienation' casts its shadow on questions of category, I mean that our likely beliefs about category are susceptible to being altered by our beliefs about how that diminution occurs. We do not expect medication to work directly on the cognitive component of alienation, just as we do not imagine there is a pill for, say, atheism or chauvinism – that sort of imagining would violate the rule that the drug we have in mind is a good deal like Prozac. Presumably, our hypothetic medication tones down obsessionality, pessimism, and social anxiety, so that, secondarily, a person feels less impelled to resist the ambient culture. It alters affective aspects of personality, where affect extends to such phenomena as sense of status in social groups.

That is to say, our premise brings into play the basis of personality. If we were certain, as many mid-century psychoanalysts were, that personality is the detailed psychic encoding of a person's experience in the world, relatively fixed but responsive to insight, then the parameters for a discussion of the pharmacologic enhancement of alienation would be clearer. Equally, if we were to discover that even minor depression is in all instances caused by a virus that deforms brain anatomy, the discussion would be stable at a different point of equilibrium. The range of philosophical arguments

* Kramer, P.: The valorization of sadness. *Hastings Center Report* **30**:13–18, 2000.

might remain similar – one can approach character armor as a medical condition and one can define living with microbes as an expectable state of human life – but in each instance we would be more inclined to entertain particular ones.

To clarify the interplay of target and technology: Setting aside Prozac, let us imagine that it is discovered that moderate doses of vitamin C decrease a person's sense of isolation. Would the taking of vitamins seem worrisome? The answer depends on how we 'listen' to the medication. We might decide that alienation of that sort was in all probability something like a vitamin deficiency. We might even decide in retrospect that our objection to cosmesis had resulted from an aesthetic assessment of the technology employed to achieve it. That is, previously (when it was a matter of using Prozac, rather than vitamins, to the same end) we had objected because the technology was artificial, scientifically complex, and manufactured and advertised by a large corporation – partaking of the very qualities we believe ought to lead to alienation, on, say, a political basis. Once vitamin C's effect was discovered, we might come to believe that Prozac had, after all, been repairing medical damage to the self. Starting with the premise that medication can mitigate alienation, it is not hard to imagine evidence in light of which alienation would be most parsimoniously understood as at least in part a psychiatric issue.

I should add that as a clinician, I find the argument by category mistake suspect because generally category mistakes are in the opposite direction from the one that perturbs Elliott. Mental illness has too often been too narrowly understood – misunderstood – as a principled response to social conditions; this error is one R. D. Laing made with regard to schizophrenia when he claimed that psychosis is a response to the absurd pressures of bourgeois family life. My own belief is that the conundrum necessarily is played out at a historical moment, ours, when the categorization of alienation remains ambiguous.

. . .

Elliott goes on to argue that alienation is circumstantially appropriate and morally valuable. Regarding personal and cultural alienation – the mismatch between particular self and the particulars of the social surround – Elliott writes that you might feel ill at ease among Milwaukee Rotarians. Elliott would disfavor your being offered Prozac in this instance because 'Some external circumstances call for alienation.'

Now I hope it is the case that no one is dispensing medication as an alternative to dropping membership in the Milwaukee Rotary. But if Elliott is at some distance from the clinical moment here, he is nonetheless successful in depicting one sort of unease, that of the sensitive person stuck in a group of philistines. Walker Percy, in a passage cited by Elliott, works the same vein as regards depression: 'Consider the only adults who are never depressed: chuckle-heads, California surfers, and fundamentalist Christians who believe they have had a personal encounter with Jesus and are saved once and for all. Would you trade your depression to become any one of these?'[3]

These examples are amusing, but I fear that because they are all of a type, they prejudice the jury. Elliott's and Percy's comments succeed, on first reading, not because we value every instance of alienation – any sort of fish out of any sort of water – but because of a cultural preference for the melancholic over the sanguine. Consider the alienation or depression of a hockey player (a potential future Rotarian) rooming with poets; we may not want him to resist integration. Or consider the sort of movie, common in recent years, where a straight-laced man is thrown into the company of a wild woman and her friends; the audience's hope is that he will overcome rather than sustain his alienation from the kooky subculture.

In *Listening to Prozac*, I addressed a similar issue – alienation from what? – in regard to mourning rituals. Those who consider the American grieving period too brief and therefore alienating to the sensitive have pointed with admiration to rural Greece, where widows mourn predeceasing husbands for five years. But enforced mourning is restrictive for resilient widows; they are the alienated in a traditional culture. If alienation means a sense of

incompatibility with the environment, then people of differing temperaments will be alienated in different settings. Do we honor both the sensitive and the resilient? Is it permissible for resilient Greek women to move to a society with shorter grieving periods? More to the point, if the sensitive move to rural Greece, will the consequent loss of alienation rob them of an aspect of their humanity? This sort of example might convince us that it is not personal or cultural alienation that we value, but the melancholic temperament or aspects of it, such as loyalty and sensitivity – and that we honor a sufferer in any setting, even one from which she is not personally or culturally alienated.

Effectively, Elliott conflates personal and cultural alienation. The notion of cultural alienation is invisibly buttressed by what I might call the Woody Allen effect. The prominently neurotic today are often political liberals, and this correlation has more or less held since the Romantic era. Soft left, hard right. But even if this conjunction is real and has an explanation (and what sort of explanation do we have in mind?), it is hardly universal. A sanguine person may be alarmed by apartheid, just as a melancholic might attribute his disaffection to the ending of apartheid. If Prozac induces conformity, it is to an ideal of assertiveness; but assertiveness can be in the service of social reform of the sort ordinarily understood as nonconformity or rebellion. The political effects of medicating the disaffected will be various.

Politics aside, we may find we have an aesthetic preference for neurosis. The melancholic temperament is the artistic temperament. Even if hearty Apollonian artists exist – Lionel Trilling and Edmund Wilson debated the point – they are less appealing than the wounded Dionysian variety.[4] The cluster of personality traits arising from the melancholic temperament (pessimism, perfectionism, sensitivity, and the rest) overlaps so strongly with our image of the intellectual that we may have difficulty crediting thinkers who are differently constituted. The pervasiveness of this valuation came home to me in the course of my writing an essay about the psychologist Carl Rogers; Rogers met all the criteria for intellectuality save one, pessimism, and on that grounds was dismissed as a lightweight.[5]

Thus concern over personal or cultural alienation comes to seem the valuation of one sort of normal person (the melancholic) over another (the sanguine). And just how far would a moralist go in this preference for alienation? Are those 25 percent of humans who lack the purported 'Woody Allen gene' morally defective? If so, we might logically favor a medication that makes them more ill at ease. It seems less a matter of mistrusting pharmacology than of valuing melancholy.

. . .

Elliott's third category is existential alienation – 'questioning' the very terms on which a life is built,' an unease such as one might suffer even on a desert island, or, as Robert Coles might put it, under any moon. Here we seem to be getting to the heart of the matter, alienation that has nothing to do with distance from a particular social surround.

We could perhaps obviate this consideration by arguing that if existential alienation is neither personal nor cultural, it should be part of being human, for all people in all times. If normal life is a project, then change qualifies as cosmetic only when life remains a project. Even for 'good responders' to medication, existence remains hedged round by death, chance, unfairness, and absurdity.

But empirically, we know that angst grabs different people differently. Some people are more constantly aware of the universal existential condition. But what is it to be aware in this sense? Even existential alienation might be intertwined with temperament. Elliott leans toward that recognition when he writes, 'Alienation of any type might go together with depression, of course, but I suspect that the two don't necessarily go hand in hand.' But that is the question at issue: to what extent is affect, such as anxiety or depression, constitutive of existential alienation? To put the matter differently: If, medicated, one retains an intellectual unease but with diminished emotional discomfort, does being in that state constitute existential alienation?

Imagine one of Walker Percy's famously alienated characters, say a commuter. He might feel bad for two reasons, because life is imperfect and because he is predisposed to feel worse than others do in response to that imperfection. If he experiences relief via medication, he might come to understand which was which, his dysthymia versus the alienation common to all humans. As a diagnostician, medication is imperfect, but neither is it simply dismissible. On a quest for authenticity, we must be open to discoveries of this sort – that what seemed carefully developed self was arbitrary, biologically based idiosyncrasy.

Elliott resists this sort of reframing when he asserts that 'there is no difference between the commuter who feels bad without knowing why and the same commuter reading a copy of DSM-IV.'[6] But that is because Elliott mistrusts the manual. Finding his condition delineated there, the commuter might decide he had formerly made a category mistake, just as, finding himself in a Walker Percy novel, a diagnosed depressive might draw a conclusion in the reverse direction. I once treated a dysthymic patient whose former psychiatrist had commanded her to 'Put away your Sylvia Plath!' Whether poetry or medication (or manual-reading) is a better means to self-discovery is in part an empirical question; a combination might prove optimal.

Another thought experiment: Imagine we have defined possible elements of existential alienation: spleen, anomie, angst, accedia, vertigo, malaise, emptiness, and the like. Now we give a medication for depression and find that some factors disappear and others remain, so that a hypothetical subject is no longer vertiginous but remains anomic. Would we have defined 'core' alienation? Dissected the existential? Well, perhaps not. Not if alienation's connection to minor depression is especially intimate. The problem of melancholic temperament cannot be made to disappear, not even by our framing the conundrum in terms of respect for existential alienation. Elliott's worry is precisely that if a medication replaces pessimism with optimism, anxiety with assertiveness, diffidence with gregariousness, it will have robbed us of a tendency to remain at a critical distance from our own existence. The affective stance is what is of value, worrying the same old bone, as Percy puts it; not mere awareness of distance but anxiety over it.

I have come to believe that much of the discussion of cosmetic psychopharmacology is not about pharmacology at all – that is to say, not about the technology. Rather, 'cosmetic pharmacology' is a stand-in for worries over threats to melancholy. That psychotherapy caused less worry may speak to our lack of confidence in its efficacy.

We do, as a culture, value melancholy. Some months ago, I attended an exhibition of the paintings of 'the young Picasso.' Seeing the early canvases, I thought, 'Here is a marvelous technician.' I turned a corner to confront the works of the Blue Period, Picasso's response to the suicide of his friend Carlos Casagemas. Instantly I thought (as I believe the curator intended): 'How profound.' That pairing – melancholic/deep – is a central trope of the culture. Or to allude to another recent museum exhibition, for years the rap on Pierre Bonnard was that his paintings were too cheerful to be important. Here is the corresponding trope: happy/superficial.

Surely the central tenet of literary criticism is Kafka's: 'I think we ought to read only the kind of books that wound and stab us. . . . [W]e need the books that affect us like a disaster, that grieve us deeply, like the death of someone we loved more than ourselves, like being banished into forests far from every one, like a suicide.'[7] This need may even be pragmatic. In his poetry (I am thinking of 'Terence, this is stupid stuff'), A. E. Housman argues that painful literature immunizes us against the pain of life's disappointments.

And here I want to lay down two linked challenges that are intentionally provocative. The first is to say that the literary aesthetic makes most sense in relation to a particular temperament (the melancholic, in which one feels great pain in response to loss) in a particular culture (one lacking technologies to prevent or diminish that pain). What if Mithradates had an antidote, so that he did not require prophylactic arsenic and strychnine? Might poetry appropriate to the antidepressant era be more like beer-drinking? And might that new art still prove authentic to the way of the world?

The second challenge is yet more provocative, call it intentionally hyperbolic: to say that there is no neutral venue for this debate over alienation or cosmesis because our sensibility has been largely formed by melancholics.

Much of philosophy is written, and much art has been created, by melancholics or the outright depressed, as a response to their substantial vulnerabilities. To put the matter only slightly less provocatively (and to return to the first challenge), much of philosophy is directed at depression as a threatening element of the human condition.

As Martha Nussbaum's *The Therapy of Desire* demonstrates in detail, classical moral philosophy is a means for coping with extremes of affect that follow upon loss.[8] The ancient Greeks' recommendations for the good life, in the writings of the Cynics and Stoics and Epicureans and Aristotelians, amount to ways to buffer the vicissitudes of attachment. If loss were less painful, the good life might be characterized not by *ataraxia* but by gusto. The connection between philosophy and melancholy continues in the medieval writings on *akdie* and then in the Enlightenment, through Montaigne, and through Pascal who writes 'Man is so unhappy that he would be bored even if he had no cause for boredom, by the very nature of his temperament.'[9] In a study of Kierkegaard, Harvie Ferguson writes, 'Modern philosophy, particularly in Descartes, Kant, and Hegel, presupposed as a permanent condition the melancholy of modern life.'[10] Even those like Kierkegaard who chide melancholics do so from such a decided melancholic position that their writing reinforces the notion that melancholy is profundity. It is Kierkegaard who inspires Walker Percy, Kierkegaard whose body of work implies that melancholy is appropriate to modernity.

As for literature, studies indicate that an astonishing percentage, perhaps a vast majority, of serious writers are depressives. Researchers have speculated on the cause of that connection – does depression put one in touch with important issues, of deterioration and loss? But no one has asked what it means for us as a culture or even as a species that our unacknowledged legislators suffer from mood disorders, or something like. If there is no inherent moral distinction between melancholy and sanguinity, then we will need to worry about the association between creativity and mood. What if there is a consistent bias in the intellectual assessment of the good life or the wise perspective on life, an inherent bias against sanguinity hidden (and apparent) in philosophy and art?

An argument of this sort is worrisome – more worrisome than the conundrum we began with. And yet can we in good faith ignore the question of who sets the values? I have been in effect proposing still another thought experiment: Imagine a medication that diminishes the extremes of emotional response to loss, imparting the resilience already enjoyed by those with an even, sunny disposition. What would be the central philosophical questions in a culture where the use of this medication is widespread?

Aesthetic values do change in the light of changing views of health and illness. Elsewhere, I have asked why we are no longer charmed by suicidal melancholics – Goethe's Werther or Chateaubriand's René or Chekov's Ivanov. Because we see major depression and affectively driven personality disorders as medically pathologic, what once exemplified authenticity now looks like immaturity or illness – as if the romantic writers had made a category error.

A final thought experiment: Imagine that the association between melancholy and literary talent is based on a random commonality of cause: the genes for both cluster, say, side by side on a chromosome. And let us further imagine a culture in which melancholy, now clearly separate from creativity, is treated pharmacologically on a routine basis. In this culture, it is the melancholics manqués who write, melancholics rendered sanguine – so that the received notions of beauty and intimacy and nobility of character relate to bravado, decisiveness, and connections to social groups, not in the manner of false cheerleading, but authentically, from the creative well-springs of the optimistic.

What would be the notion of authenticity under such conditions? Perhaps in such a culture 'strong evaluation' would find psychic resilience superior to alienation. Even today, many a melancholic looks at Panurge or Tom Jones with admiration – how marvelous to face the world with appetite! The notion of a sanguine culture horrifies those of us resonant with an aesthetics of melancholy, but morally, is such a culture inferior, assuming its art corresponds to the psychic reality? Is there a principled basis for linking melancholy to authenticity? Is there a moral hierarchy of temperaments?

. . .

I have offered an extreme version of an argument that might be more palatable in subtler form. I hope I have been convincing, or at least troubling, in one regard, the assertion that there is no privileged place to stand, no way to get outside the problem of authenticity as regards temperament.

Elliott asks whether we do not lose sight of something essential about ourselves when we see alienation and guilt as symptoms to be treated rather than as clues to our condition as human beings. The answer is in part empirical, in part contingent (on the social conditions of human life, a culture's technological resources, and such), and altogether aesthetic. If extremes of alienation are shown to arise from neuropathology, and if aspects of that pathology respond to treatment, our notion of the essential will change. And it may be that what remains of the experience and the concept of alienation will be yet more morally admirable – alienation stripped of compulsion, alienation independent of genetic happenstance, alienation that arises from free choice.

I want to end by saying that, like Percy and Elliott, in my private aesthetic, I value depression and alienation, see them as postures that have salience for the culture and inherent beauty. But the role of philosophy is to question preferences. The case for and against alienation seems to me at this moment wide open. It has become easy, in the light of the debate over Prozac, to imagine material circumstances that might cause us to reassess which aspects of alienation fall into which category. The challenge of Prozac is precisely that it puts in question our tastes and values.

References

1   P. D. Kramer. *Listening to Prozac* (New York: Viking Press. 1993).

2   C. Elliott. 'The Tyranny of Happiness: Ethics and Cosmetic Psychophamacology.' in *Enhancing Human Traits: Ethical and Social Implications*, ed. E. Parens (Washington. D.C.: Georgetown University Press. 1998), pp. 177–88, at 183.

3   W. Percy, *Lost in the Cosmos* (New York: Washington Square Press, 1983). p. 79, quoted in C. Elliott, 'Prozac and the Existential Novel: Two Therapies,' in *The Last Physician: Walker Percy and the Moral Life of Medicine*, ed. C. Elliott and J. Lantos (Durham, N.C.: Duke University Press, 1999), p. 65.

4   E. Wilson, 'Philocheles: The Wound and the Bow,' in E. Wilson, *The Wound and the Bow: Seven Studies in Literature* (Cambridge, Mass.: Riverside Press, 1941), pp. 272–95; L. Trilling, *The Liberal Imagination: Essays on Literature and Society* (New York: Viking, 1950), pp. 160–80.

5   P. D. Kramer, Introduction to *On Becoming a Person*, by C. Rogers (Boston: Houghton Mifflin, 1995).

6   See ref. 2, Elliott, 'Tyranny of Happiness.' p. 183.

7   F. Kafka, letter to Oskar Polluck, 27 January 1904.

8   M. Nussbaum, *The Therapy of Desire: Theory and Practice in Hellenistic Ethics* (Princeton: Princeton University Press, 1994).

9   B. Pascal, quoted in H. Ferguson, *Melancholy and the Critique of Modernity: Soren Kierkegaard's Religious Psychology* (London: Routledge, 1995), p. 25.

10 See ref. 7. Ferguson, *Melancholy and the Critique of Modernity*, p. 32.

11 See ref. 1, Kramer, *Listening to Prozac*, p. 297, and P. D. Kramer, 'Stage View: What Ivanov Needs Is an Antidepressant,' *New York Times*, 21 December 1997.

Pursued by Happiness and Beaten Senseless
Prozac and the American Dream*

Carl Elliott

Let us start with cases. These come from an essay by the psychotherapist Maureen O'Hara and Walter Truett Anderson. The names have been changed, but the patients, they tell us, are real.

1) Jerry feels overwhelmed, anxious, fragmented, and confused. He disagrees with people he used to agree with and aligns himself with people he used to argue with. He questions his sense of reality and frequently asks himself what it all means. He has had all kinds of therapeutic and growth experiences: gestalt, rebirthing, Jungian analysis, holotropic breathwork, bioenergetics, the Course in Miracles, twelve-step recovery groups, Zen meditation, Ericksonian hypnosis. He has been to sweat lodges, to the Rajneesh ashram in Poona, to the Wicca festival in Devon. He is in analysis again, this time with a self-psychologist. Although he is endlessly on the lookout for new ideas and experiences, he keeps saying he wishes he could simplify his life. He talks about buying land in Oregon. He loved *Dances with Wolves*.

2) Alec is forty-two, single, and for most of his life has felt lonely and alienated. He's never cared much about politics, considers himself an agnostic, and has never found a hobby or interest he would want to pursue consistently. He says he doesn't think he really has a self at all. He's had two stints of psychotherapy; both ended inconclusively, leaving him still with chronic, low-grade depression. Nowadays he's feeling a little better about himself. He has started attending a local meeting of Adult Children of Alcoholics. People at the meetings seem to understand and validate his pain; he's making friends there and believes he 'belongs' for the first time since he left the military. But he confesses to his therapist that he feels 'sort of squirrelly' about it because he's not an adult child of an alcoholic. He is faking the pathological label in order to be accepted by the community, and he's not too sure he really buys into their twelve-step ideology either.

3) Beverly comes into therapy torn between two lifestyles and two identities. In the California city where she goes to college, she is a radical feminist; on visits to her midwestern home town she is a nice, sweet, square conservative girl. The therapist asks her when she feels most like herself. She says, 'When I'm on the airplane.'[1]

Spiritual emptiness, the search for a sense of self, alienation in the midst of abundance: are there traits any more American than these? These are themes that characterize some of the most memorable American art of the middle and late twentieth century: in the poetry of T. S. Eliot and Sylvia Plath, in fiction from West and Salinger through Bellow and DeLillo, from the plays of Tennessee Williams to the documentary films of Ross McElwee, from the songs of Woody Guthrie to those of the Talking Heads. If we are to believe Tocqueville, this kind of spiritual restlessness has been with us since the early days of the republic. 'In America I saw the freest and most enlightened men, placed in circumstances the happiest to be found in the world; yet it seemed to me as if a cloud habitually hung upon their brow, and I thought them serious and almost sad even in their pleasures.'[2]

In the decade or so since the development of the selective serotonin reuptake inhibitors, many thoughtful (and some not so thoughtful) voices have urged caution, or at least a damper on our enthusiasm for the drugs, most notably in the debate prompted by Peter Kramer's splendid book, *Listening to Prozac*. Scholars have worried that *Prozac treats* the self rather than proper diseases, that it alters personality, that it feeds dangerously into the American obsession with competition and worldly success, and that it offers a mechanistic cure for spiritual problems of the sort predicted by Walker Percy in his novel *Love in the Ruins*, in which the psychiatrist Tom More treats existential ailments with his Ontological Lapsometer. But in the years since I first read Kramer's book I have begun to suspect that the problem may go deeper than Prozac; that the problem is not merely Prozac but the stance of psychiatry itself. Wittgenstein once wrote, 'The sickness of a time is cured by an alteration in the mode of life of human beings, and it was possible for the sickness of philosophical problems to get cured only through a changed mode of thought and of life, not through a medicine invented by an individual.'[3] He was talking about philosophy, not psychopharmacology, but the point is apt either way. At least part of the nagging worry about Prozac and its ilk is that for all the good they do, the ills that they treat are part and parcel of the lonely, forgetful, unbearably sad place where we live.

. . .

I am slightly reluctant to use the term 'alienation,' coming as it does with baggage that I do not necessarily want to take with me, but so be it: here, I think, it can serve a useful purpose. Alienation seems to describe at least some of the symptoms that bring people to the attention of a psychiatrist. How many patients this is, and whether Prozac actually cures them, remains to be seen. It may be very small in comparison to, say, the number who use Prozac for depression. But I take it from my psychiatric colleagues, from the case histories in Kramer's book and others, and from my many friends and acquaintances who have used the drug, that whether it affects alienation is at least an open question.

Alienation, it seems to me, differs from most of the kinds of descriptors that psychiatry ordinarily uses for psychiatric patients – descriptors like anxiety, obsessiveness, even unhappiness. These descriptors describe internal psychic states. They are about (to use a slightly misleading metaphor) what's in my own head. Relationships with things outside myself can affect my happiness or unhappiness, or for that matter, my depression or my anxiety or my obsessions; if I am in a miserable job, or if my relationship with my wife is on the rocks, or even if (as we say down South) I am not right with God, I might be more unhappy, or more anxious or depressed. But the concepts themselves are by and large measures of my internal psychic well-being.

This makes them different from alienation. Alienation generally describes an incongruity between the self and external structures of meaning – a lack of fit between the way you are and the way you are expected to be, say, or a mismatch between the way you are living a life and the structures of meaning that tell you how to live a life. Alienated people are alienated from something – their families, their cultures, their jobs, their Gods. This isn't a

* Elliott, C.: Pursued by happiness and beaten senseless. *Hastings Center Report* **30**:7–12, 2000.

purely internal matter; it isn't just in the alienated person's head. It is about a mismatch between a person and something outside himself. This, I think, is why it makes some sense (although one could contest this) to say that sometimes a person should be alienated – that given certain circumstances, alienation is the proper response. Some external circumstances call for alienation.

Alienation comes in many varieties, or so I think, many of which blur into one another. For the sake of simplicity, let me mention three, with the caveat that these divisions are artificial and overlapping. The first is a kind of personal alienation, *a sense* that you don't conform with social expectations of someone in your particular circumstances. It might be that your character doesn't quite fit into place as it should, so that you feel ill at ease among the other Princeton men or Milwaukee Rotarians or suburban high school cheerleaders. It may be that you feel alienated from the social role you are expected to occupy. You are not cut out to be a Washington political wife, or a Virginia gentleman, or the inheritor of the family hardware business. Or perhaps the direction your life is moving simply doesn't mesh with the way it's expected to move, like a New Hampshire housewife who at the age of fifty says this isn't the life for me, divorces her husband, sells the house, and goes off to Swaziland with the Peace Corps. For North Americans, these may be the most familiar kinds of alienation. They seem to be characteristic of times when a person's identity is in question or under reevaluation, such as when we are in our early twenties and are expected to decide what to do with our lives: What should I do for a living? Where should I live? Should I marry? If so, whom? Or in mid-life, when we start to look back on the decisions we have made and how they have turned out: Why did I marry him? Why didn't we have children? How in God's name did I wind up in accounting?

A second type of alienation that comes to mind, related to the first, is cultural alienation. This often involves the sense that a particular form of life is changing beneath your feet, and that you no longer have the equipment to manage in the new way. Something like this kind of alienation seems to be a motivating force behind a lot of social criticism. You step outside of your own socialization (or you are pushed) and look at your own culture from a standpoint of detachment. Perhaps the most extreme example of this kind of alienation would be characteristic of colonized and displaced peoples – Native Americans whose traditional ways of life have been erased, Hmong refugees marooned in Minnesota, Pacific Islanders colonized by the American military so that instead of fishing and harvesting tropical fruit they subsist on a diet of imported canned foods. I take it that this is also part of what Cornel West is getting at when, writing of the disappearance of traditional African American social institutions, he states that 'the major enemy of black survival in America is neither oppression nor exploitation but rather the nihilistic threat – that is, loss of hope and absence of meaning.'[4]

Walker Percy hints at this sort of alienation in *The Last Gentleman*, which takes place at a time when the old South of honor and agrarian living and racial inequality is giving way to a new, Republican, Christian South of golf clubs and subdivisions and Old Confederacy car lots. For Will Barrett, Percy's protagonist, the result is a kind of disorientation, a sense of not quite knowing how to fit into this new culture and what he is supposed to be doing there. In Barrett's family, Percy writes, 'The great grandfather knew what was what and said so and acted accordingly and did not care what anyone thought.' But over the generations Barrett's family lost its knack for action, no longer knew just what was what. Barrett's father said he didn't care what other people thought, but he cared. He wanted to act honorably and to be thought well of by others. 'So living for him was a strain. He became ironical. For him it was not a small thing to walk down the street on an ordinary September morning. In the end he was killed by his own irony and sadness and by the strain of living out an ordinary day in a perfect dance of honor.'[5]

But cultural alienation need not involve cultural change. In fact, perhaps the most recognizable symbols of American alienation are houses in the suburbs, which are seen as alienating precisely because of their static, anonymous conformity. In Richard Ford's novel *Independence Day*, the realtor Frank Bascombe says that buying a house comes with great anxiety because of that 'cold, unwelcome, built-in-America realization that we're just like the other schmo, wishing his wishes, lusting his stunted lusts, quaking over his idiot frights and fantasies, all of us popped out of the same unchinkable mold.'[6] In a society that values uniqueness and individuality, that says a fulfilled life is one in which you look inside yourself and discover your own particular values and talents, that valorizes the rule-breaking, anti-establishment, boundary-transgressing anti-hero, there is something terrifying about looking deep inside and discovering that you're no different from the guy next door. That your life is just an average life, and your story so ordinary it is not even worth telling. Anything that reminds you of this fact, anything that betrays the illusion that you are really, deep-down, quite an extraordinarily unique individual, is going to cut very close to the bone indeed. It is enough to make you think about an antidepressant.

Which leads to a third variety of alienation, one that I will call (with some trepidation) existential alienation. This kind of alienation involves questioning the very terms on which a life is built. By virtue of when, where, and to whom we are born, we inherit a sense of what it is possible to do with a human life, what kinds of lives are honorable or pointless or meaningful. To be a Southerner, a Jew, a Quebecoise, an Irishman, is to be born into a certain way of seeing and being in the world. This is part of what makes us who we are. But what happens to us, our sense of who we are, when we come to believe that the values we have are really nothing more than the values we have – not God's will, nor the inevitable consequence of history, nor the product of enlightened reason? Calling into question your own form of life involves calling into question your own values, the very stuff out of which you are built. This is not just realizing that your own particular castle is built on thin air. It is realizing you are built out of air yourself. It is radically disorienting: the ultimate, dizzying high-wire act, like Wiley Coyote after he runs off a cliff, glances down, and realizes where he is standing.

Many of the case histories surrounding Prozac, like those at the start of this essay, gesture at this kind of alienation – the sense that not only don't you know what to do with your life, you don't know what could possibly tell you what to do. The structures that might have given life its sense and meaning are now contested or in question. The result is not just the feeling that you are ill-suited for your own particular form of life, or that your form of life is fading away; rather, it is a calling into question of the foundations of any form of life. Why this job, this church, this country, this house? Why this particular way of going on when I get up in the morning? Why *any* particular way? The result of these kinds of questions can be the sense that no form of life can really have the kind of justification that you feel you need. It is a sense that there is no rhyme and reason to your form of life other than the exigencies of biology and history, that the big picture is really nothing more than a big picture.

Erik Parens has suggested to me that the account I have given here does not do justice to every sort of alienation, at least as many philosophers have understood it; that the most important sorts of alienation may be not from anything external to the self but from features intrinsic to human life. Rousseau, for example, thought that we are alienated from our sexuality. Heidegger thought that we become alienated from our essential nature as human beings when we do not face up to the fact that we will die. I think that Parens is for the most part right – and right in an especially insightful way – yet right only up to a point. There is no getting around the fact that we will all die, but alienation from our condition as mortal beings is never simply that; it is always a response to what our particular culture and age have made of our condition as mortal beings. To say, as Heidegger does, that living well requires anxiety in the face of not Being presupposes a framework of understanding that sees death as not Being (rather than, say, eternal life in the presence of God, or reincarnation, or any of the many other ways that people have thought of death). The fact that we modern Westerners are alienated from our sexuality or our mortality does not mean that all human beings at all times have been or must be alienated from them. When we are alienated from features intrinsic to human life, we are never alienated solely from those features themselves but from the meaning that our culture and age have given them.

Alienation of any type might go together with depression, of course, but I suspect that the two don't necessarily go hand in hand. I used to talk about alienation and depression with Benjy Freedman, my friend and colleague in bioethics at McGill University who died in 1997. Benjy was a loyal friend, ferociously intelligent and darkly funny, a complicated man of deep moral integrity. Yet for the first couple of years I knew him, he would periodically descend into very black moods. He would come into his office, close the door, draw the blinds and sit all day in semi-darkness. Sometimes he was irritable and would get into bitter arguments even with his close friends. I don't think Benjy would disagree with me when I say that he was probably clinically depressed. In fact, he once told me as much himself. He had recently suffered the deaths of two close family members. But Benjy was also a deeply devout Orthodox Jew. He was as secure in his faith as anyone I have ever known. He loved his family and was at home in his community. When Benjy and I talked about existential questions like these, questions about alienation from your culture and not knowing who to be or what to do with your life, he would just shake his head and laugh. He told me once he had no idea what I was talking about. These were questions with which he just couldn't connect. Which is not to say that he wasn't depressed or anxious or worried. He worried a lot about doing his duty, about whether he was doing sound intellectual work, whether he was doing a good job as a teacher. But for him, the broader structures of meaning within which these questions are located were uncontested. Unlike me: I was vaguely lost without (at least at that time) feeling particularly unhappy about it; an expatriate Southerner with a German wife living in Quebec and thus expected to be somewhat dislocated; a Walker Percy reader and thus strangely at home in the community of the alienated; undepressed, perhaps, but unlike Benjy, utterly at sea when it came to these broader structures of meaning.

. . .

What is left for those of us who are lost at sea? Apparently we have to make do with secular expertise, the professionals that Percy called the experts of the self. If we are alienated and impoverished and can't figure out why, we turn to doctors, psychologists, advice columnists, self-help authors, personal trainers, alternative healers, philosophical counselors, or (let us admit it) ethicists, who will set us on the path to righteousness, personal fitness, and sound mental hygiene. Why are you unhappy? Because you (1) are fat, (2) are shy, (3) dress badly, (4) do not own a house/sport utility vehicle/cell phone, (5) don't like to cook or keep house, (6) have never been on television, (7) are unable to converse on a variety of topics, (8) have not settled on a meaningful career, (9) do not have stimulating hobbies or fulfilling recreational activities, or (10) have not yet found the five steps to uncovering your inner capacity for childlike joy and wonderment. Experts of the self create facilities such as the Geriatrics Rehabilitation Unit in Percy's *Love in the Ruins*, where old folks often grow inexplicably sad despite the fact that their every need is met. 'Though they may live in the pleasantest Senior Settlements where their every need is filled, every recreation provided, every sort of hobby encouraged, nevertheless many grow despondent in their happiness, sit slack and empty-eyed at shuffleboard and ceramic oven. Fishing poles fall from tanned and healthy hands. Golf clubs rust. Reader's Digests go unread. Many old folk pine away and even die from unknown causes like a voodoo curse.'[7]

Here is the key to the problem psychiatry has with a notion like alienation. The measure of psychiatric success is internal psychic well-being. The aim of psychiatry is (among other things) to get rid of anxieties, obsessions, compulsions, phobias, and various other barriers to good social functioning. Within this framework, where the measure of success is psychic well-being through good social functioning, alienation is something to be eliminated. It is a psychiatric complaint. It is a barrier to psychic well-being. Whereas what I want to suggest is that maybe psychic well-being isn't everything. Some lives are better than others, quite apart from the psychic well-being of the person who is leading them. I don't mean this in any ultimate,

metaphysical sense. I'm not arguing that God prefers some lives to others, or that some lives are better than others because they are more rational or well-ordered. I just mean that the notion that some lives are better than others is part of the moral background to the way we live our lives. We all recognize that it is possible for a life to be a failure or a success, even if we aren't always able to say exactly why. Percy himself puts it this way: 'We all know perfectly well that the man who lives out his life as a consumer, a sexual partner, an "other-directed" executive; who avoids boredom and anxiety by consuming tons of newsprint, miles of movie film, years of TV time; that such a man has somehow betrayed his destiny as a human being.'[8]

Well, maybe. When I hear phrases like 'destiny as a human being' I start to squirm. But I take Percy's larger point seriously: by ignoring such matters as how a person lives his life, by steadfastly refusing to pass judgment on whether the ideals he lives by are worthy or wasteful or honorable or demeaning, psychiatry can say nothing useful whatsoever about alienation. It places itself in the position of neutrality about the broader structures of meaning within which lives are lived, and from which they might be alienated. What could a psychiatrist say to the happy slave? What could he say to an alienated Sisyphus as he pushes the boulder up the mountain? That he would push the boulder more enthusiastically, more creatively, more insightfully, if he were on Prozac?

Already I can hear the protests. Do you want to deny Prozac to Sisyphus? Who are you to criticize him for taking it? Very well then. Perhaps I spoke hastily. My purpose was not to level any moral criticism. Sisyphus may well be happier on an antidepressant. His psychic well-being will probably be improved. Certainly he is entitled to the drug, if his managed care organization will pay for it. I only wish to point out that his predicament is not simply a matter of his internal psychic well-being. Any strategy that ignores certain larger aspects of his situation is going to sound a little hollow.

Of course, taking account of the larger situation is not as simple as I make it sound. Neither pills nor psychotherapy can fix metaphysics. In his essay 'Truth to Truth' Leszek Kolakowski writes about his idea for a spiritual 'conversion agency' that would offer religious and ideological transformations for a fee. The most difficult conversions are the most expensive – say, to fundamentalist Islam or Albanian Communism. Lower fees are charged for less demanding, more comfortable belief systems, like Anglicanism or reform Judaism. The agency itself, however, needs to remain strictly neutral in order to preserve the autonomy of patients. 'Psychologists and other experts of indoctrination shall then be entrusted with the actual work, which will in no way violate the freedom of the individual. The agency itself must remain strictly neutral religiously and ideologically; it could be named Veritas, 'Truth', or Certitudo, 'Certitude' (perhaps, 'Happy Certitude.')'[9]

Kolakowski's satire points out the dilemma psychiatry has with these larger questions. Of course it makes sense to think that psychiatry should remain neutral on matters of religion and ideology. Show me a psychiatrist who sees the verities of Baptist theology as the solution to all his patients' problems and I will show you a case of psychiatric malpractice. What Kolakowski is poking fun at, though, is the notion that spiritual affairs are matters on which it is *possible* to take a truly neutral stance. Here, a neutral stance is itself an ideological stance. Any pose of strict neutrality is a masquerade. To view a change of religious frameworks as a potential means of therapy (for, say, Sisyphus) is itself a kind of ideology. In fact, it may well be an ideology that is peculiar to the postmodern condition, a stance not unlike an academic class on comparative religion. It is the stance that Stanley Hauerwas is gesturing toward when he says: 'The story of post-modernity is the story we told ourselves when we had no story.'[10] This ideology, the therapeutic world view, sees every human predicament as a problem to be fixed. (And if you disagree, that is probably because you are depressed.)

Kolakowski's conversion agency is also a satire of individualism, the myth of the self-contained, self-determining individual. Conversions like these would be impossible. A conversion could (in theory if not in actuality) bring about a change of belief, and even a change in values – but our moral horizons are much broader than this. One cannot simply escape culture and history. One cannot simply create or discard the frameworks of meaning by which a life is judged meaningful, or failed, or wasted. One cannot fix everything just by changing one's own individual outlook.

I suspect that part of the worry many people have about Prozac has less to do with the drug itself than with the enthusiasm with which Americans in particular have embraced it. Why we have embraced it (apart from the merits of the drug itself, which are not at all inconsiderable) is a matter for speculation: a multibillion dollar pharmaceutical industry, a native enthusiasm for technology, an ethic of competitive individualism, a constitutional right to the pursuit of happiness. Yet along with that enthusiasm is the suspicion that psychopharmacology alone cannot account for the predicament in which we find ourselves; that this predicament is not something that can be cured, as Wittgenstein says, with a medicine invented by an individual, but rather by a change in our manner of living. And not by my own personal manner of living, or at least not solely, but by the way we all live now, together: by what Wittgenstein might call our form of life.

Of course, it may be that antidepressants will often cure depression without touching alienation, leaving a person alienated but not depressed. Whether this would be a good state to be in or not will depend on how you see our collective situation – whether, as Percy would say, you think we are in a predicament. Yet as long as we fail to take any account of these broader frameworks of significance, we cannot take account of alienation from them. Unless we think about meaning, we cannot take the measure of meaninglessness; unless we think about home, we cannot take the measure of homelessness; unless we recognize the fact of the journey, we cannot take account of the person who is lost. If, in Clifford Geertz's famous paraphrase of Weber, we are suspended in webs of significance that we ourselves have spun, then it is only by looking closely at how we are situated in those webs that we can see how we may be trapped there, or falling, or gazing contentedly at the ceiling.

References

1   **M. O'Hara** and **W. T. Anderson**, 'Psychotherapy's Own Identity Crisis,' in *The Fontana Postmodernism Reader*, ed. Walter Truett Anderson (London: Fontana Press, 1996), pp. 166–67.

2   **A. de Tocqueville**, *Democracy in America*, tr. George Lawrence, ed. J. P. Mayer (New York: Harper and Row, 1988 [1848, 12th edition]), p. 536.

3   **L. Wittgenstein**, *Remarks on the Foundations of Mathematics*, ed. G. E. Anscombe (Oxford: Basil Blackwell, 1956), p. 57.

4   **C. West**, *Race Matters* (Boston: Beacon Press, 1993), p. 15.

5   **W. Percy**, *The Last Gentleman* (London: Panther Books, 1985 [1966]), p. 12.

6   **R. Ford**, *Independence Day* (New York: Vintage Books, 1995), p. 57.

7   **W. Percy**, *Love in the Ruins* (New York: Ivy Books, 1971), pp. 12–13.

8   **W. Percy**, *Signposts in a Strange Land*, ed. P. Samway (New York: Farrar, Straus and Giroux, 1991),p. 258.

9   **L. Kolakowski**, *Modernity on Endless Trial* (Chicago: University of Chicago Press, 1985).

10 **S. Hauerwas**, 'Sinsick,' plenary address to the annual meeting of American Society of Bioethics and Humanities, Houston, Texas, November 1998. I am quoting this from memory, which may be unreliable.

Ethical Aspects of Research and Practice of ECT*

Jan-Otto Ottosson

The postwar period has witnessed an escalated interest in the ethical foundations of medical practice and research. One major reason is the reaction in the whole civilized and democratic world against the Nazi outrage on Jews, above all in the Holocaust, but also in experiments by Nazi doctors on Jewish concentration camp prisoners, which defied every code of ethics.

Another important source of the increased devotion to medical ethics was the revelation that dissidents in the former Soviet Union were regarded as mentally ill and treated by compulsion. To the very last, the free world hesitated to accept these facts, but as time went by, the evidence became compelling.

Codes of Ethics

When the violations of human rights and dignity in Germany were disclosed at the Nuremberg trial, it filled the whole world with loathing. To prevent the recurrence of such abominable behavior, the *Nuremberg Code* was accepted in 1947. This became a forerunner of the *Helsinki Declaration* (1964, revised in Tokyo, 1975, and in Venice, 1983), which now lays down principles of experimental research on human beings.

The victimization of dissidents in the former Soviet Union was the major background of the *Hawaii Declaration* in 1977 (formal revision in 1983), the code of ethics of psychiatry. It maintains: 'The psychiatrist must never use his professional possibilities to violate the dignity or human rights of any individual or group. The psychiatrist must on no account utilize the tools of his profession, once the absence of psychiatric illness has been established.'

The *Helsinki Declaration* and the *Hawaii Declaration* are far from the only codes of ethics in medicine. The first one was the *Hippocratic Oath*, from as early as 400 BC, which is famous for its statements about benefit, harm, and justice:

I will apply dietetic measures for the benefit of the sick according to my ability and judgement; I will keep them from harm and injustice. Whatever houses I may visit, I will come for the benefit of the sick, remaining free of all intentional injustice, of all mischief and in particular of sexual relations with both female and male persons, be they free or slaves.

The *Hippocratic Oath* also has important affirmations of confidentiality, which, however, are of no special significance for ECT.

The *Hippocratic Oath* was translated into Arabic and Latin and was sworn at the European medical schools by doctors who had finished their studies of medicine and were about to enter medical practice. The *Hippocratic Oath* has had a great impact on all later codes of ethics up to the present time. In the Hippocratic spirit, the *Principles of Medical Ethics* of the American Medical Association from 1847 states:

'The principal objective of the medical profession is to render service to humanity with full respect for the dignity of man.'

The Unique Position of Psychiatry

As a medical speciality, psychiatry may to some extent rely on such common codes as the principles of the American Medical Association and analogous codes in other countries. However, some problems are more or less unique to psychiatric practice and research and therefore deserve special attention. In particular, we as psychiatrists, more often than our colleagues, have to face the following problems (Merskey, 1991):

1. Psychiatry has been entrusted with the task and responsibility of assessing whether patients can decide rationally for themselves and, if this is not the case, of making a judgment whether to deprive patients of their liberty. It is also the task of psychiatrists to administer compulsory care.

2. More than other physicians, psychiatrists have to strike a balance between the interests of the patient on the one hand and of the persons closely related and the society on the other. On both sides of the Atlantic, psychiatry has expanded, not only accepting those brought to it, but also seeking ways to help everyone in the society. The deinstitutionalization and the establishment of community mental health centers have contributed to the difficulties of defining the proper role of psychiatrists.

3. Psychiatrists have to face greater diagnostic difficulties than do other physicians. Even if the diagnostic systems such as the *ICD–10* (World Health Organization, 1992) and the *DSM–IV* (American Psychiatric Association, 1994a,b) have improved the criteria of mental disorder and facilitated the establishment of diagnoses, subjectivity is still more or less inherent in the diagnostic process.

These distinctive features give cause for special psychiatric codes. The United States was in fact ahead of the *Hawaii Declaration* with the *Principles of Medical Ethics with Annotations Especially Applicable to Psychiatry*, adopted by the American Psychiatric Association in 1973 (American Psychiatric Association, 1981). As pointed out by Musto (1991), there is an interesting difference between the *Hawaii Declaration* and the American Psychiatric Association principles. The American principles do not advocate an essentially egalitarian relationship between therapist and patient; their emphasis is rather on the need for the psychiatrist to merit and maintain the trust of patient, demonstrating the direct descent from the Hippocratic tenets. This is different from the *Hawaii Declaration*, which emphasizes an antipaternalistic stance of psychiatry (e.g., by calling for disclosure of diagnosis and discussion of alternative therapies with the patient, requiring that detained patients have an avenue of appeal, and calling for the seeking of the patients' consent to any treatment, with third-party consent in cases of patients' incompetence). By their different wordings, these two psychiatric codes of ethics reflect what is really a major ethical concern in the use of ECT.

Whereas Hippocrates was paternalistic – obviously for the good reason that his knowledge was unprecedented at the time – the modern physician has to strike a balance between contractual equality, which is natural in western

* Ottosson, J.-O.: Ethical aspects of research and practice of ECT. *Convulsive Therapy* 11:288–299, 1995.

democracies, and benevolent paternalism, which is sometimes necessary in psychiatric practice. This applies especially to psychiatrists, whose patients in some stages of their illnesses often need substitutes for good parents.

Principles of Ethics

As a common denominator of the codes of ethics, four basic principles of medical ethics have been extracted (Beauchamp and Childress, 1994): (a) beneficence, (b) nonmaleficence, (c) justice, and (d) respect for autonomy. How can these principles be applied to ECT?

Beneficence and Nonmaleficence

Beneficence and nonmaleficence are two sides of the same coin. No treatment in medicine does only good and has no side effects or risk of complications. In that respect, ECT has a very favorable risk–benefit ratio. In severe depressive disorders, it is superior to drug therapy, different modes of psychotherapy (cognitive, interpersonal), and sham ECT. In acute lethal catatonia, ECT may be lifesaving. The absence of brain damage has been convincingly shown with computed tomography (Bergsholm et al., 1989) and magnetic resonance imaging (Coffey et al., 1991). When given according to the modem standard, ECT involves only a very small risk of long-term memory impairment, which for the great majority of people, is of minimum importance compared with the suffering and hazards of depression (Merskey, 1991). In contrast, antidepressant drugs have many side effects, especially when combined with neuroleptic drugs, which have been claimed to be an alternative for ECT (Spiker et al., 1985). Still, the drug combination does not give as fast and reliable response as does ECT. In fact, few other treatments in clinical medicine are equally well examined for efficacy and safety.

Justice

Justice means equal treatment for equal cases. Mental disorders of the same kind and severity should receive the same treatment regardless of the patient's residential locality, social status, and economic capacity. Regretfully, we are far from justice as far as ECT is concerned. In the United States, ECT is more often offered in private than in public mental health care facilities (Leong and Eth, 1991). In Germany, ECT is given more often in university departments of psychiatry than in nonuniversity departments and mental hospitals. Among the heads of the German psychiatric departments, 20% have expressed fear that the use of ECT would be negative for the reputation of the department (Lauter and Sauer, 1987). In Sweden, there is a great variation in the use of ECT in different counties, the county with the highest number giving 8 times as many treatments as that with the lowest number (Socialstyrelsen, 1994). There is also an enormous variation between countries. The European continent is sparing in the use of ECT, whereas the Scandinavian countries, the United Kingdom, and Ireland have a well-established ECT tradition. In most countries, a discrepancy is common between a more positive attitude among specialists in psychiatry and a more negative attitude among patients, their relatives, general opinion, mass media, and in some cases, the legal profession. In some countries, lack of adequate training in how to administer ECT has been a limiting factor in an otherwise positive climate of opinion. For example, in England 90% of ECT treatments were given by young, less experienced doctors. Among these, 50% had received minimal instructions on the use of ECT by someone usually not more experienced, who had shown them how to press the button (Pippard and Ellam, 1981). On the whole, longer professional experience and higher level of knowledge is associated with a positive attitude to ECT (Janicak et al., 1985).

Insistence on a more rational use of ECT is not missing. In California, more than half of the psychiatrists considered that the legislation should be changed (Kramer, 1986). In Holland, a more need-adapted use of ECT has been called for (Koster, 1992).

A not unimportant factor in promoting the rational use of ECT is acceptance of ECT by the psychiatrist himself, should he have a melancholic syndrome not responding to antidepressant drugs. In a recent Swedish survey, 78% would accept ECT without hesitation, another 14% would accept with some hesitation, and only 4% would reject the option.

Respect for Autonomy

Respect for autonomy has a high priority in democratic countries. If patients can decide rationally for themselves, treatments cannot be forced on them if they, for one reason or another, do not wish to have them. If the doctor is convinced that a particular treatment (e.g., ECT) would be helpful, he should try to convince the patient, but if he does not succeed, he must respect even what he considers unwise decisions of the patients. He should offer alternative treatments, even if he considers them second best. However, respect for autonomy implies only that the patient may refuse an offered treatment, not a right to insist on a treatment that the doctor considers inappropriate according to science and experience.

At the same time, as patients who can decide rationally for themselves have a right to abstain from ECT, patients who cannot decide rationally should have a right to obtain the appropriate treatment, be it ECT or any other treatment. In such cases, doctors should act in the patients' best interests. An inability to decide rationally is obvious in delirious states (e.g., postpartum psychoses, acute lethal catatonia, and several cases of delusional depression). Refraining from using ECT in such cases, given its established superiority, would be negligent from an ethical point of view. I am not aware of a case in which legal authorities have declared negligence for not giving ECT. The day it happens will deserve an editorial in Convulsive Therapy and other psychiatric journals as well, marking the recognition of society that ECT is an indispensable part of psychiatric care.

Capacity to decide rationally for oneself is not a black-and-white issue but is often difficult to assess, especially in patients with deep depression, the major indication for ECT. As the prospects of having a favorable response to ECT increase with the severity of the depressive disorder, the difficulties also increase in getting consent from the patient and in knowing whether the consent is based on real understanding of the given information. What the doctor describes as a salubrious procedure may be perceived by the patient as putting his suffering to an end by killing him or as punishment for unforgivable sins.

Such a delusional interpretation of the real world is usually incompatible with the capacity to give informed consent. Still, as ECT is superior to other treatment modalities in such cases, the patient should be given ECT. Because jurisdiction varies among countries, the administration of ECT may require court decision, approval by a relative, commitment for compulsory psychiatric care, or more than one of these. In my country, doctors should inform relatives of patients who are not capable of making their own decisions but are alone responsible for treatment decisions. Patients or relatives may appeal against detention but not against treatment decisions. On the whole, compulsory ECT seems to be uncommon. A recent survey of Swedish ECT practice showed that treatments were given on a voluntary basis in 93%, the remaining treatment series being either compulsory throughout or compulsory from the start and voluntary as the patients began to improve (Socialstyrelsen, 1994).

A deluded state must not necessarily mean incapacity to give informed consent. I think you all recognize delusional patients who have some kind of double orientation. Instead of saying 'yes doctor,' or 'please, do whatever you find best,' we may only get a look of agreement or a silent nod on our suggestion of ECT. Sometimes we get no response at all, but the patient makes no resistance when being prepared for ECT. The degree of interference with the capacity to give informed consent is best established in a close therapeutic relationship. Gratefulness after recovery that we took more notice of the glimpses of insight than of the delusional thinking may be seen as a justification of this kind of consent. Where jurisdiction in a country does not give psychiatrists the confidence to decide, we face the difficult task of finding procedures that assess capacity to consent or refuse and that disturb the delicate doctor–patient relationship and delay effective treatment as little as possible (Martin and Bean, 1992; Martin, 1993).

There are problematic borderline cases in which the patient is ill enough for ECT to be justified but not ill enough to be incapable beyond doubt of giving informed consent. Because we cannot at the same time act in accordance with the principles of beneficence and autonomy, we have to decide which principle should have priority. In such cases, I think most of us try to give precedence to autonomy as far as possible and give drug treatment and spontaneous remission a serious chance. However, suicide may not be far away in depressive disorders and, to parody an old film title, we must not let the 'patients die with their rights on.' It requires a good deal of courage to stand up for one's beliefs against the hesitation or resistance of the patient, his relatives, and maybe even the ward personnel. After all, the psychiatrist shall serve the best interests of the patients, not those of relatives or staff.

An antiemotional attitude toward ECT in the population and in mental health care, in which ECT is regarded as part of modem psychiatric treatment options, as are drugs and psychotherapy, may promote successful trials with ECT when other treatments have failed. Responsible journalism also may be helpful, as horror-filled stories are destructive for patients' confidence in the treatment.

Whereas public insight into mental health care and the use of various treatments is a matter of course in a democratic society, it may be argued that political interference with the rational use of a specific treatment is a form of political abuse of psychiatry, not dissimilar to the political abuse of psychiatry in the former Soviet Union.

Paternalism

Should we assume a paternalistic or egalitarian attitude toward the patient? I believe we must admit that quite a few doctor–patient relationships are characterized by inequality in status, at least when more severe somatic diseases or mental disorders are concerned. Because of anxiety about the prognosis, economic hardship, and uncertainty about the future, many patients are in a disadvantaged position. They have a tendency to regress and to not behave in such a mature and responsible way as they usually do. They want to leave the decision about appropriate treatment to doctors in whom they have confidence. Any doctor who has been a patient himself knows that we may not be so interested in details of the disease or percentages of successful outcome with various treatment modalities but rather assume an attitude of trust in our doctors. We transfer the decision making to the doctors, who then function as good parents do for their children.

A paternalistic attitude should not be mistaken for an authoritarian one. To me, authoritarianism reflects lust for power and disrespect for patient autonomy and integrity, whereas paternalism means acting as good parents as long as – and only as long as – the patients cannot decide for themselves.

Ethical Aspects of ECT Research

The controlled experiment is acknowledged as the only reliable way to obtain knowledge of efficacy and safety of new methods of treatment or modifications of old methods. Only by the controlled experiment can the six unities of medical research be fulfilled: the unities of time, room, patients, procedure, attitude, and personnel (Albritton, 1956). The prevalent experimental design consists of random allocation to an experimental group and a control group, in which the control group can be either an established treatment or some kind of placebo procedure. In combination with blind assessment to avoid patient and rater bias, this design permits conclusions as to the relative merits and demerits of the new method compared with the control procedure.

These scientific demands have to be combined with the principles of ethics for medical research laid down in the *Helsinki Declaration:* 'In any medical study, every patient – including those of a control group, if any – should be assured of the best proven diagnostic and therapeutic method.'

In searching for improved modifications of ECT, the control group must get the treatment that is considered the gold standard, and there must be good reasons that the modification to be assessed has potential benefits compared with the standard procedure.

This means that it would nowadays be inconsistent with the code of ethics to study ECT modifications in which the seizure activity is restrained in one way or the other, because for all we know, self-sustained seizure activity is essential for the antidepressant effect of ECT. On the other hand, because they might have potential benefits, experiments with the prolongation of the seizure or aiming at localizing the relevant seizure activity would be consistent with the ethical demands.

It also follows from the code of ethics that experiments in which the electrical energy is increased beyond what is needed to evoke a generalized grand mal seizure would be inconsistent, because they would increase the hazards and discomfort in the form of confusion and memory disturbance. On the other hand, examination of new electrode positions (avoiding, e.g., projection over the temporal lobe) may have promise of decreasing the memory disturbance and would be perfectly ethical. The same applies to the examination of new types of current that can elicit generalized seizures with a reduced amount of electric energy. Neither would there be objections against experiments in which increased stimulus intensity aims to reach the threshold for a grand mal generalized seizure.

Looking back on my own experiments in the 1960s, in which aborted seizures and considerably suprathreshold seizures were compared with the standard procedure, they would hardly be ethically defensible today; it is hoped they once were (Ottosson, 1960, 1962). The same applies to the group of experiments in the United Kingdom, in which ECT was compared with sham-ECT. They have given us the final evidence that ECT is much more than a placebo, but they need no repetition (Freeman *et al.*, 1978; Johnstone *et al.*, 1980; West, 1981; Brandon *et al.*, 1984; Gregory *et al.*, 1985).

It goes without saying that experiments to elucidate neurochemical mechanisms of actions do not violate standard of ethics as long as they adhere to the *Helsinki Declaration* in other respects.

Informed consent is as relevant in research as in clinical practice. It is sometimes maintained that patients in compulsory care should not be enrolled in clinical experiments because they may consent under duress. It is also maintained that psychotic patients should be excluded from clinical trials because they may not understand to what they consent. Because being committed and being psychotic often coincide, there may be double reasons to exclude these patients from experiments.

From the point of view of expanding knowledge, it would be deplorable if patients with the most severe illnesses and in most need of effective treatment were not accessible to medical research. Fortunately, the *Helsinki Declaration* has taken a permissive position. For committed patients, it is recommended that the informed consent be obtained by a doctor who is neither engaged in the investigation nor involved in decisions on commitment. If mental incapacity makes it impossible to obtain informed permission, consent from the responsible relative replaces that of the subject in accordance with national legislation. In these ways, clinical research in these groups of patients may be compatible with ethical demands.

Another kind of obstacle against clinical research is erected by journalist's claiming to guard human rights but having antipsychiatric or even antiscientific purposes. By warning readers against taking part in clinical research and being used as 'human guinea-pigs,' they convey the impression that research workers take an interest only in their own scientific careers. Such irresponsible journalism is a serious impediment to recruiting patients for clinical research and can be counteracted only with information about the real aims and high ethical standard.

Concluding Words

We may go back to the Hippocratic Oath once more: 'If I fulfil this oath and do not violate it, may it be granted to me to enjoy life and art, being honored with fame among all men for all time to come.'

To be honored with fame only rarely occurs with those who advocate the proper use of ECT. However, the patients' gratitude and our own conviction of having done a good job as psychiatrists may be a sufficient reward. Taking an ethical view of ECT would seem to promote a favorable attitude toward the treatment rather than reducing confidence and acceptance. It may help people to realize the concept of risk–benefit and that the risk–benefit ratio is extremely favorable for ECT. It may also help people to object to the injustice of not having access to ECT for patients who would profit from it and to realize that the reasons for this state of affairs are not grounded in fact. An ethical analysis of ECT may also help doctors to decide when the doctor–patient relationship should be egalitarian and when a paternalistic attitude is appropriate and defensible.

Although we are sometimes attacked for being unethical by practicing ECT and doing research in ECT, we have good reasons to reply that it is unethical not to give ECT in some kinds of mental illness, and it is unethical not to do research in ECT. After all, as psychiatrists, we have an overriding ethical commitment to relieve suffering in our patients and to advance the scientific basis of our discipline.

References

Albritton EC. The six unities in medical research. *JAMA* 1956; **161**:328–33.

American Psychiatic Association. *Diagnostic and Statistical manual of mental disorders*. 4th ed. Washington, DC: American Psychiatric Press, 1994.

American Psychiatric Association. *The principles of medical ethics*. Washington, DC: American Psychiatric Press. 1981.

Beauchamp TL, Childress JF. *Principals of biomedical ethics*. 4th ed. Oxford: Oxford University Press, 1994.

Bergsholm P, Larsen JL, Rosendahl K, Holsten F. Electroconvulsive therapy, and cerebral computed tomography. A prospective study. *Acta Psychiatr Scand* 1989; **80**:566–72.

Brandon S, Cowley P, McDonald C, Neville P, Palmer R, Wellstood-Eason S. Electroconvulsive therapy results in depressive illness from the Leicestershire trial. *Br Med J* 1984; **288**:22–5.

Coffey CE, Weiner RD, Djang WT, Figiel GS, Soady SA, Patterson LJ, Holt PD, Spritzer CE, Wilkinson WE. Brain anatomic effects of electroconvulsive therapy. A prospective magnetic resonance imaging study. *Arch Gen Psychiatry* 1991; **48**:1013–21.

Freeman CPL, Basson JV, Crighton A. Double-blind controlled trial of electroconvulsive therapy (E.C.T.) and simulated E.C.T. in depressive illness. *Lancet* 1978; **i**:738–40.

Gregory S, Shawcross CR, Gill D. The Nottingham ECT study: a double-blind comparison of bilateral and simulated ECT in depressive illness. *Br J Psychiatry* 1985; **146**:520–4.

Janicak PC, Mask J, Trimakas KA, Gibbons R. ECT: an assessment of mental health professionals' knowledge and attitudes. *J Clin Psychiatry* 1985; **46**:262–6.

Johnstone EC, Deakin JFW, Lawler P, Frith CD, Stevens M, McPherson K. The Northwick Park electroconvulsive therapy trial. *Lancet* 1980; **i**: 1317–20.

Koster AM. *Views on ECT: a comparison between evaluations of patients, family members and physicians concerning electroconvulsive therapy*. Amsterdam: Thesis Publishers, 1992 (in Dutch). Reviewed by Dhossche D. *Convulsive Ther* 1993; **9**:66–8.

Kramer BA. Practice patterns of electroconvulsive therapy: a Californian perspective (1984). *Convulsive Ther* 1986;**2**:239–44.

Lauter H, Sauer H. Electroconvulsive therapy: a German perspective. *Convulsive Ther* 1987; **3**:204–9.

Leong GB, Eth S. Legal and ethical issues in electroconvulsive therapy. *Psychiatr Clin North Am* 1991; **14**:1007–16.

Martin BA. Ethics and consent. *Convulsive Ther* 1993; **9**:131–3.

Martin BA, Bean GJ. Competence to consent to electroconvulsive therapy. *Convulsive Ther* 1992; **8**:92–102.

Merskey H. Ethical aspects of the physical manipulation of the brain. In: Bloch S, Chodoff P, eds. *Psychiatric ethics*, 2nd ed. Oxford: Oxford University Press, 1991:185–214.

Musto D. A historical perspective. In: Bloch S, Chodoff P, eds. *Psychiatric ethics*. 2nd ed. Oxford: Oxford University Press. 1991:15–32.

Ottosson J-O, ed. Experimental studies of the mode of action of electroconvulsive therapy. *Acta Psychiatr Neurol Scand* 1960; 35(suppl): **145**:1–141.

Ottosson J-O. Seizure characteristics and therapeutic efficiency in electroconvulsive therapy: an analysis of the antidepressive efficiency of grand mal and lidocaine-modified seizures. *J Nerv Ment Disease* 1962; **135**: 239–51.

Pippard X, Ellam L. Electroconvulsive therapy in Great Britain. *Br J Psychiatry* 1981; **139**:563–8.

Socialstyrelsen. ECT – en behandlingsmetod i den psykiatriska vården. *Socialstyrelsen följer upp och utvärderar*. Stockholm: Socialstyrelsen 1994; **5**:1–70 (in Swedish).

Spiker DG, Weiss JC, Dealy RS, Griffin SJ, Hanin I, Neil JF, Perel JM, Rossi AJ, Soloff PH. The pharmacological treatment of delusional depression. *Am J Psychiatry* 1985; **142**:430–6.

West ED. Electric convulsion therapy in depression: a double-blind controlled trial. *Br Med J* 1981; **282**:355–7.

World Health Organization. The ICD-10 classification of mental and behavioral disorders. *Clinical descriptions and diagnostic guidelines*. Geneva: World Health Organization, 1992.

Values in Psychotherapy*

Jeremy Holmes

To state that values are important in psychotherapy can be highly provocative or entirely uncontentious. Freud, an implacable critic of religion, saw himself as a scientist, offering 'a method not a doctrine,' in search, as Rieff[1] put it, of 'truth but not "The Truth".' In this view, science and values are separate, mutually incompatible, approaches to the world. Science is descriptive and depends on verification, while ethics is prescriptive and is based on justification. But in practice, as we shall see, this neat distinction is far from the everyday realities of either science or ethics, especially as applied to psychotherapy.

Whatever their views on the scientific basis of their discipline, most psychotherapists would sharply differentiate their tasks from those of priests or politicians or other overt purveyors of values within society. Recently, however, there has been a call,[2] by no means universally accepted,[3] to recognize that therapists' personal value systems significantly influence practice[4,5] and that it might be better explicitly to acknowledge this rather than to sweep it underground.[6] It also seems absorbable to accept that therapeutic effectiveness depends on a degree of congruence between the patient's values and those of the therapist.[7]

Less contentiously, it is clear that psychotherapists, like other professionals, operate within an ethical framework comprising a set of socially prescribed values such as respect for individuals, avoidance of doing harm, alleviation of suffering, adherence to the law, and so on. It is also apparent that, at times, psychotherapists are called upon to make distinct moral choices, as, for example, when confronted with a potentially violent patient, they have to choose between preserving confidentiality and the need to protect society at large.[8]

In contrast to Freud's view of psychoanalysis as a value-free scientific activity, there are those who argue that psychoanalysis is an inherently moral discipline, albeit one of a rather unusual type. Writing about Freud, Rieff states that: 'he is not only the first completely irreligious moralist, he is a moralist without even a moralizing message.'[1] Symington finds that 'psychoanalysis is a mature natural religion.'[9] At a practical level, Lomas[10] and Smail,[11] among others, argue that what matters in psychotherapy is not 'technique,' which they see as the shibboleth of a narrow materialist culture, but the personal qualities of the therapist: her capacity for love and honesty.'

This polarization between those who view psychotherapy as a science and those who claim that it is a type of secular religion[12] needs to be qualified by recent developments within the philosophy of science and applied ethics. First, science itself, and in particular 'human science,' is never entirely value-free, in the sense that it is inevitably influenced by the prevailing mores and concerns of society.[13] To take a familiar example, Darwin's theory of evolution emerged in part from the Malthusian notion of the 'the survival of the fittest.' Second, moral viewpoints need to be supported by rational discourse to which the scientific methods of observation, classification, experimentation, and refutation can make a vital contribution. Third, a comparable practical discipline such as medicine, which looms over ethical discussion in psychotherapy as both exemplar and point of differentiation, is both science based and permeated with questions of value and ethics, many of which have psychotherapeutic reverberations – over euthanasia, abortion, the just distribution of scarce medical resources, and whether 'lifestyle' should influence eligibility for costly treatments such as transplant surgery, to take familiar examples.

The purpose of this article is to explore further some of these themes, to try to tease out some of the distinctive values embodied in psychoanalysis and psychotherapy, and to consider their relevance to psychotherapeutic practice. Due to limitations of space, these remarks are confined mainly to psychoanalysis and its psychotherapeutic derivatives.

Values and Psychoanalysis

Psychoanalytic approaches to values and ethics have gone through three distinct stages, starting with Freud's initial espousal of science and disparagement of religion. In the second phase, it became clear that not only does psychoanalysis embody a system of values but that it has important things to say about the origins of the sense of good and bad, about reparation, forgiveness, and moral maturation. Third, there have recently been attempts to link psychoanalysis with more transcendental themes of fate, beauty, chance and 'nothingness.' These stages correspond roughly with those of classicism, modernism, and post-modernism, and can likewise be mapped onto Kant's three areas of human understanding: science, ethics, and aesthetics.[13]

Psychoanalysis as an Ethical System

Phillip Rieff's[1] classic, *The Mind of the Moralist*, remains a key text in the rehabilitation of values within psychoanalysis. Rieff attempted to 'back-translate' what he saw as Freud's conversion of moral discourse into the language of science: 'Psychoanalysis is the triumph in ethical form of the modern scientific idea.' Just as nature is deceptive, its trompes-l'oeil requiring the subtlety of the scientist to yield up their secrets, so too is our inner world, requiring the probes of the psychoanalyst to reveal what is latent within our moral (and immoral) nature.

For Rieff, the 'scientific' language of psychoanalysis is a metaphor that enabled Freud to put across his moral message in a secular age. The values of truth and honesty, and their verbal expression, are central to Freud's thought. His mission was to find a language with which to describe inner experience. He believed that the power of neurosis could, like Rumpelstiltskin's, be broken if only the right words could be found to describe it:

What for Freud is "repression," psychologically understood, is "secrecy," morally understood . . . sickness may be viewed as an ingrown gesture . . . the way a patient speaks even when he is mute (p. 19).

Rieff sees psychoanalysis as an expression of the enlightenment values of autonomy and democracy as manifest within the individual psyche. Analysis leads to an enfranchisement of the unconscious, limiting the powers of the autocratic superego and educating the ego in self-government. However, as Rieff and many others have pointed out, Freud's liberalism was as conservative as it was revolutionary. He aimed to rid us of our illusions

* Holmes, J.: Values in psychotherapy. *American Journal of Psychotherapy* 50:259–273, 1996.

about the perfectibility of man: 'Men must live with the knowledge that their dreams are by function optimistic and cannot be fulfilled . . . every cure must expose him to new illness.' Rieff comments wryly on Freud's famous prescription for 'transforming . . . hysterical misery into common unhappiness'; 'It is a curious sort of promise to have attracted so many followers.'

Rieff links Freud's paradoxical ethical stance of optimistic pessimism, or active passivity (which also have their clinical resonances) with the philosophy of the Stoics and Epictetus, and Eastern religion: 'there is something Oriental in the Freudian ethic,' the aim of psychoanalytic spiritual guidance being to wean away the ego from both heroic and compliant attitudes towards the surrounding community.

Psychoanalysis as a Profession

Freud was ambivalent about the status of psychoanalysis as a discipline. He bracketed it with government and education as 'impossible professions,' 'because one can be sure beforehand of achieving unsatisfying results.'[14] Thus, he half acknowledges that psychoanalysis cannot be understood as a purely technical discipline, but depends on a sound therapeutic alliance and on the will of the analysand if it is to succeed. If we compare psychoanalysis or psychotherapy with other liberal professions, such as the law or medicine, four obvious differences stand out.

First, moral difficulties in psychotherapy arise from the fact that it is not just a treatment for psychological sickness, but that it also aims to be a prophylactic, strengthening the character against further illness. This is not just an idle claim: in the NIMH treatment of depression trial, psychotherapeutic treatments were, compared with antidepressants, on the whole *less* effective in relieving symptoms, but more useful at maintaining patients well following a period of treatment.[15]

Second, relief of symptoms – depression, anxiety, obsessionality – is much easier to define than it is to decide what constitutes 'good health,' especially good psychological health.

Third, the normal contrast between moral framework and technical content does not hold fast in psychotherapy in the same way as it does in other professions. Much of the technical content of psychotherapy is directly concerned with moral difficulties: Rieff again: 'all the issues which psychoanalysis treats – health and sickness of the will, the emotions, the responsibilities of private living, the coercions of culture – belong to the moral life.' Whereas, a patient may similarly present to a doctor or lawyer with a moral dilemma, the main business of their transaction is essentially technical – physiological or legal. Indeed, these professionals often recognize this when they recommend to a client that what he/she '*really* needs is to see a psychiatrist.'

This leads to a final problem, the lack of agreed external standards of moral development by which psychotherapists can measure a person's psychological health. Many attempts have been made to define psychological health,[16] all of which are normative in the ethical rather than the statistical sense. Some observers of psychoanalysis argue that it can provide a coherent picture of psychological maturation which has important social implications.[13] Critics, of whom Szasz[17] is perhaps the best known, point to the dangers of 'pathologizing' social transgression, so that psychotherapy provides a spurious scientific legitimization of 'illness' as an exculpation for moral turpitude.

Post-Freudian Ethics

Contemporary psychoanalysis is a pluralistic melting pot containing a number of differing perspectives, of which ego psychology, object relations theory, the interpersonal, self psychology, and Lacanianism are the most significant.[18] Each embodies a distinct ethical perspective. Shaffer[19] traces the development of Freud's thought from 'guilty man' of the Oedipus complex to 'tragic man' of the death instinct. Ego psychology presupposes a relatively benign society to which a healthy person can adapt and aims to free the ego from its conflictual contraints, leading to greater sense of freedom and autonomy.

In object relations theory, as developed by Klein and Bion, the emphasis is on relationships with oneself and others. The movement from the paranoid-schizoid to the depressive position implies a more coherent and integrated self, less dominated by the need to project unwanted feelings into others; the development of concern for the object; and the capacity to experience remorse and reparation. Only in the depressive position is real intimacy possible, both with one's true or authentic self and with the other. Object relations, especially as developed by post-Kleinians, provide a contemporary account of the nature of 'evil,' seen in terms of perverse splitting, in which the object is sequestered and terrorized by unmodulated aggression and envy. Attachment theory,[20–22] which forms the basis of interpersonal psychoanalysis, describes the developmental conditions leading to psychological health, showing how meanings arise out of the sensitivity and attunement (or otherwise) of the parental environment. Thus, as Rycroft[23] puts it, psychoanalysis is a 'biological theory of meaning.'

In the Christian tradition, pride is seen as a sinful obstacle to a good life. The psychological equivalent of pride is narcissism, which implies omnipotence and self-centeredness. Self psychology distinguishes between healthy narcissism – good self-esteem, pride in one's real achievements – and pathological narcissism, a defensive retreat in the face of an unempathic nurturing environment. Finally, Lacanian psychoanalysis is critical of the conformism implicit in ego psychology and the notion of a conflict-free area of the personality. Lacan insists on a 'return to Freud' and to the ineluctable law of the phallus – the 'no(m) du pere' – the word. However, words also contain the possibility of liberation. In the 'symbolic order,' through the expression of feelings in language, relief and maturation are possible.

Psychoanalysis, Aesthetics, and Religion

This brings us to the third phase of psychoanalytic values – the realm of the aesthetic [. . .]. As a science, psychoanalysis tries to uncover the truth about the nature of the psyche and its development. As an ethical system, psychoanalysis is Keatsian: truth is goodness and goodness means an absence of splitting – an acceptance of one's 'bad' parts without the need to deny or project them. The aesthetic dimension emphasizes the search for a form or container within which feelings can be truthfully symbolized and so objectified. This container may be the analytic relationship itself (Bion's 'thinking breast'), art in all its varied forms, or religion.

If psychoanalysis values above all the symbolic expression and containment of inner feelings, this leads to a perspective on religion very different from Freud's original critique. Symington[9] distinguishes between primitive religions whose main function is a social defense against infantile anxieties – which was the main thrust of Freud's attack – and mature religions as expressions of man's highest spiritual leanings and ethical striving. Black[24] similarly sees religions as comprising internal objects enabling the believer to 'speak more truthfully of, and relate more fully to, the larger matrix within which the human world is situated.' Symington's 'God-term'[1] (borrowing Rieff's word) is not the unconscious, but 'the Other.' Basing his approach on the Christian philosopher Macmurray, for whom 'the religious activity of the self is to enter into communion with the Other,' Symington sees psychoanalysis as a secular religion whose aim is to help its followers to find better and more satisfying relationships, not with an external deity, but with the Other.

Psychoanalysis and Post-modernism

The term 'post-modernism' attempts to capture a number of contemporary philosophical, political, and aesthetic perspectives including multiculturalism, feminism, pluralism, contextualism, narrative, and linguistics. Despite tendencies to pretentiousness and obscurity, post-modernism represents a serious attempt to characterize and theorize aspects of the fragmentation and confusion of modern, especially urban, life.

In his exploration of ethics in an era of post-modernism, Rorty[25] draws extensively on Freud:

Beginning in the 17th century, we tried to substitute a love of truth for a love of God, treating the world described by science as a quasi-divinity. Beginning at the end of the 18th century, we tried to substitute a love of ourselves for a love of scientific truth, a worship of our own deep spiritual or poetic nature, treated as one more quasi-divinity . . . [Freud] suggests that we try to get to the point where we no longer worship anything, where we treat nothing as a quasi-divinity, where we treat everything – our language, our conscience, our community – as a product of time and chance. To reach this point would be, in Freud's words, to "treat chance as worthy of determining our fate."

Rorty's heroine, or rather antiheroine, is the 'liberal ironist' who questions all the 'grand narratives' – liberalism, Marxism, science, even psychoanalysis – of the last two centuries, seeing them in relativistic terms, as languages rather than absolute truths, but who nevertheless carries on without relapsing into nihilism and despair. The typical expression of this position would be E. M. Forster's (echoing Butler): 'I disbelieve, Lord help thou my disbelief.' Freud's stoicism, coupled with its constant examination of the unconscious context of conscious thought, might make psychoanalysis a perfect candidate for the Rortyian position. But psychoanalysis as an institution struggles just as much with its transference to Freud and psychoanalysis as any other grand narrative, and certainly falls short of the Whiteheadian criterion: 'A science that fails to forget its founders is doomed.'

For Rorty, contingency and irony are key concepts for contemporary ethical theory. *Contingency* is the term that expresses the chance-based 'dedivinization of the self' which he sees as the essence of post-modernism. Here, he is very close to Freud in his sense of the dethroning of man's narcissism. We *think* we are in control of our destiny, make rational choices, and determine our fate, but in reality we are products of history, not just in the grand narrative Marxist sense, but of our unique developmental history, of the ghosts that inhabited the particular nursery in which we grew up. In the psychoanalytic view, it is not just 'Man' [sic] whose narcissism is dethroned, but each one of us, every man and woman. We have to learn first to love ('divinize') ourselves and our parents, and then to outgrow ('dedivinize') that self-love, a movement described in self psychology as 'optimal disillusionment.' In terms of attachment theory, this movement can be seen as a pathway from attachment and intimacy through detachment and autonomy to what I have characterized as non-attachment[22] (see below).

For Rorty, the self is a 'tissue of contingencies': of the random accidents of history that have made us what we are. This is the 'destiny' which Bollas[26] sees us continuously exploring and symbolizing in our lived lives. We are constantly creating a 'story,' a narrative, of that destiny. We need these stories in order to live, charts that take us through the vagaries of contingency. Psychoanalysis helps us first to be able to symbolize – to 'dream' our lives as Bollas puts it – and then to create more relevant and more subtle narratives.

What remains if all grand narratives are found wanting, if our attachment to any idea – even the idea of rational discourse – is questioned? At a philosophical level we are left with Rorty's *nothingness*. Must we then see Freud as a nihilist? No. Nothingness can be seen as an aspect of what Buddhism calls 'impermenence,' or Freud transience, and can be related to the notion of the death instinct. As an explanatory term, the death instinct may be questionable and even tautologous (to argue that we envy or destroy *because* of the 'death instinct' is to fall into the same trap as Moliere's doctor who states that a hypnotic drug makes us fall asleep *because* of its 'dormitive properties'); but, as an ethical principle, it has much in its favor, if it reminds us to see our passions and to bear our unhappiness from a more detached vantage point.

Psychoanalysis and Activism

Critics of psychoanalysis, of whom Singer[27] is one of the most articulate, have blamed psychoanalysis for its 'inward turn,' its concentration on the self, and turning away from attempts to improve the all-too-obvious inequalities and suffering of the world. Singer argues that in order to lead a more ethical life – one that is based on solidarity with the wider community of humanity – it is necessary to overcome self-centeredness and to 'take the

perspective of the universe.' But Singer takes no account of the unconscious. For him, all that appears to be needed if people are to be persuaded to act less selfishly is to present the rational arguments for humane treatment of animals, for more just distribution of resources, and to demonstrate the emptiness of a life based on consumerism, and so on. He fails to acknowledge that many consciously noble attempts to improve the world have ended in disaster, does not tackle the sense of will-sapping despair inherent in the unhappiness of the 'borderline' character often only temporarily relieved by action, and fails to recognize the need for psychological maturity if selfishness is truly to be overcome and hate and envy replaced by beneficence.

How then do we build community and solidarity out of a position that emphasizes emptiness and transience? For Rorty, a key quality of the liberal ironist is the 'skill at imaginative identification.' He sees the ethical themes for the 21st century as the personal search for autonomy and public avoidance of inflicting pain on others. Rorty sees these private and public spheres as essentially unrelated and is suspicious of attempts to link them through such soft slogans as 'the personal is the political.' But psychoanalysis provides a link between personal freedom and wider concern for the other, based on scientific investigation of the inner world of childhood and emotional disorder in adults. 'Emotional automomy'[8] – the discovery of the 'true self' – arises out of a relational context of 'good enough' mothering in which children discover their spontaneity and begin to build up a picture of the mind of the other. Post-modernism is similarly built around the crucial insight that we inhabit an inescapably *relational* linguistic universe, and that truth 'out there' is inseparable from the language we use to describe it. The Wittgensteinian view that private languages are impossible can be turned round to the idea that we inhabit a world of *others*: Winnicott's much quoted aside: 'There is no such thing as a baby, only a mother and baby together' – suggests not just a baby feeding from a mother, but also a mother and baby *communicating* with one another, albeit in the proto-language of 'babyspeak.'

What is special about psychotherapy as a moral discipline, and what makes it so relevant to the post-modernist world we inhabit, is that, without proselytizing or purveying any of the varieties of 'grand narrative,' but simply through the 'skill at imaginative identification,' therapists are helping patients to inhabit the human community more comfortably, more fully and more spontaneously. They are thus able to attach and detach themselves more authentically and autonomously. Therapists do this on the basis of their own ethical values. These comprise at one level the standard psychotherapeutic ethical principles: reliability, attentiveness, confidentiality, nonintrusiveness, and respectfulness of boundaries. At a deeper level, it requires a *texture* of moral integrity, the capacity for 'spontaneous gesture,' for love and hate and for picking up and letting go that I have tried to encapsulate in the term nonattachment. I am not saying that psychotherapists must become saints or priests or zen masters, but it does mean that psychotherapy should be seen as a discipline that requires moral development on the part of therapists, as well as acquisition of technical skills.

Values and Psychotherapy Research

Psychoanalysis is, of course, only one of many forms of psychotherapy. In the less rarified atmosphere of psychotherapy, a similar movement from a narrowly defined 'scientific' ideology to a concern with values and ethics has also taken place. In 1980, a small bombshell hit the world of empirical psychotherapy research when Bergin[4] published his paper 'Psychotherapy and Religious Values,' in which he argued that despite their reticence about admitting it, psychotherapists generally had a set of firmly held values about the constituents of a good life, which could loosely be called 'religious,' and that the existence of such values was positively correlated with mental health. Bergin's 'coming out' – religion being the 'last taboo,' after sex and death, in psychotherapy – led, he claimed, to an explosion of welcoming letters and requests for reprints and initiated intense research activity in the field of values in psychotherapy.

A number of important findings have emerged from this work. Strongly held religious beliefs are indeed protective against mental illness.[28] Psychotherapy-process researchers have investigated the question of congruence between the values held by patients and therapists which, it might seem, would be likely to be linked to favorable outcomes. In fact, the relationship between congruence and outcome is subtle. Patients do assimilate their therapists' values in the course of therapy – at least as perceived by therapists – but the best outcome arises when values shared between patient and therapist are moderately similar, neither too close nor too divergent.[8] This would be consistent with viewing autonomy as one of the central goals of therapy, since to be autonomous is to discover one's own set of values, based neither on slavish adherence to, nor rebellious rejection (Erikson's 'negative identity') of, authority.

Therapeutic Neutrality

Perhaps, the most contentious aspect of Bergin's broadside is his assault on the hallowed notion of therapeutic neutrality. He argues that this is a myth, that even the most 'non-directive' of therapists have firmly held values and that it is helpful to patients if their therapists are explicit about, for example, their valuation of: freedom, fidelity in intimate relationships, work, the need to be truthful at all times, and espousing 'higher' or spiritual values. Bergin's argument is, however, weakened by his conflation of an ethical *framework* and *technique* and by his failure to distinguish different *levels* of value judgment. Of course, psychotherapists operate within an implicit moral framework. In the context of family therapy, Boszormenyi-Nagy and his co-workers[29] bring socially accepted 'public' values, such as justice and responsibility, to bear on the 'private' inner world of the family – their techniques aim to ensure that justice is done and responsibility taken, as the family confronts its 'tasks' [. . .].

However, an essential component of the technique of psychotherapy is the suspension of judgment and the creation of an atmosphere of acceptance. A balance has to be struck between facilitating a trusting relationship, by letting the patient know that he/she and the therapist share certain values, and the need for reticence if unconscious feelings are to surface in the service of fostering the patient's autonomy. People might, for different reasons, seek out Christian counselling, feminist psychoanalysis or a therapist from the same ethnic minority as themselves. Therapist and patient need to inhabit a similar moral universe and thus to share common 'higher level' moral assumptions. But at the level of specific beliefs – that abortion is always wrong, marriage invariably disadvantageous to women, for example – the therapist's values, if they intrude, may hinder rather than foster progress.

Values and the Triangle of Attachment

It is perhaps best to see psychotherapeutic values as based on higher levels of generality than specific beliefs about, say, fidelity or the existence of a particular type of deity. For Freud, the aims and values of psychoanalysis were summarized as 'lieben und arbeiten' (to love and to work). Bergin's goals are freedom, love, identity, truth, universal values, symptom management, and work. Based on attachment theory, I have argued[22] that there is a 'triangle of attachment' comprising *autonomy, intimacy,* and *non-attachment,* which underlies the technical and ethical principles of the psychotherapies. Each of these is at a sufficiently general level to be uncontroversial and non-prescriptive. Rokeach,[30] who is credited with having devised the most reliable instrument for measuring values, distinguishes between 'terminal' and 'instrumental values' – *what* we are trying to achieve and *how* we try to achieve it. Each item in the attachment triad is both instrumental and terminal, representing both a goal and a means. They are also closely interrelated. A robust sense of autonomy, which includes the notion of taking responsibility for one's feelings and actions, is based on the internalization of intimate relationships – a secure base. True intimacy, as opposed to dependency, requires the sense of a relationship in which the other's autonomy is respected, a state of 'emotional autonomy.' Non-attachment, as opposed to isolation or denial, can be seen as an attempt to synthesize the apparently

contrasting ideals of autonomy and intimacy at a higher level and arises out of the experience of closeness to and respect for and from the Other.

Non-attachment is an ethical ideal, cognitive stance, and technical skill. As an ethical ideal derived from Buddhism, it implies an escape from the tyranny of desire that is perhaps akin to Freud's precept – 'where id was there ego shall be.' As a stage of intellectual development, it evokes the ironic stance of 'reflexive self-function,' in which one is able to see oneself from the outside, and to subject even one's most firmly held beliefs to critical scrutiny. At the level of technique, it is reminiscent of the Rogerian principle of 'non-possessive warmth,' guarding against overinvolvement with patients and their difficulties.

Values in Practice

This article has distinguished between technique, in which neutrality is a central theme, and the therapist's moral framework, in which values are of great importance. In practice, this distinction is not so clear cut. Therapists can be trained to be more honest, open, warm, and non-possessive, which suggests that 'moral' qualities are also matters of technique. An often debated question in psychotherapy circles is whether one can be both an effective therapist and morally reprehensible in one's personal life. History and common sense suggest that this is so, and one of the functions of ethical codes for psychotherapists is to scrutinize the boundary between professional and private life.

Bloch et al.[31] show how therapists approaching a family are inescapably caught up in moral choices and have to maintain a delicate balance between their personal moral framework and those of the family and the wider society. These choices exist on the fringes of practice, a faint drumbeat that draws the therapy in one direction or another, which arise out of the therapeutic context that has been created, but of which therapist and patient may be only dimly aware. For example, therapies with patients who have been traumatized or abused can assume a flavor of righteous anger and blame, in which patients are exclusively seen as passive victims of malevolent perpetrators. Other therapeutic approaches might emphasize the patients' contribution to their own continuing victimhood and stress personal responsibility and the need to leave the past behind. Others might try to help patients move from hatred and blame to understanding and acceptance. Whatever the approach, the ethical themes of suffering, retribution, forgiveness, justice, and responsibility are unavoidable.

For Freud, neurosis was a turning away from reality. But what we call 'reality' is always contestable. Therapists' expertise lies in their familiarity with the idealizations, omnipotence, denigration, cognitive distortions, and so on, that are characteristic of the inner world. Their values are embedded in their particular vision of reality. They are *advocates* of a version of reality on the basis of their *knowledge* of the workings of the mind.

If the unique feature of analytic psychotherapy as a system of expert knowledge is its emphasis on the workings of the unconscious, then therapists must strive to recognize these out-of-awareness moral influences. Values operate mainly at an unconscious level and arise out of developmental experiences that precede rational thought. Consciously held values may be undermined by, or defensive against, forces of envy, hate, and destructiveness that are the very opposite of what is overtly espoused. Therapists should make deliberate efforts to become aware of how their own values affect their work. Was I too encouraging when that patient announced that she intended to leave her husband? Did I side too openly with the adolescent in his rebellion against his rigid, militaristic father? Did I appear morally censorious, enthusiastic, or pruriently curious when this man boasted of his sexual conquests? Was there an edge of aggression in my challenge to this agoraphobic patient's fears? Was I impatient with the suspiciousness and emotional withdrawal of this person suffering from schizophrenia? Was I too enthusiastic in my attempts to rid this person of his obsessional doubts?

These everyday clinical questions may be subsumed under the heading of 'examining the ethical countertransference.' Symington[9] sees the process of self-examination as based on the Socratic principle that one cannot do something vicious and know that one is doing it at the same time, which brings us to what might be the most central psychotherapeutic value of all – the Delphic injunction to 'know yourself.'

This means that moral outcomes in psychotherapy can be quite subtle. For Bergin, marital fidelity is an absolute value to which all therapists should aspire. But the *moral* quality of 'fidelity' is exactly what might be at stake in a therapy. Thus, patients might enter therapy with sexual doubts and difficulties that at that point make them 'incapable' of being unfaithful to their partner. By the end of therapy, though, they might have achieved the sexual confidence and potency to do so, but have decided to opt for fidelity both because their current relationship is now more satisfying, and they chose not to cause pain and unhappiness, seeing that as a greater good than momentary pleasure. The key issue is not so much 'fidelity' in itself, as autonomy and capacity for intimacy, the basis of mature fidelity.

Conclusion

It is difficult, if not impossible, and perhaps even undesirable, to write about values without revealing, implicitly at least, one's own value system, or least some part of it. And yet, at the same time, one should strive for objectivity, subjecting one's own beliefs to the same critical scrutiny one devotes to those of others. In this paper, I have argued that beliefs and values are important in psychotherapy. I have suggested that as a profession, or a would-be profession, psychotherapy shares common values with other professions, typical of liberal democracies. There are also crucial differences. First, because the distinction between ethical framework and technical content of the work in psychotherapy is less clear cut than it is in, say, the law or medicine. Second, because ambiguity – or irony or paradox – is inherent in psychotherapy in that it deals with unconscious as well as conscious ideas and forces. This means that when psychotherapy becomes certain of itself or its values, it ceases to be psychotherapy and becomes something akin to a proselytizing religion. Conversely, the zeitgeist seems to have created uncertainty in the heart of religion itself, at least in its mature forms, so perhaps there is room for rapprochement. To the extent that psychotherapists hold to moral values, and inevitably they do, these should be framed at the highest level of generality so that in practice they will be open to individual interpretation and, where necessary, can be contested. Psychotherapy reflects and transmits the values of the prevailing culture; but also – for example, through its valuation of emotional autonomy, stress on the importance of the inner world, and the self-reflexive posture I have called non-attachment – makes its own unique contribution to cultural and ethical development within our pluralistic societies.

Summary

There is a tension between those who hold that psychotherapy is a scientific discipline and therefore 'value-free,' and those who believe that values are inherent in the nature of psychotherapy. Psychoanalysis has moved from a science-based ideology, through the ethical concerns of Melanie Klein, to a recognition of the 'aesthetic' dimension – the creation of suitable forms that can contain psychological distress. From this latter perspective, the antagonism between religion and psychotherapy, initiated by Freud, becomes less acute. Action-based ethical systems, which ignore the inner world, are critically scrutinized. The evidence suggesting there is a relationship between good outcome in psychotherapy and shared values between therapist and client is reviewed. It is posited that through examination of the 'ethical countertransference,' therapists should become aware of their own value systems and how they influence practice.

References

1   Rieff, P. (1959). *Freud: The mind of the moralist*. Chicago, IL: University of Chicago Press.

2   London, P. (1984). *The modes and morals of psychotherapy*. New York: Norton.

3   Walls, G. (19890). Values and psychotherapy: a comment on "Psychotherapy and religious values." *Journal of Consulting Clinical Psychology*, **48**, 640–641.

4   Bergin, A. (1980). Psychotherapy and religious values. *Journal of Consulting Clinical Psychology*, **48**, 95–105.

5   Bergin, A. (1991). Values and religious issues in psychotherapy and mental health. *American Psychologist*, **46**, 394–403.

6   Aponte, H. (1985). The negotiation of values in therapy. *Family Process*, **24**, 323–338.

7   Kelly, T., & Strupp, H. (1992). Patient and therapist values in psychotherapy. *Journal of Consulting Clinical Psychology*, **60**, 34–40.

8   Holmes, J., & Lindley, R. (1989). *The values of psychotherapy*. Oxford: Oxford University Press.

9   Symington, N. (1994). *Emotion and spirit*. London: Karnac.

10 Lomas, P. (1987). *The limits of interpretation: What's wrong with psychoanalysis*. London: Penguin.

11 Smail, D. (1988). Psychotherapy: deliverance or disablement. In G. & S. Faibairn (Eds.), *Ethical issues in caring*. Avebury: Gower.

12 Gellner, E. (1985). *The psychoanalytic movement*. London: Paladin.

13 Rustin, M. (1991). *The good society and the inner world*. London: Verso.

14 Freud, S. (1937). *Analysis: terminable and interminable*. S.E., Vol. **23**. London: Hogarth.

15 Shea, M., Pilkonis, P., Beckham, E., *et al.* (1992). Personality disorders and treatment outcome in the NIMH Treatment of Depression Collaborative Research Program. *Archives of General Psychiatry*, **49**, 782–787.

16 Valliant, G. (1977). *Adaptation to life*. Boston; Little & Brown.

17 Szasz, T. (1969). *The ethics of psychoanalysis*. New York; Dell.

18 Bateman, A., & Holmes, J. (1995). *Introduction to psychoanalysis: Contemporary theory and practice*. London: Routledge.

19 Shaffer, R. (1992). *Retelling a life*. New York: Basic Books.

20 Bowlby, J. (1988). *A secure base: Clinical applications of attachment theory*. London: Routledge.

21 Holmes, J. (1993). *John Bowlby and attachment theory*. London: Routledge.

22 Holmes, J. (1996). *Attachment, intimacy, autonomy: Using attachment ideas in adult psycotherapy*. New York: Jason Aronson. (in press)

23 Rycroft, C. (1985). *Psychoanalysis and beyond*. London: Chatto.

24 Black, D. (1993). What sort of thing is religion? A view from object relations theory. *International Journal of Psycho-Analysis*, **73**, 613–628.

25 Rorty, R. (1989). *Irony, contingency, solidarity*. Cambridge: Cambridge University Press.

26 Bollas, C. *The shadow of the object*. London; Free Associations.

27 Singer, P. (1994). *How are we to live*. London: Mandarin.

28 Bergin, A., Stinchfield, R., Gaskin, T., et al. (1988). Religious life-styles and mental health: an exploratory study. *Journal of Consulting Psychology*, **35**, 91–98.

29 Bozormenyi-Nagy, et al. (1991). Contextual therapy. In A. Gurman & D. Kniskern (Eds.). *Handbook of Family Therapy*, Vol **2**. New York: Brunner/Mazel.

30 Rokeach, M. (1973). *The nature of human values*. New York: Free Press.

31 Bloch, S., Hafner, J., Harari, E., & Szmukler, G. (1994). *The family in clinical psychiatry*. Oxford: Oxford University Press.

Psychoanalysis and Ethics – Avowed and Unavowed*

Erik H. Erikson

Robert Wallerstein [. . .] ingeniously opened this symposium by quoting a definition of science and ethics so simple that he could be sure every participant and discussant would 'take off' from it. His reward was that every speaker except the first enlarged on an ethical complexity on some borderline of psychiatric practice.

The definition, you will recall, said that science is *descriptive* and needs *verification* while ethics is *prescriptive* and seeks *justification*. But as the first speaker, Robert Michels [. . .] pointed out, we represent neither pure science nor pure ethics but a branch of the healing professions. To heal means to restore to wholeness; and we can find our ethical function only by delineating a legitimate and unique area *between* these two extreme claims – that of being a true science, objectively taught, and that of representing an ideology of healthy conduct.

In addition to the definition quoted, Robert Wallerstein offered an enumeration of concrete issues of professional ethics concerning either the rights of the patient and his family and community, or the corresponding obligations of professionals. But, again, it appeared that the panellists were interested primarily in the general relation of wider ethical concerns and professional practice; and they were not hesitant at all to discuss either sin or evil or the greatest good, and to prescribe values, whether as practitioners, researchers or educators.

Robert Lifton (*this issue*) was the most explicit in this with his term 'advocacy research.' Unwilling to let what he calls the 'absurd evil' of the Vietnam war take cover behind the hometown drama of Watergate, he spoke of his work with those veterans who now carry much of the mental burden of that war: the anti-war veterans. And as has become his chosen mission, he reminded us that psychiatry must attend to matters of existential dread as well as of sexual guilt, of mass atrocities as well as of individual perversions.

In what I wish to say, I take my cue from Robert Wallerstein's eighth question: By aspiring to heal, he said, we cannot avoid prescribing values, some 'deliberate and avowed, some unrecognized and unavowed.' If this is so, then the psychoanalytic ethos would demand that we become aware of and avow or disavow what ethics may be hidden in our work before we can, indeed, help clarify what ethics is and what we and ethics might yet do together.

I must admit that the word 'unavowed' struck a chord. For I am not only a psychoanalyst by training and practice, but also a college professor by choice. In other words, I have taught the tenets of psychoanalysis not only to practitioners who can be expected to take some systematic responsibility for their own motivational state, but to large classes of college seniors. And if to profess means to avow loudly, then psychoanalytic insight adds a new dimension and a new mandate to teaching. As we differentiate our responsibilities from those traditionally reserved for other professions – divinity, law, medicine – we must ask ourselves what it means to teach the unconscious determinants of human behaviour to the young.

Let us not overlook the fact that a deepseated resistance exists, and by no means only an unconscious one, against such enlightenment. In fact, we ourselves may well carry with us some sense of hubris about being successful practitioners and advocates of what in its beginning was and still is and must be a very intimate art-and-science. Here it is illuminating to remember that the free-thinking Einstein suggested a telling simile for the widespread fear that the influence of psychoanalysis might 'not always be salutary'. He illustrated his discomfort by pointing to the 'machinery of our legs' which, being controlled by a *hundred muscles*, could not gain in efficiency by being manoeuvred more self-consciously. As if this were not enough, he used the old story of the centipede which has a *hundred legs* and found itself stopped in its tracks when suddenly asked to anticipate, before it moved again, which leg it was going to extend first and which of the other 99 next. 'It is possible,' mused Einstein, 'that analysis may paralyse our mental and emotional processes in a similar manner.'

Up to a point, this is a convincing story. But then one begins to wonder, by what right man can compare himself to an innocent centipede, which, as far as we know, lacks not only the sense of evil and the guilt that is our existential and evolutionary heritage, but also that division into a super-consciousness and an unconscious, which makes our motivation so conflicted. In fact, when Freud spoke of man as a *Prothesengott*, almighty only by dint of having multiplied the efficiency of his faculties by adding a vast array of complex gadgetry to his limbs and senses, he made clear what a complicated variety of centipede *we* are: which explains, in turn, how much we do need a certain heightened consciousness in order to direct our motives land motions. We are, after all, the kind of centipede that studies its multiple footing from the standpoint of relativity. . . .

But history, it must be admitted, appears to validate Einstein's question. Freud, when he founded the psychoanalytic branch of enlightenment, still could take much of Western civilization for granted and was faced with the world wars and world revolutions only towards the end of his life. And he may yet have envisaged that psychoanalysis would not only be resisted and rejected by conservative consciousness – *that* he was almost proud of – but that it may be overtly accepted and, in fact, flauntingly acted out and talked out and yet remain covertly resisted in its essence. At any rate, if youth in the second part of this fast-moving century must, by an alternation of revolt and compliance, manage the memory and the mandate of all the revolutionary thought of the first part, the influence of the Freudian enlightenment is now part of that burden. True, youth often accepts the new knowledge of mankind's repressions only by displaying previously forbidden impulses, with a mixture of passion and mockery, on the very surface. Or it may challenge the unconscious precipitously with twilight states induced by drugs. But if in this stance we detect – among other things – an attempt to assimilate the insights of psychoanalysis by means of the overt enactment of behaviour previously interpreted as either repressed or only symbolically expressed, psychoanalytic enlightenment may, indeed, be faced with new Hippocratic tasks which we should, at least, attempt to envisage.

At any rate, today the relationships of the generations and the sexes cannot be approached with psychoanalytic concepts without also considering the question of the role which our concepts do, will, and should play in the cultural and ideological controversies of our time. Can we ever claim, either on our clinical homeground or in the border areas of wider application, to be merely healing our clients in offices and clinics and to be

* Erikson, E.H.: Psychoanalysis and ethics-avowed and unavowed. *International Review of Psychoanalysis* 3:409–415, 1976.

rationally enlightening our students and readers, without intervening – whether we avow it or not – in the processes by which values are formed and transmitted in our society? If such claim turns out to be both unnecessary and unlikely, it may be better to find the proper framework for teaching the tenets of psychoanalysis not only in the context of clinical training, but also in that of humanist enlightment – as Freud, above all, exemplified in his writings. To search in each setting for a form of approach which will train and enlarge consciousness even as it reveals some of the workings of the unconscious – that may well be the answer to Einstein.

The intervention of the psychiatric ethos in the values of the times becomes strikingly obvious in the era of mass communication. Yet, such intervention must be recognized as always having been implicit in the very existence and essence of professions specializing in mental healing. The new knowledge, the new insight and the new style emphasized by any therapeutic art-and-science at any given time is first of all defined by the epidemiological disturbances it was first challenged to alleviate. In establishing diagnostic and prognostic criteria for some typical and yet vexing kind of patients – be they the possessed of bygone centuries, the hysterics of early psychoanalysis or the schizoid characters of today – and in postulating an aetiology and prescribing a cure for their symptoms, such an art-and-science demarcates a vision of healthier existence. This, in turn, always includes postulates as to what must be considered normative and normal in human conduct, what men must avoid doing to each other and what they owe to each other in order to maximize each other's well-being. But then, the epidemiologically dominant neuroses and psychoses clamouring for special attention in any given period of history already represent in and by themselves a kind of inverted revolt against and challenge to the unmanageable or hypocritical values of the then existing establishment. By undertaking to cure these dominant symptoms and by publicizing what we interpret and prescribe, we, in fact, identify *with* that challenge – whether we establish that hysterics are not necessarily constitutionally inferior or urge society to modify its pressures.

What the healing professions advocate, therefore, is always part of the value struggle of the times and, whether 'avowed' or not, will be – and therefore had better be – ethical intervention.

Our patients, then, are those members of a given society who are most inactivated by the inner conflicts shared by all. And the public, obscurely aware of this, is so eager for definitions, of normal and moral conduct that it will dramatically oversimplify and will try to derive prescriptive slogans from what we conceive to be delicately scientific and therapeutic matters. We may then claim that we have been misunderstood and that all we wanted to do was to heal specific disturbances. But perhaps we should learn to take a closer look not only at the relationship of the dominant values of our (or any other) period in history to the mental disturbances typical for it, but also at the uses customarily made of the dominant terms of therapeutic enlightenment.

A few brief and simple examples will suffice. Take this matter of 'adjustment to reality.' Certain types of patients, we say, are suffering from a partial but distinct 'denial of reality'. Treatment must help them to make that denial conscious and to bring the whole person up to that level of insight and will-power which we attribute to the 'intact' part of the personality – that part which, in fact, makes the person treatable. What we really have in mind, especially with our more ambitious treatments, is *adaptive* therapy, in the sense that the cured patient, while refusing to over-adjust, should learn both to *adapt* to what is factual and inevitable and, where possible, to *adapt to himself* and others what can and should be changed in his environment. Yet, before we know it, our vocabulary is used to support a general ethical ideal of *adjustedness* to conditions which we, in fact, often do not believe a person *should* be encouraged to tolerate, especially since such adjustment may enslave the more sensitive to conditions which favour other, and often rather unethical, characters.

Or take the diagnostic emphasis on *sexual repression*. Psychoanalytic enlightenment is intended to lift infantile repressions in order to restore the capacity to make conscious choices: that is, to make it possible to do – and do with some playful abandon – what is deeply needed and truly wanted

and to renounce what is neither. Together with the ideal of adjustability, however (and with what Lifton calls 'technicism') there emerge, before long, new prescriptions of sexual conduct by which that person is considered the 'freest' who can engage in an unlimited use of others for the obsessive expression of all the whimsies suggested by the sexbooks.

Here I would like to say a word about the paper presented here by Robert J. Stoller.[1] His thesis was that a sense of sin enhances sexual incitement in that it is an indispensable aspect of the fantasies which accompany erotic arousal – but are ignored by modern researchers of sexuality. He demonstrated in the case histories of some rather far-gone perverts an overwhelming need to debase and dehumanize others in order to overcome infantile traumata by taking risks and by taking revenge – that is, always to *take* rather than to give-and-take. If Stoller goes on to indicate that we can detect in every sexual act some such tendency to subdue others and that for full satisfaction this needs to be experienced as a sinful triumph, I would wonder whether it is not – in non-perverts – a spontaneous element of playfulness which permits two partners to experience as it were, a *mutuality* of exploitation quite commensurable with love. Where this is absent, one wonders whether the prescription of a sense of sin would not soon become another technical requirement; while the very word used for the phenomenon prejudices the whole question of the existential as well as the psychological meaning 'sin' may have for the whole human being, when not acutely erotized. Stoller in his references to dehumanization does, in fact, point to a common characteristic of all sins and evils, whether they are spelled in small letters and are accessible to therapists of the mind, or whether they are capitalized for the attention of healers of the soul; and, indeed, several presentations at this symposium have expressed the apprehension that modern 'technicism', which tends to make a statistic of each person, may be aggravating a great potential Evil in our time, not the least because it can disguise itself in an ethos of efficiency and pragmatism and may desensitize man beyond any compassion – or awareness of guilt.

Finally, let me point to some consequences of our genetic habit of reconstructing the *pathogenesis* of our patients' symptoms, or what I have repeatedly referred to as our 'originological' orientation. Patients and would-be patients soon learn to derive from such causal aetiology a moral right to present themselves as victims of the generational process. Their self-accounts become self-vindications and their new autonomy is beset with vindictiveness against all progenitors and assorted other exploiters. Up to a point and in a systematic setting this may reveal important facts and may loosen forces of liberation. But without insight into the inner collusion with the exploiter, protest can exhaust itself in a habitual rage not conducive to inner nor, for that matter, outer liberation. Liberation can occur only where insight into the irresponsibility of others leads to the acknowledgement of our responsibility to ourselves.

I have deliberately concentrated here on psychoanalysis. It will be easy for the listener or reader to apply my formula to other varieties of approach such as the pharmacological one which suggests a stance of correcting the world's evils by the habitual intake of corrective dosages of some substance or another; or the behaviourist, which offers a Utopia of healthy behaviour so scheduled by implanted controls that ethical conflict is altogether unnecessary. The danger of all such interventions, 'avowed or unavowed' is that they will be absorbed by societal processes for the purposes of ethical short cuts often contrary to the initial intention of the inventors of the method. So be warned: if anyone should get the notion, say, of assigning names to the stages of life and to their conscious and unconscious crises and gains, he may soon see these names used in achievement tests and incorporated in questionnaires for self-rating.

Without the systematic vigilance of the healing professions, then, and maybe in spite of it, a society dominated by technocratic thinking is especially apt to turn every bit of new knowledge to the advantage of its prime economic and technological inclinations. All this may be 'natural' and inevitable; the question is only what, once we know it, we perceive our further function to be.

---

1 Dr. Stoller's paper was not submitted for publication. [ed.]

And here it must be said that 'unavowedly' we collude with the public's oversimplification of our findings. Psychology and psychoanalysis, by trying to keep up with the older basic sciences has tended to use terms which all too easily come to mean the opposite of what we mean. Maybe the most telling example is our habitual use of the term 'love object' to indicate the person loved as a whole person and loved with one's whole person. Freud originally spoke only of the 'object' of a hypothetical libidinal energy, even as Piaget designated as an object what the infantile senses can perceive as a coherent and persistent phenomenon. If, as happened in this very symposium, sexual experience is referred to as 'satisfaction from one's body and the outside world (one's objects)', such usage seems to advocate the 'technicist' line in sexual adjustment. Similarly, psycho-analysis, which undertook to save the vitality of Eros from the repressive sexual ethics of a mercantile and technological society, may have unavowedly contributed to an image of man which is dominated by an inner bartering system (subtracting a bit of drive here and sublimating it up there, suppressing a fantasy here and having it reappear in disguised form there) as if man were a closed entropic system performing energy transactions for the gain of 'pleasure', 'security', etc.

As it happens, the inventors of the 'mechanisms of defence' were certainly the least 'mechanical' minded in any emotional or intellectual respect. And yet, their terminology may well have contributed to the image of man as a robot of inner mechanisms. And then, of course, there is always the English term 'ego' itself, which in psychoanalysis means an orderly and ordering core in the centre of the person, but in general parlance is ego-centrism at its vainest. The term ego-identity, in turn, seems to suggest to many that one need be identical only with oneself, while it means to others that one should become totally identical with one's role. The point is that such misunderstandings are by no means only cognitive misapprehensions but are intrinsic aspects of the ethical dialectics of the times and must be studied as such.

Having said all this, I would still declare myself to be decidedly on the side of the psychoanalytic ethos. For in pointing to some of the unavowed ways which seem to make even once radical psychoanalysis subservient to major trends of the times, I have merely indicated what can and does happen to any and all revolutionary ideas: political, spiritual – and scientific. To come back to Einstein, for example, we must agree, from a dynamic viewpoint, with those who suggest that the theory of relativity, too, has been drawn into the process of *pseudo-ethical assimilation* just described, and this by being perceived as an advocacy of ethical relativism, even as older theories such as causality, the preservation of energy, or the survival of the fittest have become rationalizations of human (and inhuman) conduct. Of all fields, however, psychoanalysis has the built-in correctives for such a predicament, because it knows how to study the importance of simplified world views for the development of each person; and it can by its own methods, develop an awareness of its own historical role in such changing world images. But this also means to study the differences in method and theory between successive generations of psychoanalysts not only in terms of their apparent reliability and inner logic but also in the light of their historical relativity.

The basic paradox to be understood is that even as great thinkers detect new universal laws and thus provide new masteries for mankind, the 'rumour' of these laws awaken some basic disorientation in space and time for all but those who can affirm these laws first hand in their strictest meaning. Even the paradigms of exact science, then, need to be taught not only with logical persuasion but also with an understanding for man's deep motivational and emotional investment in conflicting world images which happen to govern the spatial and verbal metaphors conveyed through the generational process.

This brings me, in conclusion, to the evolutionary aspects of 'moral values, ethics, and psychological intervention.' Evolution connotes infinitesimally slow change; and if I speak of an evolution of ethics, I use the word in the sense postulated by Waddington when he called man 'the ethical animal.' Man, that upright creature with a highly variable *instinctual* life, the creature with stereoscopic vision and with hands that make tools, the creature marked by language and culture, also has a built-in need and capacity, during an especially long period of infantile and juvenile dependence, to learn rules of conduct – and this exactly because he is not regulated by a reliable set of *instinctive* patterns fitting a given section of nature.

One prime requirement for a psychoanalytic study of moral values and ethics is, then, the *epigenetic* point of view which postulates that the ethical need which is built into all of us phylogenetically must evolve in each of us ontogenetically, that is, through the mediation of the generational process. Morality, ideology and ethics must evolve in each person by a step-by-step development from less to more differentiated and insightful stages. And epigenetic means that even as each earlier stage lives on in all the later ones, each later stage represents a reintegration of all earlier ones. But this also bespeaks a continuing and inexorable *dynamic conflict* between the earlier and most primitive, and the later, more mature values in each person – and in all communities.

Developmentally speaking we must, in fact, differentiate between an earlier, a *moral* conscience and a later, an *ethical* one. What Freud graphically calls our superego, that part of our conscience which forever lords it over us and at times seems to crush us with guilt, serves as the internalization of early prohibitions driven into us by frowning faces and verbal threats, if not by physical punishment – and all this before we could possibly understand them. In later life, this remains our most moralistic side – that side of us which takes pleasure in condemning those who are doing what we could not dare to do and, so we claim, are endangering the moral fiber of mankind.

The more *adult* pole of our ethical nature is an affirmative sense of what man owes to man, in terms of the developmental realization of the best in each human being. There are a number of stages in between – such as the ideological one in youth – but this is not a seminar: the main point is that our most ethical and our most moralistic sides tend to make deals with each other which eventually permit us to commit or to agree to the commission of enslavement, exploitation and annihilation in the name of the highest values. It is this, above all, that psychological insight must help us resolve sufficiently to counteract the growing potentialities for cold Evil – and to match those for sympathetic progress – in a world-wide technology.

It is for us to increase the margin of ethical choice by gaining and giving insight into the blatant deals which not only virtue and vice but also the ethical and the moral are attempting to make within us and right in front of us. Let me here point only to one area of punitive moralism and of human waste which calls for the joint insight of psychoanalysts and ethicists: I mean our irrational insistence or acquiescence in the proposition that the *incarceration* of large groups of persons deemed bad or mad, including young and as yet unformed persons, is sensible and legitimate. It has, of course, some short-range advantages and even some long-range uses. But it certainly is not what it is claimed or simply assumed to be, namely corrective and, therefore, healing. I believe that insight could tell us that here we are projecting some most primitive inner 'mechanism' on the social environment at large: since we, in order to be good, had to repress parts of ourselves (i.e. create within ourselves areas out of bounds for ourselves); we believe it to be a matter of justice as well as logic that transgressors must be incarcerated and put behind bars where we can deny and forget *them*. We know or suspect that few are made better thereby and that many more will return only to poison society further with that vengeance that results from all outer as well as inner repression. And speaking of incarceration, we tend to *excarcerate* with the same primitive logic: we banish thousands of young men who resisted a war which we dared to doubt and to deplore, but not to protest against by dangerous action. Do we now not dare to face *them*?

Finally, we must develop the methodological means to study the way in which the dynamics of moral and ethical conflict is built into the values themselves. Consider only that Truth is more than not lying. Courage is more than not to be cowardly, Faith more than the mere absence of existential doubts. At any rate, the strengths which potentially emerge from each developmental crisis in life all serve the evolvement of a truly ethical sense: consonant with the facts as we know them; with the heightened reality we perceive; and with our actualization of one another.

In summary, our mandate in informing the ethicists and in being informed by them, is to gain insight into those aspects of moral and ethical man which, for phylogenetic reasons, are apt to change *very* slowly, even as we suspect that we are changing almost too fast for our own good. Mental healing and especially healing by insight into unconscious motivation has come into its own only very recently in history and, as was to be clarified by this symposium, still has difficulties in delineating itself against medical science proper, on the one hand, and religion, on the other. True, the word 'clinical' once referred to the services a priest administered at the bedside of the dying, even as healing meant to make a person hale and whole, in body, mind and soul. Ours, I think, is the specific obligation to help in the healing of persons by providing them and ourselves with some insight into the sources of irrational *anxiety* – so that they may not only gain in libidinal vitality but also be freer for the ethical choices demanded by justified *fear* and by existential *dread*.

Advocacy and Corruption in the Healing Professions*

Robert Jay Lifton

In looking at the professions one does well, I think, to hold to the old religious distinction between the ministerial and the prophetic. One should not assume, as many do, a simple polarity in which the sciences are inherently radical or revolutionary and the healing professions intrinsically conservative. The professions must minister to people, take care of them, and that is a relatively conservative process. But there are prophets who emerge from the healing ministrations of the professions – Freud is a notable example – with radical critiques and revolutionary messages. Moreover, even 'pure scientists' (in biology or physics, for example) spend most of their time ministering to the existing paradigm, doing what Thomas Kuhn (1962) calls 'normal science,' and strongly resist the breakthrough that is inevitably charted by the prophets among them. There are ministerial and prophetic elements in both the healing professions and the sciences.

But one must also distinguish between the professions, which have profound value in their capacity for continuity and renewal, and professional-ism, the ideology of professional omniscience, which in our era inevitably leads to 'technicism' and the model of the machine. The necessity for such a distinction becomes painfully clear if one looks at the situation that prevailed for psychiatrists in Vietnam. I want to take that situation as a starting point for a broader discussion of these dilemmas and their moral and conceptual ramifications. For the fact is that, in such extreme situations, the professional may be no better able than his soldier-patient to sort out the nuances of care and professional commitment on the one hand, and moral (or immoral) action on the other.

Central to my view of the present predicament of the professions is the psychology and the spirit of the survivor. The concept of the survivor derives in my work from the study I did in Hiroshima a little more than ten years ago (Lifton, 1968, ch.12) and has been fundamental to my subsequent thought. I define a survivor as one who has touched, witnessed, encountered or been immersed in death in a literal or symbolic way and has himself remained alive. Let us assume that we as professionals share the national 'death immersion' of not only Vietnam but the related Watergate-impeachment process and that our ways of surviving them can have significance for us in our work. We may then discover that we are not entirely removed from the constellation of psychological patterns that I found Hiroshima survivors to share to a rather striking degree with survivors of Nazi death camps, the plagues of the Middle Ages, natural disasters, and what Kurt Vonnegut calls 'plain old death'.

I

The concept of the survivor includes five patterns. The first is the survivor's indelible death image and death anxiety. This 'death imprint' often has to do with a loss of a sense of invulnerability. The second pattern, that of death guilt, is revealed in the survivor's classic question, 'Why did I stay alive when he or she or they died?' The question itself has to do with a sense

of organic social balance: 'If I had died, he or she would have lived'. That image of exchange of one life for another is perhaps the survivor's greatest psychological burden. A third pattern is that of desensitization or what I call psychic numbing, the breakdown of symbolic connectedness with one's environment. Numbing is a necessary protective mechanism in holocaust, but can become self-perpetuating and express itself in sustained depression, despair and apathy or withdrawal. A fourth survivor pattern has to do with the 'death-taint', as experienced by others toward survivors and by survivors themselves, resulting in discrimination against them and mutual suspicion and distrust. Central to this pattern is the survivor's 'suspicion of counterfeit nurturance', his combination of feeling in need of help and resenting help offered as a reminder of weakness. (This kind of suspicion, occurs not only in holocaust but in any situation in which 'help' is offered by the privileged to the downtrodden or oppressed, as in white-black relations; and one can readily find models for this pained interaction in parent–child relationships.)

The fifth pattern is fundamental to all survivor psychology and encompasses the other four. It is the struggle toward 'formulation' (following Langer (1942, 1967–72)) in order to be able to find form and significance in one's remaining life experience. This formulative struggle is equally visible in more symbolic experiences of holocaust, those of surviving ways of life one perceives to be 'dying'. In that sense rapid social change makes survivors of us all.

In examining our healing professions in relationship to these survivals, especially that of the psychiatric death encounter in Vietnam, we should keep in mind two general survivor alternatives. One can retreat from the issues raised by the death immersion and thereby remain bound to it in a condition of stasis (or numbing). Or one can confront the death immersion and derive insight, illumination and change from the overall survivor experience (Lifton, 1973c, ch. 13). The latter response to some kind of experience of survival has probably been the source of most great religious and political movements, and of many breakthroughs in professional life as well.

A related issue is that of advocacy, which in our profession applies both to investigation and therapy, and is crucial to issues of professional renewal. I came to my work with Vietnam veterans from two directions, from prior anti-war advocacy and from professional concern with holocaust deriving from my research in Hiroshima. In the work with veterans I sought to combine detachment sufficient to enable me to make psychological evaluations (which I had to do at every step) with involvement that expressed my own commitments and moral passions. I believe that we always function within this dialectic between ethical involvement and intellectual rigour, and that bringing our advocacy 'out front' and articulating it makes us more, rather than less, scientific. Indeed, our scientific accuracy is likely to suffer when we hide our ethical beliefs behind the claim of neutrality and that we are nothing but 'neutral screens'. The Vietnam War constitutes an extreme situation in which the need for an ethical response is very clear. But we have a tradition of great importance in depth psychology much evident in Freud, of studying extremes in order to illuminate the (more obscure) ordinary.

* Lifton, R. J.: Advocacy and corruption in the healing professions. *International Review of Psychoanalysis* 3: 385–398, 1976.

II

I want to focus now on my experience over the last three years with 'rap groups' of anti-war veterans and then to generalize from that experience about professional issues around advocacy and corruption.

The veteran's rap groups came into being because the veterans sensed that they had more psychological work to do in connexion with the war (Lifton, 1973c, ch. 3). It is important to emphasize that the veterans themselves initiated the groups. The men knew that they were 'hurting,' but did not want to seek help from the Veterans Administration, which they associated with the military, the target of much of their rage. And though they knew they were in psychological pain, they did not consider themselves patients. They wanted to understand what they had been through, begin to heal themselves and at the same time make known to the American public the human costs of the war. These two aspects of the veterans' aspirations in forming the groups – healing themselves while finding a mode of political expression – paralleled the professional dialectic of rigour and advocacy mentioned earlier. Without using those words, the veterans had that combination very much in mind when they asked me to work with them.

I called in other professionals (Chaim Shatan did much of the organizing) in the New York-New Haven area to assist us in the rap groups. I also participated with the veterans in the Winter Soldier Investigation of 1971, the first large-scale public hearing at which American G.I.'s described their own involvement in war crimes. From the beginning the therapeutic and political aspects of our work developed simultaneously. It seemed natural for us to initiate the rap groups on the veterans' own turf, so to speak, in the office of the Vietnam Veterans Against the War – and to move to the 'neutral ground' of a theological seminary when problems of space and political in-fighting developed at the V.V.A.W. office. The men wanted to meet where they were comfortable and where they could set the tone. With many stops and starts and much fluidity in general, a sizable number of these rap groups have formed, in New York City and throughout the country (Lifton, 1973c, chs. 3, 13). The one that I have been part of has been meeting continuously for three and a half years as of this writing (June 1974).

We made plans for weekly two-hour meetings, but the sessions were so intense, with such active involvement on the part of everybody, that they would generally run for three or four hours. I also interviewed many of the men individually in connexion with the research I initiated then and subsequently published. From the beginning we avoided a medical model: we called ourselves 'professionals' rather than 'therapists' (the veterans often referred to us simply as 'shrinks'), and we spoke of rap groups rather than group therapy. We were all on a first-name basis and there was a fluidity in the boundaries between professionals and veterans. But the boundaries remained important nonetheless; distinctions remained important to both groups; and in the end the healing role of professionals was enhanced by the extent to which veterans could become healers in relationship to one another and, to some degree, to professionals also. Equally important, there was an assumption, at first unspoken and later articulated, that everybody's life was at issue; professionals had no special podium from which to avoid self-examination. We too could be challenged, questioned about anything – all of which seemed natural enough to the veterans but was somewhat more problematic for the professionals. As people used to interpreting others' motivations, it was at first a bit jarring to be confronted with hard questions about our own, and with challenges about the way we lived. Not only was our willingness to share this kind of involvement crucial to the progress of the group, but in the end many of us among the professionals came to value and enjoy this kind of dialogue.

As in certain parallel experiments taking place, not only in psychological work but throughout American culture, we had a clearer idea of what we opposed (hierarchical distancing, medical mystification, psychological reductionism that undermines political and ethical ideas) than of what we favoured as specific guidelines. But before long I came to recognize three principles that seemed important. The first was that of *affinity*, the coming together of people who share a particular (in this case overwhelming) historical or personal experience, along with a basic perspective on that experience in order to make some sense of it (the professionals entered into this 'affinity', at least to a certain extent, by dint of their political-ethical sympathies and inclination to act and experiment on behalf of them). The second principle was that of presence, a kind of 'being there' or full engagement and openness to mutual impact – no one ever being simply a therapist against whom things are rebounding. The third was that of *self-generation*, the need on the part of those seeking help, change or insight of any kind, to initiate their own process and conduct it largely on their own terms so that, even when calling in others with expert knowledge, they retain major responsibility for the shape and direction of the enterprise. Affinity, presence and self-generation seem to be necessary ingredients for making a transition between old and new images and values, particularly when these relate to ultimate concerns, to shifting modes of historical continuity or what I have elsewhere called symbolic immortality (Lifton, 1973b).

I do not want to give the impression that everything went smoothly. There were a number of tensions in the group, one of them having to do with its degree of openness and fluidity. Openness was an organizing principle: in the fashion of 'street-corner psychiatry' any Vietnam veteran was welcomed to join a group at any time. Fluidity was dictated by the life-styles of many of the veterans who travelled extensively around the country and did not hold regular jobs. Professionals too were unable to attend every session. We established a policy of assigning three professionals to a group, with arrangements that at least one come to each meeting – but professionals became so involved in the process that there were usually two or all three present at a given group meeting.

When a veteran would appear at the group for the first time, obviously ill at ease, he would be welcomed by the others with a phrase, 'you're our brother.' Still, everyone came to recognize that such a policy could interfere with the probing of deep personal difficulties. A similar issue developed around the question of how accessible we would be to the media. Veterans wanted to make known the human costs of the war as part of their anti-war commitment, but after permitting a sympathetic journalist to sit in on a few of the sessions they came to recognize that group process could be interfered with by the presence of even a sensitive outsider. We eventually arrived at the policy that only veterans and professionals could be present during group sessions, but that the group could on occasion meet with interested media people after a session was over. That solution served to protect the integrity of the group while conveying to those journalists a rather vivid sense of both the impact of the war and the nature of the rap group experience.

There was also a tension among the professionals between two views of what we were doing. In the beginning a majority of the professionals felt that the essential model for our group sessions was group therapy. These professionals argued that the men were 'hurting' and needed help and that if we as therapists offered anything less than group therapy we were cheating the men of what they most needed. I held to a second model which was at first a minority view. This position, while acknowledging the important therapeutic element of what we were doing, emphasized the experimental nature of our work in creating a new institution; a sustained dialogue between professionals and veterans based on a common stance of opposition to the war in which both groups drew upon their own special knowledge, experience and needs. This model did not abolish role definitions: veterans were essentially there to be helped and professionals to help; but it placed more stress on mutuality and shared commitment.

We never resolved the tension totally between these two models in the sense of all of us coming to share a single position. The veterans tended to favour the second model but did not want to be short-changed in terms of help they wanted and needed. There was a continuing dialectic between these two ways of seeing what we were doing. But those who held to the second model – which related to other experiments taking place in American society with which the veterans identified – tended to stay longer with the project. Those professionals who conceived the effort in a more narrowly defined therapeutic way and who, I suspect, were less politically and ethically committed to an anti-war position, tended to leave.

Of course there were differences in professional style even within these two models. Some professionals were particularly skilled at uncovering the childhood origins of conflicts. I was seen as an authority on issues of death and life-continuity and on social-historical dimensions around death and survival. As a personal style, my impulse was to be something of a mediator and the group soon came to see me in that way. The group recognized and accepted differing personal styles and it was interesting to us as professionals to observe reflexions of ourselves in the responses to us not only of veterans but of other professionals sharing the experience of a particular group. The veterans began with almost no knowledge of group process but they learned quickly. The focus of the group was from the beginning on the overwhelming experience of the war and on residual guilt and rage. In the process of examining these issues the men looked increasingly at their ongoing life struggles, especially their relationships with women, feelings about masculinity and conflicts around work. There was a back-and-forth rhythm in the group between immediate life situations and war-related issues, with these gradually blending in deepening self-examination that was generally associated in turn with social and political forces in the society.

For all of us in the group there was a sense that the combination of ultimate questions (about death and survival) and experimental arrangements required that we call upon new aspects of ourselves and become something more than we had been before. Central to this process was the changing relationship between veterans and professionals. At moments the veterans could become critical of the way professionals were functioning. There was one bitter expression of resentment by a veteran who felt that the interpretations made by a professional were too conventional and tended to ignore or undercut issues very important to him. The group discussed the matter at great length. I agreed in part with the veteran, but also tried to point out that the interpretation was made in good faith. At another point one of the veterans spoke very angrily to me because I was occupied with my note-taking. I was trying to record the words of the veterans precisely because, as we had discussed earlier, I was in the group not only as a healer but also as an investigator who would write about the experience. When we discussed the matter it became clear that the veterans had no difficulty accepting that dual role. What they objected to was my not being fully 'present' with them as I focused on taking notes. I thought about that and decided they were right. I ceased my note-taking and from that point on made notes only at the end of each session, a well-established pattern in the practice of psychotherapy that I had to relearn. There were, of course, many other conflicts as well, but there was also an essential feeling of moving towards authentic insight. By taking seriously such issues as they were raised, we maintained a double level of individual-psychological interpretation and shared actuality. Taking that actuality seriously contributed to the sense of everyone's 'presence'.

One additional experience, not frequently encountered in healing endeavours, is worth mentioning. About six months after we initiated the groups a non-white veteran – we were not certain whether he was American Indian or Puerto Rican – came to a session and spoke rather movingly about his struggles to sustain himself and a baby left with him by a girlfriend who deserted him. He came to a second meeting but fled after just five minutes. We wondered at his behaviour and some weeks later discovered an explanation for it. Though he did not again appear in the group, he came to the V.V.A.W. office and confessed to another veteran that he had been an F.B.I. informer. He stayed only long enough to say that he was sorry for what he had done and felt especially badly because he had liked the rap group very much. When we discussed all this in the group, reactions varied from wondering what arcane matters the F.B.I. might have imagined we were discussing (though we concluded that he had probably been simply sent to the V.V.A.W. office and had somehow wandered into our session) to the rekindling of bitter resentment at official America, to an uneasy sense that betrayal from within – by veterans themselves (and by inference, by oneself) was all too evident a possibility.

III

The rap groups represented a struggle on the part of both veterans and psychological professionals to give form to what was in many ways a common survival, a survival for the veterans of a terrible death immersion and for the professionals of their own dislocations in relationship to the war and the society. During our most honest moments, we professionals have admitted that the experience has been as important for our souls as for theirs. For the rap groups have been one small expression (throughout the country they and related programmes have probably involved, at most, a few thousand people) of a much larger cultural struggle towards creating what I have termed animating institutions (Lifton, 1973a, c, ch. 13). Whether these emerge from existing institutions significantly modified or as 'alternative institutions', they can serve the important function of providing new ways of being a professional as well as relating to professionals. While such institutions clearly have 'radical' possibilities, they can also serve a genuinely conservative function in enabling those involved to find a means of continuing to relate, however critically, to the existing society and its other institutions, as opposed to retreating in embittered alienation, destructiveness or self-destructiveness. In this and other ways the rap group experience seemed to me a mirror on psychohistorical struggles of considerable importance throughout the society.

A compelling example was the rap group's continuous preoccupation with struggles concerning maleness. I described these struggles in a chapter of my book (Lifton, 1973c) entitled, somewhat whimsically but not without seriousness, 'From John Wayne to Country Joe and the Fish'. The men were very intent upon examining what they came to call 'the John Wayne thing' in themselves – a process actively encouraged if not required by girlfriends and wives often active in the women's movement. The essence of the issue for the veterans was their deepening realization that various expressions of super-maleness encouraged in American culture were inseparable from their own relationship to war-making. They probed unsparingly the sources and fears beneath their male bravado in enthusiastically (in many cases) 'joining up' and even seeking out the war. For the insight that gradually imposed itself on them was that only by extricating themselves from elements of 'the John Wayne thing' – notably its easy violence on behalf of unquestioned group loyalty and male mystique of unlimited physical prowess always available for demonstration – could they, in a genuine psychological sense, extricate themselves from the war. Two significant psychological alternatives were available to them from the youth culture of the 1960s: the image of a male being no less genuinely so for manifesting tenderness, softness, aesthetic sensitivity and awareness of feelings; and the overall social critique of war, war-making and the warrior ethos. It was particularly the latter that Country Joe MacDonald and his rock group (Country Joe and the Fish) gave ecstatic expression to in their celebrated song, 'I Feel Like I'm Fixin' to Die Rag'. A frenzied and bitter evocation of the absurdity of dying in Vietnam, the song propels one to the far reaches of the grotesque: 'And it's 1, 2, 3, what are we fighting for? / Don't ask me I don't give a damn. . / Well, there ain't no time to wonder why / Whoopee we're all gonna die.' And a little later in the song: 'Well, come on mothers throughout the land / Pack your boys off to Vietnam / Be the first one on your block / To have your boy come home in a box.' Ironically and significantly, the 'Fixin' to Die Rag' was probably the most frequently played song by men serving in Vietnam, and it is very likely that this expression of the other absurdity and grotesqueness of dying in Vietnam will become *the* song of the Vietnam War.

The personal transformation the veterans experience (barely suggested here) can thus be seen to have had both introspective and extrospective elements. The men constantly look inward, but they also look outward at their society both in relationship to having been drawn into the war and to what they perceived as a dubious welcome upon their return. This extrospective aspect of personal change is always important – not only in experimental institutions like the rap groups but in ordinary psychotherapy and ordinary living – but is often denied or ignored because of the implicit assumption that psychological experience, being internal, is totally self-contained. It was precisely this dual vision that enabled many veterans to develop what I came to see as an animating relationship to their sense of guilt (Lifton, 1973c, ch. 4). In contrast to static (neurotic) forms of guilt and immobilizing self-condemnation, animating guilt can provide energy towards change via the capacity to examine the roots of that guilt in both social and individual terms. I believe that these distinctions about guilt, when pursued further, have significance both for depth-psychological theory and for the ethical questions at issue in this discussion (Lifton, 1972).

IV

Guilt and rage were fundamental emotions that we explored constantly in the groups. But the men had a special kind of anger best described as ironic rage towards two types of professionals with whom they came into contact in Vietnam, chaplains and 'shrinks'. They talked about chaplains with great anger and resentment as having blessed the troops, their mission, their guns and their killing: 'Whatever we were doing – murder, atrocities – God was always on our side.' Catholic veterans spoke of having confessed to meaningless transgressions ('Sure, I'm smoking dope again. I guess I blew my state of grace again') while never being held accountable for the ultimate one ('But I didn't say anything about killing'). It was as if the chaplains were saying to them, 'Stay within our moral clichés as a way of draining off excess guilt, and then feel free to plunge into the business at hand.'

The men also pointed to the chaplain's even more direct role of promoting false witness. One man spoke especially bitterly of 'chaplains' bullshit.' He illustrated what he meant by recalling the death of a close friend – probably the most overwhelming experience one can have in combat – followed by a combined funeral ceremony–pep talk at which the chaplain urged the men to 'kill more of them'. Another who had carried the corpse of his closest friend on his back after his company had been annihilated described a similar ceremony at which the chaplain spoke of 'the noble sacrifice for the sake of their country' made by the dead. It is not generally recognized that the My Lai massacre occurred immediately after the grotesque death from an exploding 'booby trap' of a fatherly, much-revered non-commissioned officer, which had been witnessed by many of the men. That ceremony was conducted jointly by a chaplain and the commanding officer, the former blending spiritual legitimacy to the latter's mixture of eulogy and exhortation to 'kill everything in the village.' A eulogy in any funeral service asks those in attendance to carry forward the work of the person who died. In war, that 'work' characteristically consists in getting back at the enemy, thereby providing men with a means of resolving survivor guilt and a 'survivor mission' involving a sense not only of revenge but of carrying forth the task the fallen comrade could not see to completion. In Vietnam the combination of a hostile environment and the absence of an identifiable 'enemy' led to the frequent manipulation of grief to generate a form of false witness, a survivor mission of atrocity (Lifton, 1973c, ch. 2).

The men spoke with the same bitterness about 'shrinks' they had encountered in Vietnam. They describe situations in which they or others experienced an overwhelming combination of psychological conflict and moral revulsion, difficult to distinguish in Vienam. Whether one then got to see a chaplain, psychiatrist, or an enlisted-man-assistant of either, had to do with where they were at the time, who was available, and the attitudes of the soldier and the authorities in his unit towards religion and psychiatry. But should he succeed in seeing a psychiatrist he was likely to be 'helped' to remain at duty and (in many cases) to carry on with the daily commission of war crimes, which was what the ordinary G.I. was too often doing in Vietnam. Psychiatry for these men served to erode whatever capacity they retained for moral revulsion and animating guilt. They talked in the rap groups about ways in which psychiatry became inseparable from military authority.

But in their resentment of chaplains and psychiatrists the men were saying something more. It was one thing to be ordered by command into a situation they came to perceive as both absurd and evil, but it was quite another to have that process rationalized and justified by ultimate authorities of the spirit and mind, i.e. by chaplains and psychiatrists. One could even say that spiritual and psychological authority was employed to seal off in the men some inner alternative to the irreconcilable evil they were asked to embrace. In that sense the chaplains and psychiatrists formed an unholy alliance not only with the military command but also with the more corruptible elements in the soldier's psyche, corruptible elements available to all of us, whether soldier or chaplain or psychiatrist.

This 'double agent' problem arises even in wars that are more psychologically defensible (such as World War II), where the alliance between spiritual-psychological authority (chaplains and shrinks) on the one hand and the soldier's inner acceptance of killing, on the other, is buttressed by at least a degree of belief in the authenticity (or necessity) of the overall enterprise. Even then, ethical-psychological conflict occurs in everyone concerned – there is the *Catch 22* described by Heller, according to which one's very sanity in seeking escape from the environment via a psychiatric judgement of craziness renders one eligible for the continuing madness of killing and dying. But in Vietnam that alliance took on a grotesquery extraordinary even for war, as priest and healer, in the name of their spiritual-psychological function, undermined the last vestiges of humanity in those to whom they ministered.

We can then speak of the existence of a 'counterfeit universe' in which pervasive, spiritually reinforced inner corruption becomes the price of survival. In this scene the chaplains and psychiatrists were just as entrapped as the G.I.'s. For we may assume that most of them were reasonably conscientious and decent professionals – much like the writer and reader of this article – caught up in an institutional commitment in this particular war.

When the men spoke harshly in our group of military psychiatrists, we professionals of course asked ourselves whether they were talking about us. In some degree they undoubtedly were. They were raising the question whether *any* encounter with a psychiatrist, even in a context which they themselves created and into which we were called, could be any more authentic than the counterfeit moral universe psychiatrists had lent themselves to in Vietnam.

V

I want to move now to some reflexions about psychiatry in more ordinary situations. The rap group experience raised questions about the extent to which everyday work in our profession, and the professions in general, tends to wash away rather than pursue fundamental struggles around integrity – the extent to which the special armor of professionals block free exchange between them and the people they intend to serve.

In the rap group experience I found the issue of investigative advocacy more pressing and powerful than in other research I have done.[1] This was partly because veterans and professionals alike were more or less in the middle of the problem – the war continued and we all had painful emotions about what it was doing, and what we were doing or not doing to combat it.

But I also came to realize that, apart from the war, the work had important bearing upon a sense of long-standing crisis affecting all of us in the psychological professions and the professions in general – a crisis the war in Vietnam both accentuated and illuminated but by no means created. We professionals, in other words came to the rap groups with our own need for a transformation in many ways parallel to, if more muted, than that we sought to enhance in veterans. We too, sometimes with less awareness than they, were in the midst of struggles concerning living and working that had to do with intactness and wholeness, with what we have been calling integrity.

One source of perspective on that struggle, I found, was a return to the root ideas of profession, the idea of what it means to profess. Indeed, an examination of the evolution of these two words could provide something close to cultural history of the West. The Latin prefix *pro* means 'forward, towards the front, forth, out, or into a public position'. 'Fess' derives from the Latin *fateri* or *fass*, meaning 'to confess, own, acknowledge.' To profess (or be professed) then, originally meant a personal form of out-front public acknowledgment. And that which was acknowledged or 'confessed' always (until the 16th century) had to do with religion: with taking the vows of a religious order or declaring one's religious faith. But as society became secularized, the word came to mean 'to make claim to have knowledge of an art or science' or 'to declare oneself expert or proficient in an enterprise of any kind. The noun form, 'profession', came to suggest not only the act of professing, but also the ordering, collectivization and transmission of the whole process. The sequence was from 'profession' or religious conviction (from the 12th century) to a particular order or 'professed persons', such as monks or nuns (14th century) to 'the occupation which one possesses to be skilled in and follow', especially 'the three learned professions of divinity, law, and medicine' along with the 'military profession'. So quickly did the connotations of specialization and application take hold that as early as 1605 Francis Bacon could complain: 'Amongst so many great foundations of colleges in Europe, I find strange that they are all dedicated to professions, and none left free to Arts and Sciences at Large' (*Oxford English Dictionary; American Heritage Dictionary;* and Lifton, 1973c, ch. 14).

Thus the poles of meaning around the image of profession shifted from the proclamation of personal dedication to transcendent principles to membership in and mastery of a specialized form of socially applicable knowledge and skill. In either case the profession is immortalizing – the one through the religious mode, the other through works and social-intellectual tradition. And the principles of public proclamation and personal discipline carry over from the one meaning to the other – the former taking the shape of examination and licensing, the latter of study, training and dedication. Overall, the change was from advocacy based on faith to technique devoid of advocacy.[2]

To be sure, contemporary professions do contain general forms of advocacy: in law, of a body of supra-personal rules applicable to everyone; in medicine, of healing; and in psychiatry, of humane principles of psychological well-being and growth. But immediate issues of value-centred advocacy and choice (involving groups and causes served and consequences thereof) are mostly ignored. In breaking out of the premodern trap of immortalization by personal surrender to faith, the 'professional' has fallen into the modern trap of pseudo-neutrality and covert immortalization of technique. As a result our professions are all too ready to offer their techniques to anyone and anything. I am not advocating a return to pure faith as a replacement for the contemporary idea of what profession means. But I am suggesting that the notion of profession needs to include these issues of advocacy and ethical commitment. The psychiatrist in Vietnam, for example, whatever his intentions, found himself in collusion with the military in conveying to individual G.I.s an overall organizational message: 'Do your indiscriminate killing with confidence that you will receive expert medical-psychological help if needed.' Keeping in mind Camus's (1946) warning that men should become neither victims nor executioners, this can be called – at least in Vietnam – the psychiatry of the executioner. I do not exempt myself from this critique, as I served as a military psychiatrist in the Korean War under conditions that had at least some parallels to those we are discussing.

Three well-known principles of military psychiatry developed during recent wars are *immediacy* (a soldier is treated as soon as possible), *proximity* (close to the combat area) and *expectancy* (everyone under treatment is from the beginning made to expect that he will return to duty with his unit). There is a certain logic to these principles. Their use very often does eliminate or minimize the secondary gains from illness and the chronic symptomatology that would otherwise ensue when men are sent to the rear to undergo prolonged psychiatric hospitalization, as well as feelings of failure and unmanliness that become associated with eventual medical discharge from the military. One psychiatric report from Vietnam describes the use of these principles and the assumption that those requiring treatment' had run into some difficulty in interpersonal relations in their units that caused them to be extruded from these groups,' so that 'the therapeutic endeavor . . . was to facilitate the men's integration into their own groups (units) through integration into the group of ward patients' (Bloch, 1969).

The approach seems convincing, until one evaluates some of the conditions under which atrocities occurred or were avoided. I spent ten hours interviewing a man who had been at My Lai and had not fired nor even pretended he was firing. (Among the handful who did not fire most held their guns in position as if firing, in order to avoid the resentment of the majority actively participating in the atrocity.) Part of what sustained this man and gave him the strength to risk ostracism was his very distance from the group. Always a 'loner', raised beside the ocean, he had as a child engaged mainly in such solitary activities as boating and fishing. Hence, though an excellent soldier, he was less susceptible than others to group influence, and in fact remained sufficiently apart from other men in his company to be considered 'maladapted' to that immediate group situation (Lifton, 1973c, pp. 57–59). One must distinguish between group integration and integrity – the latter including moral and psychological elements that connect one to social and historical context beyond the immediate. Group integration can readily undermine integrity – in Vietnam for both the soldier and the psychiatrist who must grapple with his own struggles to adapt to a military institution with its goals of maximum combat strength, and to a combat situation of absurdity and evil. No wonder why, in Vietnam, he found little ethical space in which to move. The clear implication here is that the psychiatrist, no less than the combat soldier, is confronted with the important question of the group he is to serve and, above all, the nature and consequences of its immediate and long-range mission. To do that he must overcome the 'technicist' assumption we fall into all too easily, namely: 'Because I am a healer, anything I do, anywhere, is good.' It may not be.

VI

I wonder how many colleagues shared my sense of chilling illumination in picking up the October 1971 issue of *The American Journal of Psychiatry* and finding in it two articles by psychiatrists about Vietnam: one entitled 'Organizational Consultation in a Combat Unit' (Bey & Smith, 1971) and the other 'Some Remarks on Slaughter' (Gault, 1971). The first lives up to its title in providing a military-managerial view of the psychiatrist's task. The authors invoke a scholarly and 'responsible' tone as they describe the three principles of combat psychiatry and trace their historical development. They then elaborate their own 'workable method of organizational consultation developed and employed in a combat division in Vietnam'. The method combines these principles of military psychiatry with 'an organizational case study method' recently elaborated for industry at the Menninger Foundation and, according to the authors, has bearing on possible developments in community psychiatry. Their professional voice sounds tempered, practical and modest as they tell of their team approach (with trained corpsmen), of interviews with commanding officers, chaplains and influential 'non-coms', and acknowledge that commanders 'were far better prepared to work out solutions to their problems than we, since their area of expertise was in adminstration and fighting whereas ours was in the area of helping them to see where their feelings might be interfering with their use of these skills.'

It was enough for psychiatric consultants to serve as an 'observing ego' to the particular military unit. To back up that position they quote, appropriately enough, from an article by General W. C. Westmoreland recommending that the psychiatrist assume 'a personnel management consultation type role'. The title of that article by General Westmoreland – 'Mental Health – An Aspect of Command' – makes quite clear just whom psychiatry in the military is expected to serve.

The authors' combination of easy optimism and concern for everyone's feelings and for the group as a whole, makes one almost forget the kinds of activities the members of that group were engaged in. Reading that leading article in the official journal of the national organization of American psychiatrists gave me a disturbing sense of how far this kind of managerial 'technicism' could take a profession, and its reasonably decent individual practitioners, into ethical corruption. What is most significant about the article is that the authors never make mention of the slightest conflict – in themselves and their psychiatric team any more than the officers and men the team deals with – between group integration and personal integrity. Either they were too numbed to be aware of such conflict, or (more likely) they did not consider it worthy of mention in a scientific paper.

Gault's article, 'Some Remarks on Slaughter' was a particularly welcome antidote, even if a bit more hidden in the inside pages. As his title makes clear, Gault's tone is informed by appropriate sense of outrage. Significantly, his vantage point was not Vietnam but Fort Knox, Kentucky, where he examined large numbers of men returning from combat. He was thus free of the requirement of integration with a combat unit, and we sense immediately a critical detachment from the atrocity-producing situation.

Gault introduces the idea of 'the psychology of slaughter', combining the dictionary definition of that word ('the extensive, violent, bloody or wanton destruction of life; carnage') with a psychological emphasis upon the victim's defenselessness ('whether . . . a disarmed prisoner or an unarmed civilian'). He can 'thus . . . distinguish slaughter from the mutual homicide of the actual combatants in military battle'. He sets himself the interpretive task of explaining how 'relatively normal men overcame and eventually neutralized their natural repugnance toward slaughter'. He is rigorously professional as he picks out six psychological themes or principles contributing to slaughter, and yet his ethical outrage is present in every word. His themes are: 'the enemy is everywhere . . . [or] the universalization of the enemy'; 'the enemy is not human . . . [or] the 'cartoonization' of the victim'; the 'dilution' or 'vertical dilution' of responsibility; 'the pressure to act'; 'the natural dominance of the psychopath'; and 'sheer firepower . . . [so that] terrified and furious teenagers by the tens of thousands have only to twitch their index finger, and what was a quiet village is suddenly a slaughter-house.'

Gault sensitively documents each of these themes in ways very consistent with experiences conveyed to me during rap groups and individual interviews. He ends his article with illustrative stories: of prisoners refusing to give information being thrown out of helicopters as examples to others; of a new combat commander who refused to shoot a twelve-year-old 'dink' accidentally encountered by the company while setting up an ambush and thereby deeply jeopardized himself with his own men, who in turn saw the whole company jeopardized by the survival of someone who might, even as a prisoner, convey information about the ambush. Gault admits he does not know 'why similar experiences provoke so much more guilt in one man than in another,' and, still professionally cautious (perhaps overly so) he remains, as he says, 'unwilling to attempt to draw any large lessons from my observations'. At the end he insists only that 'in Vietnam a number of fairly ordinary young men have been psychologically ready to engage in slaughter and that moreover this readiness is by no means incomprehensible.'

One senses that these stories made a profound impact upon him, that he became a survivor of Vietnam by proxy and that the article was his way of giving form to that survival as well as resolving his own integration–integrity conflict as a morally sensitive psychiatrist in the military at the time of the Vietnam War.[3] He was able to call forth his revulsion towards the slaughter (and, by implication, his advocacy of life-enhancing alternatives) as a stimulus to understanding and to bring to bear on the Vietnam War a valuable combination of professional insight and ethical awareness.

VII

We do not have follow-up studies on psychiatrists and their spiritual-psychological state after service in Vietnam. I have talked to a number of them and my impression is that they find it no easier to come to terms with their immersion in the counterfeit universe than does the average G.I. They too feel themselves deeply compromised. They seem to require a year or more for them to begin to confront the inner contradictions they experienced. They too are survivors of Vietnam, and of a very special kind. I know of one or two who have embarked upon valuable survivor missions, parallel to and partly in affiliation with that of V.V.A.W. as an organization. But what is yet to emerge, though I hope it will before too long, is a detailed personal account by a psychiatrist of his struggles with group integration and individual integrity, and with the vast ramifications of the counterfeit that this paper only begins to suggest.

The 'technicist' model in psychiatry work something like this: a machine, the mind–body function of the patient, has broken down; another machine, more scientifically sophisticated – the psychiatrist – is called upon to 'treat' the first machine; and the treatment process itself, being technical, has nothing to do with place, time, or individual idiosyncrasy. It is merely a matter of being a technical-medical antagonist of a 'syndrome' or 'disease'. Nor is this medical-technical model limited to physicians – non-medical psychoanalysts and psychotherapists can be significantly affected by it. And the problem is not so much the medical model as such as it is the 'technicism' operating within that model.[4] The 'technicism' in turn feeds (and is fed by) a denial of acting within and upon history.

To be sure no psychiatrist sees himself as functioning within this admittedly over-drawn model. But its lingering 'technicism' is very much with us and can have the catastrophic results we have observed. Even psychological groups bent on breaking out of this 'technicism', such as some within the humanistic psychology movement (or 'third force'), can be rendered dependent upon it by their very opposition, to the point of being unable to evolve an adequate body of theory and practice of their own.

An alternative perspective, in my judgement, must be not only psychohistorical, but also psychoformative. By the latter I mean an emphasis upon the process of inwardly recreating all that is perceived or encountered (Lifton, 1973b; 1976). As in the work of Langer (1942, 1967–72) and Cassirer (1923–9, 1944) and Whitehead (1938), my emphasis is upon what can be called a formative-symbolic *process*, upon symbolization rather than any particular symbol (in the sense of one thing standing for another). The approach connects with much in twentieth-century thought, and seeks to overcome the nineteenth-century emphasis upon mechanism, with its emphasis upon breakdown of elements into component parts – an emphasis inherited, at least in large part, by psychoanalysis, as the word itself suggests (Holt, 1972; Yankelovich & Barrett, 1970; Whyte, 1944). Twentieth-century 'technicism' could be described as an aberrant (and in a sense nostalgic) re-creation of nineteenth-century mechanism. In contrast, a focus upon images and forms (the latter more structured and more enduring than the former) and upon their continuous development and re-creation gives the psychiatrist a way of addressing historical forces without neglecting intrapsychic concerns

The anti-war passions of a particular Vietnam veteran, for instance, had to be understood as a combined expression of many different psychic images and forms: the Vietnam environment and the forces shaping it; past individual history; the post-Vietnam American experience, including V.V.A.W. and the rap groups and the historical forces shaping these; and the various emanations of guilt, rage, and altered self-process that could and did take shape. Moreover, professionals, like myself, who entered into the lives of these veterans – with our own personal and professional histories, personal struggles involving the war, and much else – became a part of the overall image-form constellation.

Psychiatrists have a great temptation to swim with an American tide that grants them considerable professional status but resists, at times quite fiercely, serious attempts to alter existing social and institutional arrangements. As depth psychologists and psychoanalysts, we make a kind of devil's bargain that we can plunge as deeply as we like into intrapsychic conflicts while not touching too critically upon historical dimensions that question those institutional arrangements. We often accept this dichotomy quite readily with the rationale that, after all, we are not historians or sociologists. But the veterans' experience shows that one needs extrospection as well as introspection to deal with psychological conflicts, particularly at a time of rapid social change. And I believe that a general psychological paradigm of 'death and the continuity of life' (Lifton, 1973b) helps us to achieve this dual perspective, and to recognize the interplay of psychological and moral elements in relationship to ultimate commitments and our own involvement in that interplay.

All this points towards the need for a transformation of the healing professions themselves. In my work with veterans I restated a model of change I had elaborated in earlier work, based on a sequence of confrontation, reordering and renewal (Lifton, 1973c, 1961). The idea is worth stating at least as a model – not with any expectation of instant transformation, but with the recognition that, here and there, people are already pursuing it and will undoubtedly continue to do so in forms we have not yet imagined. Confrontation for the veterans meant confronting the idea of dying in Vietnam, often through the death of a 'buddy'. For psychiatrists it would mean confrontation of our own concerns about death, mortality and immortality, and our professional struggles with them. Reordering meant the working through of difficult emotions around guilt and rage; for psychiatry this would mean seeking animating relationships to the same emotions in ourselves and recognizing and making use of our experience of despair (Farber, 1966). Renewal for veterans meant a new sense of self and world, including an enhanced playfulness. The professional parallels are there and much can be said for the evolution of more playful modes of investigation and therapy.

I want to conclude with two quotations. The first is from Milgram, who performed controversial experiments on the willingness of people to cause pain and even endanger the lives of others when authoritatively requested to do so. Whatever one's view of the scientific and moral aspects of these 'Eichmann experiments', one of Milgram's (1967) own conclusions is worthy thinking about: 'Men are doomed if they act only within the alternatives handed down to them.'

And finally, Joseph Campbell (1956), perhaps America's most distinguished student of mythology: 'A god outgrown becomes immediately a life-destroying demon. The form has to be broken and the energies released.'

Notes

1   In contrast, my Hiroshima work, in which I also experienced strong ethical involvement, was retrospective and in a sense prospective (there were immediate nuclear problems, of course, but we were not in the midst of nuclear holocaust); my study of Chinese thought reform dealt with matters of immediate importance but going on (in a cultural sense) far away; and my work with Japanese youth had much less to do with overwhelming threat and ethical crisis (Lifton, 1961, 1970).

2   One can observe this process in the modern separation of 'profession' from 'vocation'. Vocation also has a religious origin in the sense of being 'called by God' to 'a particular function or station'. The secular equivalent became the idea of a personal 'calling' in the sense of overwhelming inclination, commitment, and even destiny. But the Latin root of vocation, *vocare*, to call, includes among its meanings and derivatives: vocable, vocation, vouch; advocate, advocation, convoke, evoke, invoke, provoke and revoke. Advocacy is thus built into the original root and continuing 'feel' of the word vocation; and vocation in turn is increasingly less employed in connexion with the work a man or woman does. If we do not say profession, we say 'occupation', which implies seizing, holding, or simply filling in space in an area or in time; or else 'job', a work of unclear origin that implies a task, activity, or assignment that is, by implication, self-limited or possibly part of a larger structure including many related jobs, but not, in essence, related to an immortalizing tradition or principle.

3   This assumption that the article was an expression of Gault's own survivor formulation, which I made originally only on the basis of reading it (and, of course, on my experience, personal and professional, with the psychology of the survivor) was strongly confirmed by a brief talk he and I had when we met as members of a panel on Vietnam veterans at a psychoanalytic meeting.

4   In this sense I am in sympathy with Szasz (1961) and Laing (1960, 1967) in their stress on the repressive uses of the medical model, but also with Osmond's (1972) defence of the enduring, human core of the medical model, which has 'stood the test of millennia' and contains still untapped resources for us. I believe that the medical model of disease and healing is still needed by psychiatrists, at least in some of our work and thought, but that it must itself be liberated from its technicist fetters.

References

Bey, D. R., Jr. & Smith, W. E. (1971). Organizational consultation in a combat unit. *Am. J. Psychiat.* **128**, 401–406.

Bloch, H. S. (1969). Army psychiatry in the combat zone – 1967–1968. *Am. J. Psychiat.* **126**, 291–292.

Campbell, J. (1956). *The Hero with a Thousand Faces.* New York: Meridian.

Camus, A. (1946). *Neither Victims nor Executioners.* Chicago: World Without War Publs, 1972.

Cassirer, E. (1944). *An Essay on Man.* New York: Doubleday Anchor.

Cassirer, E. (1923–9). *The Philosophy of Symbolic Forms.* 3 vols. New Haven: Yale Univ. Press, 1953–7.

Farber, L. (1966). The therapeutic despair. In *The Ways of the Will.* New York: Basic Books.

Gault, W. B. (1971). Some remarks on slaughter. *Am. J. Psychiat.* **128**, 450–453.

Holt R. R. (1972). Freud's mechanistic and humanistic images of man. In R.R. Holt & E. Peterfreund (eds.), *Psychoanalysis and Contemporary Science*, vol. 1 New York: Macmillan.

Kuhn, T. (1962). *The Structure of Scientific Revolutions.* Chicago: Univ. of Chicago Press.

Laing, R. (1960). *The Divided Self.* London: Penguin.

Laing, R. (1967). *The Politics of Experience.* London: Penguin.

Langer, S. (1942). *Philosophy in a New Key* Cambridge, Mass.: Harvard Univ. Press.

Langer, S. (1967–72). *Mind: an Essay on Human Feeling*, 2 vols. Baltimore: Johns Hopkins Press.

Lifton, R. J. (1961). *Thought Reform and the Psychology of Totalism: a Study of 'Brainwashing' in China*, New York: Norton.

Lifton, R. J. (1968), *Death in Life: Survivors of Hiroshima.* New York: Random House.

Lifton, R. J. (1970). *History and Human Survival.* New York: Random House.

Lifton, R. J. (1972). Questions of guilt. *Partisan Review* **39**, 524–530.

Lifton, R. J. (1973a). The struggle for cultural rebirth. *Harpers'* **246**, 84–90.

Lifton, R. J. (1973b). The sense of immortality: on death and the continuity of life. *Am. J. Psychoanal.* **33**, 3–15.

Lifton, R. J. (1973c). *Home From the War: Vietnam Veterans – Neither Victims Nor Executioners.* New York: Simon & Schuster.

Lifton, R. J. (1975). On psychohistory. In R. J. Lifton & E. Olson (eds.), *Explorations in Psychohistory: the Wellfleet Papers.* New York: Simon & Schuster.

Lifton, R. J. (1976). *The Broken Connection* (in press).

Milgram, S. (1963). Behavioral study of obedience. *J. abnorm. soc. Psychol*, **67**, 371–378.

Milgram, S. (1967). Obedience to criminal order: the compulsion to do evil. *Patterns of Prejudice* **1**, 3–7.

Osmand, H. (1972). The medical model in psychiatry: love it or leave it. *Med. Ann. District of Columbia* **41**, 171–175.

Szasz, T. (1961). *The Myth of Mental Illness.* New York: Harper & Row.

Whitehead, A. N. (1938). *Modes of Thought.* New York: Capricorn (Macmillan), 1958.

Whyte, L. L. (1944). *The Next Development in Man.* London: Cresset Press.

Yankelovich, D. & Barrett, W. (1970). *Ego and Instinct.* New York: Random House.

Psychotherapy and Religious Values*

Allen E. Bergin

The importance of values, particularly religious ones, has recently become a more salient issue in psychology. The pendulum is swinging away from the naturalism, agnosticism, and humanism that have dominated the field for most of this century. There are more reasons for this than can be documented here, but a sampling illustrates the point:

1. Science has lost its authority as the dominating source of truth it once was. This change is both reflected in and stimulated by analyses that reveal science to be an intuitive and value-laden cultural form (Kuhn, 1970; Polanyi, 1962). The ecological, social, and political consequences of science and technology are no longer necessarily viewed as progress. Although a belief in the value of the scientific method appropriately persists, there is widespread disillusionment with the way it has been used and a loss of faith in it as the cure for human ills.

2. Psychology in particular has been dealt blows to its status as a source of authority for human action because of its obsession with 'methodolatry' (Bakan, 1972), its limited effectiveness in producing practical results, its conceptual incoherence, and its alienation from the mainstreams of the culture (Campbell, 1975; Hogan, 1979).

During a long period of religious indifference in Western civilization, the behavioral sciences rose to a crest of prominence as a potential alternative source of answers to basic life questions (London, 1964). Enrollments in psychology classes reached an unparalleled peak, but our promises were defeated by our premises. A psychology dominated by mechanistic thought and ethical naturalism has proved insufficient, and interest is declining. A corollary of this trend is the series of searing professional critiques of the assumptions on which the field rests (Braginsky & Braginsky, 1974; Collins, 1977; Kitchener, 1980; Myers, 1978).

3. Modern times have spawned anxiety, alienation, violence, selfishness (Kanfer, 1979). and depression (Klerman, 1979); but the human spirit appears irrepressible. People want something more. The spiritual and social failures of many organized religious systems have been followed by the failures of nonreligious approaches. This seems to have stimulated renewed hope in spiritual phenomena. Some of this, as manifested in the proliferation of cults, magic, superstitions, coercive practices, and emotionalism, indicates the negative possibilities in the trend: but the rising prominence of thoughtful and rigorous attempts to restore a spiritual perspective to analyses of personality, the human condition, and even science itself represents the positive possibilities (Collins, 1977; Myers, 1978; Tart, 1977).

4. Psychologists are being influenced by the force of this developing zeitgeist and are part of it. The emergence of studies of consciousness and cognition, which grew out of disillusionment with mechanistic behaviorism and the growth of humanistic psychology, has set the stage for a new examination of the possibility that presently unobservable realities – namely, spiritual forces – are at work in human behavior.

Rogers (1973) posed this radical development as follows:

There may be a few who will dare to investigate the possibility that there is a lawful reality which is not open to our five senses: a reality in which present past, and future are intermingled, in which space is not a barrier and time has disappeared. . . . It is one of the most exciting challenges posed to psychology. (p. 386)

Although there has always been a keen interest in such matters among a minority of thinkers and practitioners (Allport, 1950; James, 1902; Jung, 1958: the pastoral counseling field, etc.), they have not substantially influenced mainstream psychology. But the present phenomenon has all the aspects of a broad-based movement with a building momentum. This is indicated by an explosion of rigorous transcendental meditation research, the organization and rapid growth of the American Psychological Association's Division 36 (Psychologists Interested in Religious Issues, which sponsored nearly 70 papers at the 1979 national convention). The publication of new journals with overtly spiritual contents, such as the journal of *Judaism and Psychology* and the *Journal of Theology and Psychology*, and the emergence of new specialized, religious professional foci, such as the Association of Mormon Counselors and Psychotherapists the Christian Association for Psychological Studies, and so on.

These developments build in part on the long-standing but insufficiently recognized work in the psychology of religion represented by various organizations (e.g., Society for the Scientific Study of Religion. American Catholic Psychological Association), journals (e.g., *Review of Religious Research*), and individuals like Clark Dittes, Spilka, Strunk, and others (cf. Feifel, 1958; Malony, 1977; Strommen, 1971); however, the newer positions are more explicitly proreligious and are not deferent to mainstream psychology.

The trend is therefore also manifested by the publication of straightforward religious psychologies by academicians such as Jeeves (1976), Collins (1977), Peck (1978), Vitz (1977), and Myers (1978) and by more wide-open values analyses (Feinstein, 1979; Frank, 1977). Even textbooks are slowly beginning to introduce these formerly taboo considerations. In previous years basic psychology texts rarely mentioned religious phenomena, as though the psychology and sociology of religion literature did not exist. But the new edition of the leading introductory text (Hilgard, Atkinson, & Atkinson, 1979) contains a small section called 'The Miraculous.' Although the subject is still interpreted naturalistically, its inclusion does mark a change in response to changing views.

Values and Psychotherapy

These shifting conceptual orientations are especially manifest in the field of psychotherapy, in which the value of therapy and the values that prevade its processes have become topics of scrutiny by born professionals (Lowe, 1976; Smith, Glass, & Miller, in press; Szasz, 1978) and the public (Gross, 1978).

In what follows, these issues are analyzed, as they pertain to spiritual values, in terms of six theses.

Thesis 1: Values are an inevitable and pervasive part of psychotherapy. As an applied field, psychotherapy is directed toward practical goals that are selected in value terms. It is even necessary when establishing criteria for

* Bergin, A. E.: Psychotherapy and religious values. *Journal of Consulting and Clinical Psychology* **48**:95–105, 1980.

measuring therapeutic change to decide, on a value basis, what changes are desirable. This necessarily requires a philosophy of human nature that guides the selection of measurements and the setting of priorities regarding change. Strupp, Hadley, and Gomes-Schwartz (1977) argued that there are at least three possibly divergent value systems at play in such decision – those of the client, the clinician, and the community at large. They stated that though there is no consensus regarding conceptions of mental health, a judgment must always be made in relation to some implicit or explicit standard, which presupposes a definition of what is better or worse. They asked that we consider the following:

If, following psychotherapy, a patient manifests increased self-assertion coupled with abrasiveness, is this good or a poor therapy outcome? . . . If . . . a patient obtains a divorce, is this to be regarded as a desirable or an undesirable change? A patient may turn from homosexuality to heterosexuality or he may become more accepting of either; an ambitious, striving person may abandon previously valued goals and become more placid (e.g., in primal therapy). How are such changes to be evaluated?

(Strupp et al., 1977, pp. 92–93)

Equally important is the face that

in increasing number, patients enter psychotherapy not for the cure of traditional 'symptoms' but (at least extensible) for the purpose of finding meaning in their lives, for actualizing themselves, or for maximizing their potential.

(Strupp et al., 1977, p. 93)

Consequently, 'every aspect of psychotherapy presupposes some implicit moral doctrine' (London, 1964, p. 6). Lowe's (1976) treatise on value orientations in counseling and psychotherapy reveals with painstaking clarity the philosophical choices on which the widely divergent approaches to intervention hinge. He argued cogently that everything from behavioral technology to community consultation is intricately interwoven with secularized moral systems, and he supported London's (1964) thesis that psychotherapists constitute a secular priesthood that purports to establish standards of good living.

Techniques are thus a means for mediating the value influence intended by the therapist. It is inevitable that the therapist be such a moral agent. The danger is in ignoring the reality that we do this, for then patient, therapist, and community neither agree on goals nor efficiently work toward them. A correlated danger is that therapists, as secular moralists, may promote changes not valued by the client or the community, and in this sense, if there is not some consensus and openness about what is being done, the therapists may be unethical or subversive.

The-impossibility of a value-free therapy is demonstrated by certain data. I allude to just one of many illustrations that might be cited. Carl Rogers personally values the freedom of the individual and attempts to promote the free expression of each client. However, two independent studies done a decade apart (Murray, 1956; Truax, 1966) showed that Carl Rogers systematically rewarded and punished expressions that he liked and did not like in the verbal behavior of clients. His values significantly regulated the structure and content of therapeutic sessions as well as their outcomes (cf. Bergin, 1971). If a person who intends to be nondirective cannot be, then it is likely that the rest of us cannot either.

Similarly, when we do research with so-called objective criteria, we select them in terms of subjective value judgments, which is one reason we have so much difficulty in agreeing on the results of psychotherapy outcome studies. If neither practitioners nor researchers can be nondirective, then they must accept certain realities about the influence they have. A value-free approach is impossible.

Thesis 2: Not only do theories, techniques, and criteria reveal pervasive value judgments, but outcome data comparing the effects of diverse techniques show that non-technical, value-laden factors pervade professional change processes. Comparative studies reveal few differences across techniques, thus suggesting that nontechnical or personal variables account for much of the change. Smith et al. (in press), in analyzing 475 outcome studies, were able to attribute only a small percentage of outcome variance to technique factors. Among these 475 studies were many that included supposedly technical behavior therapy procedures. The lack of technique differences thrusts value questions upon us because change appears to be a function of common human interactions, including personal and belief factors – the so-called nonspecific or common ingredients that cut across therapies and that may be the core of therapeutic change (Bergin & Lambert, 1978; Frank, 1961, 1973).

Thesis 3: Two broad classes of values are dominant in the mental health professions. Both exclude religious values, and both establish goals for change that frequently clash with theistic systems of belief. The first of these can be called clinical pragmatism. Clinical pragmatism is espoused particularly by psychiatrists, nurses, behavior therapists, and public agencies,. It consists of straightforward implementation of the values of the dominant social system. In other words, the clinical operation functions within the system. It does not ordinarily question the system, but tries to make the system work. It is centered, then, on diminishing pathologies or disturbances, as defined by the clinician as an agent of the culture. This means adherence to such objectives as reducing anxiety, relieving depression, resolving guilt, suppressing deviation, controlling bizarreness, smoothing conflict, diluting obsessiveness, and so forth. The medical origins of this system are clear. It is pathology oriented. Health is defined as the absence of pathology. Pathology is that which disturbs the person or those in the environment. The clinician then forms an alliance with the person and society to eliminate the disturbing behavior.

The second major value system can be called humanistic idealism. It is espoused particularly by clinicians with interests in philosophy and social reform such as Erich Fromm. Carl Rogers, Rollo May, and various group and community interventionists. Vaughan's (1971) study of this approach identified quantifiable themes that define the goals of positive change within this frame of reference. They are flexibility and self-exploration; independence; active goal orientation with self-actualization as a core goal; human dignity and self-worth interpersonal involvement; truth and honesty, happiness; and a frame of orientation or philosophy by which one guides one's life. This is different from clinical pragmatism in that it appeals to idealists, reformers creative persons, and sophisticated clients who have significant ego strength. It is less practical, less conforming, and harder to measure than clinical pathology themes because it addresses more directly broad issues such as what is good and how life should be lived. It embraces a social value agenda and is often critical of traditional systems of religious values that influence child rearing, social standards, and ultimately, criteria of positive therapeutic change. Its influence is more prevalent in private therapy, universities, and independent clinical centers or research institutes, and among theologians and clinicians who espouse spiritual humanism (Fromm, 1950).

Though clinical pragmatism and humanistic idealism have appropriate places as guiding structures for clinical intervention and though I personally endorse much of their content, they are not sufficient to cover the spectrum of values pertinent to human beings and the frameworks within which they function. Noticeably absent are theistically based values.

Pragmatic and humanistic views manifest a relative indifference to God, the relationship of human beings to God, and the possibility that spiritual factors influence behavior. A survey of the leading reference sources in the clinical field reveals little literature on such subjects, except for naturalistic accounts. An examination of 30 introductory psychology texts turned up no references to the possible reality of spiritual factors. Most did not have the words God or religion in their indexes.

Psychological writers have a tendency to censor or taboo in a casual and sometimes arrogant way something that is sensitive and precious to most human beings (Campbell, 1975).

As Robert Hogan, new section editor of the Journal of Personality and Social Psychology, stated in a recent APA Monitor interview,

Religion is the most important social force in the history of man . . . . But in psychology, anyone who gets involved in or tries to talk in an analytic, careful way about religion is immediately branded a meat-head; a mystic; an intuitive, touch-feely sort of moron.

(Hogan, 1979, p. 4).

Clinical pragmatism and humanistic idealism thus exclude what is one of the largest sub-ideologies, namely, religious or theistic approaches espoused by people who believe in God and try to guide their behavior in terms of their perception of his will.

Other alternatives are thus needed. Just as psychotherapy has been enhanced by the adoption of multiple techniques, so also in the values realm, our frameworks can be improved by the use of additional perspectives.

The alternative I wish to put forward is a spiritual one. It might be called theistic realism. I propose to show that this alternative is necessary for ethical and effective help among religious people, who constitute 30% to 90% of the U.S. population (more than 90% expressed belief, while about 30% expressed strong conviction about their belief; American Institute of Public Opinion, 1978). I also argue that the values on which this alternative is based are important ingredients in reforming and rejuvenating our society. Pragmatic and humanistic values alone, although they have substantial virtues, are often part of the problem of our deteriorating society.

What are the alternative values? The first and most important axiom is that God exists, that human beings are the creations of God, and that there are unseen spiritual processes by which the link between God and humanity is maintained. As stated in the Book of Job (32:8),

There is a spirit in man and the inspiration of the Almighty giveth them understanding.

This approach, beginning with faith in God, assumes that spiritual conviction gives values an added power to influence life.

With respect to such belief, Max Born, the physicist, said, 'There are two objectionable kinds of believers. Those who believe the incredible and those who believe that belief must be discarded in favor of the scientific method' (cited in Menninger, 1963, p. 374). I stand in opposition to placing the scientific method in the place of God, an attitude akin to Bakan's (1972) notion of 'methodolatry' that has become common in our culture.

Abraham Maslow, though viewed as a humanist, expressed concepts in harmony with the views presented here. He said, 'It looks as if there is a single, ultimate value for mankind – a far goal toward which men strive' (cited in Goble, 1971, p. 92). He believed that to study human behavior means never to ignore concepts of right and wrong:

If behavioral scientists are to solve human problems, the question of right and wrong behavior is essential. It is the very essence of behavioral science. Psychologists who advocate moral and cultural relativism are not coming to grips with the real problem. Too many behavioral scientists have rejected not only the methods of religion but the values as well.

(Maslow, cited in Goble, 1971, p. 92)

To quote further, 'Instead of cultural relativity, I am implying that there are basic underlying human standards that are cross cultural' (Maslow, cited in Goble, 1971, p. 92). Maslow advocated the notion of a synergistic culture in which the values of the group make demands on the individual that are self-fulfilling. The values of such a culture are considered transcendent and not relative.

Maslow's views are consistent with the notion that there are laws of human behavior. If such laws exist, they do not sustain notions of ethical relativism. Kitchener (1980) has shown, for example, that behavioristic, evolutionary, and naturalistic ethical concepts are not relativistic (cf. Bergin, 1980). He makes the important point that ethical relativism is not a logical derivative of cultural relativism. Such views are consistent with the axiom of theistic systems that human growth is regulated by moral principles comparable in exactness with physical laws. The possible lawfulness of these moral traditions has been argued persuasively by Campbell (1975). Some comparative religionists (Palmer, Note 1) and anthropologists (Gusdorf, 1976) also recognize common religious value themes across dominant world cultures. Palmer in particular has stated that 80% of the world population adhere to common value themes consistent with the theses argued here (cf. Bergin, in press). Conceivably, these moral themes reflect something lawful in human behavior.

In light of the foregoing, it is possible to draw contrasts between theistic and clinical humanistic values as they pertain to personality and change. These are my own constructions based on clinical and religious experience and are not intended to support organized religion in general. History demonstrates that religions and religious values can be destructive, just as psychotherapy can be if not properly practiced. I therefore am not endorsing all religion. I am simply extracting from religious traditions prominent themes I hypothesize may be positive additions to clinical thinking. These are depicted in Table 1 along side the contrasting views.

It should be noted that the theistic value do not come ex nihilo, but are consistent with a substantial psychological literature concerning responsibility (Glasser, 1965; Menninger, 1973), moral agency (Rychlak, 1979), guilt (Mowrer, 1961, 1967), and self-transcendence (Frankl, Note 2).

The comparisons outlined in the table highlight differences for the sake of making the point. It is taken for granted, however, that there are also domains of significant agreement, such as many of the humanistic values outlined by Vaughan (1971) that are fundamental to personal growth.

Table 1 Theistic Versus Clinical and Humanistic Values

Theistic	Clinical–Humanistic
God is supreme. Humanity, acceptance of (divine) authority, and obedience (to the will of God) are virtues.	Humans are supreme. The self is aggrandized. Autonomy and rejection of external authority are virtues.
Personal identity is eternal and derived from the divine. Relationship with God defines self-worth.	Identity is ephemeral and mortal. Relationships with others define self-worth.
Self-control in terms of absolute values. Strict morality. Universal ethics.	Self-expression in terms of relative values. Flexible morality. Situation ethics.
Love, affection, and self-transcendence are primary. Service and self-sacrifice are central to personal growth.	Personal needs and self-actualization are primary. Self-satisfaction is central to personal growth.
Committed to marriage, fidelity and loyalty. Emphasis on procreation and family life as integrative factors.	Open marriage or no marriage. Emphasis on self-gratification or recreational sex without long-term responsibilities.
Personal responsibility for own harmful actions and changes in them. Acceptance of guilt, suffering, and contrition as keys to change. Restitution for harmful effects.	Others are responsible for our problems and changes. Minimizing guilt and relieving suffering before experiencing its meaning. Apology for harmful effects.
Forgiveness of others who cause distress (including parents) completes the therapeutic restoration of self.	Acceptance and expression of accusatory feelings are sufficient.
Knowledge by faith and self-effort. Meaning and purpose derived from spiritual insight. Intellectual knowledge inseparable from the emotional and spiritual. Ecology of knowledge.	Knowledge by self-effort alone. Meaning and purpose derived from reason and intellect. Intellectual knowledge for itself. Isolation of the mind from the rest of life.

Fromm's brilliant essays on love (1956) and independence (1947), for example, illustrate value themes that must be given prominence in any comprehensive system. The point of difference is their relative position or emphasis in the values hierarchy. Mutual commitment to fundamental human rights is also assumed, for example, to those rights pertaining to life, liberty, and the pursuit of happiness specified in the Declaration of Independence. Both theistic and atheistic totalitarianism deprive people of the basic freedoms necessary to fully implement any of the value systems outlined here; therefore, clinical humanists, pragmatists, and theists all reject coercion and value freedom of choice. This basic common premise is a uniting thesis. Without it, theories of mental health would have little meaning.

Substantial harmony can thus be achieved among the views outlined, but there is a tendency for clinical pragmatism and humanistic idealism to exclude the theistic position. On the other hand, religionists have tended to be unempirical and need to adopt the value of rigorous empiricism advocated by humanists and pragmatists. My view then would be to posit what each tradition can learn from the other rather than to create an artificial battle in which one side purports to win and the other to lose. Thus, the religion-based hypotheses stated later in Thesis 6 are an open invitation to think about and test these ideas.

Thesis 4: There is a significant contrast between the values of mental health professionals and those of a large proportion of clients. Whether or not one agrees with the values I have described above, one must admit that they are commonplace. Therapists therefore need to take into account possible discrepancies between their values and those of the average client. Four studies document this point. Lilienfeld (1966) found at the Metropolitan Hospital in New York City large discrepancies between the values of the mental health staff members and their clients, who were largely of Puerto Rican, Catholic background. With respect to topics like sex, aggression, and authority, the differences were dramatic. For example, in reply to one statement, 'Some sex before marriage is good,' all 19 mental health professionals agreed but only half the patients agreed. Vaughan (1971), in his study of various samples of patients, students, and professionals in the Philadelphia area, found discrepancies similar to those Lilienfeld obtained. Henry, Sims, and Spray (1971), in their study of several thousand psychotherapists in New York, Chicago, and Los Angeles, found the values of therapists to be religiously liberal relative to those of the population at large. Ragan, Malony, and Beit-Hallahmi (Note 3) reported that of a random sample of psychologists from the American Psychological Association, 50% believed in God. This is about 40% lower than the population at large, though higher than one would expect on the basis of the impression created in the literature and at convention presentations. This study also indicated that 10% of the psychologists held positions in their various congregations, which also indicates more involvement than is predictable from the public statements of psychologists. Nevertheless, the main findings show that the beliefs of mental health professionals are not very harmonious with those of the subcultures with which they deal, especially as they pertain to definitions of moral behavior and the relevance of moral behavior to societal integration, familial functioning, prevention of pathology, and development of the self.

Thesis 5: In light of the foregoing, it would be honest and ethical to acknowledge that we are implementing our own value systems via our professional work and to be more explicit about what we believe while also respecting the value systems of others. If values are pervasive, if our values tend to be on the whole discrepant from those of the community or the client population, it would be ethical to publicize where we stand. Then people would have a better choice of what they want to get into, and we would avoid deception.

Hans Strupp and I (Bergin & Strupp, 1972) had an interesting conversation with Carl Rogers on this subject in La Jolla a few years ago, in which Carl said,

Yes, it is true, psychotherapy is subversive. I don't really mean it to be, but some people get involved with me who don't know what they are getting into. Therapy theories and techniques promote a new model of man contrary to that which has been traditionally acceptable.

(Paraphrase cited in Bergin & Strupp, 1972, pp. 318–319)

Sometimes, as professionals, we follow the leaders of our profession or our graduate professors in assuming that what we are doing is professional without recognizing that we are purveying under the guise of professionalism and science our own personal value systems (Smith, 1961), whether the system be psychodynamic, behavioral, humanistic, cognitive, or whatever.

During my graduate and postdoctoral training, I had the fortunate experience of working with several leaders in psychology, such as Albert Bandura, Carl Rogers, and Robert Sears. (Later, I had opportunities for substantial discussions with Joseph Wolpe, B. F. Skinner, and many others). These were good experiences with great men for whom I continue to have deep respect and warmth; but I gradually found our views on values issues to be quite different. I had expected their work to be 'objective' science, but it became clear that these leaders' research, theories, and techniques were implicit expressions of humanistic and naturalistic belief systems that dominated both psychology and American universities generally. Since their professional work was an expression of such views, I felt constrained from full expression of my values by their assumptions or faiths and the prevailing, sometimes coercive, ideologies of secular universities.

Like others, I too have not always overtly harmonized my values and professional work. By now exercising the right to integrate religious themes into mainstream clinical theory, research, and practice, I hope to achieve this. By being explicit about what I value and how it articulates with a professional role, I hope to avoid unknowingly drawing clients or students into my system. I hope that, together, many of us will succeed in demonstrating how this can be healthy and fruitful.

If we are unable to face our own values openly, it means we are unable to face ourselves, which violates a primary principle of professional conduct in our field. Since we expect our clients to examine their perceptions and value constructs, we ought to do likewise. The result will be improved capacity to understand and help people, because self-deceptions and role playing will decrease and personal congruence will increase.

Thesis 6: It is our obligation as professionals to translate what we perceive and value intuitively into something that can be openly tested and evaluated. I do not expect anyone to accept my values simply because I have asserted them. I only ask that we accept the notion that our values arise out of a personal milieu of experience and private intuition or inspiration. Since they are personal and subjective and are shaped by the culture with which we are most familiar, they should influence professional work only to the extent that we can openly justify them. As a general standard, I would advocate that we (a) examine our values within our idiosyncratic personal milieus: (b) acknowledge that our value commitments are subjective; (c) be clear; (d) be open; (e) state the values in a professional context without fear, as hypotheses for testing and common consideration by the pluralistic groups with which we work; and (f) subject them to test, criticism, and verification.

On this basis, I would like to offer a few testable hypotheses.[1] These are some of the possibilities that derive from my personal experience.

1. Religious communities that provide the combination of a viable belief structure and a network of loving, emotional support should manifest lower rates of emotional and social pathology and physical disease. To some extent this can already be documented (cf. Lynch, 1977).

2. Those who endorse high standards of impulse control (or strict moral standards) have lower than average rates of alcoholism, addiction, divorce, emotional instability, and associated interpersonal difficulties. For example, Masters and Johnson (1975, p. 185) found that 'swingers' at a 1-year follow-up had reduced their sexual activity and had stopped swinging.

---

1 Hypotheses like these have been tested, with ambiguous results (Argyle & Beit-Hallahmi, 1975). The reasons for the ambiguous results are analyzed in a forthcoming paper by our research group.

They apparently found that low impulse control increased the subjects' problems, and all but one couple said they were looking for an improved sense of social and personal security.

3. Disturbances in clinical cases will diminish as these individuals are encouraged to adopt forgiving attitudes toward parents and others who may have had a part in the development of their symptoms.

4. Infidelity or disloyalty to any interpersonal commitment, especially marriage, leads to harmful consequences – both interpersonally and intrapsychically.

5. Teaching clients love, commitment, service, and sacrifice for others will help heal interpersonal difficulties and reduce intrapsychic distress.

6. Improving male commitment, caring, and responsibility in families will reduce marital and familial conflict and associated psychological disorders. A correlated hypothesis is that father and husband absence, aloofness, disinterest, rejection, and abuse are major factors and possibly *the* major factors in familial and interpersonal disorganization. This is based on the assumption that the divine laws of love, nurturance, and self-sacrifice apply as much to men as to women but that men have traditionally ignored them more than women.

7. A good marriage and family life constitute a psychologically and socially benevolent state. As the percentage of persons in a community who live in such circumstances increases, social pathologies will decrease and vice versa.

8. Properly understood, personal suffering can increase one's compassion and potential for helping others.

9. The kinds of values described herein have social consequences. There is a social ecology, and the viability of this social ecology varies as a function of personal conviction, morality, and the quality of the social support network in which we exist. If one considers the 50 billion dollars a year we spend on social disorders like venereal disease, alcoholism, drug abuse, and so on, these are major symptoms or social problems. Their roots, I assume, lie in values, personal conduct, morality, and social philosophy. There are some eloquent spokesmen in favor of this point (Campbell, 1975; Lasch, 1978; and others). I quote only one, Alexander Solzhenitsyn, who said,

A fact which cannot be disputed is the weakening of human personality in the West while in the East it has become firmer and stronger. How did the West decline? . . . I am referring to the calamity of an autonomous, irreligious, humanistic consciousness. It has made man the measure of all things on earth . . . . Is it true that man is above everything? Is there no superior spirit above him? Is it right that man's life . . . should be ruled by material expansion above all? . . . The world . . . has reached a major watershed in history. . . . It will demand from us a spiritual blaze, we shall have to rise to a new height of vision . . . where . . . our spiritual being will not be trampled upon as in the Modern Era.

(Solzhenitsyn, 1978, pp. 681–684)

Conclusion

Although numerous points of practical contact can be made between religious and other value approaches, it is my view that the religious ones offer a distinctive challenge to our theories, inquiries, and clinical methods. This challenge has not fully been understood or dealt with.

Religion is at the fringe of clinical psychology when it should be at the center. Value questions pervade the field, but discussion of them is dominated by viewpoints that are alien to the religious subcultures of most of the people whose behavior we try to explain and influence. Basic conflicts between value systems of clinical professionals, clients, and the public are dealt with unsystematically or not at all. Too often, we opt for the comforting role of experts applying technologies and obscure our role as moral agents, yet our code of ethics declares that we should show a 'sensible regard for the social codes and moral expectations of the community' (American Psychological Association, 1972, p. 2).

I realize that there are difficulties in applying the notion of a particular spiritual value perspective in a pluralistic and secular society. I think it should be done on the basis of some evidence that supports doing it as opposed to the basis of the current format, which is to implement one's values without the benefit of either a public declaration or an effort to gather data on the consequences of doing so.

It is my hope that the theses I have proposed will be contemplated with deliberation and not emotional dismissal. They have been presented in sincerity, with passion tempered by reason, and with a hope that our profession will become more comprehensive and effective in its capacity to help all of the human family.

Reference Notes

1   Palmer, S. Personal communication. April 1977.
2   Frankl, V. Honors seminar lecture, Brigham Young University, November 3, 1978.
3   Ragan, C. P., Malony. H. N., & Beit-Hallahmi, B. *Psychologists and religion: Professional factors related to personal religiosity.* Paper presented at the meeting of the American Psychological Association, Washington, D.C., September 1976.

References

Allport, G. W. *The individual and his religion: A psychological interpretation.* New York: Macmillan. 1950.

American Institute of Public Opinion. Religion in America, 1977–78. *Gallup opinion index*, Report No. 145. Princeton, N.J.; Author, 1978.

American Psychological Association. *Ethical standards of psychologists.* Washington. D.C.; Author, 1972.

Argyle. M., & Beit-Hallahmi, B. *The social psychology of religion.* London: Routledge & Kegan Paul, 1975.

Bakan, C. Interview. In A. E. Bergin & H. H. Strupp (Eds.), *Changing frontiers in the science of psychotherapy.* Chicago: Aldine, 1972.

Bergin, A. E. Carl Rogers' contribution to a fully functioning psychology. In A. R. Mahrer & L. Pearson (Eds.), *Creative developments in psychotherapy* (Vol. 1). Cleveland, Ohio: Case Western Reserve University Press, 1971.

Bergin, A. E. Behavior therapy and ethical relativism: Time for clarity. *Journal of Consulting and Clinical Psychology*, 1980, **48**, 11–13.

Bergin, A. E. Conceptual basis for a religious approach to psychotherapy. In K. S. Larsen (Ed.), *Psychology and ideology* (Vol. 3). Monmouth, Oreg.: Institute for Theoretical History, in press.

Bergin, A. E., & Lambert, M. J. The evaluation of therapeutic outcomes. In S. L. Garfield & A. E. Bergin (Eds.), *Handbook of psychotherapy and behavior change.* (2nd ed.) New York: Wiley, 1978.

Bergin, A. E., & Strupp, H. H. *Changing frontiers in the science of psychotherapy.* Chicago: Aldine, 1972.

Braginsky, D., & Braginsky, B. *Mainstream psychology: A critique.* New York: Holt, Rinehart & Winston, 1974.

Campbell, D. T. On the conflicts between biological and social evolution and between psychology and moral tradition. *American Psychologist*, 1975, **30**, 1103–1120.

Collins, G. R. *The rebuilding of psychology: An integration of psychology and Christianity.* Wheaton, Ill.: Tyndale House, 1977.

Feifel, H. Symposium on relationships between religion and mental health. *American Psychologist*, 1958, **13**, 565–579.

Feinstein, A.D. Personal mythology as a paradigm for a holistic psychology. *American Journal of Orthopsychiatry*, 1979, **49**, 198–217.

Frank, J. D. *Persuasion and healing.* Baltimore, Md.: Johns Hopkins University Press, 1961.

Frank, J. D. *Persuasion and healing,* (2nd ed.). Baltimore, Md.: Johns Hopkins University Press, 1973.

Frank, J. D. Nature and functions of belief systems: Humanism and transcendental religion. *American Psychologist*, 1977, **32**, 555–559.

Fromm, E. *Man for himself.* New York: Rinehart. 1947.

Fromm, E. *Psychoanalysis and religion.* New Haven, Conn.: Yale University Press, 1950.

Fromm, E. *The art of loving.* New York: Harper & Row, 1956.

Glasser. W. *Reality therapy.* New York: Harper & Row, 1965.

Goble, F. G. *The third force: The psychology of Abraham Maslow.* New York: Pocket Books, 1971.

Gross. M. L. *The psychological society.* New York: Random House, 1978.

Gusdorf, G. P. Philosophical anthropology. *Encyclopedia Britannica,* 1976, **1,** 975–985.

Henry, W. E., Sims, J. H., & Spray, S. L. *The fifth profession: Becoming a psychotherapist.* San Francisco: Jossey-Bass, 1971.

Hilgard, E. R., Atkinson, R. L., & Atkinson, R. C. *Introduction to psychology* (7th ed.). New York: Harcourt Brace Jovanovich, 1979.

Hogan, R. Interview. *APA Monitor,* April 1979, pp. 4–5.

James, W. *The varieties of religious experience,* Garden City, N.Y.: Doubleday, 1902.

Jeeves, M. A. *Psychology and Christianity: The view both ways.* Leicester, England: Inter-Varsity Press. 1976.

Jung, C. G. *The collected works: Vol. II. Psychology and religion: West and East.* New York: Pantheon, Books, 1958.

Kanfer, F. H. Personal control, social control, and altruism: Can society survive the age of individualism? *American Psychologist,* 1979, **34,** 231–239.

Kitchener, R. F. Ethical relativism and behavior therapy. *Journal of Consulting and Clinical Psychology,* 1980, **48,** 1–7.

Klerman, G. L. The age of melancholy? *Psychology Today,* April 1979, pp. 36–42; 88–90.

Kuhn, T. S. *The structure of scientific revolutions* (2nd ed.). Chicago: University of Chicago Press. 1970.

Lasch, C. *The culture of narcissism.* New York: Norton. 1978.

Lilienfeld, D. M. The relationship between mental health information and moral values of lower class psychiatric clinic patients and psychiatric evaluation and disposition (Doctoral dissertation, Columbia University, 1965). *Dissertation Abstracts,* 1966, **27,** 610B-611B. (University Microfilms No. 66–6941).

London, P. *The modes and morals of psychotherapy,* New York: Holt, Rinehart & Winston. 1964.

Lowe, C. M. *Value orientations in counseling and psychotherapy: The meanings of mental health* (2nd ed.). Cranston, R.I.: Carroll Press, 1976.

Lynch, J. J. *The broken heart: The medical consequences of loneliness.* New York: Basic Books, 1977.

Malony, H. N. (Ed.). *Current perspectives in the psychology of religion.* Grand Rapids, Mich.: Eerdmans, 1977.

Masters, W. H. & Johnson, V. E. *The pleasure bond.* New York: Bantam Books, 1975.

Menninger, K. *The vital balance: The life process in mental health and illness,* New York: Viking Press, 1963.

Menninger, K. *Whatever became of sin?* New York: Hawthorn Books, 1973.

Mowrer, O. H. *The crisis in psychiatry and religion,* Princeton, N.J.: Van Nostrand, 1961.

Mowrer, O. H. (Ed.) *Morality and mental health.* Chicago: Rand McNally, 1967.

Murray, E. J. A content-analysis method for studying psychotherapy. *Psychological Monographs,* 1956, **70** (13, Whole No. 420).

Myers, D. G. *The human puzzle: Psychological research and Christian belief.* New York: Harper & Row, 1978.

Peck, M. S. *The road less traveled: A new psychology of love, traditional values, and spiritual growth.* New York: Simon & Schuster, 1978.

Polanyi, M. *Personal knowledge: Towards a post-critical philosophy.* Chicago: University of Chicago Press. 1962.

Rogers, C. R. Some new challenges. *American Psychologist,* 1973, **28,** 379–387.

Rychlak, J. F. *Discovering free will and personal responsibility.* New York: Oxford University Press, 1979.

Smith, M. B. 'Mental health' reconsidered: A special case of the problem of values in psychology. *American Psychologist,* 1961, **16,** 299–306.

Smith, M. L., Glass, G. V., & Miller, T. I,. *The benefits of psychotherapy.* Baltimore, Md.: Johns Hopkins University Press, in press.

Solzhenitsyn, A. A world split apart: The world demands from us a spiritual blaze. *Vital Speeches of the Day,* 1978, **45,** 678–684.

Strommen, M. P. *Research on religious development: A comprehensive handbook.* New York: Hawthorn Books, 1971.

Strupp, H. H., Hadley, S. W., & Gomes-Schwartz. B. *Psychotherapy for better or worse: The problem of negative effects.* New York: Aronson, 1977.

Szasz, T. S. *The myth of psychotherapy: Mental healing as religion, rhetoric, and repression.* Garden City, N.Y.: Doubleday, 1978.

Tart, C. *Transpersonal psychologies.* New York: Harper & Row, 1977.

Truax, C. B. Reinforcement and nonreinforcement in Rogerian psychotherapy. *Journal of Abnormal Psychology,* 1966, **71,** 1–9.

Vaughan, J. B. Measurement and analysis of values pertaining to psychotherapy and mental health (Doctoral dissertation, Columbia University, 1971). *Dissertation Abstracts International,* 1971, **32,** 3655B–3656B. (University Microfilms No. 72–1394)

Vitz, P. C. *Psychology as religion: The cult of self-worship.* Grand Rapids, Mich.: Eerdmans, 1977.

The Negotiation of Values in Therapy*

Harry J. Aponte

WHEN THERAPIST and family engage in therapy, they embark upon a personal relationship that is framed by the professional parameters of therapy. This is particularly true in the more therapist-active modalities such as family therapy in which therapists, in some degree, give opinions, share judgments, make suggestions, and assume overt relational positions vis-à-vis family members for the purpose of trying to influence family relationships.

Therapists draw upon both their professional training and personal life experience to understand and intervene with families. The human problems that families present have common elements with the issues therapists have had and are currently dealing with in their own lives. Both therapists and families define and interpret their respective personal issues through diverse dimensions, including their emotional experiences and personal values.

Values frame the entire process of therapy. They are the social standards by which therapists define problems, establish criteria for evaluation, fix parameters for technical interventions, and select therapeutic goals. All transactions between therapist and family or individual about these aspects of therapy involve negotiations about the respective value systems that each party brings into the therapeutic relationship.

These values, whether moral, cultural, or political, are the standards by which a person directs his actions and defines, interprets, and judges all social phenomena. A person's values are drawn from family life, social networks, educational experiences, and community and sociopolitical organizations. These multiple standards converge into the complex configurations that become the dynamically evolving value systems of the therapist and the families and individuals in treatment.

Society's values are propagated through its social structures, including therapy, which is one of society's means for helping people manage their lives within its value framework. The founders, teachers, and practitioners of therapy, including the institutions they represent, all infuse therapy with their values.

Therapy is shaped by the interaction of the personal values of therapists with the values of societal institutions such as social agencies, psychiatric clinics and hospitals, along with government, insurance companies, professional associations, and academic and training facilities. These institutional representatives of society systematically, and often in coordination, set regulations for the practice of psychotherapy. They define what psychotherapy is, who is eligible to receive it, and who is qualified to practice it. They also decide the conditions for which and the extent to which psychotherapy will be subsidized financially, whether through direct insurance payments or tax deductions, and which patients (families, couples, or individuals), and practitioners will be approved for these supports. In making these determinations, societal representatives implement their values about the nature of mental illness, family pathology, and treatment. They thereby institutionalize their views about society's relationship to these human difficulties and their alleviation.

These complexes of values are then filtered in a variety of ways and forms through the therapist to the individuals and families exposed to therapy. Values conveyed by the therapist confront the individual's and family's own values in the therapeutic process. Therapist and patient negotiate the value framework within which problems are interpreted, goals are defined, and approaches to solutions are selected.

Depending, in part, upon their school of therapy, there is a myth among many therapists that their work is 'technical,' 'scientific,' or perhaps even 'artistic,' but in any case, free of moral and social value biases. This is patently not only untrue, but impossible.

Some therapists acknowledge the values inherent in their therapeutic approaches; most do not. Consider some of these quotes. First, from an individually oriented, psychoanalytic therapist: 'This concept of good [for a patient] must derive from what I want for myself together with an identification with the human community . . . [while] the therapist . . . functions not only as 'good parent,' but also as a representative of the community' (6, p. 37). One family therapist states that the 'cornerstone' of his therapy is a concern for 'the long-term preservation of an oscillating balance among family members, whereby the basic interests of each are taken into account by the others . . . .' (3, p. 160). Another family therapist approaches family problems involving children by assuming that 'the hierarchy in the family is in confusion' and proceeds to advise a strategy by which 'the therapist should side with the parents against the problem young person, even if this seems to be depriving him or her of individual choices and rights' (7, p. 45). Finally, another family therapist from a different school of thought views emotion as impeding the intellect in the functioning of families, as evidenced by his statement that 'as the intellectual system gains more separateness from emotional influence, it is freer to define principles and beliefs based on objective assessments of available knowledge' (12, p. 238).

Since relatively few therapists explicitly acknowledge and identify the values underpinning their theories and methods, it is difficult to compare their implicit values on the same continuum. The preceding quotes offer glimpses and clues about the variety of values represented by therapists. Values are inherent in the theoretical level of therapy as well as in its practical application. To illustrate the pervasiveness of values in therapy, even at an abstract theoretical level, take the concept of 'circularity,' a concept drawn by family therapists from the work of Gregory Bateson. The circular model is opposed to the linear, with the former assigning no beginning or end to a complex of circular loops of interactions, whereas the latter speaks in terms of cause and effect in human transactions.

In recognizing the systemic nature of human relationships, the circular model throws light on the nature of the linkage in social transactions. Consider one interpretation of the implications for therapy of the concept of circularity in social systems:

The therapist can no longer be seen as 'impacting' on the client or family . . . . The therapist is not an agent and the client is not a subject. Both are part of a larger field in which therapist, family, and any number of other elements act and react upon each other in unpredictable ways.

[9, p. 8]

Circularity would appear to stand as a principle free of social bias, but this interpretation of the concept also seems to negate the personal responsibility

---

* Aponte, H. J.: The negotiation of values in therapy. *Family Process* **24**:323–338, 1985.

of therapists, individuals, and families in their transactions in therapy. If there is no cause and effect in a transaction, then how can one assign or assume responsibility? There are a variety of responses to this question, but the intention here is not to resolve the issue. It is to demonstrate how an apparently value-free theoretical principle in therapy may imply values of significant social import to the professional and the family in the therapeutic relationship.

At a practical level, values are an important issue even in such an elemental matter as the selection of the object of therapy. For example, theorists and practitioners in the field of family therapy consider the object of therapy, the family, to be many different things, including the nuclear family, the extended family, or even the family and its social network. A therapist's decision about what 'parents' to include in the therapy, whether a biological parent, a stepparent, or a live-in adult partner of a biological parent, may have socially sanctioning or disqualifying implications, whatever the therapist's rationale or intentions.

Take, for instance, the value perspectives inherent in Keith and Whitaker's(11) discussion about their work with Ed, who had separated from his wife, Molly, and was living with Linda while trying to decide about divorcing Molly. The therapists included Linda and, apparently, Ed's children from his marriage in sessions with Molly and Ed.

Molly and Linda noted with amusement how they would sometimes pair to mother Ed. The children steered clear of Linda. They orbited mainly around Ed and Molly. The two women, however, were the best weekend parent set for the boys.

[p. 125]

Ultimately, the therapist's value system defines the social unit or network that is to assume responsibility for defining the 'family' problem and for working with the therapist to settle on goals and the means to those goals. This same issue is contained in Elkaïm's(4) thesis that the problems of an individual or family may be the result of society's relationship to them; therefore, the appropriate intervention in such a case must aim at a change in the sociopolitical context of families by working with the families to change their community(4). In these examples, the therapists' determinations about who constitute the 'family' for the theater of therapy and what components of society make up the proper object of change in therapy conveyed distinct social values.

Again, from a practical standpoint, the question of values is also central to assessment and evaluation in therapy. One cannot evaluate without standards. If evaluative standards are drawn from society's determination of what is functional and appropriate in personal and social adjustment, then they are rooted in the society's value framework. If one could disassociate symptomatic behavior from its social context, an argument could be made about its being unencumbered by social significance and, therefore, values. However, once a problem is recognized as a facet of the social transaction in which it is born and nurtured, whether family, work, or school, the structure of its social context (with its value systems) becomes part of the essence and significance of the symptomatic behavior.

How would a therapist assess the personal autonomy of an Italian man, the 'father of two adolescents,' who 'went to his mother's home (next door) for dinner rather than eat with his nuclear family?' (14, p. 346). As Rotunno and McGoldrick(14) assert, 'It is not unusual for parents and grandparents to maintain daily contact' with their offspring in a traditional Italian family; 'separation from the family is not desired, expected, nor easily accepted' (p. 346).

Culture, ethnicity, race, and even socioeconomic status are bearers of systems of values through which people interpret their reality and guide their behavior. Although therapists are often unconscious of these aspects of human functioning in their assessments, they nevertheless operate through them in the biases inherent in the therapies they use, their own personal life experience, and the policies and organization of the institutions through which they treat families.

What has been said about values in the designation of the object of therapy and in the evaluation of problems can similarly be said about values in relation to technical interventions. In writing about Jewish families, Herz

and Rosen(8) argue that given that 'Jewish Americans value verbal ability' (p. 371) and 'self-expression' (p. 372), it is not surprising that Jewish families may seek analytic, individual therapies....Brief goal-oriented therapy with a specific plan and with right and wrong ways of operating spelled out are less likely to seem satisfying to Jewish families' (p. 387).

On the other hand, in talking about poor Puerto Rican families, Garcia-Preto(5) asserts that 'the therapist's influence in the system will automatically increase if the family is able to relate to him or her as they would do to a *comadre* or *compadre*' (p. 179). Her statement reflects the value that Puerto Rican families traditionally place on personalizing relationships. She further states that 'the therapist's willingness to meet the family's request for concrete services and to act as their advocate is an important vehicle for establishing a trusting relationship' (p. 180). She recommends structural family therapy because the 'emphasis that the approach places on engaging the family in such a relationship is a reason for its success with Puerto Ricans' (p. 183).

While one set of authors postulates that Jewish families need the therapist to use a more verbal and analytic approach, the other writer advocates more practical and personal methods of intervention with traditional, poor, Puerto Rican families. Whatever one's opinion about the writers' conclusions, they demonstrate the kinds of values and biases that influence therapists' choices of intervention with families.

With respect to values in the determination of therapeutic goals, we see this issue arising in practical, day-to-day ideals that therapists communicate to families, as well as in therapeutic objectives with broad sociopolitical implications. As an example of the former, consider a transcript of an interview conducted by Salvador Minuchin(13) with the family of a 7-year-old obese boy:

The grandfather and mother, who cannot deny him anything, express their love by giving him food. The grandmother thinks that this approach is destructive for the child.
Grandmother: That's two against one.
Minuchin: But you are right and they are wrong. Even if they are two, you are still right.
Grandmother: Well I just don't believe in giving a child everything.

[p. 280]

Minuchin stands with the grandmother in aiming for different child-rearing practices from those advocated by the grandfather and the mother.

In the broader arena, we have those therapists who are proponents of setting therapeutic goals that would alter traditional family structures or community structure in relátion to families. James and McIntyre(10) come from a feminist perspective when they contend that 'family therapists need to be more cognizant of the social content of psychological distress they confront' and should seek to broaden and revise 'both theoretical models and therapeutic interventions with particular focus on their social and political implications' (p. 128). Although they do not fully spell out the implications of their proposals for therapy, it is evident that their ideals for the family and society would translate into therapeutic goals that represent feminist values.

Our contention here is that value biases are pervasive in all aspects of therapy and the question is not one of *whether* the therapist's values will confront those of the family but *how*. The task that remains to be addressed is how therapists can work with their professional and personal values in ways that benefit the families they treat.

The Nature of the Negotiations

The negotiation of values is an issue that is more central to the process of therapy in today's society than ever before. Less is accepted on the strength of tradition and precedent and more is open for debate and discussion. The rapidity of technological and social changes is greater today than at any previous period in human history. Additionally, people are more active than ever in determining the terms of these changes.

A major reason for this progressive acceleration of social change is the explosion in the amount and quality of information available through schools, the media, telephones, computers, and more accessible travel. It has played a prime role in escalating the rate of change of traditional relationships between races, socioeconomic groups, age groups, the sexes, and other social networks.

The intensification of these systemic feedback loops has opened the entire ecostructure[1] of society to rapid and pervasive change. Walls collapse and options multiply. Traditions, customs, and roles within social relationships are forced to contend with mounting pressure to change. They resist, accommodate, mutate, or vanish within this swirl of social movement.

With the expansion of information available, people gain greater autonomy, flexibility, and power over their own lives and in relation to the rest of society. Such personal freedom has been formally sanctioned by society through legislative and judicial decisions asserting the respective rights of all segments of society. Increasingly, this phenomenon has created more individual choices and thus also more sources of personal stress. Therapy is one of the means that society uses to assist people to negotiate more successfully this social evolution in the personal context of their lives.

A fundamental premise for understanding the nature of this negotiating process is that the evolution of society depends upon continual negotiation among the systemic components of society's structures (the organization and patterns of relationships), its values (operational standards), and its functions (the operations through which society carries out its purposes). The structures, values, and functions of society are interdependent, with structure mediating the relationship of society's values to its functioning.

When therapists engage with individuals and families to help them change their functioning, they work at reordering internal psychic and social structures of people within some value framework. Change in structure and functioning is always effected in relation to the evolving values of people in a continually changing social context.

A therapist can understand an individual and his family only in the value framework of their ecostructural context. This means understanding *what* they are doing (function) and *how* (structure) in reference to the values that are guiding them, which, for example, include their cultural standards. In modern society, however, individuals and families are being bombarded by influences from the varied and changing cultural values of their social environment.

Part of the development of their relationship with this environment involves negotiating with society (i.e., accepting, accommodating, resisting, attempting to change) the values that frame their relations with the host community. Family members are also negotiating with one another about what they as a family will hold as their operating values. And the individuals are debating (negotiating) with themselves, in light of all their community and family influences, what their values will be and how they will express them in their social behavior.

For example, a Hispanic family and its members in a predominantly non-Hispanic society are being exposed to Anglo values in all their encounters with the broader community. The parents need to make decisions about the extent to which they will maintain their traditional values about rearing their children in an environment with which their children will probably identify more than their parents. Each family will resolve the issue differently. Within the family, individuals will also assume different courses from one another about cultural assimilation. These decisions will also be in a continual state of review, debate and change, which will be mostly an unconscious process. Learning about the cultural standards of Hispanics, blacks, Italians, WASPs and other groups is to identify the dominant outlines of evolving patterns of their value frameworks. These patterns of values become part of what characterizes people within these groups, and, unfortunately, by which they may also be caricatured.

For a therapist to understand the process of value negotiations, he must take into account that he, too, is undergoing his own evolution of social values. Moreover, the family the therapist is treating is yet another force in his social context that influences his own value system. Viewed in this way, the negotiation of values between the therapist and the family is a dynamic process requiring that the therapist deal not only with the family's values but also with his own in relation to the family's issues.

The process is further complicated by the reality that while therapist and family are engaging in a mutually influencing relationship, the therapist is in a special position of power. Society's sanction of the therapist's authority, along with the personal helping posture of the therapist, give the therapist considerable moral leverage in the therapist-family negotiations. Along with the multiple implications for the therapeutic process, such leverage places on the therapist the responsibility of certain ethical concerns: what values to communicate and how to exert his influence in negotiating the values between himself and the family.

Clinicans' Application of Values

In practice, the therapist who does not actively attend to and manage the negotiations between his values and those of the family is not assuming responsibility for the influence of his values on the family. Moreover, without attention to the transactions over values between him and the family, the therapist cannot gain mastery over one of the fundamental forces shaping the therapeutic process.

Negotiations over values are held at different levels of abstraction. They range from 'parents should love their children' (general principle) to 'this parent should love her child' (particular implication) to 'in these circumstances this parent should demonstrate her love for her son in this particular way' (operational application).

The more abstract the value level, the more likely the agreement between therapist and family. Naturally, the odds in favor of agreement also improve to the extent that the parties involved share similar personal backgrounds, including socio-economic, racial, cultural, and religious heritage. However, the closer one gets to the operational applications of a value or the greater the background differences between therapist and family, the greater the value differences are likely to be.

The model of therapy, the characteristics of the clientele, and the professional and personal styles of the therapist will all influence the degree and level of involvement a therapist has in the family's values. Problem-solving approaches to therapy, such as the structural, utilize practical action to achieve therapeutic results. Consequently, these tend to involve therapists in judgments and decisions about the operational applications of value principles.

With regard to the characteristics of the family, when, for example, any therapeutic approach is employed with low-income families whose emotional problems are intrinsically linked to their social and economic conditions, therapists are necessarily drawn into more practical life issues. Moreover, these families are more likely to suffer from some degree of underorganization necessitating the therapist's assistance to encourage further development and refinement of the structure of the relationships among the family members and for the family within its social context. The therapist is thereby more likely to become involved with the family in the application of value principles to practical operations related to the formation of hierarchies, subsystems, rules, etc.

When the therapist is active in the treatment process, either because of the therapeutic model or personal style, the work is also more likely to proceed at a level of operational applications of values. In the structural approach, therapists, for instance, may actively align themselves with different members of a family around particular issues in order to alter stable, dysfunctional family coalitions. Therapists whose personal style leads to the communication of their personal values through self-disclosure are also likely to lean in the direction of operationalizing values. In any case, all therapists working with any and all therapies are engaged at some level in the negotiation of values in the process of the therapy they conduct.

Values, Structure, and Function

Values, structure, and function are the three formative factors of a social system. A social unit is an aggregate of people who join together in patterned structures to carry out a function or complex of functions in accord with a framework of standards or values.

Structure is the pattern of organization of relationships within a system. The three organizational dimensions along which people in a system relate to one another are: boundary (what defines a social unit, including identity, role, hierarchy, inclusion, and exclusion), alignment (joining together through affection, alliances, cooperation, etc., or opposing one another), and power (indicating who in a social system have the greater or the lesser influence in determining the outcome of a social transaction).

Function is the purpose for which the social system is organized, therefore, the reasons for its actions. An ad hoc system may be organized around a single function, such as people extemporaneously forming some sort of line in preparation to board a bus. A family, on the other hand, has such a complex of functions for which its members come together and society supports it that one is hard put to identify them all. As stated earlier, values are the standards by which the members of a system guide the organizing of their relationships and the actions that flow out of the organization.

Though, logically, structure is the outgrowth of a social system attempting to carry out its functions in accord with its values, we are dealing with circularly impacting factors that are affected by their relationships with other systems in the broader ecosystem with their own values, structures, and functions. Changes in functions in families, for example, affect structure and values of the family. So, if for the sake of more family income, a woman relegates homemaking to a secondary function in the home and joins the work force outside the home, the shift in the priorities of her functions at home will reorganize the family. If the rest of the family is also wanting her to dedicate her efforts to drawing in more income, there will be a shift in what the family members will value in the woman's accomplishments. Any change in one of these factors will likely have an impact upon the other two. In reality, these changes are taking place continuously as a family evolves through time.

For a therapist to be more competent about the negotiation of values, he needs to be able to distinguish values from structure and function and must understand their relationships. One must appreciate, among other things, that for any social function a variety of structures and sets of values are possible. So, for example, to generate children (a social function), there are such structural possibilities as conception through sexual union in marriage or out of marriage, along with artificial insemination within a marital relationship or outside of it. There are also a number of rules (reflecting the values) relevant to the generation of children, and these are legal, cultural, and religious, with some reinforcing one another and others conflicting, often within the same person or family. Some people, and institutions, hold values that view the conception of children as an essential purpose of marriage and other people consider conception incidental to marriage. The values held by some people treat conception, and its termination, as a decision belonging to the woman, whereas others see it as an issue belonging equally to the woman and the man. When dealing with termination of a pregnancy, the state, for example, includes itself in the decision about the procedure by setting legal parameters.

Thus, people making decisions about something as *functionally* basic as conception have *structural* and *value* choices to make. With more complex sets of functions, like how to raise a child, those options multiply considerably. A therapist addressing any social function will be dealing with a broad range of structural and value choices at a variety of levels within the family and its societal context.

The therapist's primary responsibility is to assist with the improvement of function. The clearer a therapist is about the functions being addressed in therapy, the more readily identifiable will be the structural and value options. However, the distinctions among function, structure, and value are not simple to make because semantics can confuse the presentation of the concepts. The phrase, 'ensuring that a child attend school regularly,' can represent a function, a value or a structure. As a *function*, the phrase would stand for the intent to have the child attend. As a *value*, it would reflect the conviction that a child ought to attend. As a *structure*, the phrase would signify the way people organize themselves to act with the child about his attending school.

Furthermore, because of the complex interdependence of systems, it is difficult to abstract from any operation[2] the values, structures, and functions involved. For example, in an operation in which a mother is helping her son with his homework, as a parent she may be helping to educate him, whereas as an individual she may be exercising her intellectual skills. At the same time, the boy may be, among other things, not only learning academic material, but also exercising the personal function of asserting his own autonomy in relation to his mother. The two of them, moreover, may be using the operation as a medium through which to share affection and intimacy. Taking only these functions as a starting place, the combinations of structures and values related to these functions would be many. The conceptual dissection of a social operation can uncover an almost unlimited number of components. Therapists will often struggle with families over identifying the problem, setting therapeutic goals, evaluating behavior, or choosing solutions, because they and the family are looking, unawares, at different functions, values, and structures of the same issue rather than because of any essential differences of opinion.

Case Example

In an actual case, Mr. and Mrs. A came into therapy with the objective of helping Mrs. A overcome her depression, a problem that appeared to have begun after she discovered she was pregnant. As they explored the significance of the depression, it became apparent that although they perceived their family life as harmonious, they had areas of conflict they were hiding from themselves and one another.

The husband and wife wanted to relieve the wife's depression to enable her to resume her functioning. They did not anticipate having to change the structure of the family's relationships. The couple also basically shared the same values – namely, that the husband assume the role of provider, leader, and overall protector of the family and the wife be the caretaker of the home and the emotional life of the family. The structure of their relationship was consistent with their values. He controlled the family money and financial information, and the wife managed their home life, including the children. Moreover, their values and relational structures reflected their individual emotional needs by allowing the man the rationale and opportunity to escape emotional intimacy at home, which because of his insecurity he found threatening. The woman could avoid the world outside their home, which, because of her personal shyness, she feared.

It was apparent that the woman was having considerable difficulty handling alone the day-to-day emotional turmoil of raising three children with yet another child on the way. She also had to organize her life around her husband's efforts to avoid and contain his chronic anxiety, which he did by drinking heavily and not confiding in her his personal insecurity and sense of failure. This meant that the husband avoided allowing his wife to share her personal fears with him and withheld himself from any substantial involvement with the children's emotional problems and needs.

Because of Mrs. A's values about family roles and her husband's need to shield himself emotionally, the woman could see no way to relieve her burden by asking more of him at home. This bind pushed her into a depression, which, paradoxically, effectively put her on a strike at home and forced her husband to organize his life around her and her emotional illness.

In contrast to the couple, the therapist chose to address the depression by working to change the structure of Mr. and Mrs. A's relationship so that the couple could better share the responsibility for one another's personal needs within their family life. The values the therapist brought into the therapy reflected a more egalitarian notion of husband-wife relationships. This value stance translated into the therapist envisioning that Mrs. A would grow strong enough not only to insist on her husband's help but also to support him in a way that would make him feel safe to be vulnerable with her and allow him greater personal intimacy with her. This therapy, like all therapies, would challenge all parties, including the therapist, to negotiate the terms of change.

The wife was painfully shy and generally had a poor sense of her own self-worth. She had accepted her inferior position vis-à-vis her husband, who was a successful businessman, in exchange for his creating a protective barrier around her from the outside world. Mr. A gave his wife anything he could stretch their resources to buy and cushioned her in an atmosphere of personal flattery away from the world. These trappings served the function of propping Mrs. A's fragile sense of self-esteem but did not protect her from feeling inadequate to assume responsibility for the domestic and personal travails of all family members.

In this case, the therapist concluded that the values of this couple, which called for the full burden of the domestic and emotional life of the family to be borne by the wife, were contributing to the emotional breakdown of this woman. Her psychological frailty, based on her low self-esteem, had made her accept these values that enabled her to avoid stress from the world outside the family and effectively complemented her husband's efforts to escape personal and domestic involvement. Their three children pushed Mrs. A to her emotional limit, and the prospect of the fourth had tipped her over the edge into depression. Their family structure, justified and supported by their values, had locked the woman into a dysfunctional pattern that was becoming increasingly pathological. The therapist decided that at the same time he addressed their emotional needs, he would attempt to alter their ideals (values) about family life to facilitate change in the family.

From a strategic standpoint, the therapist could not directly attack the family's values and their corresponding relational structures. He began the negotiations with the couple over their values by using as leverage their intense distress over the woman's depression. He leaned on the entrenched value of the family that the husband should be his wife's protector and appealed to the husband to encourage her, for her sake, to voice all her complaints about their family life.

The problem this presented for the husband was that it violated the family rules that he was not to be troubled with their domestic concerns. But the therapist was not overtly asking him to become involved in solving the wife's domestic problems. He was only to listen supportively to her complaining about them. Therefore, the function being elicited (to listen) was just short of his greater fear (domestic intimacy), and their way of carrying out the function was also within their pattern (structure) for handling certain problems, namely, that he could take charge of the task.

Of course, once he took on the task and his wife responded, everything began to change; when he became party to unlocking the cap on the pressure his wife was struggling with, he was swept into engaging with her about her distress. The force with which the woman voiced her complaints made some changes compelling. She needed more of his personal assistance with the children and the problems they bore. The opportunity to express herself began to set the terms of his involvement in their domestic life and increased her power in the family and, thus, her self-confidence. This change eventually led to her wanting more say about their finances and less reliance upon the gossamer fence with which her husband was protecting her. She became able to support him in ways more productive both for him and for her, and he reciprocated. Her ideals about what a husband-wife relationship should be began to change, and some of his traditional views also softened. Their values were in the process of changing in line with alterations in their relational patterns.

My thesis is that the therapist's responsibility is to assist the family with the evolution of those values that correspond to the relational structures that are essential to improving the family's functioning. The negotiation of values pertains to the therapy when the therapist judges that some change in the family's values is necessary to the solution of their problem. Where that contingency between values and a solution does not exist, the therapist would be going outside the pale of his responsibility if he were to seek a change in the family's values.

A change in values is essential to change when (a) a conflict about values between members of a family or between a family and its community is a significant pathological force in the dysfunction being addressed in the therapy. Examples of these are easy to imagine and are evident, for example,

in marriages in which the partners are in conflict because they come from different ethnic, racial, religious, or socioeconomic backgrounds, or when a family has problems because it lives in a neighborhood where it represents a racial minority that is discriminated against.

However, conflicts in values commonly serve as the outer skin to a deeper emotional conflict in a family problem and contribute varying weights of force to the emotional issues. People most often adopt dysfunctional relational patterns for primarily psychological reasons and attempt to rationalize their behavior by selectively drawing from their sociocultural framework of values. Families may present a value conflict as their principal concern to defend against confronting the emotional forces embedded in a structural conflict. An adolescent and parent, for example, may articulate a conflict over values about dating, whereas the underlying struggle derives from tension over the growing emotional distance between them due to the adolescent's developing separation from the family. Still, although the emotional conflict may be the primary source of the family problem, the value conflict related to it, however secondary, may also bring energy of its own to the problem and demand attention from the therapist.

A change in values is also an issue when (b) the family's values are not compatible with the function the family intends to carry out or the structures through which it is to operate. The lack of fit between the values of the family and its functions or structures is likely to emerge from evolutionary changes in the family or its social circumstances. For example, a family may place an overriding value on centering the lives of its members on the children because the parents cannot manage personal intimacy between themselves. At the point their children mature and move away from home, this priority will no longer be an adequate standard by which to organize their relationship to one another. With respect to a change in the family's social context, the standards parents use in one country to guide their adolescents may not be adaptive to the social demands of a different culture. For instance, in a move from a culture in which higher education of a daughter is discouraged to one in which it is encouraged, not only will there be incompatibility between the family and its society, but there may also be conflict between the parents and their daughter should she develop aspirations for advanced education.

A change in values is relevant to the therapy (c) if the family or its members have not developed the values necessary to guide the evolution of structures necessary to deal with the functional issues with which the family is contending. The underorganized(1) family is commonly a family that not only is lacking structural organization, but also does not have a well-elaborated, cohesive, or flexible framework of values. The development of a value framework influences how well organized the structure of a family's relationships will be. A family that has a primitively developed, inconsistent, conflicted, or rigid set of values will find it difficult to establish effectively functional relationships among its members.

Finally, values are in issue in the process of therapy (d) to the extent that the family and the therapist are struggling to agree on a value framework for addressing the family's dysfunction. For example, take the case a therapist presented to her supervisor in which a couple with two children were facing the wife's ongoing affair with another man. The therapy had stalled, and the therapist was dissatisfied with her approach to the couple, which was to offer mostly technical assistance to the couple's decision-making process. The therapist could not see how to incorporate the family's underlying emotional issues into this process. What she lacked was a framework of values to lend definition and direction to her therapeutic approach to the couple's emotional struggle.

An exploration with the therapist of her own family of origin revealed that her father had carried on a long-term affair with her mother's knowledge while the therapist was a child. The affair ended only when her father committed suicide. As a child, the therapist had an inkling of the affair when she found herself sharing a variety of recreational outings with her father and his woman friend and received gifts from the woman. She became part of her own family's conspiracy of silence. In her current life, the therapist had been seriously hurt by the infidelities of a lover, and she herself had not been able to establish a relationship with anyone founded on an enduring, exclusive commitment. She could not decide for herself what fidelity she had a right to expect of a partner in a love relationship or marriage and therefore she did not have a personal reference point from which to respond to the confusion of the couple she was treating about their respective expectations of marital fidelity. Moreover, the therapist, who had not adequately dealt with her own childhood experience, did not even think to consider the effect of the client-mother's infidelity on the couple's 5- and 9-year-old children. Without a value framework forged out of a resolution of her own personal life experiences, she was approaching the family's dilemma without a personal rudder of values to guide her therapeutic interventions.

Preparing Therapists to Negotiate Values

Most professional training aims at inculcating in therapists the need to respect the values of families but does not prepare them to negotiate and deal with the family's values. Considering the significance values play in the formation and functioning of families, focus on values as part of the training of therapists is indicated. There are four elements one might want to include in such training:

1   An identification, differentiation, and understanding of the relationships among values, structures, and functions in the problems of the families

2   An awareness of their own personal and professional values and an ability to utilize them with respect to the problems and values of the families

3   Knowledge and understanding of the sociocultural value frameworks of the families

4   Clinical skill in managing the negotiation of values between the therapist and family

We have already discussed the difficulties in discerning the distinctions among values, structures, and functions of the family system. The therapist's task is to understand the relationships among these three dimensions with respect to the family's problems. The therapist will need to understand both how each factor relates to the existence of the problem and how to work with the elements to bring about change in the family.

Therapists' awareness of their personal and professional values is not easy to come by, not only because values are often subliminal to their consciousness, but also because therapists may be unclear and conflicted about their values. Moreover, therapists often have not examined their values with respect to the issues and circumstances presented by families. Most therapists require specifically focused training while conducting therapy to be able to recognize how their values come into play in therapy. (2) Training should provide the therapist with a baseline, with all its ambiguities and contradictions, of his personal and professional value framework. The training should also help the therapist resolve issues he has about both personal and professional values. His effort to resolve his more personal questions may require that he not only deal with himself but also with his own family of origin and current family. Whatever the degree of resolution he achieves about his evolving framework of values, the goal of the training will be to free and empower him to actively manage his values in his work with families.

Understanding the values of a family involves acquiring knowledge of how the family and its members are currently dealing with the dialectics of the evolution of their values in relation to the issues they bring to therapy. When the family's framework of values is alien to the therapist, he may need to learn about the family's social group, as well as gain first-hand experience in its community. In general, the therapist needs to develop a sensitivity to values and their evolutionary process that will facilitate detecting values in the communications and behavior of families without explicitly asking people to state them. Commonly, what people say they believe in and what they actually operate from may be quite different.

Developing clinical skill in value negotiations with families means that therapists are able to observe and monitor, over the course of the therapy, conflicts and mutations of their own and the family's values with regard to the issues they are addressing. This skill also implies that therapists learn to allow for differences and for the mutual exercise of power between the family and themselves and be prepared to work within this mutuality when negotiating values with the family. If the family cannot exercise power with the therapist, they cannot have a say in the outcome of their transactions. The therapist's respect for the family and its values will permit the family to assume different positions from him and to assert these differences. The therapist's knowledge of and respect for his own values will facilitate his exercising his power and influence with the family with more ease and conviction.

The basic premise is that *the therapist should attempt to exercise no more influence over the family's values than is required adequately to address the family's problems.* Although it is true that it is impossible to divorce the therapist's values from the therapy, there are degrees of influence that the therapist can choose to exercise. At the minimal end of the spectrum, the therapist concentrates on offering the family technical help in evaluating and adjusting their own values. A simple example is seen when the therapist assists members of the same family to negotiate values among them, with the therapist coaching the family on how to negotiate. At the other end of the spectrum is the therapist who makes a conscious effort to influence the family's values, as a therapist might do who tries to convince a parent that severe physical discipline is not in the best interest of his child, even if the parent's family tradition so advocates.

A therapist will need to develop not only awareness but discipline and skill to handle such negotiations. The awareness opens the therapist's eyes to the juxtaposition of his own and the family's values in the therapeutic relationship. The discipline assists the therapist to work at the point in the spectrum of influence that he considers proper and useful for the family. The skill enables the therapist to integrate the awareness of his own personal and professional values into his work to help the family to utilize a value framework that will facilitate a solution to their problems. Again, training and supervision that specifically targets these skills could be profitable for most therapists.

All this still leaves the ethical issue of how a therapist concludes that he is free to assert some influence over a family's values. The issue is easily addressed in a situation in which the family *consciously* understands the relationship of the suggested values to the resolution of its problems and chooses to reject or adopt the proposed values. The sanction for the therapist to exert this influence may also be relatively forthright when the therapist represents a social institution that openly advocates certain values, such as sectarian counseling services, or an organization that has the legal right and responsibility to enforce public law, such as a court or a public child welfare department.

More difficult are the situations in which the therapist simply believes that he has a way of looking at matters that is an improvement over the family's value perspective and more beneficial to the family. Here, the therapist depends upon the integrity of the therapeutic process that calls for him to assume the minimal posture of influence over the family's values that the therapist judges necessary to assist the family with its functioning while still allowing the family the maximum ability to exercise its own options and power in making determinations.

More difficult yet is the situation in which the therapist disagrees on purely ethical grounds with the value framework the family is using in dealing with a problem. The position of minimal therapist influence and maximum family influence will usually permit a therapist to disassociate himself from the moral decisions made by a family when the family chooses a course he is not able to support. When the therapist cannot allow himself even a remote association with the family's moral decision, he has the option to discontinue therapy with the family and refer them elsewhere.

Training therapists to understand and utilize their own values in their transactions with families about the family's values is a complex task. In their training, therapists are more accustomed, and find it more acceptable, to deal with their personal emotions than with their values. Trainers have their own values and will have to deal with the trainees about the differences in values between them and the trainees. This process between trainer and trainees will serve as a model for the therapeutic process trainees will engage in with the families they treat.

The training around values is best conducted within a small group so that issues that arise can be viewed less as specific to the particular trainer and trainee and more as part of a group process. The group facilitates the delicate work on values because it offers a variety of perspectives on the same issue and a variety of human resources for dealing with them. The trainer is responsible not only for the work with each trainee but also for the process through which the trainees help one another.

The work on values cannot be done in isolation from training that deals with the therapist's emotional and family life. The trainee's values and emotional life are as intertwined with each other as are the family's values with their problems. The therapist's handling of his own values can be worked on by the trainer both implicitly and explicitly during the training in connection with the personal family issues that the therapist brings into the process.

Since the work with the therapists' values, as well as emotional and family life, is primarily to enhance their effectiveness as therapists, it needs to be done in relation to clinical work. Training on the person of the therapist will undoubtedly focus therapists on themselves, and time and energy will explicitly be directed to helping them understand, resolve, and learn to deal with personal family issues. Nevertheless, therapists will work on their issues not only within the training group but also during the supervision of their therapy with families.

Summary

Values are integral to all social systemic operations and therefore to the heart of the therapeutic process. For the therapist, values are an essential component in defining and assessing a problem, determining goals, and selecting therapeutic strategy. Therapists do not have a choice about whether they need to deal with values in therapy, only about how well.

The training of therapists about their values needs to be integrated with the training about their own emotional and family issues. This training should be carried out in the context of treating families and have as its primary focus the relationship of the therapists' personal issues to the conduct of their therapy with families. Personal insight and mastery over handling their own values and family issues will maximize therapeutic effectiveness.

Notes

1 Ecostructure is defined as the relational patterns among interdependent social systems that constitute the fabric of society, including individuals, families, communities, and all societal entities.

2 An operation is any action of a system through which the system carries out its functions.

References

1 **Aponte, H.**, 'Underorganization in the Poor Family,' in P. J. Guerin, Jr. (ed.), *Family Therapy: Theory and Practice*, New York, Gardner Press, 1976.

2 **Aponte, H.**, 'The Cornerstone of Therapy: The Person of the Therapist,' *The Family Therapy Networker*, **6** (2): 19–21, 1982.

3 **Boszormenji-Nagy, I.** and **Ulrich, D. N.**, 'Contextual Family Therapy,' in A. S. Gurman and D. P. Kniskern (eds.), *Handbook of Family Therapy*, New York, Brunner/Mazel, 1981.

4 **Elkaïm, M.**, 'Broadening the Scope of Family Therapy or From the Family Approach to the Socio-Political Approach,' *Psychologic Und Gesellschafskritik*, No. 9–10; 82–101, 1979.

5 **Garcia-Preto, N.**, 'Puerto Rican Families,' in M. McGoldrick, J. K. Pearce, and J. Giordano (eds.), *Ethnicity and Family Therapy*, New York, Guilford Press, 1982.

6 **Graham, S. R.**, 'Desire, Belief and Grace: A Psychotherapeutic Paradigm,' *Psychother. The. Res. Pract.* **17**: 370–371, 1980.

7 **Haley, J.**, *Leaving Home*, New York, McGraw-Hill, 1980.

8 **Herz, F. M.** and **Rosen, E. J.**, 'Jewish Families,' in *Ethnicity & Family Therapy*, op. cit.

9 **Hoffman, L.**, *Foundations of Family Therapy* New York, Basic Books, 1981.

10 **James, K.** and **Mcintyre, D.**, 'The Reproduction of Families: The Social Role of Family Therapy?,' *J. Mar. Fam. Ther.* **9**: 119–129, 1983.

11 **Keith, D. V.** and **Whitaker, C. A.**, 'The Divorce Labyrynth,' in P. Papp (ed.), *Family Therapy: Full Length Case Studies*. New York, Gardner Press, 1977.

12 **Kerr, M. E.**, 'Family Systems Theory and Therapy,' in *Handbook of Family Therapy*, op. cit.

13 **Minuchin, S.** and **Fishman, H. C.**, *Family Therapy Techniques*, Cambridge, Harvard University Press, 1981.

14 **Rotunno, M.** and **Mcgoldrick, M.**, 'Italian Families,' in *Ethnicity & Family Therapy*, op. cit.

6 Special Clinical Populations

Arguably, all psychiatric patients are special in the sense of being unique. Thus, when an ethical aspect of their illness and treatment emerges as warranting the clinician's attention, this should also be regarded as unique. On the other hand, certain areas of clinical practice generate a set of distinctive ethical issues. Forensic psychiatry, for instance, as we discuss in Chapter 7, is especially problematic in relation to the practitioner's complex role as expert witness in a legal proceeding.

We have mulled over this question long and hard and determined, albeit with a degree of arbitrariness, that children and adolescents at one end of the life cycle and the elderly at the other constitute clinical populations which, on occasion, present ethically challenging questions of a circumscribed type. Similarly, women, racial minorities and indigenous peoples present certain moral properties which call for a particular focus.

We have therefore delineated this section on special clinical populations. The snag is the paucity of written work on the ethical dimension of women's mental health and ill-health. We have therefore woven pertinent comments on this subject into two other sections – the psychiatrist-patient relationship (see Chapter 2) and diagnosis (see Chapter 3).

You will also note the brevity of the section on children and adolescents. Here, we need to mention that two topics replete with ethical interest – treatment of ADHD and the link between selective serotonin reuptake inhibitor antidepressants and suicide in young people – have been incorporated, for convenience, into the section on treatment and mental health services (see Chapter 5).

Children and adolescents

Jonathan Green and Anne Stewart[1], two British child and adolescent psychiatrists, have put it most succinctly: 'Special ethical problems in child and adolescent psychiatry relate to the nature of the child as a developing being, with changing morals, cognitions and emotions, and as a dependent being, reliant on adults – whether parents or professionals.'

In the past, the law has come to the rescue of medicine, including psychiatry, by determining chronologically based milestones. Thus, for instance, in the UK, a child under 10 cannot be charged with a criminal offence and in many Western countries, an 18-year-old is deemed responsible to vote. On the other hand, the law may be too insensitive to the psychological and social dimensions of child development and fail to guide mental health professionals when they encounter tricky ethical quandaries.

The child and adolescent psychiatric terrain is replete with them. Consider the following as illustrative. Parents are accorded the responsibility to raise their offspring but this is not regarded as a right. The State can, through its statutory authorities, and by recruiting psychiatry and other mental health professions in the process, intervene to protect the child who is subject to physical or sexual abuse or emotional neglect. A single mother, overwhelmed by paranoid ideas, as part of a schizophrenic illness, may lack the wherewithal to bring up her son. A severely depressed new mother may be unable to respond empathetically to her baby. Even worse, she may harbour infanticidal urges and fear acting on them. An adolescent may be coping dismally at her studies as a result of struggling desperately to save her parents' marriage.

In these variegated circumstances, legal provisions may serve the psychiatrist in a broad-brushstroke way but often fail to do justice to the human predicaments of the protagonists. Ethical considerations then have a decisive role to play, and in a form that is distinguishable from their place in psychiatric practice with adults.

Green and Stewart's focus is central in this regard – the young person is a developing being in crucial respects and, necessarily, dependent on others – both family and professional – for a whole range of decisions and their implementation.

These ethically driven qualifications are dynamic, having changed radically over time, and will, undoubtedly, be subject to continuing re-evaluation. Philipe Aries'[2] pioneering contribution to the social history of childhood demonstrates this dynamism; de Mause offers a further perspective[3]. Indeed, childhood as a social construction has a relatively brief history. For centuries, children were ready victims of infanticide and other killings, as well of enslavement and forms of brutality. During the industrialized era, purportedly a period of enlightenment, children were subject to harrowing labour conditions – little more than an essential workforce to keep the wheels of capitalism moving (this still applies in many parts of the developing world).

Only in the aftermath of the Second World War, amid the ruins of European and other societies, and with millions of innocent children slaughtered or orphaned, did the international community assume active steps to safeguard children's status and recognize their need to grow, develop and mature under specified social conditions[4].

It still took another four decades before the Convention on the Rights of the Child was ratified, in 1959, by the United Nations. This proclaimed that children should be regarded as persons in their own right and, at the same time, have the need of protection and guidance in the light of their initial stage of dependence.

Alongside this profound milestone is the passage of national legislation in several countries that stipulates the needs and interests of children. The Children Act 1989 in the UK, for instance, accords specific rights to children vis-à-vis statutory authorities.

This brief historical context brings us to self-determination, a prominent issue in the sphere of young people's psychiatric ethics.

Consent and competence

A number of psychiatrists working with young people have highlighted the ethical challenge of how to determine their competence to consent to procedures and treatment, in both clinical and research settings. We have dealt with the latter in the section on research (see Chapter 9); instead, we will focus on the routine clinical context.

Given its clarity and pragmatism, an editorial in the *British Journal of Psychiatry* is our first selection. Professor Pearce[5] contextualizes the topic in referring to the much-quoted Gillick case. In essence, the highest British court determined that if a child 'is of sufficient understanding to make an informed decision', his or her consent should be obtained when embarking on any medical assessment or treatment[6]. Age should not be the determining factor. More specifically, the judgement indicated criteria such as 'sufficient maturity to understand what is involved'. Reference was also made to 'intelligence'.

Gillick also unpacked the issue of refusal to consent, rather than merely withholding it. The aforementioned 1989 Children Act grasped this nettle when stating that a child with sufficient understanding to make an informed decision could 'refuse to submit to a medical or psychiatric examination or other assessment'. We need to bear in mind, however, that the court still retains the right to enforce treatment against a young person's wishes, for example an emergency protection order.

Pearce[5] articulates helpfully how to assess competence to consent, covering such elements as young people appreciating their own needs and those of others, understanding the nature of their condition and the rationale for treatment and being able to weigh up risks and benefits of having or not having particular treatments, including over time. A tabulated 'consent checklist' embodies these aspects as well as posing related questions: the quality of the parent-child and doctor-patient relationships, sources of influence on the child (e.g. teacher, grandparent) and the possibility that more time and/or information are needed to arrive at a consensus. Agreement may be readily achieved by a Gillick-competent child, parents and professionals in which event the ethics are relatively clear cut. In the case of a clash in views, the young person's competence to consent becomes pivotal and Pearce's pragmatism most appealing.

Pragmatism, however, has its limitations. We need to address a caveat in positing an ethically acceptable remedy in the face of colliding viewpoints on the need for assessment or treatment. The complexity of the child's decision-making process comes into play. Two British experts, Donna Dickinson and David Jones[7] raise the tantalizing question of how we can be confident that the young person's express decision reflects his true wishes. It could be argued that children and adolescents are less rational, have a less secure identity and are less autonomous than adults. The authors are more than aware that an adult may also not necessarily express his true wishes on the grounds of irrationality, insecure identity or lack autonomy. Dickinson and Jones tackle their topic in the light of a range of English legal cases, arguing that it is preferable to test out carefully a child or adolescent's true wishes regarding treatment than to adopt a rigid boundary between children and adults. The clinician assumes a crucial function by using multiple forces of information, with the aim of ascertaining their patient's wishes.

The two authors reinforce their view when echoing John Eekelaar's[8] thesis that if we are to grant a set of rights to children, they should be offered the opportunity to learn, 'under guidance', how to 'constitute their own interests' and appreciate that this occurs in a setting where others are pursuing their own interests. The underlying principle is clear – the capacity to select and further one's interests is an intrinsic good[9].

Conclusion

Many other ethical challenges arise in the practice of young people's psychiatry, *inter alia*, confidentiality, dual agency, behavioural control, values, compulsory treatment, diagnostic labelling – but since the issues underlying them are, in their essence, not dissimilar to those pertaining to the adult, we have not dealt with them here but refer the reader to the relevant chapters of the anthology.

The elderly

A range of ethical challenges faces the clinician who assesses and treats elderly people with psychiatric conditions, and their families[10]. A large proportion of these are similar to those arising in adult clinical psychiatry and include informed consent, respect for autonomy, confidentiality, involuntary treatment, restraints, imposing values, resource allocation,

specificity of diagnosis, dual agency, suicide and research, and do not require separate discussion here.

Noteworthy in the elderly clinical population, and a topic we do cover in this introduction, is that of competence with its multi layered ramifications such as the nature of personhood, truth telling, decision-making capacity, surrogate decision-making, advanced directives and ethical burdens in the relative as caregiver. Given the centrality of chronic degenerative brain disorders in psychogeriatric practice, our principal focus will be on autonomy and dementia.

Autonomy and dementia

As people live longer and longer lives they become increasingly prone to a range of diseases that affect their capacity to know, and express, what is in their best interests. The dementias are prominent in this regard since their prevalence rises substantially as people enter their ninth decade, they are incurable as well as commonly progressive, and core mental functions are lost.

A key issue arises in those in the throes of dementia – to what extent can they be considered to retain a measure of autonomy. The corollary follows: should we regard them as competent to handle decisions that affect their lives, both long term and day to day? Diverse views have been expressed on these interrelated questions, leading to a limited consensus, and difficulty in dealing with both dementia patients and family carers.

The eminent philosopher, Ronald Dworkin[11], has advanced an argument in this context (which is clearly laid out in our selection 'Autonomy and the demented self'; see also his book *Life's dominion: An argument about abortion, euthanasia, and individual freedom*[12]). An initial premise revolves around the principle that in order to promote the well-being of people, we should accord them a general right to autonomy and allow them to act in what they consider to be their best interests. Moreover, we should respect this right even when the action is, as far as one can judge, contrary to their interests. An obvious example is continuing to smoke in the wake of chronic lung disease. On this view, people retain the right to autonomy since they are responsible for their own lives in the light of an overall, coherent conception of how they wish to live these lives. Dworkin refers to this as an integrity or authenticity position on autonomy.

In the case of people with dementia, the right to autonomy can still be granted where 'the capacity to direct [their] life in accordance with a recognised and coherent scheme of values, that is capacity for integrity and authenticity' is preserved. This may apply to the 'mildly' demented person in whom there is a perceptible continuity with a pre-dementia self.

On the other hand, in the more advanced case, where 'choices' are 'incoherent', 'contradictory' and 'discontinuous', autonomy should be viewed as lacking and competence, correspondingly, defective. Dworkin carefully distinguishes here between the 'overall' ability to act authentically and making a limited, task-based decision.

A final step in his argument relates to the place of precedent autonomy in treating the severely demented person. If we are confident that we know what conception they had of their lives (e.g. through an advanced directive) it should be possible to suggest that past choices constitute evidence of current desires. Contrariwise, if evidence of pre-dementia attitudes is lacking, we cannot resort to precedent autonomy in making contemporary decisions (see Buchanan[13] for a comprehensive and coherently argued account of the relationship between Alzheimer's disease and personal identity).

Rebecca Dresser[14], whose paper is another selection, adopts a contradictory position to Dworkin, especially in relation to the relevance of choices made prior to the onset of dementia. The case of Margo, a woman with Alzheimer's disease, is skilfully woven into her argument. Margo has clearly lost the capacity to experience 'genuine meaning and coherence' in her life and therefore is not in a position to satisfy her fundamental interests (Dworkin refers to these interests as 'critical' in that a person would be worse off overall if she did not recognize them). On the other hand, she does manifestly enjoy music and painting and thus can satisfy her experiential interests (another Dworkin term covering those aspects of life which we enjoy the experience of carrying out).

Dresser asserts that Margo's critical interests, that she once enjoyed as an autonomous woman but now does not care about, should be overridden by her experiential interests which bring her satisfaction and pleasure. Thus, we should do what we can to enhance her 'subjective' state of well-being and not exclude her from the 'moral community'. For Dresser, we 'owe her our concern and respect in the present'.

Steven Post[15] echoes this emphasis on subjective experience when positing that such Western society's values as activity and productivity are unduly limited in their scope and fail to take into account internal psychological states which could be satisfying to, 'and have redeeming features for, the person with dementia'. Like Dresser, Post draws on a clinical case, pointing out that Mrs G may have lost all memory function but remains emotionally responsive and is 'always pleased to interact in conversation no matter how incoherent'. Is society too 'rationalist', he asks rhetorically, to 'value the affections?'

Diligent observation of dementia patients rather than a restriction to theoretical considerations appears to appeal to several participants in the debate on how we should conceptualise autonomy and related competence. Julian Hughes[16], a Consultant in Old Age Psychiatry, with a deep interest in the ethical dimension of clinical care, puts forward the premise that any notion of the person in the context of dementia must 'square with clinical experience'. The implications are clear-cut – his patients warrant respect, and assessment and treatment is a 'human experience of a certain kind', which involves the '. . . whole hurly-burly of human actions, the background against which we see any action' (Hughes is quoting Wittgenstein here).

Hughes then proposes a 'situation-embodied agent' view of the person whereby he interacts in a specific socio-cultural and historical context with physical, emotional and cognitive dimensions. The patient with dementia remains a self-embodied agent in this respect. For instance, if he signs an advanced directive when coherent, this act should be seen as valid given the continuity of the person through 'embodiment'. This conceptual approach is in direct contradistinction to one that claims that in order for a demented person to be seen as a personal identity, they have to exhibit a psychological connectedness or continuity through memory, beliefs, preferences and intentions. This is the essence of the philosopher Derek Parfit's[17] position in his landmark book *Reasons and persons* – if the demented patient has no links with his past psychological self we have no choice but to conclude that he is a different person entirely. Parfit draws on such philosophers as John Locke and David Hume in fashioning his argument.

We should, for completeness sake, cite Soren Holm's[18] argument that the question of autonomy and competence in dementia patients is so complex and so ill-defined as to preclude setting explicit rules in how to care for them. The principal factor in this position is the prevailing continuum of competence which does not have 'clear-cut points'. Therefore, no criteria are currently available to determine when a clinical or therapeutic intervention is legitimate or not. An ethical implication follows – the obligation to assess the authentic preferences and judgements in the *individual* case as carefully as possible and then to work out which to support. In terms of theoretical underpinning, we could regard Holm's approach as consonant with care ethics (see Chapter 1). Holm's conclusion appears less helpful than it might but he does in fact offer the clinician a series of useful guidelines.

Bart Collopy's[19] systematic account of the potential hurdles in assessing autonomy in the long term care of the elderly in general is more detailed as it is pragmatic. He differentiates six polarities within autonomy which pose a risk for the patient; possible correctives are offered in each case. The polarities and their correctives are, in summary:

1   confusing the making of decisions and their implementation – the clinician enables the patient to continue the former even if their independent execution is not possible;

2   confusing direct autonomy and delegation to others – the clinician enables appropriate allocation of decisions and/or actions to relevant care givers;

3   confusing competence and incapacity – the clinician avoids global and superficial assessments of incompetence;

4   confusing authentic and inauthentic patient choices– the clinician appreciates the patient's values to facilitate authentic decisions. Agnieszka Jaworska[20] has advanced the thesis that the potential for autonomy is mainly associated with 'the capacity to value', and that this is not entirely disrupted in dementia. The capacity to value in effect facilitates a 'basic level of autonomy', but one that can be enhanced by helping the patient to live 'according to her remaining values, to the extent that this is still feasible'. Moreover, Jaworska differentiates valuing from desiring, suggesting that the former is linked to one's sense of self-worth, that is how one values oneself 'in terms of how well [one] lives up to [one's] values'. She illustrates her case with Mrs D, a woman with severe memory impairment through dementia who was able however to volunteer often as a research subject out of a sense of altruism. Dr B, similarly afflicted, also exhibited an eagerness to participate in a research project, given his judgement that the research was sound and appropriate 'real good, big project . . . a sort of scientific thing.';

5   confusing immediate and long-range autonomy – the clinician recognises that current considerations may override future ones; and

6   blurring negative and positive aspects of autonomy – the clinician balances negative claims to non-interference and positive claims to entitlement.

Tom Kitwood[21] has also contributed systematically to the goal of optimizing ethically based care of dementia patients, although he suggests that the means to achieve this is hermeneutic rather than through moral philosophy. He does, however, bring together, in a wide-ranging analysis, the orthogonal dimensions of power and opportunity; the ideal pattern of caring is one of low domination and high opportunity. How the interaction with the patient promotes personal identity and well-being is at the heart of Kitwood's approach. Thus the care-giver acknowledges the patient as a unique being, consults with him about his preferences and needs, collaborates rather than imposes, helps the patient to be spontaneous, relates through the body as well as through cognitive understanding (e.g. massage), promotes a sense of relaxation, validates the patient's experience principally through empathy, serves as a psychological 'container' for any distress and facilitates action by providing what is missing.

Kitwood also lists 17 kinds of interaction that undermine the personhood; they include deception, disempowerment, infantilization, inducing fear, labeling, stigmatizing, invalidating, objectifying, imposing, belittling and disparaging.

It could be argued that Kitwood's account of optimal care-giving by health-care professionals applies equally to family care-givers. Baldwin and colleagues[22] have taken the preliminary step of ascertaining how relatives who occupy the role of carer for a person with dementia consider ethical aspects. What emerges from interviews of 62 such care-givers is (a) the need to add an 'ethical burden' to the physical and emotional burdens customarily experienced; (b) the absence of a clear moral framework in trying to judge what is the 'right thing to do'. The ethical hurdles they face (in as many as 39 areas, e.g. confidentiality, informed consent, truth-telling, life issues, competing demands, advanced directives and resource allocation) are not necessarily consonant with moral convictions they have held previously or the same challenges facing the professional. The study raises basic questions about the role of professionals in assisting the family to grapple with ethical challenges at the same time as they themselves have to deal with their own moral agenda. The caveat of professionals not imposing their values or solutions is an obvious corollary.

Truth-telling is an excellent example of an ethical burden for the family as carer. Traditionally, the dementia patient has not been told that they have the condition and what is likely to ensue. The majority of the relatives have not wanted the patient to be given the diagnosis (paradoxically, most of them would want to know the truth if they themselves were afflicted)[23]. Yet patients *do* want to know. For instance, in a study of 30 dementia patients[24] the majority indicated that no one had ever spoken with them about their condition. A similar proportion wanted more information. Importantly, nine patients did not want to know what was wrong with them.

Despite the latter finding, some practitioners are convinced that the truth should always be told. As in oncology where the position has altered radically such that virtually all cancer patients are given their diagnosis, so the dementia patient should be informed, this on the basis of respect for autonomy. Pinner and Bouman[25] are of this view in stating that ' it is not a question of whether to disclose or not: we must be truthful to our patients'. The process involved should be determined with patient as partner. Clearly the timing is crucial – disclosure needs to occur at an early stage when the patient is still competent and has the opportunity to make choices about the future, including giving informed consent regarding new drug treatments.

Three scenarios are possible upon asking the patient if they want information about their state: patient and relatives agree about this, the patient declines the offer, the patient wants information but the relatives do not wish this to occur (invariably to protect then from becoming unduly distressed or losing hope). Pinner and Bouman modestly recommend an ethically grounded approach to truth-telling, based on the patient's right to know in which ascertaining, as a matter of routine, whether the patient wants relevant information is paramount. They call for further research (presumably along the lines of Baldwin et al.) to learn how to optimize the process of disclosing relevant information. Paradoxically, the Fairhill guidelines[26], published in 1995, which stemmed from the testimonies of patients and relatives about the ethical dimension of dementia care, include the recommendation that in the case of 'mild' dementia, the diagnosis should be disclosed to the patient. This enables then to be counselled with regard to such feelings as self-blame, anxiety and depression and to determine and express wishes concerning vital matters like wills and advanced directives.

Conclusion

Decision-making capacity in the practice of psychogeriatrics, particularly in the context of dementia, remains a thorny ethical matter. Fortunately, both clinician and ethicist have begun to examine its complexity and thereby shed light on how to wrestle with this major ethical challenge[27]. We hope that our own account and selection of pertinent articles will also contribute to its further clarification.

Racial minorities and indigenous peoples

The association between racism and psychiatry has had a long and unsavoury history. As far back as the 1840s, Edward Jarvis, a Kentucky physician, concluded from his study of the rates of insanity in Negroes and Whites that slavery had protected the 'coloured' man since it had a '. . . wonderful influence upon the moral faculties . . .' and spared him '. . . some of the liabilities and dangers of active self-direction . . . Where there is the greatest mental torpor, we find the least insanity'[28]. Jarvis' reasoning was derived from the higher prevalence of mental illness he found in blacks in the free states compared to the slave states.

He was in good company when it came to such blatant prejudice. Even philosophers of the stature of David Hume and Immanuel Kant opined that coloured people were inferior to whites. Hume for example propounded that '. . . there was never a civilised nation of any other complexion than white . . . No ingenious manufacturers amongst them (coloured people), no arts, no sciences'[29].

Negro slaves, according to Jarvis, may have been spared insanity but they were, according to other physicians of the day, prone to specific mental disorders. For instance, a new diagnosis, that of *Drapetomania*, was formulated to explain the phenomenon of runaway slaves; *Dysaesthesia aethiopica* was devised to describe rascal behaviour[30]. In 1913 a psychiatrist advanced the thesis that blacks had '. . . learned no lessons in emotional control, and what they had obtained during their few generations of slavery left them

unstable . . .'. They were thus vulnerable to '. . . deterioration in the emotional sphere . . .'[31].

It was only in the second half of the twentieth century that American psychiatry confronted the issue of racism in mental health in a systematic and scientific way. Benjamin Pasamanick[32], director of research at the Columbus Psychiatric Institute in Ohio, carefully scrutinized a number of epidemiological studies, particularly investigations conducted in Baltimore, and was able to determine that rates of psychosis and neurosis for blacks and whites were similar. He suggested that findings of interracial differences reported earlier were a function of inadequate diagnostic procedures and, possibly, the result, in part, of biases in the examiner. He concluded that previous hypotheses proposing that blacks had an increased rate of psychosis due to racial discrimination and their effort to deal with it were untenable.

Pasamanick's conclusions were supported by other data, assembled and evaluated by Joel Fischer[33] in the late 1960s. He demonstrated how poor the epidemiological studies were, including even those carried out by prominent investigators like Benjamin Malzberg in New York State. Rates of mental illness were not elevated in blacks according to several studies and there was no evidence for a causal association between race and psychiatric disorder. Fischer also strongly advocated the abandonment of using hospital rates and related inaccurate measures to examine the relationship between race and mental illness. Only more sophisticated measures like community surveys were acceptable. Furthermore, the myth of an increased rate of mental illness in blacks should be utterly demolished to spare its victims from indignity and other psychological harms.

We need to remind ourselves that the 1960s saw the expansion of the civil rights movement in the US. It is not surprising therefore that apart from such trenchant critiques as those of Pasamanick and Fischer, psychiatrists became more aware of, and sensitive to, institutional white racism within their professional orbit. Melvin Sabshin and his colleagues[34] painted a dismal picture of such racism. This encompassed not only the perpetuation of the aforementioned myths regarding rates of illness but also discrimination against blacks – both adults and children – in terms of access to mental health services, and racial stereotyping, even to the point of caricature, like rage, promiscuity, psychological insensitivity and self-deprecation. They ended their paper with a call for a concerted effort to eliminate racism in psychiatry.

Three decades later, the Surgeon-General of the US Department of Health and Human Services was still highlighting the differential access of blacks and whites to mental health services[35]. The former were less likely to receive treatment and, when they did, it was more likely to be of an inferior standard. Although several cogent factors were cited for the disparity, the 'historical and present day struggle with racism and discrimination' constituted one impediment to racial minorities seeking care. Moreover, the inherent stress of suffering discrimination elevated the risk of ethnic and racial minorities to such states as depression and anxiety.

The authors of the report were no doubt influenced by the findings of Kessler et al.[36] which showed in a survey of over 3,000 adult American respondents that 'perceived major discrimination was reported by 50 per cent of Afro-Americans compared to a third of whites'. Day to day perceived forms of prejudice were mentioned as occurring 'often' by a quarter of blacks but only by three per cent of whites. In both racial groups such perceived experiences correlated with psychological stress and diagnoses of anxiety and depression (see also Thompson)[36].

Our comments hitherto have been confined to the US. Psychiatry in other Western countries has also been affected by cultural and racial bias. Annu Thakur[37] in her presidential address in 2004 to the Canadian Psychiatric Association quoted the work of Lawrence Kirmayer, a leading figure in Canadian transcultural psychiatry, who had found evidence of '. . . incorrect diagnosis, inadequate or inappropriate treatment, and failed treatment alliances' in the wake of cultural misunderstanding[38].

In the UK, Lewis et al[39]. detected racial bias in a study of a group of British psychiatrists. Faced with a case vignette of a psychiatric illness in which only the race of the patient was varied, the respondents regarded

Afro-Caribbean men as more likely to act violently, with criminal proceedings as more appropriate, than an identical white case. The authors were concerned that this racial stereotyping could have 'harmful consequences, especially where it interferes with clinical judgement', and suspected that bias was widespread among British clinicians.

A decade later, in 2001, Minnis and her colleagues[40] replicated the study in order to ascertain whether racial stereotyping still prevailed. The picture had changed fortunately, with only minimal differences in approach to treatment for the two racial groups. The authors however were not fully reassured, given the findings of other contemporary investigators that, *inter alia*, involuntary hospitalization of young black men was occurring more commonly than their white counterparts and diagnostic differences persisted despite robust epidemiological research data to the contrary.

The influence of race in these, and other, respects has been carefully considered by two prominent figures in the field in the UK, Drs Dinesh Bhugra and Kamaldeep Bhui[41]. They note, for example, under-diagnosis of depression (and neurosis generally) in black people (see also Adebimpe[42] for a view of this aspect by an American black psychiatrist), over-diagnosis of schizophrenia, a greater use of medication (higher doses for longer periods) as well as of ECT and, conversely, a lower rate of counselling and psychotherapy, the latter on the assumption that blacks are not adequately 'psychologically sophisticated'.

Several commentators on the adverse affects of racial stereotyping have recommended remedial action. Psychiatrists need, first and foremost, to appreciate that racism exists in society and that they themselves may perpetuate it within their own institutions. Culturally sensitive clinical services are regarded as vital to improve the situation. They incorporate, for example, well trained interpreters (see Swartz[43] for a vivid account of the 'politics of interpretation'), public health education directed at ethnic minorities (see, for example, Marwaha and Livingston[44]), collaboration between mental health professionals and voluntary community organizations of ethnic minorities, promoting access to psychiatric programs including the psychotherapies, training in order to enhance multicultural sensitivity and skills (see Ridley et al.[45]) and application of distinctive models of mental health care such as the therapeutic community (see Dolan et al.[46]) to meet the needs of minority ethnic groups.

We can only hope that these steps are being taken and that institutional racism in psychiatry will be consigned before long to the history books.

Psychiatry and indigenous peoples

Blacks and other ethnic minorities may be stereotyped, with adverse repercussions, but the position of indigenous peoples is, at the beginning of the new millennium, nothing short of calamitous. As Alex Cohen[47] has meticulously documented in an international overview of the mental health of indigenous peoples for the World Health Organisation, their needs and rights were of minimal concern to the colonial powers for centuries. On the contrary, the indigenous were systematically brutalized and dehumanized.

Indigenous peoples are usually defined in terms of this pattern of colonization – a group is subjugated and marginalized by invaders of their territory who are racially and culturally different from themselves. An indigenous people can also be regarded as sharing a language, and a sense of identity through a shared history and culture.

The points we made earlier with reference to cultural sensitivity in treating ethnic minorities apply to indigenous people in the context of the latter definition. Less obvious is the need to incorporate into their care their history of victimization at the hands of the colonizer. Cohen highlights this feature in the conclusion to his report, arguing that psychiatric interventions cannot ignore socio-economic and historical forces like poverty, genocide and disempowerment.

Swan and Raphael[48], in their report on indigenous mental health in Australia, echo this view when asserting that psychiatric treatment must recognize the tragic legacy of the Aboriginal community – the history of invasion, loss of land and the enduring effects of colonization. Mental health services need to 'deal with the particular and extensive effects of trauma and grief'. In similar vein, Garvey et al.[49] refer to the history of Aboriginal dispossession and continuing racism and exploitation, leading to a pervasive sense of loss and grief.

The aforementioned Lawrence Kirmayer[38] highlights social factors influencing mental health in Canadian aboriginal peoples. Again a legacy of colonization has led to cultural dislocation, political marginalization and a pervasive sense of personal and communal trauma.

Cohen calls for treatment programs which deal with individual as well as community suffering in the light of the unique experience of indigenous peoples. Espousal of such a value-based approach is superbly demonstrated by the family therapy program of Charles Waldegrave, Wahiri Campbell and Kiwi Tamasese – white, Maori and Samoan respectively[50]. Working in a non-governmental family agency in Wellington, New Zealand, they operate on the premise that problems confronting the families they treat are 'imposed by broader social structures' rather than stemming from within the family group itself. Prominent in this regard is the continuing injustice suffered by the indigenous Maori, a community marginalized by a dominant white culture since the beginning of the British colonial era.

The authors invite us to consider this scenario

A country is colonised; her indigenous people made to live in the periphery and enforced to ape the 'civilization' of the dominant culture. They are then told that they will never make the grade anyway. Their histories, distorted/erased/dismissed, are left untold[51].

The authors also quote the Samoan novelist, Albert Wendt, who has summarised this sort of history succinctly and poignantly 'We are what we have lost'.

'Just therapy' is an intervention which emerges logically from such reflections, the term designed to convey the sense of its central goal – to bring to prominence the injustice meted out to the Maori family for generations and the need for it to be redressed. Such a position could readily be misinterpreted as a form of paternalism, the professional taking on the role of social advocate for the family. But this is not the case in the Wellington group. Kiwi Tamasese links the original colonizer and the contempory therapist when noting that the latter may imperil the autonomy of the family unwittingly: 'I think of colonization no longer with the might of the sword, no longer with decimation through disease, but through the gentle conversion of the therapist assuming the rightness of her/his value system.'

Just therapy encourages family members to give meaning to their experience and to create their own 'reality'. They examine their current circumstances including, necessarily, a social and political agenda in addition to a family one. Therapists take considerable care to encourage the emergence of 'silenced meanings'. The stories of the families are respected, honoured and then reflected upon. This process paves the way for instilling hope and offering liberating possibilities. A key value in this work is to regard the therapeutic dialogue as nothing less than sacred.

Conclusion

Frantz Fanon (1925–1961), the Martinique-born psychiatrist who worked in Algeria when it was under oppressive French colonial rule, used a psychoanalytic, Marxist and phenomenological framework in his contention that dehumanization by the colonizer of indigenous peoples contributed to their psychiatric maladies. As he put it:

Because it is a systematic negation of the other person and a furious determination to deny the other person all attributes of humanity, colonialism forces the people it dominates to ask themselves the question constantly: 'In reality who am I?[52]

Fanon also saw a Eurocentric form of psychiatry in Algeria as contributing to institutionalized racism. The result was that blacks internalized their status as inferior into their culture and transmitted it to subsequent generations. He concluded that the struggle for national freedom was an essential prerequisite to recover a sense of humanity.

Some psychiatrists might bristle at such a blatantly politicized view of psychiatric illness and treatment. All they need to do is peruse the classic text on ethnic minorities and psychiatry, *Aliens and alienists*, by Roland Littlewood and Maurice Lipsedge[53]. There they will read accounts of many, diverse instances of the pathogenic effects of prejudice. Psychiatrists are ethically obliged to consider seriously the particular circumstances of ethnic minorities and indigenous people in an endeavour to care for the mentally ill among them, and to promote their overall psychological well-being.

References

1　Green, J. and Stewart, A.: Ethical issues in child and adolescent psychiatry. *Journal of Medical Ethics* **13**: 5–10, 1987.

2　Aries, P.: *Centuries of childhood. A social history of family life*. New York, Vintage, 1962.

3　De Mause, L.: (ed.) *The history of childhood. The evolution of parent-child relationships as a factor in history*. London, Souvenir Press, 1974.

4　Bowlby, J.: *Maternal care and mental health*. Geneva, World Health Association, 1951.

*5　Pearce, J.: Consent to treatment during childhood. The assessment of competence and avoidance of conflict. *British Journal of Psychiatry* **165**:713–716, 1994.

6　*Gillick v. West Norfolk and Wisbech Area Health Authority*. 1986. 1 Appeal Cases 112–207.

7　Dickenson, D. and Jones, D.: True wishes: The philosophy and developmental psychology of children's informed consent. *Psychology, Psychiatry and Philosophy* **2**:287–303, 1995.

8　Eekelaar, J.: The interests of the child and the child's wishes: The role of dynamic self-determination. *International Journal of Law and the Family* **8**:42–61, 1994.

9　Batten, D.: Informed consent by children and adolescents to psychiatric treatment. *Australian and New Zealand Journal of Psychiatry* **30**:623–632, 1996.

10　Oppenheimer, C.: Ethics in old age psychiatry. In *Psychiatric ethics*, 3rd edn, ed. S. Bloch, P. Chodoff and S. Green. Oxford, Oxford University Press, pp. 317–343, 1999.

*11　Dworkin, R.: Autonomy and the demented self. *Milbank Quarterly* **64**:4–16, 1986.

12　Dworkin, R.: *Life's dominion: An argument about abortion, euthanasia and individual freedom*. New York, Knopf, 1993.

13　Buchanan, A.: Advance directives and the personal identity problem. *Philosophy and Public Affairs* **17**:277–302, 1988.

*14　Dresser, R.: Dworkin on dementia: Elegant theory, questionable policy. *Hastings Center Report* **25**:32–38, 1995.

15　Post, S.: Severely demented elderly people: A case against senicide. *Journal of the American Geriatrics Society* **38**:715–718, 1990.

16　Hughes, J.: Views of the person with dementia. *Journal of Medical Ethics* **27**:86–91, 2001.

17　Parfit, D.: *Reasons and persons*. Oxford, Oxford University Press, 1984.

18　Holm, S.: Autonomy, authenticity, or best interest: everyday decision-making and persons with dementia. *Medicine, Health Care and Philosophy* **4**:153–159, 2001.

*19　Collopy, B.: Autonomy in long term care: Some crucial distinctions. *Gerontologist* **28**:10–17, 1988.

20　Jaworska, A.: Respecting the margins of agency: Alzheimer's patients and the capacity to value. *Philosophy and Public Affairs* **28**:105–138, 1999.

21　Kitwood, T.: Toward a theory of dementia care: Ethics and interaction. *Journal of Clinical Ethics* **9**:23–34, 1998.

22　Baldwin, C., Hope, T., Hughes, J., Jacoby, R. and Ziebland, S.: Ethics and dementia: the experience of family carers. *Progress in Neurology and Psychiatry* **8**:25–28, 2004.

23　Barnes, R.: Telling the diagnosis to patients with Alzheimer's disease: relatives should act as proxy for patient. *British Medical Journal* **317**:375–376, 1997.

24　Marzanski, M.: Would you like to know what is wrong with you? On telling the truth to patients with dementia. *Journal of Medical Ethics* **26**:108–113, 2000.

25　Pinner, G. and Bouman, W.P.: To tell or not to tell: On disclosing the diagnosis of dementia. *International Psychogeriatrics* **14**:127–137, 2002.

26　Post, G. and Whitehouse, P.J.: Fairhilll guidelines on ethics of the care of people with Alzheimer's disease: A clinical summary. *Journal of the American Geriatrics Society* **43**:1423–1429, 1995.

27　Eisemann, M., Richter, J., Bauer, B., Bonelli, R. and Porzsolt, F.: Physicians' decision making in incompetent elderly patients: A comparative study between Austria, Germany (East, West), and Sweden. *International Psychogeriatrics* **11**:313–324, 1999.

28　Cited in Pasamanick, B.: Some misconceptions concerning differences in the racial prevalence of mental disease. *American Journal of Orthopsychiatry* **33**:72–86, 1963.

29　Cited in *Racism and mental health*. ed. K. Bhui. London, Jessica Kingsley, p. 12, 2002.

30　Cited in Thomas A., and Sillen, S.: *Racism in psychiatry*. New York, Brunner Mazel, 1972.

31　Evarts, A.: Dementia praecox in the coloured race. *Psychoanalytical Review* **1**:338–403, 1913.

32　Pasamanick, B.: Some misconceptions concerning differences in the racial prevalence of mental disease. *American Journal of Orthopsychiatry* **33**:72–86, 1963.

33　Fischer, J.: Negroes and whites and rates of mental illness: reconsideration of a myth. *Psychiatry* **32**:428–446, 1969.

34　Sabshin, M., Diesenhaus, H. and Wilkerson, R.: Dimensions of institutional racism in psychiatry. *American Journal of Psychiatry* **127**:787–793, 1970.

35　*Mental health: Culture, race, ethnicity – supplement. A report of the Surgeon-General*. Washington DC, Office of the Surgeon-General, US Department of Health and Human Services, 2001.

36　Kessler, R.C., Mickelson, K.D. and Williams, D.R.: The prevalence, distribution and mental health correlates of perceived discrimination in the United States. *Journal of Health and Social Behaviour* **40**:208–230, 1999; also see Thompson, V. Perceived experiences of racism as stressful life events. *Community Mental Health Journal* **32**:223–233, 1996.

37　Thakur, A.: Culture and mental health: Not a minor matter. *Bulletin of the Canadian Psychiatric Association* **36**:3–7, 2004.

38　Kirmayer, L.: The mental health of aboriginal peoples: Transformations of identity and community. *Canadian Journal of Psychiatry* **45**:607–616, 2000.

39　Lewis, G., Croft-Jeffreys, C. and David, A.: Are British psychiatrists racist? *British Journal of Psychiatry* **157**:410–415, 1990.

40　Minnis, H., McMillan, A., Gillies, M. and Smith, S.: Racial stereotyping: survey of psychiatrists in the United Kingdom. *British Medical Journal* **323**:905–906, 2001.

*41　Bhugra, D. and Bhui, K.: Racism in psychiatry: paradigm lost – paradigm regained. *International Review of Psychiatry* **11**:236–243, 1999.

42　Adebimpe, V.R.: Overview: white norms and psychiatric diagnosis of black patients. *American Journal of Psychiatry* **138**:279–285 1981.

43　Swartz, L.: The politics of black patients' identity: ward-rounds on the 'black side' of a South African psychiatric hospital. *Culture, Medicine and Psychiatry* **15**:217–244, 1991.

44　Marwaha, S. and Livingston, G.: Stigma, racism or choice. Why do depressed ethnic elders avoid psychiatrists? *Journal of Affective Disorders* **72**:257–265, 2002.

45　Ridley. C.R., Chih, D.W. and Olivera, R.J.: Training in cultural schemas: An antidote to unintentional racism in clinical practice. *American Journal of Orthopsychiatry* **70**:65–72, 2000.

46　Dolan, B., Polley, K., Allen, R. and Norton, K.: Addressing racism in psychiatry: Is the therapeutic community model applicable? *International Journal of Social Psychiatry* **37**:71–79, 1991.

47　Cohen, A.: *The mental health of indigenous peoples. An international overview*. Geneva, World Health Organisation, 1999.

48　Swan, P. and Raphael, B.: 'Ways forward': national consultancy report on Aboriginal and Torres Strait Islander mental health. Canberra, Australian Government Publishing Service, 1995.

49 **Garvey, G., Towney, P., McPhee, J.R., Little, M.** and **Kerridge, I.H.**: Is there an aboriginal bioethic? *Journal of Medical Ethics* **30**:570–575, 2004.

*50 **Waldegrave C.** and **Tamasese, K.**: Some central ideas in the 'Just Therapy' approach. *Australian and New Zealand Journal of Family Therapy* **14**:1–8, 1993.

51 **Tamasese, K.** and **Waldegrave, C.**: Cultural and gender accountability in the 'Just Therapy' approach. *Journal of Feminist Family Therapy* **5**:29–45 1993.

52 **Fanon, F.**: *The wretched of the earth*. New York, Grove, 1963.

53 **Littlewood, R.** and **Lipsedge, M.**: *Aliens and alienists*, 2nd edn. London, Unwin Hyman, 1989.

Consent to Treatment During Childhood

The Assessment of Competence and Avoidance of Conflict*

John Pearce

Recent rulings by the Court of Appeal (re R, 1991; re W, 1992) have again highlighted the complexity of the decisions that have to be made if a child under the age of 16 is to give consent to treatment. This has stimulated healthy debate, reflecting the free society that we live in. The issue is not a simple one, and the arguments for and against children giving consent to treatment tend to be unhelpfully polarised. Giving consent is often seen as an all or nothing ability, where a person is either able to give consent or is incompetent to consent. It makes little sense to have a magic age when children suddenly become competent to give consent. Indeed, in England and Wales the age of majority moved downwards from 21 to 18 years as a result of the Family Law Reform Act 1969, and subsequently many adult rights have been given to children aged 16 years or even younger. For example, the United Nations Convention on the Rights of the Child, now formally adopted by the British government, proposes that every child should have the right to self-determination. This is rather confusing because the child's age is not specified and no account is taken of children who have delayed cognitive development or who are emotionally immature.

The Department of Health and Welsh Office (1990) have proposed a helpful definition of consent, which is the voluntary and continuing permission of the patient to receive a particular treatment, based on adequate knowledge of the purpose, nature, likely effects and risks of that treatment, including the likelihood of its success and any alternatives to it. This definition of consent is the one used here.

Giving and refusing consent

In 1986 the House of Lords decided in the Gillick case that children under the age of 16 could give valid consent to treatment if they had 'sufficient maturity to understand what is involved'. Lord Scarman stated that 'parental right yields to the child's right to make his own decisions when he reaches a sufficient understanding and intelligence' (Law Report AC 112, 1986). This has sometimes been taken to mean an immediate transfer of rights once the critical age has been reached. However, the use of the word 'yield' might imply a more gradual process. Subsequently the 1989 Children Act of England and Wales stated that 'if the child is of sufficient understanding to make an informed decision he may refuse to submit to a medical or psychiatric examination or other assessment'. The implications of the Children Act (1989) in relation to child psychiatric practice has been helpfully discussed by Jones (1991). The Act moved the argument away from giving consent to the much more challenging position of refusal to give consent. Devereux *et al* (1993) have argued that there should be no difference between giving and withholding consent because the right to give consent is worthless if it is not accompanied by the right to refuse consent. The logic of this position is clear, but it assumes that consent can be conceived in absolute terms and can be

considered in isolation from the context in which it is either given or refused. If a child declines to give consent for treatment it might reasonably be assumed that treatment has been refused. However, the refusal could be due to the child's feelings of anxiety or anger. On the other hand the refusal might be related to a limited capacity to understand the nature of the request or simply a misunderstanding about what is required.

The consequences of withholding consent to treatment are usually much more significant and potentially dangerous than simply giving consent – unless one believes that most treatments are either unnecessary or are likely to be more dangerous than the condition for which they were prescribed. Refusal to consent to treatment suggests that the patient has knowledge or beliefs that conflict with expert medical advice. Thus it can be argued that refusing to give consent is a higher order of decision-making than merely giving consent (MaCall-Smith, 1992). A more stringent test should therefore be applied when assessing a child's ability to refuse consent than when assessing competence to consent. This approach allows a child to learn about giving consent before progressing on to the potentially dangerous and highly responsible decision to withhold consent.

The difference between giving and refusing consent has been recognised in rulings at the Court of Appeal by Lord Donaldson (re R, 1991; re W, 1992). In both cases the Judge ruled that young people under the age of 18 years have no absolute right to give or refuse consent to treatment. Parents, local authorities and others with parental responsibilities also have the right to give and refuse consent. For example an emergency protection order under the Children Act (1989) allows local authorities to exercise the right to give consent on behalf of a child, even if this is against the parents' wishes. Ultimately the inherent jurisdiction of the court gives it the right to impose treatment against a person's wishes. Thus there are shared responsibilities where children and young people are concerned. This means it is possible for a 17-year-old who has sufficient understanding of the issues, and is therefore 'Gillick competent', to refuse treatment and then be overruled by the teenager's parents, the local authority or the court. The rulings by the Court of Appeal have been seen by many as going against the earlier ruling in the Gillick case and they have been strongly criticised (Lawson, 1991; Douglas, 1992).

The whole area of consent in childhood would seem to be in a state of some confusion (Shield & Baum, 1994). In addition to the purely legal, ethical and clinical arguments, there are liberal views that are in marked conflict with the more traditional views about what children should or should not be allowed to do. Rather than pursue this debate here, the focus of this article will be on the more practical clinical issues concerned with assessing a child's competence to give consent to treatment.

The process of giving consent

No doubt there will always be situations where the court has to be asked to decide on treatment issues in difficult cases, but this should be avoided as

* Pearce, J.: Consent to treatment during childhood. The assessment of competence and avoidance of conflict. *British Journal of Psychiatry* **165**:713–716, 1994.

far as possible (Neville, 1993). There is a tendency for the law to view an issue as if it were frozen in time, whereas the reality is that people keep changing and medical conditions can vary greatly from day to day, especially where children are concerned. In any case, the courts will always have to be advised by clinicians about the nature of the treatment and whether or not a child has a satisfactory understanding. The role of the court should be to set a framework within which children, parents and their doctors can reach their own agreements about treatment.

Children, their parents and doctors all have rights and responsibilities. In addition to the competent child's right to give consent and take responsibility for their own treatment, parents have a responsibility to protect their children from harm. Parents also have the right to give their children guidance and support. At the same time, clinicians would claim the right to provide the best possible treatment for their patient and they certainly have a responsibility to guide patients towards treatments that they believe are in that person's best interest. Clearly these rights and responsibilities will sometimes be in conflict with each other.

Thus there are inherent contradictions and complexities to be taken into account when young people consent to treatment. Nevertheless, this should not prevent a consensus being achieved. Clinicians are in a key position to lead children and parents towards the goal of effective treatment by providing clear information and communicating it in such a way that it can be adequately understood. However, the mere provision of information is not enough. It needs to be given within the context of a supportive and trusting relationship. Poor communication and a notable absence of trusting relationships between the child, the parents and the doctor is usually at the heart of disputes about consent.

Assessment of competence to consent

A number of factors must be taken into account when assessing a child's ability to consent to treatment. The central issue concerns the child's stage of cognitive development. In order to give valid consent, children must have reached the stage of maturity where they have a clear concept of themselves in relation to other people, including an ability to recognise their own needs and the needs of others. Competent children will have an ability to understand the nature of their disorder and know why treatment is deemed to be necessary. They should be able to understand the significance of the risks and benefits of having or not having the treatment. In addition, the competent child will be able to understand these issues in relation to the passage of time and be fully aware of what might happen in the future as a result of having or foregoing the treatment. Most children below the age of eight years have not yet developed a good understanding of time, nor have they gained a clearly defined self-concept. It is therefore inappropriate to give any responsibility for consent to treatment to children below this age. Children of around 14 years of age are normally able to grasp the more subtle and wider aspects of giving consent and the effect that this might have on themselves and other people. But whatever their age and level of maturity, the views of school-age children should always be sought and taken into account when treatment decisions are made.

It is between the ages of eight and sixteen years where difficulties can arise when deciding if a child has sufficient understanding to give consent. The context in which consent to treatment is given or refused is of critical importance. The quality of the relationship between the parent and the child is highly influential, as is the doctor-patient relationship. The majority of young people will normally go along with their parents' wishes and do what they advise, but some children will deliberately do the opposite. Which way this goes will be chiefly influenced by the child's emotional state at the time. Relatives and others who play a significant role in the child's life may also be very influential. Grandparents, teachers, other patients, and non-medical staff sometimes play a crucial role in shaping a child's thinking. Consequently it is essential to try to secure a consensus from all the relevant adults concerned about the proposed treatment before obtaining consent from the child. Unless the child's

carers are able to reach a reasonable level of agreement, there is an ethical, moral and possibly legal risk of giving a treatment to which the child alone has consented. This risk recedes as children approach adulthood and independence.

Balancing risks and benefits

The next aspect to consider is the nature, risks and benefits of the treatment for which permission is being sought. An emergency procedure for a life-threatening illness is very different from a planned intervention for a cosmetic problem. It follows that the implications of giving or withholding consent will vary according to the risk of significant harm. Alderson investigated 120 school-age children who were to have orthopaedic operations. She concluded that children younger than ten years old were able to grasp the concepts of treatment and the consequences quite well. Indeed, they were sometimes better informed and more able to give informed consent than their parents (Alderson, 1993). However, none of the operations was life-saving and the consequences of refusing consent would have had no immediate adverse effect. Nevertheless, Alderson highlights the risk of underestimating children's abilities to make wise and sensible choices. By excluding young people from the decision-making process, children as young as four or five years old may feel resentful and angry as they grow older, and have to live with the consequences of decisions in which they had no involvement. An interesting finding from Alderson's study was that children put the maturity threshold for consent at 14 years. This was in marked contrast to professionals who put it at 10.3 years.

Clearly, a delicate balance has to be struck between the need for children to be in control of what happens to them and the need to do what is deemed to be in the child's best interest. There is a danger of using 'in the best interests of the child' as an excuse for poor communication and for failing to take the necessary time to explain the proposed treatment properly. At the same time there is also a risk of placing an unacceptably high level of responsibility on the child which can release parents from their own duty of care; a trend that appears to be increasing in frequency.

In the majority of cases there is unlikely to be much difficulty in deciding what contribution a child can reasonably make to the process of giving consent. Problems only arise if the child or the parents withdraw their consent. Then the key factor is whether or not the child is competent to give consent. A 'Gillick competent' child should be able to override a parent's opinion if the criteria listed above have been carefully assessed and it is concluded that the child does indeed have the ability and the emotional maturity to arrive at a well reasoned and balanced decision. But what if the competent child refuses consent for treatment that could be life-saving? In the case of psychiatric treatment there should be no problem because there is no age bar to the use of the Mental Health Act (1983) England and Wales, (1984) Scotland, although clearly it is less appropriate for children who do not have sufficient understanding to give consent. In the case of children who are not 'Gillick competent' the parents should explain the issues to their children and after listening carefully to what the children have to say on the matter, either give or withhold consent. The responsibility of parents and clinicians to involve children in the decision-making process and to give clear explanations is exactly the same whether a child is at home, subject to a care order, a residence order or subject to guardianship under the terms of mental health legislation.

There will always be cases where conflict arises or where it is unclear whether or not a child below 16 years has sufficient understanding to refuse consent to treatment. In these cases it will be helpful to run through a 'consent checklist' (Table 1) to consider the child's cognitive and emotional state, their relationships, the nature of the illness and its treatment. Every effort should be made to reach a consensus, however protracted this process may be – so long as this does not involve taking unacceptable risks with the child's future health. Failure to obtain consent to treatment does not necessarily mean that treatment has to be given by force. It is usually better to delay treatment until attitudes and relationships have changed – which could just as easily be the professional's attitude as the patient's. If this approach proves to be unsuccessful, it may be helpful to request a second opinion from a senior and experienced clinician. If at all possible, the involvement of the courts is best avoided. Nevertheless, the inherent jurisdiction of the High Court in England and Wales is always available to decide the most complex ethical dilemmas. Ultimately, the clinician's common law duty to treat a patient who requires emergency treatment as a life-saving measure [. . .] precedence over all other considerations. What [. . .] happens, there can be no substitute for explanations, patience and compassion.

Table 1 A consent checklist

1. The child's stage of *cognitive development*
   Does the child have a satisfactory understanding of:
   The nature of the illness?
   Their own needs and the needs of others?
   The risks and benefits of treatment?
   Their own self-concept?
   The significance of time: past, present, future?

2. The *parent-child relationship*
   Is it supportive and affectionate?

3. The *doctor-patient relationship*
   Is there trust and confidence?

4. The *views of significant others*
   Whose opinion influences the child and how?

5. The *risks and benefits of treatment*
   What are the risks of treatment or no treatment?

6. The *nature of the illness*
   How disabling, chronic of life-threatening?

7. The *need for consensus*
   Is more time or information needed?
   Is a second opinion required?

References

Alderson, P. (1993) *Children's Consent To Surgery.* M [. . .] Keynes: Open University Press.

Department of Health and Welsh Office (1990) *A Guide Consent for Examination or Treatment.* London: DoH [. . .] Management Executive.

Devereux, J. A., Jones, D. P. H. & Dickinson, D. L. (1993) children withhold consent to treatment? *British Medical Jour* [. . .] **306**, 1459–1461.

Douglas, G. (1992) Limiting Gillick. *Bulletin of Medical Eth*[. . .] **75**, 34–35.

Jones, D. P. H. (1991) Working with the Children Act: tasks a[. . .] responsibilities of the child and adolescent psychiatrist. *Proceedings of the Children Act 1989 Course*, Royal College Psychiatrists' Occasional Paper OP12, pp. 23–41. London Royal College of Psychiatrists.

Law Report AC 112 (1986) *Gillick v. West Norfolk and Wisbe*[. . .] *Health Authority & The DHSS.* WLR 830.

Lawson, E. (1991) Are Gillick rights under threat? *Childright*, **8**, 17–21.

MaCall-Smith, I. (1992) Consent to treatment in childhood *Archives of Disease in Childhood*, **67**, 1247–1248.

Neville, B. G. R. (1993) Letter – Children's consent to treatment *British Medical Journal*, **307**, 260.

re R (1991) (A Minor) (Wardship: Consent to Treatment) 3WL[. . .] 592.

re W (1992) 4 All ER 627.

Shield, J. P. H. & Baum, J. D. (1994) Editorial – Children'[. . .] consent to treatment. *British Medical Journal*, **308**, 1182–1183

Autonomy and the Demented Self*

Ronald Dworkin

CONSIDER THE RIGHTS, NOT OF SOMEONE WHO WAS born and always has been demented, but of someone who was competent in the past. We may think of that person, as the putative holder of rights, in two different ways: as a demented person, in which case we emphasize his present situation and capacities, or as a person who has become demented, in which case we emphasize that his dementia has occurred in the course of a larger life whose whole length must be considered in any decision about what rights he has. We shall have to face a series of problems that seem to contrast, in different ways, the interests of the person conceived in one of these two ways with his interests conceived in the other.

Does a competent person's right to autonomy include, for example, the power to dictate that life-prolonging treatment be denied him later, even if he, when demented, pleads for it? Should what is done for a demented person be in his contemporary best interests, that is, such as to make the rest of his life as pleasant or comfortable as possible? Or in the best interests of the person who has become demented, that is, such as to make his life judged as a whole a better life? (Suppose a demented patient wants care and treatment that would make him a serious burden to other members of his family, and we think that people lead better lives when they are not a serious burden to others. Is it in his best interests, overall, to allow him to become the burden he is now anxious to be?) Someone's dignity seems connected, in some central way, to his capacity for self-respect. Should we care about the dignity of a dementia patient if he has no sense of his own dignity left? That seems to depend on whether the dignity of a competent person is in some way still implicated in how he is treated when he has become demented. (If it is, then we may take his former capacity for self-respect as requiring that he be treated with dignity now: we may say that dignity is necessary to show respect for his life as a whole.) Should the resources available to a demented patient depend on what his competent predecessor has actually put aside by way of insurance for his own care in that event, or at least would have put aside if insurance were available on a competitive and realistic basis? Insurance schemes, both private schemes and mandated public schemes, play an important part in the way we provide resources for catastrophes of different sorts. But is the insurance approach, as I shall call it, the proper model to use in thinking about provision for the demented? That must depend on whether a competent person has the requisite concern for himself in a later demented stage: whether he has what I shall call a *prudential* concern.

Many of the most prominent issues, then, about the rights of the demented, seem to call for a study of how their interests relate and connect to the interests and decisions of their past competent selves. But every aspect of that claim rests on an assumption I must now acknowledge: that it is *correct* to regard a demented person in the way I said we can, as a person who has become demented. That conception of him supposes that the competent and demented stages of life are stages in a single life, that the competent and demented selves are parts of the *same* person. I relied on that assumption in the various suggestions I just made about how the interests and decisions of a competent person might affect his treatment when

demented. I assumed, for example, that the control a competent person might seek to exercise over how he is treated when demented is correctly described as autonomy rather than paternalism, that is, that it is the kind of control people seek to have over the course of their own lives. I assumed, in describing the problem raised by beneficence, that it makes sense to treat the different kinds of interests I mentioned – the interest of the demented person in comfort and of the competent person in not being a burden – as competing interests of the same person, so that someone trying to act in that person's best interests would, therefore, have a conflict to resolve. I raised the question whether a competent person's dignity might be still at stake after he has become demented, which would not be a possibility unless his demented stage was part of his life, and whether a competent person can have prudential concern for the demented person he becomes, which would be out of the question unless he remained the same person throughout.

Many philosophical theories about personal identity, however, challenge the assumption that identity survives serious and permanent dementia. They argue that personal identity requires psychological continuity, so that a person who becomes seriously demented, and has no important connections of memory and personality with his former self, has ceased to exist, and the demented person he has become must be treated as a new person altogether. So the question of personal identity, in this context at least, is not a mere academic, philosophical issue or a barren semantic question. It must be faced, and resolved, in any competent theory about the rights of the demented. My own view, argued elsewhere (Dworkin 1987) is that personal identity does survive even the most serious dementia. If my claims about personal identity are wrong, and identity does not survive dementia, many of my arguments and conclusions about the rights of the demented would have to be abandoned.

Rights to Autonomy: Contemporary Autonomy

It is a familiar idea in political philosophy that adult citizens of normal competence have a right to autonomy, that is, a right to make decisions about the character of their lives for themselves. Except in very special circumstances, we reject paternalism – forcing people to act in what the government deems to be their best interest – because paternalism denies that right to autonomy. So competent adults are free to make poor investments, provided others do not deceive or withhold information from them, and smokers are allowed to smoke in private, though cigarette advertising must warn them of the dangers of doing so. Autonomy is often at stake in medical contexts (see Buchanan and Brock 1986). A Jehovah's Witness, for example, may refuse blood transfusions necessary to save his life because he believes transfusions offensive on grounds of religious conviction. Or a patient whose life can be saved only if his legs are amputated, but who prefers to die soon rather than to live longer in what he would regard as intolerable circumstances, is allowed to refuse the operation. American law

* Dworkin, R.: Autonomy and the demented self. *Milbank Quarterly* **64**:4–16, 1986.

quite generally recognizes the patient's right to autonomy in circumstances like these (see Annas and Glantz 1986).

How far do the demented have a right to autonomy? How far, that is, do they have a right to make decisions for themselves that others would deem not in their best interests? (See appendix note 1.) Should they be allowed to spend or give away their money as they wish, or to choose their doctors, or to refuse prescribed medical treatment, or to decide which of their relatives will be appointed as their guardian? How far does this depend on the importance of the decision, and the degree of their incompetence? There may, of course, be some other reason, beyond autonomy, for allowing them to do as they please. They may become so agitated, for example, if prevented from doing as they wish, that though the decision they make is not itself in their interest, we do them more harm than good by opposing them. Our present question is whether we have reason to respect their decision even when this is not so, even when we think it would be in their best interest, even all things considered, to take some decisions out of their hands.

We cannot answer that question without reflecting on the *point* or value of autonomy, that is, on why we should ever respect the decisions people make when we believe these are not in their interests. One popular answer might be called the *evidentiary* view: it holds that we should respect the decisions people make for themselves, even when we think these decisions imprudent, because as a general matter each person knows what is in his own best interests better than anyone else does (see Buchanan and Brock 1986). We often think that someone has made a mistake in judging what is in his own interests, that we know better than he does what is good for him. But experience teaches us, according to this argument, that in most cases we are wrong to think this. So we do better for people's well-being, in the long run, by recognizing a general right to autonomy, which we always respect, than by reserving the right to interfere with their lives whenever we think they have made a mistake. If we accept this evidentiary account of autonomy, we will not extend the right of autonomy to decisions made by the seriously demented. For it is very implausible to assume that someone who is demented, who has lost the power to appreciate and engage in reasoning and argument, even generally knows what is in his own best interests as well as trained specialists, like doctors, do. In some cases that assumption would be incoherent, when, for example, as is often the case, the wishes and decisions of a demented person change radically from one bout of lucidity to another.

But the evidentiary view of the point of autonomy is very far from compelling. For autonomy requires us not only to allow someone to act in what he takes to be his best interests but to allow him to act in a way he accepts is not in his interests at all. (See appendix note 2.) This is sometimes a matter of what philosophers call 'weakness of the will.' Many people who smoke would prefer not to; they do not think that smoking, all things considered, is in their best interests, but they smoke anyway. If we believe, as we do, that autonomy requires allowing them to act in this way, we cannot accept that the point of autonomy is to protect an agent's welfare. Sometimes people act against what they believe to be their own best interests for more admirable reasons. Someone who refuses medical treatment he knows he needs because he believes others, who would then have to go without, need it more, acts out of convictions we admire even if we would not act the same way. If autonomy requires us to respect such decisions, then once again autonomy is poorly explained on the view that the right to autonomy actually promotes the welfare of people making apparently imprudent decisions.

This suggests that the point of autonomy must be, at least to some large degree, independent of the claim that people know their own best interests better than other people can, and in that case it would not follow, just from the fact that a demented person will often be mistaken about his own best interests, that others are entitled to override the choices he makes. So perhaps the demented have a right to autonomy after all. The most plausible alternate view of the point of autonomy emphasizes, however, not the welfare of the choosing agent, but his *integrity*. The value of autonomy, on this view, lies in the scheme of responsibility it creates: autonomy makes each of us responsible for shaping his own life according to some coherent and distinctive sense of character, conviction, and interest. It allows us to lead our own lives rather than being led along them, so that each of us can be, to the extent a scheme of rights can make this possible, what he has made himself. This view of autonomy focuses not on individual decisions one by one, but the place of each decision in a more general program or picture of life the agent is creating and constructing, a conception of character and achievement that must be allowed its own **distinctive integrity**. We allow someone to choose death over radical amputation, or even blood transfusion, if that is his informed wish, because we acknowledge his right to a life structured by his own values even when these values are not ours.

The integrity view of autonomy does not, of course, assume that normally competent people, whose autonomy we must respect, have thoroughly consistent values or always make thoroughly consistent choices. It recognizes that people often make choices that reflect weakness, indecision, caprice, or plain irrationality: that some people otherwise fanatical about their health continue to smoke, for example. So any plausible integrity-based theory of autonomy must distinguish between the general point or value of autonomy and its consequences for any particular person. Autonomy encourages and protects the capacity competent people have to direct their own lives at least generally in accordance with a scheme of value, each has recognized and chosen for himself or herself. The principal value of that capacity is *realized*, in any particular life, only when that life does, in fact, display a general, overall integrity and authenticity. But autonomy protects and encourages the capacity by allowing people who have it themselves to choose how far and in what form they will seek to realize its value in that way, and some people will partly or largely waste it.

If we accept this integrity view of autonomy, our judgment about whether some patient has a right to autonomy will turn on the degree of that patient's capacity to direct his or her life in accordance with a recognized and coherent scheme of value, that is, capacity for integrity and authenticity. When a mildly demented person's choices are reasonably stable, reasonably continuous with the general character of his life before he became demented, and inconsistent only to the rough degree the choices of fully competent people are, he can be seen as still in charge of his life, and he has a right to autonomy for that reason. But if his choices and demands, no matter how firmly expressed one by one, systematically contradict one another, or reflect no coherent character whatever, or perhaps even if they are radically discontinuous with the values of his previous life, then he has presumably lost the capacity that it is the point of autonomy to protect. Recognizing a continuing right to autonomy for him would be pointless. So he has no right that his choice of a guardian, or choices about the use of his property, or about his medical treatment, be respected for reasons of autonomy. He still has the right to beneficence, that is, the right that decisions on these matters be made in his best interests, and his preferences may, for different reasons, be important in deciding what his best interests are. But he has no right, as competent people do, himself to decide contrary to those interests.

I should emphasize that the decision whether a particular patient is sufficiently competent to have a right to autonomy, on the integrity view of that right, must be a *general* judgment about his overall capacity to seek integrity and authenticity, not a specific, task-sensitive judgment. I have in mind the following contrast. 'Competence' is sometimes used in a task-specific sense to refer to the ability to grasp and manipulate information bearing on a particular problem. Competence, in that sense, always varies, sometimes greatly, even among ordinary, nondemented people; I am more competent than you at making some decisions, perhaps, but probably much less competent at others. The literature concerning surrogate decision making for the demented points out, perfectly properly, that competence, in that task-specific sense, is relative to the character and complexity of the decision in question (Buchanan and Brock 1986; see also appendix note 3). A patient who is not competent to administer his complex business affairs may nevertheless be able to grasp and appreciate information bearing on a decision whether to remain at home or to enter an institution, for example. Competence in the overall sense presupposed by the right to autonomy is a very different matter, however. It means, not the capacity to grasp particular information or solve particular problems, but the more diffuse and general capacity for integrity: the capacity to see and evaluate particular decisions in the structured context of an overall life organized around a coherent conception of character and conviction. There will, of course, be hard cases, in which we will be unable to say, at least with any confidence, whether a particular dementia patient is competent in that overall sense. But the question of autonomy requires that overall judgment, not some combination of judgments about specific task-capability. (See appendix note 4.) Patients suffering from serious dementia have plainly lost the necessary general capacity for integrity, and, as I said, have no right that *any* decision be respected just out of concern for their autonomy.

Precedent Autonomy

So neither the evidentiary view of autonomy, not the more plausible integrity view, recommends any right to autonomy for the seriously demented. But we have so far been considering the contemporary autonomy of a demented person; we must now consider the precedent autonomy of the person he was before. Suppose a patient is now incompetent in the general, overall sense just discussed, but that, years ago, when perfectly competent, he executed a 'living will' providing that he was not to be kept alive by expensive medical treatment if he became permanently demented, or that his property was to be given *to* charity rather than used for his care. Does autonomy now require that such provisions be respected by those in charge of the patient if they think them against the patient's best interests? If we accept the evidentiary view of autonomy, we will think the case for respecting such precedent choices very weak. People are not the best judges of what their own best interests would be under circumstances they have never encountered, and in which their preferences and desires will undoubtedly have changed. If we accept the integrity view, on the other hand, we will be drawn to the view that precedent autonomy must be respected, because it seems essential to someone's control of his whole life that he be able to dictate what will happen to him when he becomes incompetent. A competent person, making a living will providing for his treatment if he becomes demented, is making the kind of judgment that autonomy, on the integrity view, respects, a judgment about the overall shape or character of the kind of life he wants to have led.

But it might now be objected that the right to autonomy is *necessarily* contemporary: that it is only a right that someone's *present* decision be respected. Certainly that is the normal force of recognizing autonomy. Suppose that a Jehovah's Witness, whose religious convictions so require, has signed a formal document stipulating that he is not to receive blood transfusions even if he, our of weakness of will, requests them when he will otherwise die. He wants, like Ulysses, to be tied to the mast of his faith. But when the moment comes, and he needs a transfusion, he pleads for it. We would not think ourselves required, out of respect for his autonomy, to disregard that plea to honor his former, formal request. We can interpret that example in two different ways, however, and the difference becomes important when we consider whether autonomy requires enforcing prior decisions about one's treatment when demented. We can say, first, that the later plea countermanded the original decision because the plea expressed a contemporary desire. On that view, it is right to defer to past decisions only when we have reason to think that the agent still wishes what he chose then; we treat the past decision, that is, as evidence of present wish, and disregard that decision when we have reason to think it is not, in fact, good evidence of that. On this view precedent autonomy is an illusion: we attend to past decisions only as rebuttable evidence of contemporary preference or choice. Second, we can say that the later plea countermands the original decision because the later plea counts as a fresh exercise of autonomy, that if we disregarded it we would be treating the person who pleads as no longer in charge of his own life. The difference between these two accounts of the force of autonomy is crucial when the conditions of autonomy no longer hold when someone changes his mind. Suppose that the same accident that made a transfusion medically necessary for the Jehovah's Witness also deranged him and, while still plainly deranged, he demands the transfusion. On the first view, we would not violate his autonomy by administering it; but on the second we would.

Which view of autonomy is right? Suppose we were confident that the Jehovah's Witness, if he receives the transfusion and lives, will become competent again, and will then be appalled at having had a treatment he believes was much worse for him than dying. In those circumstances, I believe, we would be violating his autonomy by nevertheless giving him the transfusion while he is deranged. That argues for the second view of autonomy, the view that endorses precedent autonomy. The deranged Jehovah's Witness does not object to the transfusion: he wants it. This is not, that is, like the case in which someone who objects to a treatment is asleep or unconscious when he needs it; in that case we can say (using a dispositional sense of objecting) that he continues to object then. If we withhold the transfusion from the deranged Jehovah's Witness, we withhold it in spite of the fact that he wants it then. We are relying on the fact that he does not have the capacity necessary for his wants to count in countermanding what he wanted when he was competent, and that means we are relying on the second view of autonomy's point. Someone might object that we are actually relying, not on any lack of capacity, but on the assumed fact that the Jehovah's Witness will regret the transfusion, if he receives it, when he becomes competent again. But we would take a different view if the Jehovah's Witness had not become temporarily deranged. Suppose he pleads for the transfusion at the moment when he needs it, not because he is temporarily deranged, but just because he finds he wants to live at that moment, though we are confident that he will change his mind and be appalled at his decision tomorrow. If we would accede to his request for the transfusion when he wants it (as I believe we should), that shows that we are not relying, in the case when he has become deranged, just on the fact that we predict he will have a different opinion when he recovers his senses. That fact seems important, in that case, only because it confirms that he had not changed his mind when he was still competent to do so.

Our argument, then, supports the idea of precedent autonomy. A competent person's right to autonomy requires that his past decisions, about how he is to be treated if he becomes demented, be respected even if they do not represent, and even if they contradict, the desires he has when we respect them, provided he did not change his mind while he was still in charge of his own life. If we refused to accept precedent autonomy, and instead insisted that past decisions made when competent will not be enforced unless they represent the present wishes of the incompetent patient, we would be violating the point of autonomy on the integrity view. For competent people, concerned to give their lives the structure integrity demands, will naturally be concerned about how they are treated when demented. Someone anxious to insure that his life is not then prolonged by medical treatment is anxious exactly because he thinks the character of his whole life would be compromised if that life were prolonged in that way. This argument has austere consequences, however. Many would be outraged by the prospect of denying an incompetent patient life-prolonging care he pleads for, of allowing someone to the who very much wants to live, just because, years earlier, he signed a document requiring this. I have been arguing that his right to autonomy – the right of the person he has been and remains – unambiguously requires that his pleas now be denied; he is not like the imagined Jehovah's Witness who changed his mind when he knew he was dying. (See appendix note 5.) We may be unable to deny him. We may think that people who refuse pleas for life for any reason are inhumane. Or we may have other good reasons for treating him as he now demands. But if so these are reasons that violate, rather than enforce, his autonomy.

I end this discussion of autonomy with one final distinction. We must distinguish the precedent autonomy we have now recognized from other ideas with which it may easily be confused. Commentators and judges have said, for example, that crucial decisions affecting the care of dementia patients should reflect the decisions the patient probably would have made himself if he were competent.[1] (So a patient's family succeeded in persuading a judge to terminate his care by arguing that he had been, when

---

1 See, e.g., *In Re Quinlan*, 355 A.2d 647, *cert. den.* 429 U.S. 922 (N.J., 1976).

competent, a vital person who very much enjoyed physical activity of which he was no longer capable, which suggests that he would not wish to continue living were he competent to make that choice.)[2] Speculation about what a demented person would have preferred under assumed conditions of competence may be relevant to determining what is in that person's best interests, and so what he or she is entitled to have under a right to beneficence. (See appendix note 6.) But any appeal to a right to precedent autonomy requires evidence of an actual past decision contemplating the circumstances the patient is now in. It is not enough to argue that a particular conviction (for instance, the desire not to have one's life prolonged) would be more consistent with the patient's former habits and patterns of life than any contrary conviction. The point of autonomy, on the integrity view, is to allow an agent to construct his own life and character according to his own lights, not to allow others to make, for him, a life they think most consistent in ideal or character. So for the great majority of dementia victims who have made no such actual decision the right to precedent autonomy plays no part in any contemporary decision made by others on their behalf.

Appendix Notes

1   I am assuming, in this discussion, that it can be in a person's overall best interests, at least sometimes, to force him to act otherwise than as he wants – that it can be in a person's overall best interests, for example, to be made not to smoke, even if we count the fact that his autonomy is to some degree compromised, considered in itself, as against his interests.

2   There is an important debate in the economic literature on the question whether it can be rational to act against one's own best interests. The better view is that it can be. See, e.g., Amartya, S. 1977. Rational Fools: A Critique of the Behavioral Foundations of Economic Theory. *Philosophy and Public Affairs* 6 (4).

3   Questions of task-sensitive competence are plainly relevant to the issues considered in the Buchanan and Brock article. But when the argument against surrogate decision making relies on the autonomy of the demented person affected by these decisions, the overall, nontask-sensitive sense of competence is also relevant.

4   Problems are presented, for this judgment of overall integrity capacity, when a patient appears only periodically capable of organizing his life around a system of desires and wishes. He seems able to take command of his life sometimes, and then lapses into a more serious stage of dementia, becoming lucid again only after a substantial intervening period, at which time the desires and interests he expresses are very different, or even contradictory. It would be a mistake to say that such a patient has the capacity for autonomy 'periodically.' The capacity autonomy presupposes is of necessity a temporally extended capacity; it is the capacity to give structure to a continuing life.

5   I am assuming, in this contrast, that at least some cases of what the philosophers call weakness of will – failing to abide by settled convictions in a moment of great temptation – are nevertheless exercises of autonomy. It would be, I think, a serious mistake to conflate two very different situations: when someone has the general capacity to bend his life to his convictions, and does not exercise this, and when he has become demented and so lost the capacity altogether.

6   Since such speculation has only evidentiary value, it may be somewhat misleading to treat 'substituted judgment' and 'best interests' as two different, independent rests of what may or should be done to or for a demented person. See also Annas and Glantz 1986.

References

Annas, G.J., and **L.H. Glantz.** 1986. The Right of Elderly Patients to Refuse Life-sustaining Treatment, *Milbank Quarterly* 64 (Suppl. 2):95–162.

Buchanan, A., and **D.W. Brock.** 1986. Deciding for Others. *Milbank Quarterly* 64 (Suppl. 2):17–94.

Dworkin, R. 1987. Philosophical Issues in Senile Dementia. (Forthcoming.)

---

2 See *In Re Spring*, 405 N.E.2d 115 (Mass. 1980). See the discussion of this decision, and of *In Re Quinlan, supra,* and *Superintendent of Belchertown State School v. Saikewicz*, 373 Mass. 728, 755 (1977), in the Buchanan and Brock article in this volume. That report identifies the confusion noticed in the text.

Dworkin on Dementia

Elegant Theory, Questionable Policy*

Rebecca Dresser

In his most recent book, Life's Dominion: An Argument About Abortion, Euthanasia, and Individual Freedom,[1] Ronald Dworkin offers a new way of interpreting disagreements over abortion and euthanasia. In doing so, he enriches and refines our understanding of three fundamental bioethical concepts: autonomy, beneficence, and sanctity of life. It is exciting that this eminent legal philosopher has turned his attention to bioethical issues. Life's Dominion is beautifully and persuasively written; its clear language and well-constructed arguments are especially welcome in this age of inaccessible, jargon-laden academic writing. Life's Dominion also is full of rich and provocative ideas; in this article, I address only Dworkin's remarks on euthanasia, although I will refer to his views on abortion when they are relevant to my analysis.

Professor Dworkin considers decisions to hasten death with respect to three groups: (1) competent and seriously ill people; (2) permanently unconscious people; and (3) conscious, but incompetent people, specifically, those with progressive and incurable dementia. My remarks focus on the third group, which I have addressed in previous work,[2] and which in my view poses the most difficult challenge for policymakers.

I present Dworkin's and my views as a debate over how we should think about Margo. Margo is described by Andrew Firlik, a medical student, in a Journal of the American Medical Association column called 'A Piece of My Mind.'[3] Firlik met Margo, who has Alzheimer disease, when he was enrolled in a gerontology elective. He began visiting her each day, and came to know something about her life with dementia.

Upon arriving at Margo's apartment (she lived at home with the help of an attendant), Firlik often found Margo reading; she told him she especially enjoyed mysteries, but he noticed that 'her place in the book jump[ed] randomly from day to day.' 'For Margo,' Firlik wonders, 'is reading always a mystery?' Margo never called her new friend by name, though she claimed she knew who he was and always seemed pleased to see him. She liked listening to music and was happy listening to the same song repeatedly, apparently relishing it as if hearing it for the first time. Whenever she heard a certain song, however, she smiled and told Firlik that it reminded her of her deceased husband. She painted, too, but like the other Alzheimer patients in her art therapy class, she created the same image day after day: 'a drawing of four circles, in soft rosy colors, one inside the other.'

The drawing enabled Firlik to understand something that previously had mystified him:

Despite her illness, or maybe somehow because of it, Margo is undeniably one of the happiest people I have known. There is something graceful about the degeneration her mind is undergoing, leaving her carefree, always cheerful. Do her problems, whatever she may perceive them to be, simply fail to make it to the worry centers of her brain? How does Margo maintain her sense of self? When a person can no longer accumulate new memories as the old rapidly fade, what remains? Who is Margo?

Firlik surmises that the drawing represented Margo's expression of her mind, her identity, and that by repeating the drawing, she was reminding

herself and others of that identity. The painting was Margo, 'plain and contained, smiling in her peaceful, demented state.'

In Life's Dominion, Dworkin considers Margo as a potential subject of his approach. In one variation, he asks us to suppose that

years ago, when fully competent, Margo had executed a formal document directing that if she should develop Alzheimer's disease . . . she should not receive treatment for any other serious, life-threatening disease she might contract. Or even that in that event she should be killed as soon and as painlessly as possible. (p. 226)

He presents an elegant and philosophically sophisticated argument for giving effect to her prior wishes, despite the value she appears to obtain from her life as an individual with dementia.

Dworkin's position emerges from his inquiry into the values of autonomy, beneficence, and sanctity of life. To understand their relevance to a case such as Margo's, he writes, we must first think about why we care about how we die. And to understand that phenomenon, we must understand why we care about how we live. Dworkin believes our lives are guided by the desire to advance two kinds of interests. Experiential interests are those we share to some degree with all sentient creatures. In Dworkin's words:

We all do things because we like the experience of doing them: playing softball, perhaps, or cooking and eating well, or watching football, or seeing Casablanca for the twelfth time, or walking in the woods in October, or listening to The Marriage of Figaro, or sailing fast just off the wind, or just working hard at something. Pleasures like these are essential to a good life – a life with nothing that is marvelous only because of how it feels would be not pure but preposterous. (p. 201)

But Dworkin deems these interests less important than the second sort of interests we possess. Dworkin argues that we also seek to satisfy our critical interests, which are the hopes and aims that lend genuine meaning and coherence to our lives. We pursue projects such as establishing close friendships, achieving competence in our work, and raising children, not simply because we want the positive experiences they offer, but also because we believe we should want them, because our lives as a whole will be better if we take up these endeavors.

Dworkin admits that not everyone has a conscious sense of the interests they deem critical to their lives, but he thinks that 'even people whose lives feel unplanned are nevertheless often guided by a sense of the general style of life they think appropriate, of what choices strike them as not only good at the moment but in character for them' (p. 202). In this tendency, Dworkin sees us aiming for the ideal of integrity, seeking to create a coherent narrative structure for the lives we lead.

Our critical interests explain why many of us care about how the final chapter of our lives turns out. Although some of this concern originates in the desire to avoid experiential burdens, as well as burdens on our families, much of it reflects the desire to escape dying under circumstances that are out of character with the prior stages of our lives. For most people, Dworkin writes, death has a 'special, symbolic importance: they want their deaths, if possible, to express and in that way vividly to confirm the values they believe most important to their lives' (p. 211). And because critical interests are so personal and widely varied among individuals, each person must have the right to control the manner in which life reaches its conclusion. Accordingly,

* Dresser, R.: Dworkin on dementia: Elegant theory, questionable policy. Hastings Center Report 25:32–38, 1995.

the state should refrain from imposing a 'uniform, general view [of appropriate end-of-life-care] by way of sovereign law' (p. 213).

Dworkin builds on this hierarchy of human interests to defend his ideas about how autonomy and beneficence should apply to someone like Margo. First, he examines the generally accepted principle that we should in most circumstances honor the competent person's autonomous choice. One way to justify this principle is to claim that people generally know better than anyone else what best serves their interests; thus, their own choices are the best evidence we have of the decision that would most protect their welfare. Dworkin labels this the *evidentiary* view of autonomy. But Dworkin believes the better explanation for the respect we accord to individual choice lies in what he calls the *integrity* view of autonomy. In many instances, he contends, we grant freedom to people to act in ways that clearly conflict with their own best interests. We do this, he argues, because we want to let people 'lead their lives out of a distinctive sense of their own character, a sense of what is important to them' (p. 224). The model once again assigns the greatest moral significance to the individual's critical interests, as opposed to the less important experiential interests that also contribute to a person's having a good life.

The integrity view of autonomy partially accounts for Dworkin's claim that we should honor Margo's prior choice to end her life if she developed Alzheimer disease. In making this choice, she was exercising, in Dworkin's phrase, her 'precedent autonomy' (p. 226). The evidentiary view of autonomy fails to supply support for deferring to the earlier decision, Dworkin observes, because '[p]eople are not the best judges of what their own best interests would be under circumstances they have never encountered and in which their preferences and desires may drastically have changed' (p. 226). He readily admits that Andrew Firlik and others evaluating Margo's life with dementia would perceive a conflict between her prior instructions and her current welfare. But the integrity view of autonomy furnishes compelling support for honoring Margo's advance directives. Margo's interest in living her life in character includes an interest in controlling the circumstances in which others should permit her life as an Alzheimer patient to continue. Limiting that control would in Dworkin's view be 'an unacceptable form of moral paternalism' (p. 231).

Dworkin finds additional support for assigning priority to Margo's former instructions in the moral principle of beneficence. People who are incompetent to exercise autonomy have a right to beneficence from those entrusted to decide on their behalf. The best interests standard typically has been understood to require the decision that would best protect the incompetent individual's current welfare.[4] On this view, the standard would support some (though not necessarily all) life-extending decisions that depart from Margo's prior directives. But Dworkin invokes his concept of critical interests to construct a different best interests standard. Dworkin argues that Margo's critical interests persist, despite her current inability to appreciate them. Because critical interests have greater moral significance than the experiential interests Margo remains able to appreciate, and because 'we must judge Margo's critical interests as she did when competent to do so' (p. 231), beneficence requires us to honor Margo's prior preferences for death. In Dworkin's view, far from providing a reason to override Margo's directives, compassion counsels us to follow them, for it is compassion 'toward the whole person' that underlies the duty of beneficence (p. 232).

To honor the narrative that is Margo's life, then, we must honor her earlier choices. A decision to disregard them would constitute unjustified paternalism and would lack mercy as well. Dworkin concedes that such a decision might be made for other reasons – because we 'find ourselves unable to deny medical help to anyone who is conscious and does not reject it' (p. 232), or deem it 'morally unforgiveable not to try to save the life of someone who plainly enjoys her life' (p. 228), or find it 'beyond imagining that we should actually kill her' (p. 228), or 'hate living in a community whose officials might make or license either of [Margo's] decisions' (pp. 228–29). Dworkin does not explicitly address whether these or other aspects of the state's interest in protecting life should influence legal policy governing how people like Margo are treated.

Dworkin pays much briefer attention to Margo's fate in the event that she did not explicitly register her preferences about future treatment. Most incompetent patients are currently in this category, for relatively few people complete formal advance treatment directives.[5] In this scenario, the competent Margo failed to declare her explicit wishes, and her family is asked to determine her fate. Dworkin suggests that her relatives may give voice to Margo's autonomy by judging what her choice would have been if she had thought about it, based on her character and personality. Moreover, similar evidence enables them to determine her best interests, for it is her critical interests that matter most in reaching this determination. If Margo's dementia set in before she explicitly indicated her preferences about future care, 'the law should so far as possible leave decisions in the hands of [her] relatives or other people close to [her] whose sense of [her] best interests . . . is likely to be much sounder than some universal, theoretical, abstract judgment' produced through the political process (p. 213).

Life's Dominion helps to explain why the 'death with dignity' movement has attracted such strong support in the United States. I have no doubt that many people share Dworkin's conviction that they ought to have the power to choose death over life in Margo's state. But I am far from convinced of the wisdom or morality of these proposals for dementia patients.

Advance Directives and Precedent Autonomy

First, an observation. Dworkin makes an impressive case that the power to control one's future as an incompetent patient is a precious freedom that our society should go to great lengths to protect. But how strongly do people actually value this freedom? Surveys show that a relatively small percentage of the U.S. population engages in end-of-life planning, and that many in that group simply designate a trusted relative or friend to make future treatment decisions, choosing not to issue specific instructions on future care.[6] Though this widespread failure to take advantage of the freedom to exercise precedent autonomy may be attributed to a lack of publicity or inadequate policy support for advance planning, it could also indicate that issuing explicit instructions to govern the final chapter of one's life is not a major priority for most people. If it is not, then we may question whether precedent autonomy and the critical interests it protects should be the dominant model for our policies on euthanasia for incompetent people.

Dworkin constructs a moral argument for giving effect to Margo's directives, but does not indicate how his position could be translated into policy. Consider how we might approach this task. We would want to devise procedures to ensure that people issuing such directives were competent, their actions voluntary, and their decisions informed. In other medical settings, we believe that a person's adequate understanding of the information relevant to treatment decisionmaking is a prerequisite to the exercise of true self-determination. We should take the same view of Margo's advance planning.

What would we want the competent Margo to understand before she chose death over life in the event of dementia? At a minimum, we would want her to understand that the experience of dementia differs among individuals, that for some it appears to be a persistently frightening and unhappy existence, but that most people with dementia do not exhibit the distress and misery we competent people tend to associate with the condition. I make no claims to expertise in this area, but my reading and discussions with clinicians, caregivers, and patients themselves suggest that the subjective experience of dementia is more positive than most of us would expect. Some caregivers and other commentators also note that patients' quality of life is substantially dependent on their social and physical environments, as opposed to the neurological condition itself.[7] Thus, the 'tragedy' and 'horror' of dementia is partially attributable to the ways in which others respond to people with this condition.

We also would want Margo to understand that Alzheimer disease is a progressive condition, and that options for forgoing life-sustaining interventions will arise at different points in the process. Dworkin writes that his ideas apply only to the late stages of Alzheimer disease, but he makes implementation of Margo's former wishes contingent on the mere development of the condition (pp. 219, 226). If we were designing policy, we would want to ensure that competent individuals making directives knew something about the general course of the illness and the points at which various capacities are lost. We would want them to be precise about the behavioral indications that should trigger the directive's implementation. We would want them to think about what their lives could be like at different stages of the disease, and about how invasive and effective various possible interventions might be. We would want to give them the opportunity to talk with physicians, caregivers, and individuals diagnosed with Alzheimer disease, and perhaps, to discuss their potential choices with a counselor.

The concern for education is one that applies to advance treatment directives generally, but one that is not widely recognized or addressed at the policy level. People complete advance directives in private, perhaps after discussion with relatives, physicians, or attorneys, but often with little understanding of the meaning or implications of their decisions. In one study of dialysis patients who had issued instructions on treatment in the event of advanced Alzheimer disease, a subsequent inquiry revealed that almost two-thirds of them wanted families and physicians to have some freedom to override the directives to protect their subsequent best interests.[8] The patients' failure to include this statement in their directives indicates that the instructions they recorded did not reflect their actual preferences. A survey of twenty-nine people participating in an advance care planning workshop found ten agreeing with both of the following inconsistent statements: 'I would never want to be on a respirator in an intensive care unit'; and 'If a short period of extremely intensive medical care could return me to near-normal condition, I would want it.'[9] Meanwhile, some promoters of advance care planning have claimed that subjects can complete directives during interviews lasting fifteen minutes.[10]

We do not advance people's autonomy by giving effect to choices that originate in insufficient or mistaken information. Indeed, interference in such choices is often considered a form of justified paternalism. Moreover, advance planning for future dementia treatment is more complex than planning for other conditions, such as permanent unconsciousness. Before implementing directives to hasten death in the event of dementia, we should require people to exhibit a reasonable understanding of the choices they are making.[11]

Some shortcomings of advance planning are insurmountable, however. People exercising advance planning are denied knowledge of treatments and other relevant information that may emerge during the time between making a directive and giving it effect. Opportunities for clarifying misunderstandings are truncated, and decisionmakers are not asked to explain or defend their choices to the clinicians, relatives, and friends whose care and concern may lead depressed or imprudent individuals to alter their wishes.[12] Moreover, the rigid adherence to advance planning Dworkin endorses leaves no room for the changes of heart that can lead us to deviate from our earlier choices. All of us are familiar with decisions we have later come to recognize as *ill-suited* to our subsequent situations. As Dworkin acknowledges, people may be mistaken about their future experiential interests as incompetent individuals. A policy of absolute adherence to advance directives means that we deny people like Margo the freedom we enjoy as competent people to change our decisions that conflict with our subsequent experiential interests.[13]

Personal identity theory, which addresses criteria for the persistence of a particular person over time, provides another basis for questioning precedent autonomy's proper moral and legal authority. In *Life's Dominion*, Dworkin assumes that Margo the dementia patient is the same person who issued the earlier requests to die, despite the drastic psychological alteration that has occurred. Indeed, the legitimacy of the precedent autonomy model absolutely depends on this view of personal identity. Another approach to personal identity would challenge this judgment, however. On this view, substantial memory loss and other psychological changes may produce a new person, whose connection to the earlier one could be less strong, indeed, could be no stronger than that between you and me.[14] Subscribers to this view of personal identity can argue that Margo's earlier choices lack moral authority to control what happens to Margo the dementia patient.

These shortcomings of the advance decisionmaking process are reasons to assign less moral authority to precedent autonomy than to contemporaneous autonomy. I note that Dworkin himself may believe in at least one limit on precedent autonomy in medical decisionmaking. He writes that people 'who are repelled by the idea of living demented, totally dependent lives, speaking gibberish,' ought to be permitted to issue advance directives 'stipulating that if they become permanently and seriously demented, and then develop a serious illness, they should not be given medical treatment except to avoid pain' (p. 231). Would he oppose honoring a request to avoid all medical treatment, including pain-relieving measures, that was motivated by religious or philosophical concerns? The above remark suggests that he might give priority to Margo's existing experiential interests in avoiding pain over her prior exercise of precedent autonomy. In my view, this would be a justified limit on precedent autonomy, but I would add others as well.

Critical and Experiential Interests: Problems with the Model

What if Margo, like most other people, failed to exercise her precedent autonomy through making an advance directive? In this situation, her surrogate decisionmakers are to apply Dworkin's version of the best interests standard. Should they consider, first and foremost, the critical interests she had as a competent person? I believe not, for several reasons. First, Dworkin's approach to the best interests standard rests partially on the claim that people want their lives to have narrative coherence. Dworkin omits empirical support for this claim, and my own observations lead me to wonder about its accuracy. The people of the United States are a diverse group, holding many different world views. Do most people actually think as Dworkin says they do? If I were to play psychologist, my guess would be that many people take life one day at a time. The goal of establishing a coherent narrative may be a less common life theme than the simple effort to accept and adjust to the changing natural and social circumstances that characterize a person's life. It also seems possible that people generally fail to draw a sharp line between experiential and critical interests, often choosing the critical projects Dworkin describes substantially because of the rewarding experiences they provide.

Suppose Margo left no indication of her prior wishes, but that people close to her believe it would be in her critical interests to die rather than live on in her current condition. Dworkin notes, but fails to address, the argument that 'in the circumstances of dementia, critical interests become less important and experiential interests more so, so that fiduciaries may rightly ignore the former and concentrate on the latter' (p. 232). Happy and contented Margo will experience clear harm from the decision that purports to advance the critical interests she no longer cares about. This seems to me justification for a policy against active killing or withholding effective, nonburdensome treatments, such as antibiotics, from dementia patients whose lives offer them the sorts of pleasures and satisfactions Margo enjoys. Moreover, if clear evidence is lacking on Margo's own view of her critical interests, a decision to hasten her death might actually conflict with the life narrative she envisioned for herself. Many empirical studies have shown that families often do not have a very good sense of their relatives' treatment preferences.[15] How will Margo's life narrative be improved by her family's decision to hasten death, if there is no clear indication that she herself once took that view?

I also wonder about how to apply a best interests standard that assigns priority to the individual's critical interests. Dworkin writes that family members and other intimates applying this standard should decide based on their knowledge of 'the shape and character of [the patient's] life and his own sense of integrity and critical interests' (p. 213). What sorts of life narratives would support a decision to end Margo's life? What picture of her critical interests might her family cite as justification for ending her life now? Perhaps Margo had been a famous legal philosopher whose intellectual pursuits were of utmost importance to her. This fact might tilt toward a decision to spare her from an existence in which she can only pretend to read. But what if she were also the mother of a mentally retarded child, whom she had cared for at home? What if she had enjoyed and valued this child's simple, experiential life, doing everything she could to protect and enhance it? How would this information affect the interpretation of her critical interests as they bear on her own life with dementia?

I am not sure whether Dworkin means to suggest that Margo's relatives should have complete discretion in evaluating considerations such as these. Would he permit anyone to challenge the legitimacy of a narrative outcome chosen by her family? What if her closest friends believed that a different conclusion would be more consistent with the way she had constructed her life? And is there any room in Dworkin's scheme for surprise endings? Some of our greatest fictional characters evolve into figures having little resemblance to the persons we met in the novels' opening chapters. Are real-life characters such as the fiercely independent intellectual permitted to become people who appreciate simple experiential pleasures and accept their dependence on others?

Finally, is the goal of respecting individual differences actually met by Dworkin's best interests standard? Although Dworkin recognizes that some people believe their critical interests would be served by a decision to extend their lives as long as is medically possible (based on their pro-life values), at times he implies that such individuals are mistaken about their genuine critical interests, that in actuality no one's critical interests could be served by such a decision. For example, he writes that after the onset of dementia, nothing of value can be added to a person's life, because the person is no longer capable of engaging in the activities necessary to advance her critical interests (p. 230). A similar judgment is also evident in his discussion of an actual case of a brain-damaged patient who 'did not seem to be in pain or unhappy,' and 'recognized familiar faces with apparent pleasure' (p. 233). A court-appointed guardian sought to have the patient's life-prolonging medication withheld, but the family was strongly opposed to this outcome, and a judge denied the guardian's request. In a remark that seems to conflict with his earlier support for family decisionmaking, Dworkin questions whether the family's choice was in the patient's best interests (p. 233). These comments lead me to wonder whether Dworkin's real aim is to defend an objective nontreatment standard that should be applied to all individuals with significant mental impairment, not just those whose advance directives or relatives support a decision to hasten death. If so, then he needs to provide additional argument for this more controversial position.

The State's Interest in Margo's Life

My final thoughts concern Dworkin's argument that the state has no legitimate reason to interfere with Margo's directives or her family's best interests judgment to end her life. A great deal of *Life's Dominion* addresses the intrinsic value of human life and the nature of the state's interest in protecting that value. Early in the book, Dworkin defends the familiar view that only conscious individuals, can possess interests in not being destroyed or otherwise harmed. On this view, until the advent of sentience and other capacities, human fetuses lack interests of their own that would support a state policy restricting abortion. A policy that restricted abortion prior to this point would rest on what Dworkin calls a *detached* state interest in protecting human life. Conversely, a policy that restricts abortion after fetal sentience (which coincides roughly with viability) is supported by the state's *derivative* interest in valuing life, so called because it derives from the fetus's own interests (pp. 10–24, 168–70). Dworkin believes that detached state interests in ensuring respect for the value of life justify state prohibitions on abortion only after pregnant women are given a reasonable opportunity to terminate an unwanted pregnancy. Prior to this point, the law should permit women to make decisions about pregnancy according to their own views on how best to respect the value of life. After viability, however, when fetal neurological development is sufficiently advanced to make sentience possible, the state may severely limit access to abortion, based on its legitimate role in protecting creatures capable of having interests of their own (pp. 168–70).

Dworkin's analysis of abortion provides support, in my view, for a policy in which the state acts to protect the interests of conscious dementia patients like Margo. Although substantially impaired, Margo retains capacities for pleasure, enjoyment, interaction, relationships, and so forth. I believe her continued ability to participate in the life she is living furnishes a defensible basis for state limitations on the scope of her precedent autonomy, as well as on the choices her intimates make on her behalf. Contrary to Dworkin, I believe that such moral paternalism is justified when dementia patients have a quality of life comparable to Margo's. I am not arguing that all directives regarding dementia care should be overridden, nor that family choices should always be disregarded. I think directives and family choices should control in the vast majority of cases, for such decisions rarely are in clear conflict with the patient's contemporaneous interests. But I believe that state restriction is justified when a systematic evaluation by clinicians and others involved in patient care produces agreement that a minimally intrusive life-sustaining intervention is likely to preserve the life of someone as contented and active as Margo.

Many dementia patients do not fit Margo's profile. Some are barely conscious, others appear frightened, miserable, and unresponsive to efforts to mitigate their pain. Sometimes a proposed life-sustaining treatment will be invasive and immobilizing, inflicting extreme terror on patients unable to understand the reasons for their burdens. In such cases, it is entirely appropriate to question the justification for treatment, and often to withhold it, as long as the patient can be kept comfortable in its absence. This approach assumes that observers can accurately assess the experiential benefits and burdens of patients with neurological impairments and decreased ability to communicate. I believe that such assessments are often possible, and that there is room for a great deal of improvement in meeting this challenge.

I also believe that the special problems inherent in making an advance decision about active euthanasia justify a policy of refusing to implement such decisions, at the very least until we achieve legalization for competent patients without unacceptable rates of error and abuse.[16] I note as well the likely scarcity of health care professionals who would be willing to participate in decisions to withhold simple and effective treatments from someone in Margo's condition, much less to give her a lethal injection, even if this were permitted by law. Would Dworkin support a system that required physicians and nurses to compromise their own values and integrity so that Margo's precedent autonomy and critical interests could be advanced? I seriously doubt that many health professionals would agree to implement his proposals regarding dementia patients whose lives are as happy as Margo's.

We need community reflection on how we should think about people with dementia, including our possible future selves. Dworkin's model reflects a common response to the condition: tragic, horrible, degrading, humiliating, to be avoided at all costs. But how much do social factors account for this tragedy? Two British scholars argue that though we regard dementia patients as 'the problem,' the patients

are rather less of a problem than *we. They* are generally more authentic about what they are feeling and doing; many of the polite veneers of earlier life have been stripped away. *They* are clearly dependent on others, and usually come to accept that dependence; whereas many 'normal' people, living under an ideology of extreme individualism, strenuously deny their dependency needs. *They* live largely in the present, because certain parts of their memory function have failed. *We* often find it very difficult to live in the present, suffering constant distraction; the sense of the present is often contaminated by regrets about the past and fears about the future.[17]

If we were to adopt an alternative to the common vision of dementia, we might ask ourselves what we could do, how we could alter our own responses so that people with dementia may find that life among us need not be so terrifying and frustrating. We might ask ourselves what sorts of environments, interactions, and relationships would enhance their lives.

Such a 'disability perspective' on dementia offers a more compassionate, less rejecting approach to people with the condition than a model insisting that we should be permitted to order ourselves killed if this 'saddest of the tragedies' (p. 218) should befall us. It supports as well a care and treatment policy centered on the conscious incompetent patient's subjective reality; one that permits death when the experiential burdens of continued life are too heavy or the benefits too minimal, but seeks to delay death when the patient's subjective existence is as positive as Margo's appears to be. Their loss of higher-level intellectual capacities ought not to exclude people like Margo from the moral community nor from the law's protective reach, even when the threats to their well-being emanate from their own former preferences. Margo's connections to us remain sufficiently strong that we owe her our concern and respect in the present. Eventually, the decision to allow her to the will be morally defensible. It is too soon, however, to exclude her from our midst.

Acknowledgment

I presented an earlier version of this essay at the annual meeting of the Society for Health and Human Values, 8 October 1994, in Pittsburgh. I would like to thank Ronald Dworkin and Eric Rakowski for their comments on my analysis.

References

1 **Ronald Dworkin**, *Life's Domination: An Argument About Abortion Euthanasia, and Individual Freedom* (New York: Alfred A. Knopf, 1993.)

2 See, for example, Rebecca Dresser, 'Missing Persons: Legal Perceptions of Incompetent Patients,' *Rutgers Law Review* 609 (1994): 636–47; Rebecca Dresser and Peter J. Whitehouse, 'The Incompetent Patient on the Slippery Slope,' *Hastings Center Report* 24, no. 4 (1994): 6–12; Rebecca Dresser, 'Autonomy Revisited: The Limits of Anticipatory Choices,' in *Dementia and Aging: Ethics, Values, and Policy Choices*, ed. Robert H. Binstock, Stephen G. Post, and Peter J. Whitehouse (Baltimore, Md.: Johns Hopkins University Press, 1992), pp. 71–85.

3 **Andrew D. Firlik**, 'Margo's Logo,' *JAMA* 265 (1991): 201.

4 See generally Dresser, 'Missing Persons.'

5 For a recent survey of the state of advance treatment decisionmaking in the U.S., see 'Advance Care Planning: Priorities for Ethical and Empirical Research,' Special Supplement, *Hastings Center Report* 24, no. 6 (1994).

6 See generally 'Advance Care Planning.' The failure of most persons to engage in formal end-of-life planning does not in itself contradict Dworkin's point that most people care about how they die. It does suggest, however, that people do not find the formal exercise of precedent autonomy to be a helpful or practical means of expressing their concerns about future life-sustaining treatment.

7 See generally Dresser, 'Missing Persons,' 681–91; Tom Kitwood and Kathleen Bredin, 'Towards a Theory of Dementia Care: Personhood and Well-Being,' *Ageing and Society* 12 (1992): 269–87.

8 **Ashwini Sehgal** *et al.*, 'How Strictly Do Dialysis Patients Want Their Advance Directives Followed?' *JAMA* 267 (1992): 59–63.

9 **Lachlan Forrow, Edward Gogel**, and **Elizabeth Thomas**, 'Advance Directives for Medical Care' (letter), *NEJM* 325 (1991): 1255.

10 **Linda L. Emanuel** *et al.*, 'Advance Directives for Medical Care – A Case for Greater Use,' *NEJM* 324 (1991): 889–95.

11 See Eric Rakowski, 'The Sanctity of Human Life,' *Yale Law Journal* 103 (1994): **2049, 2110–11.**

12 See Allen Buchanan and Dan Brock,'Deciding for Others,'in *The Ethics of Surrogate Decisionmaking* (Cambridge: Cambridge University Press, 1989), at 101–7 for discussion of these and other shortcomings of advance treatment decisionmaking.

13 See generally Rebecca Dresser and John A. Robertson, 'Quality-of-Life and Non-Treatment Decisions for Incompetent Patients: A Critique of the Orthodox Approach, '*Law Medicine & Health Care* 17 (1989): 234–44.

14 See Derek Parfit, *Reasons and Persons* New York: Oxford University Press, pp. 199–379.

15 See, e.g., Allison B. Seckler *et al.*, 'Substituted Judgment: How Accurate Are Proxy Predictions?' *Annals of Internal Medicine* 115 (1992): 92–98.

16 See generally Leslie P. Francis, 'Advance Directives for Voluntary Euthanasia: A Volatile Combination?' *Journal of Medicine & Philosophy* 18 (1993): 297–322.

17 Kitwood and Bredin, 'Towards a Theory of Dementia Care,' 273–74.

Autonomy in Long Term Care: Some Crucial Distinctions*

Bart J. Collopy

Within long term care few ethical issues prove more problematic than those involving personal autonomy. When care impinges on the freedom and independence of the elderly, as it frequently does, a nettlesome question arises: Should the self-determination of the elderly or the decisions and standards of caregivers have priority? Beneath this question lurk primal philosophical and experiential tensions: between freedom and best interest, self-determination and dependence on others, individual choice and the pressures of collective care. When these tensions are resolved chiefly by caregivers and chiefly in favor of best interest, dependency, or collective concerns, the result can be ethically ironic. Care can slide toward control, not from malevolence but simply from the dynamic of powerful and resourceful professionals interacting with vulnerable and resource-weak clients.

Furthermore, precisely when care is beneficent, intrusions upon autonomy can go unchecked, unscrutinized, even unobserved behind the curtain of good intentions. Helping interventions are often judged by the motivations and goals of the helpers, not by the preferences and life projects of those helped (Buchanan, 1981; Gaylin et al., 1981; Veatch, 1981). In short, beneficent intentions can breed unchecked authority over those who are served or helped. To the extent, therefore, that it fails to pursue rigorous examination of autonomy issues, the long term care profession risks conceptual and philosophical naivete about its own ethical foundations.

Defining Autonomy

Although the etymological roots of autonomy suggest the compact definition *self-rule* (autonomous), the conceptual contents of such a definition belie its neatness. As Beauchamp and Childress (1983) pointed out, autonomy is rich in paraphrase, loose in definition. It translates into a whole family of value-laden ideas: individual liberty, privacy, free choice, self-governance, self-regulation, moral independence. Focusing on just this latter paraphrase, Dworkin (1978) suggested seven different meanings for moral independence. In similar fashion, Thomasma (1984), suggested five different types of freedom which function within the ambit of autonomy.

With an eye to this conceptual plasticity, in the following discussion autonomy is defined as a notional field, a loose system of inter-orbiting concepts that trace out the varied paths of self-determination. Accordingly, autonomy is understood as a cluster of notions including self-determination, freedom, independence, liberty of choice and action. In its most general terms, autonomy signifies control of decision-making and other activity by the individual. It refers to human agency free of outside intervention and interference.

The scope of such agency is, of course, quite varied. It includes the freedom to shape long range goals and purposes, to determine life priorities and commitments, to control the content and direction of personal history. In more particular terms, it includes the freedom to manage the short range, ad hoc aspects of life, the mundane realities that measure self-determination on a day-to-day basis. It should be noted, too, that in this definition the autonomous person is not a lone, isolated, atomistic agent making decisions without ties to other people, social institutions, and traditions of thought and action (Callahan, 1984; Cohler, 1983; Dworkin, 1976, 1978; MacIntyre, 1981). Finally, autonomy does not require that an individual be master of all circumstances or be entirely untouched by outside influence and constraint. Even the autonomous person knows the bounds of time and space, history and biology, society and personality. Thus, truly autonomous decision-makers recognize and respond to external determinations, precisely by freely choosing and accepting them.

Tensions and Polarities within Autonomy

A good deal of attention has been paid to paternalism as an external threat to autonomy (Childress, 1982b; Dworkin, 1972,1983; Reamer, 1982, 1983; Van De Veer, 1986). But autonomy is an internally problematic concept, bristling with distinctions and polarities that can be ethically perplexing even in settings where professionals are committed to client self-determination. By way of preview, Chart 1 indicates six such polarities, the ethical risks they create for client autonomy, and potential responses to these risks from caregivers.

As exploratory probes these polarities do not offer the only possible conceptual mapping of autonomy, nor do they reveal immediate solutions to the complex problems of autonomy in long term care. They can be used, however, to suggest directions for research, policy formulation, and canons of practice. Accordingly, the following explication and analysis of these polarities offer practical case illustrations, as well as focal questions about philosophy of practice and research agendas in long term care.

Decisional Autonomy and Autonomy of Execution

Decisional autonomy, as the name implies, consists in the ability and freedom to make decisions without external coercion or restraint. Autonomy of execution consists in the ability and freedom to act on this decisional autonomy, that is, to carry out and implement personal choices.

In full measure, autonomy should be decisional and executional. But it is not always so. Decisional autonomy can exist without the ability or freedom to execute decisions. Individuals can be intellectually and volitionally autonomous, and yet be incapacitated, constrained, or otherwise prevented from acting. For the elderly in long term care, this is, then, a pivotal distinction. With advancing frailty, autonomy of execution frequently shrinks or disappears completely. Consequently, if autonomy is defined principally in terms of execution, the frail elderly will be relegated to non-autonomous status. But autonomy is a broader concept and includes decisional modes which can remain quite intact, even when execution becomes limited or dependent on others.

The distinction between decisional autonomy and autonomy of execution is ethically critical, therefore, because it provides an incremental and conservationist mapping of self-determination. It challenges, unitary, act-oriented, all-or-nothing notions of autonomy. It contends that loss of physical performance does not automatically signal or justify loss of decisional autonomy. In fact, as the outward reach of autonomy shrinks,

* Collopy, B.: Autonomy in long term care: Some crucial distinctions. *Gerontologist* **28**:10–17, 1988.

Chart 1. Polarities *Within Autonomy*: Risk and Response in *Long Term Care*

Polarity	Inherent risks	Possible correctives
Decisional vs. Executional: having preferences, making decisions vs. being able to implement them or carry them out.	Decisional autonomy too easily abrogated whenever autonomy of execution is diminished or lost.	*Enabling the elderly to continue* making *decisions in activities* (ADL, IADL) *where they need assistance.*
Direct vs. Delegated: deciding or acting on one's own vs. giving authority to others to decide/act for one.	Only direct autonomy fully recognized and respected; delegation effectively reduced to surrender or forfeiture of autonomy.	Developing norms for delegation of decisions/ activity to caregivers; developing explicit, mutually acceptable maps of what authority is retained by the elderly, what delegated to caregivers.
Competent vs. Incapacitated: reasonably and judgmentally coherent choice/activity vs. that which exhibits rational defect or judgmental incoherence.	Labeling of the elderly as incapacitated because of: (1) the sheer difficulty and complexity of competency assessments; (2) decisions made by the elderly which challenge institutional goals, professional expectations, societal norms.	Avoiding global and perfunctory judgments of incompetency; recognizing the often partial, context-specific nature of competency; respecting elderly individuals' own norms for what constitutes reasonable, logical or coherent choice.
Authentic vs. Inauthentic: choices/actions which are consonant with character vs. those which are seriously out of character.	Defining autonomy solely in terms of rationality; ignoring or over-riding the elderly individual's own personal values, moral career, goals, and motivations in favor of caregivers' value system.	Developing an understanding of and protective response to the value histories of elderly clients; documenting a value inventory to aid caregivers in identifying authentic choices (particularly those which are highly idiosyncratic).
Immediate vs. Long Range: present or limited expressions of autonomy vs. future or wide-ranging expressions.	Defining autonomy only in terms of a rigid rights perspective which unquestioningly allows immediate freedom to work against long-range autonomy; conversely, defining autonomy only in terms of long-range considerations, thereby giving wide latitude to paternalistic intervention and interference.	Admitting the inherent tensions between immediate and long-range autonomy; recognizing that for the elderly long-range considerations may often be secondary to immediate ones; developing a calculus of care that counter-balances present/ limited with future/global autonomy.
Negative vs. Positive: choice/activity that claims a right only to non-interference vs. that which claims positive entitlement, support, capacitation.	Defining autonomy only in terms of non-interference, thereby encouraging a laissez-faire response to harmful choice and behavior; defining autonomy in positive terms that do not recognize scarcity of resources; defining enhancement as a license for intervening in spheres where the elderly themselves want only a non-interfering commitment to their autonomy.	Developing balanced interplay between positive and negative notions of autonomy; admitting and protecting the primacy of the negative definition (non-interference); moving beyond this minimum to explore caregiver obligations to enhance autonomous choice and activity among the elderly.

its inner decisional core becomes a last and therefore most crucial preserve of self-determination. From an ethical perspective, then, loss of execution argues for greater protections for decisional autonomy, precisely because the physically dependent elderly are increasingly vulnerable to external coercion. The following case indicates how such coercion may develop.

Case 1. – Mrs. A., 79 years old, shares a two family house with her married son and family. She is quite frail and needs assistance in a number of daily life activities and the tasks instrumental to them. She cannot dress herself without assistance, cannot do her laundry, shopping, or most of her cooking. She has regular homemaker assistance, and her daughter-in-law gives her a good deal of daily help.

Even though she depends on this assistance, Mrs. A. has become increasingly frustrated and depressed by its effect on her independence. She feels that her daughter-in-law treats her like a child as she helps her dress and, automatically, chooses clothes for her every day. In addition, because Mrs. A. depends on others for shopping and meal preparation, she feels she has lost even more control over her daily life. She swings between arguing with her caregivers and depressively accepting their ministrations. In her view, care comes at a biting price. 'My helpers have taken over,' she says.

As suggested here, loss of autonomy can slide inexorably from execution to decisionmaking. When frail elderly are no longer able to act independently in certain spheres, they can lose decisional control over those spheres. From an ethical vantage point, this suggests a number of questions for future research and conceptualizing, as well as for ethical guidelines and policy: Within the dynamics of care, is physical dependency interpreted as a sign of decisional dependency? Is loss of autonomy presumptively extended from levels of execution to levels of decisionmaking? Are there specific zones of autonomy in which this is most likely to happen for the

frail elderly (e.g., autonomy with regard to medication and medical treatment, autonomy in daily life style and schedule, autonomy with regard to finances, living arrangements, personal care)?

Direct and Delegated Autonomy

Direct autonomy is a matter of unmediated, hands-on agency. In such autonomy, long term care patients decide and act as individual, independent, self-sufficient agents with strong authorial control over their choices and actions. In delegated autonomy, on the other hand, individuals freely accept decisions and activities supplied for them by others. Here, care recipients authorize others to make decisions and carry out activities in their place. They no longer stand alone but instead depend on the agency of surrogates and sustainers.

If this distinction is not recognized, autonomy is liable to be understood in direct terms only. In such an understanding, delegation is seen as surrender or forfeiture of autonomy. All decision-making or activity given over to others therefore constitutes dependency, evidence of ineffectual or failed autonomy. Although such a definition would narrow the scope of autonomy in any setting, it is particularly straitening within long term care. It suggests that to remain autonomous the elderly must steadfastly resist any delegation of decisions or activity to others. In a world of direct autonomy only, the elderly are therefore left with a stark choice: loss of autonomy or lone and unsupported autonomy.

In contexts fixated on direct autonomy, the elderly must perform with high autonomy or else be relegated to the ranks of the non-autonomous. Such oversimplification can, however, be checked by notions of delegated autonomy. For the frail elderly, self-determination may be supported and survive longer when there are opportunities to delegate certain activity and decisions to others. When delegation is recognized as a valid form of autonomy, the elderly are clearly positioned as agents and active participants, indeed as authorizers of the circumstances and processes of care. Moreover, caregivers become not merely managers of care but true surrogates, supportive proxies, for their elderly clients. Thus, delegated autonomy directs attention to the inherently moral dimensions of long term care: its reciprocal nature, its response to vulnerability, its highly charged interplay between power and frailty, control and freedom (Childress, 1982a; May, 1975, 1982).

The notion of delegated autonomy does not, of course, solve the ethical problems of autonomy in long term care. Transference of agency to others is fraught with potential misunderstandings between the elderly and their caregivers. Indeed, delegation of autonomy can be injurious to personal freedom and independence, not only within institutions (Bennett, 1963; Goffman, 1960), but within any setting where autonomy is pre-empted by those who provide care. Consider, for example, the following cases.

Case 2. – Mr. B., a 72-year-old widower, has not fared well since his wife's death. He does not eat properly, misses doctors' appointments, and fails to take his blood-pressure medication regularly. He cares less and less about personal grooming and appearance. Troubled by this downhill course, his daughter finally prevails upon him to move in with her, her husband, and their two teenage sons.

Things do not go well, however. Mr. B. argues frequently with his two teenage grandsons, begins drinking heavily, is often withdrawn and reclusive. He regularly refuses to eat with the family, snacking instead on crackers and sardines in his room. His daughter claims that he is more trouble than her two teenage sons. 'I feel he is deteriorating right before my eyes, and I can't get him to do anything about it.' Finally, she confronts him with an accumulated list of grievances about his behavior. 'This is my home, and I won't stand by and just let you fall apart,' she tells him. 'If I want to fall apart, I will. I'm not one of your children,' he retorts.

Case 3. – Mrs. C. and Mr. D., both of whom have lost their spouses, have been residents in the same nursing home for a number of years. Unable to manage independently outside the home, they are, nonetheless, mentally alert and emotionally robust. In the course of the last 2 years they have developed a close and intimate relationship, one that becomes highly problematic when a nurse's aide, coming unexpectedly into Mrs. C.'s room, finds them in bed together.

Word of the discovery spreads, and a senior staff member confronts the two, telling them that their behavior is inappropriate. Mr. D. keeps angry silence, refusing to discuss the matter at all. Mrs. C. tells the staff member that her relationship with Mr. D. is none of the staff's business, that their privacy should be respected. 'The home is not in charge of our sexual relations,' she says.

Mrs. C.'s son, who pays for part of his mother's care and visits her weekly, learns of the incident from a staff member. He reacts very negatively and goes to the home's administrator demanding that Mr. D. be 'kept away' from his mother.

Both of these cases exhibit conflicts about the autonomy of the frail elderly and the authority of those who care for them. From the caregivers' vantage point, entry into a care setting can imply that the elderly have surrendered to others a determining role in certain areas of personal choice and behavior. The elderly, on their part, may feel that they retain direct control, that they have delegated very little of this autonomy to others. The resulting conflict suggests some leading questions for both theory and practice: Can long term care develop a well-defined, feasible principle of delegated autonomy? What ethical problems result when delegation of authority remains assumed, tacit, global, not negotiated mutually by the elderly and their caregivers? When should delegation of authority be mandated by the necessities of care and when should it be determined by the elderly themselves?

Competent and Incapacitated Autonomy

This is the most highly sanctioned and widely discussed distinction in the area of autonomy. Competent autonomy is choice or behavior that is

informed, rationally defensible, and judgmentally effective in choosing appropriate means to desired ends. Incapacitated autonomy consists in choice or activity that is substantially uninformed, unreasonable, or judgmentally unsound. The distinction is crucial because incapacity, when it leads to harmful choice, provides defensible grounds for intervening in the choice and behavior of the elderly.

The interrelation of competency and autonomy is treated extensively in a separate section of this supplemental issue. Thus, it is sufficient, perhaps, to indicate that the principal ethical challenge involves determining when the exercise of autonomy is so incapacitated that others may justifiably intervene. For the elderly in long term care, this determination can be absolutely definitive for autonomy, as suggested by the following case.

Case 4. – Mrs. E., 82 years old, has been a resident in a nursing home for 4 years. An alert, relatively vigorous and active woman, she has recently undergone surgery for the removal of a malignant ovarian tumor. Her surgery and post-surgical convalescence prove to be more protracted, painful, and emotionally draining than she had anticipated. After surgery she begins a chemotherapy regimen, but she experiences extreme nausea and weakness from the first treatment. She refuses to continue with chemotherapy, telling her son. 'First, the awful surgery, and now this. I've never been so sick. I don't want any more chemo. If the cancer comes back, I'll deal with it.'

Her physician and others try to convince her to continue with the treatment, but she remains adamant. 'It makes sense for younger people, but not for me.' Mrs. E's son is very troubled by this decision. He tells the physician that he thinks his mother's decision is tragically unreasonable. He urges that everything possible be done to change her mind and even asks whether there is some way they can 'press' his mother into continuing with chemotherapy. In response, the physician arranges a psychiatric consult for Mrs. E.

As this case illustrates, refusal of care easily serves as the decisional gate for challenges to competency (Drane, 1985). But if the social, institutional, and professional canons which determine 'indicated' care are not checked by the principle of self-determination, competency can come to mean little more than obedience to the value system of caregiving institutions and professions. In such a situation, the elderly run the risk of being judged decisionally incapacitated simply by being sharply and singularly individual, by being decisionally irregular. On the other hand, if idiosyncratic and harmful decisions are automatically honored under the rubric of autonomy, there is real danger that truly incapacitated choice and behavior will work grievous harm to the elderly.

Given the import of the competency versus incapacity distinction on the autonomy of the elderly, the long term care profession faces a number of pressing questions: Are the ethical problems connected with assessments of competency fully admitted and examined? Is there sufficient attention to the problems of borderline competency, intermittent and context-specific competency? In cases where refusal of care instigates doubts about competency, is reasonableness defined as a client-centered norm? In such cases, are professional, institutional, and other communal biases clearly held in check?

Authentic and Inauthentic Autonomy

Competency has long been the standard measure for determining when, on psychological, philosophical, and moral grounds, autonomy has a valid claim against intervention. But competency is not the only factor used to define and enforce this claim. Although autonomy obviously includes rationality and judgmental coherence, it goes far beyond this. In full measure, autonomy is the active expression of human identity, intention, and history. Thus, any thoroughgoing discussion must move beyond issues of rational competency to those which involve the wider repertoire of the self: individuality, character, personal integrity and coherence.

Authenticity moves beyond rational mechanisms to the characterological elements of autonomy: issues of life history, moral career, value priorities and dispositions, relational and ideological commitments, decision-making habits, precisely as all of these are rooted in personal identity, integrity, and responsibility (Dworkin, 1976). Authentic autonomy therefore consists in choices and behavior that are deeply in character, that flow from past moral career and ethical style, as well as from present values and immediate self-shaping. Inauthentic autonomy consists in choices and activities that are seriously out of character, discontinuous with personal history and present values, lacking self-possession and self-understanding.

Although authenticity widens the conceptual and empirical scope of autonomy, it does not make autonomy any more tractable from an ethical point of view. In long term care, for example, elderly individuals may express their deepest selves, act in utmost accord with their personal history and values, and yet make choices which caregivers find ambiguous, harmful, unacceptable and, therefore, dilemma-ridden. Conversely, the elderly may, under coercion, behave quite reasonably by common standards, and yet be acting in sharp discord with their authentic selves.

To make judgments about authenticity, then, caregivers must give careful attention to elderly individuals' moral careers, their past preferences, commitments, and value priorities, as well as their present motivations, options, and situations (Donchin, 1984; McCullough & Wear, 1985). Obviously, judgments about authenticity can probe autonomy on levels that are not as publicly available as those revealing competency (which explains, perhaps, why competency tends to be the primary norm in testing autonomy). Furthermore, the moral-psychological components of authenticity are mutable and historical. Authenticity can be built from a shifting history of decisions and choices, consents and refusals. It can involve alteration as well as constancy, wavering as well as decisiveness, tentative inchings and trials, and all manner of consonance between past and present (Cassell, 1978; Childress, 1982b).

Distinguishing between authentic and inauthentic autonomy can be, therefore, quite daunting. But the very recognition of this challenge is salutary. It prevents authenticity from being employed as a handy device either for quickly overriding idiosyncratic choices or underwriting harmful ones. Simply because authenticity is not readily available to scrutiny and easy assessment, it protects autonomy by building cautions around it. But those cautions can create ethical tension and perplexity, as is, perhaps, demonstrated in the following cases.

Case 5. – Mr. F. is 72 years old and suffers from Parkinson's disease. He had always been a proud, highly independent, self-sustaining individual, but since the death of his wife 2 years ago, he has had to depend more and more on his two married daughters and their families for assistance and care. He has a close and warm relationship with all of them, and they very willingly respond to his needs, but he feels that he has become increasingly burdensome to them.

After much brooding about this, Mr. F. tells his oldest daughter that he has decided to sell his house and disperse all his capital to his grandchildren, keeping only enough to support himself in a small apartment until he can qualify for Medicaid. At that time he will apply for admission to a nursing home and so cease being a burden to his daughters and their families.

His daughter protests, but Mr. F. tells her that he has pondered all his options carefully. His plan is eminently reasonable and carefully calculated. That it is, she admits, but it is also very disturbing. To her mind, the plan represents a terrible surrender, a self-wounding, for this proud and independent man. She cannot imagine her father living in a small apartment, spending down into poverty, finally entering a nursing home bereft of resources. 'It's just not him,' she says to herself.

Case 6. – Mrs. G., 83 years old, has been a resident at a nursing home since she suffered a serious stroke 6 years ago. Within the last year she has become increasingly frail and non-communicative, and a bout with pneumonia, necessitating a 2-week hospital stay, leaves her only more frail.

Upon her return to the nursing home, the staff finds that Mrs. G. refuses all solid food. Sustained mainly by liquid nourishment which she intermittently takes, she continues to grow weaker. She becomes more quiet and withdrawn, almost never speaks, except to say 'hello' or 'thank you' to the staff who care for her. Mrs. G.'s daughter visits almost daily. Her mother smiles and greets her. She holds her daughter's hand, listens to her, but rarely says anything in reply. On one occasion when her daughter asks her

why she doesn't talk, or eat, or respond more actively, Mrs. G. simply responds: 'There's no need.'

After some hard reflection, Mrs. G.'s daughter decides that her mother has chosen to accept death and struggle no longer to extend her life. The daughter speaks to a nurse who has cared for her mother for a number of years. 'I think my mother has reached the point where she is waiting, willingly, for her death. If she continues to refuse food, I don't want her to be forced to eat or artificially fed.' The nurse feels that Mrs. G.'s daughter has read the situation correctly. She also knows that, according to usual practice, the nursing home will very soon undertake intravenous feeding of Mrs. G. She sees potential conflict ahead, but for the time being she says nothing.

In both of these cases, the question of intervention hinges on notions of authenticity. For Mr. F.'s daughter, the possibility that her father's decision is deeply out of character could be grounds for intervening against the plan he has so single-mindedly and rationally proposed. In this case authenticity would pull against competency. The characterological oddness of Mr. F.'s plan, its failure to fit who he is and has been, would undercut its logic and rationality. But because authenticity and rationality do not mesh, any decision (to accept Mr. H.'s plan or to intervene against it) will face ethical risk and ambiguity. In case 6, Mrs. G.'s daughter faces the possibility that her mother's refusal to eat represents an authentic choice about the end of her life. If this is so, then the claims of her autonomy should not be summarily overridden. Those responsible for her care face probing questions and difficult weighing of options and responsibilities. If Mrs. G.'s refusal to eat is authentic, and if she is competent (her silence and withdrawal are not automatic denials of this), then her autonomy looms large as a value to be respected and protected.

In dealing with ethical dilemmas involving authenticity and inauthenticity, a number of focal questions might prove helpful: Are the controversial choices or troublesome behavior of the frail elderly scrutinized not only for reasonableness, but also for authenticity? Does authenticity protect choices that appear unreasonable but are idiosyncratically personal? Conversely, do signs of inauthenticity warn that individuals may be under coercion because they are acting against their own personal history and values? How thorough are attempts to understand the value history, personal goals, life plan, and present motivations of the elderly whose autonomy is at stake? Is authenticity recognized as an added empowerment to competency, so that interventions against competent and authentic decisions are faced with exceedingly grave burdens of justification?

Immediate and Long Range Autonomy

The ethics of long term care is frequently complicated by conflict between immediate and long range autonomy. Immediate autonomy refers to present freedom or freedom in a specific, limited sphere of choice and behavior. Long range autonomy is a matter of future freedom or wide-ranging, global areas of decision-making and action.

It is the very nature of autonomy that individuals are able, ironically, to choose against themselves. Present choice can delimit or thwart future choice; autonomous action in one area of life can foreclose on such action in another area. This opposition is, of course, a chief incentive to paternalistic intervention. To the extent that long term care professionals are primarily committed to long range autonomy for the elderly, immediate choice or behavior which threatens this autonomy will seem ripe for well-intentioned intervention (Weiss, 1985).

Furthermore, those who define long range autonomy (in many cases, not the elderly but their caregivers) will, in the very act of definition, determine the grounds for intervening in immediate choice. For example, if the ultimate goal of medical treatment is long range autonomy (Komrad, 1983), then patient resistance or non-compliance can be viewed as merely an immediate and short range expression of autonomy. The future and more comprehensive goals of care can easily override such specific and narrow expressions of autonomy.

On the other hand, if the moral force or autonomy is primarily housed in its immediate forms, that is, in present choice, then every autonomous choice and act creates moral constraints against intervention (Nozick, 1974). The major weakness of this position is that it can nullify social responsibility for destructive choices and acts. It does this precisely by its act-centered framework, its atomistic definition of autonomy. In such a definition, the contradictions and harm of autonomous choice are simply the risks of private responsibility. Thus, if this definition protects autonomy, it also isolates it, creating very short moral linkage between caregivers and their clients. For long term care practitioners, this presents particular problems, because it can create a kind of laissez-faire attitude, a passive, uninvolved model of moral agency for caregiving.

The tension between immediate and long range autonomy derives, in large measure, from competing conceptualizations. Long range autonomy envisages self-determination as a final, ultimate good. In immediate autonomy, on the other hand, self-determination is perceived as an instrumental, immediate right (Nozick, 1974). Thus, the opposition between the two is formal and structural. Given the elemental nature of this opposition, it is important to sustain the tension between immediate and long range autonomy, rather than release it by giving priority to one over the other. A case example illustrates the problem.

Case 7. – Mr. H., 83 years old, is in a nursing home where he is recuperating from a hip fracture. He receives physical therapy but is making very slow progress in his ability to walk. One evening, trying to maneuver the few steps from the wheelchair to his bed, he falls. He is not hurt, but the next day he gets up from his wheelchair and falls again. Told not to leave his wheelchair without assistance, he persists in his short journeys. After a third fall in which he suffers a cut on his head, the decision is made to restrain him in the wheelchair. Mr. H. reacts vigorously against this, constantly pulling at the restraint and pleading with staff, even with visitors, to untie him.

Mr. H.'s son initially accepts the protective rationale offered for the restraint, but when his father continues to be agitated by the restraint he finally goes to the charge nurse and asks that the restraint be removed for the sake of his father's freedom. The nurse tells him that this would be a mistake. 'If he falls again and really hurts himself, what freedom will he have? You should consider his long term status. He might be restrained now, but it's only for the sake of his future mobility.'

In this case, caregivers intervene against present autonomy in the name of future or long range autonomy. Yet neither the priority nor the substance of long range autonomy is defined by the elderly client. Mr. H. seems to prefer risk-laden independence now rather than more secure independence later. His caregivers, following their own value systems, define independence in terms of future, fuller, and fall-free mobility. But although their view, that long range autonomy trumps immediate autonomy, creates ethical conflict, the reverse prioritization is by no means free of ethical problems. If immediate autonomy is granted strict priority over long range autonomy, then caregivers can remain unconcerned about choices that work against long range autonomy. Mr. H. can simply take his own chances at walking and falling.

Rather than opt, programmatically, for either immediate or long range autonomy, the surer ethical course might be for caregivers to admit dilemma and ethical bind, to struggle with the moral equivalent of Mr. H.'s physical restraint. Again, some exploratory questions might indicate the nature of this restraint and the ethical deliberations it would provoke. Within the dynamics of care is the immediate freedom of the elderly protected against absorption into long range autonomy (especially as defined and imposed by caregivers)? Conversely, are the elderly protected from isolation and unconcern when they choose immediate paths that diminish future autonomy? Do conflicts between immediate and long range autonomy provide an opportunity for everyone involved (the elderly, their families, and their caregivers) to realize how they are all entangled in the coils of mutual responsibility and freedom, of shared conflicts and crossed intentions?

Negative and Positive Autonomy

This last binary description of autonomy is developed from the philosophical discussion of rights and liberty. Such discussion commonly distinguishes between negative claims to non-interference and positive claims to entitlement (Beauchamp & Childress, 1983; Fried, 1978; Young, 1986). Accordingly, a negative liberty or right is a claim against invasion and interference. It prevents restraint, forbids coercion and control, and builds barriers around spheres of agency. Bluntly put, it announces that an individual agent should be left alone.

A notion of negative autonomy, developed along similar lines, would forbid interference or intervention in an individual's self-determination. It would oblige others to stand back, not to overrule, block, or even meddle in the free choice and action of an individual. In effect, negative autonomy would set off human agency as something posted against trespass, even beneficent and well-intentioned trespass.

On the other hand, with positive liberties and rights, claims are levied for empowerment, for support and enhancement beyond the negative minimum of non-interference. A positive right proclaims entitlement, obliges others not simply to stand back and refrain from interference, but to step forward and provide resources, to offer instrumental means. Consequently, positive autonomy could be used to assert a claim to opportunity, to assistance and resources that would operationalize choice and enable it to reach at least some minimal potential. Given a positive definition, response to autonomy becomes a matter of advocacy, of mounting barricades to press freedom forward, not merely building barricades to protect its present forms.

Within the long term care system, positive notions of autonomy involve a much more comprehensive, interactive, and time-consuming process than do negative notions (Gadow, 1979, 1980). In contrast to the dictum-like guideline of negative autonomy ('do not interfere'), positive definitions of autonomy raise a wide-ranging series of questions about how elderly individuals ought to be supported and strengthened in their autonomous choices and actions. The tensions between these quite different notions of autonomy can be exemplified by a case example:

Case 8. – Mr. J., in his late seventies, has been in a nursing home for 2 years. Three months ago, weakened from a bout with pneumonia, he was given a wheelchair as a temporary means of mobility. As matters turned out, he adapted very well to the wheelchair, finding that it meant certain prerogatives and special attention from staff. In fact, he so valued these 'rewards' that he showed little inclination to walk on his own, as his recuperation progressed.

At present, Mr. J. routinely refuses to go to physical therapy sessions, and most staff members have begun to treat him as wheelchair-bound. In fact, moving him about by wheelchair is in many ways less troublesome than trying to get him to walk even a few steps. Mr. J.'s wife, who visits him daily, presses the staff to get him back on his feet. She is very distressed that more isn't being done to make him ambulatory. The staff explains that her husband cannot be physically coerced or intimidated into walking. Moreover, they do not see his wheelchair status as a serious problem.

In this case Mr. J.'s caregivers contend that he should be left alone. His wife, on the other hand, holds a strongly positive view of autonomy, one that requires staff members to draw out and enlarge her husband's dormant mobility. In this latter view, respecting autonomy goes beyond mere non-intervention to active involvement and encouragement. Caregivers ought to call autonomy forward, ought to prompt and capacitate self-dependence, particularly when an individual is passive and unduly dependent on others. Thus, in the case of Mr. J., caregivers are especially obligated to encourage independence because the reward system of the institution may have induced and encouraged his non-mobility. (Those who advance positive notions of autonomy would be very sensitive to instances of iatrogenic dependency, to learned helplessness that might go unchallenged by those applying only negative definitions of autonomy).

But if negative notions of autonomy can be used to justify care that is non-involved, non-responsive, and minimally custodial, positive notions of autonomy are also ethically problematic. Are there, for example, any limits to entitlement? To what lengths must staff go in efforts to rehabilitate an uncooperative Mr. J.? Given scarce resources and multiple, competing claims on them, caregivers cannot face absolutely open-ended obligations. Autonomy might be an ever-expanding possibility in the life of an individual, but it cannot be used to levy limitless obligations on others. An additional problem with positive autonomy is that it can encourage interference with the choice and behavior of the elderly in the name of enhancing autonomy. Thus, in the name of expanding autonomy, caregivers might be prompted to intervene quite freely in client choices which they consider too narrow and limiting.

The two extremes which threaten autonomy (non-interference that constitutes neglect and care that constitutes control) can be checked by cautionary questions: Are the risks of negative autonomy fully recognized (i.e., isolation and separation of the elderly; non-involvement on the part of caregivers)? At the same time, are positive definitions of autonomy scrutinized for unrealistic, promissory notions of entitlement, for the risk that caregivers might too readily intervene in the name of enhancing client autonomy?

Conclusion

Autonomy can be a source of persistent and serious ethical conflict between the frail elderly and those institutions, agencies, and individuals who provide care to them. To the extent that care subordinates or suppresses autonomy, its benefits come at dubiously high cost of human individuality and freedom. To the extent that individuality and freedom run counter to the dictates of care, autonomy can seem an ambiguous benefit.

Steering a course through this underlying dilemma is more than a matter of good will. Autonomy is a philosophically complex and ethically problematic value, thick with distinctions, polarities, and interpretive variation. Kept in full view, this multiplicity of elements reveals the range and fertile dynamics of self-determination. Fixation on a particular aspect or interpretation of autonomy can lead, however, to a narrow constraining or a tyrannical enlargement of this value. To avoid both extremes, long term care theory, research, and practice must develop the fullest possible account of autonomy, its conceptual and empirical complexity, its relative priority as a value, its conflictual potency and pervasiveness.

References

Beauchamp T., & Childress, J. (1983). *Principles of biomedical ethics*. New York: Oxford University Press.

Bennett, R. (1963). The meaning of institutional life. *The Gerontologist*, **3**, 117–125.

Buchanan, A.E. (1981). Medical paternalism. In M. Cohen, T. Nagel, & T. Scanlon (Eds.), *Medicine and moral philosophy*. Princeton, NJ: Princeton University Press.

Callahan, D. (1984). Autonomy: A moral good, not a moral obsession. *Hastings Center Report*, **14**, 40–42.

Cassell, E. (1978). Self-conflict in ethical decisions. In H. T. Engelhardt, Jr. & D. Callahan (Eds.), *Morals, science and sociality*. Hastings, NY: Hastings Center.

Childress, J. (1982a). Metaphors and models of medical relationships. *Social Responsibility: Journalism, Law, Medicine*, **8**, 47–70.

Childress, J. (1982b). *Who should decide? Paternalism in health care*. New York: Oxford University Press.

Cohler, B. J. (1983). Autonomy and interdependence in the family of adulthood: A psychological perspective. *The Gerontologist*, **23**, 33–39.

Donchin, A. (1984). Personal autonomy, life plans, and chronic illness. In D. H. Smith (Ed.), *Respect and care in medical ethics*. Lanham, MD: University Press of America.

Drane, J. F. (1985). The many faces of competency. *Hastings Center Report*, **15**, 17–21.

Dworkin, G. (1972). Paternalism. *The Monist*, **56**, 64–84.

Dworkin, G. (1976). Autonomy and behavior control. *Hastings Center Report*, **6**, 23–28.

Dworkin, G. (1978). Moral autonomy. In H. T. Engelhardt & D. Callahan (Eds.), *Morals, science and sociality*. Hastings, NY: Hastings Center.

Dworkin, G. (1983). Paternalism: Some second thoughts. In R. Sartorius (Ed.), *Paternalism*. Minneapolis, MN: University of Minnesota Press.

Fried, C. (1978). *Right and wrong*. Cambridge: Harvard University Press.

Gadow, S. (1979). Advocacy nursing and new meanings of aging. *Nursing Clinics of North America*, **14**, 81–91.

Gadow, S. (1980). Medicine, ethics, and the elderly. *The Gerontologist*, **20**, 680–685.

Gaylin, W., Glasser, I., Marcus, S., & Rothman, D. J. (1981). *Doing good: The limits of benevolence*. New York: Pantheon.

Goffman, E. (1960). Characteristics of total institutions. In M. R. Stein, A. J. Vidich, & D. M. White (Eds.), *Identity and anxiety: Survival of the person in mass society*. Glencoe, IL: Free Press.

Komrad, M. S. (1983). A defense of medical paternalism: Maximizing patient autonomy. *Journal of Medical Ethics*, **9**, 38–44.

MacIntyre, A. (1981). *After virtue*. Notre Dame, IN: University of Notre Dame Press.

May, W. F. (1975). Code, covenant, contract, or philanthropy? *Hastings Center Report*, **5**, 29–38.

May, W. F. (1982). Who cares for the elderly? *Hastings Center Report*, **12**, 31–37.

McCullough, L., & Wear, S. (1985). Respect for autonomy and medical paternalism reconsidered. *Theoretical Medicine*, **6**, 295–308.

Nozick, R. (1974). *Anarchy, state, and utopia*. New York: Basic Books.

Reamer, F. (1982). *Ethical dilemmas in social service*. New York: Columbia University Press.

Reamer, F. (1983). The concept of paternalism in social work. *Social Service Review*, **57**, 254–271.

Thomasma, D. C. (1984). Freedom, dependency, and the care of the very old. *Journal of the American Geriatrics Society*, **32**, 906–914.

Van De Veer, D. (1986). *Paternalistic intervention: The moral bounds of benevolence*. Princeton, NJ: Princeton University Press.

Veatch, R. (1981). *A theory of medical ethics*. New York: Basic Books.

Weiss, G. (1985). Paternalism modernized. *Journal of Medical Ethics*, **11**, 184–187.

Young, R. (1986). *Personal autonomy: Beyond negative and positive liberty*. New York: St. Martin's Press.

Racism in Psychiatry: Paradigm Lost – Paradigm Regained*

Dinesh Bhugra and Kamaldeep Bhui

Introduction

Racism has played an important role in the subjugation of ethnic minorities in certain societies and cultures. Sometimes it has been linked with the historical, social and economic contexts in which ethnic minority groups have survived. In addition psychiatry has been often seen as a tool of the state and psychiatrists encouraged to detain people who appear to be a threat to themselves or others – thus being 'saved' from themselves or 'saving' others. In psychiatry, more than in many other disciplines of medicine, 'prejudice' is asserted to explain variations in the management of ethnic minority patients.

Although diverse cultural groups mingle at various social, political, and spiritual contexts, for example, through trade, migration or conquest, the benefits of any one group's cultural advantage does reach others eventually. However, this passage to equality of opportunity is hard won at many levels of society. Therefore, racism in its functionality, and existence in its entirety, cannot be treated simply from a single theoretical perspective, or from a simple individualistic approach.

Historical and economic contexts are important. The structures of society play an important role in the development and maintenance of racial prejudices and racism in society. All pervasive state regulations that structure social and economic processes have to be taken into account. When comparing psychological and cultural variables across cultures Bagley & Verma (1979) reported that although personality factors such as neuroticism, psychological rigidity and poor self-esteem were contributing to prejudiced attitudes in Britain and the Netherlands, prejudice was in overall terms much less prevalent in the Netherlands which the authors attributed to a lack of cultural tradition of racism in that country. In this paper we link individual and group factors that contribute to the emergence and persistence of racism. We then go on to study these in relation to psychiatry and we conclude by identifying the practical, clinical and research implications of racism.

Definitions

Race and the use of this word has multiple meanings and is often emotionally loaded. Often a distinction between biological and social concepts of race muddles the issue further. Even though racial characters should be seen on a continuum, race is defined as a socially defined group for which membership is based on a combination of cultural heritage, historical circumstance and/or the presence of distinguishable physical features such as skin colour. It can be applied to nation states, languages, families, tribes, minorities and is seen as a phenotypically distinct group. Often, race itself is used as a derogatory term – identifying groups which may be seen as economically or culturally vulnerable and the term used to identify such a group.

* Bhugra, D. and Bhui, K.: Racism in psychiatry: paradigm lost – paradigm regained. *International Review of Psychiatry* 11:236–243, 1999.

Racism

Racism is as old as mankind itself. Cicero (100 BC) had advised Atticus not to get slaves from Britain because they were stupid and incapable of learning. Racism can be described as an ideology or belief that helps maintain the *status quo* and more specifically it refers to the belief that one race is superior to other races in significant ways and that the superior race is seen as being entitled, by virtue of its superiority, to dominate other races and to enjoy a share of society's wealth and status. These advantages are related to health care, education, employment, wealth and power hence there is no reason to change any of society's institutionalized ways of doing things. Rex (1983), while defining racism and race prejudice, suggested that the concepts of race as biologists used it had no relevance to the political differences among men and sought to indicate problems of race relations. He proposed three elements:

(a) that it was necessary but not a sufficient condition of a race relations situation that there should be a situation of severe competition, exploitation, coercion or oppression;

(b) that this situation occurred between groups rather than individuals, with only limited possibilities of mobility from one group to the other;

(c) that the inter-group structure so produced was rationalized at the ideological level by means of a deterministic theory of human attributes, of which the most important type historically had been based upon biological and genetic theory.

UNESCO, following a meeting of biologists and social scientists concluded:

(a) Race is a taxonomic concept of limited usefulness as a means of classifying human beings but probably less useful that the more general concept of population. The former term is used to refer to 'groups of mankind showing well-developed and primarily heritable physical differences from other groups' and the latter – 'groups whose members marry other members of the group more frequently than people outside the group' and hence have a relatively limited and distinctive range of genetic characteristics.

(b) It is agreed that observable human characteristics are, in nearly all cases, the result of biological and environmental factors.

(c) Various characteristics commonly grouped as racial are in fact transmitted either independently or in varying degrees of association.

(d) All men living today belong to a single species and are derived from a common stock.

(e) It may not be desirable to deny a particular national group as a race but rather to affirm that it is not justifiable to attribute cultural characteristics to the effects of genetic inheritance.

(f) Human evolution has been affected to a unique degree as compared with evolution of other species by migration and cultural evolution.

As Rex (1983) concludes, taking into account all of the above, the concept of race as used by the biologists has no relevance to the political differences among men.

Types of racism

The persistence of racism in society can be understood at different levels and in different categories. Richardson & Lambert (1985) identified three associated aspects of racism: as ideology, as practice and as a social structure. Racism may operate through overt beliefs and actions of the individual (active racism) or through less conscious attitudes in society as a whole, for example, not offering housing, education or care to ethnic groups (aversive racism) (Dolan *et al.*, 1991). The aspect of racial actions taking place, in an 'unwitting' manner has recently been given credence in the UK by the enquiry into the murder of the teenager Stephen Lawrence. Yet, such an accusation produces, not rational thought, but narcissistic rage.

Rattansi (1992) argues that racism must be distinguished from racial discrimination. The former is restricted to discourses about grouping human populations into 'races' on the basis of some biological signifier – for example, 'stock' – with each 'race' being regarded as having essential characteristics or a certain essential character (e.g. the 'British' character or in attributions to races of laziness, rebelliousness or industriousness) and where inferiorization of some 'races' may or may not be present. Such views may shade off into ethnocentrism – where ethnic groups are defined primarily in cultural terms and are regarded as having essential traits. Nationalism therefore can be seen as a form of ethnocentrism in which cultural groups, and their essential characteristics, are defined by nationality and cultural attributes of one or more nations regarded as inherently superior or inferior. Nationalism may also contain racial elements in so far as particular nations may be regarded as deriving from specific racial stocks, and biologically defined communities may be regarded as the prime source of cultural characteristics.

Institutional racism can be defined as enforcement of racism and maintenance by the legal, cultural, religious, educational, economic, political, environmental and military institutions of society – racism then becomes an institutionalized form of (personal) attitude. As Feagin & Sikes (1994) suggest, the majority of Whites appear to view 'racism in the head'. The majority of Whites in response to African-Americans see serious racism as the prejudices and actions of extreme bigots who are not considered to be representative of the White majority and these authors assert that the Whites can thus see these attacks of racial discrimination with detachment which makes it easier for them to deny the reality of much of the racism reported by Blacks. Racism therefore is not only a combination of prejudices and discrimination to the recurring ways in which White people dominate Black people in every major area of the society.

The economies within the capitalist system were political and not national economies and such economies went on to shape the capitalist system. The enslaving of Africans and Asians, the use of Asians as indentured labour, and the particular forms of racist ideologies constructed to rationalize such activities were embedded in earlier forms of organization of labour within European societies. Giddens (1986) argues that the employment of immigrant workers from poorer countries in the affluent societies of Western Europe has led to ethnic oppression. The differences in the way in which European and African migrants to the US were treated have led to differences in assimilation which, according to Feagin & Sikes (1994), reflect the differences experienced by middle-class African-Americans. Such ethnic oppression is not exclusively associated with capitalist systems but in the context of understanding such expressions historical and economic factors are important. It can be argued that the British efforts to recruit Asian and African-Caribbeans to fill the lowly paid menial jobs and the lure of working for the mother country were nothing less than an oppressive act to colonize the minds of the economically disadvantaged.

Racism has been classified into several types – a mixture of prejudice, power and identity. It can be dominative – where hatred is turned into action and the stereotype of racial bigot is met. It could be aversive racism which accepts the superiority of the White but cannot act on it and avoids conflict by avoiding any kind of action. It can be *regressive*. Other types of racism which have been identified have included pre-reflecting gut – (fear of strangers and need to feel superior to others), post-reflecting gut – (rationalization and justification), cultural (leisure, social customs, manners, religious and moral beliefs), *institutional* – (already discussed above), *paternalistic* (White majority decide for Black) or colour-blind (acceptance of differences is seen as racially divisive). New racism is the variety where as a symbol it is couched in values like individualism in America, where affirmative action is objected to; special favours are criticized and on-going racism is criticized on grounds of present achievements.

Psychiatry is reflecting dominant social values; discriminating these values in the pervasive form of so-called scientific statements and providing an asocial human image of the human being which portrays the individual as essentially independent from his socio historical context. Racist experiences of patients affect help-seeking, diagnosis, compliance with treatment and attitudes towards mental illness, psychiatry and the psychiatric profession. It impinges on the clinician's attitudes, the way help is provided and diagnosis and management. It affects society by inducing feelings of rebellion, alienation, poor membership and the need for increased resources.

Institutional levels of racism pertain to 'establishment' which at a macro level decides on the values important for society and members of the society. Thus, patterns of language use including use of grammar and accent, educational systems which stream pupils and cause misalignment, inculcating feelings of superiority on the basis of some artificial factors. The legal system by virtue of class, upbringing, background and symbolized and invested powers means that the system encourages individuals to set themselves aside. Thus the police, political systems and financial services form an 'elite' that less familiar ethnic minorities have to negotiate. On an individual level, the notions of racial superiority are then subliminally expressed and sanctioned, although racist thoughts may not translate into racist attitudes and behaviour. Yet at some level, there occurs a transformation (see Figure 1).

Why racism?

Racism in society plays a role in allowing the majority to identify 'the other' who can thus be pitied, looked down upon, hated or marginalized. Such a concept makes the majority society feel pure about itself. This set of 'skills' allows one group to identify factors which give it a sense of superiority and survival. Two caveats must be borne in mind – firstly that such differences are often institutionalized and the individuals may not see it as a problem and secondly that such views are not static. Despite prevailing 'social science' approaches which depict people as creatures of their surrounding environment, or as victims of social institutions

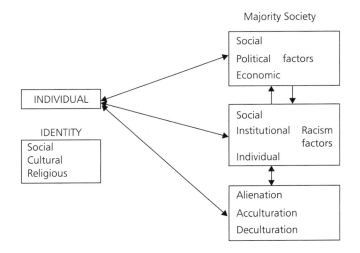

Figure 1

immediately impinging on them, both emigrants and conquerors have carried their own skills and behaviours – their cultures – to the farthest regions of the planet in the most radically different societies, and these patterns have often persisted for generations or even centuries (Sowell, 1994). The concepts of racism often involve the conqueror and the vanquished.

Immigrant workers in all the countries concerned share the same basic position: they have the poorest and lowest status in every social sphere and the immigrants are furthermore highly concentrated in a limited range of occupations and industries and are over-represented in the lowest categories of socio-economic class. They experience great difficulties in obtaining housing which then reflects in serious health problems (Castles & Kosack, 1973). This proletariat is also a focus of nationalism where the employers (or the majority society) tend to control the housing, health, education, legal standing and other institutional aspects of control. The central location of such institutions deals with the majority whereas immigrants, ethnic minorities or 'the other' identified by sexual orientation, gender, skin colour, religious values are on the periphery. The central zone partakes of the nature of the sacred and the central value system is not the whole of the order of values and beliefs espoused and observed in the society and these value systems are regarded as being distributed along a range. The central value system has primary and secondary values and legitimizes the existing distribution of roles and rewards to persons possessing the appropriate qualities which in various ways symbolize degrees of proximity to authority. The central institutional system therefore is legitimized by the central values. Although there may be a sense of consensus in maintaining the central institutional system, this emerges from the majority who have a vested interest in the *status quo*. There is of course a limit to consensus and it can never be all embracing. Although Rex (1961) proposes that central values are dictated by central conflict – the balance of power within such conflict does not always shift rapidly. The 'other' is therefore required to maintain such a control and balance of power and is associated with keeping the outsider out, just in case he/she becomes a threat from within. While the 'other' is outside such an individual is far easier to define and identify. Thus from this necessarily brief discourse, it would appear that if psychiatry is at the periphery of the medical society, the psychiatric patient too is at the periphery. To complicate things even further the ethnic minority mentally ill patient is at the periphery of the mentally ill patients bearing the weight of double jeopardy.

Ethnic and cultural identity

The word identity is fraught with difficulties – it often means different things depending upon how it is being conveyed. It may include the self, religious identity, sexual orientation or occupational identity. Psychologists have long been aware of the highly complex process of identity formation and of the critical role played by race and ethnicity in this process. Early research was grounded on the assumption that out-group orientation as measured by doll-preferences and other paradigms was interpretable in terms of psychopathology. At the level of adulthood, out-group-identification, self-hatred and psychopathology were conceptually merged and interpreted in the historical context of slavery, segregation and the cultural disenfranchisement of the Negro in America (Harris *et al.*, 1994). The self-hatred gave way to pride and positive identity during and after the Civil Rights Movement. The distinction between group and individual identity comprise functionally distinct domains within the individual (Cross, 1991). Cross (1978) has developed a multi-stage model of identity development that analyses the psychological process of coming to terms with one's racial identity. Racial and ethnic identity is not static and is in a constant state of development and reworking in the adult.

Racism in clinical situations

The impact of racism and its influence on the institutional practice as well as individual diagnostic patterns can be investigated at the one-to-one level in clinical encounters.

Misdiagnosis. Psychiatric diagnostic systems deal with categories which have been developed with Western nosological categories in mind. This means that individual differences get lost in the diagnostic encounter. Although ICD-10 and DSM-IV have both started to take the impact of culture into account, day-to-day interactions may not be affected at all. Individual diagnostic patterns and impressions of interactions contribute to the therapeutic encounter. Chess *et al.* (1953) had highlighted the deterministic nature of behaviour within a group membership, thereby reflecting different psychodynamics in individuals' functioning in different situations and in individuals from different cultural backgrounds. On the other extreme, there is often a temptation to make sweeping generalizations concerning culturally-determined differences in behaviour patterns which are not backed up by evidence but are arrived at by apparently rigid preconceptions of the author. The fact that such a discrepancy may reflect lack of ability on the part of the diagnosing physician or clinician to bridge the culture gap is often ignored. Both underdiagnosis and overdiagnosis are often a result of ignorance and are a result of the observer's lack of effort in making any attempt to understand the cultural norms and gaps. The whole concept of diagnosis in psychiatry and its stability has to be looked at again (see Clare, 1973, for some of the arguments).

Underdiagnosis. For a long time it was considered likely that depression if existed in Africa and in India it was of fleeting nature and the stereotype of the noble and happy savage persisted ignoring the clinical evidence and relying on rather inadequate epidemiological data (see Bhugra, 1996, for a review). The psychological conflicts of the Negro group seemed of a more simple, elementary nature, resulting in the less complex type of symptomatology typical of sociopathic behaviour, emotional instability, inadequate personality, simple maladjustment and temperamental unsuitability. The tortuous, intricately structured mechanisms typical of psychoneurosis seemed to be less common. There appeared to be a conspiracy of collective conviction among psychiatrists who, having believed that depression was rare among savages, did not care to look any deeper or anywhere else relying on epidemiological data collected in psychiatric hospitals rather than from the community. The possibility that this difference may not be a real or significant one but rather a reflection of a lack of rapport and understanding between the two participants in the therapeutic encounter did not appear to occur to the clinician.

Culture-bound syndromes. Culture-bound syndromes are a classical example of Western methods of looking at the esoteric, exotic and the rare, sometimes ignoring the social and cultural contexts altogether. The ongoing debate between Simons (1985) and Kenny (1985) on the concepts of *latah* is an excellent example of the divide between the anthropologist and the psychiatrist and between the universalist and the relativist positions. There is also an underlying question about the validity of such syndromes. The whole concept arose out of social anthropological discipline which is blamed on the colonial administration in the UK at least. The exotic and slightly crazy native who had to be sorted out by the colonial master is reflected in the criteria for diagnosis and also legal changes the colonial administrators brought in to deal with these syndromes (e.g. *amok*).

The development of these syndromes and the maintenance of such categories are linked with diagnostic environments and have to be seen in that context.

Management. Clinical management in psychiatry reflects that prevailing clinical practice and it can be argued that where there is a pressure to be colour blind in managing psychiatric conditions and underlying racist streak exists. Such clinical practices may be encouraged and endorsed by the establishment.

Medication. There is plenty of clinical evidence to suggest that people from ethnic minorities are often given higher doses of medication without clear indicators and also for longer periods (see Bhugra & Bhui, 1999, for a review). Not only are the ethnic minorities more likely to be treated compulsorily, they are also more likely to be given ECT and higher doses of neuroleptics, minor tranquilisers and anti-depressants. Limited research data is available on pharmacokinetics and pharmacodynamics of these drugs in ethnic minority groups.

Psychoanalysis. Freud developed his theories of psychoanalysis in nineteenth century Vienna and these, although universally accepted, adopted and applauded, remain tied to the culture of a specific period. Psychoanalysis itself has been branded racist on the grounds that some analysts have adapted it blindly for application to other cultures and groups ignoring the advice of many authors including Chess *et al.* (1953) who maintain that unless the social milieu in which the patient functions is understood and given adequate consideration, significant errors in psychiatric management and prognostic factors will occur.

Psychotherapies. Patients from ethnic minorities are frequently not offered counselling or psychotherapy on the premise that such individuals are not psychologically sophisticated or psychologically minded. Therein lies another fallacy because psychological concepts practised and taught in the West are very culture-bound and the indigenous psychologies and psychological interventions are ignored. There is plenty of clinical evidence to suggest that in spite of language barriers, group therapy works in ethnic minorities and with appropriate modifications family therapy can be undertaken successfully (Bhugra & Bui, 1997).

The clinical management of ethnic minorities' health care needs is in the context of social, economic, political and health care systems and the trends which lead to application of the standard psychiatric criteria for diagnosis, treatment and prognosis. We have not discussed problems associated with psychological testing and the decisive influence of cultural and environmental factors in determining test results and their interpretation. The concepts of underlying personality also vary across cultures and personality itself is not a static phenomenon and needs to be assessed accordingly.

Research and racism

There is often evidence in research publications of the underlying streak of racism. The individual researchers do not often set out to be racist but due to naivety and ignorance, the findings can be misinterpreted.

Findings. One of the commonest errors is the interpretation of findings which are often seen as a result of academic research with little thought paid to the consequences of the findings – how the community would respond to these – e.g. if schizophrenia is found to be high in one group – the media and other groups may see it as a pathology and highlight it. However, the community may well see it as a result of poor social conditions. In an ideal world, both these interpretations need to find a place in the report.

Interpretations. As mentioned earlier, interpretation of the data is one of the problems but it is not only simple reading of the date, it is also essential that the implications of the data are discussed before proceeding with publication. These need to be discussed with the community, community leaders, researchers from the same ethnic background and other interested parties. It does not mean that the researchers have an opportunity of discussing the most obvious results which may well determine resources and management. Secondly, the interpretations may need to be put into context – a lot of papers presented earlier in this century were in the social context (and prejudices) of that time but nowhere was it suggested that this was the case.

Service implications. Any kind of clinical research has to be linked very closely with provision of service. If, after repeated studies the results are ignored by health authorities, trusts, primary care providers, the community's perceptions of the racist establishment are confirmed and not only that they withdraw their support and resent researchers and clinicians. They are then more likely to not cooperate with the researchers simply because there are no tangible observable changes at the end of it. Certainly, for clinical research with ethnic minorities, the clinician must be absolutely certain of the service implications of the research which must be incorporated in the research planning.

Practical implications of racism

For the society. Here the focus may well be on relationships between different groups of people and social categorization and the cognitive processes which affect social categorization and the cognitive consequences of group divisions.

As noted earlier, stereotype of individuals confirms for the observer a lazy way of not dealing with diversity and individual differences. Such a process of simple and basic pigeonholing also allows individuals to ignore racism at an individual level and racism therefore becomes a part of the limitations of rational mental organization and ignoring emotional, motivational and ideological factors altogether. Thus, in a way, the individual observer gets away from his/her responsibility and thereby consolidates institutional racism. As stereotypes are sets of physical or behavioural traits attributed to social groups anyone who dares not fit into the standard stereotype becomes 'exception to prove the rule'. Such an exception is even more threatening rather than actual stereotype and the society may therefore find ways of dealing with it. Although the beliefs may be classified in a hierarchical manner, they do not necessarily provide a hierarchical behavioural setting. Quite often the society chooses not to deal with these cognitions and the argument put forward may be that individuals are too powerless to do anything but the society itself cannot decide where to begin to dismantle these processes.

For the patient. If the patients are buried heavily with the load of society's perceptions and behaviour on racist lines then not only their significant other are being affected but their ideas, beliefs, and values on the one side but also materials and objects on the other (Figure 2).

These interconnecting features are affected by various social and establishment as well as political systems and both the individual and social cognitions contribute to this interaction. The impact of prejudice and racism is not static and does not happen once and the patient tends to forget it but it goes on for a considerable period and may well have features of post traumatic stress disorder. The patients' set of assumptions, strategies and questions about behaviours meted out to them are crucial in making any interaction – therapeutic or other – possible.

For the clinician. As noted earlier, the clinician's experiences and specialist interest will affect racism and vice versa. The dimensions of institutional racism do produce an impact on the clinician and the clinical practice. There are both implicit and explicit aspects of institutionalized racism. The implicit aspects may be absorbed in the medical school or specialist training and explicit aspects reflect the structural aspects. When confronted with crises in Black-White relations most White psychiatrists tend to focus on the helping role that they can play in resolving these conflicts for *other* organizations rather than looking closely at the ways that psychiatry has perpetuated myths of Black inferiority (Sabshin *et al.*, 1970). Under these circumstances the clinician may not have realistic concerns. Black patients have been stereotyped. Institutional racism has been linked with individual

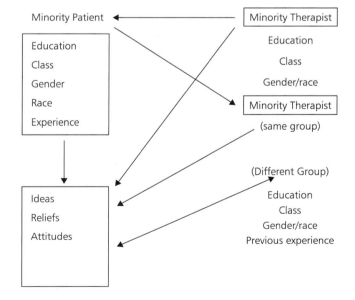

Figure 2

clinician's blind spots, stereotype images, reactive guilt as well as unconscious prejudice. For a long time, a lack of clinical data was seen as a reflection of the institutionalized racism but the relationship of inappropriate research and inadequate interpretation continues to confirm these processes (of institutionalized racism). A lack of appropriate services affects the patient and the clinician alike. The pathways into care for ethnic minorities may thus be blocked. As Sabshin *et al.* (1970) observed, 'unfortunately, greater attention has been paid by White psychiatrists to extending mythical definitions of Black psychopathology than to providing psychiatric services for actual Black patients'. Psychiatrization or medicalization of social issues for ethnic minorities does contribute to clinicians' behaviour which may be inappropriate.

Models of management

The first step in attempting to deal with racism is to recognize its existence and then develop models of organizational management which will include ways and means of dealing with individual stereotypes and encourage community and clinicians to work together. Some of the recommendations are listed in Table 1. The underlying desire to scapegoat individuals must be addressed.

Race should be considered as a social label or category rather than a biological fact. Lock (1993) suggests that race be seen as a politically motivated category which allows for an inherent racial difference and thereby reinforces a continuing ghettoization of ethnic groups. Individual biology needs to be correlated with population biology. Useful generalizations are possible some of which may well assist in clinical practice (e.g. in remembering that pharmacodynamics and pharmacokinetics may well differ across ethnic groups). Quantitative biological differences need to be linked with qualitative, culturally constructed categories of race (Lock, 1993). However, recognition of an ongoing dialectic between culture and biology in which both are recognized as fluid entities will contribute to dealing with individual as well as institutionalized racism. Wade (1993) argues that once racism is embedded within the structures of society, the prejudice of individuals is no longer the main problem.

Three psychological approaches – individual, interpersonal and intergroup – need to be understood and developed in order to deal with racism. There is obviously a likelihood that on an individual level personality differences (akin to authoritarian personality) may contribute to individualized racism. The interpersonal approach will deal with what goes on within social groupings and individual's links with other members is related to the in-group identity. Such an approach attempts to discover the extent to which people conform to the dominant values of a particular social situation. Such a management model therefore can deal with intra-group and individual as well as inter-group situations (where relationships between social groups play an important role).

Thus social psychological explanations of prejudice and conflict sensitize clinicians and patients alike to the evils of racism and to a certain extent

ignore the social context such as culture, social, economic factors and the historical background. Therefore as a clinician planning to set up management of clinical situations in ethnic minorities also has the influence but he/she has to put all the above mentioned factors into an appropriate context.

Conclusions

Institutional and individual racism are a result of three levels or approaches – individual, intra-group and intergroup. The experiences that a patient brings along to the clinical encounter have to be seen in a historical and macro-economic as well as social context. Training for clinicians has to consider aspects of both institutional and individual racism so that clinicians are able to recognize the impact of such a phenomena and deal with it appropriately. The emphasis on biological race needs to be shifted on to qualitative aspects of individual's functioning and the therapeutic encounter must take broader factors into account.

References

Bagley, C. & Verma, G.K. (1979).*Racial prejudice, the individual and society*. Farnborough: Saxon House.

Bhugra, D (1996). Depression across cultures, *Primary Care Psychiatry*, **2**, 155–165.

Bhugra, D. & Bhui, K.S. (1997). Cross-cultural psychiatric assessment. *Advances in Psychiatric Treatment*, **3**, 103–110.

Bhugra, D. & Bhui, K.S. (1999). Ethnic and cultural factors in psychopharmacology. *Advances in Psychiatric Treatment*, **5**, 89–95.

Castles, S. & Kosack, G. (1973). *Immigrant workers and class structure in western Europe*. Oxford: Oxford University Press.

Chess, S., Clark, K. & Thomas, A. (1953) .The importance of culture evaluation in psychiatric diagnosis and treatment, *Psychiatric Quarterly*, **27**, 102–114.

Clare, A. (1973). *Psychiatry in dissent*. London: Tavistock.

Cross, WE. (1978). The Thomas and Cross models on psychological nigrescence: a literature review. *Journal of Black Psychology*, **4**, 13–31.

Cross, WE. (1991). *Studies of Black: diversity in African-American identity*. Philadelphia: Temple University Press.

Dolan, B., Polley, K., Allen, R. & Norton, K. (1991). Addressing racism in psychiatry. *International Journal of Social Psychiatry*, **37**, 71–79.

Feagin, J. & Sikes, M. (1994). *Living with racism: the Black middle class experience*, Boston, MA: Beacon Press.

Giddens, A. (1986). *Sociology: a brief but critical introduction*. London: MacMillan.

Harris, E., Blue, E. & Griffith, E. (1994). Introduction. In: E. Harris, E. Blue & E. Griffith (Eds), *Racial and ethnic identity*. New York: Routledge.

Kenny, M. (1985). Latah: paradox lost. In: C.C. Hughes & R. Simons (Eds), *Culture-bound syndromes*. Dordrecht: D. Reidel.

Lock, M. (1993). The concept of race: an ideological construct, *Transcultural Psychiatry Research Review*, **30**, 203–227.

Rattansi, A. (1992). Changing the subject? Racism, culture and education. In: J. Donald & A. Rattansi (Eds), *Race, culture and difference*. London: Sage.

Rex, J. (1961). *Key problems in sociological theory*. London: Routledge & Kegan Paul.

Rex, J. (1983). *Race relations in sociological theory*. London: Routledge & Kegan Paul.

Richardson, J. & Lambert, J. (1985). *The sociology of race*. Lancaster: Causeway Press.

Sabshin, M., Diesenhaus, H. & Wilkerson, R. (1970). Dimensions of institutional racism in psychiatry. *American Journal of Psychiatry*, **127**, 787–793.

Simons, R. (1985). Latah: paradox. In: C.C. Hughes & R.C. Simons (Eds), *Culture-bound syndromes*. Dordrecht: D. Reidel.

Sowell, T. (1994). *Race and culture: a world view*. New York: Basic Books.

Wade, J.C. (1993). Institutional racism: an analysis of the mental health system. *American Journal of Orthopsychiatry*, **63**, 535–544.

Table 1 Recommendations for change

1. Organizations take the lead
2. Understand social and individual racism
3. Set up local groups to deal with research and clinical services
4. Suggest means of eliminating stereotypes
5. Encourage equal opportunities
6. Clinicians must provide leadership
7. Clinicians report success and failures of their services
8. Researchers report success and failures of their projects and interpret data in discussion with the community
9. Clinicians made aware if their every day practices perpetuate institutional racism
10. Clinicians to sanction and support efforts to provide culturally appropriate services

Some Central Ideas in the 'Just Therapy' Approach*

Charles Waldegrave and Kiwi Tamasese

Kiwi's greeting

E muamua ona ou ta le vai afei ma ou faatalofa i le paia o le fonotaga nei.n
  I le paia o tagata nuu ole motu nei – Talofa lava!
  I le paia lasilasi o Ausetalia ma ana faiganuu ese ese Talofa lava!
  I le paia o Aotearoa ma ona sui usufono o le fonotage nei. Talofa lava!

We draw from the waters of tranquillity hoping that in its soothing waters we meet each other today. The waters of tranquillity are of the Pacific. The very waters from whom birthed Hawaii to the north, Papua and New Guinea to the West, Marquesas to the East, and to the South, The Land of the Dreamtime-Australia and Aotearoa-New Zealand.

This body of soothing water from whom we were born has touched our different shores, scripting for us different cultures, gifting to us different voices and lies in waiting for our speaking, our naming of her.

Do we give name to the sacredness of her people's cultures
crafted over thousands of years in her different
shores?
Do we give name to their decimation?
Do we give name to the sacredness of their courage?
Do we give name to their survival and their daily struggles?
Do we give name to all or do we in our non-naming of her and her peoples transform her soothing waters into a pool of tears mourning our *neglect*?
Naming is indeed an act of courage, a political act, a costly act, an act ascribing belonging, drawing on sacredness.
Naming is a powerful act of defining.
Naming, if it gives life, is an act of liberation.

To you the People of Koorie, we bring with us Greetings and Sacred Love from the people of the shores from whence we come, Samoa and Aotearoa. The waters of our births break in waves of blood on our shores telling us of your sorrow.

In your Greeting of us, you spoke of Healing of the Past and your dream of a brighter future. In your courage of naming and the sacredness of your journey, we greet you.

To the land and the shores of this island of the Dreamtime we bring you greetings.

To all you peoples of Australia and your various communities and their sacred stories of pain and hope we bring you greetings.

To you people of the Island of America and of Finland we bring you greetings.

To you the people of Aotearoa, Maori and Pakeha who struggle daily with issues of families and communities, we greet you in those struggles!

To you Elders and Practitioners of this discipline who bring life and wholeness to families, Charles Waldegrave and myself join with our colleagues here, Flora Tuhaka and Richard Sawrey and all our colleagues at

the Family Centre and its extended *aiga/whanau* in extending our Greetings to you.

May the waters of the Pacific in waves crest and break bringing in hope, bringing in wholeness to many families as a result of our meeting throughout these days.

Charles's greeting

It takes us rather a long time to say hello in New Zealand!

I come from a team of women and men from three different cultures. And it's our custom on these occasions to greet people in a Pacific way. First in Maori, the indigenous first people of our land of *Aotearoa* (New Zealand).

Whakamoemiti kite Atua mo nga manaakitanga me nga awhina kia matou.
Te tangata whenua a Ahitereiria, koutou te tangata Koorie tena koutou. Nga mihinui kia koutou.
Nga kaiwhakahaere o tenei hui tena koutou.
Nga rangatira me nga whanau awhina, Tena koutou Tena koutou Tena koutou katoa.

Firstly, I thanked the source and spirit of life for the many ways we have been helped, and the hospitality of this gathering.

Secondly, I greeted the indigenous people of this land, particularly the Koorie people in Victoria after the honour of their welcome this morning. Thirdly, I acknowledged the organisers of this conference, and finally I greeted you as elders and chiefs who bring health to families.

In Samoan
  E faatalofa atu i le paia lasilasi ua faatasimai.

I've greeted you in the deepest sacrificial sense of love, acknowledged your own sacredness, and wished you as elders the fullness of Pacific life.

And in our third language, which I assume all of you can understand, greetings to you all from our colleagues at the Family Centre. We would like to thank the organisers of this conference for the invitation to give this plenary address on social justice.

Charles's address

We never planned to develop a 'Just Therapy'. We simply worked in our community. We reflected upon our experience with families. We began to accord meaning to the events we experienced differently from other therapists. We started asking different questions in therapy. We began to understand people's problems in alternative ways. This led us to work with a broader range of workers, families, cultures and socio-economic groups.

It was risky, though. So we developed an action/reflection approach to our work. We learned to monitor it carefully by accounting to each other and our communities. We developed procedures to account to the cultural communities and to the women associated with the Family Centre.

After a period, we began to share the work. To our surprise, people appeared really interested. This was followed by the highs and lows of challenge and encouragement that new work often brings. We nearly

* Waldegrave C. and Tamasese, K.: Some central ideas in the 'Just Therapy' approach. *Australian and New Zealand Journal of Family Therapy* 14:1–8, 1993.

abandoned taking it further. It was a number of Australians as a matter of fact, and some colleagues at home, who encouraged us to write it up, teach more and get it out. We took their advice, and published the *Just Therapy* monograph (Waldegrave, 1990).

Since then, we have taken the ideas to different parts of the world. Colleagues here and there have required us to reflect deeply on our work, sharpen it up and account for its history.

Let me point to three windows into our history that have changed the meanings we give events.

1. **The Beginnings**

We have always worked from an action/reflection base, as I noted earlier. We tried to monitor the things we did. So we developed a time every six months (which we euphemistically call a retreat) where the field work staff go away to a quiet lake in the country to reflect for five days. There, away from the Centre, away from our families and the telephone, we reflect on and analyse our work of the past six months, and set out goals for the next six months.

It was at the third of these retreats, 18 months after we began, that we realized many families coming to us located the onset of their problem with events external to the family. I refer to events like unemployment, bad housing or homelessness, racist or sexist experiences. We were treating their symptoms as though they were the symptoms of family dysfunction, when in fact our analysis informed us that they were really not the symptoms of family dysfunction, but the symptoms of poverty, of unjust economic planning, of racism and sexism.

We had families approach us with a range of problems as a result of these injustices. They included psychosomatic illnesses, violence, depression, delinquency, marital stress, psychotic illnesses, parenting problems and so on. And we did what most therapists continue to do today. We treated those problems as though they were the result of internal family dysfunction.

So people came to us depressed in bad housing, and, were sent away undepressed to the same conditions. After all, we were only therapists! We sent them away to be happy in poverty! As we reflected on this, we realized that we were unintentionally, but nevertheless very effectively, adjusting people to poverty. And we realized that's what most therapists do with most families in the lowest 30 percent of income levels in most Northern and Western countries. This is a very large group of people. I've estimated in Australia we're talking about 4 million people, and in my own country, over a million.

We further reflected that we and most other therapists were acting politically for the State by unwittingly silencing the victims of unjust social policies. By not relating our therapeutic work directly to the political, economic, gender, social and cultural structures, we were colluding with those systems in society that oppress, deprive and dehumanize families.

Furthermore, by implication we were encouraging in the families the belief that they, rather than the unjust structures, are the authors of their problems and failures. We did this despite our knowledge of structured unemployment in most modern industrial countries, despite our knowledge of the physical and psychological pathologies associated with inadequate housing and despite our knowledge of the patriarchal determinants of violence and sexual abuse.

These reflections led us into new conversations with families. For example, when we discovered that a family was referred to us from another institution with the label 'multi-problem' and they had been in serious housing need for 6 months or more, we congratulated them. We congratulated them for having survived the housing crisis. A crisis not of their own making. A crisis many city dwellers in Western countries are subjected to because of the failure of economic and social planners to provide adequately for all their citizens.

We have been quite amazed by the ability of many families to heal with this sort of change of meaning. We should not have been surprised, because there is a lot of research that indicates the psychological and physical pathologies associated with inadequate housing (Rosenberg, 1982; Murie,

1983; Waldegrave & Coventry, 1987 and Kearns, Smith & Abbott, 1991). When you think of it, there is actually nothing much more basic to a family than a home. Most of us would probably develop a few problems ourselves if we had to double up with another family because there was no other choice.

When we admire their ability to survive, and place responsibility where it more appropriately belongs, families cease to blame themselves and gain courage from their strength. Furthermore, we cease colluding with flawed social policy under the guise of clinical practice.

2. **Cultural Knowledge**

I remember working with my colleague Warihi Campbell in the early days of our Centre. He was developing therapeutic work with Maori families. In those days, unlike now, he had no other Maori colleagues at the Centre. He worked as a cultural consultant whenever there was a Maori family. We had made an absolute commitment we would never override a direction he made concerning culture with Maori families by using social science or other arguments. We would simply act on his advice.

One of the first Maori families we saw was referred by the Family Court because of a custody and access dispute. The couple had separated, and the father was living in the family home with the 3 children. The mother wanted to move back into the house, and wanted the father to move out. Both were capable parents with good relationships with their children.

It became clear that the father was quite happy to move out. The problem was that the maternal grandmother did not want this to happen. The therapist, who was *Pakeha* (European), eventually suggested that as both parents agreed, it would be sensible for the mother to move back to the house and for the father to move out. They could then explain their decision to the grandmother later.

Warihi, behind the one way mirror, became very concerned about this and spoke to us. He stated that traditionally in Maoridom the prime relationship is between grandparent and *mokopuna* (grandchild), not parent and child as for most white cultures. If this couple go against the stated wishes of the grandmother, they run the risk of alienating themselves from the *whanau* (extended family). She will have reasons for acting in this way.

The therapist was instructed to return to the family and pass on what Warihi had said. The couple immediately understood and agreed, because they were Maori. It was like wise advice about something they knew but had overlooked. The custody and access dispute was resolved immediately and amicably. Both parents arranged a lot of time with their children.

As we reflected on this, we realised that in this family it would have been as unjust to have gone with the parents' wishes and not the grandmother's wishes as it would be in a *pakeha* family to go with a grandparent's wishes and not the parents. As we thought more about it, we realised this was something we were never taught in a psychology class. The implications became very significant.

Had Warihi not been there, we would have severely ruptured the extended family support that offered the most natural healing and resolution to the problem. With the best of intentions, we would have continued ever so subtly the colonial imposition of a 'better way'. We learned that day that social science knowledge should sit humbly alongside cultural knowledge in therapeutic settings.

We have become very critical of the dominance of social science in the health and welfare sectors of modern industrial States. This dominance has subjugated cultural knowledge to a peripheral, voluntary and nonprofessional status.

Increasingly, we refer to social science as a particular cultural way of describing events. It is not value free. It has been developed in countries where individualism and individual human rights are viewed as central concepts of health and well-being. The prime goal of practically all modern psychotherapies is individual self worth. Most cultures do not relate to concepts of individualism in this way. Communal and extended family based cultures tend to define health and well-being in relational terms.

These concepts are very different, as some writers have noted (McGoldrick, Pearce and Giordano, 1982; Durie, 1986; Gurnoe and Nelson, 1989; Boyd-Franklin, 1989; Waldegrave, 1986, 1990). So too are approaches to spirituality. For many cultures health and well-being are essentially spiritual concepts. Social science constructs are fundamentally suspicious of that which is unmeasurable and unverifiable. It is therefore not surprising that counselling and psychotherapy have had very little success or patronage outside the cultures (and often the class) from which they evolved.

Even the post-modern approaches to therapy that emphasise the deconstruction of oppressive narratives are, generally speaking, culturally bound. With the exception of some excellent gender theory and practice, most meaning change has centred around symptoms or sicknesses. They are primarily individualistic, and do not draw upon the depth of belonging from which people come. This is particularly true if you come from a culture that is dominated in your society.

If you are from a dominated culture in your country, then you need a liberating therapy that addresses the problem and the colonising context that in many cases created the problem in the first place. When therapy is given by a person of your culture, who understands and can draw upon the deep sense of belonging and relationship in your culture – using your words, your concepts and your history – then the therapy is not only addressing the symptomatic problem, but the colonising context that usually creates the problem as well.

This is real post-modern meaning change. We know of very few family therapists who are prepared to address these levels of meaning.

This might not be such a problem, if it wasn't for the statistical fact that those most in need of the health and welfare resources in modern industrialised States are usually people whose culture is dominated in those States. In other words the decision makers, the processes and the institutional rules are all decided by people whose ways are different from yours. This in turn increases your likelihood of developing the problems that will require health and welfare resources.

3. Gender Experience

The third window into our history relates to our gender work. From our inception in 1979, the Family Centre worked closely with the survivors of abuse referred by the local Women's Refuges. The women and the families came, for example, if they were having problems with their children, hassles and demands from their ex-partner, or if they planned to live with their partner again.

Because we were trained as therapists to resolve conflicts and encourage harmony, we naturally endeavoured to accomplish the same with these families. We tried to find points of agreement, order highly charged discussions and encourage new ways of relating. We often worked in teams as female and male therapists.

A number of women, including staff, clients and Refuge workers, over a period of time had the courage to criticise aspects of our work. They said that we were often too nice and too keen to resolve conflicts in therapy, and that this frequently silenced their experience. The family harmony we achieved together with their families was at their cost. Although elements of violence were always addressed, the extent of it and other forms of abuse got lost in the quest for family solutions. This left a number of women feeling resentful and even betrayed.

As we reflected on these criticisms, the women on our staff sensitised us much more to the primacy of women's experience in families. Although until recently most of the psychotherapeutic texts were written by men, women sustain and participate in families more than men. Women's stories are different and we needed to hear them.

It became clear as we continued to struggle with the criticisms, that at times we were inadvertently encouraging women to adjust to male power. We did this by compromising the full extent of their stories of abuse in order to get everyone co-operating again. This often made it easier for

children in the short term, because of their need to have stability as soon as possible. The long term consequences were far more serious.

Some women felt silenced after all they had been through. And in some families the violence recurred, because it had not been adequately addressed in the first place. We learned to listen for all the stories that were relevant, particularly those of the women and the meanings they gave to events. That helped us to distinguish much more clearly the different ways women and men attribute meaning (Walters, Carter, Papp & Silverstein, 1988; Luepnitz, 1988; Kamsler, 1990; Goldner, 1985, 1992).

An outgrowth of this work led to a challenge to the men in the Centre. Refuge workers, other women in the community and women staff at the Centre asked the men to start working with men who were violent and develop a practice that would stop the violence. They wanted us to change the behaviour by addressing the patriarchial context.

We started working with the men. We learned to expose individually and in groups the meanings men give to women, and the blessings and encouragement society gives those attitudes. We helped men to become self conscious about their violence and confront it, helping each other. They learned to listen to women and understand, often for the first time, the meaning women gave those events.

In time, separate Maori and Pacific Island men's groups emerged as a result of needs in their own communities. These were run each on quite different lines, as they addressed the gender arrangements in their own cultures in liberating ways. Throughout this process all gender work, and all work with men in the Centre, was made accountable to the women.

This set up a structure for authentic dialogue that enabled men and women to work against the destructive effects of patriarchy in a manner that inspired trust between them. It also provided us men with the educating experience of surrendering the oversight of our work to women. Through these processes, we learned how to take much more responsibility for the destructive side of the collectivity of men.

Weaving Meaning

These are three windows into our history. They are symbols of so many events, and reflections on events, that led to the development of our 'Just Therapy' approach. For us, a just therapy is one that adequately addresses the cultural, gender and socio-economic contexts of therapy.

We learned to sidestep the scientific positivist search for objective diagnoses, causes, explanations and cures. Often such an approach creates pathology, defines and entrenches it. All such naming is a creation of the therapist and is full of meaning. Even to refer to someone as a patient or to name a sickness gives a certain status that creates its own expectations.

Instead we have developed our own metaphors that create different meanings. When describing therapy, we often use the analogy of weaving. Although the symbolism of weaving is international, it is particularly appropriate in this context because it evokes the activity of many women in the South Pacific Ocean. People come with problem-centred patterns, and the therapist's task is to weave new threads of meaning and possibility that give new colour and new textures. The task of the therapist is to loosen the tight and rigid problem-centred pattern, enabling new and liberating weavings of resolution and hope.

Another metaphor we often use is that of spirituality. By spirituality, we are not referring to christian institutionalism, but something more akin to the sacredness of life or 'soul' in music. For us the therapeutic conversation is a sacred encounter, because people come in great pain and share their story. The stories they share are nearly always deeply personal and very exposing. These are the sort of stories people normally only share with their closest friends and family.

For us, the story is like a gift, a very personal offering to the therapist given in great vulnerability. It has a spiritual quality. It is not a scientific pathology that requires removal, nor is it an ill-informed understanding of the problem that requires correction. It is rather a person's articulation of events, and the meaning given to those events, which has become problematic.

The therapist truly honours the story. The story needs to be respected in a manner not dissimilar from that of a trusting friend exposing their own pain or sorrow. The therapist listens for the story and helps its articulation. S/he helps people say the difficult bits, go back to the missed out bits, ensuring its totality and all its pain.

Then in return for the story, the therapist offers a reflection deeply from the family's story of belonging. The reflection is designed to inspire resolution and hope. In the best traditions of spirituality, it offers liberating meanings usually around a central metaphor of the family's culture. We view this as a sacred exchange of meaning that draws authentically on the images and traditions of womanhood and manhood in the culture.

In this sense spirituality is a metaphor to describe the therapeutic conversation. The metaphor encourages the highest levels of respect and humanity, qualities the medical and social science metaphors have failed to do. Furthermore, because it is sacred it encourages a sense of belonging. Soul is associated with one's roots and liberation.

We are now centring this work around three primary concepts: BELONGING; SACREDNESS; and LIBERATION. Belonging refers to the essence of identity, sacredness to the deep respect for the humanity of people's stories and liberation to the freedom and wholeness people seek in therapy. We are interested in the interdependence of these concepts. For example, not all stories of belonging are liberating, and some experiences of liberation are neither sacred nor in harmony with one's culture.

These ideas are expressed beautifully in a song called *Irish Heartbeat* by Van Morrison (it sounds better with the music):

> Oh won't you stay,
> Stay a while with your own ones.
> Don't ever stray,
> Stray so far from your own ones.
> For the world is so cold,
> Don't care nothing for your soul
> You stay with your own ones.
>
> Don't rush away,
> Rush away from your own ones
> One more day
> One more day with your own ones.
> Yes the world is so cold,
> Don't care nothing for your soul
> You stay with your own ones.
>
> There's a stranger and he's kneeling by your door.
> Might be your best friend,
> Might be your brother,
> You may never know.
>
> I'm going back,
> Going back to my own ones,
> Back to talk
> Talk awhile with my own ones.
> This whole world is so cold
> Don't care nothing for your soul.
>
> This whole world is so cold
> Don't care nothing for your soul.
> You stay with your own ones.
>
> Da da dadada dada . . .

In this context 'my own ones' refers to the essence of identity, our sense of belonging as women and men in our cultures. As Van Morrison puts it for himself and his people, 'Irish Heartbeat'. Although most people have access to their culture, for some their sense of belonging has been destroyed by war, political oppression, migration or whatever. This often provides the key to why there is so much pain.

So much therapy has been 'so cold', because it cared 'nothing for your soul'. And we take from the song, the implication that he found liberation with his 'own ones'.

So in developing a 'Just Therapy', we are changing the language. We are changing the metaphors. We are encouraging the silenced meanings to come forth and tutor us. The cultural stories, the women's stories and the stories of those who struggle to survive offer critical contexts to our work.

Kiwi's address

Van Morrison in his yearning reminds us of the centrality of belonging. 'Of your own ones'.

Cultures with their baseline of values and the expressions of these in structures, rituals and arrangements are at the heart of a people's sense of belonging. Cultures define identity. Cultures and their positioning within each society define who and what we are.

Achebe (1958), an African novelist quoting Yeats' *The Second Coming*, reminds us of the futility of a people losing the centrality of their belonging – their culture.

> Soaring and soaring
> In a widening gyre
> The falcon cannot hear
> The falconer
> Things fall apart
> The centre cannot hold
> Mere anarchy is
> Loosed upon the world.

How and when did the soaring away from the centrality of belonging begin? Who designed the spirals and how further away was the taking of our people? The stories of the peoples of the Pacific are similar yet different depending on who and what the conditions of colonial arrangements were. The end result is the scars that the present generations bear that lead them to many a therapist's door today.

I share with you a reflection I wrote while working with a Samoan family who was referred to the Family Centre. This reflection is a symbol of similar stories borne out by the peoples of the Pacific as a result of Colonialism. This reflection is about this family, it is about my culture and our people's journey, it is about family therapy – a continuation of the colonial process defining people away from their centre of belonging. I leave that for all of us here today to reflect upon.

My reflection was triggered by the following poem of a Samoan poet called Ruperake Petaia (1972).

> *I Think Of It*
> On our talking about it,
> my plight as a dedicated public servant
> for five years or so now,
> always pleases my father,
> 'you are doing fine son', he says
> 'Dedication and faithful service
> paves the way to success.'
>
> 'Think of the many Samoans
> now dressed in brass shoes
> and knee high stockings;
> all with respectable
> future guaranteed jobs.
>
> 'Think of the many Samoans
> each with a freehold
> piece of the land
> a new car and
> a big *papalagi** house.   *European
>
> 'Think of them and their lives,
> That is progress son;
> the educated way
> just like *papalagis*'.
>
> I think of it and agree.
> Yes, all so true father,
> the brass shoes,
> knee high stockings
> and respectable jobs;
> the freehold land,

new cars and *papalagi* houses
just like *papalagis* alright.

But,
have you thought of what
I have to lose to become
a successful *papalagi*?
Do you know that in the process
I may lose you father?'

My reflection from behind the one-way mirror was penned in Krakow, Poland in 1990. The courage and the history of the Polish people inspired it.

I think of it!
I think of the culture of your origin,
I think of the values of your culture from which structures grew out.
I think of the structures in your culture that ensured the survival of these values,
I think of *faaaloalo*/respect,
I think of *alofa*/love
I think of *paia*/sacredness
I think of *feagaiga*/covenant
I think of the way these values informed your relationships with your sisters, your brothers, your parents, your ancestors, your *aiga* (family),
I think of the way these values informed your relationship to the land,
I think of collectivity that springs from these values that ensured
your lands'survival, your family's survival and ultimately your survival,
I think of you now, as you sit with your family across the one-way mirror, in the absence of these values.

I think of it.
I think of me as a family therapist.
I think of the value base of this discipline.
I think of individualism, of materialism, of scientific rationality,
I think of secularism, of objectivity, of linear time frames, of modernity,
I think of the living out of its definitions,
I think of postmodernity and its reluctance to look at power difference and to consider families in history.
I think of the imposition of these values on families of other cultures tearing them away from their natural support systems, leaving them vulnerable to 'helping professions' like my own, leaving them vulnerable to state provision of services like my own.
I think of colonisation, no longer with the might of the sword, no longer with the decimation through disease, but through the gentle conversation of a therapist assuming the rightness of her/his value system, or, more dangerously, assuming that the discipline is scientific, therefore value-free, therefore intercultural and international.

I think of it.
I think of you as you sit with your *aiga* in the presence of a family therapist,
I think of your body language, your eyes turned down, your head lowered, showing your respect.
I think of the therapist's meaning to this.
I think of your mother torn away from the house of womanhood through colonialism, another ism and ism.
I think of the loudness of her silence/*musu* – a state of temporary or permanent silence signaling 'I need space to work this out. I am in too much pain.'
I think of the therapist and her/his meaning to this.
I think of your father and the patriarchal nature of New Zealand society making him a factory worker only to produce this patriarchy in the four walls of your house.
I think of the leaving of his village so he could fulfil through you the prescribed dreams of the colonists.
I think of his long speech, acknowledging the embrace of God, acknowledging the presence of the therapist acknowledging the 'failure' of your family.
I think of the therapist's meaning to this.
I think of your letting your sister speak when you were asked a question.
I think of the conferring of your right of voice to her through the sister/brother covenant/*feagaiga*,
I think of the therapist's meaning to this.
I think of your family, a part of the larger *aiga*, the fear they hold of the therapist's inappropriate disclosure of information, bringing shame not only to you but to the many who are connected to you.

I think of you as the therapist walks in dressed in jeans, another confirmation of your failure, after all, your 'failure' does not deserve respectable attire.
I think of you trying to reciprocate to the relief of pain in your family.
I think of your story, the culmination of a story which began a long time ago.
I think of when the first missionaries arrived and declared you uncivilised.
I think of their nationalities, European of English and of French descent.
I think of the classes they came from.
I think of the values they brought, the Protestant Work Ethic, the disconnectedness of body and soul – sensuality/spirituality.
The image of Mary and of Eve that your women were supposed to live out.
I think of their swiping away of your Gods, declaring them pagan.
I think of the traders that came in.
I think of the diseases they brought, the forced settling of land they began.
I think of the message they brought: the land is a commodity to be bought and sold – Man did not belong to land – land belonged to Man.
I think of the three Great Powers that vied for you – America wanting you for your harbours, of Germany wanting you for cotton plantations, and for Great Britain, another expansion of her empire.
I think of the way they manipulated your leaders.
I think of the way they failed at an agreement and brought their warships into your harbour.
I think of the hurricane that destroyed their warships.
I think of you braving the hurricane to save them from drowning in their folly.
I think of them returning to Berlin to sign the Berlin Act of 1889 dividing you amongst themselves.
The Western part to Germany.
The Eastern part to United States in return for these countries' non interference in Great Britain's affairs in Africa and other parts of the Pacific.
I think of the definition through this of you as aliens when you visit your family members across the seas.
I think of the German colonisation of you.
I think of the message you received: 'Where the eagle struck its claws, the land is German, and Germany shall remain'.
I think of your resolve to resist Germanisation which led to the exile of your elders.
I think of the First World War, the European War of 1914–1918.
I think of the so-called 'brave' New Zealand men who saved you from the Germans.
I think of them walking on the beach towards a flagpole putting you on the map as the first Allied Conquest of the War.
I think of the New Zealand Dream of materialism and puritanism that was infused in you through education, another of the colonial processes.
I think of you as you struggled for your independence from New Zealand and attaining this in 1962.
I think of you now as you and your *aiga* gently confronts us – that you are subjects of history no longer to carry the stories of the victors.
I think of you as you teach us to redirect our discipline, enriching our profession.
I think of my colleagues who in the beginning were involved in this redirection.
I think of Sui Neemia and her struggles to find sense through the pain.
I think of Tessa Siolo and her struggle to come to terms with the conflicts of cultures.
I think of Albert Umaga and his recollections of part stories.
I think of Charles today, presenting with me as he tries to make sense of our and his world view.

Any group of people made to live in the periphery of a dominant culture holds within themselves a knowledge piece. The periphery offers not only a view of one's own culture but also a view of the centre culture, the dominant one. One grows up knowing that there is a plurality of cultures, of meaning systems. One too grows up knowing that while there may be a plurality of meaning systems, there certainly is a power difference amongst these. The centre culture defines how and when the resources are to be expended. They define the type and placements of homes, your peoples are going to receive. They define how much money you live on and when you receive it.

Slowly or abruptly, depending on the situation, they start defining how one should see the world and how one should see one's own culture. Education and religion are the mighty swords of colonialism and assimilation. More dangerously the helping professions, because they are usually defined by the centre culture along its meaning system, impose both therapy and models on people of other cultures tearing them away from the centre of their belonging, their culture.

Family therapy is no different from other helping professions. We need to examine the theories and the models we use and how these define people into either their own centre of belonging or leave them soaring like Yeats' falcon, in a widening gyre.

The post-modernists and their influence on family therapy are acknowledging the knowledge piece of the peoples of the periphery. There is no one meaning. However, we of the periphery know that he who holds the purse strings certainly has more definition of whose meaning it is that one acquires either through Education, Religion or Family Therapy.

The experience of women at the hands of family therapy is similar. We invite you to our workshop in which we will be examining the Interface of Culture and Gender much more thoroughly.

In our hands are the many lives, that seek relief of their pain from us the family therapists. Are we the continuation of a colonial story and become the 1992 claws that tear people away from their sense of belonging, or are we the mature searching and knowing therapists that enable healing, and belonging?

> Name your name
> Name your culture
> Name its positioning within our societies
> Name your history
> Name your losses
> Name your dead

We name Jack, son of Janie Waldegrave who last year passed on from us, and Masiofo Noue Tupua Tamasese who died this week. Samoan poet Albert Wendt (1984) in naming it said 'Our dead are the splendid robes our souls wear'.

> Name our discipline
> Name its shortcomings
> Name its strengths,
> Name its drawing of people into belonging.
> Naming is indeed an act of courage, a political act, a costly act, an act ascribing belonging, drawing on sacredness.
> Naming is an act of liberation.
> Naming is indeed a therapeutic act.

References

Achebe, C., 1958. *Things Fall Apart*, Heinemann.

Boyd-Franklin, N., 1989. *Black Families in Therapy: A Multisystems Approach*, N.Y., Guilford.

Durie, M.H., 1986. *Maori Health: Contemporary Issues and Responses*, Mental Health Foundation of New Zealand.

Goldner, V., 1985. Feminism and Family Therapy, *Family Process*. 24: 31–47.

Goldner, V., 1992. Making Room for Both/And, *The Family Therapy Networker*, **16**: 2, March/April.

Gurnoe, S. and Nelson, J., 1989. Two Perspectives on Working with American Indian Families: A Constructivist-Systemic Approach, in E. Gonzales-Santin (ed.), *Collaboration: The Key*, Arizona State University School of Social Work, Tempe.

Kamsler, A., 1990. Her-Story in the Making: Therapy with Women who were Sexually Abused in Childhood, in White, C. and Durrant, M. (eds.), *Ideas for Therapy with Sexual Abuse*, Adelaide, Dulwich Centre Publications.

Kearns, R.A., Smith, C.J. & Abbott, M.W., 1991. *The Stress of Incipient Homelessness*, Mental Health Foundation of New Zealand.

Luepnitz, D.A., 1988. *The Family Interpreted*, N.Y., Basic Books.

McGoldrick, M., Pearce, J.K. & Giordano, J. (eds.), 1982. *Ethnicity and Family Therapy*, N.Y. Guilford.

Murie, A., 1983. *Housing Inequality and Depression*, Heinemann.

Petaia, R., 1972. 'I Think of It', in Wendt, A. (ed.) *The Blue Rain*, Suva Press.

Rosenberg, A., 1982. High Population Densities in Relation to Social Behaviour, *Ekistics*, 296 Sept/Oct.

Waldegrave, C. & Coventry, R., 1987. *Poor New Zealand: An Open Letter on Poverty*, Platform Publishing.

Waldegrave, C.T., 1986. Mono-cultural, Mono-class, and So-called Non-political Family Therapy, *Australian & New Zealand Journal of Family Therapy*, **6**: 4, 197–200.

Waldegrave, C.T., 1989. Weaving Threads of Meaning and Distinguishing Preferable Patterns, *Plenary Papers, First Australia & New Zealand Family Therapy Conference*, Christchurch.

Waldegrave, C.T., 1990. Just Therapy, *Dulwich Centre Newsletter*, **1**: 5–46.

Walters, M., Carter, B., Papp, P. & Silverstein, O., 1988. *The Invisible Webb*, N.Y. Guilford.

Wendt, A., 1984. 'Parents and Children', in Wendt, A. (ed.) *Shaman of Vision*, Auckland University Press.

7 Forensic Psychiatry

Introduction

The subspecialty of psychiatry now known as forensic psychiatry has its roots in the need for civilized society to distinguish between criminal acts committed with or without conscious intent. Acceptance of this moral obligation has been considered a hallmark of civilization since ancient times. A commentary on the Hebrew Scripture in the sixth century BC explored the role of responsibility in the commission of unlawful acts, and the Greek philosophers, as far back as the fifth century BC, considered the distinction between culpable and nonculpable acts to be among 'the unwritten laws of nature supported by the universal moral sense of mankind'.[1] Determinations of responsibility became more of a medical function during the Middle Ages and Enlightenment. And in modern times, the M'Naghten ruling[2] inaugurated the era of a still contentious and unresolved debate concerning the role of insanity in criminal circumstances. The case was largely responsible for the appearance of medico-legal specialists in nineteenth century America known as 'alienists', a group primarily concerned with assessing mental competence. These practitioners eventually lost their separate identity, becoming incorporated into psychiatry as the profession broadened its scope under the impact of modern thinkers emerging from the Freudian era. Nevertheless, the problems that alienists dealt with have persisted in the expanded borderland of psychiatry and the law.

Forensic psychiatry was established as a distinct sub-specialty in the US by the American Board of Psychiatry and Neurology in 1992, though as Applebaum[3] notes, *The principles of medical ethics with annotations especially applicable to psychiatry*[4] 'neglects the forensic realm almost completely'. The American Academy of Psychiatry and the Law was founded in 1969, and adopted its first Code of Ethics in 1987 (subsequently updated in 1995).[5] Although highly useful these codes, separately and in tandem, fail to fully resolve ethical dilemmas that arise in forensic psychiatry.

Practitioners are continually challenged to offer judgments in clinical situations requiring a delicate weighing of the interests of individuals suffering from mental illness against those of society at large. This section will discuss that core issue as it arises in the context of varied psychiatric services that, as discussed by Gutheil,[6] encompass civil, criminal, correctional, and legislative matters, and involve forensic psychiatrists in testimony before such bodies as courts, licensing boards, and ethics committees of professional organizations.

Theoretical foundations

A firm moral underpinning for all medical practitioners, including psychiatrists, is *primum non nocere*, 'first of all, do no harm'. Questions about adhering to this principle that may arise whenever it conflicts with the demands of justice or societal needs are intrinsic to forensic practice and have prompted different positions as to the proper ethical response. In the selection 'The ethics of forensic psychiatry: a view from the ivory tower', Stone[7] advocates forcefully for primacy of the fiduciary nature of the doctor-patient relationship. He argues that clinicians lose sight of known ethical guidelines when they afford greater weight to the cause of justice than to patients' welfare, and expresses grave concerns about the 'ambiguity of the intellectual and ethical boundaries of forensic psychiatry'. For example, he fears the forensic psychiatrist might 'go too far and twist the rules of justice and fairness to help the patient' or, contra wise, might 'deceive the patient in order to serve justice and fairness'. Stone articulates five relevant ethical debates, including the fact-value distinction and the role of free will versus determinism, that support his adherence to the purist position: psychiatrists cannot achieve a neutral scientific posture from which to decide legal-moral questions. Though acknowledging individual practitioners might resolve these dilemmas to their own satisfaction, he doubts any would claim forensic psychiatry has achieved consensus on the issues. Stone reviews, then challenges, standards offered by others to counteract his opposition to psychiatric involvement in legal matters. In response to the claim that he has 'failed to recognize the avowedly adversarial nature of forensic testimony', Stone reiterates his basic thesis that psychiatrists cannot simply adjust to that system and remain true to their calling as physicians. (He backs his theoretical argument with a personal decision of never testifying in forensic cases.)

Applebaum[3] directly rebuts Stone's position in the selection 'The parable of the forensic psychiatrist: ethics and the problem of doing harm'. His two-pronged argument begins with the claim that the principles of beneficence and nonmaleficence are not central to forensic psychiatry, given the absence of a consensus that they should govern the clinician-patient interaction in that context. As Applebaum points out, offering such a promise 'would undermine the very basis of the forensic process, dependent as it is on the psychiatrist's revelation of the data from his evaluation and the resulting conclusions, regardless of the consequences.' He sees no intrinsic wrong, perceiving physicians as agents whose obligatory primary duties are not beneficence and nonmaleficence, noting that 'as human beings [they] enter into a variety of relationships outside the medical setting where doing good and avoiding harm' are not the guiding determinants of their behavior. Applebaum's second, and possibly more controversial, claim is that 'the forensic psychiatrist in truth does not act as a physician', given that the 'essence of the physician's role is to promote healing and/or to relieve suffering' while the forensic psychiatrist 'operates outside the scope of that role'. He concludes that it might be more appropriate to use a different term to denote clinicians in the field, suggesting 'forensicist', which underscores a nonmedical role with its own set of ethical values. He suggests that the move frees evaluators who apply knowledge of psychiatric diagnosis to assist the legal system from the need to consider the people they examine as patients to be dealt with in accordance with the standard bioethical principles of beneficence and nonmaleficence. He believes a comprehensive understanding of forensic psychiatry's ethical underpinnings begins at this point of departure from medical ethics.

Applebaum pursues this line of thought in the selection 'A theory of ethics for forensic psychiatry',[8] which argues that the primary value of forensic work is 'to advance the interests of justice', and that the two principles on which that effort rests are truth-telling and respect for autonomy. He rejects what he terms a 'theory of mixed duties', namely a theoretical justification that retains some measure of obligation to the principles of beneficence and nonmaleficence within the forensic arena. He argues that such a course leaves vague whether the primary goal of forensic psychiatry is pursuit of justice or of health, a situation that promotes the problem of double agency (see Chapter 2) by allowing the creep of therapeutic principles into forensic duties.

Applebaum's proposed theory warrants the skepticism posed by Stone[9], who has little confidence 'the principle of truthfulness that applies in the courtroom situation will . . . prevent any slide into ethical chaos'. He questions the validity of some expert testimony, as subjective truth varies with what a witness genuinely believes, while objective truth requires acknowledgments of limitation that are rarely offered in court. Indeed, he believes most forensic psychiatrists and trial lawyers acknowledge the widespread problem that many expert witnesses are, as Morse[10] says, 'hired liars'. In Diamond,[11] 'The psychiatric expert witness: honest advocate or "hired gun" '?, comprehensively reviews the debate concerning legitimacy of forensic testimony.

In 'The role of traditional medical ethics in forensic psychiatry', Weinstock, Leong and Silva[12] present a theoretical perspective different from Stone's and Applebaum's. The selection offers an historical and philosophical review of the evolution of psychiatric ethics, detailing the tension between the Hippocratic tradition and the clinician's role in the legal system. The authors suggest that guidelines specific to forensic work generally are 'no solution for complex ethical problems' that may confront the practitioner whose role in protecting the public good can impose unfair harm to the individual, and review varied approaches for resolving that moral dilemma. They note the approach of Hundert,[13] a psychiatrist who employs a type of Rawlsian[14] 'reflective equilibrium' that weighs 'competing values as they arise from the particular facts of a problematic case'. Baruch Brody,[15] the philosopher, has a similar approach in which 'conflicting appeals' are balanced against one another, with the knowledge that it is unlikely a particular appeal 'will always take precedence over all others'. Drawing on these and other accounts of moral decision-making, Weinstock, Leong and Silva conclude that a strong case exists for retaining traditional medical ethical values in the forensic sphere, as particular circumstances require different levels of attention to needs of the public and the individual. They recognize that lack of consensus as to how to balance these claims raises a degree of subjectivity concerning the emphasis various forensic practitioners would afford the Hippocratic values, possibly re-enforcing Applebaum's concern about confusing legal and therapeutic goals.

Candilis, Martinez and Dording[16] also propose a synthesis of ethical perspectives as the grounding for forensic work. In the selection 'Principles and narrative in forensic psychiatry: towards a robust view of professional role', they acknowledge the need for a principle-based ethics, as argued by Applebaum[8], but additionally embrace Griffith's[17] belief that forensic work sometimes requires a complementary narrative approach in order to incorporate distinctive 'historical elements' of the medical profession. Candilis, Martinez and Dording believe the two approaches converge in a professional role that embraces bioethical principles guiding physicians' personal integrity, as well as 'socially determined' standards of professional integrity. They envision 'personal and traditional physicianly values' as being 'contextualized' by the narrative of specific cases, permitting 'greater flexibility in the discussion of what constitutes a true forensic interaction'. The approach suggests that a theory of ethics for forensic psychiatry should combine the principle- and virtue-based perspectives (see Chapter 1).

Evaluators versus Treaters

The Stone-Applebaum debate highlights a conflict among American forensic psychiatrists as to whether or not their role is exclusively that of evaluator or if they may additionally function as treater. An extensive literature explores the possibility of separating these two roles, and the clinical and ethical implications of each position.

In the selection, 'On wearing two hats: role conflict in serving as both psychotherapist and expert witness', Strasburger, Gutheil and Brodsky[18] emphatically advocate for separation of these roles whenever possible. They base their argument in discussion of the nature of the physician's alliance that varies with the different goals of clinical and forensic work. Like Stone they view psychological benefit of the patient as the purpose of the treatment alliance, in order to promote healing by enlarging an individual's self-awareness, responsibility, choice and welfare. The forensic context, on the other hand, is directed towards social benefit 'by promoting fair dispute resolution through the adversarial legal system'. The authors explore aspects of the clinical alliance (e.g., empathy, neutrality, and anonymity) and indicate how each adheres differently in therapeutic and forensic work because of their different goals. For example, therapists employ considerable anonymity when helping patients accept greater personal responsibility in an effort to achieve psychological growth, while forensic consultants may display outright partisanship during expert testimony. They then discuss different ethical guidelines for the alliance in the therapeutic and forensic arenas. Strasburger, Gutheil and Brodsky conclude by articulating the risks for clinicians who simultaneously wear the hats of treaters and evaluators, and warn against the practice that they conceive of as a 'boundary violation' due to its potential for compromising therapy.

Miller[19] offers a contrary view. In the selection 'Ethical issues involved in the dual role of treater and evaluator' he emphasizes the practicalities of forensic work, noting how it is sometimes difficult to separate the two roles. Offering an historical perspective concerning the evolution of psychiatry from the public sector into the academic sphere and private practice, he describes how the ethical codes of professional organizations emphasized the individual psychotherapy approach, a trend reflected in the forensic Ethical Guidelines of the American Academy of Psychiatry and the Law[5] as articulated in Guideline IV:

A treating psychiatrist should generally avoid agreeing to be an expert witness or to perform an evaluation of his patient for legal purposes except in minor matters. The demands of a forensic evaluation may require that other people be interviewed and testimony can adversely affect the relationship.

Miller faults the guideline for not adequately addressing issues of public psychiatry, and offers an approach to forensic practice that responds to this concern.

Given the complexity of the debate, he divides discussion into a series of 'dichotomies', such as civil versus criminal practice or the type of treatment involved (e.g., pharmacotherapy versus psychotherapy). The approach highlights common clinical situations that oblige psychiatrists to wear two hats. For example, some jurisdictions afford clinicians statutory authority for civil commitment without a judicial hearing, as well as the right to appeal a patient's right to refuse treatment. The duty to protect third parties, established by the *Tarasoff* decisions,[20] squarely places therapists in the positions of dual agents, as do laws obliging the report of child abuse. Moreover, psychiatrists in publicly supported state forensic hospitals are required to serve as treaters and evaluators. All these activities exempt clinicians from legal consequences though, as Miller points out, they sometimes fail to resolve moral dilemmas confronting individual practitioners, those matters of conscience that Diamond classifies as 'personal ethics' (e.g., refusal by a clinician to evaluate the sanity of death row prisoners if it could result in certification of fitness for execution) (12, p. 38).

However, Miller argues that in certain circumstances serving as treater and evaluator is not only ethically sound both personally and professionally, but advantageous both to the patient and society. These include such situations as prediction of future behavior, treatment refusal, and dealing with unusual clinical conditions (e.g., multiple personality disorder) where fulfilling the dual role often improves clinicians' abilities to provide relevant and helpful information required for specific legal determinations. He feels the approach is most applicable to situations where interests of the state and individuals coincide, even though 'some patients may feel betrayed' and subsequently invest less trust in the therapeutic relationship. Though Miller believes it is often desirable to separate the roles of treater and evaluator, he stresses that even in simple situations, like a standard forensic evaluation, 'it is frequently impossible to avoid some aspects of the dual role, even if only in the mind of the evaluatee'. Nor does he believe the issue of dual agency is resolved 'if only we practiced ethically', and presses for recognition of that reality in order to promote discussion that would sensitize the profession, the judiciary and legislative bodies to policy positions that respond to the ethical nuances of dual agency.

Halleck[21] also advocates a 'compromise position', as related in the selection 'The ethical dilemmas of forensic psychiatry: a utilitarian approach', arguing that the roles of treater and evaluator converge or diverge depending on the particular circumstances. Like Miller, he believes there may be merit to psychiatrists serving in a double agent role (e.g., informing society about 'deviant citizens'), as long as that action outweighs potentially serious, unjust consequences to a patient. He proposes measures to maximize benefits and minimize harms in forensic work, such as fully informing patients as to the process and potential outcome of a forensic interview, or ensuring that the psychiatrist's report is not employed as a *de facto* mandate for administrative decisions, and uses the ethics of civil commitment as an illustrative example of his methodology. Halleck believes the approach is applicable to all controversial legal roles involving psychiatrists, as it permits them to 'define conditions under which their services are likely to create the least harm and do the most good'.

An all too common situation that may reflect Halleck's utilitarian approach – though not necessarily by design – is the child custody consultation. As outlined in the *Practice parameters for child custody evaluation* by the Academy of Child and Adolescent Psychiatry,[22] lack of separation of the roles of therapist and forensic evaluator is 'inappropriate and complicates both the therapy and the evaluation'. The guidelines emphasize how 'the aim of the forensic evaluation is not to relieve suffering or to treat the child but to provide objective information and informed opinions to help the court render a custody decision'. Nevertheless, the process of custody consultations sometimes makes it difficult to avoid conflation of the treater and evaluator roles for a variety of reasons including, as Schetky[23] discusses, attempts by attorneys to seek specific recommendations from a child's therapist.

Billick and Perry[24] describe how the current 'best interest of the child' standard in custody determinations requires more psychological assessment than in the past, prompting more court-ordered psychiatric evaluations. The authors note that models for conducting these evaluations differ depending on how they are triggered (e.g., the request of two opposing attorneys, a guardian *ad litem*, or a child care agency), and describe questions that must be addressed in the course of each. As outlined by the American Psychiatric Association,[25] these enquiries review the quality of the reciprocal attachment between parent and child, the child's needs and the adults' parenting capacities, and relevant family dynamics. If such information is required to make an ethically based custody recommendation, it seems the potential is ever-present that clinicians must, at least to some degree, conflate the roles of treater and evaluator as the data garnered can compel opinions on such issues as visitation, parental qualification, or the need for psychiatric treatment for child or either parent.

An even more tangled ethical thicket may arise in what Miller[19] deems unusual clinical situations, such as the therapist treating an individual diagnosed with multiple personality disorder attributed to repressed memories of childhood sexual abuse. He would argue that the treating clinician is well-suited to serve the interests of some patients by contributing to legal proceeding that may arise during therapy (e.g., suing accused parents), and Schetky[23] sets forth specific guidelines that he believes allow for a therapist's ethical consultation with the defense in cases of alleged sexual abuse. Others hold precisely the opposite view. Gutheil and Simon,[26] for example, believe the therapist's role in these circumstances is no different from all other clinical work – 'to explore, understand, and work through with the patient the issues raised by these memories'. They view the pursuit of other goals, such as trying to validate childhood memories via input from third parties, as ill-advised countertransference problems. Moreover, that course may induce patients to interpret a therapist's doubts about reported

material as failure of empathy, an assault on the therapeutic alliance that ultimately proves harmful to a patient's welfare. Underlying their thorough review of the various factors that must be considered in these cases, the authors emphasize the ethical principles that should govern the therapist's conduct, principally maintenance of neutrality and treatment boundaries, respect for patient dignity and autonomy, and the avoidance of patient exploitation through therapist ambition. Gutheil and Simon maintain that issues involving recovered memories 'should be worked out in therapy, not in court', and clinicians should appreciate that danger to their patients and themselves if they fail to separate their clinical and forensic roles.

It should be noted that the treater-evalutaor debate is practically non-existent in Great Britain, as demarcation between the two roles rarely obtains. As Taylor[27] observed in a comprehensive review of forensic readings, of the many psychiatrists treating offender patients few would 'even by choice, avoid writing reports for a criminal or civil court, or for a Mental Health Act Review Tribunal or other statutory body'. The demand for clinical services has emphasized treatment and management as primary goals for forensic psychiatry training, in contrast to more academic pursuits. A practical consequence of this shift positions the British perspective on the treater-evaluator debate in line with Miller's model.

Culpability

An issue that formed a nidus of the long process leading to the present subspecialty of forensic psychiatry is captured in the question, To what extent, if at all, does mental illness exculpate or mitigate responsibility for a criminal act? The so-called insanity defense – which might better be called the 'mental irresponsibility' defense to avoid such invidious implications of a person's 'wildness', 'childishness' or 'madness' – rests on the premise that it does. As mentioned in the introduction to this section, the moral need to grapple with this issue has been central in defining some of society's legal practices.

The modern era of concern over criminal responsibility dates from 1843 when Daniel M'Naghten was acquitted by reason of insanity for murdering Sir Robert Peel's private secretary. The House of Lords formulated the M'Naghten test of insanity in the following terms:

It must be clearly proved, that at the time of the committing of the act, the party accused was laboring under such a defect of reason, from disease of the mind, as not to know the nature and quality of the act he was doing; or if he did know it, that he did not know what he was doing wrong.[2]

As Bonnie discusses in the selection 'The moral basis of the insanity defense',[28] this position is grounded in the cognitive prong of the defense, the belief that an individual can be found 'not guilty by reason of insanity' if some mental disease causes substantial lack of capacity to understand or appreciate the legal or moral significance of his actions. However, a Model Penal Code[29] proposed by the American Law Institute additionally includes a volitional prong of the defense, an understanding that an individual's inability to conform his conduct to the requirements of law also excuses unlawful actions on the basis of insanity. The complexity of evaluating cognitive and volitional components of criminal behavior in order to assess responsibility of will in the presence of mental illness has generated misunderstanding and dissatisfaction over the years. Queen Victoria remarked of the M'Naghten verdict, 'The law may be perfect, but how is it that whenever a case for its application arises, it proves to be of no avail?'.[1] Public indignation in the United States about the Hinckley verdict prompted similar discussion about the validity and scope of the insanity defense.

Bonnie's discussion of the issue supports retention of the insanity defense on the grounds that 'it is essential to the moral integrity of the criminal law', but advocates narrowing its scope by shifting to the defendant the burden of proof that mental illness rendered him unable to appreciate his wrongful conduct. His position, consistent with the M'Naghten standard, eliminates the volitional prong because of its potential to heighten 'risks of fabrication and "moral mistakes" . . . when experts and the jury are asked to speculate whether the defendant had the capacity to "control" himself or whether he could have "resisted" the criminal impulse.' Bonnie's position is based in the notion that no objective basis exists for distinguishing between offenders who were 'undeterrable and those who were merely undeterred, between the impulse that was irresistible and the impulse not resisted, or between substantial impairment of capacity and some less impairment'. He believes the volitional prong of the insanity defense can only be determined by 'moral guesses', a standard he is unwilling to support when grappling with the consequences of criminal culpability in the face of mental illness. He proposes as the sole test of legal insanity whether or nor a defendant can 'appreciate the wrongfulness of his conduct'. In response to criticism that this standard fails to adequately respond to those suffering psychotic deterioration, Bonnie replies that his test of insanity is broad enough to include that group, as the term 'appreciate' encompasses affective, as well as cognitive, dimensions of mental illness.

Morris aggressively takes the opposite position in a debate with Bonnie as to whether or not the insanity defense should be abolished.[30] Characterizing it as a 'hypocritical tribute to a feeling that we had better preserve some rhetorical elements of moral infrastructure of the criminal law', he criticizes attempts to formulate it as being engulfed in a sea of words without real resolution, leading only to confusion. Morris marshals multiple arguments against its retention, concluding that it is false psychologically, morally, politically and (possibly) symbolically. His doubt as to its psychological validity comes from the belief – which he feels is shared by many – that most prisoners found not guilty by reason of insanity are not the most seriously psychologically disturbed. Rather, they are individuals who, because of particular circumstances, society pretends to acquit by placing them in a special legal category. The argument is closely connected to his contention that the insanity defense is morally flawed in two respects. First, it is based in the assumption that whether or not someone is responsible for a wrongful act is a simple yes-no determination, 'when obviously it is on a continuum and poses a difficult problem of linedrawing'. Second, he challenges the claim that insanity is the only situation that excuses individuals from the blame of willful acts, and cites 'other pressure on human behavior' that presses individuals towards criminality; for example, he contends that economic and sociological deprivation foster social adversity that is 'much more criminogenic than psychosis'. Bonnie counters that the whole issue of establishing innocence by reason of insanity 'boils down to one of moral intuition' of the community elaborated by juries, a task Morris believes 'surpasses human competence'.

The currently accepted standards for forensic assessment of culpability are contained in *Practice guidelines: forensic psychiatric evaluation of defendants raising the insanity defense*[31]. Beginning with a comprehensive historical and legal review of this issue they address diverse conditions, with sections devoted to substance abuse and so-called 'non-traditional' mental conditions, such as PTSD.

Psychiatry and the death penalty

One possible result of establishing culpability in the mentally ill is to expose patients to the risk of capital punishment. Freedman and Halpern,[32] among others, oppose psychiatric assessment of condemned prisoner's because of its potential for intimate connection to an execution. Bonnie,[33] on the other hand, contends there is no difference in principle from pretrial assessment of a capital defendant's competence to stand trial and testifying in a capital sentence hearing, as each 'can be used to establish a legally necessary predicate for . . . a death sentence'. Given that forensic participation in the earlier stages of a capital case is ethical, he concludes 'a properly structured assessment of competence for execution would also seem to be ethically acceptable, as long as the process is invoked on the prisoner's behalf and as long as the ultimate decision maker is a judge'. Stone[34] offers another argument supporting this position in his commentary on the U.S. Supreme Court decision, *Atkins vs. Virginia*,[35] which ruled unconstitutional the execution of a mentally retarded man. Stone suggests the case illustrates

how psychiatric assessment of the condemned can advance nonmaleficence and benevolence, as a clinical diagnosis, in this instance mental retardation, becomes 'a constitutional bar to execution'. Moreover, he sees this as a possible first step in the argument against execution of the mentally ill.

The disturbing nature of this debate is intensified when a psychiatrist is called upon to treat someone who, at the point of regaining competency, could then be executed. *The principles of medical ethics with annotations especially applicable to psychiatry*,[4] states 'a psychiatrist should not be a participant in a legally authorized execution', a position that generates little controversy if interpreted to mean that, like any other physician, he or she should not inject a lethal substance into the vein of the condemned. However, this apparently simple injunction has generated a fiery debate among forensic psychiatrists as to whether or not it is ethical to treat a mentally incompetent criminal whose clinical improvement would result in removing the sole barrier to execution?

Differing positions are presented in a forum discussion of the issue beginning with the selection 'A crisis in the ethical and moral behavior of psychiatrists', in which Freedman and Halpern[32] take the absolutist stand that such treatment is equivalent to allowing physicians to participate in an execution. Citing the World Psychiatric Association Congress of Madrid,[36] Bloche's[37] notable discussion of capital punishment, and the 1992 guidelines of the Royal College of Psychiatrists,[38] they reject Applebaum's 'forensicist' argument that clinicians who act as 'advocates of justice' are not bound by the ethical principle to 'do no harm'. A consequence of their position is to condemn, as morally wrong, any actions that expose mentally ill persons to death, such as restoring competence. Freedman and Halpern[39] present a fuller exposition of their views in a strongly argued article 'The psychiatrist's dilemma: a conflict of roles in legal execution.'

Commenting on Freeman and Halpern's position, Bloche[40] skillfully explicates the tension generated in forensic psychiatrists who must balance the Hippocratic tradition against expectations of the state. He believes that forensic psychiatrists acknowledge both commitments and generally 'accept a healthy measure of restraint on their service to the state'. Absent that moderation, they can too readily by manipulated into promulgating political abuses, such as those imposed on dissidents in the former Soviet Union. Bloche argues against clinical work that 'too provocatively and dramatically breaks with society's faith in doctors' benevolence'. He believes restoration of competence for execution is best viewed in this perspective, and that serving as an agent of the state's punitive apparatus is an unacceptable social role for physicians. On the other hand, he believes Freedman and Halpern are too categorical in their prohibition against treating a condemned prisoner, as it may sometimes be necessary to alleviate torment and suffering, such as symptoms of severe psychosis.

A final point relates to Freedman and Halpern's criticism of Applebaum's 'forensicist' argument. Bonnie[33] bluntly states, 'Nobody argues that psychiatrists serving forensic roles are not bound by psychiatric ethics.' He clarifies a position he shares with Applebaum, namely that 'ethical principles governing forensic psychiatry cannot be derived from the therapeutic ethic that governs that physician-patient relationship'. He acknowledges the challenge of formulating principles

designed to govern this particular social role . . . while being rooted in the professional aspirations of medicine, and while forbidding the sorts of abuses that arise when doctors surrender their professional identity and allow themselves to become agents of the state

Indeed, this is what Applebaum attempts in his previously cited essay.[8]

Confidentiality, Dangerousness and Third Parties

The issues of confidentiality and dangerousness, central to the tension between the forensic clinician's role as treater and evaluator, are discussed in detail in Chapters 2 and 4. However, we wish to briefly note here that medico-legal developments triggered by the *Tarasoff*[20] decisions, respectively promulgating duties to warn and to protect, have generated considerable ethical debate. Anfang and Applebaum[41] survey a tangled twenty-year history of legal interpretation since the *Tarasoff* verdicts and offer advice on how clinicians should conduct themselves when faced with the stark conflict between obeying state laws or breaking confidentiality when dealing with a potentially violent patient (This essay is included as a selection in Chapter 4). They note the unease engendered in psychiatrists when, in the pursuit of an ethically correct course, they are obligated to endorse intrusion into the protected psychotherapeutic environment.

The dangerousness issue has taken a different turn in Great Britain, following a proposal by the Home Office[42] to preventively detain individuals deemed to be suffering from a 'dangerous severe personality disorder' (DSPD). McMillan[43] frames the issue by first discussing the overriding concept regarding compulsory treatment, namely an individual's 'responsibility or lack thereof'. He believes such treatment is warranted when mental illness impairs a person's ability to 'autonomously choose and act on a treatment decision' when 'significant harm to others or self' is involved. He praises the 1992 New Zealand Mental Health Act for making the link between responsibility and civil commitment explicit, so that 'both dangerousness that results from diminished autonomy and diminished autonomy are necessary for justifiable compulsory treatment'. In contrast he believes Great Britain's Mental Health Act of 1983 is ethically suspect because it technically allows compulsory treatment of competent persons and, in turn, preventative detention of individuals diagnosed with DSPD. McMillan recognizes that dealing with these individuals involves 'a delicate balancing of their interests, the extent to which their ability to act autonomously is impaired, and the seriousness of the danger they present to other persons'; however, he concludes the Home Office proposal can only be justified in the face of proven diminished autonomy. In contrast, Adshead's[44] discussion of the issue focuses on the principle of nonmaleficence. Acknowledging that detention in the name of public safety is common in criminal justice settings, he maintains it makes little sense in health settings where the patient's welfare is morally and legally the object of professional duty and care. As a result he views doctors involved in preventative detention as doing their patients 'both a wrong and a harm'. Adshead recognizes that forensic psychiatrists have a duty to third parties in certain circumstances, but 'not an overall duty to protect the public'.

Conclusion

Morality comprises a society's values and beliefs about questions of right and wrong, while the law is the agency empowered to render operational decisions on these questions – to paraphrase the playwright Arthur Miller, law is a metaphor for the moral order of men. All psychiatrists must be mindful of these matters, but the professional task of applying psychiatric principles to the law specifically falls to the forensic clinician. The selected articles and references cited in this section record how they have dealt with the ethical conflicts arising in their complex work.

References

1   *ABA Criminal Justice Mental Health Standards*. Washington, D.C., American Bar Association, 1989, pp. 324–325.

2   *M'Naghten Case*. 8 Eng. Rep. 718, 722 (1843).

*3   Applebaum, P.: The parable of the forensic psychiatrist: ethics and the problem of doing harm. *International Journal of Law and Psychiatry* 13:249–259, 1990.

4   American Psychiatric Association: *The principles of medical ethics with annotations especially applicable to psychiatry*. Washington, D.C., American Psychiatric Association, 2001.

5   American Academy of Psychiatry and the Law, Ethics Committee: *Ethical guidelines for the practice of forensic psychiatry*. Newsletter American Academy of Psychiatry and Law 12:16–17, 1995.

6   Gutheil, T.: Ethics and forensic psychiatry, in *Psychiatric ethics*, 3rd edn, ed. S. Bloch, P. Chodoff and S. Green. Oxford, Oxford University Press, 1999, pp 345–362.

*7   Stone, A.: The ethics of forensic psychiatry: a view from the ivory tower, in *Law, Psychiatry and Morality*. Washington, D.C., American Psychiatric Press, Inc., 1984, pp. 57–75.

*8   Applebaum, P.: A theory of ethics for forensic psychiatry. *Journal of the Academy of Psychiatry and Law* 25:233–247, 1997.

9   Stone, A.: Revisiting the parable: truth without consequences. *International Journal of Law and Psychiatry* 17:79–97, 1994.

10   Morse, S.: Reforming expert testimony. *Law and Human Behavior* 39:6–19, 1982.

11   Diamond, B.: The psychiatric expert witness – honest advocate or 'hired gun'?, in *Ethical practice in psychiatry and the law*, eds. R. Rosner and R. Weinstock. New York, Plenum Press, 1990, pp. 75–84.

*12 Weinstock, R., Leong, G. and Silva, J.: The role of traditional medical ethics in forensic psychiatry, in *Ethical practice in psychiatry and the law*, ed. R. Rosner and R. Weinstock. New York, Plenum Press, 1990, pp. 31–51.

13   Hundert, E.: A model for ethical problem solving in medicine with practical applications. *American Journal of Psychiatry* 144:839–846, 1987.

14   Rawls, J.: *A theory of justice*. Cambridge, Massachusetts, Harvard University Press, 1971.

15   Brody, B.: *Life and death decision making*. New York: Oxford University Press, 1988.

*16 Candilis, P., Martinez, R. and Dording, C.: Principles and narrative in forensic psychiatry: towards a robust view of professional role. *Journal of the American Academy of Psychiatry and the Law* 29:167–173, 2001.

17   Griffith, E.: Ethics in forensic psychiatry: a cultural response to Stone and Applebaum. *Journal American Academy of Psychiatry and Law* 26:171–184, 1998.

*18 Strasburger, L., Gutheil, T. and Brodsky, A.: On wearing two hats: role conflict in serving as both psychotherapist and expert witness. *American Journal of Psychiatry* 154:448–456, 1997.

*19 Miller, R.D.: Ethical issues involved in the dual role of treater and evaluator, in *Ethical practice in psychiatry and the law*, ed. R. Rosner and R. Weinstock. New York, Plenum Press, 1990, pp. 129–150.

20   *Tarasoff v. Regents of the University of California*. 529 P.2d 553 (Cal 1974); 551 p. 2d 533 (Cal 1976).

*21 Halleck S.: The ethical dilemmas of forensic psychiatry: a utilitarian approach. *Bulletin of the American Academy of Psychiatry and Law* 12:279–288, 1984.

22   Academy of Child and Adolescent Psychiatry. *Practice Parameters for child custody evaluation. Journal of American Academy of child and Adolescent Psychiatry* 36:57S-68S, 1997.

23   Schetky, D.: Ethical issues in forensic child and adolescent psychiatry. *Journal of the American Academy of Child and Adolescent Psychiatry* 31:403–407, 1992.

24   Billick, S. and Perry, C.: Role of the psychiatric evaluator in child custody disputes, in *Principles and practice of forensic psychiatry*, ed. R. Rosner. New York, Chapman and Hall, 1994, pp 271–281.

25   American Psychiatric Association. *Child Custody Consultation*. Washington, D.C., American Psychiatric Association, 1988.

26   Gutheil, T. and Simon, R.: Clinically based risk management principles for recovered memory cases. *Psychiatric Services* 48:1403–1407, 1997.

27   Taylor, P.: Readings in forensic psychiatry. *British Medical Journal* 153:271–278, 1988.

*28 Bonnie, R.: The moral basis of the insanity defense. *American Bar Association Journal* 69:194–197, 1983.

29   American Law Institute: *Model Penal Code*. Philadelphia, PA, American Law Institute, 1962.

30   Morris, N. and Bonnie, R.: Should the insanity defense be abolished. *Journal of Law and Health* 1:113–140, 1986–87.

31   American Academy of Psychiatry and the Law. *Forensic psychiatric evaluation of defendants raising the insanity defense. Journal of the American Academy of Psychiatry and the Law* 30(Suppl):S1–S40, 2002.

*32 **Freedman, A.** and **Halpern, A.**: Forum – Psychiatrists and the death penalty: some ethical dilemmas. a crisis in the ethical and moral behaviors of psychiatrists. *Current Opinion in Psychiatry* **11**:1–2, 1998.

33 **Bonnie, R.**: Forum – Psychiatrists and the death penalty: some ethical dilemmas. a crisis in the ethical and moral behaviors of psychiatrists. Comments. *Current Opinion in Psychiatry* **11**:5–7, 1998.

34 **Stone, A.**: Supreme Court decision raises ethical questions for psychiatry, *Psychiatric Times* **19**(9):1, 2002.

35 **Atkins v.** Virginia 536 U.S. 304, 122 S. Ct. 2242 (2002).

36 The World Psychiatric Association's 1996 Declaration of Madrid, in 3rd edn, Ed. S. Bloch, P. Chodoff and S. Green *Psychiatric ethics*, Oxford, Oxford University Press, 1999, pp 517–519.

37 **Bloche, M.**: Psychiatry, capital punishment and the purpose of medicine. *International Journal of Law and Psychiatry* **16**:301–357, 1993.

38 Royal College of Psychiatrists London, 1992.

39 **Freedman, A.** and **Halpern, A.**: The psychiatrist's dilemma: a conflict of roles in legal executions. *Australian and New Zealand Journal of Psychiatry* **33**:629–635, 1999.

40 **Bloche, M.**: Forum – Psychiatrists and the death penalty: some ethical dilemmas. a crisis in the ethical and moral behaviors of psychiatrists. Comments. *Current Opinion in Psychiatry* **11**:9–10, 1998.

41 **Anfang, S.** and **Applebaum, P.**: Twenty years after *Tarasoff*: reviewing the duty to protect. *Harvard Review of Psychiatry* **4**:67–76, 1996.

42 Home Office/Department of Health. *Managing dangerous people with severe personality disorders: proposals for policy development.* London: Home Office/Department of Health, 1999.

43 **McMillan, J.**: Dangerousness, mental disorder, and responsibility. *Journal of Medical Ethics* **29**:232–35, 2003.

44 **Adshead, G.**: Care or custody? ethical dilemmas in forensic psychiatry. *Journal of Medical Ethics* **26**:302–304, 2000.

The Parable of the Forensic Psychiatrist
Ethics and the Problem of Doing Harm*

Paul S. Appelbaum

In his presidential address to the American Psychiatric Association, Alan Stone (1980) told a story he called 'the parable of the black sergeant.' The sergeant, who was being court-martialed for stealing government property, had been sent to an Army psychiatrist to determine whether his behavior had been driven by kleptomaniacal impulses. After a thorough examination, the psychiatrist 'concluded that the sergeant did not have kleptomania or any other mental disorder that should excuse him from responsibility,' and so testified.

Nonetheless, at trial, the psychiatrist – who we discover at the end of the parable was Alan Stone himself – was deeply disturbed about his testimony. As he faced the court, he averted his eyes from the sergeant, 'who sat there in his dress uniform with his medals, his wife, and their small children.' When the court passed its sentence of five years at hard labor, the powerful feeling that something terrible had happened overcame Stone, a feeling so potent that '[e]ach time my mind takes me back to that occasion I have a sense of dismay that will not be dissipated.'

Why this intense reaction? In the course of evaluation, the sergeant revealed that the roots of his crime lay not in kleptomania, but in his bitterness over the fate of a black man in a discriminatory society. In Stone's words, '[H]e stole with a sense of entitlement and reparation in protest of the racist world that had deprived him of his hopes.' Yet, Stone apparently chose not to describe these motives to the court, relying on a narrowly psychopathological model of explanation. His courtroom analysis was restricted to a consideration of the presence or absence of the syndrome of kleptomania. Though information about the social origins of the sergeant's actions would not have been exculpatory in a legal sense, Stone believes that it might have induced leniency in sentencing by the Army judges, and faults himself for omitting it. This parable forms the basis for an important discussion by Stone of the difficulties modern, eclectic psychiatry has in integrating its conceptual models.

I believe, however, that there is more to learn from this story. It might equally well have been entitled 'the parable of the forensic psychiatrist,' since either of its protagonists could have served as tragic hero. The tale of the black sergeant driven to take revenge on a racist society is no more poignant than the description of an anguished psychiatrist haunted by the spectre of the harm to which he contributed. In fact, if my colleague and friend will permit me to speculate on his reactions, I think it probable that the infliction of harm, as much as the more abstract problem of selecting among conceptual models, lies at the core of Alan Stone's discomfort, both past and present.

Stone's visceral response to the court's verdict, his sympathetic descriptions of the defendant and his family, and his subsequent publicly avowed unwillingness to become involved in court proceedings are all understandable as the reaction of a morally sensitive man to a situation that confounded his ethical intuitions. How could a psychiatrist – whose calling is to help humanity – contribute to a process that resulted in an already abused person being sentenced to five years at hard labor? How could he have done harm to that man?

* Applebaum, P.: The parable of the forensic psychiatrist: ethics and the problem of doing harm. *International Journal of Law and Psychiatry* **13**:249–259, 1990.

Three years later, in his address to the American Academy of Psychiatry and the Law, Stone elaborated on his concerns regarding these issues, particularly the justification of doing harm (Stone, 1984):

The crucial word for me is 'justify': when the psychiatrist's goal is to do the best he/she can to ease the patient's suffering, he/she has a powerful justification. It is the justification for every physician who did not wait for science and theory to be perfected. Do whatever you can to help your patient and *primum non nocere*, first of all do no harm . . . [A]s physicians we know what the ethical struggle is. We know the boundaries of the ethical debate. When we turn our skills to forensic psychiatry, when we serve the system of justice, we can no longer agree on the boundaries of the debate.

Stone's parable is important because it reflects more than just the ethical struggles of a single psychiatrist. It describes the central ethical enigmas of forensic psychiatry. If psychiatrists are committed to doing good and avoiding harm, how can they participate in legal proceedings from which harm may result? If, on the other hand, psychiatrists in court abandon medicine's traditional ethical principles, how do they justify that deviation? And if the obligations to do good and avoid harm no longer govern psychiatrists in the legal setting, what alternative principles come into play?[1]

Psychiatric Ethics versus Forensic Ethics

A prior question must be addressed before considering these dilemmas. Are psychiatrists in general bound by the principles of beneficence and non-maleficence – doing good and avoiding harm – as Stone assumed? A decade ago the question might have seemed strange. From the time of the Hippocratic oath, these two values have been seen as central to the practice of medicine. Most commentators today continue to give them primary importance in their ethical schemata (see e.g., Beauchamp & Childress, 1979). But the most recent revision of the American Medical Association's *Principles of Medical Ethics* makes no reference to these principles (AMA, 1980). Instead, the AMA emphasizes what one ethicist characterizes as a 'contractual' approach to doctor-patient relationships (Veatch, 1981). Would Stone have seen things differently today in light of the current 'Principles?'

I think not. The 'Principles' themselves consist of a concise preamble and seven single-sentence statements of 'conduct which define the essentials of honorable behavior for the physician.' This brief exposition of medical ethics cannot be seen as exhaustive, nor can it be read out of historical context. When the AMA (1980) says, as it does in the first section of the 'Principles,' 'A physician shall be dedicated to providing competent medical service with compassion and respect for human dignity,' that statement can only be understood, in the framework of two millenia of medical ethics, as incorporating the principles of beneficence and nonmaleficence. Certainly, if one asked the majority of physicians about the ethical values that guide their behavior, those two would almost always be endorsed. If one asked most patients what they expect of their physicians, the answer would be the same.

Thus, our original questions are valid. We must be concerned with the applications of these principles to forensic psychiatry. Can a case be made that beneficence and nonmaleficence are not central to forensic ethics, that is, that the ethical principles guiding forensic psychiatrists differ from those adhered to by their clinical colleagues? Not only do I believe it can, but as we shall see, that the failure clearly to make this distinction leads to untold mischief.

Beneficence and nonmaleficence have the status of goods in themselves regardless of context. Like other goods, however, they often need to be balanced against competing values, and sometimes against each other. When goods conflict, the decision rules used to determine which, if any, takes precedence, are context specific. In the doctor-patient relationship, beneficence and nonmaleficence are given primacy (though even here they may be modified by other values, such as respect for persons (Burt, 1979)) because they form an intrinsic basis for the healing relationship. Physicians, often explicitly but always implicitly, promise to adhere to these values as a means of encouraging persons in need of medical care to entrust their bodies and well-being to them. In the absence of a belief that physicians will act to benefit patients and attempt to avoid harm, only foolish patients indeed would seek medical care.

Although the status of beneficence and nonmaleficence as moral goods in themselves is not dependent on this implicit medical promise, they become obligatory, primary goals for physicians when doctor-patient relationships are established with the presumption that they will control. Nor has the modern practice of informed consent, with its contract-like procedures, altered the importance of these principles. Patients remain dependent on physicians for the information and advice on which their choices depend. If patients in general come to doubt that physicians are offering information and advice solely with the intent of seeking their benefit and avoiding harm to them, even our consent-based medical system will rapidly fall apart.

But does such an analysis apply to the forensic setting, that is, where the task is not healing, but evaluation for the purpose of testimony in court to advance the general interests of justice? Beneficence and nonmaleficence remain goods, of course, but in the absence of a promise that they will govern the relationship, they do not attain primacy for the forensic psychiatrist. To give such a promise would undermine the very basis of the forensic process, dependent as it is on the psychiatrist's revelation of the data from his evaluation and the resulting conclusions, regardless of the consequences. Even in the absence of a promise to adhere to those values that predominate in therapeutic contexts, were a psychiatrist to seek to aid or avoid harm to an evaluee as primary goals, the evaluation process would lose its value for the justice system. The possibility that a result harmful to the evaluee might flow from the evaluation is the very feature that endows it with value. Of course, if it is possible to aid the evaluee in ways that are compatible with the primary purpose of the evaluation (e.g., by recommending psychiatric treatment, when that is indicated) that remains a good – as it does for all people in all situations. So, too, does the avoidance of gratuitous harm, (e.g., avoiding disclosure of irrelevant information obtained from an evaluee that may be embarrassing or harmful). But these goals must be subordinated to the purpose of the evaluation.

Is there something intrinsically wrong with a physician participating in a function in which beneficence and nonmaleficence are not the obligatory primary duties? Certainly physicians as human beings enter into a variety of relationships outside the medical setting where doing good and avoiding harm are not the major principles guiding their behavior. Negotiating the sale of a house, for example, is a situation in which no one could quarrel with the right of a physician to seek to maximize his own gain rather than others'. Even nonmaleficence might legitimately fall by the wayside when a physician seeks to undercut the fees of a competitor, though knowing that to do so will deprive him of income or perhaps drive him out of business. In short, we have no basis for objecting to physicians foregoing primary adherence to the principles of beneficence and nonmaleficence when they act other than as physicians.

Although not usually conceptualized in this way, the forensic psychiatrist in truth does not act as a physician either. If the essence of the physician's role is to promote healing and/or to relieve suffering, it is apparent that the forensic psychiatrist operates outside the scope of that role. To say this is not to denigrate the evaluative function that forensic psychiatrists perform.

Society values highly – and in many respects increasingly – the application of psychiatric expertise in legal contexts. But to apply that expertise is not to practice psychiatry, at least not in any ethically meaningful sense of the term. Perhaps it would be better if we even used a different term to denote the role played by the evaluator who applies knowledge of psychiatric diagnosis and psychological functioning to assist the legal system in reaching legally useful conclusions. Were we to call such a person a 'forensicist,' or some similar appellation, it might more easily be apparent that a different – nonmedical – role with its own ethical values is involved.

The existing, sparse, but growing literature on the ethics of forensic psychiatry reveals an occasional but unclear and sometimes ambivalent recognition of these differences. The major ethical code for psychiatrists, the American Psychiatric Association's 'Annotations' to the AMA's 'Principles,' neglects the forensic realm almost completely (APA, 1989). Recognizing this, the largest organization of American forensic psychiatrists, the American Academy of Psychiatry and the Law (1987) adopted 'Ethical Guidelines for the Practice of Forensic Psychiatry.' The four substantive sections of these 'Guidelines' address confidentiality, consent, impartiality and objectivity, and the qualifications of forensic psychiatrists. No attempt is made, however, to develop principles underlying these guidelines, much less to distinguish them from those governing therapeutic encounters. While the existence of a separate set of guidelines in itself may suggest some recognition that the ethical underpinnings of forensic psychiatry differ from those of general psychiatry, the final section of the 'Guidelines' undercuts that presumption. It states that complaints against forensic psychiatrists will be referred to the American Psychiatric Association (APA) for adjudication, though the APA relies exclusively in ethics complaints on its own 'Annotations.'[2]

The unofficial literature on ethics in forensic psychiatry has gone a bit further in drawing distinctions between forensic and clinical psychiatric ethics. Rappeport (1981, 1982), for example, has considered the differences between general and forensic psychiatrists (or more properly between psychiatrists filling clinical and forensic roles) based on the absence of doctor-patient relationships in the latters' work (see also, Modlin, 1984). He does not, however, directly address the implications of this distinction for the ethical principles to which forensic psychiatrists should adhere. Rather, like most other writers in this area (see e.g., Watson, 1984; Zonana, 1984), he foregoes an explicit discussion of principles, moving instead to address rules that govern in circumstances peculiar to forensic settings.

Questions of the relative primacy of ethical principles were considered most directly in two sources. First, the 1984 report of the APA Task Force on the Role of Psychiatry in the Sentencing Process recognized the potential conflict between seeking information to promote justice, and adhering to beneficence and nonmaleficence, but argued that neither set of principles ever exists in pure culture.[3] 'Since some compromise between these two [sets of values] is inevitable, the only question is at what point to strike the balance' (APA, 1984, p. 8). The Task Force answered the question by giving priority to the need to promote justice. Once having satisfied this obligation to society, however, it concluded that the psychiatrist should then seek the good of and avoid harm to the evaluee. This statement of the ethics of forensic work comes close to the argument of this paper, but does not quite bite the bullet: it fails to acknowledge openly that forensic evaluation and testimony may cause harm that cannot be ameliorated. Instead, it stresses the residual role of the principles of beneficence and nonmaleficence. For example, at a later point in the report, the Task Force falls back on nonmaleficence as a basis for urging psychiatrists to avoid direct recommendations for disposition to the court, since this might place the psychiatrist in the position of doing harm to an evaluee for whom he believes incarceration is appropriate.

The Criminal Justice Mental Health Standards formulated by the American Bar Association (1989) also come close to embracing the approach to forensic ethics presented here:

When professionals function as either evaluators or consultants, they establish no therapeutic or habilitative relationships with defendants and thus owe them no loyalty. However, if a treatment or habilitative relationship commences, a professional owes loyalty to the person undergoing treatment or habilitation. (p. 13)

Although the meaning of the term 'loyalty' is obscure in this statement, and the basis for the conclusion is uncertain, the conclusion appears to echo the one advanced above.

The issue of a qualitatively different basis for forensic ethics, although approached in some sources, has been largely unaddressed and unjustified in the literature on the ethics of psychiatry, and its implications are wholly unexplored.

The Implications of a Distinct Forensic Ethics

Before considering some of the implications of this analysis, it might be beneficial to recognize the artificiality of examining two ethical principles, as I have done so far, in isolation from the many other values relevant to forensic psychiatry. To place the discussion in an adequate context, however, would require the development of a comprehensive theory of forensic ethics, a task yet to be undertaken and well beyond my objectives here. Nonetheless, I believe that there is value in this narrower focus, both because the question at issue is a pivotal one, and because this argument may offer some stimulus to the formulation of a more complete theory.

It is fair to ask at this point, therefore, about the implications of the lack of primacy of beneficence and nonmaleficence in forensic psychiatry. Consider the question, for example, whether it is legitimate for psychiatrists to participate in criminal proceedings, especially on behalf of the prosecution, when their testimony may result in a defendant being convicted of a crime and punished. This question arises most directly when the forensic psychiatrist presents negative evidence concerning an individual's defense of not guilty by reason of insanity, as in the parable. It may also be implicated, however, when psychiatrists assess and testify about defendants' competence to have waived their rights (e.g., in giving a confession or allowing a search to take place); competence to stand trial; history and prognosis as they relate to considerations in sentencing; and post-trial competencies (e.g., competence to waive appeal). Many psychiatrists feel this issue with particular acuity in capital cases, where the punishment that may result is death.

Some psychiatrists avoid criminal courtroom work altogether in an effort to avoid doing harm. Others will work only for the defense, in the hope that their testimony will thereby never be harmful to the defendant. Given the difficulty of determining the likely effect of testimony on juries, however, it may be difficult to guarantee that even evidence the psychiatrist believes is helpful will not redound to the detriment of the defendant (Bonnie, 1990). The possibility that adverse information will be elicited on cross-examination further increases the possibility that harm will result. In some jurisdictions, psychiatrists who have examined a defendant for the defense but are not called by the defense at trial – presumably because they discovered information adverse to the defendant – can be subpoenaed by the prosecution and compelled to testify. As a strategy to comport with the principles of nonmaleficence, a decision to work only for the defense is imperfect at best.

If taken seriously, therefore, the duty of nonmaleficence would appear to preclude psychiatrists from involvement in almost all aspects of criminal trials. Courts would be forced to make determinations involving questions of defendants' mental states without any psychiatric input. The principles can also be recruited selectively, as some authors do, to denounce participation in particular forensic roles, such as predictions of dangerousness to establish aggravating circumstances at death penalty hearings (Ewing, 1982). Such a technique allows an advocate to argue for the exclusion of psychiatrists from almost any forensic function, without having to consider the general implications of the argument.

For persons who believe that psychiatric expertise has little to offer to the criminal courts, loss of these functions would not be mourned (Morse, 1982). On the other hand, if diagnostic and psychodynamic formulations are viewed as having some value, as they are increasingly in criminal law,

(*Ake v. Oklahoma*, 1985; Bonnie & Slobogin, 1980) this is a serious loss to the pursuit of justice. It is also, as our analysis makes clear, an unnecessary loss. The intuition of many forensic psychiatrists that their participation is not ethically problematic because their role in court differs from their therapeutic functions is supported by the recognition that nonmaleficence and beneficence do not have a primary claim on their ethical loyalties in forensic settings.

This is not to say, of course, that no behavior of forensic psychiatrists in court can be called unacceptable, an argument ironically advanced by Stone (1984), who sees in the fall from primacy of beneficence and nonmaleficence a slide into ethical chaos. ('[F]orensic psychiatrists seem to be without any clear guidelines as to what is proper and ethical.' p. 58) In so far, for example, as witnesses' behavior is incompatible with the principle of truthfulness (e.g., the psychiatrist lies about the data derived from his examination, or misrepresents existing psychiatric knowledge (Appelbaum, 1984b)), it violates the ethical framework of the courtroom. Thus, prediction of long-term propensities for violence is ethically problematic not because it may lead a jury to impose the death penalty – though that consequence may call for extra caution – but because it cannot be done in an accurate fashion, and to pretend otherwise is to falsify one's testimony (Appelbaum, 1984a).

The problem of nonmaleficence is not limited to criminal contexts. Most civil litigation involves two or more competing parties, one of whom will be harmed by an unfavorable judgment; these include claims of psychic trauma and disputes over civil competencies. If no distinction were to be drawn between therapeutic and forensic ethics, nonmaleficence as a primary value would preclude psychiatrists' testimony in those cases as well.

A second set of controversies to which our analysis can be applied may be the most difficult ethical conundra facing psychiatrists today: the questions of whether to participate in proceedings related to the assessment of persons thought incompetent to be executed and in the treatment of those found incompetent. Like the insanity defense, competence to be executed is an issue that may be more important for its heuristic value than for the frequency with which it is raised. Since the right not to be executed while incompetent was given new prominence and constitutional status by the U.S. Supreme Court in 1986 (*Ford v. Wainwright*), the best estimates are that only a handful of death-row prisoners have been assessed for competence. Nonetheless, the legal and ethical problems have stimulated a steady flow of papers on the subject, and the issue has also attracted the attention of the lay press (see e.g., Finkel, 1986; Radelet & Barnard, 1986, 1988; Salguero, 1986; Ward, 1986).

One set of positions on psychiatric participation argues for abstention from assessment and treatment of incompetence on the grounds that to take part would violate the principles of beneficence and nonmaleficence (Ewing, 1987; Sargent, 1986). It is argued that the ultimate purpose of both assessment and treatment, even if a finding of incompetence as a result of the former may postpone execution, is to remove an obstacle to the prisoner's death. This violates general proscriptions against doing harm: '[A] physician should not engage voluntarily in behavior that will bring about the death of a patient who does not want to die and who, but for the physician's intervention, would not' (Sargent, 1986). Sometimes this argument is linked more directly to a provision of the AMA's 'Principles' that applies the principle of nonmaleficence to the death penalty context: 'A physician, as a member of a profession dedicated to preserving life when there is hope of doing so, should not be a participant in a legally authorized execution' (AMA, 1980). Both assessment and treatment are deemed to violate this prohibition.[4]

In contrast, there are those who argue that participation in neither function is precluded by psychiatric ethics. Mossman (1987), for example, appeals to Kant's justification of punishment: '[W]hen responsible individuals commit crimes, they thereby commit themselves to suffer the consequences of not obeying the law.' This leads to the conclusion that a psychiatrist who removes obstacles to a prisoner's execution is actually effectuating his wishes. Relying next on Hegel, Mossman (1987) argues that execution may even constitute a benefit to prisoners, since permitting execution to proceed 'allows them to receive the punishment to which their humanity entitles them.'

Neither of these extreme positions is defensible once we begin to separate therapeutic from forensic contexts and to apply the appropriate ethical analysis to each. The assessment of competence to be executed is quintessentially a forensic function. To use Pollack's (1974) classical definition of forensic psychiatry, its involves 'the application of psychiatry to legal issues for legal [not therapeutic] ends.' As such, the argument that the principle of nonmaleficence will be violated if harm results to the evaluee is irrelevant. As long as the psychiatrist conducts and reports an evaluation in keeping with other applicable ethical standards (e.g., truthfulness, respect for persons, etc.), the assessment itself does not raise ethical concerns.

How then do we account for the disquiet that many psychiatrists feel about such evaluations? One psychiatrist reported to me his experience of being called to another state to evaluate a prisoner's competence to be executed. Only after disembarking from the airplane did he focus on the consequences that would ensue if he reached the conclusion that the prisoner was likely to be competent. At that point, he refused to perform the evaluation and returned home. Surely a good deal of anxiety about this issue relates to mistaken attempts to apply the principle of nonmaleficence. Beyond that, however, the immediacy and degree of harm to which the prisoner is subject heighten ethical concerns. But this may simply be a case of being closer to the consequences of one's actions. As Bonnie (1990) has argued:

[I]f we focus on the outcome-effect of the clinician's opinion, rather than on its timing, the case against participation in a capital sentencing evaluation would seem to be stronger than the case against participation in an execution competency evaluation. (p. 80)

Treatment of prisoners found incompetent to be executed, however, is a different matter. As a treating physician, the psychiatrist's therapeutic ethics are implicated. Treatment should not be undertaken unless the demands of beneficence and nonmaleficence can be satisfied. Sargent's (1986) belief that treatment of an incompetent death row prisoner carries overwhelmingly negative consequences holds much greater weight here. Successful treatment will result in the prisoner/patient's death. Although it can be argued that a condemned prisoner has the right to have a competent request for such treatment honored – on the basis that he prefers relief of the immediate pain of psychosis, even if that hastens his death, to indefinite continuation of the psychotic state (Bonnie, 1990) – it is difficult to find an ethical basis for the treatment of unwilling prisoners or those incapable of making competent judgments.

This argument against treatment is not free of problems, foremost among them the question of whether an injunction against treatment of incompetent prisoners means that no psychiatric therapy can be offered on death row. The problem here is that any severe psychiatric disorder holds the potential for rendering the prisoner incompetent if it remains untreated. Does not any effort at treatment then remove a potential obstacle to execution? I think this argument fails since the evidence suggests that only a tiny percentage of prisoners will become severely ill enough to meet the generally strict standards for incompetence. Thus, the balance of risks and benefits is very different for a prisoner for whom the question of incompetence has not been raised, but who may be in need of psychiatric care. Whether or not this response is sufficient to support the position of those who oppose involvement in treatment, the basis on which the question of treatment must be decided is clear: does treatment satisfy the demands of beneficence and nonmaleficence?

Mossman's position is inadequate in this context. It may be philosophically tenable to argue that prisoners will their punishment by means of an implicit social contract. However, it does not follow that physicians legitimately can or must become the agents of that punishment. Mossman fails to recognize that societal role differentiation involves ethical differentiation as well. Although some person or profession may be justified in inflicting punishment, physicians – whose ethics are based on doing good and avoiding harm – are not.

The Parable Reconsidered

What then of the psychiatrists who agonize over the harms their testimony may cause the persons they have evaluated? Although their anguish is understandable, particularly when the harms are severe, it cannot justifiably be ascribed to a failure to conform to ethical norms. For psychiatrists operate outside the medical framework when they enter the forensic realm, and the ethical principles by which their behavior is justified are simply not the same. Concern over violating the principles of beneficence and nonmaleficence is misplaced. There may be other reasons for anguish, including the failure to portray the results of their evaluations as best they can in the difficult quest for truth, perhaps a legitimate basis for Alan Stone's regrets about the case of the black sergeant. But the possibility of failing to do good and of contributing to harm – while serving other, valid ends – is an inherent and justifiable element of forensic work. Attempts to fashion a comprehensive theory of the ethics of forensic psychiatry must begin here.

Notes

1 I have chosen to focus this paper on *psychiatric* ethics, while recognizing that other mental health professions, especially psychology, have come to play as significant a role as psychiatry in forensic work. Nonetheless, psychologic ethics differ in history and in particulars from psychiatric ethics. It may be that an argument identical to the one that I make in this paper could be applied to forensic psychology. Alternatively, it may be that the origin of psychology as an academic discipline derived from philosophy, rather than as a clinical art and science, presents a very different ethical perspective. To distinguish between these possibilities would require a detailed effort that I make no attempt here to undertake.

2 Ethics complaints against forensic psychiatrists are, as far as I can determine, infrequent. This may be because the kinds of behaviors that would serve as a focus of complaint are simply unaddressed in the APA's ethical code. Perhaps this omission represents a tacit acknowledgement that forensic evaluation lies outside the usual scope of psychiatric practice. Should the APA attempt to formulate ethical standards for forensic psychiatrists? My argument suggests that confusion would be avoided between the ethics of clinical and forensic roles were that task left to another, subspecialty group. Efforts on the part of the latter to avoid responsibility in this regard are unfortunate.

3 I served on the Task Force and was a coauthor of the report.

4 In the early stages of thinking through this problem, this was precisely the position that I held and argued for in the media and public debates (Appelbaum, Bonnie, Dietz, & Thorup, 1987; *Nightline*, 1986).

References

Ake v. Oklahoma, 105 S. Ct. 1087 (1985).

American Academy of Psychiatry and the Law (1987). *Ethical Guidelines for the Practice of Forensic Psychiatry*. Baltimore: Author.

American Bar Association (1989). *ABA Criminal Justice Mental Health Standards*. Washington, DC: Author.

American Medical Association (1980). *Principles of Medical Ethics*. Chicago: Author.

American Psychiatric Association (1989). *The Principles of Medical Ethics, with Annotations Especially Applicable to Psychiatry*. Washington, DC: Author.

American Psychiatric Association (1984). *Psychiatry in the Sentencing Process: A Report of the Task Force on the Role of Psychiatry in the Sentencing Process*. Washington, DC: Author.

Appelbaum, P. S. (1984a). Hypotheticals, psychiatric testimony and the death sentence. *Bulletin of the American Academy of Psychiatry and the Law*, **12**, 169–177.

Appelbaum, P. S. (1984b). Psychiatric ethics in the courtroom. *Bulletin of the American Academy of Psychiatry and the Law*, **12**, 225–231.

Appelbaum, P. S., Bonnie, R. J., Dietz, P. E., & Thorup, O. A. (1987). The death penalty: Dilemmas for physicians and society – a panel discussion. *Pharos*, **50** (3), 23–27.

Beauchamp, T. L., & Childress, J. F. (1979). *Principles of Biomedical Ethics*. New York: Oxford University Press.

Bonnie, R. J. (1990). Dilemmas in administering the death penalty: Conscientious abstention, professional ethics, and the needs of the legal system. *Law and Human Behavior*, **14**, 67–90.

Bonnie, R. J., & Slobogin, C. (1980). The role of mental health professionals in the criminal process: the case for informed speculation. *Virginia Law Review*, **66**, 427–522.

Burt, R. A. (1979). *Taking Care of Strangers: The Rule of Law in Doctor-Patient Relations*. New York: Free Press.

Ewing, C. P. (1982). 'Dr. Death' and the case for an ethical ban on psychiatric and psychological predictions of dangerousness in capital sentencing proceedings. *American Journal of Law and Medicine*, **8**, 407–428.

Finkel, D. (1986). Dilemmas abound in hospital for inmates. *St. Petersburg Times*, July 27, p. B-1.

Ewing, C. P. (1987). Diagnosing and treating 'insanity' on death row: legal and ethical perspectives. *Behavioral Sciences and the Law*, **5**, 175–187.

Ford v. Wainwright, 106 S. Ct. 2595 (1986).

Modlin, H. C. (1984). The ivory tower v. the marketplace. *Bulletin of the American Academy of Psychiatry and the Law*, **12**, 233–236.

Morse, S. J. (1982). Failed explanations and criminal responsibility: experts and the unconscious. *Virginia Law Review*, **68**, 971–1084.

Mossman, D. (1987). Assessing and restoring competency to be executed: should psychiatrists participate? *Behavioral Sciences and the Law*, **5**, 397–409.

Nightline (1986). Catch-22: Curing prisoners . . . to die. ABC television broadcast, March 6.

Pollack, S. (1974). Forensic psychiatry – a specialty. *Bulletin of the American Academy of Psychiatry and the Law*, **2**, 1–6.

Radelet, M. L., & Barnard, G. W. (1986). Ethics and psychiatric determination of competency to be executed. *Bulletin of the American Academy of Psychiatry and the Law*, **14**, 37–53.

Radelet, M. L., & Barnard, G. W. (1988) Treating the mentally incompetent death row inmate: ethical chaos with only one solution. *Bulletin of the American Academy of Psychiatry and the Law*, **16**, 297–308.

Rappeport, J. R.(1981). Ethics and forensic psychiatry. In S. Bloch & P. Chodoff (Eds.), *Psychiatric Ethics* (pp. 255–276). New York: Oxford University Press.

Rappeport, J. R. (1982). Differences between forensic and general psychiatrists. *American Journal of Psychiatry*, **139**, 331–334.

Salguero, R. G. (1986). Medical ethics and competency to be executed. *Yale Law Journal*, **96**, 167–186.

Sargent, D. A.(1986). Treating the condemned to death. *Hastings Center Report*, **16**(6), 5–6.

Stone, A. A. (1980). Presidential address: Conceptual ambiguity and morality in modern psychiatry. *American Journal of Psychiatry*, **137**, 887–891.

Stone, A. A. (1984). The ethical boundaries of forensic psychiatry: a view from the ivory tower. *Bulletin of the American Academy of Psychiatry and the Law*, **12**, 209–219.

Veatch, R.(1981). *A Theory of Medical Ethics*. New York: Basic Books.

Ward, B. A. (1986). Competency for execution: problems in law and psychiatry. *Florida State University Law Review*, **14**, 35–107.

Watson, A. S.(1984). Response from a straw man. *Bulletin of the American Academy of Psychiatry and the Law*, **12**, 221–224.

Zonana, H. (1984). Forensic psychiatry: critique of a critique. *Bulletin of the American Academy of Psychiatry and the Law*, **12**, 237–241.

The Ethics of Forensic Psychiatry

A View from the Ivory Tower*

Alan A. Stone

At a recent meeting of 60 federal judges from around the country, one of the trial judges defined the essence of the distinction between trial and appellate judges. 'Trial judges,' he said, 'are in the front lines of legal warfare; they are foot soldiers involved in bloody hand-to-hand combat. Appellate judges, in contrast, sit on a safe hill overlooking the battlefield. When the fighting is over, the appellate judge comes down from his position of safety and goes about shooting the wounded.' Similarly one could describe forensic psychiatry as a kind of hand-to-hand combat, and now as never before, the troops are wounded and bloody. Scholarly criticism has been blistering,[1] and after the trial of John Hinckley, the media have been unrelenting in their attacks. Now, when forensic psychiatrists need encouragement, healing balms, and soothing treatment, I have come down from my ivory tower to 'shoot the wounded.'

But forensic psychiatrists need not be afraid: like the trial judges, they will survive to fight again. In fact, though wounded and bloody, they are paradoxically stronger than ever before. The legal assault on psychiatry of the past two decades had one consistent result. It took discretionary authority away from the psychiatrist and handed it over to the courts. But the courts, in order to take on this burden responsibly, require more, not less psychiatric testimony. The more they distrust forensic psychiatrists, the more they need them. Whatever the reasons forensic psychiatry, though condemned and repudiated, seems nonetheless to be flourishing. There is an array of related journals,** new organizations and subspecialty boards, a remarkable number of well-trained competent practitioners, and an increasingly sophisticated intellectual dialogue. In a stagnant psychiatric economy, forensic psychiatry is one of the few growth stocks. The sudden boom in forensic psychology gives further evidence of the strength and attractiveness of the market.

Although I have spent the past 20 years teaching, studying, and writing about Law and Psychiatry, I am not a forensic psychiatrist. The reasons why I am not are in fact what I shall here discuss. What has kept me out of the courtroom is my concern about the ambiguity of the intellectual and ethical boundaries of forensic psychiatry. At the outset, let me state what I think the boundary problems are.

First, there is the basic boundary question. Does psychiatry have anything true to say to which the courts should listen?

Second, there is the risk that the forensic psychiatrist will go too far and twist the rules of justice and fairness to help the patient.

Third, there is the opposite risk that the forensic psychiatrist will deceive the patient in order to serve justice and fairness.

Fourth, there is the danger that forensic psychiatrists will prostitute the profession, as they are alternately seduced and assaulted by the power of the adversarial system.†

Finally, as one struggles with these four issues (Does one have something true to say? Is one twisting justice? Is one deceiving the patient? Is one prostituting the profession?), there is the additional problem that forensic psychiatrists seem to be without any clear guidelines as to what is proper and ethical. In this regard I shall be commenting on (1) the good clinical practice standard; (2) the scientific standard; (3) the truth and honesty standard; and (4) the adversary standard. For now I shall simply assert that the American Medical Association's *Principles of Ethics with Annotations for Psychiatrists*[2] are irrelevant as guidelines for forensic psychiatrists. Eventually, I shall test this proposition by examining the ethical complaints that have been voiced against forensic testimony for the prosecution as considered by the Supreme Court in the *Barefoot v. Estelle*[3] case. I will argue that there is no neutral general principle by which such testimony can be called unethical.

Psychiatry and Truth

The most basic question is whether psychiatrists have true answers to the legal and moral questions posed by the law. Immanuel Kant, who after centuries is still a dominant figure in the landscape of moral philosophy, had strong opinions about this question. He wrote, 'concerning the question whether the mental condition of the agent was one of derangement or of a fixed purpose held with a sound understanding, forensic medicine is meddling with alien business.'[4] Kant would give a different meaning to the ancient designation of the forensic psychiatrist as an *alienist*. Kant also wrote, 'physicians are generally still not advanced enough to see deeply into the mechanisms inside a human being in order to determine the cause of an unnatural transgression of the moral law.'[5]

Kant's opinion was both that our science was inadequate and that, as to moral questions, alienists were meddling in alien business. A century later, Freud echoed Kant's sentiments in a new vocabulary: '[T]he physician will leave it to the jurist to construct for social purposes a responsibility that is artificially limited to the metapsychological ego.'[6] Since Freud's time some psychoanalysts have attempted to generate a theory of moral responsibility not limited to the metapsychological ego. But Freud's most authoritative interpreter – certainly his most orthodox – Heinz Hartmann, in his monograph Psychoanalysis and Moral Values,[7] drew a sharp clear line: psychoanalysis could say something about why people come to hold the values and morality they hold but could say nothing substantive about those values and morals.

This purist position of Kant-Freud-Hartmann would suggest that even today the forensic psychiatrist outside the therapeutic context is meddling in alien business. Given the basic premise of these purists, the attempt to delineate the ethical boundaries of forensic psychiatry is vacuous. Psychiatrists are immediately over the boundary when they go from psychiatry to law. To ask what are the ethical boundaries for this practice would be rather like asking what are the ethical boundaries for an imposter. From this purist perspective the problem with forensic psychiatry is not the adversarial process and its use of adversarial experts, which distorts the 'science.' Rather, purists think it is as absurd for psychiatrists to decide legal-moral questions and questions of social justice as neutral scientific friends of the court as it is for them to be adversarial witnesses.

* Stone, A.: The ethics of forensic psychiatry: a view from the ivory tower, in *Law, Psychiatry and Morality*. Washington, D.C., American Psychiatric Press, Inc., 1984, pp. 57–75.
** *Bulletin of the American Academy of Psychiatry and the Law; Criminal Justice and Behavior; International Journal of Law and Psychiatry; International Journal of Offender Therapy and Comparative Criminology; Journal of Forensic Sciences; Journal of the Forensic Science Society; Journal of Psychiatry and Law; Law and Human Behavior; Law and Psychology Review; Mental Disability Law Reporter*.
† Different problems arise when the psychiatrist testifies as *amicus* to the court. Although many psychiatrists prefer this role, it is, from the point of view of Anglo-American law, employing the procedures of the inquisitional process. The difficulties in making inquisitional exceptions to the adversarial process go far beyond the scope of this essay, and indeed of psychiatric testimony.

The purist position can be reached by different kinds of reasoning. Intellectually, there seem to be five strands that make up the purist position. I shall briefly allude to them and suggest their relevance to forensic psychiatry.

The Intellectual Chasm

First, there is the problem of the fact–value distinction. This is the philosophical line followed by Hartmann. It assumes that there is a sharp distinction between facts in the objective sphere of science and values in the subjective sphere of morality and law and that the gap between them is unbridgeable. The purist sees forensic psychiatrists as simply confusing the two spheres or as failing to recognize their distinctions. Forensic psychiatrists present their values as though they were scientific facts.

Two lines have been taken here. One is Hartmann's, and according to it the psychoanalyst has nothing to say about moral questions, except possibly to explain how people come to hold their particular moral values, and that is the end of the matter. The second line says that psychoanalysts should acknowledge their own value preferences – for example, a belief that our society should place the interests of children above those of adults – and then in light of the psychoanalytic facts develop particular legal policies. This is the familiar strategy adopted by Goldstein, Freud, and Solnit in formulating a variety of legal rules having to do with the interests of children.[8] Since such views have had considerable acceptance and influence, they merit more detailed, though still too brief, considerations among the five strands of the purist position.

When one looks at what these authors offer as psychoanalytic facts, one must question whether the purported facts are not themselves tainted by value judgments. Goldstein, Freud, and Solnit offer as a psychoanalytic fact the claim that events affecting young children are more important than those affecting older children.

Children, in this conception, are like a biological system. When exposed to a trauma at an early point they are more apt to be harmed than when trauma happens at a later date. This is the implicit assumption behind the authors' psychoanalytic 'fact,' and although the analogy is intuitively appealing, it is in essence unwarranted biological reductionism – unwarranted by empirical observation and by psychoanalytic theory itself. This implicit biological reductionism creates the illusion that the authors are talking about facts rather than values.

They argue, for example, that given their explicit value preference for children over adults and given these psychoanalytic facts, the law should keep a small child with his psychological parents rather than make him suffer the separation trauma inherent in handing him over to his biological parents-even if at a later time the decision to deprive him of his biological parents may be troubling. But in fact the empirical studies of separation trauma have to do with the unreplaced loss of the psychological parent, not transfer to a biological parent who is eager to become a psychological parent – a transfer in which the psychological parent could assist under the best circumstances.

Even if there were empirical evidence that the trauma of such transfer is apparent in the short run, there is no evidence that in the long run the trauma of transfer is worse than the trauma of deprivation of one's biological parents. The latter depends on a multitude of variables, including the meaning of the transfer and the meaning of having biological parents.[9] The issue of meaning suggests the fallacy in their reductionistic concept of trauma.

Trauma in psychoanalysis is psychic trauma. Psychic trauma involves an interactive event plus its meaning and its conscious and unconscious significance. Indeed, the meaning and significance of an observable event over time may well determine whether that event was a trauma or a helpful emotional experience. Whether or not these criticisms are entirely correct, they show [. . .] perils of trying to separate facts and values, even when those making the [. . .] are acutely aware of the difficulty. Indeed, it is possible to argue that Goldstein Freud, and Solnit can best be understood as having a value preference not for children, but for adults who devote themselves to

children, that is, psychological parents. One can argue about the pros and cons of such a value preference, but one should not claim it is an argument about psychoanalytic facts.

The second problem area is that of free will vs. determinism. The debate has never been resolved by psychiatrists. It is relevant to every question of volition and responsibility. It is a principal theme in Professor Morse's lengthy and detailed attack of the fallacies of psychodynamic testimony in criminal trials.[10] Without a resolution of the problem it is impossible to evaluate the significance of the psychiatrist's testimony. If his account of a party's condition is presented in terms of deterministic causal forces which preclude the party's being responsible for his own actions, then we may draw one conclusion.

If the account is one which outlines deterministic causes which somehow leave untouched a sphere of free will (as Kant might have said), one need not draw the same conclusion. If the psychiatric account should be understood as something other than a deterministic causal account, its implications could again be different.

A third area is the deconstruction of the self: without the unity of the self, moral reasoning becomes impossible. It is the deepest, most basic theoretical dilemma of modern psychiatry, and it is not just the work of psychoanalysis and the metapsychological ego. It is an issue in behavioral and biological psychiatry. It is specifically relevant to claims about how the criminal law should deal with multiple personality, dissociative reactions, and unconscious forces in general.

Without an understanding of when the self retains its unity and how that unity is essential to moral conduct, we cannot assess the relevance of psychiatric accounts for moral-legal questions concerning how the law should deal with the party to whom the psychiatric accounts apply. Freud implicitly acknowledged this problem when he wrote about 'a responsibility that is artificially limited to the metapsychological ego.' The moral theorist would argue that Freud 'artificially' divided the self into the ego, the superego, and the id. But this deconstruction of the self is characteristic of modern thought. The self, like Humpty Dumpty, has been shattered, and all the king's philosophers and all the king's lawyers cannot put Humpty Dumpty together again.

The fourth area is the mind-brain problem.[11] The mind-brain problem plagues all our endeavors to account for human actions. It is particularly pertinent to alcoholism, to drug abuse, and to recent theories of violence. Whatever understanding science may offer of the nature and functions of the brain, we cannot assess its relevance to the law's proper disposition of a particular party's case without taking a position on the mind-brain problem. If mental states are somehow reducible to brain states, then scientific accounts of the brain could in principle provide full accounts of human psychology. But on any other hypothesis about the mind-brain problem, the very relevance of information about the brain is less clear. If there is somehow a mind-brain interaction, its relevance depends on the nature of that interaction; if there is minimal or no mind-brain interaction, its relevance is minimal or nonexistent. If this is too abstract, think of the *Torsney*[12] case in which a white police officer's unprovoked killing of a black youth was attributed to temporal lobe epilepsy resulting in a verdict of not guilty by reason of insanity. A chapter in my book *Law, Psychiatry, and Morality* offers examples from the Hinckley trial, and the reader will see how important the mind-brain problem is to forensic psychiatry. Professor Michael Moore has demonstrated, to my satisfaction, that America's most influential forensic psychiatrist, Isaac Ray, got lost in the mind-brain trap and never got out.[13]

Last, there is the chasm that has opened up between what Kuhn[14] would call 'normal science,' and morality – a chasm which characterizes almost all of modern thought and, particularly, behavioral sciences. The chasm can be seen in terms of some of the preceding strands. Science is the realm of fact, while morality is the realm of value, so that the gap between fact and value contributes to the distance between science and morality. Similarly, science is the attempt to discover causal explanations of behavior, while morality may seem to presuppose the absence of such explanations of behavior.

The apparent incompatibility of free will and determinism thus further splits science and morality. Finally, science, particularly 'bench science,' seems to be well equipped to study the brain, but it cannot apply its methods directly to the study of the mind. The mind is an essential aspect of the domain where morality has its more ready application. The mind-brain question thus also contributes to the chasm between morality and normal science. It is that chasm which forensic psychiatry tries to bridge. I shall touch on some of these strands, but here let me say only that the purist position is not easily dismissed – it raises serious questions about the basic legitimacy of forensic psychiatry.

Each forensic psychiatrist may have resolved the five intellectual problems in his or her own mind, but I doubt that any of us would claim that forensic psychiatry has achieved a consensus on these issues. Philosophers[15] and lawyers[16] might also claim to have resolved these questions, but it seems that they have no more consensus as to these problems than do psychiatrists. The conceptual problems which have been outlined are not limited to psychodynamic testimony. They apply equally to behavioral, biological, and social psychiatry. They apply even to what many would consider the hard science part of psychiatry.

The Good Clinical Practice Standard

Now it can be argued against my position that all that I have said is applicable to everything psychiatrists do and not just to forensic psychiatry. This counterargument leads to the good clinical practice standard, the argument made by my colleague and friend, Andrew Watson. He believes that psychiatrists are constantly making value judgments and expressing moral convictions implicitly, if not explicitly. He would acknowledge all of the difficult intellectual problems I have enumerated, but he would say they are just as relevant to clinical practice as to forensic psychiatry. Finally, he would say, if we do it in our office why can't we do it in the courtroom? We even make predictions about future dangerousness in our office. Do we believe in the practice of psychiatry or don't we? I shall accept Doctor Watson's 'good clinical practice' argument so that we can cross the first boundary into the law.

But I shall first take you back almost two centuries to enter the courtroom. From this safe vantage point we can consider twisting justice, deceiving the patient, and prostituting the profession. Let me quote the interrogation of a 'forensic' psychiatrist that took place in 1801. It is reported by Nigel Walker in his treatise on crime and insanity in England.[17] The trial involved a Jew who had been caught stealing spoons.

The Jews of the London community had set up a society for visiting the sick and doing charitable deeds. The society employed a Doctor Leo, who three times testified at the Old Bailey on behalf of his Jewish patients. On all three occasions, his patients had been accused of shoplifting. This was his third appearance. First Doctor Leo was questioned by the court.

COURT: Are you particularly versed in this disorder of the human mind?

LEO: I am.

COURT: Then you are what is called a mad doctor? [Walker adds, 'no doubt there was laughter in the court at this sally.']

Then he was cross examined by the prosecutor.

THE PROSECUTOR: Have you ever given evidence before?

LEO: [Walker adds, 'almost losing his temper.'] I believe that I have. Is that any matter of consequence?

THE PROSECUTOR: Upon your oath, have you or have you not been examined as a witness here before?

LEO: I never took any notice.

THE PROSECUTOR: Have you not been here twice?

LEO: Yes.

PROSECUTOR: Have you not been here more than three times?

LEO: I cannot say.

THE PROSECUTOR: Have you not been here before as a witness and a Jew physician, to give an account of a prisoner as a madman, to get him off upon the ground of insanity?

The nastiness with which Doctor Leo was treated by these English contemporaries of Immanuel Kant (who shared their anti-Semitism) cannot be attributed to their intellectual position, but their examination of the witness strikes two notes which resonate even today in the halls of Congress and our state legislatures – namely, that the psychiatrist is a bad joke in the courtroom, and that forensic psychiatrists are there to get defendants off.[18]

The question I would pose to Doctor Watson is, what could he say today in defense of Doctor Leo's testimony? He could tell the prosecutor, as I would, that anti-Semitism is vile and repugnant, particularly so in an officer of the court. But could he argue, given the primitive state of psychiatry in 1801, that Doctor Leo had a good clinical understanding of what he called 'the mania' of his patient for stealing spoons? Could he say that his purpose in testifying was other than to help a fellow Jew escape what the law of the day considered just punishment? Was he not twisting justice and fairness to help his patient and prostituting his profession to do so?

Doctor Watson might say that my example is ridiculous and far-fetched, but I ask him and those who share his view to imagine some psychiatric historian 200 years from now examining the good clinical practice and the clinical diagnostic concepts advanced by the psychiatrists on either side of the Hanckley trial. Is there much chance that the historian of our profession would conclude that those psychiatrists, to use Kant's language, 'saw deeply into the mechanisms inside the human being in order to determine the cause of an unnatural transgression of the moral law?'[19] Or would the historian more likely comment on the primitive state of clinical psychiatry in 1982: its incomplete understanding of the brain and the mind and its bizarre diagnostic categories as set out in DSM-III?

The Scientific Standard

Another of my friends and colleagues, Loren Roth, is of the view that what should guide ethical forensic psychiatrists is their commitment to the standards of science. As I understand his view, he wants to set a higher standard than Andrew Watson's 'good clinical judgment.' I think Loren Roth shares my view that 'good clinical judgment' is a precariously egocentric standard.

I once assisted in some empirical research on humor. It turned out that every subject I gave the 'Mirth Response Test' to thought he or she had a very good sense of humor.[20] Similarly, it seems to me that every psychiatrist thinks he has very good clinical judgment. Doctor Roth wants to find a brighter line. He would limit his testimony to what he knows to be scientific. Based on that standard, he would not allow forensic psychiatrists to answer ultimate legal questions which have no scientific answers. But I would claim that if forensic psychiatrists limited themselves to the standards of bench scientists, not only would they not testify about ultimate legal questions; their lips would be sealed in the courtroom.

Psychiatry is still closer to social science than to physical science, and Max Weber's statement about social science applies to us. We must expect that what we believe to be right will soon be proved wrong.[21] It is no disgrace to work at a primitive science. As Jonas Rappeport asks, 'Are we embarrassed to let the public know that the state of our art is such that we do not know everything and that there are different schools and theories in psychiatry?'[22] The hubris in psychiatry has come from passing it off as scientific certainty or claiming that we know things beyond a reasonable doubt. But if psychiatry is an art, as Rappeport's candor suggests, how do we adhere to Roth's standards of science?

The relevant difference between clinical practice and forensic practice has sometimes been discussed under the heading of the psychiatrist as double agent. I do not want to rehearse that discussion, although it is a valuable way to analyze these problems. A forensic examination for the other side confronts the psychiatrist with problems of being a double agent – problems which otherwise often go unnoticed.

Rappeport's solution to the thorny dilemma of examining a patient for the other side is for the interviewer to recognize the potential for abuses of confidentiality and always to inform the patient which side he or she is serving.[23] But I agree with Seymour Halleck that informing the examinee of the fact that you are a double agent is necessary but not sufficient to resolve the conflict of interests. There are two reasons for this conclusion; I put off one until my discussion of testimony in capital punishment. Skilled interviewers like Doctors Halleck, Roth, and Watson will create a relationship in which the examinee can readily forget that he has been warned. It is no accident that good clinicians are often emotionally seductive human beings who inspire personal trust. Emotionally seducing a schizophrenic to reach him in his autistic withdrawal may or may not be bad technique, but it is certainly easier to justify as a parameter of treatment than as a method of obtaining information to determine whether he should have visitation rights with his children.

The Ethical Dialectic of Psychiatry

The crucial word for me in what I have just said is 'justify': when our goal as psychiatrists is to do our best to ease a patient's suffering, we have a powerful justification. It is the justification for every physician who did not wait for science and theory to be perfected. Do whatever you can to help your patient and *primum nil nocere*, first of all do no harm.[24] These contradictory claims constitute the ethical dialectic of the physician's practice. We have not yet found the synthesis of this thesis and antithesis; our fate is to struggle within this contradiction. But as physicians treating patients, we know what the ethical struggle is. We know the boundaries of the ethical debate. When we turn our skills to forensic psychiatry, when we serve the system of justice, we can no longer agree on the boundaries of the debate.

A few words about the adversary system and how it bears on this ethical dialectic. Let me return to Doctor Leo at the Old Bailey in 1801. Doctor Leo is typical of a certain kind of psychiatrist who goes to court: the psychiatrist who knows very little about the law but who goes to court out of sympathy for a client or for a cause. To some forensic psychiatrists these are the real villains, and amateurs who do not recognize that forensic psychiatry is a professional subspecialty.

But it is not the amateur's naïveté about the law which interests me; rather, it is his impulse to help the patient or to serve some cause which the patient represents. The amateur, it seems to me, is still trying to act according to the basic ethical calling of the physician – he is trying to relieve suffering, he is still struggling within the ethical dialectic of the healer.

It is my impression that this impulse has not been limited to amateurs. Many distinguished forensic psychiatrists have felt more comfortable acting on behalf of criminal defendants than on behalf of the prosecution. The current professional attitude of forensic psychiatry is to provide testimony for both sides, in part because otherwise the forensic psychiatrist runs the risk of being pilloried by the prosecution as a defense-biased witness. But it seems to me there has long been a very comfortable ideological fit between being a forensic psychiatrist and being against capital punishment, being therapeutic rather than punitive, being against the prosecution and what was seen as the harsh status quo in criminal law. This ideological fit has begun to come apart in recent history. But during the days when Judge David Bazelon and American psychiatry had their love affair the fit was real. Those were the halcyon days when the concept of treatment and the concept of social justice were virtually indistinguishable.

Here we confront what I believe is still a lingering confusion in the enterprise of forensic psychiatry. The problem is that helping the patient – which is the ethical thesis of the practitioner – becomes the ethical temptation in the legal context. What principle does the forensic psychiatrist have to restrain himself against this temptation? What is his equivalent to the therapist's antithesis of do no harm, particularly when he is cajoled by the lawyers, dazzled by the media spotlight, and paid more than Blue Cross/Blue Shield? I have already suggested that I believe Doctor Watson's good clinical practice is a precariously egocentric standard for self-administered ethical restraints. One only needs to hear forensic psychiatrists criticizing each other's ethics to see how precarious it is. Doctor Roth's scientific standard would, in my opinion, lead to a vow of silence.

The Standard of Truth

My colleague and friend, Paul Appelbaum, has suggested that the standard of truth should govern the forensic psychiatrist. In a moral dialogue it seems to me that this is a very appealing standard, but like Kant's categorical imperative it is much more convincing as an abstract statement than it is useful as a practical guide to conduct. I assume that Paul Appelbaum's standard of the truth is not the same as the one I raised at the beginning of this chapter – the truth in some absolute sense. That kind of absolute truth keeps the psychiatrist out of the courtroom. What Doctor Appelbaum means, I think, is closer to honesty: the forensic psychiatrist must honestly believe what he says and should not allow his views to be distorted by the media spotlight, by the lawyers, or by the money. He should be an honest, good clinical practitioner. Let us consider how this standard fares in the adversarial context.*

The adversarial system, of course, requires psychiatrists for both sides. That was one of he complaints against the old lineup of concerned psychiatrists for the defense: psychiatry was not being fair to the adversarial system. My late friend and colleague Seymour Pollack was particularly concerned about this issue,[25] and even Judge Bazelon lamented the lack of competent psychiatrists on both sides. Bazelon wanted psychiatrists to recognize and accede to the higher ethical framework of the adversarial system's search for justice.[26] The problem he failed to consider was how the psychiatrists would square the ethical imperative of the healing profession with the adversarial goals of criminal prosecution.

Testifying for the Prosecution in Capital Punishment

To illuminate that problem I want to examine what I take to be the most challenging case – Doctor Grigson's practice of testifying for the prosecution in capital punishment cases, such as *Barefoot v. Estelle*. At the outset, let me say that I disagree with those who would claim that such testimony is unethical.* By that I mean that it does not violate the American Psychiatric Association's canons of ethics as I would interpret them, it does not violate the good clinical practice standard, and it does not violate the truth as honesty standard. It may violate Doctor Roth's scientific standard, but again I claim that almost everything but a vow of silence would violate his standard.

The practice in question is as follows. The defendant had been found guilty of a capital offense. The court then heard testimony from Doctor Grigson, who had never personally examined the defendant. (A prior decision by the Supreme Court had dealt with an earlier practice in which psychiatrists who had examined defendants for some other purpose then testified against them at this capital punishment stage.[27] This decision is discussed at length in other chapters.) Here, there had been no prior professional contact and therefore no possible allegation could be made that Doctor Grigson had violated the rights of the defendant. Doctor Grigson was asked a series of hypothetical questions relevant to the defendant's history and criminal behavior. His answers, expressed with almost absolute clinical conviction, were that such persons are sociopaths: they are and will be very dangerous, and they do not experience remorse. Dangerousness and lack of remorse are two of the criteria which are relevant to the death penalty.

Now what is unethical about such testimony? I assume that Doctor Grigson believes what he is saying. One certainly has no basis to assume otherwise just because he almost always testifies for the prosecution, and in favor of the death penalty. I assume he is as honest and sincere and as much

---

* But, *see* Rappeport, *op cit*, pp 258–259. Rappeport believes it is possible to testify honestly and effectively. He argues that the limits of our knowledge will be made evident, so long as we do not try to confuse the issues or suggest that we have knowledge which we in fact lack

* Nor did the Court in *Barefoot* state that such testimony was unethical. Rather, it upheld the practice of allowing psychiatrists to respond to hypothetical questions about a person they had never examined

committed to the good clinical practice standard as the forensic psychiatrists who almost always testify against the death penalty or who go around the country urging verdicts of not guilty by reason of insanity.

After all, Doctor Grigson and the other psychiatrists testify under oath, they are sworn to tell the truth. 'You do solemnly swear to testify to the truth the whole truth, and nothing but the truth. So help you God.'[28] I may not have done justice to Doctor Appelbaum's standard – he may have been thinking along different lines (I shall return to this matter of sworn testimony). But if I have made my friends into strawmen, it was to make clear to you that my ideas are part of an intellectual dialogue with them.

Let me turn briefly and finally to examine Doctor Grigson's testimony in light of the APA's own Principles of Ethics. Here the language is specific. What annotations could one cite if one wished to make an ethical complaint against such testimony in capital punishment cases? One might allege that he gave diagnostic opinions about a patient he never examined.

The relevant annotation, annotation 3 of section 7, clearly is not aimed at courtroom testimony. It was added by the APA after the Goldwater fiasco.[29] Hundreds of psychiatrists were willing to fill out questionnaires and diagnose Barry Goldwater as mentally ill during the Presidential elections of 1964. The incident, which says something about the fact-value problem in psychiatry, embarrassed the psychiatric establishment, resulting in the addition of this annotation. I opposed this change at the time as a denial of free speech and of every psychiatrist's God-given right to make a fool of himself. If the psychiatric establishment banned everything that embarrassed them, they would ban forensic psychiatry. And if annotation 3 of section 7 were strictly enforced, forensic psychiatrists could never write or lecture relying on decided case law and the trial transcripts which present relevant clinical aspects of 'patients' like Hinckley, Sirhan, Poddar, Torsney, etcetera. Parts of this book would be unethical.

Furthermore, if Doctor Grigson violated annotation 3 then it is also regularly violated when forensic psychiatrists routinely answer hypothetical questions about testamentary capacity long after a person they never examined has died.

Testifying to hypothetical questions in court is not unethical, at least as I interpret the language and the history of annotation 3 of section 7. The procedure is used by Doctor Grigson, of course, to escape the double-agent conflict I mentioned earlier. Never having examined the patient, there is no doctor-patient relation, no false expectation, no deception, and no conflict of interest.

To object to Doctor Grigson's procedure is to attempt to deprive the prosecution of a legitimate adversarial witness. Forensic psychiatry has no general neutral principle for doing that. We have the intuition that such testimony in death penalty cases is unethical because of our basic practical ethical guideline to do all we can to ease the suffering of our patients. Ironically, this basic guideline is no longer part of the American Medical Association's ethical guidelines – nor is 'first of all do no harm.' If we were to take this basic guideline very seriously, how could we ever be zealous advocates for the prosecution in death penalty cases? And if the legal system thought we were bound by this practical ethical guideline, how could we serve the adversarial system of criminal justice? The Supreme Court seems to share these views. It upheld the constitutionality of Doctor Grigson's hypothetical testimony despite a dissenting opinion that raised the ethical questions.[30] If there are problems with Doctor Grigson's testimony, as I believe there are and as I try to demonstrate in my book *Law, Psychiatry, and Morality*, the fault lies not in his professional integrity but in forensic psychiatry.

The Appeal to Nonmedical Values

When we object to the ethical conduct of Doctor Grigson as the prosecution's expert, it is because we want to have our cake and eat it too. We want to be doctors who are healers and we want to serve the adversary system. My colleague and friend. Laurence Tancredi, has commented that to many moral philosophers, justice is itself a beneficence. He is certainly correct, but justice is a beneficence to a society of unidentified persons – that is, to

the general good. In contrast, the doctor's practical ethical duty is to ease the suffering of particular identified patients. Medicine has not yet solved the problem of how to balance the particular good of the identified patient against the general good of the unidentified masses. We lose our practical ethical guidelines when we try to serve such greater good in the courtroom.

Consider in this regard the Soviet psychiatrists whom we have condemned for the unethical political abuse of psychiatry. If one has a dialogue with these Soviet forensic psychiatrists, one of the first points they make is that for them, the revolution is the greatest good for the greatest number. The greatest piece of social justice in the twentieth century is the greatest beneficence imaginable. It is when these psychiatrists act in the service of that beneficence that we believe their ethical compass as psychiatrists begins to wander. The scandals in medical research in this country demonstrate the same theme.[*] The advancement of science is a noble goal; you may prefer it to the revolution, or to the American system of justice, but when doctors give it greater weight than helping their patients or doing no harm they lose their ethical boundaries.

The Adversarial Standard

It is sometimes said by forensic psychiatrists that all of the supposed ethical problems which have been rehearsed here do not exist because I have failed to recognize the avowedly adversarial nature of forensic testimony. These forensic psychiatrists would argue that they openly accept the fact that they have been selected in a biased fashion to be partisan expert witnesses. They have no ethical problems because they openly accept the responsibility of putting forward the best possible case for their side. Furthermore, they could argue that the ethics and value of such adversarial testimony is in fact as intelligible as it is for lawyers. But their assumption must be that this practice is ethical because, just as is the case with lawyers, it is understood by all of the participants in the system of Justice and no one is misled.

But does the jury clearly understand this partisan role of the forensic psychiatrist? After all, they watch as the forensic psychiatrist takes an oath to tell the truth, the whole truth, and not the partisan truth. The psychiatrist does not begin by revealing to the jury that he or she has been retained to make the best case possible. Rather, he or she is introduced to the jury with an impressive presentation of distinguished credentials to establish expertise, not partisanship or bias.

Nor does the judge instruct the jury that they should keep in mind, in weighing the expert testimony, that the forensic psychiatrists have an 'ethical' responsibility to be biased. The jury is not told that even the most prestigious and convincing expert should be understood as having attempted to present the best case possible. Until there is this kind of candor in the courtroom, it will be impossible to sweep the ethical problems of psychiatry under the rug of intelligible adversarial ethics. And if the forensic psychiatrist is an explicit adversarial witness, think of how the intellectual problems will be solved! This may be an intelligible solution of the ethical boundaries, but it will certainly expose the limitations of our scientific and intellectual boundaries.

None of these are simple matters and I do not mean to suggest that they are or that I have any answers. What I have tried to do in this chapter is to suggest that from the vantage point of the ivory tower, the intellectual and the ethical problems are inescapably linked.

Forensic psychiatry is caught on the horns of an ethical dilemma. It is a painful position to be in, but the greater danger is to think that one has found a more comfortable position: that one can simply adjust to the adversarial system or remain true to one's calling as a physician. The philosophers say life is a moral adventure; I would add that to choose a career in forensic psychiatry is to choose to increase the risks of that moral adventure.

---

[*] *See, e.g.,* discussion of cancer research in Katz, J: *Experimentation with Human Beings: The Authority of the Investigator, Subject, Profession and State in the Human Experimentation Process*, Russell Sage, 1972.

References

1   Morse: Failed Explanations and Criminal Responsibility. *Va Law Review* 1982, **68**:971–1084.

2   American Psychiatric Association: *The Principles of Medical Ethics with Annotations Especially Applicable to Psychiatry.* Washington, DC, APA, 1981.

3   *Barefoot v Estelle*, 103 S. Ct. 3383, 1983.

4   Kant I: *Anthropology from a Pragmatic Point of View*, Dowdell, VL (trans), Southern Illinois University Press, 1978, p 111.

5   Id.

6   Freud S: Moral Responsibility for the Content of Dreams, cited in Katz, Goldstein and Dershowitz, *Psychoanalysis, Psychiatry and Law.* New York, Free Press, 1967, p 127.

7   Hartmann H: *Psychoanalysis and Moral Values.* New York, International Universities Press, 1960.

8   Goldstein J, Freud A, Solnit A: *Beyond the Best Interests of the Child.* New York, Free Press, 1973 and *Before the Best Interests of the Child*, Free Press, 1980.

9   Furman E: *A Child's Parent Dies.* New Haven, Yale University Press, 1974.

10 *Op. Cit. 1.*

11 Hook S (ed): *Dimensions of Mind: A Symposium.* New York, New York University Press, 1960.

12 *Matter of Torsney*, 412 N.Y.S. 2d 914, rev'd 420 N.Y.S.2d 192, 394 N.E.2d 262

13 Moore MS: Legal Conceptions of Mental Illness in Brody B, Englchardt T (eds): *Mental Illness: Law and Public Policy.* Kluwer Academic, 1980.

14 Kuhn T: *The Structure of Scientific Revolutions.* Chicago, University of Chicago Press. 1970. p 2.

15 Hudson WD (ed): *The Is/Ought Question.* New York, St. Martins Press. 1970.

16 Moore MS: Responsibility and the Unconscious. *So Cal Law Rev*, 1980, **53**:1563–1675.

17 Walker N: *Crime and Insanity in England.* Edinburgh, Scotland. Edinburgh University Press, 1968, p 82.

18 Ashbrook J: The insanity defense. *Congressional Record*, November 17, 1981, E 5365–6.

19 *See Ref* 4.

20 Redlich F, Bingham J: *The Inside Story: Psychiatry and Everyday Life.* New York, Knopf. 1953.

21 Weber M: Objectivity in Social Science and Social Policy. *The Methodology of the Social Sciences*, translated by Shilis E and Finch H. New York, Free Press, 1949.

22 Rappeport J: Ethics and Forensic Psychiatry in Bloch S and Chodoff P (eds): *Psychiatric Ethics.* New York. Oxford University Press, 1981, p 259.

23 *Id.* at p 264.

24 Dedek J: *Contemporary Medical Ethics.* Sheed and Ward, 1975, p 6.

25 Pollack S: *Forensic Psychiatry in Criminal Law.* University of Southern California Press. 1974.

26 Bazelon: The Role of the Psychiatrist in the Criminal Justice System. *Bull Am Acad Psychiatry Law* 1978, **6**:139–146.

27 *Estelle v Smith*. 451 U.S. 454, 1981.

28 Oath of Affirmation of Governing Principles, Form 161, Oath of Witness, *25 Am. Jur. Pl. and Pr. Forms* (revised), pp 356–357.

29 The Unconscious of a Conservative: A Special Issue on the Mind of Barry Goldwater. *Fact Magazine* 1964, **1**:3–64.

30 *See Ref* 3.

A Theory of Ethics for Forensic Psychiatry*

Paul S. Appelbaum

In 1982, at the annual meeting of the American Academy of Psychiatry and the Law (AAPL), Alan Stone posed a stark challenge to the moral legitimacy of forensic psychiatry.[1] Casting a skeptical eye on the ethical principles forensic psychiatrists might use to guide their behavior. Stone rejected them all. The competing possibilities, he charged, were either internally inconsistent or useless in practice. Indeed, so chaotic was the state of ethics in forensic work that forensic psychiatrists 'are without any clear guidelines as to what is proper and ethical.'

If correct, as Stone's audience grasped immediately, this conclusion has some fairly troubling implications for forensic psychiatry. A field that is unable to distinguish the proper from the improper, the ethical from the unethical, must tolerate all behaviors equally, since no neutral principle exists for accepting some and condemning others. There can be no good practices and no bad practitioners. The formulation of standards of behavior is beyond the profession's reach. It is difficult to imagine another occupation about which a similar statement may be made: even thieves, after all, are said to have honor among them. Forensic psychiatry, in this view, is a quintessentially lawless activity.

Had Stone merely been describing the contemporary state of ethics in forensic psychiatry, his portrayal might have been taken as a challenge. Organized forensic psychiatry was relatively young at that point, its major organization, the AAPL, having been founded only 13 years earlier. If insufficient attention had been paid to ethics so far, that was unfortunate, but remediable. But Stone's judgment was more pessimistic still, preempting the possibility of future advances. Not only had no guiding principles for forensic work been identified to date – the task was hopeless. The bedrock principles of beneficence and nonmaleficence, to which medicine had looked historically, were inapplicable outside the clinical realm. Without these compass points to steer by, forensic psychiatry was condemned to wander in an ethical waste land, permanently bereft of moral legitimacy.

In the years since Stone's speech, many commentators have challenged his nihilism regarding forensic ethics, pointing to principles that might constitute starting points for an ethical framework for forensic psychiatry.[2–4] The AAPL itself has formulated a code for its members that, although far from comprehensive, offers generally accepted guidelines for behavior.[5] The organization has begun issuing opinions of its Ethics Committee to 'flesh out' the bare bones of the guidelines, much the way other specialty groups in medicine have done.[6] Indeed, Stone himself, in his more recent writing, seems less despairing of being able to identify some operational principles and is even willing to offer suggestions for minimizing ethical conflicts.[7]

If the situation was never as bleak as Stone's portrayal, and if considerable attention has been given in the intervening years to formulating more clearly the profession's ethical foundations, there is one respect in which we might yet legitimately be criticized. Forensic psychiatry still lacks a theory of ethics by which to shape its behavior. By theory I mean the justification of a set of principles that constitute the ethical underpinnings of forensic work, based on which operationalized guidelines can be formulated in a consistent fashion. Such a theory would enable us to resolve conflicts regarding the applicability

of various ethical principles to forensic psychiatry, as well as assist us in more precisely crafting ethical guidelines for particular circumstances.

To be sure, various commentators, myself included, have addressed one or another principle that might constitute components of a theory of forensic ethics.[2 4, 8–10] But none has linked these principles to a more comprehensive schema. I suspect that inarticulated elements of such a theory exist among forensic practitioners. Indeed, it would otherwise be difficult to account for the widespread agreement in the field about so many aspects of forensic ethics.[11, 12] The task that remains is to make explicit those moral judgments that lie just below the surface of consciousness and to provide a justification for them.

I propose in this article to develop the outlines of a theory of ethics for forensic psychiatry. It seems inevitable that such a theory will be in some ways incomplete and that adjustment will be required. The likelihood of some degree of imperfection, however, is insufficient reason to avoid beginning the work.

Why 'Professional' Ethics?

In attempting to construct an ethical theory for forensic psychiatry, we must confront a basic question about professional ethics in general. Professionals, whether teachers, engineers, accountants, or psychiatrists, are all members of a broader society. If we accept that certain ethical norms are binding on everyone, what justification is there for allowing discrete occupational groups to create separate rules for themselves? To press the point, if the norms embodied in professional ethics are identical to those more widely subscribed to, there would appear to be little reason to construct a distinct ethical framework for the professions. On the other hand, if professional ethics differ from – and therefore have the potential for being in conflict with – general norms, how can we justify such deviations?

To answer this question requires some reflection on the nature and application of moral principles.* Moral philosophers recognize two types of principles that guide our behavior. Bernard Gert calls them 'moral rules' and 'moral ideals.'[13] Moral rules are generalizable maxims that proscribe behavior likely to cause harm to other people. 'Thou shall not kill' is a classic example of a moral rule. We are always obligated to follow a moral rule, unless, as Gert suggests, 'an impartial rational person can advocate that violating it be publicly allowed.' Thus, a person who deviates from the moral rule against killing in order to save his or her own life would generally be acknowledged as having engaged in a justifiable violation of the rule.

Violations of moral rules, in fact, are an inevitable consequence of the complexity of life. Situations frequently arise in which two moral rules, each seemingly absolute, are in conflict with each other. Resolving that conflict requires balancing, among other morally relevant factors, the nature of each imperative, the benefits and harms likely to flow from its violation, and the alternative means of achieving the desired end. A parent, for example, who bears a moral duty to care for a child, might be justified in

* Appelbaum, P.: A theory of ethics for forensic psychiatry. *Journal of the Academy of Psychiatry and Law* 25:233–247, 1997.

* Following the practice of most contemporary ethicists. I use the terms 'moral' and 'ethical' interchangeably in this article.

breaking a promise to help a friend move her belongings if the child were sick and needed the parent's care. Keeping promises is a moral rule, but in this context, the moral responsibility to care for a child takes precedence.

In contrast to moral rules, moral ideals 'encourage people to act so as to prevent and relieve the suffering of others.'[13] Although usually worthy of praise, such behavior is not ordinarily required of persons. Were that not the case, people might well feel morally compelled to expend all of their time and resources helping other people, to the utter neglect of their own aims in life. Giving charity embodies a moral ideal, usually to be encouraged, but not compelled. The legal philosopher Lon Fuller uses the felicitous term 'morality of aspiration' to describe this kind of moral principle, in contrast to the binding 'morality of duty.'[14] Moral rules generally outweigh moral ideals, but not always: Gert offers the example of a person who, by breaking a promise (thereby violating a moral rule) can save a life (which only represents a moral ideal), in this case the morally appropriate choice.

With this background in moral theory, we can return to the question of how one can justify a distinct code of ethics for any subgroup in society. Clearly, it would be difficult to rationalize any profession's blanket abrogation of moral rules precluding harm to others, and that is not the function of professional ethics. But a society that desires to promote certain important moral values, as the ethicist Benjamin Freedman[15] suggests, might well elect to allow professions dedicated to those values to weight particular moral rules more heavily than others. 'Professional morality,' in Freedman's words, 'sins a sin of zealousness rather than laxity.'[15]

For example, to promote the value of health, society might permit physicians to elaborate an ethical code that gave primacy to rules congruent with that purpose. Keeping confidences, which Freedman sees as a corollary of the duty of nonmaleficence (familiar to physicians in its Latin form, *primum non nocere*—first do no harm), may be a moral rule for all people, but for physicians, especially for psychiatrists, it achieves elevated status. Recognition of this can be seen in the recent decision of the U.S. Supreme Court in *Jaffee v. Redmond*, which held that psychiatrists and other psychotherapists could not be compelled to give testimony in federal court when doing so would mean violating the confidences of their patients.[16] The usual primacy of the value of justice, and of the rule that every person must help in the pursuit of justice, even if it requires breaching confidences, was abrogated for the sake of promoting the treatment of persons with mental disorders.

Moreover, as Gert indicates, professional codes of ethics may transform the goals of moral ideals into moral rules, binding on the members of a profession.[13] Relieving pain is one such moral ideal, the goal of which becomes a duty incumbent on physicians, nurses, and other health professionals when they accept responsibility for a particular patient. This is a second way in which professional ethics "sins a sin of zealousness," in Freedman's term.

How do we know on which moral rules a profession should confer preeminence or which moral ideals should be translated into duties? The answer should be fairly apparent by now. Creating an ethical code for a profession must begin with identification of the values that society desires the profession to promote. Of course, those values must in themselves be morally legitimate. Health is such a value: discrimination on the basis of race, religion, or sexual orientation is not. Then, relative dominance is conferred on those moral rules that support that value, and the moral ideals that act similarly may be transmuted into binding duties. If the work is undertaken correctly, the ethics of any profession differ from ethical standards more generally applied only insofar as is necessary to advance the value in question.[17]

The Necessity for a Distinct Set of Ethics for Forensic Psychiatry

Even with the justification clear in our minds for professional ethics in general, there is an additional obstacle that must be overcome before we can outline the principles of ethics for forensic psychiatry *per se*. It might be objected that a framework to guide the ethical thinking of forensic psychiatrists already exists. Since every forensic psychiatrist is a physician, and the principles of medical ethics are widely subscribed to by members of the profession, the work of elaborating a distinct set of ethical principles for a medical subspecialty is unnecessary. To discern the moral obligations of forensic psychiatrists, or of physicians in any other role, we need only examine the principles of medical ethics.

As a rejoinder to this claim, I note that the assumption that all activities of physicians must be governed by the same ethical principles is clearly fallacious. The ethics of medicine, focused as they are on the principles of beneficence – to do good for one's patients, whenever one can – and nonmaleficence – to avoid doing harm if at all possible – derive from the usual clinical setting.[18] When patients come to physicians for diagnosis and treatment of medical problems, patients seek and are appropriately reassured by physicians' nearly single-minded fidelity to their interests. Fried refers to this as the principle of 'personal care.'[19] This commitment to personal care has served medicine well, and it constitutes the bedrock on which the structure of medical ethics has been constructed.

Imagine for a moment, however, a physician who selects by chance for his or her patient a medication of uncertain efficacy at a dosage that bears no relation to the patient's own needs, all the while refusing to tell the patient which medication the patient is actually receiving. Indeed, the physician herself remains deliberately ignorant of what the patient is taking, complicating evaluation of the patient's situation, including puzzling changes in the patient's state, which may or may not be due to medication side effects. To what extent does this behavior measure up to the usual standards of ethical medical care? Not in the least. Are we then willing to condemn the physician's actions as unethical? Perhaps not quite yet. Indeed, we might conclude that the physician is acting ethically after all.

For in our example, the physician is caring for the patient as part of a research protocol. The procedure involves comparing the efficacy of two medications, assigned at random, and administered on a double-blind basis. Dosages are determined in advance and standardized, to permit clearer estimation of the comparative efficacy and side effects of the medications. Although the research physician has turned aside from medicine's usual dedication to patients' interests (we might more accurately refer to patients here as 'research subjects'), he or she would not be condemned for this behavior. Rather, it would be generally acknowledged that the ethics of the research setting differ substantively from those that apply in ordinary clinical work.[19]

This premise is true in two respects. Certain obligations that usually would be binding in clinical medicine are abrogated in research studies. Research physicians are expected to give primary attention to the production of valid, generalizable data, rather than to meeting patients' individual needs. They may even subject patients to procedures that are unlikely to benefit them and hold some degree of risk, if that course advances the research.[†] Beneficence and nonmaleficence toward the individual patient are not their principal obligations. On the other hand, although research physicians might not owe primacy to patients' interests, they assume additional duties, including the obligation of obtaining a valid informed consent from their research subjects, which involves disclosure of just how the research process differs from ordinary clinical care. The justification of their behavior is based, in part, on their subjects' knowing and voluntary acceptance of these altered conditions of treatment.

Differentiation of ethical principles applicable to physicians according to the functions they are performing is in keeping with the rationale we considered above for the existence of professional ethics as distinct from general ethical norms. To determine which moral rules and ideals a group of professionals ought to observe with particular zealousness, we look to the values that society desires that profession to promote. It is not unusual,

---

[†] Of course, in keeping with generally accepted ethical principles, the degree of risk to which subjects are exposed must be proportionate to the expected benefits of the research; and if unexpected harms occur or it becomes clear that subjects are foregoing important benefits, research projects may be stopped premsturely to protect subjects interests.

however, for professionals to be charged with pursuing different values at different times, depending on the roles they are fulfilling. A physician may work in a general outpatient clinic in the morning, where fidelity to patients' interests (that is beneficence and nonmaleficence) is the over-riding moral imperative. Later in the day, he or she may move to a research unit, where the advancement of knowledge, rather than the pursuit of health, takes priority. There is no reason to be uncomfortable with the notion that as' one's role changes, so also do the ethics to which one is committed.

A similar argument, it should be evident by now, can be made for forensic psychiatry. Whereas clinical medical ethics are rooted in a physician-patient relationship, no such nexus is established in the forensic setting.‡ Forensic psychiatrists who conduct evaluations for legal purposes do not enter into a physicianpatient relationship, and therefore the ethical principles that apply in the latter situation are different from those in the former. As numerous commentators have recognized, were forensic psychiatrists to be charged with pursuing subjects' best interests and avoiding harm – as are their clinical colleagues – their evaluations would be worthless to the courts.[4,22] They would be no more than advocates: junior lawyers doing their best to win a case for their clients. Inherent in the value of the forensic evaluation for the courts is the idea that information adverse to the subject's interests might well be derived from the evaluation and that the forensic expert will truthfully present such data when they are relevant to the legal issue at hand.

Forensic psychiatrists, therefore, like all other physicians whose roles may sometimes depart from the paradigm of the treatment setting, require a distinct set of ethical principles to guide their work. There is no shame in this reality, just as clinical researchers ought to feel no compunctions about observing a code of ethics distinct to their role. Indeed, Stone recognized the inevitability of this conclusion in his chastisement of forensic psychiatry for lacking ethical bearings.[1] His error came in suggesting that it is not possible to identify an alternative set of principles to take the place of those that function in the clinical realm. It is to that task that I now turn.

Principles of Ethics for Forensic Psychiatry

Recalling that the underlying premise for all professional ethics is that society has an interest in advancing certain important moral values, we must begin by asking which values forensic psychiatry is intended to promote. It seems clear that society prizes psychiatric testimony in court because of its potential to advance the interests of justice: the fair adjudication of disputes and the determination of innocence or guilt. Psychiatrists provide information that helps the courts to determine who ought not to be tried at a given point in time, because they are incapable of assisting in their defense; who should not be punished for the acts they have committed, because they lack moral responsibility; who have been subject to psychological injury as the result of others' negligence; and who are so impaired as to be reasonably

unable to work. Testimony on these and other subjects is sought from forensic experts because jurists believe that when they are in possession of that testimony they are better able to reach accurate judgments on these very difficult issues.

If justice is the value to be advanced by forensic psychiatrists, what does that imply about the ethical principles that should guide their work? Two primary ethical principles can be derived from this functional analysis. A strong hint with regard to the first principle comes from the oath to which witnesses swear as they prepare to testify: '. . . to tell the truth, the whole truth and nothing but the truth.'[23] *Truth-telling* is the first principle on which the ethics of forensic psychiatry rest. As I have suggested elsewhere, '[t]he primary task of the psychiatrist in the courtroom is to present the truth, insofar as that goal can be approached, from both a subjective and an objective point of view.'[24]

Subjective truth-telling implies something akin to the concept of honesty, i.e., saying what one believes to be true. Is this enough, however, for the forensic expert? What about the forensic psychiatrist who, willfully or by neglect, remains ignorant of the professional literature, knowledge of which might well alter the opinions he or she provides? What about the expert who, although truthful in his or her testimony, as far as it goes, fails to tell the court that his or her conclusions are based on a theory held by only a small minority of peers, or that much evidence exists contradicting the conclusions reached? When the courts ask forensic psychiatrists to tell 'the truth, the whole truth . . .'. I submit that they are asking for something more.

Here is where the objective component of truth-telling comes into play. The psychiatric witness who is being objectively truthful will acknowledge, insofar as possible, the limitations on his or her testimony, including those due to the limits of scientific or professional knowledge, as well as those specific to a particular case (e.g., due to inability to locate records or directly to examine the subject of the evaluation).[25] Moreover, when the witness' testimony is based on an idiosyncratic theory or interpretation of the literature, the minority status of those views will be made clear. Failure to do so, deliberately or by neglect, will mislead finders of fact about the *prima facie* weight they should give to the expert's testimony and violate the obligation of truthfulness.

Although of critical importance, expressing the limits on one's testimony is not always a simple matter. Forensic psychiatrists operate in an adversarial system in which the attorneys who have hired them may have strong interests in minimizing the extent to which they express uncertainty about their own opinions or about the state of knowledge in the field.[25] Since attorneys and not witnesses are in control of courtroom testimony, questions may be framed in a way so as to discourage experts from making such remarks. But expert witnesses are not helpless in this regard. Experts can set as a condition of their participation an agreement by the attorneys who engaged them to allow them to state the essential limits on their testimony. An expert's ultimate recourse is always to walk away from a case if he or she feels that continued participation will compromise professional ethics.

The second moral rule on which the ethics of forensic psychiatry rests is *respect for persons*. Were truth the only desideratum of the justice system, the police would be permitted to torture suspects to obtain confessions and to search premises on the mere suspicion that illegal activity is occurring. Courts could compel defendants to testify, even against their interests, and district attorneys could reopen the prosecution of acquitted defendants when new, apparently incriminating evidence became available. Under the American constitutional system, none of this is permitted. Rather, we temper our justice system's pursuit of truth with the recognition that sometimes other values must take precedence. Although one might conceptualize the values underlying the exclusion of probative evidence in a variety of ways, I think it is fair to construe them as representing society's commitment to a respect for persons, even when those persons are suspected of having committed crimes.

The implications of the moral rule of respect for persons differ for the various actors in the criminal justice system, because their roles place them at risk for violating this principle in different ways. For the police, their entitlement to use physical force to protect social order creates the risk that

---

‡ When I speak of forensic psychiatry and the forensic setting. I refer to the evaluation of subjects for the purpose of generating a report or testimony for an administrative or legal process. This is in keeping with Pullack's well-known definition of forensic psychiatry as 'the application of psychiatry to legal issues for legal ends.'[20] This is distinct from other functions that persons who consider themselves forensic psychiatrists sometimes fulfill, such as treatment of persons in the correctional system. Psychiatrists providing such treatment fill a role much closer to the one usually played by physicians, and thus – although the particular circumstances of, for example, prison psychiatry, may alter some of the usual ethical rules (e.g., concerning confidentiality) observed in a general treatment setting – they are more tightly bound by the duties associated with beneficence and nonmaleficence. The ethics of correctional psychiatry would benefit from a careful analysis, but I do not intend to offer one in this article.

Forensic psychiatrists sometimes also act as consultants to attorneys, assisting them with strategic and tactical decisions, but not directly testifying themselves. In a brief treatment of this role. I have suggested that its ethical contours may differ somewhat from the ethical parameters associated with the role of expert witness.[21] Although a more detailed consideration of this function is warranted, that is not the focus here

unnecessary force may be used.[26] For prosecutors, the discretion afforded in deciding what charges to file or whether to seek the death penalty creates the potential for the intrusion of illegitimate factors such as the defendant's race or sexual orientation into their decisions.[27] In the case of forensic psychiatrists, the major risk is that subjects of forensic evaluations will assume that an evaluating psychiatrist is playing a therapeutic role and, therefore, that the usual ethics of the clinical setting apply. 'This person is a physician,' they may reason. 'Surely she is here to help me, and at least will do me no harm. I am safe in speaking freely about whatever I choose.'

Respecting persons means acting to negate the risks associated with one's role. Thus, the police must avoid use of unnecessary force, and prosecutors must strive to exclude racial and other personal characteristics of defendants from influencing their decisions. Forensic psychiatrists, in turn, must undercut subjects' beliefs that they, acting in the usual way that physicians act, are placing subjects' interests above all other considerations. Although allowing subjects to hold such beliefs might be an effective means of gathering information, it is inherently deceptive and exploitive, and fails to respect subjects as persons.

Forensic psychiatrists, to avoid violating the rule of respect for persons, must make clear to the subjects of their evaluations who they are, what role they are playing in the case (including which side they are working for), the limits on confidentiality, and – of particular importance – that they are not serving a treatment function.[28] Just as in the research setting, where the fidelity of a physician to the interests of the research subject is similarly altered, care must be taken to insure that the subject is aware of the different parameters of this situation.[§]

This dimension of the obligation to respect persons sometimes goes by the rubric of 'informed consent.' Insofar as use of that phrase implies an identity with informed consent in clinical contexts, I think the term is misleading. Subjects often submit to forensic examinations under coercion and, in some settings, forensic psychiatrists may perform their assessments even over the objections of the evaluee (e.g., a competence to stand trial evaluation of a belligerent prisoner). To refer to these situations as embodying informed consent distorts the accepted meaning of the term. Nonetheless, subjects at a minimum can elect to withhold their cooperation from the evaluation – albeit often at some cost[‖] – and respecting them as persons means giving them sufficient information to allow them to decide whether or not to do so.[¶]

Respect for persons also underlies the adherence of forensic psychiatrists to maintaining the confidentiality of the evaluation, except to the extent that disclosure is necessary to fulfill the forensic function. Even when a blanket warning is given that nothing said by the subject will be considered confidential, the implication is that information may be revealed as part of the legal process. Outside that process, however, as in conversations with the news media, revelation of the information communicated by the subject manifests a serious lack of respect for the subject as a person.

Between them, truth-telling and respect for persons appear to provide sufficient foundation for most generally accepted ethical intuitions regarding

the behavior of forensic psychiatrists, including those embodied in the AAPL guidelines. But are they the only moral rules or ideals to which forensic psychiatrists must be sensitive? What about beneficence and nonmaleficence, for example, those mainstays of medical ethics? Here, it is important to return to the general justification for professional ethics. Recall that although a code of professional ethics may intensify the obligation of professionals to uphold particular moral rules or ideals, it cannot entirely negate their duty to conform to the moral rules (usually injunctions not to harm others) that bind all citizens – although it may alter the balance among those rules when they come into conflict one with another. Nor does subscription to a professional code diminish the virtue associated with acting according to moral ideals, as long as they do not conflict with professional functions.[13,15]

Thus, forensic psychiatrists – not as professionals, but as citizens – have the same duties as other people to behave nonmaleficently, except when acting within the legitimate scope of their professional roles, thereby advancing the pursuit of justice. Moreover, they cannot avoid the obligation of determining whether the actions they are being asked to perform in fact promote justice. Assisting in the torture or abusive interrogations of prisoners would fail that test, not as a matter of professional ethics, but by virtue of ordinary moral reasoning. To accept the pursuit of justice as a basis for forensic ethics is not to say that forensic psychiatrists thereby surrender the right to determine with what actions it is appropriate to become involved, or that they avoid the opprobrium associated with participating in morally reprehensible acts.

In a similar vein, with regard to the moral ideal or aspiration of acting beneficently toward persons, such actions by forensic psychiatrists may be praiseworthy, even though they cannot be said to be part of their professional role. Conversely, although forensic psychiatrists may win acclaim for performing beneficent acts (e.g., diagnosing a melanoma in a subject they are interviewing), they should not be subject to professional sanction for failing to do so.

An Alternative Approach

What other ways might there be to think about ethics in forensic psychiatry, and how do they compare with the theory presented here? The leading alternative, embraced by several authors, although never fully elaborated or justified at the theoretical level, might be called a theory of mixed duties. According to this framework, forensic psychiatrists retain some (usually unspecified) measure of obligation to the principles of beneficence and nonmaleficence that underlie clinical ethics, in addition to whatever duties may be specific to the forensic arena.

Various commentators differ on the degree of priority these clinical principles demand. Some argue that they obligate psychiatrists only to the extent that psychiatrists can fulfill the duties of beneficence and nonmaleficence without interfering with their forensic functions.[28] Others, however, hold open the possibility that clinical duties may take center stage, maintaining that '[t]raditional medical values should be one factor in the balancing process' used by forensic psychiatrists to resolve ethical dilemmas, 'given varying weight by individual practitioners in different circumstances.'[30] Perhaps the most radical view is offered by a philosopher, who claims, 'In spite of the other things that they are called on to do [referring specifically to forensic evaluations], psychiatrists and other doctors must surely be seen *primarily* as healers, with *primum non nocere* as their guiding light.'[31]

The problems with this model of mixed duties are evident at the levels of both theory and practice. On the theoretical plane, as should be clear from the discussion above, the justification for professional ethics lies in its capacity to promote a distinct set of values that are embedded in the functions of the professionals in question. Ethical principles relevant to the forensic role, therefore, cannot legitimately be drawn from the clinical realm, because the values that underlie each function are so different: clinicians seek to promote health, while forensic evaluators seek to advance the interests of justice. As the medical philosopher Edmund Pellegrino has

---

[§] A variety of suggestions have been made as to how to respond if it appears that the subject has not grasped the difference between a forensic and a clinical evaluation, or loses an appreciation of the differences during the course of the evaluation. These suggestions range from reinforcing the subject, to stopping the evaluation, to consulting with the subject's attorney or the judge, to excluding any testimony derived from the evaluation.[. . .]

[‖] Defendants who desire to plead not guilty by reason of insanity, for example, but refuse to submit to an evaluation by the psychiatrist working for the prosecution will typically be precluded from introducing expert testimony of their own regarding their state of mind at the time of the offense.

[¶] What impact a subject's lack of competence might have on the evaluating psychiatrist's obligations is a complex question worthy of more consideration than I can offer in this article. Note the suggestion of the APA Task Force on the Role of Psychiatry in the Sentencing Process: 'When it appears that the defendant is incompetent to give informed consent [sic], the psychiatrist should stop the examination, inform the party who requested the evaluation of the defendant's condition, and allow the legal system to arrive at a solution to the problem. It should be noted that the law is unclear as to whether a substituted consent is permissible in such circumstances, and if it is, who is authorized to provide it.'[28]

noted, "[t]he subject-physician relationship [i.e., in the forensic evaluation context] does not carry the implication or promise of primacy for the patient's welfare that [is] intrinsic to a true medical relationship."[18] Principles based on the pursuit of health, therefore, have no logical nexus with forensic ethics.

What then is the appeal of a theory of mixed duties? Many forensic psychiatrists, I suspect, are reluctant to relinquish their attachment to the ethical principles imbued during their training, which motivate so many aspects of their professional lives. It is difficult for them to accept that, when they perform forensic functions, they have entered into an arena in which these principles are not dominant. Moreover, some forensic psychiatrists may share Stone's concern – that having eliminated beneficence and nonmaleficence as ethical touchstones, we are left with no principles at all to guide our actions. I hope that this discussion has eased those fears.

Other advocates of a model of mixed duties have a different agenda. They are opponents of the death penalty, looking for some way to block psychiatrists from participating in one or another aspect of the adjudication of capital cases.[10, 31] They clearly hope that principles drawn from clinical ethics will make it more difficult to justify participation by forensic psychiatrists, as the tension between the principles of justice and nonmaleficence 'strains the contradictory ethical framework of forensic psychiatry to the breaking point.'[10] But the tension to which this commentator was referring arises only as a result of his inappropriate introduction of principles properly confined to the clinical realm. As is often the case when teleological reasoning prevails, the attempt to shape the ethics of forensic psychiatry to impede use of the death penalty is ultimately illogical and unsatisfactory.

A final group of supporters of the role of 'traditional medical ethics' in forensic work fails to distinguish forensic from therapeutic functions. One example comes from the writings of the philosopher Phillipa Foot, who was cited above to the effect that *primum non nocere*, the principle of nonmaleficence, must be physicians' ethical 'guiding light.'[31] She suggests that the principle might help psychiatrists to determine at what stages of capital proceedings they ought not to participate. But the only example she offers is that psychiatrists should decline to treat a defendant (presumably she means a prisoner) on death row to restore his competence to be executed; this is a treatment function outside of the forensic realm, which legitimately should be governed by ordinary medical ethics.

A similar example comes from a report of surveys of forensic psychiatrists that is said to show support for the relevance of the principles of clinical ethics in forensic psychiatry.[30] The examples cited, however, such as psychiatrists' rejection of a request to write a seclusion order solely to support prison discipline, almost all relate to treatment rather than forensic examination. Those few items that pertain to the forensic context – for example, respondents' agreement with the statement that they should not reveal embarrassing information acquired in an evaluation that could be used to press the evaluee for a settlement – are consistent with principles such as respect for persons that inhere in forensic ethics *per se*. The survey results offer no persuasive evidence that forensic psychiatrists support the blurring of the boundaries between clinical and forensic ethics.

When we turn from the theoretical to the practical level, an additional good reason appears to shun the model of mixed duties. Many writers have worried about the 'double agent problem' in forensic work. Stone, for one, has come to see 'the intermingling of the roles of expert and therapist' as one of the major issues in forensic ethics.[7] He is concerned that the forensic psychiatrist might take advantage of the subject's tendency to view the evaluator as a treater (i.e., to develop a therapeutic transference), in order to extract information that will later be revealed in court to the subject's detriment. His proposal is that 'forensic psychiatrists should as a first principle eschew any overlap between their clinical and evaluative functions.' Indeed, if the evaluation begins to take on therapeutic overtones, Stone would demand that the forensic psychiatrist withdraw from testifying on the basis of the information obtained.[#]

The extent of the double agent problem, that is, the frequency with which subjects in forensic evaluations develop therapeutic transferences, is an open empirical question. Nonetheless, as I noted above. I consider failure to address this issue as constituting a deception of the subject, which violates the principle of respect for persons. Stone's key insight, I think, is that double agency is a matter of countertransference as well as transference. That is, when the forensic psychiatrist approaches the subject as a treater would, the subject responds accordingly. The first task in combatting the problem is to persuade both parties that the situation in which they find themselves bears no relationship to the therapeutic setting. The psychiatrist is not present to help the subject; his or her job is to ascertain the truth relevant to the legal issue at hand.

The most deleterious effect of the insistence on holding on to therapeutic principles of ethics in forensic work, therefore, may be its consequences for psychiatrists' and subjects' perceptions of the evaluators' role. If forensic psychiatrists persuade themselves that they maintain a residual duty – of a professional nature – to benefit and not to harm evaluees, they are likely to communicate that to their subjects.[**] The psychiatrist, for example, who believes he has a duty to evaluate the efficacy of a subject's current treatment, when that is irrelevant to the legal issue in dispute, will ask the kind of questions that treating psychiatrists ask, and should not be surprised to receive the same kind of answers. Both parties may be misled into thinking that this is a quasi-therapeutic encounter. In this process of mutual deception, it is the subject who will be betrayed and potentially hurt.[††]

If we are serious about ridding ourselves of the problem of double agency, we must begin with the code of ethics to which we adhere. When we allow therapeutic principles to creep in to our thinking, we open the door to profound confusion over the psychiatrist's role. A clear advantage of deriving the professional ethics of forensic psychiatry from the pursuit of justice, rather than of health, is the message that it sends regarding the distinction between the forensic and therapeutic roles.

Conclusion

The success of any moral theory depends on how well it satisfies its audience, accounting for their ethical intuitions and providing useful guidance in resolving ethical dilemmas. The extent to which this theory meets those *desiderata* will only be known over time. It is my hope, however, that this effort to describe and justify a theory of ethics in forensic psychiatry will provide a stimulus for a thorough examination of the ethical foundations of our behavior.

Acknowledgments

Earlier drafts of this article were reviewed by Kenneth Appelbaum, MD. Richard Bonnie. JD, Philip Candilis, MD, Thomas Grisso, PhD, Steven K. Hoge, MD, Rose Zolick-lick, LLB. LLM. Jay Katz, MD, and Alan Stone, MD.

[#] Unfortunately, Stone never specifics how one might determine when an evaluation 'has turned into a therapeutic encounter,' clearly the key question on which the implementation of his proposal depends.

[**] A similar phenomenon, which I have called the 'therapeutic misconception.' occurs for much the same reason between clinical researchers and their subjects. Potential research subjects enter discussions over participating in research with the expectation that physician-investigators will manifest that same loyalty to their personal care that they have experienced in ordinary clinical settings. Researchers, often uncomfortable with the different ethical framework under which they are operating, may encourage these beliefs through the words they use and the attitudes they convey. When subjects and family members, however, discover that subjects interests have not been given primacy by the researchers, they feel angry and betrayed[32] Clarifying prospectively the actual scope of researchers ethical duties is the only way to prevent this unfortunate outcome.

[††] Shuman focuses on a different aspect of the examiner-subject interaction, the deliberate use of empathic techniques by the forensic psychiatrist, especially 'reflective empathy,' defined as 'the communication of a 'quality of felt awareness' of the experiences of another person;'[33] (e.g., 'Oh, that must have been a horrible experience for you. I can imagine how frightened you felt.') To the extent that these techniques are employed, they reinforce the false image in the mind of the subject that the current interaction is akin to those that he or she may have had previously in therapeutic settings. Allowing practitioners to believe that they have residual beneficent duties toward subjects increases the risk that they will use empathic techniques.

The author is extremely grateful for their assistance, but assumes full responsibility for the sentiments expressed herein.

References

1 **Stone AA**: The ethical boundaries of forensic psychiatry: a view from the ivory tower. *Bull Am Acad Psychiatry Law* **12**:209–19, 1984

2 **Rappeport JR** (editor): Special issue on ethics in forensic psychiatry. *Bull Am Acad Psychiatry Law* **12**:205–302, 1984

3 **Rosner R**, **Weinstock R** (editors): *Ethical Practice in Psychiatry and the Law*. New York, Plenum Press, 1990

4 **Appelbaum PS**: The parable of the forensic psychiatrist: ethics and the problem of doing harm. *Int J Psychiatry Law* **13**:249–59, 1990

5 **American Academy of Psychiatry and the Law**: *Ethical Guidelines for the Practice of Forensic Psychiatry – 1987* (rev 1995). Bloomfield. CT: AAPL, 1996

6 **American Academy of Psychiatry and the Law**: *Opinions by AAPL's Committee on Ethics: Additional Opinions*. Bloomfield, CT: AAPL, 1995

7 **Stone AA**: Revisiting the parable: truth without consequences. *Int J Law Psychiatry* **17**:79–97. 1994

8 **Mossman D**: Is expert psychiatric testimony fundamentally immoral? *Int J Psychiatry Law* **17**:347–68, 1994

9 **Pellegrino ED**: Societal duty and moral complicity: the physician's dilemma of divided loyalty. *Int J Psychiatry Law* **16**:371–91, 1993

10 **Bloche MG**: Psychiatry, capital punishment, and the purposes of medicine. *Int J Psychiatry Law* **16**:301–57, 1993

11 **Weinstock R**. Controversial ethical issues in forensic psychiatry: a survey. *J Forensic Sci* **33**:176–86, 1988

12 **Weinstock R**: Perceptions of ethical problems by forensic psychiatrists. *Bull Am Acad Psychiatry Law* **17**:189–202, 1989

13 **Gert B**: Morality, moral theory, and applied and professional ethics. *Prof Ethics* **1**:5–24, 1992

14 **Fuller L**: *The Morality of Law*. New Haven: Yale University Press, 1964

15 **Freedman B**: A meta-ethics for professional morality, in *Moral Responsibility and the Professions*. Edited by Baumrin B, Freedman B, New York: Haven Publications, 1982

16 **Jaffee v**. Redmond, 116 S. Ct. 1923 (1996)

17 **Goldman AH**: *The Moral Foundations of Professional Ethics*. Totowa, NJ: Rowman and Littlefield, 1980

18 **Pellegrino ED**: Toward a reconstruction of medical morality. *J Med Philos* **4**:32–56, 1979

19 **Fried C**: *Medical Experimentation: Personal Integrity and Social Policy*. New York: American Elsevier. 1974

20 **Pollack S**: Forensic psychiatry – a specialty. *Bull Am Acad Psychiatry Law* **2**:1–6. 1974

21 **Appelbaum PS**: In the wake of *Ake*: the ethics of expert testimony in an advocate's world. *Bull Am Acad Psychiatry Law* **15**:15–25, 1987

22 **Rosner R**: Forensic psychiatry: a subspecialty, in *Ethical Practice in Psychiatry and the Law*. Edited by **Rosner R. Weinstock R**. New York: Plenum Press, 1990

23 **Saks MJ**: Expert witnesses, nonexpert witnesses, and nonwitness experts. *Law Hum Behav* **14**:291–313, 1990

24 **Appelbaum PS**: Psychiatric ethics in the courtroom. *Bull Am Acad Psychiatry Law* **12**:225–32, 1984

25 **Katz J**: 'The fallacy of the impartial expert' revisited. *Bull Am Acad Psychiatry Law* **20**:141–52, 1992

26 **Davis M**: Do cops really need a code of ethics? *Crim Justice Ethics* **10**:14–28, 1991

27 **Baldus DC. Pulaski C, Woodworth G**: Comparative review of death sentences: an empirical study of the Georgia experience. *J Crim Law Criminol* **74**:661–753, 1983

28 Task Force on the Role of Psychiatry in the Sentencing Process: *Psychiatry in the Sentencing Process*. Washington. DC: American Psychiatric Association. 1984

29 **Appelbaum PS, Gutheil TG**: *Clinical Handbook of Psychiatry and the Law* (ed. 2). Baltimore: Williams and Wilkins. 1991

30 **Weinstock R, Leong GB, Silva JA**: The role of traditional medical ethics in forensic psychiatry, in *Ethical Practice in Psychiatry and the Law*. Edited by Rosner R, Weinstock R. New York: Plenum Press. 1990

31 **Foot P**: Ethics and the death penalty: participation by forensic psychiatrists in capital trials, in *Ethical Practice in Psychiatry and the Law*. Edited by **Rosner R, Weinstock R**. New York: Plenum Press, 1990

32 **Appelbaum PS, Roth LH, Lidz CW, Benson P, Winslade W**: False hopes and best data: consent to research and the therapeutic misconception. *Hastings Cent Rep* **17**:20–24. 1987

33 **Shuman DW**: The use of empathy in forensic examinations. *Ethics Behav* **3**:289–302, 1993

The Role of Traditional Medical Ethics in Forensic Psychiatry*

*Robert Weinstock, Gregory B. Leong and
J. Arturo Silva*

Introduction

Traditional medical ethics originated with Hippocrates and a small group of reform-minded physicians in ancient Greece. The concepts of helping and not harming have permeated medical ethics for centuries and have remained a core foundation for the special professional obligations of physicians. The tradition of helping and not harming is most strongly stated in the Latin, *primum nil nocere*, or, first of all, do no harm.

Several years ago, psychiatrist Seymour Pollack formulated a definition of forensic psychiatry which concluded with a statement that the forensic psychiatrist applied psychiatry to legal issues for legal purposes and ends.[1] The forensic psychiatrist was supposed to be ethically neutral in providing consultation to the legal system, and Pollack's definition implied that it was not relevant for the forensic psychiatrist to question the legal purposes or ends in his professional capacity. Such issues were considered appropriate for his 'personal morals' or beliefs as a citizen, but not for professional ethics. However, it is far from clear that a definition settles this issue, since definitions can be arbitrary and other definitions are possible. Moreover, surveys of American Academy of Forensic Science (AAFS) psychiatry and behavioral science section members,[2,3] and the tri-state chapter of the American Academy of Psychiatry and the Law (AAPL)[4] have suggested that the majority of forensic psychiatrists, at least in the groups studied, do retain traditional medical values as a consideration in their functioning as forensic psychiatrists.

The American Board of Forensic Psychiatry recognized the need for forensic psychiatry to have its own ethics independent of those of attorneys or courts' requirements.[5] The board concluded its definition of forensic psychiatry with a statement that 'forensic psychiatry should be practiced in accordance with guidelines and ethical principles enunciated by the profession of psychiatry.' The board recognized the need for forensic psychiatry to develop its own ethical guidelines, consistent with medical and psychiatric ethics and not by default to leave the professional ethics of forensic psychiatry to the vagaries of the legal system.

A set of ethical guidelines which do address some fundamental ethical problems has been adopted by AAPL.[6] Although some issues consistent with traditional medical ethical values are addressed in these guidelines, many others found to present ethical problems in surveys of forensic psychiatrists[2–4] are not addressed. The new definition of forensic psychiatry adopted by the board and reiterated in AAPL's ethical guidelines does clarify that the current prevailing view is that the profession itself should determine what is ethically proper for the forensic psychiatrist and not relegate it to the legal system.

Psychiatrist Bernard Diamond[7] recently conceptualized the proper role of the forensic psychiatrist as that of a fiduciary to the legal system. Much as the individual physician and psychiatrist do not provide whatever treatment a particular patient desires, but only what the practitioner agrees would be helpful and consistent with his own values, the forensic psychiatric practitioner should participate only in such a way that he agrees can

be useful, promotes better understanding, and functions in a manner consistent with his professional and personal values. In this model, the forensic psychiatrist would not blindly do the legal system's bidding but would do his best to participate only when he could do so honestly in a fiduciary manner, consistent with the profession's values. Such a model could also recognize the autonomy of the legal system much as the current informed-consent model allows for patient autonomy. Negotiation could occur. However, the forensic psychiatrist would not participate in ways he considers harmful or not consistent with his ethics, any more than an individual practitioner would feel obligated to treat an individual patient in such a manner, merely to conform to the patient's wishes. Most psychiatrists, for example, would not wish to treat a corporation executive who wishes to feel less guilty about embezzling money from his company or drug dealer who wishes to experience less conflict in selling drugs to children.

Psychiatrist Alan Stone[8] has described forensic psychiatrists as facing serious ethical dilemmas and conflicts for which medical and psychiatric ethics provide no resolution. He states that a psychiatrist cannot simply adjust to the adversarial system or remain true to one's calling as a physician. Doing whatever possible to help the patient and *primum nil nocere*, constitute the ethical dialectic of the physician's practice. Stone believes that although we know the boundaries of the ethical debate as physicians treating patients, 'When we serve the system of justice, we can no longer agree on the boundaries of the debate.' He believes this problem exists in all situations in which we go beyond the individual doctor-patient relationship. In his opinion, doctors lose their ethical boundaries when they give other factors such as justice, advancement of science, or political causes greater weight than helping their patients or doing no harm. Moreover, Stone notes that the practical ethical guideline to do everything we can to ease the suffering of our patients is no longer part of the American Medical Association's (AMA's) medical ethics nor is 'first of all do no harm.' Consequently, there is no current ethical principle by which to declare actions unethical which go contrary to these traditional medical ethical standards.

Origins of Traditional Medical Ethics

A review of the origin of traditional medical ethical values is crucial in an analysis of the ethical problems. According to medical ethics professor Robert Veatch,[9] physicians have been seen as a 'profession' in the sense that besides having a body of specialized knowledge they 'were committed to a special ethic that bound the members of the profession to special norms, duties and virtues.' Physicians have had an ethical tradition that dates back to Hippocrates in ancient Greece and the Hippocratic oath. According to psychiatrist Allen Dyer, 'patients and physician alike – with only the vaguest notions of what the oath might actually entail – think of the oath as something morally binding on the physician and requiring obligations to the patient. The oath and the name of Hippocrates still remain in the popular mind as the highest symbol of the physician's dedication to healing and . . . the oath continues to encourage a fundamental bond of trust among the patient, the physician, and the medical profession' (p 29).[10]

* Weinstock, R., Leong, G. and Silva, J.: The role of traditional medical ethics in forensic psychiatry, in *Ethical practice in psychiatry and the law*, ed R. Rosner and R. Weinstock. New York, Plenum Press, 1990, pp. 31–51.

The Hippocratic school of physicians lived and worked on the Greek Island of Cos and emerged about the fifth century B.C. with Hippocrates as its head. The school produced a large body of scientific and ethical writings, but not all writings were authored by Hippocrates. In Rome at the time of physician Galen, 130–200 A.D. , there were disputes over authorship.[9] There also are disputes over the date and origin of the oath, but Western physicians trace the foundations of their ethics to Hippocrates and the oath.

Ludwig Edelstein, a scholar on ancient Greece, believed that Hippocrates and the oath were significantly influenced by the Pythagoreans who had a special interest that no harm or injustice be done to people as a result of immoderate or unhealthy eating habits.[11] The oath, according to Edelstein, is almost a pure transcription of Pythagorean ethics (asceticism) with injunctions against abortion, euthanasia (poisons), and surgery as well as strict sexual mores and the keeping of confidences.[12]

The Latin, *primum non nocere*, or, first, do no harm, has become the best-known formulation of traditional Hippocratic medical values. However, many scholars have tried to discover the origin of this formulation without success. Some even consider it to be a revision of the original version.[13] However, related concepts are expressed in the oath and *Epidemics* (Book I, section XI) – a work in the Hippocratic corpus. Their exact meaning differs depending upon the translation from the Greek.

Edelstein's translation of the relevant section of the oath is the most restrictive and reads, 'I will apply dietetic measures for the benefit of the sick according to my ability and judgment; I will keep them from harm and injustice.'[11] Helping and harming are of equal value and solely dietetic measures for the sick are involved. However, philosopher Paul Carrick and others believe this section refers to other areas of medical practice as well, and not just to dietetics.[11] Another translation of this section is: 'I will use treatment to help the sick according to my ability and judgment; I will keep them from harm and injustice.' It also has been translated, 'I will use treatment to help the sick according to my ability and judgment, but I will never use it to injure or wrong them.' This last version gives added strength to the second half of not harming.[13]

The translation by J. Chadwick and W. N. Mann of the Hippocratic oath includes: 'I will use my power to help the sick to the best of my ability and judgment; I will abstain from harming or wronging any man by it.'[14] A later section of the oath reads, 'Whenever I go into a house, I will go to help the sick and never with the intention of doing harm or injury.' According to this translation, the oath is not restricted to the physician's treatment of patients but refers to any use of medical powers. Such an interpretation is consistent with seeing medical ethics as pertinent to all aspects of the physician's work.

Chadwick and Mann's translation of the *Epidemics* (Book I, section XI) reads, 'Practice two things in your dealings with disease: either help or do not harm the patient.'[14] This section has also been translated 'as to diseases make a habit of two things – to help – or to do no harm.' In one translation it reads, 'to help or at least to do no harm.'[13] The latter translation with the addition of 'at least' comes close to, first, do no harm, with the avoidance of harm as a minimum and necessary characteristic of professional ethical behavior.

Medical ethics professor Albert Jansen agrees that the origin of *primum non nocere* is obscure.[15] However, he states that 'do no harm' admonishes physicians that they enter a moral enterprise and exhorts them to 'focus their skills on the well-being of patients.'

The wider interpretation and translation of the Hippocratic requirement would seem to apply to all uses of medical powers and not merely to the treatment of patients. Such a wider interpretation would include evaluations such as those performed by forensic psychiatrists.

According to Carrick,[11] under no circumstances did the physician's profession 'morally permit him to be an accomplice to murder. There are several considerations that render this wider meaning acceptable. First, it is a documented fact that in the Greco-Roman era it was popularly believed that the physician who is skillful at curing, by virtue of this knowledge could also kill. One can find Plato echoing this suspicion in his *Republic*. In book one, Socrates asks Polemarchus: 'Who then is the most able when they are ill to benefit friends and harm enemies in respect to disease and health?' to which Polemarchus replies, 'The physician.'

Anthropologist Margaret Mead considered the Hippocratic oath as marking the first time in history that there was a complete separation between killing and curing. Throughout the primitive world the doctor and the sorcerer were the same person. The person with the power to kill also had the power to cure, including undoing his own killing activities. It marked the first time that the 'power to heal was vested in a practitioner who was not also a shaman with the power to harm.'[10] Dyer states that the Hippocratic oath was unique among ancient codes in making the healing of patients the single overriding feature. By contrast, an ancient Indian code, the *Charaka Samhita*, obliges the physician to deny services to enemies of his rulers, unattended women, or evildoers. It thereby subsumes the physician's obligations to the interests of the state.[10] In the Hippocratic oath there is to be 'equal treatment for males and females, free and slave.' The physician must subsume self-interest to what is good for the patient.[10]

The Hippocratic oath thereby required a stricter morality for Hippocratic physicians than was established by Greek law, and was not the norm among medical practitioners at the time. There is no record of any analogous oath or work directed to medical ethics in ancient times. The Babylonians were the first civilization to record laws regulating medical practice in approximately 1727 B.C. under the Code of Hammurabi. This code set forth stiff fines for surgical malpractice but only for those of certain social status.[11] It does not provide a single standard of care for all patients and is not a work about ethics. There is nothing in the code comparable to Hippocratic ethics.

The lack of licensing and regulation of medicine in Greece provided opportunities for charlatanism and abuse and injury of patients. Medicine was merely a craft, and the oath affirms the importance of the physician being committed to and responsible for the welfare of patients who trustingly and naively seek medical help and the technical competence of himself and his peers.[11] The oath expresses a desire and resolve to make oneself and the profession the best they can be: 'To be a professional in this sense, is to profess competence and personal integrity not merely at the moment of entry into the ranks of trained healers, but every day of one's working life.'[11]

The image of the good physician in the 'Hippocratic corpus underwent some transformation in ancient times, from a craftsman's ethic of work done well to the stoic ethic of duty and obligation to mankind and humanity.'[12] There is therefore some debate about whether the Hippocratic oath dates back to the time of Hippocrates or whether it is a later development, as late as the second century A.D. Hippocratic writings make no mention of the oath in any other sections.

Medicine was first referred to as a profession in the first century A.D. when Scribonius Largus, a physician at the time of Claudius, so referred to it in his treatise *On Remedies*. He also made the earliest reference to details of the oath. Scribonius, following the middle stoa of Panaetius, with origins also in Cicero's *De Officiis*, said that each profession has its own ethics, and we 'must play the role required by our profession – one which we choose voluntarily.' This concept is more demanding than that of the physician as craftsman, and implies a certain nobility of dedication. Perceiving a profession as a special calling is reflected later in Galen's *De Placitis* and in the 18th-century code of Thomas Percival, as well as the original AMA Code of 1848.[12] The later modern view of a profession differed from the earlier stoical one in that it promulgated the image of a special calling with prerogatives of authority and paternalism. Percival saw the physician as 'courteous, kind, yet firm, interested yet objective, taking his patient's concerns into account and acting on his behalf. His comportment must be proper; he should inspire confidence.' These ideas are similar to some in the Hippocratic corpus. What is new is the concept of medicine as a gentlemanly profession, with the idea of privilege rather than the specific obligations emphasized by Scribonius.

One of the characteristics of a profession which developed is to have its own code of ethics enforced by the profession. Special knowledge was considered necessary to evaluate practitioners and its special ethics was the justification for self-regulation. Increasing professional liability litigation has reduced the justification for these procedures, but does not negate the value of a profession trying to police itself to maintain its standards.

Traditional medical ethics as perceived by physicians and patients alike traces its origins back to the Hippocratic oath and the Hippocratic corpus. These traditions were reintroduced in the 10th century A.D. into Western Europe under the influence of the Christian church. References to the Greek gods were replaced by an infusion not only of Christian religious values, but also the Fifty Admonitions to Physicians of Isaac Israeli and the Code of Ishaq Ibn Ali Al-Ruhawi, both of the ninth century.[12] Hippocratic tradition was rediscovered after obtaining works from Moslem and Jewish sources. In the early Middle Ages the ethics of the Hippocratic oath were first universalized. Its sources were refurbished by the humanism of the great religions and served as a well-spring for much of 19th-century American medical ethics.[12] After the Christianization of Europe, other Greek ethical systems had lost favor, but the Hippocratic ethic was preserved because of its similarity to Christian ethics.[9] The importance of Hippocratic ethics increased in the 10th century, when many Greek writings were recovered from Arabic sources.

Interest in the Anglo-Saxon world in medical ethics did not revive until the 18th century. It had undergone an earlier revival in France and the Continent where medicine had a higher status and the Catholic church had greater influence. In fact, in France confidentiality was seen as absolute, much as in the Hippocratic oath. Thus, the concept of the 'professional secret' developed which would not allow testimony in court even with the patient's consent.[16] The value of confidentiality and the professional secret was considered so important for society that no individual patient would be permitted to sacrifice it even voluntarily in a courtroom setting. Only recently have some exceptions developed in France. In contrast, English common law did not contain even a physician-patient privilege.

It was not until the 18th century that interest in medical ethics was revived in the Anglo-Saxon world, when John Gregory published his *Lectures on the Duties and Qualifications of a Physician* based on concepts of Scottish moralists such as David Hume and Frances Hutcheson. In 1789 in Manchester, England, an epidemic struck which overworked the infirmary staff and caused disputes. Thomas Percival was asked to help prevent such disputes, and he wrote his *Medical Ethics*, which presented a scheme for professional conduct which had many features in common with the Hippocratic oath,[9] and became a model for ethical codes in the United States.

In the United States, a dispute among several schools of physicians led orthodox practitioners to found the AMA in 1847. A code of medical ethics that was patterned after Thomas Percival's scheme was developed.

According to Dyer,[10] 'traditions at least as old as the cults of Aesculapius and the oath of Hippocrates stress the fiduciary character of medical practice. The fundamental warrant of medical practice is the trust placed in the physician, based on the physician's competence and intention to help or benefit the patient. But being traditional, these ideals are largely unarticulated and inherently ambiguous. In recent years ever more explicit codification has supplemented the received traditions' (p. 47).[10] Dyer's concept seems to imply that more recent ethical codifications supplement traditional medical ethics. However, their absence from any recent codification does not and should not necessarily negate their traditional importance and influence, at least for some of the most basic core characteristics, such as beneficence and non-maleficence.

Relevant Philosophical Concepts

Distinctions are sometimes made between professional ethics and morals. However, such distinctions are not generally useful since the terms 'ethics' and 'morals' have been used interchangeably and in differing contexts. The word 'ethics' is derived from the Greek *ethika*, meaning 'of or for morals.'[11] Philosopher Philippa Foot states that rather than distinguishing between 'ethics' and 'morals' it is useful to focus on the source of obligations and restrictions of conduct. She distinguishes between professional ethics which stem from special professional obligations and ethical obligations which would apply to any person.[17]

Philosopher Ruth Macklin states that 'ethics embraces professional and applied ethics, theoretical concerns in ethics, philosophical and conceptual questions and whatever your group means by 'morals.' Some people construe 'morals' to mean codes of conduct to guide individual or group actions, while 'ethics' is taken to refer to the principle of right action. In the secular philosophical tradition in which I was educated, 'ethical' and 'moral' are virtually synonymous. The difference is only a matter of etymology . . . It is folly to think that one can rule out an area of conduct as 'inappropriate' simply by defining it one way or another . . . The fact that your group could probably not reach consensus . . . does not mean it is therefore a matter of 'morals' rather than ethics.'[18]

Psychiatrist Paul Appelbaum has stated, 'I have always considered professional ethics to have as their scope consideration of the moral principles that underlie the actions taken by professionals in their professional capacities. The implication of this definition for the issues raised in your letter is that no behavior of psychiatrists as psychiatrists is outside the realm of psychiatric ethics. It may be, of course, that no consensus is possible among psychiatrists as to which principles are relevant to a given professional function (e.g., participation in capital cases), or as to how they should be applied; but that is different from saying that these behaviors are not susceptible to ethical analysis.'[19]

Diamond[20] has suggested a division into organizational professional ethics and personal professional ethics:

Organizational professional ethics are the minimal standards of conduct (ethical, moral, or whatever) below which the practitioner is unacceptable to his peers and, perhaps, assumes legal liability for his conduct. This standard is applicable to all members of the profession, regardless of sex, race, religion, school of thought, training, etc. Examples: sex between therapist and patient, false charges, and deliberately deceiving patients as to need for therapy. Also included here are standards applicable to all members who practice in certain specialized areas. Examples: entering into excessive social or business relationships with patients in psychoanalysis or deep psychotherapy and a forensic psychiatrist who conceals a conflict of interest.

A subcategory of organizational ethics are ideal standards of practice which should be, but are not yet enforceable. That is, standards of ethical practice of the professional leaders, most highly competent practitioners, etc., but which are not enforceable by the professional organization (or the law) because of a lack of consensual agreement that they should represent the general standard of practice. These may be presented as desirable guides for professional practice rather than requirements. Organizational standards of ethical practice sometimes do not distinguish between those which are absolutely required by all, in all circumstances, and those which are guidelines for desirable practice.

The second division of ethics concerns ethical standards accepted by individuals or particular groups of practitioners who for their own personal reasons feel obligated to follow special ethical standards. For example, Catholic psychiatrists may consider it unethical for them to participate in abortion decisions. If one opposes capital punishment one might consider it unethical to evaluate the sanity of a death row prisoner if such evaluation were to be used to certify that he is fit to be executed. The second group may be very strongly held and serve as powerful guides to clinical practice for the persons who subscribe to them, but they cannot be enforced upon all practitioners, even though one might wish to do so, and certainly should not be required of the entire membership of an organization. One must be careful at this point, for frequently strong demands are made for adoption of ethical requirements when, in fact, the ethical concept properly belongs only to a special group of individuals.

In some cases, reason, it would be hoped, can be used to resolve problems in professional ethics. Reason can be most useful when important principles or facts have been overlooked or inconsistencies not appreciated. Difficulties can be most problematic or even impossible to resolve when different values are involved or differing priorities are given to the various values.

Consequentialist or teleological reasoning appeals to consequences such as doing the most good for the most people, e.g., utilitarian philosophy. At the other pole sits deontological reasoning which come from the Greek *deon*, meaning duty, or that which is binding. It appeals not to something extrinsic but to something intrinsic to the situation. For illustration, the pursuit of a worthy utilitarian goal, the patient's health, is constrained by a deontological value, the right to give informed consent.[21] An extreme strict utilitarian position would justify killing an innocent man, if it would be beneficial to society to have someone punished for the crime. It requires deontological values to explain why most people would consider executing an innocent man unethical.

Ethical guidelines are an important start in professional ethics. The latest extensive 1980 revision of the AMA's Principles of Medical Ethics states that the principles 'are not laws but standards of conduct which define the essentials of honorable behavior for the physicians' and are 'intended as guides to responsible professional behavior, but they are not presented as the sole or only route to medical morality.'[22] Philosopher Stephen Toulmin[23] has stated that moral principles, theories, and rules need interpretation to be useful. If guidelines are too highly specific they are not likely to allow the discretion necessary for all sorts of situations. However, if they are so general that they cover every kind of case, they are unlikely to offer clear direction about what to do. Toulmin[23] recommends rules that allow for discretion, since to do otherwise is a denial of uncertainty, because it presupposes that in forming rules and principles, we can think of every kind of situation that could come before us.[24] Psychiatrist Jay Katz[25] has said that people generally have difficulty acknowledging uncertainty and the extent to which it pervades our daily lives. However, such acknowledgment is a prerequisite for careful ethical analysis in complex cases rather than rigid application of an inappropriate rule and an inability to consider other competing values.

When values conflict, and it is impossible to follow one rule or pursue one good without violating another, a moral dilemma is created. Dyer states, 'Modern medicine seldom offers us the clear-cut alternatives that could neatly be dissected as *either* good *or* bad, or *either* right *or* wrong. Instead we are offered complex situations in which any course of action compromises certain ethical principles.'[10]

Psychiatrist Edward Hundert states that in a moral dilemma, moral values in each side of a case are in conflict because there are a multiplicity of values we hold dear. We can do the right thing by weighing and balancing the scale and acting in the way it tips. The values which are outweighed produce anxiety.[26]

Dyer sees ethics as a process of reflecting on the value judgments we make. He sees analogies to clinical judgment. Much like psychotherapy, he has found that when ethical reflection becomes abstract and remote it is useful to ask 'Where is the affect?' as a way of locating ethical conflict.[10]

Hundert has stated that medicine is not value-neutral. It is dedicated to the relief and prevention of suffering. It is therefore not surprising that medicine and law can have conflicting values which can come into conflict since 'medicine gives more weight to considerations of welfare than to considerations of justice as compared to the legal profession.'[27]

Hundert also believes that what is most needed for medical ethics is to teach physicians a way to think about moral dilemmas. Ethical guidelines are only a start and are insufficient when values and principles are in conflict. Our consciences need to compute how much each value is worth in terms of each of the competing values. These resulting moral principles evolve with our moral experiences in dynamic 'reflective equilibrium.' He states, 'The moral actions we take are determined by the ultimate balance of relative weights assigned to all of the competing values as they arise from the particular facts of a problematic case.' Each new dilemma enables us to develop and refine our principles by introducing new patterns of conflicting values. Hundert's model dismisses the simplistic position of those who believe their moral principles are defined in terms of adherence to a consistent action, by emphasizing that consistency applies not at the level of actions but at the level of principles. The patterns of value balancing 'characteristics of medicine as a profession gives rise to what is commonly called "medical ethics" – an ethics that may conflict with that of other institutions within which doctors must make moral decisions.'[27]

Philosopher Baruch Brody has developed a model for dealing with moral dilemmas with some similarities to Hundert's model, which he calls the

model of conflicting appeals.[28] In his model, various conflicting appeals must be balanced. He states that there are several ways to do this. One model involves a lexical ordering of appeals. Examples are political philosopher John Rawls' system, in which justice (the equal distribution of liberty) should take precedence over a principle justifying some social or economic inequity. Another such system is Veatch's, which states that non-consequentialist principles, such as promise-keeping, autonomy, honesty, avoiding killing, and justice have lexical priority over the consequentialist principle of beneficence. Beneficence, according to philosopher Tom Beauchamp, is defined as 'a directive to help others further their important and legitimate interests when we can do so with only minimal risk or inconvenience to ourselves.'[29]

However, as stated by Brody, it is difficult to think of any moral appeal which always takes precedence over all others. In order to avoid beneficence always swamping all other appeals, one need only allow that non-consequentialist or deontological principles should sometimes take precedence. In addition, if in a hierarchical approach, a moral appeal always took precedence over any other appeal alone, it is highly unlikely that it also should always take precedence over all other appeals jointly.[28]

Brody also refers to a scale approach to conflict which is very similar to Hundert's approach insofar as each moral appeal is given a differing weight in different circumstances. We then add up all the appeals favoring one action and all the appeals favoring another and come to a conclusion in the given case about which set of appeals takes precedence. The main difficulty Brody has with this approach is that 'we have no reason to believe that it is possible to do all the things it requires us to do. Its first task, indicating when a given moral appeal has greater or lesser significance in a particular case is perhaps possible. The second task, constructing a common scale so that we can add the strengths of the various appeals on each side is a different matter' (p. 77).[28]

Brody proposes a modification which he calls the judgment approach. It agrees with the scale approach that we need to develop a theory about when a given moral appeal has greater or lesser significance in a given case and identify all the moral appeals relevant to a given case (which can include both deontological and utilitarian appeals). However, Brody states that moral theory can take us no further, since we have no common measure to use in weighing conflicting appeals. The last process he claims is a process of judgment rather than weighing. Otherwise it is the same as Hundert's approach. It also can include a theory of the significance of a given appeal which ranks the differing 'uses of the appeal in terms of likelihood to override other appeals, *all other things being equal*' (p 77).[28] However, judgment is necessary in the last step whose parameters cannot be spelled out consistently by any theory; but the specific circumstances in a specific case must be considered.

This process admittedly is complex and does not produce the simple clear-cut solutions one would like from ethics. Simple problems, of course, can be addressed with simple ethical rules. However, complex problems with values and principles in conflict have no easy solution, which is why they are moral dilemmas.

The judgment approach according to Brody is disturbing because (1) after noting the significance of differing moral appeals the decision maker will often still be unsure what decision to make and would like guidance from moral theory which the judgment approach cannot provide; (2) people's judgments may disagree, although they agree upon the relevant appeals and their significance; and (3) it is open to abuse by those interested in justifying a pre-chosen alternative. However, the reasons Brody gives for accepting it are: (1) by default, because of the problems with other approaches; and (2) it seems to do justice to the reality of moral ambiguity, since good people, after careful examination of the relevant issues, often disagree. A complex model may be what is needed for complex cases.[28]

Issues in Forensic Psychiatry

The forensic psychiatrist functions at the interface of the medical and the legal systems which have different and sometimes competing ethical values. Justice David Bazelon, who wanted psychiatrists to 'recognize and accede to the higher ethical framework of the adversarial system's search for justice,' according to Stone, failed to consider 'how the psychiatrists would square the ethical imperative of the healing profession with the adversarial goals of criminal prosecution.'[8] As a result of the ethical challenges, Stone[8] stated, 'Forensic psychiatry is caught on the horns of an ethical dilemma.'

Philosopher Jay Kantor states that the legal system implies that only some persons should not be punished but the implication of the psychological deterministic tradition is that no persons should be punished for their behavior.[30] Psychotherapeutic treatment, according to Kantor, tries to be nonjudgmental and warmly to help a patient overcome feelings of guilt. In contrast, the criminal justice system coldly tries to bring a felon's feelings of guilt to the surface so that he can suffer over them. Kantor gives as the most striking example of the moral inadequacy of trying to separate 'objective' medical judgment from their eventual nonobjective use is that of concentration camp physicians in Nazi Germany who gave objective determinations about the fitness of inmates to work in the camp, or by default to be fit only to be exterminated.

Recent works have emphasized the importance of physicians to the Nazi killing.[31,32] Genetic theories about purifying the race, by respected German physicians and scientists who wished to compensate for the recent absence of natural selection in humans resulting from the care given to 'genetically inferior' individuals by society, gave intellectual sanction to the killing first of the mentally retarded, then of mental patients, and lastly of Jews and dissidents who were blamed for Germany's loss in World War I. After March 9, 1943 a medical license was required of those making the selections on the railway ramps and supervising the killing in Auschwitz and other extermination camps. Lifton documents the active participation of psychiatrists in the killing of their patients paradoxically described as treatment insofar as it put 'life that was not worth living' out of its misery, as well as the doubling process in which a part of a person serves as a whole and which allowed ordinary people who often were not sadistic monsters to do outrageous things.[31] Of course this analogy is not to suggest that current forensic psychiatrists are ever this evil, but only to call attention to what can happen in a system in which fundamental Hippocratic ideals are forgotten and in which physicians separate technical competence from any concern about the outcomes of their endeavors, performed without any consideration of the relevance of traditional medical ethics.

Kantor raises a question about the ethics of a Nazi physician who would have lied about a person's fitness for work or a person's Jewish origin. Such lying would certainly be consistent with doing no harm. Kantor also asks about the ethics of a physician who opposed the death penalty who tried to 'save as many condemned as possible from execution, doing anything from giving his evaluees the "benefit of the doubt" about their competence to outrightly lying about his evaluation.'[30] Kantor states that such a physician risks in the microcontext having his judgment no longer trusted by the courts and in the macrocontext 'breeding distrust of psychiatry in general.' The Nazi physician who would have lied created a more problematic moral dilemma in which most people probably would consider lying ethically appropriate.

Poet Ezra Pound who faced charges of treason illustrates a similar dilemma. In order to save him from harm, a psychiatrist reportedly evaluated Pound as incompetent to stand trial even though the psychiatrist's professional judgment was that Pound was competent. Pound was saved from trial and possible execution because the evaluating psychiatrist, in playing God, believed that Pound was a great poet who deserved special treatment.[30]

Stone similarly raises a question about the ethics of Dr. Leo who testified routinely in order to help Jewish defendants in the Old Bailey in England in approximately 1801. He apparently did so because of the harsh legal system, but became the laughingstock of the court. His frequent participation in court as well as his evasiveness about this fact seem to have been interpreted as automatically undermining his credibility.[8] Stone also has questioned the proper role for psychiatry in his parable of the black army sergeant in which Stone's testimony resulted in the man's conviction and lengthy prison sentence for stealing small items in a system which gave no consideration to racism. Stone believes he was wrong to consider psychiatry 'objective' under those circumstances.[33]

Proposed Resolution to Ethical Problems

Although conflicting values of the medical and legal systems can produce ethical dilemmas, ethical solutions probably usually exist. These solutions already are recognized by most forensic psychiatrists in an implicit, if not explicit manner, as shown by their responses to the previously mentioned surveys.[2–4]

In many situations, there is no conflict between values. Helping a defendant in a criminal case may be completely consistent with Hippocratic values. Testifying for the prosecution in a case where the defendant is dangerous and treatment will be offered also may not present significant conflict for most forensic psychiatrists, considering the restrictions posed by current mental health laws. It is true that Hippocratic medical values involved treatment of individual patients, and not efforts to help society. However, it is not a significant extension or departure from the core values of traditional medical ethics to consider the welfare of society as well as of the individual.[34] The 1957 Revision of the AMA's Principles of Medical Ethics included responsibility to society.[9] Later revisions have continued to include this aspect; although, the ethics of becoming societal agents of social control can be complex.[35] Moreover, in resolving financial disputes between parties or child custody suits or preventing someone from succeeding with a false disability claim, or succeeding with a valid disability claim – all do not necessarily involve ethical dilemmas. In only a relative minority of cases does participation on one side or the other significantly conflict with traditional medical ethics. In fact, Appelbaum's[36] standard of truth 'to present the truth, insofar as that goal can be approached from both a subjective and an objective point of view,' can usually be followed with minimal ethical conflict. Appelbaum[36] recommends that an objective approach to truth requires the psychiatrist to make evident the limitations on his or her conclusions. Subjectively, to present the truth as he or she sees it, the psychiatrist should gather the maximum possible amount of relevant data.

According to Stone,[37] claiming clinical certainty in predictions of dangerousness as routinely done by Texas psychiatrist Grigson in death penalty cases arguably is unethical because it disregards the empirical evidence. Becoming an avid prosecution advocate in death penalty cases, or those in which the recommended punishment appears excessive, can provide ethical problems for many forensic psychiatrists. Nevertheless, honest participation for the defense in these cases could be considered appropriate,[17] and there is no reason for psychiatrists opposed to capital punishment to withdraw from all such cases. It even is possible to support capital punishment in some cases as a citizen yet believe that to advocate it professionally violates traditional Hippocratic ethics.

It sometimes is believed that the only way to appear to be honest in the courtroom is to testify for both sides in different cases and to be prepared to testify for either side if the facts of the case so warrant. Although many people are of this opinion, this recommendation does not obviate the rare 'hired gun' who will sell testimony to the highest bidder even if it involves stretching or distorting the truth. The 'hired gun' may be prepared to testify for whatever side pays a sufficient fee. Therefore the absence of an ideological motivation or bias does not preclude a financial motivation or bias. The 'hired gun' issue was considered the number-one problem by forensic psychiatrists who responded to the first AAFS survey.[2]

As Diamond points but, the crucial distinction between advocacy and a 'hired gun' is that the advocate is honest but the 'hired gun' is dishonest.[38] The honest advocate still can have an ideological motivation and accept only cases where the facts fit his social philosophy, are consistent with medical ethics, or consistent with what he considers an appropriate fiduciary role to the legal system. The crucial issue is that he is totally honest and turns down cases in which truthful honest testimony does not fit his social agenda or coincide with his personal and professional ethics. He does not twist the facts to help an evaluee or further his social agenda, but tries his best not to participate if he cannot do so in a way that is consistent with his ethics. He is not on one side's payroll or always makes the best case possible for one side regardless of his honest opinion. If his attempt not to participate is unsuccessful because of subpoenas and court rulings and he achieves in an isolated case the opposite result from what was intended, that still does not negate the ethical value of the attempt.[17] Advocacy is therefore not necessarily inconsistent with professional ethics, but dishonesty is, since it destroys respect for the profession in the courtroom as well as in society. There is no reason that ideological motives automatically should lead to dishonesty any more than financial motives.

Respondents to the ethical surveys appear to consider traditional medical Hippocratic values in their functioning as forensic psychiatrists.[2-4] They considered the following to be ethical problems: reporting prison marijuana use despite a promise; writing a seclusion order solely to support prison discipline; or not respecting a competent, not civilly committable prisoner's right to refuse psychiatric treatment. In these situations, traditional Hippocratic ethics seem relevant. Additional situations considered unethical include the following: committing to a position before examining the person, records, or facts; performing a forensic evaluation without attempting to ascertain relevant legal criteria; performing a forensic evaluation without attempting to obtain significant material; or telling only a portion of the truth on the witness stand despite the oath. In this section respondents seem to be opposed to the 'hired gun' and to sloppy, incompetent, superficial work.

However, with other forensic issues, traditional medical ethical concerns appear to be even more relevant. Respondents believed there was a duty to protect both the defendant and society regardless of who paid their fee, and not to reveal irrelevant embarrassing material which could be used to press for a settlement.

Regarding death penalty issues there were suggestive trends. A majority did not feel it was an ethical problem to evaluate a defendant's competency to be executed and a slight majority even saw no ethical problem in treating individuals to restore their competency to be executed. Nevertheless, a substantial minority of psychiatrists would consider such treatment as presenting ethical problems or as being contrary to their personal ethical standards as shown by the close vote on this issue. A large majority clearly believed it presented ethical problems not personally to examine a defendant yet give an opinion in a death penalty case despite the United States Supreme Court opinion about its legal acceptability.[39] Respondents apparently recognized that the profession can declare this procedure unethical despite the court declaring it legal. As psychiatrist Howard Zonana states, psychiatric ethics currently require a personal examination for civil commitment.[40] Section 7, Annotation 4 of the APA Annotations[41] states, 'the psychiatrist may permit his/her certification to be used in the involuntary treatment of that person.' It is, however, ethical to testify in other situations, such as testamentary capacity, without examining the defendant, or to help draw up a psychological profile of a mass murderer without a personal examination. Opinion 7A of the APA Ethics Committee[42] also considers it ethical to testify for the state in a criminal case about the competency of a defendant based on criminal records, without examining the defendant or obtaining approval to render an opinion. However, the death penalty is a problem for which relevant testimony should require special care and caution, considering the extreme importance of the accuracy of such testimony. To quote Zonana, 'Is the death penalty less demanding than civil commitment? . . . The need for reliability might argue for ethical if not legal guidelines regarding the nature and minimal basis for psychiatric testimony.'[40]

Respondents to the survey saw an ethical problem in specifically recommending a death penalty verdict or expressing an opinion amounting to a death penalty recommendation. They also agreed with the APA position of not being a participant in a legally authorized execution and saw a need to treat the death penalty differently because of its special seriousness. The earlier survey showed a difference of opinion regarding the ethics of contributing in any way to a death penalty verdict.[2] This difference of opinion suggest that contributing to a death penalty in any way produces ethical problems for approximately half the members of the groups surveyed. Active direct advocacy for the death penalty is problematic ethically for most members; the death penalty is an act of retribution in which the wishes of the law most clearly can come into conflict with traditional Hippocratic ethics.

Consistent with traditional medical values, respondents clearly saw no ethical problems in performing a forensic consultation on a former patient even in a major case, despite the discouragement of this practice in AAPL's current guidelines.[3,4] Psychiatrist Robert Miller discusses this issue further.[43]

The most consistent way to view these findings is that most forensic psychiatrists consider traditional medical ethics as one value that they bring to their consultations to the legal system. Differing practitioners clearly weigh these values differently, but most forensic psychiatrists appear to balance traditional medical values among other values when they consult to the legal system.

The survey results suggest that forensic psychiatrists use methods similar to those recommended by Hundert or to the model of conflicting appeals by Brody, even though these evaluations are more likely to have been made on a preconscious basis by doing what seems or 'feels' right. They appear informally to consider traditional medical ethics as one value in this balancing process. Appelbaum[44] has stated that the forensic psychiatrist uses his Hippocratic medical injunction of doing no harm and non-maleficence before and after his evaluation of the forensic issue in question, but not in his evaluating role as a forensic psychiatrist. Perhaps a more appropriate model would consider traditional medical values as one factor even in the evaluation process of the forensic issue insofar as they influence how the evaluation is conducted and how the results are permitted to be used; although, they may be even more relevant in other aspects of the encounter. Even in clinical work, a truthful diagnosis such as antisocial personality may be harmful to a patient.[45]

Although traditional Hippocratic values or biases should not operate in the attempt to reach a truthful honest opinion, they should operate in the decision about whether to participate or in how the opinion will be used – at least to the degree that the forensic psychiatrist has any control over this process. If he determines that some harm would be done to the defendant but good would be done to society, most forensic psychiatrists would probably see no ethical conflict. Other circumstances may differ. For example, if a truthful evaluation would lead to a death penalty verdict, a forensic psychiatrist has the option of trying to withdraw from the case if he believes such participation violates either organizational or his personal professional ethics, even if he might support the death penalty in some cases as a private citizen. Moreover, presentation of mitigating factors in the penalty phase of capital cases can be quite appropriate. Relevant aspects of mental illness may be pertinent in those states which require balancing of aggravating and mitigating factors. Aspects which explain why a person committed the crime may be relevant here even if the legal criteria for an insanity defense are not met. Both the AMA and APA consider it unethical 'to be a participant in a legally authorized execution.'[41] This section of the Principles of Medical Ethics with Annotations has been narrowly interpreted to refer only to the actual killing. Opinion 1 of the APA Ethics Committee potentially is broader stating that 'the overriding meaning of this principle is that the physician-psychiatrist is a healer, not a killer, no matter how well-purposed the killing may be.'[42]

Objections sometimes are raised that medical ethics apply only to patients and not forensic evaluees. In addition to the survey results, the *Current Opinions* of the AMA Council on Ethical and Judicial Affairs state: 'Ethical standards of professional conduct and responsibility may exceed but are never less than nor contrary to those required by law . . . In the ethical tradition of Hippocrates and continually offered thereafter, the role of the physician has been a healer . . . A physician's responsibilities to his patient are not limited to the actual practice of medicine. . . .'[46] In a situation analogous to forensic evaluations, i.e., a preemployment physical examination by a physician hired by the employer, 'no physician-patient relationship exists between the physician and the examinee.' Nonetheless, the information 'obtained by the physician as a result of such examinations is confidential and should not be communicated to a third party, without the individual's prior written consent unless it is required by law. If the individual authorizes the release . . . the physician should release only that information which is reasonably relevant to the employer's decision regarding that individual's ability to perform the work required by the job.'[46] Hippocratic ethical tradition is mentioned directly in this section. Also, it is clear that some aspects of medical ethics apply even when evaluees are not patients. Similarly, aspects of medical ethics could apply in a forensic evaluation. The psychiatric profession, of course, can set a higher ethical requirement than the minimum required by law.

There have also been objections that the Hippocratic oath and ethics are outdated. They no longer appear directly in the AMA Principles of Medical Ethics even though they do in the AMA's *Current Opinions*.[46] Abortion today is frequently practiced and even mercy killing is being considered. The Hippocratic oath even prohibited surgery, since Hippocratic physicians were not trained in its practice. Moreover, it has been said that physicians have participated in torture, Nazi death camp selections, and may have even cheered at the Inquisition when souls who were 'saved' were burned at the stake. Additionally, recent trends have turned physicians into mere employees with no special ethics. Physician beneficence and paternalism have been replaced by patient autonomy and informed consent with Hippocratic traditions gradually becoming antiquated. Moreover, some believe that medical ethics outside the doctor-patient relationship remain nebulous.

According to ethicist Edmund Pellegrino and coauthor David Thomasma, what is most significant is the ethos and not a formally developed ethic of the physician-patient relationship: 'That ethos which is still the dominant influence on how physicians see themselves is that of the benign authoritarian dedicated and competent craftsman who acts in the interest of his patient out of motives as practical as a good reputation and as lofty as a love of mankind' (p 203).[12] They also view some degree of effacement of self-interest as always having been understood as part of a physician's duty, as in the treatment of contagious diseases.[47] Furthermore, they view the fiduciary model as best describing the physician-patient relationship in that the whole person is treated, and that the values of the patient must also be part of the dialogue about medical treatment.[47] Paternalism, although often considered a regressive authoritarian element of Hippocratic ethics, is not necessarily bad. It is not, strictly speaking, always unduly authoritarian, though the Hippocratic physicians may have had little respect for patient autonomy. Paternalism can be considered analogous to the responsibility of a good parent towards a dependent child – namely to promote growth and autonomy when the person is unable to make these judgments.[10] A weak form of paternalism involves making decisions for people only when they are unable to make their own judgments.[29]

Even if much of Hippocratic ethics has become antiquated, the central concepts are not. They still appear to have influenced survey responses of forensic psychiatrists. Those departures from traditional medical ethics, as in Nazi Germany, are unfortunate and tragic aberrations. They are well combatted by traditional ethics much as in the law where unwritten common law continues to exert influence. While military psychiatrists as 'double agents' may inadvertently contribute to the death of their patient by sending him back into battle, as Foot states, there is an important distinction and moral difference between inadvertently killing someone and doing something directly and intentionally to produce the killing.[17] Opposing something wrong is the proper ethical action even if it produces no immediate good result. It may have some good consequence eventually, though, even if no immediate good result is seen.[17]

Although abortion was prohibited by the Hippocratic oath, as was euthanasia, new knowledge has raised questions about the exact point where life begins. Nevertheless, many Catholics as well as others still oppose abortion. Giving a terminal patient the means to kill himself or allowing a terminal patient to refuse life-sustaining treatment is not the same as a physician 'giving a fatal draught to anyone' if asked,[14] or deciding himself who warrants euthanasia. Although some aspects of Hippocratic ethics are debatable or have changed, for many centuries, the fundamental aspects

have continued to resurface and guide medicine's nobler actions. It still remains a part of the AMA's Opinions.[46]

Unfortunately, knowledge of ethics does not in itself lead to ethical action. Ethical behavior is more complex. An individual physician must also have the will to be ethical. Virtue in physicians has recently received attention in medical ethics as well as what is involved in a physician being virtuous.[48,49] This emphasis marks a resurgence of Aristotelian ethics focusing on excellence in human activity, as in integrity and character.[50] Knowing the ethical thing to do does not help if a physician or anyone else decides to ignore this knowledge.

Moreover, the appropriateness of judging ethical knowledge and behavior by adherence to guidelines or to ethical principles, such as justice, has been criticized by developmental psychologist Carol Gilligan.[51] She states that the morality of caring is at least as important, which takes into account relationships and loyalties and not theoretical justifications based on principles, as emphasized by psychologists Jean Piaget and Lawrence Kohlberg. Gilligan believes that women score lower on many morality tests because women emphasize caring, but that such considerations are not part of the tests. She believes these considerations are not sex-dependent and need more emphasis. As can be seen, the philosophical justifications for professional ethics also can be quite complex.

Much like Diamond,[20] Dyer has written about the two functions of ethics: 'Ethics in the upward perspective functions by means of the ego ideal, and ethics in the downward perspective functions by means of the superego. One is beckoned upward by the highest standards of moral perfection, but restricted from falling below certain minimal standards by means of superego strictures, if internalized, and by the possibility of external punishment if necessary' (p 121).[10] Both aspects of professional ethics are helpful and useful. Ethics can serve to guide the motivated practitioner who is striving to find a solution to a complex ethical problem. It also can specify the minimum behavior acceptable to the profession – violation of which could result in ethical sanctions by the profession, and thereby police the actions of practitioners.

Ethical guidelines therefore are the starting point, not the end point, of medical ethics. They often are of no help in complex moral dilemmas with competing ethical values. They are the bare minimum, not the upper limit of ethics in forensic psychiatry, and are far from the last word. Moreover, the presence or absence of a consensus does not, in and of itself, necessarily settle all ethical questions. In fact, it is important to be cautious that the majority are not tyrannical towards a legitimate minority by enforcing its will on the minority if the minority has good reasons for its behavior. Exceptions must be allowed if there are competing and overriding ethical values. An individual forensic psychiatrist also can have his own personal ethical standards which may be more stringent than those required by the profession.

Conclusion

A strong case remains for the retention of traditional medical ethical values in the functioning of the forensic psychiatrist. Training in the ethical model of Hundert and the model of conflicting appeals by Brody should be an important part of forensic psychiatric (and general psychiatric) training. Simple guidelines generally are no solution for the complex ethical problems sometimes encountered by the forensic psychiatrist; although they may be helpful in most ordinary cases. Traditional medical values should be one factor in the balancing process – given varying weight by individual practitioners in different circumstances.

If the survey respondents are at all reflective of forensic psychiatrists generally, the results suggest that members informally and on their own already are considering factors such as those discussed in this chapter. Such considerations probably operate when forensic psychiatrists have a moral sense of the ethical thing to do when problems arise. Training in forensic psychiatry should encourage continued consideration of traditional medical ethics as one factor in determining a proper ethical course of action and not dismiss such considerations as 'therapeutic bias.'[52] Much like values such as public safety, Hippocratic ethics should remain a consideration. However, because of a current lack of consensus, traditional Hippocratic values currently would be given differing emphasis and importance by various practitioners. Some issues such as evaluating death penalty cases without a personal examination achieve a general consensus and warrant inclusion in ethical guidelines.

Rather than being inconsistent, or inappropriately influenced by 'therapeutic bias,' forensic psychiatrists generally already seem to appreciate the value of retaining traditional core medical values as one consideration in their functioning as forensic psychiatrists. This appreciation should be fostered and encouraged.

References

1 Pollack S: *Forensic Psychiatry in Criminal Law*. Los Angeles, University of Southern California, 1974.

2 Weinstock R: Ethical concerns expressed by forensic psychiatrists. *J Forensic Sci* 1986; **31**:596–602.

3 Weinstock R: Controversial ethical issues in forensic psychiatry: A survey. *J Forensic Sci* 1988; **33**:176–186.

4 Weinstock R: Perceptions of ethical problems by forensic psychiatrists. *Bull Am Acad Psychiatry Law* 1989:**17**:189–202.

5 Actions of the American Board of Forensic Psychiatry, May 1985.

6 American Academy of Psychiatry and the Law Ethical Guidelines, for the Practice of Forensic Psychiatry. Revised version in Appendix of this volume.

7 Diamond BL: The psychiatrist: Consultant vs activist in legal doctrine. Presented at the 19th Annual Meeting, American Academy of Psychiatry and the Law, San Francisco, October 20, 1988.

8 Stone AA: The ethics of forensic psychiatry: A view from the ivory tower, in Stone AA: *Law, Psychiatry, and Morality*. Washington, D.C., American Psychiatry Press, 1984. Reprinted in Rosner R, Weinstock R (eds): *Critical Issues in American Psychiatry and the Law*, Vol 7, Ethical Practice in Psychiatry and the Law. New York, Plenum, 1990, pp 3–18.

9 Veatch RF: Medical ethics – An introduction, in Veatch RF (ed): *Medical Ethics*. Boston, Jones and Bartlett, 1989.

10 Dyer AR: *Ethics and Psychiatry*. Washington, DC, American Psychiatric Press, 1988.

11 Carrick P: *Medical Ethics in Antiquity*. Dordrecht, Netherlands, D. Reidel, 1985.

12 Pellegrino ED, Thomasma DD: *A Philosophical Basis of Medical Practice*. New York, Oxford University Press, 1981.

13 MacKinnon B: On not harming: Two traditions. *J Med Philos* 1988; **13**:313–328.

14 Lloyd GER (ed.): *Hippocratic Writings*. New York, Viking-Penguin, 1978.

15 Jansen AR: Do no harm, in Veatch RF (ed): *Cross-Cultural Perspectives in Medical Ethics*. Boston, Jones and Bartlett, 1989.

16 Shuman DW, Weiner MF: *The Psychotherapist-Patient Privilege: A Critical Examination*. Springfield, IL, Charles C. Thomas, 1987.

17 Foot P: Ethics and the death penalty: Participation by forensic psychiatrists in capital trials, in Rosner R, Weinstock R (eds): *Critical Issues in American Psychiatry and the Law*, Vol 7, Ethical Practice in Psychiatry and the Law. New York, Plenum, 1990, pp 207–218.

18 Macklin R: personal communication, April 19, 1988.

19 Appelbaum PS: personal communication, April 19, 1988.

20 Diamond BL: personal communication, April 25, 1988.

21 Callahan JC: *Ethical Issues in Professional Life*. New York, Oxford University Press, 1988.

22 American Medical Association: *Principles of Medical Ethics*. Chicago, American Medical Association, 1980.

23 Toulmin S: The tyranny of principles. *Hastings Cen Rep* 1981; **11**:31–39.

24 Koppelman LM: Moral problems in psychiatry, in Veatch RF (ed): *Medical Ethics*. Boston, Jones and Bartlett, 1989.

25 Katz J: Why doctors don't disclose uncertainty. *Hastings Cen Rep* 1984; **14**:25–44.

26 Hundert EM: Competing medical and legal ethical values: Balancing problems of the forensic psychiatrist, in Rosner R, Weinstock R (eds): *Critical Issues in American Psychiatry and the Law*, Vol 7, Ethical Practice in Psychiatry and the Law. New York, Plenum, 1990, pp 53–74.

27 Hundert EM: A model for ethical problem solving in medicine with practical applications. *Am J Psychiatry* 1987; **144**:839–846.

28 Brody BA: *Life and Death Decision Making*. New York, Oxford University Press, 1988.

29 Beauchamp TL: *Philosophical Ethics: An Introduction to Moral Philosophy*. New York, McGraw Hill, 1982.

30 Kantor JE: Psychiatry in the service of the criminal punishment system: Some conceptual and ethical issues, in Rosner R, Harmon RB (eds): *Critical Issues in American Psychiatry and the Law*, Vol 6, Correctional Psychiatry. New York, Plenum, 1989.

31 Lifton RJ: *The Nazi Doctors*. New York, Basic Books, 1986.

32 Müller-Hill B: *Murderous Science*, Fraser G (trans). New York, Oxford University Press, 1988.

33 Stone AA: Morality for psychiatry, in Stone AA: *Law, Psychiatry, and Morality*. Washington, DC, American Psychiatric Press, 1984.

34 Mills MJ, Sullivan G, Eth S: Protecting third parties: A decade after *Tarasoff*. *Am J Psychiatry* 1987; **144**:68–74.

35 Leong GB: The expansion of psychiatric participation in social control. *Hosp Community Psychiatry* 1989; **40**:240–242.

36 Appelbaum PS: Psychiatric ethics in the courtroom. *Bull Am Acad Psychiatry Law* 1984; **12**:225–231.

37 Stone AA: Psychiatry and the Supreme Court, in Stone AA: *Law, Psychiatry, and Morality*. Washington, DC, American Psychiatric Press, 1984.

38 Diamond BL: The honest advocate, in Rosner R, Weinstock R (eds): *Critical Issues in American Psychiatry and the Law*, Vol 7, Ethical Practice in Psychiatry and the Law. New York, Plenum, 1990, pp 75–84.

39 Barefoot v Estelle, 103 S Ct. 3383 (1983).

40 Zonana HV: Critique of a critique. *Bull Am Acad Psychiatry Law* 1984; **12**:237–241.

41 American Psychiatric Association: *Principles of Medical Ethics with Annotations Especially Applicable to Psychiatry*. Washington, DC, American Psychiatric Association, 1989.

42 American Psychiatric Association: *Opinions of the Ethics Committee on the Principles of Medical Ethics with Annotations Especially Applicable to Psychiatry*. Washington, DC, American Psychiatric Association, 1985.

43 Miller RD: Ethical issues involved in the dual role of treater and evaluator, in Rosner R, Weinstock R (eds): *Critical Issues in American Psychiatry and the Law*, Vol 7, Ethical Practice in Psychiatry and the Law. New York, Plenum, 1990, pp. 129–150.

44 Appelbaum PS: The problem of doing harm. Presented at the 19th Annual Meeting, American Academy of Psychiatry and the Law, San Francisco, October 20, 1988.

45 Weinstock R, Nair M: Antisocial personality – Diagnosis or moral judgement? *J Forensic Sci* 1984; **29**:557–565.

46 American Medical Association: Current Opinions of the Council on Ethical and Judicial Affairs (History and sections 5.08, 5.09, 9.08). Chicago, American Medical Association, 1989.

47 Pellegrino ED, Thomasma DD: *For the Patient's Good: The Restoration of Beneficence in Health Care*. New York, Oxford University Press, 1988.

48 Putnam DA: Virtue and the practice of modern medicine. *J Med Philos* 1988; **13**:433–444.

49 Veatch RF: The danger of virtue. *J Med Philos* 1988; **13**:445–446.

50 Brody H: The physician/patient relationship, in Veatch RF (ed): *Medical Ethics*. Boston, Jones and Bartlett, 1989.

51 Gilligan C: *In a Different Voice*. Cambridge, Harvard University Press, 1982.

52 Pollack S: Psychiatry and the administration of justice in Curran WJ, McGarry AL, Petty CS (eds): *Modern Legal Medicine, Psychiatry, and Forensic Science*. Philadelphia, FA Davis Co. 1980, pp. 655–674.

Principles and Narrative in Forensic Psychiatry: Toward a Robust View of Professional Role*

Philip J. Candilis, Richard Martinez, and Christina Dording

Ethics theories of forensic psychiatry have struggled between applying classical clinical ethics and developing new theories for forensic practice.[1–4] Principles of beneficence and nonmaleficence, which attain primacy in clinical practice, may be insufficient to direct the ethics aspects of forensic work because of obligations to forces outside the traditional dyadic patient-professional relationship – namely, the judicial system.[5–9] Nowhere is the tension of clinical and forensic ethics more evident than in discussions of the incompatibility of being both therapist and forensic expert for the same individual. This is exemplified in the courtroom testimony of clinical caregivers on behalf of their patients seeking disability, damages, or defense from legal sanction. A strict principlist approach, such as that of Appelbaum,[3] which orders justice above traditional physicianly principles, consequently may differ from a narrative approach, such as that of Griffith,[4] which criticizes ethics models that do not explicitly value the narrative of historically disadvantaged cultures within society. We offer a case for analysis that underscores the conflict between clinical and forensic roles but offers a reconciliation of current principlist and narrative approaches to forensic ethics. We construct a model of forensic ethics that synthesizes both views, with a place for principled theory enriched by narrative application to specific cases. (Case material has been disguised to protect the identity of the participants.)

The Case of Ms. George and the Forensic Expert

Ms. George was a vibrant, athletic, and strong-willed woman in her mid-40s who suffered a catastrophic brain-stem stroke that left her almost completely paralyzed. She was a college-educated entrepreneur who had managed a business and valued close contact with her relatives. Her family was deeply involved in her care, applying both the immigrant parents' southern European sensibilities and the values of American-born children to daily clinical matters. Family meetings had always been, and remained, boisterous affairs with dramatic arguments, rifts, and just as dramatic – and predictable – reconciliations.

Now, this family star and former triathlete could only raise her eyebrows to communicate her needs. As she struggled through two years of rehabilitation to maintain basic muscular tone and respiratory support, she could not penetrate the severe paralysis that had trapped an active mind in an unresponsive body. Indeed, her treaters considered it miraculous that she had even regained consciousness; she was not expected to recover further.

Ms. George ultimately was transferred to a nursing facility, having taken advantage of all that specialty rehabilitation could offer. She remained active in meeting with visitors, listening to music, watching films, and even learning advanced mathematics on videotape. She refined and memorized a communication system that used an alphabet board pasted above her bed.

Two and a half years after her stroke, Ms. George began to request help from family and health-care staff alike to end her life. Her current condition was untenable, she reported, and she preferred to be allowed to die. Indeed, she began to refuse the regular tube feedings she received. The facility's psychiatric consultant endorsed the 'competence' of her decision to refuse nutrition and hydration but requested consultation by a forensic specialist because the institution lacked an ethics committee or similar body to address staff discomfort with the decision. Because her family split vehemently over her request, Ms. George asked the local probate court to appoint a legal guardian to advocate for her position. She did not wish for delays caused by the maelstrom of opinions surrounding her.

The probate court appointed a forensic psychiatrist to assess Ms. George's 'current psychological/psychiatric functioning and its relevance to her decision to fast for the purpose of ending her life.' The court noted that the appointment was for 'the limited purpose of conducting a forensic evaluation relative to the competence of the ward.'

Guided by the court's warning of family discord, the consultant's first effort was an extended family meeting, without Ms. George, to gather information, explain the forensic role, and to offer family members the opportunity to be heard. A number of concerns were vehemently and painfully expressed. One parent with conservative Eastern Orthodox views opposed her daughter's choice of 'suicide' on religious grounds. One brother expressed Adventist views on his sibling's behalf, explaining that the patient had been baptized by the sect while paralyzed and that the decision to fast would be considered sinful. A second brother expressed holistic medical views, interpreting movements described as reflexive by physicians as potential evidence of a missed diagnosis or inaccurate prognosis. Another family member expressed concern that Ms. George was unduly influenced by a friend who stood to gain from the will. Although the evaluation ultimately would proceed along common clinical guidelines, a good deal of work would be required to address relevant family, religious, and financial influences.

Conflicting Roles

The issue of conflicting forensic and clinical roles has only recently been addressed in the clinical literature. Paul Appelbaum notes that during his training it was commonplace for psychiatrists to act as both psychiatrist and forensic expert.[10]

Recently, however, psychiatrists and other physicians have found themselves thrust unwillingly into this role of 'double agent.' This particular brand of double agency confuses whether the expert acts as an agent (or advocate) of the patient or of the court. A few common scenarios include the psychiatrist who is asked to testify on damages to a patient being treated for posttraumatic stress disorder or the psychiatrist asked to render an opinion on the parental fitness of a patient in a custody dispute.

Strasburger, Gutheil, and Brodsky[11] illustrate paradigmatic differences between the two roles. Although the treating psychiatrist generally undertakes a psychodynamic approach with an emphasis on the patient's psychological perceptions and distortions, the forensic expert generally adopts a descriptive

* Candilis, P., Martinez, R. and Dording, C.: Principles and narrative in forensic psychiatry: towards a robust view of professional role. *Journal of the American Academy of Psychiatry and the Law* **29**:167–173, 2001.

approach with an emphasis on objective diagnosis and classification. The treating psychiatrist is interested in the patient's truth, a form of 'narrative' or interpretative truth that is influenced invariably by internal psychological experiences. Narrative truth in this context is a search for meaning rather than objective fact. It represents the patient's 'inner personal reality, albeit colored by biases and misperceptions.' This truth may be reflected on and altered as the patient gains insight and personal understanding during the course of therapy, but courts of law generally are not interested in the patient's psychic advancement. The forensic expert is concerned with factual, objective information and indeed would be worthless to a court of law otherwise.

The treating psychiatrist is obligated, in the words of Candilis and Appelbaum, 'not to advance justice, but to provide good care, grounded in therapeutic process, confidentiality, and the traditional principles of beneficence and non-maleficence.'[6] However, the responsibility of the *forensic* psychiatrist is more a societal one, with allegiance to the law, the courts, and society as a whole. The forensic psychiatrist serves society's interest in the delivery of expert testimony that advances the interests of justice: 'the fair adjudication of disputes and the determination of innocence or guilt.' One prominent theory of forensic ethics consequently places social principles of justice, truthfulness, and respect for persons above personal obligations of beneficence and nonmaleficence.[3]

Furthermore, in a therapeutic relationship confidentiality generally is maintained unless patients are a danger to themselves or others. This promise of confidentiality allows patients to reveal intimate, embarrassing, or painful details from their personal lives. When patients enter a legal setting, these same intimate revelations may become damaging public knowledge. In the forensic role, psychiatrists are not focused on protecting patients from harm. Indeed, the effect of their testimony may be more than embarrassing; it may be punitive and psychologically destructive.

In the case of Ms. George, familial strife amid a tragic situation called for more than an aseptic assessment of capacity to refuse nutrition and hydration. Ignoring the family's conflict, their lack of information, and the potential loss of emotional resolution and comfort at a critical time would be unacceptable on a human level. A compassionate professional involvement would necessarily include clinical elements of education, counseling, conflict resolution, and spiritual guidance. To do otherwise would abrogate responsibilities to an individual and family in profound distress. From an ethics perspective, a strict adherence to forensic role responsibilities would fail all parties.

As the court's expert, the forensic consultant was appointed to inform the judicial process about a fluid clinical situation requiring forensic expertise. However, once involved as an 'expert,' the consultant was confronted with a complex family drama. New professional responsibilities and obligations emerged, requiring a more flexible and complex approach. Although ethics principles and strict adherence to forensic role responsibilities allowed the capacity assessment to be completed, a broader conceptualization of professional role, framed within a detailed narrative of the situation, would be needed to address the larger and more ambiguous aspects of professional involvement in the case.

Beyond Roles: Professional Integrity

In forensic psychiatry, professionals are viewed as 'in a role.' Role morality guides professionals in their expert activity,[12] identifying both the responsibilities of the professional and the limits of professional activity. Often, however, in defining limits of activity, role morality espouses professional behavior that incorporates minimum obligations to the evaluee. Such a narrow adherence to the professional role can lead to exclusion of other important ethics considerations. In some cases, frank harm to both the evaluee and the relationship may result. A broader view of professionalism, a view that considers internal norms of the profession and professional aspirations toward moral ideals, may be useful. Although contrary to current views of forensic roles, we argue for a model of professional role that includes personal morality of the individual professional and historical elements of the medical profession. We believe this integrated approach can help clarify the moral ambiguity often found in complex situations.

Role dilemmas in forensic psychiatry reveal much about the tension between personal and professional morality. A view of professional integrity that is helpful for this discussion of forensic roles is offered by Miller and Brody.[13] These authors construct a robust view of professional roles first by defining personal integrity and then offering a conceptualization of *professional* integrity. Personal integrity is tied to one's identity, the activity that affects trust, and the qualities of wholeness and intactness. Three elements are necessary for integrity: (1) a set of well-regarded personal principles that remain somewhat stable over time and are coherent; (2) verbal expression of those values and principles; and (3) consistency between what one says and what one does. Coherence and integration of personal and professional spheres are espoused by this model.

Although personal integrity is tied closely to individual identity, professional integrity and professional identity are more socially determined. Both professional integrity and identity are tied to the community – a community that defines expectations and places restrictions on individual expression. Professional integrity, then, encourages a more dynamic understanding of the interplay of personal and professional morality than strict views of the forensic role allow. Currently, strict interpretation of the forensic role elevates the professional's obligations to the court over personal values and traditional professional obligations. In fact, the current view of the forensic role would appear to require a careful discrimination between professional and personal values. However, because professional integrity is tied to the community and its values, the community may legitimately expect a broader, more traditional physicianly approach from its experts.

In addition, professions possess an internal set of duties, values, and ideals that are essential for professional identity and integrity. Intrinsic values and activities of professions define the profession and operationalize the meaning of professional integrity. *Just* as personal integrity generates a certain consistency over time, a profession possesses tradition and a *historical narrative* of its goals, duties, values, and ideals.[13] This historical narrative anchors the profession in those values that resist the vagaries of social and situational forces, especially when these forces influence the professional to behave contrary to the historical narrative.

Strict views of the forensic role may fail to balance adequately the tension between the historical narrative of the medical profession and the need to offer objective analysis in complex cases such as that of Ms. George. Rigid adherence to an objective 'expert' role in complex relationships such as this may conceivably harm individuals and their loved ones.

In forensic psychiatry, we contend that the historical narrative of the specialty, as in any professional activity, is still emerging. One approach has been to view the forensic psychiatrist through role theory and social psychology, narrowly defining professional activity as an agency of society and the court.[3,11] Others have argued for application of traditional clinical ethics to the dilemmas of forensic psychiatry.[1,2] We are closer to this latter view in proposing that broader views of professional integrity – that include the historical narrative of medical practice – permit greater flexibility in the discussion of what constitutes a true forensic interaction. This view permits personal and traditional physicianly values to inform the forensic role. Although it has been difficult to admit traditional values such as beneficence and nonmaleficence into the strict view of forensic expertise, a view that replaces professional role with the concept of professional integrity may allow exactly that. This conceptualization of professional integrity then can be applied to individual cases by describing the narrative in which the expert and the evaluee find themselves.

Finally, the choice of proper professional action must be coupled with the question of what kind of professionals we wish to be. In forensic work, for many of us, it is not possible, much less desirable, to detach forensic consultations from our traditional commitments to patients. Our profession is a large part of who we are and is deeply connected to the larger community that contains and supports us. David Luban, in his book *Lawyers and Justice, An Ethical Study*,[14] provides insight into why we must link individual and professional integrity. He writes, '. . . commitments to the duties of a profession, to a career, or to major social situations. . . . These can be, they frequently are, among the deepest loyalties and commitments in our lives; and it cannot be right to ask us to reconsider them, to trade them off, again and again.'

The Narrative Context

One final element is necessary for our move toward a robust view of professional role: the use of personal narrative. The concept of narrative entered medicine through medical ethics. Initially, narrative, along with casuistry, phenomenology, the ethics of care, and virtue theory were offered as criticism of the principle-based approach that dominated medical ethics.[15] Proponents of narrative argue that the traditional principles of medical ethics – autonomy, beneficence, nonmaleficence, and justice – fail to guide us in the often complex and ambiguous aspects of moral problems in medicine.[16–19] Griffith, for example, has argued powerfully that principlism is not sufficient to address the reality of a nondominant group whose narrative is not adequately valued by society.[4] Indeed, principles alone may be limited in addressing the motives and intentions of those involved in clinical and legal relationships. Finally, as we have argued, because a strict view of professional role may be inadequate for situations such as that of Ms. George and the forensic expert, narrative may permit an alternative understanding of professional obligations and responsibilities, inform the interplay of personal and professional morality, and provide a methodology for examining the larger moral aspects involved in all human dramas.

Narrative offers an approach by which medical knowledge is seen as storytelling knowledge. The individual's predicament is the telling of a story, with empathy and compassion elevated using humanistic language. In addition, narrative ethics is a methodology that increases sensitivity to the particulars of cases. It fortifies our moral deliberations by heightening our appreciation of the nuance and subtlety intrinsic to human dilemmas. Narrative includes such forms of communication as news, gossip, anecdote, history, drama, and fiction. Broader views accept all forms of human expression as narrative. Visual arts, film, dance, and music become texts that can be deconstructed to reveal hidden meanings and intentions. What is left out of the 'text' becomes as important as what is included.

In medicine, as in other professions, moral dilemmas arise from the details of human drama. The narrative approach allows attention to those elements of language and storytelling that actively permit reflection on the intricacies of morality. In this sense, the narrative approach becomes a methodology for describing the situations that raise moral questions. How are we to provide guidance for moral dilemmas if we cannot adequately describe the problems we hope to solve?

However, this is not to say that narrative works alone in describing the ethics landscape. Justification of right action still requires use of principles to represent the ideals of objectivity and generalizability in reaching reasoned ends. Principles work at the theoretical level to create a framework for right action.[15] Then, narrative can operationalize theory in a practical manner, describing the individual's unique path toward the forensic encounter.

In the case of Ms. George and the forensic expert, then, can we incorporate the language of suffering; appreciate moral ambiguity in the intentions and motives of the people involved; struggle with the tension between therapeutic engagement and expert detachment; and consider the place of witnessing, affirming, and validating?

Narrative and the Case of Ms. George

At first glance, the case of Ms. George and the forensic expert involves a competence determination. The methodology of competence assessment (more accurately, decision-making capacity) has become routine practice when patients make requests that are in conflict with the values or wishes of caregivers and families. However, the case of Ms. George requires more from the forensic expert than the mere report to the court on the state of her decision-making. From the perspective of professional integrity and narrative ethics argued for this case, several themes become apparent.

First, although principles and forensic role responsibilities generally are adequate to direct capacity assessments, the doctrine of informed consent that undergirds these assessments is poorly served by the narrow approach. Decision-making capacity and its determination are processes by which we ensure that the doctrine of informed consent has integrity. For the purposes of informed consent to be realized, certain conditions must be present. One of these conditions is that individuals should be involved in medical decisions from a position of increased power; that is, they should be informed and supported in their capacity to evaluate, communicate, and understand choices. The risk here is that a strict view of the forensic role will meet only minimum standards of informed consent, failing to support its larger purposes.

The importance of informed consent lies in its ability to create, facilitate, encourage, and if necessary, require a kind of conversation between the individual and the professional – a conversation that serves to reduce the power differential between vulnerable individual and powerful professional. This conversation diminishes parentalism and increases the likelihood that the decisions reached are truly the voluntary informed decisions of an autonomous person. What is intended by informed consent doctrine is the creation of a process that embraces its full spirit.[20,21] For the forensic expert in this case to ignore this larger view would be to undermine the moral integrity of informed consent.

Second, limiting professional obligations to the strict forensic role fails to address larger professional obligations. Although it is clear under the principle of autonomy that Ms. George has a right to her competent decision, other morally ambiguous aspects of her case remain unclarified. What is the obligation of the professional toward the family and toward the individual after her decision-making capacity becomes clear? The dynamics of moral agency, of so-called 'expert testimony' in the midst of human tragedy, must be expanded if we are to appreciate fully the place of experts in such situations.

A third related theme is the tension between principles of autonomy and beneficence. In the language of law, one might argue that individual rights and the duties created by such rights are to be practiced stringently. This practice is supported within our political-philosophical tradition. Individuals and courts respect autonomy and self-determination – as they should – and the presumption is that the dignity of Ms. George is supported. However, respect for autonomy may be operationalized inappropriately as a form of 'pseudoempathic' medical practice, in which the professional acts as if the only obligation is to assess the individual and then leave her alone. In such cases, the doctrine of informed consent is implemented as a kind of 'Miranda' warning.[20,21] The forensic consultant is particularly vulnerable to such an approach.

Stringent adherence to the autonomy principle without considering the rich context surrounding Ms. George may marginalize the professional and family voices intimately connected to the case. A narrow focus on principles can foster a compartmentalization of professionalism, in which the voice of the expert is confined to the purposes of the court but fails the larger moral commitment to the individual and the family. In the case of refusal of treatment, Sullivan and Youngner point out the dangers of this approach: 'Reluctance to explore the reasons for refusal can be particularly dangerous when combined with a superficial adherence to the ideal of patient autonomy and respect for the 'right' to refuse treatment.'[22] These authors agree that a more complicated involvement of the expert is necessary.

This use of professional integrity and narrative to contextualize a specific case has its pitfalls no doubt. But in the view argued here, the neglect of evaluee and family that might result from a rigid adherence to principlism and a narrow view of professional role is of greater harm than the inclusion of all voices involved in the drama. In our view, the activity of the forensic consultant that includes clinical therapeutic involvement is not disrespectful of the patient's right to decide but honors the complexities and ambiguities of the case.

Professional Integrity, Narrative, and Moral Agency

The narrative approach, then, considers the humanistic elements in such cases. The uncertainties of suffering – the impact of the patient's decision on her family, on the doctors and nurses involved in her care, and on the expert witness and the court itself – are enhanced when a robust view of the forensic role drives the interaction. The tradition of disengaged and objective involvement would be troubling here. Objectivity and distance, like other values of the enlightenment, are intended to serve the goals of both evaluees and professionals. However, in the case of Ms. George emphasizing objectivity and distance may undermine the involvement necessary if professionals are to consider their obligations humanely. In the postmodern age, when we know to be skeptical of the 'objective' and 'disengaged' position, we must create a language for those dramas that is larger than the language of law and the courts alone. The inevitability of shared suffering requires the expert consultant to engage the sorrow and grief of the participants. Moral process in forensic psychiatry, unlike legal process alone, requires a professional integrity that is robust, humane, and resistant to forces that would overly restrict professional behavior.

This approach broadens moral agency in forensic work. As physicians called to these tasks, is it justifiable to be merely agents of the court carrying out a technical procedure? The tension between different professional roles, the blurring of the proper uses of medical knowledge (i.e., therapeutic versus forensic), and the tension between the professional's personal morality and professional role are evident here. However, without the humanistic language of narrative to clarify moral ambiguity, the language of the courts alone trumps our attempt to improve participation in the larger moral context.

In the narrative tradition, in which all medical and legal dramas are viewed from the perspective of characters in a play, the process itself is moral agency. The participants cocreate a moral tale, and in their shared decisions, in their dialogue and actions, develop a moral outcome. Ms. George's decision and its effects involve difficulties from which legal and medical language cannot protect the participants. The particulars of human struggle and suffering should be the origin of the ethics analysis of this case. How did the forensic expert struggle with his engagement at the bedside and in the court? How did his personal values and private feelings come into play? How did personal and professional ideals inform the conduct of the forensic evaluation? Clearly, the consultant is pulled toward a 'therapeutic relationship' while performing an 'expert role.' But the arbitrary division of functions – an expert in one place, a clinician in another, a complete person at home – although desirable in a theoretical sense, is not consistent with the particulars of human drama and the manner in which most of us experience our lives. Such an approach fails to capture the richness of our experience.

Conclusion

In the case of Ms. George, the complete consultation ultimately did include elements of counseling, education, conflict resolution, and referral for spiritual guidance. Although it is plausible that a forensic-therapeutic split could be conducted humanely, the consultant did not include another outsider in the emotionally charged and time-pressured setting. The consultant's own Eastern Orthodox upbringing served to penetrate and resolve cultural tensions between immigrant parents and their American-born daughter. Ms. George's narrative was explored to clarify the motivations to refuse treatment and her family's resistance to her choice. With her family's reluctant support and the court's acquiescence, Ms. George died quietly and comfortably some 10 days into her fast.

The case of Ms. George illustrates the need for a richer method to examine the ethics dilemmas that naturally arise in complicated forensic cases. A view of professional integrity that includes personal and traditional physicianly values and that is contextualized by narrative argues for a new approach toward cases such as this. Not only are new professional obligations and responsibilities elucidated, but also aspirations toward professional ideals are supported and encouraged.

Although the strict view of the forensic role attempts to prevent harm to evaluees and patients, role dilemmas also can be intimate moments when the professional's moral and clinical capacities are joined. The movement toward creative thought, discernment, and judgment shapes this moment. Consequently, for the practitioner who aspires to professional ideals, the robust view of role responsibility is an opportunity to balance the needs of the individual and society and derive greater meaning from the work.

References

1   Weinstock R, Leong GB, Silva JA: The role of traditional medical ethics in forensic psychiatry, in *Ethical Practice in Psychiatry and the Law*. Edited by Rosner R, Weinstock R. New York: Plenum Press, 1990.

2   Foot P: Ethics and the death penalty: participation by forensic psychiatrists in capital trials, in *Ethical Practice in Psychiatry and the Law*. Edited by Rosner R, Weinstock R. New York: Plenum Press, 1990.

3   Appelbaum PS: A theory of ethics for forensic psychiatry. *J Am Acad Psychiatry Law* 25:233–47, 1997.

4   Griffith EEH: Ethics in forensic psychiatry: a cultural response to Stone and Appelbaum. *J Am Acad Psychiatry Law* 26:171–84, 1998.

5   Appelbaum PS: The parable of the forensic psychiatrist: ethics and the problem of doing harm. *Int J Law Psychiatry* 13:249–59, 1990.

6   Candilis P, Appelbaum PS: Role responsibilities in the conflict of clinic and courtroom. *Ethics and Behavior* 7:382–5, 1997.

7   Stone AA: Ethical boundaries of forensic psychiatry: a view from the ivory tower. *Bull Am Acad Psychiatry Law* 12:209–19, 1984.

8   Ciccone JR, Clements CD: The ethical practice of forensic psychiatry: a view from the trenches. *Bull Am Acad Psychiatry Law* 12:263–77, 1984.

9   Shuman DW, Greenberg S, Heilbrun K, Foote WE: An immodest proposal: should treating mental health professionals be barred from testifying about their patients? *Behav Sci Law* 16:509–23, 1998.

10 Appelbaum PS: Ethics in evolution: the incompatibility of clinical and forensic functions. *Am J Psychiatry* 154:445–6, 1997.

11 Strasburger LH, Gutheil TG, Brodsky A: On wearing two hats: role conflict in serving as both psychotherapist and expert witness. *Am J Psychiatry* 154:448–56, 1997.

12 Hardimon MO: Role obligations. *The Journal of Philosophy* 91:333–63, 1994.

13 Miller FG, Brody H: Professional integrity and physician-assisted death. *Hastings Cent Rep* 25:8–17, 1995.

14 Luban D: *Lawyers and Justice: An Ethical Study*. Princeton, NJ: Princeton University Press, 1988, p. 142.

15 Beauchamp TL, Childress JF: *Principles of Medical Ethics* (ed 4). New York: Oxford University Press, 1994.

16 Pellegrino ED, Thomasma DC: *The Virtues in Medical Practice*. New York: Oxford University Press, 1993.

17 MacIntyre A: *After Virtue* (ed 2). Notre Dame, IN: University of Notre Dame Press, 1984.

18 Zaner RM: *Troubled Voices: Stories of Ethics and Illness*. Cleveland, OH: The Pilgrim Press, 1993.

19 Nelson HL (ed): *Stories and Their Limits: Narrative Approaches to Bioethics*. New York: Rutledge, 1997.

20 Katz J: *The Silent World of Doctor and Patient*. New York: The Free Press, A Division of Macmillan, Inc. 1984.

21 Meisel A, Kuczewski M: Legal and ethical myths about informed consent. *Arch Intern Med* 156:2521–6, 1996.

22 Sullivan MD, Youngner SJ: Depression, competence, and the right to refuse lifesaving medical treatment. *Am J Psychiatry* 151:971–8, 1994.

On Wearing Two Hats: Role Conflict in Serving as Both Psychotherapist and Expert Witness*

Larry H. Strasburger, Thomas G. Gutheil, and Archie Brodsky

Should psychotherapists serve as expert witnesses for their patients? Psychotherapists of all disciplines need to confront the potential clinical, legal, and ethical problems involved in combining the roles of treating clinician and forensic evaluator. As clinicians find themselves drawn into proliferating, often ambiguously defined contacts with the legal system, clarity in role definitions becomes crucial.

Definitions

The term 'therapist' refers to a clinician hired by the patient or the patient's family to provide psychotherapy; therapists treat 'patients' or 'clients.' A 'fact witness' testifies as to direct observations that he or she has made; a fact witness does not offer expert opinions or draw conclusions from the reports of others. Thus, a therapist who serves as a fact witness testifies as to observations of the patient during therapy and the immediate conclusions (such as diagnosis and prognosis) drawn from those observations. These conclusions are offered not as an opinion but simply as a report of what the therapist thought, did, and documented during therapy.

An 'expert witness' (who may also act as a forensic consultant) is a paid consultant who chooses to become involved in the case and is retained by an attorney, judge, or litigant to provide evaluation and testimony to aid the legal process. Unlike a fact witness, an expert may offer opinions about legal questions. This role typically involves participation in a trial. Forensic experts deal with 'examinees' or 'evaluees' rather than with patients or clients. They do not attempt to form a doctor-patient relationship with their subjects.

Common Scenarios

Several common scenarios may prompt a clinician to wear the two hats of treater and expert on behalf of the same person. A patient may have suffered a traumatic incident (such as a criminal assault or an automobile accident) during or before therapy, and litigation may ensue. A patient may become involved in child custody litigation. A referral may come from an attorney ostensibly seeking treatment for a client but actually seeking to document psychiatric damages or obtain favorable testimony in a custody dispute. An individual may be referred by an attorney to a single clinician for both treatment and forensic evaluation because the attorney is simply unaware of the incompatibility of these two procedures. Finally, there may be only one practitioner available to provide both psychotherapy and forensic services.

Role conflict may not be immediately apparent to attorneys, patients, or clinicians. Attorneys may believe that by enlisting the treating clinician as a forensic expert, they are making efficient use of the most knowledgeable source of information. After all, who is closer to the patient than his or her own therapist? Moreover, current ethical opinions of the American Medical Association state, 'If a patient who has a legal claim requests a physician's assistance, the physician should furnish medical evidence.'[1] The attorney may also want to save money: 'Why bring in a new person, who probably charges even higher fees than the treating psychotherapist, for an evaluation the therapist can easily perform?' The patient, too, may object to a separate forensic evaluation: 'Why must I repeat a painful story, and to someone I don't already know and trust?' The therapist, in the throes of countertransference[2] as well as anxious to spare the patient needless suffering, may readily endorse this reasoning. Clinicians who lack forensic training may think it natural to extend the mission of supporting the patient in therapy to advocating for the patient in court.

The Core Conflicts

It is prudent for clinicians to resist both the external pressures emanating from the attorney or patient or both and the internal pressures from the therapist's felt allegiance to the patient. The legal process is directed toward the resolution of disputes; psychotherapy pursues the medical goal of healing. Although these purposes need not always be antithetical and may even be congruent, the processes themselves typically create an irreconcilable role conflict.

In essence, treatment in psychotherapy is brought about through an empathic relationship that has no place in, and is unlikely to survive, the questioning and public reporting of a forensic evaluation. To assume either role in a particular case is to compromise one's capacity to fulfill the other. This role conflict, analyzed in detail later in this article, manifests itself in different conceptions of truth and causation, different forms of alliance, different types of assessment, and different ethical guidelines.[3] Therefore, although circumstances may make the assumption of the dual role necessary and/or unavoidable, the problems that surround this practice argue for its avoidance whenever possible.

Writing in 1984, Miller[4] noted that concern about this form of dual relationship 'has seldom appeared in the literature' (p. 826). Even now, it is remarkable how little critical attention this major ethical issue has received, even in articles and texts purporting to offer comprehensive expositions of the ethics of forensic practice.[5] A brief review of the professional literature shows the need for a more definitive analysis.

Historical Overview – A Slowly Emerging Issue

Role conflict has come to preoccupy the psychotherapeutic professions as the legal, economic, and social ramifications of their work have multiplied. An early expression of this concern was Stanton and Schwartz's exploration of the therapist-versus-administrator dilemma.[6] In the 1970s the term 'double agent,' both in psychotherapy[7] and in medicine,[8] came to signify the clinician's joint responsibilities to the patient and the state.

These early critiques, however, generally neglected to ask whether the evaluee's treating therapist is the right person to perform a forensic evaluation. Even in the early forensic psychiatric literature, clear linguistic distinctions between a forensic and a clinical examination[9] and between a

* Strasburger, L., Gutheil, T. and Brodsky, A.: On wearing two hats: role conflict in serving as both psychotherapist and expert witness. *American Journal of Psychiatry* 154:448–456, 1997.

forensic evaluee and a patient[10] were not always maintained. As late as 1987, a major textbook on forensic evaluation[11] did not directly address the treater-as-expert question.

An emerging emphasis on separating the clinical and legal roles was articulated in Stone's 1983 advice to therapists who learn that a patient may have been sexually abused by another therapist.[12] Stone recommended that the therapist discharge the ethical responsibilities of confidentiality and neutrality by engaging a consultant to pursue legal and administrative remedies on the patient's (and the public's) behalf. The following year, Halleck made the most explicit mention to date of the treater/expert role conflict in the literature on the double agent.[13] Since then, a few clear warnings about such role conflict have appeared in the literature of forensic psychiatry[14,15] and forensic psychology,[16] but these have been oases in a desert.

Ethics Codes

The problematic treater/expert relationship differs from the dual relationships commonly proscribed in ethics codes of professional organizations[17] in that it represents a conflict between two professional roles rather than between a professional and a nonprofessional one. This particular role conflict is addressed most directly by the American Academy of Psychiatry and the Law in its *Ethical Guidelines for the Practice of Forensic Psychiatry*:

A treating psychiatrist should generally avoid agreeing to be an expert witness or to perform an evaluation of his patient for legal purposes because a forensic evaluation usually requires that other people be interviewed and testimony may adversely affect the therapeutic relationship.[18]

Sound as they are, these guidelines not only lack detailed elaboration, but are unenforceable, since the American Academy of Psychiatry and the Law refers ethics complaints to APA, which has not adopted the Academy's ethical guidelines. APA has, however, issued a comparable position statement with respect to employment-related psychiatric examinations.[19]

For psychologists, the ethical boundary is less sharply drawn. The American Psychological Association's code of ethics[20] allows psychologists to serve simultaneously as consultant or expert and as fact witness in the same case, provided that they 'clarify role expectations' (p. 1610). Guidelines developed specifically for forensic psychologists by the American Psychology-Law Society and Division 41 of the American Psychological Association[21] address the 'potential conflicts of interest in dual relationships with parties to a legal proceeding' (p. 659). These guidelines, however, allow broader latitude than those of the American Academy of Psychiatry and the Law.

Surveys of Forensic Psychiatrists

Surveys of forensic psychiatrists' ethical concerns reveal a surprising lack of consensus on the treater/expert role conflict. In a 1986 survey of forensic psychiatrists who belonged to the American Academy of Forensic Sciences, two-thirds considered 'conflicting loyalties' a significant ethical issue, yet only three of 51 respondents specifically mentioned the treater/evaluator role conflict.[22] In 1989, with the ethical guidelines of the American Academy of Psychiatry and the Law recently in place, members of both the American Academy of Forensic Sciences and the American Academy of Psychiatry and the Law rated the treater/expert scenario least significant among 28 potential ethical problems listed.[23] (Only 14.5% of the members of the American Academy of Forensic Sciences perceived this situation to represent an ethical problem, while 71.0% did not.)

In 1991, among 12 controversial ethical guidelines proposed for consideration, members of the American Academy of Psychiatry and the Law gave least support to extending the Academy's warning against performing forensic evaluations on current patients to include former patients as well.[24] The authors of the survey attributed this opposition, as well as continuing disagreement even about the impropriety of evaluating current patients, to a 'recognition of the dual treater-evaluator role sometimes being both necessary and appropriate' (p. 245). Thus, during the past decade, any increased scrutiny of this dual role has confronted the reasoning that 'multiple agency and a balancing of values have become a necessary part of all current psychiatric practice, not only for forensic psychiatry' (p. 246).

Contexts and Complications

The resistance of highly trained specialists to such an ethical principle becomes understandable when set against the changing landscape of psychotherapy. Limited reimbursements are making extended psychodynamic exploration a luxury. Moreover, with many patients' problems being seen as manifestations of extrapsychic (environmental, institutional, economic, legal, or political) conditions, the therapist is becoming a social worker, mobilizing resources on the patient's behalf; a gatekeeper, unlocking the doors of managed care; a detective, obtaining useful information; or an agent of social control, protecting others from the patient. The therapist, thus placed in an advocate's or case manager's role, is expected to influence external outcomes rather than simply accompany the patient on an inner exploration.

Mental health services today are commonly delivered in public institutions (such as state hospitals and prisons) where therapists are accountable to society as well as to the patient. In these settings confidentiality may be breached from the outset, and therapy often has a built-in forensic component. Even private psychotherapy takes on a forensic dimension in the case of reportable offenses or threats to third parties. To some degree, then, the treater/expert role conflict has become incorporated into the therapist's job description. 'Pure,' disinterested psychotherapy is compromised as legal, economic, and social responsibilities multiply and fewer clinicians really practice independently. More and more, the therapist is working for institutions, corporations, and society.

Given these conditions, rigorous separation of the treater and evaluator roles in public practice has been called unworkable and even inadvisable.[25] Nonetheless, a strong reaffirmation of role clarity is still called for, especially in light of an epidemic of aggressive legal advocacy by therapists. The proliferation of cases of 'recovered memory,' for instance, with their dubious methodologies and controversial outcomes, shows that some therapists are losing sight of the essential distinction between subjective experience and historical reconstruction.[26] These therapists, perhaps driven by unexamined countertransference,[2] step out of role when they urge their patients to take court issues that might better be resolved in therapy.

For didactic clarity, the following discussion is cast in the language of traditional psychotherapy. Nonetheless, it applies to many forms of psychiatric and psychological treatment, including psychopharmacological, behavioral, and cognitive therapies. Since questions of trust, rapport, and confidentiality enter into all clinical treatment, the evaluator's role of gathering and reporting information from multiple sources external to the dyad is always in conflict with the treater's role.

Truth and Causation

Clinical and forensic undertakings are dissimilar in that they are directed at different (although overlapping) realities, which they seek to understand in correspondingly different ways.

Psychic Reality Versus Objective Reality

The process of psychotherapy is a search for meaning more than for facts. In other words, it may be conceived of more as a search for narrative truth (a term now in common use) than for historical truth.[27] Whereas the forensic examiner is skeptical, questioning even plausible assertions for purposes of evaluation,[28] the therapist may be deliberately credulous, provisionally 'believing' even implausible assertions for therapeutic purposes. The therapist accepts the patient's narrative as representing an inner, personal reality, albeit colored by biases and misperceptions. This narrative is not expected to be a veridical history; rather, the therapist strives to see the world 'through the patient's eyes.' Personal mythologies are reviewed, constructed, and remodeled as an individual reflects on himself or herself and his or her functioning.

Although the therapist withholds judgment and does not rush to reach (let alone impose) a conclusion, the ultimate goal is to guide the patient to a more objective understanding. Nonetheless, the achievement of insight, one of the principal goals of psychotherapy, is not a fact-finding mission and cannot be reliably audited by an external source. What emerges with insight often cannot be objectively corroborated, confirmed, or validated so as to meet legal standards of proof.

One possible consequence of the clinician's tactical suspension of disbelief in the patient's subjective reality is that a plaintiff's psychotherapist may fail to diagnose malingering.[29] If the patient's agenda, conscious or unconscious or both, includes building a record for future court testimony, a psychotherapeutic goal will not be achieved, whether or not the therapist eventually testifies. Distortions of emphasis and a withholding of information, affect, and associations will likely compromise both the therapy and the testimony. Therefore, in cases that may have legal ramifications, the limits of the therapist's role with respect to forensic evaluations and court testimony should be made clear as part of the treatment contract. Of course, the therapist cannot always anticipate the litigable issues that may emerge in therapy or assume that an initial disclaimer will dispose of the patient's unconscious agendas.

Descriptive Versus Dynamic Approach

Whereas the treating clinician looks out from within, the forensic expert, who must adhere to an ethical standard of objectivity,[18] looks in from outside. Thus, whereas the treater might appropriately take a psychodynamic perspective, with its emphasis on conflict and the role of the unconscious, the forensic evaluator's view is more likely to be a descriptive one. The objective/descriptive approach to psychiatry, with its emphasis on classification and reliable diagnosis, tends to be favored by forensic practitioners because the law is interested in categorization. Diagnosis A may be compensable or potentially exculpatory, while diagnosis B may not be.

This is not to say that the stereotypical forensic psychiatrist, who reconstructs an individual's inner world (if at all) only from tangible (e.g., crime scene) evidence, is truly representative of this specialty. It may well be that forensic psychiatry is best practiced by those who can immerse themselves in the evaluee's inner world and then exit that world with useful observations and testable hypotheses in a search for corroboration or lack of corroboration. For the most part, however, the law sees human beings as operating consciously, rationally, and deliberately.[30] Although it allows for mental state defenses and gives selective attention to particular dynamic mechanisms, such as transference in sexual misconduct litigation,[31] the law has little interest in the unconscious.

On the other side of the coin, although a therapist may have a high degree of confidence in a patient's clinical diagnosis, this determination is not to be confused with the forensic evaluator's effort to document an accurate historical reconstruction. A therapist must tolerate ambiguity to such a degree as to be often unable to answer a legal question with the 'reasonable degree of medical certainty'[32] required of an expert opinion. To say, 'I am reasonably certain that this person is presenting with posttraumatic stress disorder,' is not to say, 'It is my opinion, to a reasonable degree of medical certainty, that the trauma was caused by the sexual abuse she says she suffered at her father's hands.' Equating these two statements is a damaging mistake that clinicians unfamiliar with the courts often make when they move into the legal arena.

The Nature of the Alliance

The clinical and forensic situations differ with respect to the nature and purpose of the relationships formed within them. Involvement in litigation inevitably affects the empathy, neutrality, and anonymity of the clinician.

Psychological Versus Social Purpose

Like the psychotherapist and patient, the forensic evaluator and evaluee jointly undertake a task. But the two tasks are not the same. In treatment,

the purpose of the alliance is the psychological one of benefiting the patient by promoting healing and enlarging the sphere of personal awareness, responsibility, choice, and self-care. In the forensic context the purpose is the social one of benefiting society by promoting fair dispute resolution through the adversarial legal system. At its best, the forensic psychiatric evaluation has been characterized as sharing some qualities of a working alliance but only for the limited purpose of conducting the evaluation.[28]

Because amelioration through civil law usually takes the form of financial compensation, the contrast between the two alliances is, in one sense, that of making whole psychologically versus making whole economically. These separate restitutions only sometimes overlap. The respective outcomes may also be thought of as insight versus justice, as changing primarily the internal world rather than the external world. In the course of a therapeutic alliance the patient must often accept personal responsibility as a condition of change. This contrasts strongly with the plaintiff's quest to assign responsibility to others in order to achieve recompense, cost sharing, or equity-as well as vindication. In therapy, the patient frequently must learn to understand and forgive; these considerations are largely irrelevant to the forensic evaluee and antithetical to the retributive thrust of litigation.

In building a treatment alliance the psychotherapist attempts to ally with that part of the patient that seeks to change, to give up psychopathological symptoms, and to resume or develop healthy adaptations.[33] The perspective is future oriented; troubles should be ameliorated for a better, happier life. Entitlements may have to be discarded so that one can cope with everyday existence. One must accept that life is hard and often unjust and assume responsibility for one's role.

The forensic evaluator, on the other hand, may be allied with (or else opposed to) that part of the evaluee which seeks concrete redress for injury, exculpation from responsibility, or avoidance of responsibility through a finding of incompetence. The evaluator's approach may emphasize psychopathology, in contrast to the normalizing approach of the psychotherapist. The attention paid to a psychopathological slice of past life, without any hope-giving search for renewal and remediation, may foster a depressive rather than an encouraging outlook.

People often bring legal action in the belief that it will be therapeutic and empowering. Sometimes it is, but it can also be traumatic. Moreover, the sense of entitlement fostered by an unremitting quest for justice tends to harden characterological defenses, thereby making constructive change more elusive. In such cases, litigation may be said to bring about a developmental arrest or regression antithetical to therapeutic growth. Given such risks, the proper role of a treating therapist is not to encourage a lawsuit or to be the patient's legal advocate. Rather, it is to assist the patient in deciding whether or not to bring suit and to provide support in going through the legal process, if that be the decision. The therapist ought to stand at the same distance from the lawsuit as from any other significant event in the patient's life.

Empathy

Empathy, when used as a therapeutic technique, enables the patient to feel understood and facilitates the achievement of insight. Contrary to stereotype, empathy is not necessarily absent from the forensic evaluation, since a skilled evaluator creates an atmosphere in which the evaluee feels free to speak within the limits set by the absence of confidentiality.[28] However, even the legitimate use of empathy can lead to a quasitherapeutic interaction that ultimately leaves the evaluee feeling betrayed by the evaluator's report.[34]

The clinician's habit of empathic identification, if not balanced by objectivity, can bias a forensic evaluation even in the absence of a treating relationship. Stone[35] argues, therefore, that forensic evaluators must be prepared to withdraw from the forensic role when a forensic evaluation turns into a therapeutic encounter. How much greater, then, the likelihood of bias in the case of a treating therapist, whose mission of promoting patient welfare calls for deliberate identification (at the risk of overidentification) with the patient.

Neutrality

Therapeutic neutrality[36] – that posture of helping the patient listen to himself or herself without critical judgment, and fostering self-knowledge through the emergence of hidden feelings and attitudes – is undermined when the clinician acts as a forensic consultant to the patient or attorney; judgmental assessments are inevitable in that role, and serious real – world consequences may turn on every utterance of the patient. The crucial therapeutic posture of expectant listener, to whom anything may be said without consequence or penalty, is compromised. Free access to the patient's inner world is impeded as each disclosure is weighed, not just against 'What will she [or he] think of me?' but also 'How will what I say affect the outcome of my case?' Neutrality vanishes as the therapist assumes the consultant's role of advocacy for an opinion supporting the patient's cause,[37] a role assumed in the U.S. Supreme Court's Ake decision.[38] Both patient's and therapist's rescue fantasies are activated, with their potential for idealization of the therapist and regression and infantilization of the patient. Patient autonomy and responsibility correspondingly diminish.

Anonymity

The anonymity of the psychotherapist, which aids in the development and interpretation of transference[39] and the mobilization of clinically useful projections onto the therapist, is clearly compromised by the legal process. Such anonymity, which may be a key to the residual attitudes of the patient's relationships with important figures in his or her past, is contaminated when the therapist steps out of the transference relationship and into the patient's present, external world. The patient who sees his or her therapist on the witness stand may have strong reactions, not only to the testimony itself, but to whatever is exposed about the clinician's professional background, character, or personal history. Problems also arise if the patient sees the therapist embarrassed by a vigorous and effective cross-examination. Will confidence and trust not be diminished by fears of the therapist's vulnerability?

Assessments

Further incompatibilities between the roles of treater and expert become apparent when we consider how each obtains, evaluates, and interprets information. A clinical assessment is not the same as a forensic assessment.

Evidence Gathering and the Use of Collateral Sources

Therapeutic assessments tend to rely much less on collateral sources of information than do forensic evaluations. While spouses and other family members may be interviewed (with the patient's permission) as part of a clinical assessment – particularly for hospitalized or substance – abusing patients – a forensic evaluation routinely requires meticulous examination of multiple sources of information, such as medical, insurance, school, and occupational records, as well as interviews with family members, co-workers, employers, friends, police officers, and eyewitnesses. Such far-ranging scrutiny by a psychotherapist, especially in outpatient treatment, would be highly unusual. Indeed, were a therapist to seek external 'truth' so diligently, the patient might well exclaim, 'Doctor, don't you believe me?'

In practice, forensic assessments may also include observing the evaluee in the home, the workplace, the courtroom, and other nonclinical settings. Except in some types of couple or family therapy, comparable behavior by a psychotherapist would likely be perceived by the patient as highly intrusive (and hence destructive of confidence and trust) or as a therapeutic boundary violation.[40]

Interview Strategies

Psychotherapists and forensic psychiatrists approach their patients/evaluees with divergent interviewing strategies. The forensic psychiatrist begins with an explicit legal question to be answered by marshalling relevant psychiatric data.[41] For the psychotherapist this external question would be a distraction from the patient's inner world and therapeutic goals. Moreover, the direct probing necessary for forensic evaluation is inconsistent with the 'evenly hovering attention'[42] (pp. 111–112) of the dynamic psychiatrist. Using an open-ended approach, the psychotherapist starts with the problem as perceived by the patient and proceeds to collect an associative anamnesis[43] intended to yield a dynamic understanding of the issues. The language of the therapist deliberately emulates that of the patient, who is encouraged to tell his or her own story in his or her own way.

In contrast, the forensic evaluator's gaining informed consent to the interview opens with a defining statement of purpose. While the forensic examiner's initial inquiries may be phrased open-endedly to encourage the interviewee's participation, the questioning becomes increasingly structured in keeping with implicit legal standards, if not the actual statutory issue and vocabulary. (In some jurisdictions, such as New York, the evaluee is permitted to have a lawyer present, giving the interview the cast of a legal deposition rather than a clinical interview.) If such an examination is undertaken by the treating psychotherapist, it may well be experienced by the patient as a failure of empathy.

Psychological Defenses

Psychotherapy, the 'talking cure,' requires that thoughts and feelings be put into words in order to effect change. While enactments of various past and present conflicts inevitably occur and, indeed, are often instructive when they can be explored, verbal communication is the mode of choice. In any psychotherapy, resistances and defenses may impede the work. Litigation tends to enhance these defensive maneuvers: it may provide a defense against experiencing affect or a distraction from considering meaningful aspects of the past. Thus, a therapist who is drawn into a patient's litigation is participating in an enactment or acting out.

Time

Time limitations also differentiate forensic from treatment evaluations, except for certain deliberately short-term therapeutic techniques. A sense of urgency and a need to move toward closure, while characteristic of managed care settings, are not inherent to traditional psychotherapy. Except in an emergency, the treating psychiatrist usually has some leeway to wait for material to emerge in its own time or to wait to intervene until the moment is right. The intrinsic schedule is that of the patient, not that of the court. The forensic specialist usually does not have this luxury. 'Having one's day in court' requires respect for deadlines and inevitably leads to temporal closure, whether or not clinical end points have been reached.

Ethical Guidelines

Problems occur when the ethic of healing (doing 'individual good') collides with the ethic of objectively serving the legal system (doing 'social good'). The following are some of the ethical dilemmas that arise when one attempts to serve one client in two arenas.

'First, Do No Harm'

The ethical dictum of primum non nocere, by which treating physicians are bound, does not apply directly in the courtroom.[44] An evaluee may suffer substantial harm from a forensic expert's testimony, not only through lost self-esteem, financial loss, or deprivation of liberty, but even through loss of life in capital sentencing. Moreover, the damage done by inadequate or ineffective testimony resulting from a therapist's incomplete understanding of the legal system may be financially as well as emotionally costly.[45] Even when the testifying expert is a qualified forensic specialist, the experience of hearing one's intimate life revealed and analyzed in court may be exceedingly traumatic.[46]

Mossman[47] opines that honest forensic evaluations and testimony, even when they do immediate harm to individuals, confer long-range benefits on all concerned (including those adversely affected) by up-holding the fairness of the justice system. Nonetheless, that way of doing good is not part of the treating physician's role. A person who suffers harm from adverse or painful testimony should not suffer the additional pain of having that testimony emerge from a doctor-patient relationship.

Reimbursement

Another ethical issue arises when the psychotherapist goes to court. If a prognosis is offered that a patient will require long-term treatment, the therapist, as treater, stands to benefit directly from this statement.[29] This financial stake in the outcome may destroy the credibility of the therapist's testimony. It places the therapist in the position of testifying for a built-in contingency fee, which is unethical for forensic psychiatrists[18] and forensic psychologists[21] – and, by extension, for treaters who testify.

Agency

Clear disclosure of whose 'agent' one serves as – i.e., whom one is working for – is required in both the clinical and forensic arenas. Barring an emergency, including danger to others or 'public peril,' a therapist works only for the patient. Such an 'agency statement' is usually implicit in a contract between psychiatrist and patient for individual psychotherapy.[33] In the forensic context, however, the combined therapist/expert witness must serve two masters, the patient/examinee and the law. When the therapist thus blurs his or her role, the patient's claim to sole allegiance is compromised.

The biasing effect of agency on forensic evaluations, a matter of concern to forensic specialists,[48] is called forensic identification – a process by which evaluators unintentionally adopt the viewpoint of the attorneys who have retained them.[49] If agency biases forensic opinion, agency conflict, or double agency, must influence both the evaluator (therapist) and evaluee (patient).

Confidentiality

The question of confidentiality goes hand in hand with that of agency. Who is listening? What will be revealed and where? The privacy of the consulting room, protected by law, is essential to frank communication during which a patient suspends self-judgment. In its Jaffee v. Redmond decision in 1996,[50] the U.S. Supreme Court gave unequivocal protection to the confidentiality of the psychotherapeutic relationship. Given the Court's reaffirmation of the primacy of therapeutic confidentiality, over and above other vital interests of society, clinicians would be unwise to compromise this right by carelessly crossing the boundary into the forensic arena.

A patient who puts his or her mental condition at legal issue and thereby waives privilege loses that privacy. Although the patient may consent to breaching privacy for the purpose of litigation, the prior confidential relationship may be incapable of being restored after the litigation is over. Moreover, the patient's consent to reveal treatment records may not constitute informed consent to full disclosure in court to family members, the press, or curious bystanders.[46] A warning that the adversarial discovery process may reveal closely held personal details may not address the full extent of the exposure that occurs and its emotional consequences.

These hazards of litigation are present whether or not the therapist actually testifies. If the therapist agrees to act as a forensic evaluator, the hazards intensify. While a treating therapist may sometimes successfully appeal to exclude intimate material because of its irrelevance, the forensic evaluator is less likely to be able to withhold anything learned in the course of an evaluation.

Risks for the Clinician who acts in a Dual Role

At a time when forensic experts have been held liable for negligence in evaluation,[51] the therapist who attempts to combine the roles of treating clinician and forensic evaluator embarks on especially treacherous waters. Even a clinician who testifies as a fact witness may find this seemingly unambiguous role compromised.[50] In court, the fact witness may face pressure to give an expert opinion without receiving an expert witness's fee.[52] Worse, a therapist whose factual testimony displeases the patient may later be charged with negligence for having failed to carry out the investigatory tasks of a forensic expert.[53]

These problems are best avoided by offering the patient's treatment records in lieu of testimony. The clinician who does testify as a fact witness should rigorously maintain role boundaries by declining to perform the functions of an expert witness, such as reviewing the reports or depositions of other witnesses. A therapist who is asked to give expert testimony about a patient can respond to an attorney's request, a subpoena, or (at last resort) courtroom questioning with a disclaimer such as this: 'Having observed the patient only from the vantage point of a treating clinician, I have no objective basis for rendering an expert opinion, with a reasonable degree of medical certainty, on a legal as opposed to a clinical question.'

Caveats

1 *Ruling out this form of dual relationship is not meant to limit the expert role to a small group of specialists.* Any professional can serve as an expert witness within the limits of his or her expertise. A psychiatrist without specialized credentials in forensic psychiatry can still perform evaluations and testify as an expert in psychiatry.

2 *Separating the roles of treater and expert implies no denigration of clinical expertise.* 'Expert witness' is a legal term that describes the particular role a person plays in the legal process. To insist that the role of an expert witness is incompatible with that of a treating clinician is not to imply that clinicians are any less expert in their own realm.

3 *Treating clinicians do have legitimate roles in legal proceedings.* Treating clinicians properly participate in certain legal determinations as part of their clinical responsibilities. For example, the assessment of competence to give informed consent to treatment is inherently part of the clinical interchange. Similarly, the clinician who petitions a court for involuntary commitment of a patient usually testifies as a fact witness – an involved party, a partisan for safety and patient health – about his or her observations of the patient during therapy. There is, however, an inherent ambiguity in this role in that legal conclusions are being reached on the basis of the testimony. Although the clinician's temporary assumption of an oppositional role in court for the patient's benefit may strain the therapeutic alliance, inpatient treatment can restore the patient's insight, so that the patient comes to understand why hospitalization was necessary and the treatment alliance can resume.

4 *Sometimes the dual role is unavoidable.* Institutional policies increasingly force clinicians to wear two hats with the same patient. Similarly, in commitment hearings and disability determinations the clinician may be drawn into a quasi-expert role. Geography can also be a limiting factor; in a small town or rural area there may be only one practitioner available with the requisite credentials to perform a forensic evaluation.[54] Even in less than ideal circumstances, however, one should be vigilant to avoid compromising one's role, especially through unnecessary breaches of confidentiality.[50]

Conclusions

The psychotherapist's wish to help the patient too often carries over into more direct, active forms of 'helping' that (however well-motivated) are contrary to the therapeutic mission. In particular, a therapist's venturing into forensic terrain may be understood as a boundary violation that can compromise therapy as surely and as fatally as other, more patently unethical transgressions. For the numerous reasons detailed previously, such dual agency is unsound and potentially damaging both to the evaluee/patient and to the evaluator/clinician. As the psychotherapist's role boundaries widen, there is a proportional increase in the intensity of ethical conflict and legal liability. Notwithstanding the growing pressures from the complex clinical/legal marketplace to perform simultaneously in multiple roles, two heads are better than one only if they really are two distinct heads, each wearing its own hat.

References

1   American Medical Association, Council on Ethical and Judicial Affairs: Code of Medical Ethics: *Current Opinions With Annotations*. Chicago, AMA, 1994, p 138.

2   Long BL: Psychiatric diagnoses in sexual harassment cases. *Bull Am Acad Psychiatry Law* 1994; **22**:195–203.

3   Hundert EM: Competing medical and legal ethical values: balancing problems of the forensic psychiatrist, in *Ethical Practice in Psychiatry and the Law*. Edited by Rosner R, Weinstock R, New York, Plenum, 1990, pp 53–72.

4   Miller RD: The treating psychiatrist as forensic evaluator. *J Forensic Sci* 1984; **29**:825–830.

5   Golding SL: Mental health professionals and the courts: the ethics of expertise. *Int J Law Psychiatry* 1990; **13**:281–307.

6   Stanton A, Schwartz M: *The Mental Hospital*. New York, Basic Books, 1954.

7   Gaylin W: In the Service of the State: *The Psychiatrist as Double Agent: Hastings Center Report Special Supplement*. New York, Institute of Society, Ethics and Life Sciences, 1978.

8   Lomas HD, Berman JD: Diagnosing for administrative purposes: some ethical problems. *Soc Sci Med* 1983; **17**:241–244.

9   Watson AS: On the preparation and use of psychiatric expert testimony: some suggestions in an ongoing controversy. *Bull Am Acad Psychiatry Law* 1978; **6**:226–246.

10 Rappeport JR: Differences between forensic and general psychiatry. *Am J Psychiatry* 1982; **139**:331–334.

11 Melton GB, Petrila J, Poythress NG, Slobogin C: *Psychological Evaluations for the Courts*. New York, Guilford Press, 1987.

12 Stone AA: Sexual misconduct by psychiatrists: the ethical and clinical dilemma of confidentiality. *Am J Psychiatry* 1983; **140**:195–197.

13 Halleck SL: The ethical dilemmas of forensic psychiatry: a utilitarian approach. *Bull Am Acad Psychiatry Law* 1984; **12**:279–288.

14 Group for the Advancement of Psychiatry, Committee on Psychiatry and Law: *The Mental Health Professional and the Legal System: Report 131*. New York, Brunner/Mazel, 1991.

15 Epstein RS: *Keeping Boundaries: Maintaining Safety and Integrity in the Psychotherapeutic Process*. Washington, DC, American Psychiatric Press, 1994.

16 Shapiro DL: *Forensic Psychological Assessment: An Integrative Approach*. Boston, Allyn & Bacon, 1991.

17 Rinella VJ, Gerstein AI: The development of dual relationships: power and professional responsibility. *Int J Law Psychiatry* 1994; **17**:225–237.

18 American Academy of Psychiatry and the Law: *Ethical Guidelines for the Practice of Forensic Psychiatry*. Bloomfield, Conn, AAPL, 1991.

19 American Psychiatric Association: Position statement on employment-related psychiatric examinations. *Am J Psychiatry* 1985; **142**:416.

20 American Psychological Association: Ethical principles of psychologists and code of conduct. *Am Psychol* 1992; **47**:1597–1611.

21 Committee on Ethical Guidelines for Forensic Psychologists: Specialty guidelines for forensic psychologists. *Law and Human Behavior* 1991; **15**:655–665.

22 Weinstock R: Ethical concerns expressed by forensic psychiatrists. *J Forensic Sci* 1986; **31**:596–602.

23 Weinstock R: Perceptions of ethical problems by forensic psychiatrists. *Bull Am Acad Psychiatry Law* 1989; **17**:189–202.

24 Weinstock R, Leong GG, Silva JA: Opinions by AAPL forensic psychiatrists on controversial ethical guidelines: a survey. *Bull Am Acad Psychiatry Law* 1991; **19**:237–248.

25 Miller RD: Ethical issues involved in the dual role of treater and evaluator, in *Ethical Practice in Psychiatry and the Law*. Edited by Rosner R, Weinstock R. New York, Plenum, 1990, pp. 129–150.

26 Gutheil TG: True or false memories of sexual abuse? a forensic psychiatric view. *Psychiatr Annals* 1993; **23**:527–531.

27 Spence DP: *Narrative Truth and Historical Truth: Meaning and Interpretation in Psychoanalysis*. New York, WW Norton, 1982.

28 Bursztajn HJ, Scherr AE, Brodsky A: The rebirth of forensic psychiatry in light of recent historical trends in criminal responsibility. *Psychiatr Clin North Am* 1994; **17**:611–635.

29 Simon RI: Toward the development of guidelines in the forensic psychiatric examination of posttraumatic stress disorder claimants, in *Posttraumatic Stress Disorder in Litigation: Guidelines for Forensic Assessment*. Edited by Simon RI. Washington, DC, American Psychiatric Press, 1995, pp. 31–84.

30 Morse SJ: Brain and blame. *Georgetown Law J* 1996; **84**:527–549.

31 Gutheil TG: Some ironies in psychiatric sexual misconduct litigation: editorial and critique. *Newsletter of the Am Acad Psychiatry and Law* 1992; **17**:56–59.

32 Rappeport JR: Reasonable medical certainty. *Bull Am Acad Psychiatry Law* 1985; **13**:5–16.

33 Gutheil TG, Havens LL: The therapeutic alliance: contemporary meanings and confusions. *Int Rev Psychoanal* 1979; **6**:467–481.

34 Shuman DW: The use of empathy in forensic examinations. *Ethics & Behavior* 1993; **3**:289–302.

35 Stone AA: Revisiting the parable: truth without consequences. *Int J Law Psychiatry* 1994; **17**:79–97.

36 Hoffer A: Toward a definition of psychoanalytic neutrality. *J Am Psychoanal Assoc* 1985; **33**:771–795.

37 Diamond BL: The fallacy of the impartial expert. *Arch Criminal Psychodynamics* 1959; **3**:221–236.

38 Ake v Oklahoma, 105 S Ct 1087 (1985).

39 Freud S: Observations on transference – love: further recommendations on the technique of psycho-analysis, III (1915 [1914]), in *Complete Psychological Works*, standard ed, vol 12. London, Hogarth Press, 1958, pp. 157–173.

40 Gutheil TG, Gabbard GO: The concept of boundaries in clinical practice: theoretical and risk-management dimensions. *Am J Psychiatry* 1993; **150**:188–196.

41 Rosner R: A conceptual framework for forensic psychiatry, in *Principles and Practice of Forensic Psychiatry*. Edited by Rosner R. New York, Chapman & Hall, 1994, pp. 3–6.

42 Freud S: Recommendations to physicians practising psychoanalysis (1912), in *Complete Psychological Works*, standard ed, vol 12. London, Hogarth Press, 1958, pp. 109–120.

43 Deutsch F, Murphy WF: *The Clinical Interview, vol I: Diagnosis: A Method of Teaching Associative Exploration*. New York, International Universities Press, 1955.

44 Appelbaum PS: The parable of the forensic psychiatrist: ethics and the problem of doing harm. *Int J Law Psychiatry* 1990; **13**:249–259.

45 Carmichael v Carmichael, Washington, DC, Court of Appeals Number 89-1524.

46 Strasburger LH: 'Crudely, without any finesse': the defendant hears his psychiatric evaluation. *Bull Am Acad Psychiatry Law* 1987; **15**:229–233.

47 Mossman D: Is expert psychiatric testimony fundamentally immoral? *Int J Law Psychiatry* 1994; **17**:347–368.

48 Rogers R: Ethical dilemmas in forensic evaluations. *Behavioral Science and Law* 1987; **5**:149–160.

49 Zusman J, Simon J: Differences in repeated psychiatric examinations of litigants to a lawsuit. *Am J Psychiatry* 1983; **140**:1300–1304.

50 Jaffee v Redmond et al. 1996 WL 315841 (US).

51 Weinstock R, Garrick T: Is liability possible for forensic psychiatrists? *Bull Am Acad Psychiatry Law* 1995; **23**:183–193.

52 Brun v Bailey, Number CO11911, Court of Appeal of California, Third Appellate District. 27 Cal App 4th 641; 1994 Cal App LEXUS 833; 32 Cal Rptr 2d 624.

53 Althaus v Cohen and WPIC, Federal Civil Action Number 92-2435.

54 Boundary issues take on new meanings when you're the only psychiatrist around. *Psychiatric News*, Nov 17, 1995, p. 6.

Ethical Issues Involved in the Dual Role of Treater and Evaluator*

Robert D. Miller

Of all the medical specialties, psychiatry has the longest history of accepting the dual role of providing individual treatment to patients and providing expert opinions and management of persons perceived to be dangerous to society. For much of its history, the majority of psychiatrists in the United States were employed in prisons and public mental hospitals, where their major roles were perceived (at least by their employers) as serving the interests of the state in resolving criminal cases and protecting the public.[1,2] With the growth of academic psychiatry and the differentiation of private, individual psychotherapy from public psychiatry in the 1940s, an increasing number of psychiatrists have left the public sector for a more traditionally medical, autonomous private practice.[3,4]

As private and academic practitioners began to predominate within psychiatry, the ethical codes developed by their professional organization emphasized an individual psychotherapy approach to areas such as confidentiality.[5] Critics began to point out the ethical dilemmas involved in the public sector when psychiatrists practiced in a 'society-oriented' as opposed to a 'client-centered' mode.[6-9]

As the trend toward individual practice extended to the subspecialty of forensic psychiatry,[10] the modal forensic interaction also came to be conceptualized as a private evaluation done at the request of an attorney or judge. Since the great majority of such evaluations are undertaken voluntarily by private practitioners, the recent forensic Ethical Guidelines developed by the American Academy of Psychiatry and the Law[11] reflect that discontinuous relationship.[11] The Commentary to Guideline IV (Confidentiality) states:

A treating psychiatrist should generally avoid agreeing to be an expert witness or to perform an evaluation of his patient for legal purposes except in minor matters. The demands of a forensic evaluation may require that other people be interviewed and testimony can adversely affect the therapeutic relationship.

While such a blanket position may be appropriate for the majority of private evaluations, it does not adequately take into account the continuing exigencies of legitimate public practice, particularly in forensic hospitals which have the dual responsibility to evaluate and to treat patients; it creates a double standard of practice by ignoring clinical reality in a variety of public practice situations; and it does not deal with a number of particular issues which have arisen recently, such as duties to report a variety of patient behaviors considered to pose threats to society. This chapter will use the still embryonic professional ethical guidelines which are relevant to forensic practice to analyze the question of the potential for dual agency inherent in combining the treatment and evaluation roles from a number of aspects, and attempt to differentiate those situations in which treating psychiatrists should avoid providing expert testimony about their patients from those in which such activities are appropriate and even preferred. I will divide the issues into a series of dichotomies for greater simplicity of analysis, realizing that there is considerable overlap among the various categories.

* Miller, R.D.: Ethical issues involved in the dual role of treater and evaluator, in *Ethical practice in psychiatry and the law*, ed. R. Rosner and R. Weinstock. New York, Plenum Press, 1990, pp. 129–150.

Private Versus Public Practice

The majority of forensic psychiatrists practice in private or academic settings,[3,10,12] and thus professional ethical guidelines have reflected their practices and ideologies. There is a significant difference in the degree of autonomy characteristic of private versus public practice. Private practitioners, whether in individual, group, or academic practice settings, are essentially free to choose the type of services they provide, and the types of patients or agencies to whom they provide those services. They are therefore usually able to 'avoid agreeing to be an expert witness' if they choose to do so. In the case of evaluations requested concerning persons whom they are not already treating, private psychiatrists are of course free to decline, and the great majority of them do. Those who specialize in forensic practice may choose to accept such referrals, but they are free not to, and can thus ensure that they do not mix their roles as treaters and evaluators if they choose not to do so.

There are exceptions, of course, even for private practitioners. Patients who come for clinical psychotherapy may subsequently end up in court in a variety of situations, such as child custody conflicts or after alleging psychic trauma. In such situations, private psychotherapists may find themselves subpoenaed to testify as to their client's or former client's mental state at some past time. While some judges have held that the confidentiality of the psychotherapeutic relationship protects the clinician who declines to testify without his patient's consent,[13] most have ruled that the court's need for relevant evidence overrides confidentiality, and have compelled testimony under threat of contempt.[14,15] Presumably, psychiatrists who testify under court order would not be considered to have violated any official ethical principles, as all professional ethical codes provide exceptions for legally mandated duties. However, many therapists would still object strongly to such court orders, based on what Diamond[16] calls 'personal ethics,' a matter of individual conscience, as opposed to 'professional ethics,' that which an organized profession has determined to impose on all its members.

Clinicians in the public sector generally do not have the freedom of choice available to private practitioners, although their personal moral preferences may be the same. Clinicians employed at state forensic facilities in particular are usually required as part of their jobs to provide both treatment and evaluation for the same patients, and staffing rarely permits the luxury of separating the roles by having different staff perform them. Despite significantly greater variety in severity of criminal charges in which defendants' mental states are called into question than had previously been the case,[17] the majority of patients in forensic facilities are still charged with serious crimes, not 'minor matters,' and public employees thus are placed in a potentially greater bind by ethical prohibitions designed essentially for private practitioners who have choices to exercise. In addition, while the consequences of evaluation itself may be less severe in the case of 'minor matters,' the impact on the therapeutic relationship might be equally deleterious.

Economic factors also frequently differentiate the two practice settings. Because of the contingency fee system common in civil practice, there are stronger financial incentives for evaluators in civil cases to produce opinions useful to their referral sources than exist in criminal evaluations, the great majority of which are performed by salaried public practitioners.[18]

While it might be argued (and has been in the analogous case of the quality of care provided by state civil mental hospitals prior to the reforms of the 1970s[19]) that ethical clinicians should simply refuse to practice in such situations, such simplistic solutions avoid rather than address the issues. If the 'ethical' practitioners abandoned the public system, they might feel better as individuals, but the system would go on, and without the benefit of internal critics who are in the best position to effect what changes are possible.

While such arguments may appear to be merely utilitarian, or what Modlin[20] calls situational or marketplace ethics, they assume that the ethical prohibitions against the dual role are appropriate; as I shall argue subsequently, I believe that this is also a simplistic answer to the problem which ignores both reality and the potential benefits available when the same clinicians provide both evaluation and treatment.

Civil Versus Criminal Practice

The nature of the dual role of treater and evaluator also may differ, depending upon whether it exists within a criminal or civil framework. In many ways, the potential problems are fewer with criminal evaluations. First, the rights of criminal defendants are much more carefully spelled out in statutes and court decisions, and procedures for protecting those rights are correspondingly more explicit, than is the case with civil procedures.[21] Virtually all psychiatric evaluations of criminal defendants are prospective in the sense that the court orders a particular clinician or facility to perform an examination of the defendant's mental state as it relates to competency to perform a specified set of actions (such as to understand Miranda rights, to plea-bargain, or to proceed to trial), or as it relates to the defendant's mental state at the time of the alleged crime. The scope of the evaluation is thus somewhat limited, and thus easier both to perform and to explain to the subject. The distinction between treatment and evaluation is thus easier for both the clinician and the defendant to understand, and the potential for blurring the roles is thus reduced. In addition, the adversarial nature of the legal process is also more easily understood by criminal defendants than by civil litigants, and defendants are less likely to become confused about the role of the evaluator.

Civil evaluations typically involve more complex issues, such as psychic trauma or child custody, in which the issues to be considered more closely resemble those typical in more standard psychiatric evaluations, and thus pose a greater likelihood that the evaluatee will believe that the evaluator is operating in a traditional physician's role with a patient, despite any warnings given by the evaluator.

Thus, the parameters of the relationship with a criminal defendant are usually specified prior to the initial contact, permitting the clinician to inform the evaluatee at the outset of the nature of the evaluation (see Section 10, below). Although a clinician who has been treating a patient in conventional private psychotherapy occasionally becomes involved unexpectedly in a criminal case,[22,23] such involvement is quite unusual, and is much more frequent in civil cases.

There is some inevitable conceptual overlap with the previous dichotomy between private and public practice, since virtually all civil evaluations are performed privately,[12] while the majority of evaluations performed by forensic psychiatrists in the public system are criminal, either inpatient or outpatient. But the clearer adversarial framework and the more explicit procedural rules established by courts and legislatures for criminal evaluations make it easier to separate the roles of evaluator and treater in such situations.

On the other hand, the court-mandated treatment of forensic patients (both to restore competency to stand trial and after a finding of insanity) is almost invariably carried out in the public sector, often in forensic hospitals,[18,24] and thus frequently requires a combination of treatment and evaluation to be provided by the same clinicians.

Type of Treatment Involved

Psychotherapy

The major problem cited by critics of combining the roles of treater and evaluator is misrepresentation or betrayal of the confidentiality of the therapeutic relationship, with damage potentially accruing to the patient through the impact of the forensic opinion itself, as well as more generally damage to the ability of clinicians to provide effective treatment due to the destruction of the trust which is essential for psychotherapy.[7–9,25]

While these are certainly significant concerns, their impact is somewhat contextual, depending upon the nature of the therapy in question. There is no doubt that traditional long-term psychotherapy, both insight-oriented and supportive, requires considerable trust between patient and therapist. In such situations, it is clear that the role confusion and potential conflicts of interest involved in the dual role of treater and evaluator present serious difficulties.

Such conflicts are more frequent in the context of the treatment of forensic patients, chiefly because the possibilities of the therapist being called upon to provide expert testimony are more numerous. Some of these situations will be discussed in more detail below; but they typically involve predictions of future dangerousness based on information gained during therapy. While it is clear from the standpoint of society and its judicial representatives that treating therapists have the most comprehensive knowledge of their patients, and are therefore presumably in the best position to make accurate predictions, it is equally clear from the standpoint of the patient's treatment (which may be essential for the ultimate reduction of the dangerousness about which society is legitimately concerned) that patients cannot be expected to be appropriately self-disclosive if they have cause to fear that their revelations will be used against them by their therapists.[26]

In nonforensic treatment, while there is less risk of having to testify against one's patient, there is also less likelihood that the patient will have been informed of the possibility of such testimony at the beginning of therapy. In addition, the problem of overidentification with a patient who has been in treatment for some time might cause a therapist to err on the side of supporting a patient's wishes against professional judgment.[27] Another possible consequence of overinvolvement arises when patients are involved in civil litigation which could result in their receiving compensation which therapists consider both justified and necessary for them to regain control over their lives. Although a recent study indicates that there is little objective evidence to support the assertion that such situations significantly influence the course or outcome of therapy,[28] the danger exists in individual cases nevertheless.

Pharmacological Therapy

Although it has been argued that there is no evidence to support the assertion that psychotropic medication is effective when administered involuntarily,[29] most psychiatrists who have experience treating committed patients would probably agree that it is quite effective when used for appropriate clinical indications, whether the patient consents or not. It may be, therefore, that the conflicts introduced by the dual role may be less problematic with patients who require psychotropic medication, particularly antipsychotic medication, as an essential part of their treatment.[26] Since the majority of forensic patients in treatment under court orders suffer from major psychoses,[30,31] the problems inherent in the dual role may again be less with such patients, since their trust and cooperation is not as essential for the efficacy of psychopharmacological treatment.

It must be pointed out, however, that although medications can be administered without a patient's cooperation in inpatient facilities and in some outpatient settings, the establishment of trust in therapists is often essential over the long term to ensure that patients continue taking their medication once court jurisdiction is removed. The type of therapeutic alliance which may be jeopardized by the therapist acting as evaluator as well as treater may not even be possible with many acutely psychotic patients; but once the medication has exerted its maximum effects, if therapy is to extend beyond pharmacology, its efficacy will depend upon patients' confidence and trust in their therapists.

Therefore, even within the class of medication treatment of forensic patients, it will make a difference whether or not the therapy is to be long-term, with the goal of restoration of the capacity to return to relatively independent community living (such as in the treatment of insanity acquittees or sex offenders) or whether the treatment goals are more limited, as in the case of restoration of competency to stand trial. In the latter case, the assumption by the clinician of both roles may be less destructive, as no therapeutic relationship has been established, and the patient is unlikely to return to the same clinician for subsequent treatment. The problem of generalization from experience with one therapist to subsequent treatment remains, however.

The Order of Assumption of the Roles

The impact of combining treatment with evaluation frequently depends upon the order in which the roles are assumed. Most problematic is the situation in which an ongoing relationship has been established solely on a treatment basis and the therapist is unexpectedly required to provide an expert opinion concerning the patient. As mentioned previously, one such category of evaluations includes situation in which the patient's mental state becomes an issue in litigation, such as child custody or psychic trauma. Another category which has become prominent in the literature (if not in the courtroom) more recently is that of the protection of society from dangers posed by patients. This latter category will be addressed in more detail below.

When therapy is sought for purely clinical reasons, and the therapist's initial evaluation has not turned up any reason to suspect a subsequent need for expert testimony (such as previous dangerous behavior, a troubled marriage, or a recently accident allegedly resulting in emotional problems), there is little likelihood that the patient will have been warned at the beginning of therapy that the therapist might be called to testify about him or her, and the greatest potential danger to the therapeutic alliance exists.

In the forensic context, the order is often reversed, with evaluation for competency to stand trial or criminal responsibility preceding treatment. Since evaluations are (or *should* be) always preceded by explicit warnings of the purpose and potential outcomes of the evaluation, and given before a therapeutic alliance has formed, and often to patients whose severe mental disorders preclude the formation of such an alliance at that time, the damage in practice is often less.[26]

Wisconsin has recognized this distinction in its civil commitment statutes; the evaluation done within 3 days of admission and presented at the probable cause hearings are performed by hospital staff, while the subsequent evaluations for the final commitment hearings held within 14 days of admission are performed by evaluators independent of the hospital.[32]

There are problems, however, even when the evaluation role precedes treatment. Some patients will develop such a strong negative transference to the evaluating clinician that it will be impossible subsequently to establish an effective working relationship, even if the initial treatment (particularly with medications) is effective.

Another type of problem may arise if a clinician who initially evaluates a person privately for legal purposes subsequently assumes the role of treater. If the outcome of the legal procedure was unsatisfactory to the prospective patient, he or she may blame the evaluator, consciously or unconsciously, and be unable to develop an appropriate alliance during treatment. Even if the therapy itself proceeds effectively, the appearance of conflict of interests or 'ambulance-chasing' can pose significant ethical problems for the clinical professions, even if the patients in question do not object.[33]

Treaters as Decision Makers

An even more difficult ethical and therapeutic dilemma arises when clinicians are called upon not just to offer opinions to courts or other judicial decision makers, but to preside over hearings and actually make the decisions in question. Such roles exist almost exclusively in forensic contexts, and are less common than formerly, when courts officially deferred to clinical judgment much more often than is the case today. Nevertheless, they continue to exist in many jurisdictions in a variety of forms.

Obviously, the potential for damage to a therapeutic relationship is significantly increased when therapists serve as the final decision makers, rather than as advisers. Legislatures and regulatory bodies have recognized this problem, and have generally prohibited clinicians serving as decision makers from being directly involved in the patient's treatment.

Involuntary Civil Commitment

Examples of such roles include those jurisdictions in which clinicians have the statutory authority (and increasingly, the responsibility) to hospitalize patients involuntarily under civil commitment without a judicial hearing, such as California.[34] In such situations, the admitting clinicians are also often called upon to provide testimony at the initial judicial hearing, held within a few days of admission. Not only do such procedures create an even more adversarial relationship between therapists and patients then mere testimony, but the potential exists for greater destruction of therapeutic potency if the court overrules the clinician's original decision to hospitalize.

Sexual Psychopath Laws

A number of states created statutory schemes in the 1950s and 1960s to permit diversion of certain types of recidivist criminals into the mental health system. Called sexual psychopath or defective delinquent laws, they accepted current clinical thinking that treatment would both rehabilitate the criminals and provide greater protection for the public.[35] Since such schemes were conceived as therapeutic rather than as punitive, the decision-making power was often delegated to clinicians, an abdication which has been criticized by Halleck.[36] While the majority of such programs, and the statutes that established them, have been abolished, some remain.

In one such system, the Wisconsin Sex Crimes Law (which was repealed in terms of new commitments, but not in terms of continuing authority over those convicted prior to 1980) provides two release procedures. One is a modified parole board with an independent psychiatrist, a law professor, and a member of the state parole board. The other involves staff from the treating facility serving as hearing officers, and making their recommendations to the Secretary of the state Department of Health and Social Services.[37] While the regulations prohibit treating clinicians from serving as hearing officers, because patients are transferred between units in the Forensic Center, it is often difficult to find a hearing officer who has not had some treatment or administrative responsibility over the patient at some time. One patient went so far as to file a lawsuit over this very issue.[38]

When the hearing officer is not permitted to make autonomous decisions, but rather is instructed for policy reasons not even to recommend release, as has happened under the Wisconsin system,[36] the ethical problems go beyond the potential damage to individual therapeutic relationships, and place hearing officers in the position of appearing to apply clinical judgment when in reality they are totally agents of social control. The American Psychiatric Association Ethics Committee has issued an opinion that it is unethical for psychiatrists to participate in such hearings under such circumstances.[39]

Pacht and Halleck,[27] referring directly to the Wisconsin sex crimes procedures, also point out that the pressures on therapists to recommend release (and thus to adopt the usual therapist's role of supporting patients) is strong and makes it difficult to make an objective decision, particularly when the burden of proof lies on the patient to prove that he is no longer dangerous.

Right to Refuse Treatment

Although they have seldom been explicitly pointed out in the clinical literature, potential conflicts also exist when clinicians attempt to treat committed patients against their wills. Most states now recognize a qualified right for competent patients to refuse treatments such as psychosurgery, aversive conditioning, electroconvulsive therapy, and psychotropic medication.[40] All provide, however, mechanisms for challenging such refusals through determination of incompetency to make treatment decisions. While some states provide for full judicial hearings, most permit the decisions to be made by clinicians, either ones independent of the facility,[41] or even clinicians from the same facility as long as they are not directly involved with a patient's treatment.[42]

Although most clinicians who have written on the subject clearly prefer clinical to judicial decision making with respect to overriding patients' rights to refuse medication,[43] it has not previously been conceptualized as another example of the dual role of treater and evaluator. In all systems of determination of patients' competency to refuse treatment, treating clinicians serves as initial evaluators, and their recommendations are presented to the decision makers quite analogously to expert opinions in other types of legal decision making. In fact, that role is clearest in those jurisdictions with judicial determinations, since in most of those jurisdictions, in addition to the role as initial evaluator, treating psychiatrists are also appointed in effect as guardians for their patients who are found incompetent to make treatment decisions.

Explicit Duties to Warn or to Protect

The General Duty to Protect Third Parties

As if there were not enough problems with situations in which therapists are required to respond to requests for information and expert opinions about their patients, recent legal developments have established that therapists may also have duties to take action without waiting for requests. Because of the recently discovered 'special relationship' between therapists and patients,[44] society now looks upon therapists as protectors of the public from the behavior of patients in treatment, and, most recently, from other therapists. Although courts for many years have found therapists liable for acts committed by hospitalized patients,[45] the *Tarasoff* decision[44] and its progeny in other states have extended that responsibility to outpatient clinicians as well.[46-49]

The duty to release confidential information without patient consent to prevent danger to the public has been a part of the ethical codes of the American Psychiatric Association,[5] the American Psychological Association,[50] and the National Federation of Societies for Clinical Social Work[51] for some time, without any significant outcry in the professional literature. But once the courts and legislatures began to define the duty themselves and to hold therapists financially liable for its breach, therapists forget their own ethical codes and complain that externally mandated breaches of confidentiality are unethical and will surely lead to the extinction of psychotherapy as we know it.[46] Once again a double standard is applied; when private and academic practitioners find themselves held to the same standard which has applied to public and hospital-based practitioners for years, the cries of ethical dilemmas are suddenly heard in the land.

The Duty to Report Child Abuse

Another duty, which psychotherapists share with a number of other professionals, is that of reporting suspected child abuse. While this duty raised ethical questions when it was first created in every state in the 1960s, it has become generally accepted as necessary and effective in preventing further abuse. In the situation contemplated by the originators of such statutes, there is technically no duality, since the report is made concerning the child who is abused. Critics pointed out, however, that while the child might technically be the identified patient, the legally responsible persons were the parents, who were most likely to be the subject of the reports. It was argued that reporting suspected child abuse violated the rights of the parents, and also that the threat of reporting might prevent parents from bringing their injured children in for treatment, whether they had been abused or not.[52]

While those arguments have died out in the last decade as reporting has become accepted, there is a subset of cases which continue to raise troubling ethical problems. While most child abuse comes to light through examination of the injured children, it may also come to the attention of therapists who are treating the abusers themselves. It is thus similar to the more general duty to warn, with the significant difference that most statutes require reporting past abuse even when there is no danger of future abuse (such as when the children have already been removed from the parents, or in the case of child sexual molesters who have been removed from their victims by the courts and are in treatment in inpatient forensic facilities[53]).

In the case of the treatment of sex offenders, it is certainly possible to warn them at the outset of treatment that reports will have to be made of any child abuse they have caused for which they have not already been prosecuted, and most forensic facilities do so by policy.[53] But there remains the significant dilemma of encouraging patients to be appropriately self-disclosive in therapy while warning them at the same time that 'anything they say may be held against them.'

The Duty to Report Sexual Abuse by Previous Therapists

A growing number of states have created a newer duty, modeled after the established child abuse reporting statutes, under which psychotherapists are encouraged or required to report sexual abuse by previous therapists which is reported to them by their current patients.[54] The rationales of the two sets of statutes are similar, in that both attempt to prevent future abuse by removing the abuser from a situation in which further abuse can occur, although the second main purpose of child abuse reporting laws, to ensure treatment for the victims, is unnecessary in the case of sexually abused patients who are already in therapy.

The few statutes that have been enacted to date differ from each other in one important area: some, like the Minnesota statute,[55] can be interpreted to *require* therapists to report sexual abuse revealed during therapy, even without their patients' consent, or over their objections. Such statutes track child abuse reporting statutes, which are also mandatory rather than permissive, and obviously value prevention of future abuse over the rights of an already abused patient. The obvious dilemma created by such statutes is that they may require therapists to force a patient who has already been abused once to submit to the consequences of an investigation she or he may not be psychologically prepared to handle, and thus further complicate the course of therapy, particularly since she has not been abused by another therapist.[54]

By contrast, statutes such as that recently passed in Wisconsin,[56] are permissive in that they require therapists to obtain informed consent from their patients before making reports, even reports that omit the name of the alleged victim. While such procedures will perhaps be less effective in identifying abusers, they have the advantage of eliminating the ethical dilemmas posed by their mandatory counterparts.

Prosecution of Mental Patients

When persons with mental disorders that do not significantly impair their responsibility for their behaviors commit illegal acts while under the control of clinicians (as while involuntarily hospitalized), those clinicians may feel compelled to behave more like police than therapists.[57,58] Although therapists are not required by any statutes or regulations to report past criminal acts by their patients, there are times when it appears, for any of a number of reasons, that initiation of criminal prosecution is the most appropriate course of action for a therapist to take.

In some cases, prosecution is appropriate because the 'patient' has chosen to assume that role in preference to accepting appropriate and justified responsibility for his actions, and to permit him to hide behind the shield of a simulated mental disorder would be to grant him virtual carte blanche to commit crimes without consequences. By initiating criminal charges, the therapist not only refuses to condone the actions of a calculating criminal, but also opposes the type of blatant misuse of process which jeopardizes the chances of genuinely mentally disordered persons to avail themselves of the legitimate protections of the criminal law.

In other cases, the patient's mental disorder is genuine, but the therapist feels that it is necessary for treatment to progress that the patient accept responsibility for those of his actions over which he does in fact have control, including criminal ones. Bringing criminal charges (which in such cases are rarely carried through) may be clinically necessary in order to force the patient to accept that responsibility.

In the first type of situation, therapists may appear to be clearly violating their duties to their patients by initiating criminal charges; but I would argue[58] that when such 'patients' attempt to take advantage of the patient role for nontherapeutic purposes, they have relinquished any rights they may have had to benefit from the professional duties of therapists, and cannot expect the protections of therapeutic support and confidentiality available to those genuinely in need of such protections.

And in the latter case, prosecution (or the threat of prosecution) becomes an integral part of treatment itself, is done solely for the patient's benefit (as is clearly demonstrated by the reluctance of police and prosecutors to follow through on the criminal complaints), and thus is not a true example of dual agency, although patients may initially perceive it as such.

Advantages of Combining Treating and Evaluating

While the presence of legal duties to perform both roles, such as the *Tarasoff* duty, the duty to report abuse of children or patients, and the combined duties to evaluate and treat which exist in most state forensic facilities, might exempt clinicians from any legal professional consequences of combining the roles, that does not mean that the personal ethical dilemmas are also eliminated. There are, however, some situations in which I would argue that the same clinician serving both as treater and evaluator not only violates no ethical guidelines, personal *or* professional, but is actually more appropriate both for the patient and for society.[60]

Halleck[36] argues that the double-agent role may be beneficial in situations in which the state and the patients' overt interests coincide, and even when a patient initially disagrees with the results (such as is frequently the case in involuntary civil commitment). But he also points out that some patients may feel betrayed by the results of such interactions, and this distrust may generalize to future therapeutic relationships.

Unusual Clinical Conditions

One such situation is that in which the clinical condition is unusual, requiring special expertise to diagnose and to treat, particularly in the forensic context. Such conditions as posttraumatic stress disorder,[61] multiple personality disorder,[62] pathological gambling,[63] pathological intoxication,[64] and pedophilia[65] have perhaps been overrepresented in forensic populations since their acceptance in DSM-III,[66] and other proposed diagnoses, such as paraphiliac rapist, would also be likely to be utilized frequently in court if included in a future Manual.

There are several reasons why these diagnoses are increasingly found (or at least claimed) in forensic populations. By their very nature, persons with these disorders are more likely than those with most other disorders to commit criminal or tortious acts, and therefore many defense attorneys have become sufficiently knowledgeable about them to raise the issues when their clients appear to fit in one of the categories. Since experts on these conditions have generally argued that they are underdiagnosed in part because they are not suspected by general psychiatrists, attorneys represent another group with motive to suggest the presence of such conditions.

Because of the higher incidence of diagnosis (even if not actual occurrence) of these disorders in forensic populations, the clinicians assigned to evaluate and treat persons suffering from them have the opportunity to develop a level of expertise which is not readily available to the general psychiatrist.

Prediction of Future Behavior

A related justification for combining the roles of evaluator and treater is that the combination should be expected to improve clinicians' abilities to provide the courts with certain types of legally relevant predictive opinions. In what has become the most common situation, private evaluators make predictions about a variety of issues, including restoration of competency to stand trial, future dangerousness, and response to treatment, often without sufficient personal experience with the treatment of forensic patients to form the basis for accurate opinions.[10]

Continuity of Care

Another potential advantage of the combined role is that it can provide continuity of treatment for forensic patients, and help to integrate the legal and clinical facets of their experience. Strasburger[67] argues that it can be devastating for mentally disordered persons to hear the opinions derived from forensic evaluations for the first time in court, without the opportunity for the evaluators to explain them and to discuss them with the patients. I would certainly agree, and have pointed out[68,69] that the best solution to the dilemma is for evaluators to share their opinions and the reasons for their conclusions with those they have evaluated at the time of the evaluation. Strasburger[70] has pointed out that such discussions may not be possible in the case of private evaluations, particularly those performed at the request of opposing counsel, in which legal strategic reasons may prevent evaluators from disclosing their opinions to patients lest the information become available to opposing counsel. This reality provides another example of the advantages that can accrue when evaluations are performed in the context of an ongoing clinical as well as legal relationship, which is usually possible with inpatient evaluation and treatment, but often logistically or procedurally difficult with outpatient evaluations.

Also, in contrast to the more usual view that adversarial legal proceedings can disrupt a therapeutic alliance,[71] Ensminger and Liguori[72] have pointed out that the alliance may actually be strengthened by such proceedings (assuming that the court accepts the treating clinician's recommendations) when the patient realizes that an objective, independent decision maker reinforces the clinical position.

The Right to Refuse Treatment

The various legal and clinical issues surrounding the right to refuse treatment provide another example of the advantages of combining evaluation and treatment. Jurisdictions that have accepted the right have established various procedures for the determination of a patient's competency, several of which require evaluation and decisionmaking by independent clinicians.[43] But in all cases, it is clinically as well as legally important that those responsible for the patient's treatment plan provide the basic information concerning the need for the proposed treatment and the patient's capacity to understand the need for that treatment.[73] It would be difficult for independent evaluators in necessarily limited evaluations to determine patients' competency to make treatment decisions, and inappropriate for them to attempt to convince patients to accept such treatment, a necessary step in most procedures for determining patients' competency to refuse treatment.

Separation of Treatment from Evaluation

Despite the potential advantages of combining the roles discussed in the previous section, it is clear that in many situations there advantages in separating them. Some states have attempted to address the problem (although generally in response to perceived conflicts of interest, not out of concern for preservation of therapeutic alliances) by statutorily separating the roles, as Wisconsin has done in the case of civil commitment,[32] pretrial evaluations for criminal responsibility,[74] and evaluations for release from commitments following insanity acquittals.[74] Even if treaters are required to provide clinical information to decision makers, it may be possible to minimize the negative effects of such testimony by refraining from asking ultimate questions (such as whether the patient is ready for release).[27]

Such separation may also be established procedurally within a treatment facility. If it can be predicted from initial contacts that a forensic evaluation and resulting testimony will permanently disrupt a therapeutic alliance, it may be possible to assign an evaluating therapist different from the one who will ultimately provide treatment. Additionally, it may be possible to separate the administration of psychotropic medications and/or disciplinary functions, (typically the most contentious parts of treatment) from psychotherapeutic approaches by assigning different therapists to those roles. Such a separation may be particularly important if the patient suffers from a disorder which requires specific 1expertise both to evaluate and to treat (such as multiple personality disorder or certain types of sexual disorders).

Unfortunately, even such attempts to separate the roles may not be completely successful in achieving the desired results in terms of preservation of therapeutic alliances. Even if treating clinicians do not testify directly in legal proceedings, independent evaluators usually consult previous and current clinical records as part of their evaluations, so the supposed separation of treatment and evaluation, even where it is explicitly established, is seldom complete in practice. Patients will learn at their hearings that some of the information upon which the evaluator's opinion is based was derived from clinical records from his treaters, and the same problems will exist. And while avoidance of answering ultimate questions has been recommended on a variety of theoretical grounds,[27] even its most ardent supporters admit that in practice it is frequently impossible to present comprehensive clinical information without essentially answering ultimate questions in the process, even if only indirectly.[75] If such legal fictions do not deceive judges and juries, it is not surprising that they also fail to convince patients that their treating clinicians are not directly (and adversely) involved in the decision-making process.

Even if attempts at separation are made through using different clinicians for evaluation and treatment, patients, particularly if they have paranoid disorders, may still generalize from one clinician to all. It may therefore not be possible to separate the roles completely in practice; but such efforts as have been presented here are still effective in many cases, and should be attempted whenever ongoing therapeutic relationships have been established.

Warnings to Patients at the Beginning of a Relationship

Warnings at the Outset of a Forensic Evaluation

It might seem that explicitly informing patients at the outset of a formal evaluation for legal purposes might help to separate the roles of evaluator and treater. It is well established that clinicians evaluating criminal defendants have a legal[21] as well as an ethical[5,11] duty to inform those they evaluate of the purpose of the evaluation and the disposition of any report generated in advance of the evaluation.

Unfortunately, the distinction is often lost on patients in practice, for several reasons. First, as Halleck[36] points out, in order to inform the patient as to the purpose of the evaluation, the evaluator must understand it, and frequently does not, either because the referring source has not made the request sufficiently clear ('Evaluate Mr. X's mental state,' or 'Perform a psychiatric evaluation'), or because the evaluator is unfamiliar with the legal definitions of the conditions to be evaluated, and confuses the criteria for one evaluation with those for another.[76] In such situations, evaluators may end up testifying on issues different from those they explained to the patients they evaluated, as happened most notoriously in *Estelle v Smith*.[21]

Secondly, even if the request is exact, the evaluator understands it completely, and explains it carefully and accurately to the patient, it is clear from empirical studies of Miranda warnings in the criminal justice system[77,78] and similar warnings to patients facing civil commitment,[79] that few persons, either criminal defendants or mental patients, fully

understand what they are being told. There is even some evidence[79,80] that complete disclosure of the purposes of evaluation may even have the unintended and paradoxical effect of inducing the misapprehension in patients that they are in fact involved in a confidential treatment relationship rather than a legal evaluative one. Thus, while such warnings are absolutely required, both legally and on the basis of professional ethics, they may in practice be ineffective. Evaluators must therefore continue to monitor the evaluation process carefully, and to give additional warnings if they perceive patients to be disclosing information which appears to be counter to their expressed interests.

Third, evaluators can no longer necessarily assume that even private evaluations done at the request of the patient's attorney will be protected by the attorney-client privilege, particularly in criminal cases. Although the U.S. Supreme Court has held that criminal defendants with apparent mental disorders are entitled not only to expert evaluations of their competency to stand trial and criminal responsibility, but also expert consultation in the preparation of the defense case,[81] it has so far avoided ruling on the larger issue of discoverability by the prosecution of expert opinions provided to the defense. Because of the nationwide trend toward a retrenchment from individual rights and greater consideration for protection of the public, prosecutors are increasingly pressing for access to the results of evaluations done for the defense but not presented by the defense at trial (which would almost guarantee that the opinions generated would be supportive of the prosecution's case).[82] As they have been successful in some of their efforts, evaluators must be careful in the guarantees that they give patients being evaluated, and aware of the applicable statutory and case law in the jurisdiction in which the evaluation is being done.

Warnings during the Course of Clinical Practice

All these problems exist even in the relatively simple situation in which a clinician knows in advance of contact with a patient that at least one purpose of that contact will be to provide a legal opinion to a third party. Unless clinicians are prepared to read a lengthy and complicated list of hypotheticals to every new patient they see (which would most probably serve either to confuse or frighten most of them away), it is unlikely that patients coming in voluntarily for clinical treatment can effectively be warned about all the circumstances under which the clinician might be called upon to provide expert opinions about them to courts or other third parties. Perhaps the best that clinicians can do under the present circumstances is to be alert for signs that such opinions might be sought (such as threats of violence, difficulty disciplining a child, or serious marital strife), and to warn patients immediately upon recognizing such signs that expert opinions might well be called for in such situations.

The Special Case of Competency for Execution

Although ethical principles do not usually depend on the circumstances of particular cases, or on the consequences of rendering particular opinions, it cannot be denied that the finality of the death penalty places clinical participation in the decisions surrounding it on a different level of ethical discourse. While it is clear that actual direct participation in the execution itself is out of bounds for all physicians, there is no professional consensus on related issues, such as whether mental health professionals should participate as expert witnesses in any or all phases of a capital prosecution. At one pole, Resnick[83] argues that there is no ethical distinction between treating a condemned inmate who has been found incompetent for execution and evaluating that defendant's competency to stand trial. The National Medical Association also adopts a consistent position which finds no ethical problems in evaluating and treating condemned but incompetent inmates, reasoning that clinicians have an ethical responsibility to provide treatment to all persons in need of it, regardless of the subsequent nonclinical consequences.[84] Others[85] would support evaluation of competency for execution but not treatment to restore such competency; while still others[86] would provide evaluations of competency to stand trial and criminal responsibility, and even provide opinions in capital sentencing hearings in capital cases, but not become involved in the issue of competency for execution itself.

Unlike other types of treatment under involuntary circumstances, such as civil commitment, treatment to restore competency to stand trial, or treatment of persons committed after findings of not guilty by reason of insanity or under sexual psychopath laws, a significant number of clinicians would refuse to provide treatment to restore competency for execution under any circumstances. Even those who would provide the treatment generally refuse also to provide subsequent legal evaluation of their patients' competency to the courts.[87]

Clinicians at Florida State Hospital, which has had the greatest experience with the dilemma, have developed an uneasy division of labor, under which hospital clinicians provide the treatment, but are not called upon to provide opinions or testimony on the issue of competency, which is provided by independent clinicians (who, however, have access to the hospital's treatment records, thus again preventing in practice the complete separation of treatment and evaluation).[88,89]

The only legal approach which deals satisfactorily with the clinical dilemma is that found in Maryland[90] and Great Britain,[91] both of which require automatic and permanent commutation of a death penalty to life imprisonment without the possibility of parole upon a finding of incompetency for execution. Such a provision relieves clinicians of the special problems inherent in treatment which, if successful, would have the effect of removing the last barrier to execution; but it of course at the same time makes the prospect of malingering even greater than would be the case if temporary incompetency would result only in temporary delay in execution.

Conclusions

As long as the mental health professionals are perceived to have unique information of value to legal decision makers, and unique skills in dealing with the mentally disordered which are of use to society in general, some degree of double agency is inevitable. Even in the simplest situation, involving an explicit request for a specified forensic evaluation, with no treatment relationship required, it is frequently impossible to avoid some aspects of the dual role, even if only in the mind of the evaluatee.

It is not useful to pretend that such conflicts do not exist, or that we could somehow avoid them altogether if only we practiced 'ethically.' While it is true that many of the more overt dilemmas can be avoided by eschewing practice in public, especially forensic, systems, I would argue that such a course would merely turn us into a profession of ostriches, righteously burying our heads in the sands of 'pure' clinical practice while ignoring the real, practical problems that will continue to exist around us. If those who have well-developed ethical senses choose to leave the fray, it can only mean that it will be left to practitioners who are less sensitive to the problems, and would be therefore a type of abandonment of patients for whom we can provide the best (if imperfect) protections from misuse by an adversarial system often more interested in protecting the dignity of its own practices than providing justice to our patients.

It is essential that we acknowledge the reality of dual agency at all levels of current clinical as well as forensic practice, and continue to discuss them within our professions as well as to advocate for such changes as would have significant impact in reducing or eliminating unnecessary conflicts. Those practices that appear to be unacceptable to the great majority of practitioners, such as failing to warn persons being formally evaluated for the courts of the purpose of the evaluation, or perhaps serving as both treater and evaluator of condemned inmates found incompetent for execution, should be incorporated into what Diamond[16] calls 'professional ethics,' where they might ultimately form a sufficiently powerful consensus to permit changes to be made in statutes or court decisions. More controversial issues, which Diamond would classify as falling under 'personal ethics' need to be

continuously debated, if for no other reason than to educate clinicians who have not recognized them to be problems.

It is essential that ethical principles be developed with the strong input of those who practice on the front lines as well as those who recline in ivory towers and view the fray from afar. We should not attempt premature closure on difficult questions by codifying abstract theory into rigid principles that do not fit the everyday reality of clinical and forensic practice in *all* types of settings.[92]

It is also essential that such discussions permeate our training programs, which have perhaps heretofore had too much of a tendency to be satisfied with providing pat answers, rather than raising the difficult and ultimately unanswerable questions which reflect the reality of our practices.

References

1   Halleck SJ: American psychiatry and the criminal: An historical review. *Am J Psychiatry* 1965; **121**:Supplement i.

2   Smith CE: Psychiatry in corrections. *Am J Psychiatry* 1964; **120**:1045–1049.

3   Dietz PE: Forensic and non-forensic psychiatrists: An empirical comparison. *Bull Am Acad Psychiatry Law* 1978; **6**:13–22.

4   Knesper DJ: How psychiatrists allocate their professional time: Implications for educational and manpower planning. *Hosp Comm Psychiatry* 1981; **32**:620–624.

5   American Psychiatric Association: *American Medical Association Principles of Medical Ethics With Annotations Especially Applicable for Psychiatry*. Washington DC, American Psychiatric Association, 1978.

6   Szasz TS: *Law, Liberty and Psychiatry*. New York, Macmillan, 1963.

7   Hollender MH: Privileged communication and confidentiality. *Dis Nerv System* 1965; **26**:169–175.

8   Hastings Center: In the service of the state: the psychiatrist as double agent. *Hastings Cen Rep*, special suppl, April 1978.

9   Monahan J (ed): *Who is the client? The ethics of psychological intervention in the criminal justice system*. Washington DC, American Psychological Association, 1980.

10 Kaplan LV, Miller RD: The courtroom psychiatrist: Expertise at the cost of wisdom? *Int J Law Psychiatry* 1986; **9**:451–468.

11 American Academy of Psychiatry and the Law, Ethics Committee: Ethical Guidelines for the Practice of Forensic Psychiatry. *Newsletter Am Acad Psychiatry Law* 1987; **12**(1); 16–17.

12 Miller RD: The harassment of forensic psychiatrists outside court. *Bull Am Acad Psychiatry Law* 1985; **13**:337–343.

13 *In re Roth*, 394 A.2d 419 (Pa. Sup. Ct. 1978).

14 *In re Lifschutz*, 2 Cal.3d 415, 85 Cal.Rptr. 829, 467 Pac.2d 557 (1970).

15 *Caesar V Mountanos*, 542 F.2d 1064 (9th Cir. 1976).

16 Diamond B: in Rosner R, Weinstock R (eds.) *Critical Issues in American Psychiatry and Law*, vol 7. New York, Plenum Medical Books, 1990, p. 38.

17 Rachlin S, Stokman CLJ: Incompetent misdemeanants – Pseudocivil commitment. *Bull Am Acad Psychiatry Law* 1986; **14**:23–30.

18 Miller RD, Germain EJ: Inpatient evaluation of competency to stand trial. *Health Law in Canada* 1989; **9**(3):74–78, 92.

19 Solomon H: Presidential address to the American Psychiatric Association. *Am J Psychiatry* 1958; **115**:1–9.

20 Modlin HC: The ivory tower v. the marketplace. *Bull Am Acad Psychiatry Law* 1984; **12**:233–236.

21 *Estelle v Smith*, 451 U.S. 454, 101 S.Ct. 1866 (1981).

22 Hudgins RW: Murder by a manic-depressive. *Int J Neuropsychiatry* 1965; **1**:381–383.

23 Ratner RA: Mania, crime, and the insanity defense: A case report. *Bull Am Acad Psychiatry Law* 1981; **9**:23–32.

24 Wisconsin Statutes Chapters 971.14(5) and 971.17.

25 Gutheil TG: Prosecuting patients (ltr). *Hosp Comm Psychiatry* 1985; **36**:1320–1321.

26 Miller RD: The treating psychiatrist as forensic evaluator in release decisions. *J Forensic Sci* 1987; **32**:481–488.

27 Halleck SJ, Pacht AR: The current status of the Wisconsin Sex Crimes Law. *Wis Bar Bull* 1960:17–26.

28 Modlin HC: Compensation neurosis. *Bull Am Acad Psychiatry Law* 1986; 14:263–271.

29 Cole R: Patients' rights vs. doctors' rights: Which should take precedence? Paper presented at conference, *Refusing Treatment in Mental Health Institutions: Values in Conflict*. Boston, November 10, 1980.

30 Pasewark RA, Pantle ML, Steadman HJ: Characteristics and disposition of persons found not guilty by reason of insanity in New York State, 1971–1976. *Am J Psychiatry* 1979; 136:655–660.

31 Heller MS, Traylor WH, Ehrlich SM, Lester D: Intelligence, psychosis and competency to stand trial. *Bull Am Acad Psychiatry Law* 1981; 9:267–274.

32 Wisconsin Statutes Chapter 51.

33 Sadoff RL, Tanay E: Should the forensic evaluator be the treater? Panel presented at the 15th Annual Meeting of the American Academy of Psychiatry and the Law, Nassau, Bahamas, October 27, 1984.

34 California Welfare and Institutions Code ## 5000-5404, 1967, effective 1969 (Lanterman-Petris-Short Act).

35 Weiner BA: Sexual psychopath laws. In Brakel SJ, Parry J, Weiner BA (eds): *The Mentally Disabled and the Law*, ed 3, Chicago, American Bar Foundation, 1985.

36 Halleck SJ: The ethical dilemmas of forensic psychiatry: A utilitarian approach. *Bull Am Acad Psychiatry Law* 1984; 12:279–288.

37 Miller RD: The Terry hearings to determine the release of offenders committed under Wisconsin's Sex Crime Law. *Wis Bar Bull* 1988; 61(1): 17–19.

38 *State v Post*, Case No. I-7439 (Milwaukee Cty. Cir. Ct., September 1984).

39 American Psychiatric Association Ethics Committee: Opinion, expressed in a letter to the author from William L. Webb, Jr., M.D., Chair, APA Ethics Committee, April 18, 1986.

40 Miller RD: *Involuntary Civil Commitment of the Mentally Ill in the Post-Reform Era*. Springfield, IL, Charles C. Thomas, 1987, pp 129–170.

41 Bloom JD, Faulkner LR, Holm VM, Rawlinson RA: An empirical view of patients exercising their right to refuse treatment. *Int J Law Psychiatry* 1984; 7:315–328.

42 Zito JM, Lentz SL, Routt WW, Olson GW: The treatment review panel: A solution to treatment refusal? *Bull Am Acad Psychiatry Law* 1984; 12:349–358.

43 Appelbaum PS: The right to refuse treatment with antipsychotic medications: retrospect and prospect. *Am J Psychiatry* 1988; 145:413–419.

44 *Tarasoff v Regents of the University of California*, 118 Cal. Rptr. 129, 529 P.2d 553 (1974); 17 Cal.3d 425, 551 P.2d 334 (1976).

45 Miller RD, Doren DM, Van Rybroek GJ, Maier GJ: Emerging problems for staff associated with the release of potentially dangerous forensic patients. *Bull Am Acad Psychiatry Law* 1988; 16:309–320.

46 Stone AA: The *Tarasoff* case and some of its progeny: Suing psychotherapists to safeguard society, in *Law, Psychiatry and Morality*. Washington DC, American Psychiatric Press, 1984.

47 Appelbaum PS, Meisel A: Therapists' obligations to report their patients' criminal acts. *Bull Am Acad Psychiatry Law* 1986; 14:221–230.

48 Felthous AR: Liability of treaters for injuries to others: Erosion of three immunities. *Bull Am Acad Psychiatry Law* 1987; 15:115–125.

49 Weinstock R: Confidentiality and the new duty to protect: The therapist's dilemma. *Hosp Comm Psychiatry* 1988; 39:607–609.

50 American Psychological Association: Ethical principles of psychologists. *Am Psychol* 1981; 36:633–638.

51 National Federation of Societies for Clinical Social Work: Responsibilities of clinical social workers. Cited in Loewenberg F, Dolgoff R: *Ethical Decisions for Social Work Practice*. Itasca, IL, F.E. Peacock Publishers, 1985.

52 Newberger EH: The helping hand strikes again: Unintended consequences of child abuse reporting. *J Clin Child Psychol* 1983; 12:307–311.

53 Miller RD, Weinstock R: Conflict of interest between therapist-patient confidentiality and the duty to report sexual abuse of children. *Behav Sci Law* 1987; 5:161–174.

54 Gartrell N, Herman J, Olarte S, Feldstein M, Localio R: Sexual abuse of patients by therapists: Strategies for offender management and rehabilitation. *Hosp Comm Psychiatry* 1988; 39:1070–1074.

55 Minn. Stat. Ann. Secs. 148A.01-148A.06, Supp. 1987.

56 1987 Wisconsin Act 380, published May 2, 1988, amending Wisconsin Statutes Chapter 940.22.

57 Hoge SK, Gutheil TG: The prosecution of psychiatric patients for assaults on staff: a preliminary empirical study. *Hosp Comm Psychiatry* 1987; 38:44–49.

58 Miller RD, Maier GJ: Factors affecting the decision to prosecute mental patients. *Hosp Comm Psychiatry* 1987; 38:50–55.

59 Appelbaum PS, Meisel A: Therapists' obligations to report their patients' criminal acts. *Bull Am Acad Psychiatry Law* 1986; 14:221–230.

60 Miller RD: The treating psychiatrist as forensic evaluator. *J For Sciences* 1984; 29:825–830.

61 Apostle DT: The unconsciousness defense as applied to post traumatic stress disorder in a Vietnam veteran. *Bull Am Acad Psychiatry Law* 1980; 8:426–430.

62 Kluft RP: The simulation and dissimulation of multiple personality disorder. *Am J Clin Hyp* 1987; 30:104–108.

63 McGarry AL: Pathological gambling: A new insanity defense. *Bull Am Acad Psychiatry Law* 1983; 11:301–308.

64 Perr IN: Pathological intoxication and alcohol idiosyncratic intoxication – Part I: Diagnostic and clinical aspects. *J Foren Sci* 1986; 31:806–811.

65 Resnick PR: Necrophilia, murder and insanity. Presented at the 18th Annual Meeting of the American Academy of Psychiatry and the Law, Ottawa, Canada, October 16, 1987.

66 American Psychiatric Association: *Diagnostic and Statistical Manual of Mental Disorders*, ed 3, revised. Washington DC, American Psychiatric Press, 1987.

67 Strasburger LH: Crudely, without any finesse: The defendant hears his psychiatric evaluation. *Bull Am Acad Psychiatry Law* 1987; 15:229–233.

68 Miller RD: Forensic testimony (Letter). *Newsletter Am Acad Psychiatry Law* 1988; 13(1):24.

69 Miller RD: Should forensic evaluators be informed of evaluators' opinions prior to trial? *Bull Am Acad Psychiatry Law*, 1989; 17:53–59.

70 Strasburger LH: Response (Letter). *Newsletter Am Acad Psychiatry Law* 1988; 13(1):24.

71 Amaya M, Burlingame W: Judicial review of psychiatric admissions: The clinical impact on child and adolescent patients. *J Am Acad Child Psychiatry* 1981; 20:761–776.

72 Ensminger JJ, Liguori TD: The therapeutic significance of the civil commitment hearing: An unexplored potential. *J Psychiatry Law* 1978; 6:5–44.

73 Miller RD, Bernstein MR, Van Rybroek GJ, Maier GJ: The impact of the right to refuse treatment in a forensic patient population: Six-month review. *Bull Am Acad Psychiatry Law* 1989; 17:107–119.

74 Wisconsin Statutes Chapter 971.17.

75 Melton GB, Petrila J, Poythress NG, Slobogin C: *Psychological Evaluation for the Courts: A Handbook for Mental Health Professionals and Lawyers*. New York Guilford Press, 1987.

76 Bukatman BA, Foy JL, DeGrazia E: What is competency to stand trial? *Am J Psychiatry* 1971; 127:1225–1229.

77 Bursten B: Voluntariness of waiver of Fifth Amendment rights. *Bull Am Acad Psychiatry Law* 1979; 7:352–362.

78 Grisso T, Manoogian S: Juveniles' comprehension of Miranda warnings. In Lipsitt PD, Sales BD (eds): *New Directions in Psycholegal Research*. New York, Van Nostrand Reinhold, 1980.

79 Miller RD, Maier GJ, Kaye M: The right to remain silent during psychiatric evaluation in civil and criminal cases – A national survey and an analysis. *Int J Law Psychiatry* 1986; 9:77–94.

80 Gutheil TG, Appelbaum PS: *Clinical Handbook of Psychiatry and the Law*. New York, McGraw-Hill, 1982.

81 *Ake v Oklahoma*, 470 U.S. 68, 105 S.Ct. 1087, 84 L.Ed.2d 53 (1985).

82 Friedenthal JH: Discovery and use of an adverse party's expert information. *Stanford Law Rev* 1962; 14:455–488.

83 Resnick P, Discussion at the Spring Scientific Meeting of the Midwest Chapter of the American Academy of Psychiatry and the Law, Cincinnati, April 4, 1987.

84 National Medical Association Section on Psychiatry and Behavioral Sciences: Position statement on the role of the psychiatrist in evaluating and treating 'death row inmates,' Washington DC, undated.

85 Rappaport J, Roth LH: Resolved: It is unethical for psychiatrists to diagnose or treat condemned persons in order to determine their competency to be executed. Debate presented at the Annual Scientific Meeting of the American Psychiatric Association, Chicago, May 13, 1987.

86 Appelbaum PS, Sargent DA: Resolved: It is unethical for psychiatrists to diagnose or treat condemned persons in order to determine their competency to be executed. Debate presented at the Annual Scientific Meeting of the American Psychiatric Association, Chicago, May 13, 1987.

87 Miller RD: Evaluation of and treatment to competency to be executed: A national survey and an analysis. *J Psychiatry Law* 1988; **16**:67–90.

88 McClaren H: A model mental health system for death row – Evaluation of competency for execution following *Ford v Wainwright*. Presented at the 18th Annual Meeting of the American Academy of Psychiatry and the Law, Ottawa, Oct 18, 1987.

89 Radelet ML, Barnard GW: Treating those found incompetent for execution: Ethical chaos with only one solution. *Bull Am Acad Psychiatry Law* 1988; **16**:297–307.

90 Annotated Code of the General Public Laws of Maryland, 1987 Cumulative Supplement, Article 27, Par. 75A(9)(d)(3).

91 Duff R: *Trials and Punishments*, 1986, p 15.

92 Hundert EM: A model for ethical problem solving in medicine, with practical applications. *Am J Psychiatry* 1987; **144**:839–846.

The Ethical Dilemmas of Forensic Psychiatry
*A Utilitarian Approach**

Seymour L. Halleck

The problem of defining a set of ethical principles that will guide mental health practitioners in their interactions with patients is not limited to forensic psychiatry. All aspects of psychiatric practice have ethical implications, and these are particularly complex when the psychiatrist's allegiances are not directed entirely toward the patient. Any psychiatric function that obligates the psychiatrist to evaluate patients for purposes that serve the interests of social or private agencies may support actions on the part of agencies that patients perceive as harmful. There are obvious ethical problems for members of a healing profession who participate in activities that may harm their patients. The problems are similar whether that harm is created by courtroom testimony or by virtue of the psychiatrist submitting a written or oral report to an agency.

The first part of this article is an effort to define general principles that might assist psychiatrists in assessing the ethical dimensions of all types of forensic and social functions. In elaborating on these principles, I emphasize that process of procedural aspects of our social and forensic functions must be given special attention in dealing with ethical conflicts. Once defined and discussed, these principles will then be considered as they apply to one of psychiatry's most important social and forensic roles, the involuntary commitment of dangerous patients.

The 'Double-Agent' Role

The ethical problems of social and forensic psychiatry were eloquently described by Thomas Szasz in the early 1960s when he distinguished contractual from institutional psychiatry.[1] In contractual psychiatry, patients volunteer for treatment. Nothing is done to or for them without their consent. Information they disclose to psychiatrists is protected from the scrutiny of others. In institutional psychiatry, psychiatrists are employed by the government or some agency. The agency employed psychiatrist relates to a patient primarily to serve some need of that agency. This is the major reason for the physician-patient interaction. In the course of the examination interview, the psychiatrist may have some concern with the needs of the patient. It is never clear, however, where the psychiatrist's allegiances really lie. The psychiatrist may attempt to be the agent of the institution or the state and the agent of the patient at the same time. (Szasz described the psychiatrist in this role as a double agent.) According to Szasz, the psychiatrist will inevitably lean toward meeting the needs of whoever pays his or her salary or fee. This means that the patient may experience harm as a result of participating in the evaluation process.

Some examples involving use of the double-agent role are interviewing patients for the purpose of civil commitment, examining offenders in the process of sentencing, examining applicants for an insurance policy, or examining students who have been mentally ill to see if they can be allowed to return to school. One of the most significant ways in which the double-agent role differs from the traditional practice of psychiatry is that it is not accompanied by any guarantee of confidentiality. Psychiatrists who take on

* Halleck S.: The ethical dilemmas of forensic psychiatry: a utilitarian approach. *Bulletin of the American Academy of Psychiatry and Law* **12**:279–288, 1984.

the double-agent role usually are obligated to report to someone else much of what their patients tell them. As a result of the psychiatrist's findings, the patient may be given a longer prison sentence; may be committed to a mental institution; may be deprived of a job, an opportunity to enter school, or a license to engage in his or her profession. This poses an obvious moral question for the physician who is trained in the doctrine of 'primum non nocere.'

There are ethical problems other than the risk that the psychiatrist may hurt the patient. Whatever harm results from a psychiatric evaluation is occasioned by the psychiatrist using skills designed to help people. In a commitment evaluation, a sentencing evaluation, or an insurance evaluation, the psychiatrist is obligated to learn about the patient's disability. This can be done only if the patient communicates in a verbal or nonverbal fashion. If the psychiatrist is to report accurately, it is important that the patient's communication be as complete and reliable as possible. The patient must disclose behavior, thoughts, or feelings that would not be revealed in most social situations. To obtain honest self-disclosure, the psychiatrist uses certain skills. He or she tries to be straightforward, friendly, reinforcing, and, above all, empathic. Without use of these skills, the psychiatrist is not much more efficient than a lay person. It is almost impossible for a competent psychiatrist to conduct a psychiatric examination without being selectively reinforcing and empathic. Herein lies the most difficult aspect of the ethical dilemma posed by the double-agent role. Is it morally justified to use skills originally developed for the sole purpose of helping patients in order to derive information that ultimately may be used to hurt them?

The Szaszian position on this question is a clear and resounding 'No.' I and others have adopted more of a compromise position.[2,3] The common argument of those of us who urge a more temperate approach is that each double-agent role should be evaluated on its own merits. Such evaluation requires the use of some type of conceptual framework that helps the psychiatrist consider which factors must be evaluated in each role. The easiest way to develop such a framework is to first examine the potential harms and benefits of double-agent roles in general. Specific roles can then be evaluated in terms of their possible harms, their benefits, and to what extent the process by which they are entered into can be modified so as to maximize benefit and minimize harm.

Reducing Harm and Increasing Benefits

There are certain general advantages to the double-agent role. First of all, society may be helped by knowing more about its deviant citizens and sometimes only psychiatry can provide the kind of help that society is looking for. Second, the patient may be helped. There are many instances in which society and the patient can be helped at the same time. Certainly, many patients who are involuntarily committed are later grateful for what has been done to them. It can even be argued that a person who is given a longer prison term as a result of psychiatric intervention may be spared the aversive consequences that would follow committing a new crime, including the possibility of an even longer period of incarceration. Help also may be provided in the course of the evaluation interview. A skilled psychiatrist may be able to comfort or counsel a patient in the course of a single examination. Third, the double-agent role can be helpful to the psychiatric profession. It can provide psychiatrists with power, a certain amount of prestige, and, at times, considerable financial remuneration.

The most serious objection to any double-agent role is, of course, the harm it may cause to the patient. There also may be harm to the psychiatric profession. Insofar as psychiatrists begin to be looked on as agents of oppression rather than as helping individuals, their public image suffers. There also may be significant harm to the doctor-patient relationship. This may be both specific and general. A patient may be aware that he or she may be harmed by the doctor's actions and will not fully cooperate. Or the patient actually may experience harm as a result of the double-agent role and will not trust that doctor in subsequent interactions. In both instances the patient's treatment is compromised, and a specific harm is created. Other patients who begin to learn about and fear this apparent psychiatric duplicity will come to distrust any psychiatrist who takes on an institutional role and perhaps all psychiatrists. This is a general harm that can be created.

There are certain procedural aspects of institutional psychiatric practice that have significant potential harmfulness. The manner in which these roles are assumed can have enormous influence in increasing or decreasing their risks. Double-agent roles are least controversial under the following conditions:

1 The psychiatrist has a clear idea of what kind of evaluation is being requested. It would seem that such clarity would be routine. Unfortunately it is not. Legal and social agencies often are unclear as to why they request a psychiatric evaluation.[4] Sometimes it is the psychiatrist who is confused. Psychiatrists still confuse requests to evaluate competence to stand trial with requests for evaluation of insanity. Most disturbing, psychiatrists not uncommonly will predict dangerousness when such a prediction is not even called for.[5] The harm engendered by such lack of clarity has been poignantly illustrated in the *Smith v Estelle* case in which a psychiatrist's prediction of dangerousness made in the course of a competence evaluation was later used to justify a capital sentence.[6] Social agencies and courts should define as specifically as possible what information they are looking for. Psychiatrists should ascertain they understand the request and should respond to it as precisely as possible. They should not provide information unrelated to the issue consideration.

Clarity is, of course, increased when the terms used in the agency's request are defined as precisely as possible. Two examples of words usually not defined or defined imprecisely are 'dangerousness' and 'treatability.' Dangerousness in our society has become almost a term of art and can refer to any undesirable conduct from having a greater than average tendency to shoplift to having qualities that lead to a high probability of committing homicide. Treatability implies many goals ranging from reducing chances of recidivism, to removing symptoms, to restructuring the personality. To the extent these terms are not defined, psychiatrists must construct their own definitions. The predictions they make based on these private definitions are not likely to provide the social or forensic agency with meaningful information.

2 The information requested by the agency is of a variety that the psychiatrist is able to obtain on the basis of his or her clinical skills. In general, psychiatrists are skilled in evaluating the personality structures and emotional cognitive capacities of their patients. They have less skill in evaluating specific task-oriented capacities such as capacities to drive, to be a student, or to be an air traffic controller. Because they usually are not experts in fields such as education, driving, or air traffic safety, they cannot do much more than speculate as to how various emotional or cognitive incapacities are likely to influence the patient's task performance.

Psychiatrists also have quite limited skills in predicting future violence. There are circumstances in which they can predict the probability of violence on the part of a given individual living in a given environment over a given time span.[7] As a rule, however, psychiatrists do not have sufficient clinical skills that allow for a meaningfully accurate prediction of violence. Many of the predictions of violence they are asked to make (usually framed in the context of predicting dangerousness) are beyond their clinical expertise.

3 The psychiatrist's report is not a de facto mandate for an administrative decision. Agencies must make difficult decisions as to whether to allow their clients certain privileges (such as entering a university or being given a driver's license). Courts must decide difficult issues such as competence to stand trial, dangerousness, or insanity. Many moral, social, and political considerations go into these decisions. Too often, agencies or courts try to bypass the moral and social dimensions of decision making by simply accepting the recommendations of the psychiatrist. This makes the psychiatrist more of an ethical decision maker than an expert. Psychiatric participation in double-agent roles is least controversial when the psychiatrist's report or testimony is scrupulously reviewed by social or judicial agencies and when it is weighed as only one of many factors involved in making a final decision.

4 Patients are provided with thorough information as to the process and potential outcome of the interview. Many individuals who are subject to the double-agent role do not know that the doctor is also obligated to an agency. They may view the physician solely as their helper and not as a person who can do them harm. Sometimes they may know that the doctor is functioning in a double-agent role but may be so accustomed to viewing doctors as helping individuals that they may suppress their awareness of the agency employed psychiatrist's function. Many psychiatrists, including myself, have admonished psychiatrists who function in this role to explain clearly to their clients all the potential risks of communication or noncommunication in the interview process.[8] Patients so informed are unlikely to perceive themselves as having been misled into revealing information that is later used against them.

The Ethics of Civil Commitment

I would like to apply the criteria I have listed to one specific social and forensic role: the psychiatrist's involvement in civil commitment of patients dangerous to others. Much of what I say probably is relevant to other forms of civil commitment, but the case is much easier to make when considering the dangerous mentally ill. The statutes that control them were not drafted with beneficence toward patients in mind. The psychiatrist who participates clearly is involved in a social control function.

I wish to emphasize that I am not arguing against civil commitment. I believe society has a right to involuntarily detain individuals who are mentally ill and dangerous to others. My primary concern is with the current psychiatric role in that process of detention. I will argue that in its current use the role does not effectively serve the interests of either the patient, society, or the psychiatrist and that participation in this role seriously compromises the ethical position of the psychiatrist.

There are several ways in which the psychiatrist becomes involved in detaining the dangerously mentally ill. Sometimes a psychiatrist in a walk-in or emergency clinic interviews a patient who has voluntarily appeared or who comes under duress from the family, and the psychiatrist reluctantly concludes that the patient is a severely ill person who could do harm to others. The patient may reject the psychiatrist's recommendation for voluntary hospitalization. In this situation the psychiatrist usually has begun the interview in an empathic manner. The issue of involuntary commitment is not raised until the patient has been substantially exposed to an empathic interviewer and has probably disclosed a great deal of information about himself or herself. There is no semblance of informed consent here. Once the psychiatrist appreciates that commitment is necessary, there must be a considerable amount of maneuvering to preserve the safety of all involved parties. Often the patient is not told he or she is to be committed until security officers have been notified. This is hardly a gratifying medical function and is painful to all involved.

More commonly, the psychiatrist in the emergency room is presented with a patient brought by the sheriff, and the initial petition for commitment has been made by family, friends, or social agencies. Here, the psychiatrist may provide a brief explanation of the purposes of the interview, but it is usually not very elaborate. A more serious problem for all concerned parties is that the psychiatrist's evaluation in the emergency room situation is hampered by a very confusing factual situation. The petition form may simply say that the patient threatened to kill his wife. The patient may deny this.

At this point the psychiatrist is in the unfortunate position of trying to investigate whether a violent act did occur. The wife may have disappeared by the time the patient has arrived at the evaluation center. The police may simply note that the patient has always been a peaceful citizen. If the other criteria of civil commitment are met, the psychiatrist is, in effect, placed in the role of becoming a detective. The psychiatrist has no particular skill in this role and is further handicapped by an absence of investigatory resources. Telephone calls may be made trying to gain information as to exactly how the patient did behave. These time-consuming operations often reveal little. The psychiatrist has no certainty as to the reliability or even the identity of the person who is called. The psychiatrist who becomes involved in the difficult process of trying to gain facts about past behavior may also find there is no one to be called. Here, the only source of information is a client who has no wish to be cooperative. I believe this kind of detective role, especially one that imposes so many handicaps on the seeker of truth, is inappropriate for a member of a helping profession.

Whether serving as both petitioner and examiner or simply as an examiner in the commitment process, the psychiatrist is called on to make a judgment whether the patient is mentally ill (and this part is usually easy) and whether the risk of that patient being dangerous is sufficient to justify his or her restraint. The latter task is made somewhat easier in states where dangerousness is at least defined as a threat of bodily harm, or an attempt to inflict bodily harm. Even when dangerousness is defined, however, the statutes provide little guidance as to what degree of probability the patient will commit a violent act constitutes dangerousness.

There may well be good reasons for keeping such statutes vague. In every instance when an individual is civilly committed as dangerous to others, some decision must be made as to whether the type of harm that individual threatens, and its likelihood of occurring in a given time frame, is sufficiently threatening to society to justify restraining that individual. The public's interest in self-protection must be balanced against a need to consider the individual's rights. Society must decide how many it will restrain unnecessarily to protect us from the one person who might hurt us. This is purely a moral and political issue that must be left to the conscience of the community.

It is the vagueness of the term dangerousness that allows the court to interpose community values on the commitment process. In this sense, dangerousness does not exist and cannot exist until it is legally designated. If the psychiatrist signs a form stating that he or she believes an individual is dangerous before the court has decided that individual is dangerous, the psychiatrist can only be guessing as to the conscience of the community. The psychiatrist is then assuming the role of the judge rather than that of the medical expert.

In dealing with emergency room commitments, the psychiatrist is, in effect, invested with a great deal of judicial power. It can be argued the psychiatrist's initial recommendations to detain a patient until a hearing can be held are reviewed by a magistrate. In most states, this is a perfunctory review. It is extremely uncommon for a magistrate to overturn a psychiatrist's recommendation for initial restraint. Until a formal hearing is held, the psychiatrist is, for the most part, the patient's sole judicial tribunal. Psychiatrists naturally abhor such a role and avoid it when they can. Most frequently the role is thrust on those who might be considered the underclass of the psychiatric profession. The overwhelming majority of commitments in the United States are done by psychiatric residents and public sector psychiatrists who often are foreign medical graduates.

Once the initial petition for commitment has been sustained, hospital psychiatrists also may become involved in the process of commitment. Sometimes they may be asked to testify at the formal hearing as to the patient's current mental status. In addition, any psychiatrist who is caring for the hospitalized patient has the legal power to release the patient at any time in the process of commitment. This means that the psychiatrist who may be treating the patient has a tremendous degree of control over the patient's freedom. Such power may impair the doctor's and patient's capacity to form a therapeutic relationship. On the one hand, the psychiatrist is telling the patient to be open, honest, and frank. On the other hand, to the extent that the patient has recovered his or her sanity, the patient will appreciate that honest self-disclosure to the physician may put him or her in jeopardy of continued deprivation of freedom. This situation impairs, sometimes drastically, the quality of therapy that can be performed with civilly committed patients.

In reviewing the process of civil commitment, it is useful to reflect on the inconsistent manner in which the court apportions power to psychiatrists. Psychiatrists are given power to release any patient at any time. They are given a great deal of power subject only to the approval of a magistrate to restrain patients until a formal hearing is held. They are given much less power in the process of formally committing patients at the time of the judicial hearing. It seems courts have less trust in psychiatrists' judgments that result in patients being deprived of liberty (the exception here is when psychiatrists' recommendations for detention prior to a formal hearing are only briefly reviewed by a magistrate) than they do in psychiatrists' judgments that result in the release of potentially dangerous patients.

Is it possible that the courts are more interested in protecting the rights of patients than in protecting the public? It would seem unlikely that society would take such a cavalier attitude toward its own protection. Certainly, current practices save money insofar as they allow one professional to make judicial as well as treatment decision, but is this savings worth the risk to public safety? A possible consideration here is that our courts are relying on psychiatrists to be more conservative in releasing than in hospitalizing patients. One reason the courts may anticipate such conservatism is that the fear of being sued for releasing a patient who later harms someone is quite prevalent (and realistically so) among psychiatrists.

Summary

How does the current role of psychiatrists in the commitment of dangerous patients stack up in terms of its potential harmfulness to all concerned parties?

1 Do current statutes provide clear criteria for the determination of dangerousness? The answer is a definite no. Often even definitions of mental illness in commitment statutes are unclear insofar as they include elements of dangerousness to self or others.

2 Do psychiatrists have skills enabling them to determine whether individuals should be committed as dangerous? The answer is a qualified but definite no. Psychiatrists, as noted, have some skills in predicting violence. The best they can do, however, is to make a probability statement as to the likelihood a violent act will occur in a given period of time under certain circumstances. Usually that probability is quite small. It also should be emphasized that the factual or data base on which predictions of dangerousness are made in the civil commitment process is likely to be inadequate.

3 Is there sufficient judicial review of the psychiatrist's reporting so as to ascertain he or she does not become a de facto decision maker? The answer is that this is true only in certain aspects of the commitment process. Most of the time the psychiatrist assumes unwanted and unnecessary power.

4 Is good informed consent provided in the commitment process? Most of the time it is not.

5 Is it likely the current system of commitment provides maximum protection for the rights of patients and the safety of other citizens? There is no definitive way of answering this question absent research comparing the current system with a different one. It would seem likely, however, that commitment based on imprecise requests for information, on misguided perception of expertise, on blurring of expert and social roles, and on insufficient attention to informed consent cannot be very efficient in protecting either patients or society.

6   Does the current commitment process complicate the subsequent treatment of patients? It is reasonable to assume that in situations in which the doctor has total control over the patient's freedom, therapeutic trust and rapport are compromised.

7   Does the current commitment process harm the image of psychiatrists? It is hard to see how it could avoid hurting our image. Many of the most powerful attacks on the profession of psychiatry are based on a critique of the civil commitment role.

8   Does the role give psychiatrists power? Yes, but that power is accompanied by responsibilities that make psychiatrists more susceptible to lawsuits.

9   Does it give psychiatrists prestige or money? No.

On the basis of this review and summary, it would appear that the current role of psychiatrists in civil commitment of dangerous patients creates too many harms and too few benefits to be ethically justified.

Proposals for Change

While the ethical problems involved in the psychiatrists' participation in the civil commitment process never can be eradicated, they certainly can be minimized by adhering to procedures that provide greater protection for all concerned parties. The following recommendations for statutory change illustrate this point:

1   Psychiatrists should be allowed to petition for the commitment of patients suspected of being both mentally ill and dangerous to others if their patients do not enter the hospital voluntarily. This petition should not be viewed as a formal psychiatric examination. Once it is made, the petitioning psychiatrist should have no further role in the commitment process. (In this role the psychiatrist's function would be similar to that of any other citizen. The ethical problems raised around the issue of informed consent, however, still remain.)

2   Once the petition has been filed with the clerk of court, the sheriff should be instructed to bring the patient to a forensic psychiatrist employed by the state. The forensic psychiatrist must provide the patient with full informed consent as to the nature of the examination. Under no circumstances should this psychiatrist institute any type of treatment (absent a life-threatening emergency) either during or after the examination. The psychiatrist should be a fully trained professional who is paid a substantial fee for conducting the examination. Once the examination is completed, the psychiatrist's report must immediately be presented to a judicial officer who is on call 24 hours a day.

3   The psychiatrist's report should be restricted to listing evidences of mental illness, evidences of potential violence, and a probability statement as to the likelihood that the individual would be violent in a certain period of time under various circumstances. The psychiatrist should make no statement as to the patient's dangerousness. The ultimate decision for even the initial brief detention must be made by a judicial officer, who will conduct a relatively formal hearing.

4   No psychiatrist who is treating a patient should be allowed to testify at the patient's commitment hearing. Only forensic psychiatrists employed by the state for this specific purpose should be allowed to testify at any commitment hearing.

5   No treating psychiatrist should have the power to release a committed patient. Only the court should have this power after having heard the opinions of state-employed forensic psychiatrists. Again, the state-employed psychiatrist in this situation should be paid an adequate fee.

The above recommended changes provide certain advantages to all concerned parties. First, they define each participant's role accurately and honestly. No professional is required to go beyond his or her expertise. Decisions are made by judicial agencies. Second, they are likely to result in improved treatment of civilly committed patients, since treating physicians will have nothing to do with restraining patients. Third, they should enhance the image of psychiatry. Fourth, by putting this function in the hands of skilled forensic psychiatrists, residents in psychiatry would be relieved of a painful and unrewarding task. Fifth, they allow psychiatrists to collect money for a service that is now provided free of charge. Sixth they would curtail malpractice suits against psychiatrists for releasing patients who harm others. (A judge who releases a patient who commits harm cannot be sued.)

An obvious disadvantage of these changes is that they would require much more of the courts. Some judicial officers, just like physicians, would have to be on call 24 hours a day. This would add extra economic costs to the process. Paying for forensic psychiatrists is also likely to add to the economic burden. Finally, it is likely that new costs would be incurred as a result of an increase in the number of judicial procedures. All the additional costs, however, might be more than balanced by the savings associated with a more efficient system. The long-range benefits to patients and society might make the overall increase in costs trivial.

Conclusion

The analysis I have presented of psychiatrists' role in the civil commitment of dangerous patients can be applied to every controversial, social, and legal role psychiatrists assume. Usually, such analysis will suggest changes that make for a less conflictive ethical role. Sometimes these changes can be negotiated between the examining psychiatrist and the agency to which he or she reports. Sometimes they require legislative intervention. Psychiatrists cannot, as a rule, control the conditions by which they function in social and forensic roles. They can, however, define conditions under which their services are likely to create the least harm and do the most good. To the extent they do this and also seek to create these conditions, they will begin to resolve many of the ethical problems of psychiatric practice.

References

1   Szasz T: *Law, Liberty and Psychiatry*. New York, MacMillan, 1963.

2   Halleck SL: *The Politics of Therapy*. New York, Science House, 1971.

3   Robitscher J: *The Powers of Psychiatry*. Boston, Houghton Miflin, 1980.

4   Farmer L: *Observation and study: Critique and recommendations on federal procedures*. Unpublished report, Federal Judicial Center, Washington, DC, 1977.

5   Geller S and Lister E: The process of criminal commitment for pretrial psychiatric examination: An evaluation. *Am J Psychiatry* **135**:53–60, 1978.

6   Smith v Estelle, 78–1839, Fifth Circuit Court of Appeals, September 31, 1979.

7   Monahan J: *The clinical prediction of violent behavior. Crime and Delinquency Issues*, U.S. Department of Health and Human Services, Rockville, MD 1981.

8   Halleck SL: *Psychiatry and the Dilemmas of Crime*. New York, Harper and Row, 1967.

The Moral Basis of the Insanity Defense*

Richard J. Bonnie

Two fundamentally distinct questions are intertwined in discussions of the insanity defense. One concerns the moral issue of responsibility, a question looking backward to the offender's mental condition at the time of the offense. The other is essentially dispositional and looks forward in time: what should be done with mentally disordered offenders, including those who are acquitted by reason of insanity, to minimize the risk of future recidivism?

This article addresses the issue of responsibility. Sweeping proposals to abolish the insanity defense should be rejected in favor of proposals to narrow it and shift the burden of proof to the defendant. The moral core of the defense must be retained, in my opinion, because some defendants afflicted by severe mental disorder who are out of touch with reality and are unable to appreciate the wrongfulness of their acts cannot justly be blamed and do not therefore deserve to be punished. The insanity defense, in short, is essential to the moral integrity of the criminal law.

But there are several observations to be made about the dispositional issues now receiving legislative attention.

First, the present dissatisfaction with the insanity defense is largely rooted in public concern about the premature release of dangerous persons acquitted by reason of insanity. Increased danger to the public, however, is not a necessary consequence of the insanity defense. The public can be better protected than is now the case in many states by a properly designed dispositional statute that assures that violent offenders acquitted by reason of insanity are committed for long-term treatment, including a period of postdischarge supervision or 'hospital parole.'

Second, a separate verdict of 'guilty but mentally ill,' which has been enacted in several states, is an ill-conceived way of identifying prisoners who are amenable to psychiatric treatment. It surely makes no sense for commitment procedures to be triggered by a jury verdict based on evidence concerning the defendant's past rather than present mental condition and need for treatment. Decisions concerning the proper placement of incarcerated offenders should be made by correctional and mental health authorities, not by juries or trial judges. Of course, the 'guilty but mentally ill verdict' may not reflect dispositional objectives so much as it does a desire to afford juries a 'compromise' verdict in cases involving insanity pleas. If so, it should be rejected as nothing more than moral sleight of hand.

Third, it is often said that the participation of mental health professionals in criminal proceedings should be confined to the sentencing stage. Clinical expertise is likely to be most useful on dispositional rather than on responsibility questions, and, indeed, most clinical participation in the criminal process now occurs at the sentencing stage. Expert witnesses, however, cannot be excluded from the guilt stage so long as the defendant's mental condition is regarded as morally relevant to his criminal liability.

This brings the inquiry back to the issue of criminal responsibility.

The historical evolution of the insanity defense has been influenced by the ebb and flow of informed opinion concerning scientific understanding of mental illness and its relation to criminal behavior. But it is well to

remember that, at bottom, the debate about the insanity defense and the idea of criminal responsibility raises fundamentally moral questions, not scientific ones. As Lord Hale observed three centuries ago, in *History of Pleas of the Crown*, the ethical foundations of the criminal law are rooted in beliefs about human rationality, deterrability, and free will. But these are articles of moral faith rather than scientific fact.

Some critics of the insanity defense believe that mentally ill persons are not substantially less able to control their behavior than normal persons and that, in any case, a decent respect for the dignity of those persons requires that they be held accountable for their wrong-doing on the same terms as everyone else. On the other hand, proponents of the defense, among whom I count myself, believe that it is fundamentally wrong to condemn and punish a person whose rational control over his or her behavior was impaired by the incapacitating effects of severe mental illness.

Few would dispute this as a moral claim. The question is how best to describe the moral criterion of irresponsibility and to minimize the number of cases in which the defense is successfully invoked by persons who should properly be punished.

Criminal responsibility: the options

Putting aside details concerning the drafting of various tests, there are, in principle, three approaches to the insanity defense.

1 **The Model Penal Code.** One option is to leave the law as it now stands in a majority of the states and, by judicial ruling, in all of the federal courts. Apart from technical variations, this means the test proposed by the American Law Institute in its Model Penal Code. Under this approach, a person whose perceptual capacities were sufficiently intact that he had the criminal 'intent' or mens rea required in the definition of the offense nonetheless can be found 'not guilty by reason of insanity' if, by virtue of mental disease or defect, he lacked substantial capacity either to understand or appreciate the legal or moral significance of his actions, or to conform his conduct to the requirements of law. In other words, a person may be excused if his thinking was severely disordered – the so-called cognitive prong of the defense – or if his ability to control his behavior was severely impaired – the so-called volitional prong of the defense.

2 **Revival of M'Naghten.** The second option is to retain the insanity defense as an independent exculpatory doctrine – independent, that is, of mens rea – but to restrict its scope by eliminating the volitional prong. This approach would revive the M'Naghten test as the sole basis for exculpation on ground of insanity. This is the approach I favor, although I would modify the language used by the House of Lords in 1843 in favor of modern terminology that is simpler and has more clinical meaning. M'Naghten is now distinctly the minority position in this country. Fewer than one third of the states use this approach, although it is still the law in England.

3 **Abolition: the mens rea approach.** The third option is the 'mens rea' approach, which has been adopted in two states and has been endorsed by the Reagan administration. Its essential substantive effect is to abolish any

* Bonnie, R.: The moral basis of the insanity defense. *American Bar Association Journal* **69**:194–197, 1983.

criterion of exculpation, based on mental disease, that is independent of the mens rea elements of particular crimes. Instead, mentally ill (or retarded) defendants would be treated like everyone else.

Case against the mens rea approach

If the insanity defense were abolished, the law would not take adequate account of the incapacitating effects of severe mental illness. Some mentally ill defendants who were psychotic and grossly out of touch with reality may be said to have 'intended' to do what they did but nonetheless may have been so severely disturbed that they were unable to understand or appreciate the significance of their actions. These cases do not arise frequently, but when they do a criminal conviction, which signifies the societal judgment that the defendant deserves to be punished, would offend the basic moral intuitions of the community. Judges and juries would be forced either to return a verdict of conviction, which they would regard as morally obtuse, or to acquit the defendant in defiance of the law. They should be spared that moral embarrassment.

The moral difficulty with the mens rea approach is illustrated by a case involving Joy Baker, a 31-year-old woman who shot and killed her aunt. According to her account – which no one has ever doubted – she became increasingly agitated and fearful during the days before the shooting; she was worried that her dogs, her children (ages eight and 11), and her neighbors were becoming possessed by the devil and that she was going to be 'annihilated.' On the morning of the shooting, after a sleepless night, she ran frantically around the house clutching a gun to her breast. Worried about what the children might do to her if they became demonically 'possessed' and about what she might do to them to defend herself, she made them read and reread the 23d Psalm. Suddenly her aunt arrived unexpectedly. Unable to open the locked front door, and ignoring Mrs. Baker's frantic pleas to go away, the aunt came to the back door. When she reached through the broken screening to unlock the door, Mrs. Baker shot her.

The aunt then fell backward into the mud behind the porch, bleeding profusely. 'Why, Joy?' she asked. 'Because you're the devil, and you came to hurt me,' Joy answered. Her aunt said, 'Honey, no, I came to help you.' At this point, Mrs. Baker said, she became very confused and 'I took the gun and shot her again just to relieve the pain she was having because she said she was hurt.'

All the psychiatrists who examined Mrs. Baker concluded that she was acutely psychotic at the time she killed her aunt. The police who arrested her and others in the small rural community agreed that she must have been crazy because there was no rational explanation for her conduct. She was acquitted. Yet, had there been no insanity defense, she could have been acquitted only in defiance of the law. Although she was clearly out of touch with reality and unable to understand the wrongfulness of her conduct, she had the 'criminal intent' or mens rea required for some form of criminal homicide. If we look only at her conscious motivation for the second shot and do not take into account her highly regressed and disorganized emotional condition, she, was technically guilty of murder (euthanasia being no justification, of course). Moreover, even if the first shot had been fatal, she probably would have been guilty of manslaughter because her delusional belief that she was in imminent danger of demonic annihilation was, by definition, unreasonable.

These technical points, of course, may make little practical difference in the courtroom. If the expert testimony in Joy Baker's case were admitted to disprove mens rea, juries might ignore the law and decide, very bluntly, whether the defendant was 'too crazy' to be convicted. The cause of rational criminal law reform, however, is not well served by designing rules of law in the expectation that they will be ignored or nullified when they appear unjust in individual cases.

The case for narrowing the defense

While I do not favor abolition of the 'cognitive' prong of the insanity defense. I agree with critics who believe the risks of fabrication and 'moral mistakes' in administering the defense are greatest when the experts and the jury are asked to speculate whether the defendant had the capacity to 'control' himself or whether he could have 'resisted' the criminal impulse. I favor narrowing the defense by eliminating its so-called volitional prong or control test.

Few people would dispute the moral predicate for the control test – that a person who 'cannot help' doing what he did is not blameworthy. Unfortunately, however, there is no scientific basis for measuring a person's capacity for self-control or for calibrating the impairment of that capacity. There is, in short, no objective basis for distinguishing between offenders who were undeterrable and those who were merely undeterred, between the impulse that was irresistible and the impulse not resisted, or between substantial impairment of capacity and some lesser impairment. Whatever the precise terms of the volitional test, the question is unanswerable, or it can be answered only by 'moral guesses.' To ask it at all invites fabricated claims, undermines equal administration of the penal law, and compromises its deterrent effect.

Sheldon Glueck of the Harvard Law School observed in *Menial Disorder and the Criminal Law* (1925) that the 19th century effort to establish irresistible impulse as a defense met judicial resistance because 'much less than we know today was known of mental disease.' He predicted 'that with the advent of a more scientific administration of the law – especially with the placing of expert testimony upon a neutral, unbiased basis and in the hands of well-qualified experts – much of the opposition to judicial recognition of the effect of disorders of the . . . impulses should disappear.' He added that 'expert, unbiased study of the individual case will aid judge and jury to distinguish cases of pathological irresistible impulse from those in which the impulse was merely unresisted.'

The opposition to the control test did not disappear in Professor Glueck's generation. In 1955, when the Model Penal Code was being drafted, *M' Naghten* still constituted the exclusive test of insanity in two thirds of the states. Advances in clinical understanding of mental illness in the 1940s and 1950s, however, inspired a new era of optimism about the potential contributions of psychiatry to a progressive and humane penal law. This renewed optimism was reflected in the model code's responsibility test that included 'substantial' volitional impairment as an independent ground of exculpation.

The Model Penal Code has had an extraordinary impact on criminal law. For this we should be thankful, but I believe the code approach to criminal responsibility should be rejected. Psychiatric concepts of mental abnormality remain fluid and imprecise, and most academic commentary within the last ten years continues to question the scientific basis for assessment of volitional incapacity.

The volitional inquiry probably would be manageable if the insanity defense were permitted only in cases involving psychotic disorders. When the control test is combined with a loose or broad interpretation of the term 'mental disease,' however, the inevitable result is unstructured clinical speculation regarding the 'causes' of criminal behavior in any case in which a defendant can be said to have a personality disorder, an impulse disorder, or any other diagnosable abnormality.

For example, it is clear enough in theory that the insanity defense is not supposed to be a ground for acquittal of persons with weak behavior controls who misbehave because of anger, jealousy, fear, or some other strong emotion. These emotions may account for a large proportion of all homicides and other assaultive crimes. Many crimes are committed by persons who are not acting 'normally' and who are emotionally disturbed at the time. It is not uncommon to say that they are temporarily 'out of their minds.' But this is not what the law means or should mean by 'insanity.'

Because the control test, as now construed in most states, entitles defendants to insanity instructions on the basis of these claims. I am convinced that the test involves an unacceptable risk of abuse and mistake.

It might be argued, of course, that the risk of mistake should be tolerated if the volitional prong of the defense is morally necessary. The question may be put this way: Are there clinically identifiable cases involving defendants whose behaviour controls were so pathologically impaired that they ought to be acquitted although their ability to appreciate the wrongfulness of their actions was unimpaired? I do not think so. The most clinically compelling cases of volitional impairment involve the so-called impulse disorders – pyromania, kleptomania, and the like. These disorders involve severely abnormal compulsions that ought to be taken into account in sentencing, but the exculpation of pyromaniacs would be out of touch with commonly shared moral intuitions.

A proposed test

The sole test of legal insanity should be whether the defendant, as a result of severe mental disease, was unable 'to appreciate the wrongfulness of his conduct.' My statute would read:

'Defense of [Insanity] [Nonresponsibility Due to Mental Disease].

'A. A person charged with a criminal offense shall be found [not guilty by reason of insanity] [not guilty only by reason of insanity] [not responsible due to mental disease] [guilty of a criminal act but not responsible due to mental disease] if he proves, by the greater weight of the evidence, that, as a result of mental disease or mental retardation, he was unable to appreciate the wrongfulness of his conduct at the time of the offense.

'B. As used in this section, the terms mental disease or mental retardation include only those severely abnormal mental conditions that grossly and demonstrably impair a person's perception or understanding of reality and that are not attributable primarily to the voluntary ingestion of alcohol or other psychoactive substances.'

This language, drawn from the Model Penal Code, uses clinically meaningful terms to ask the same question posed by the House of Lords in *M' Naghten* 150 years ago. It is a necessary and sufficient test of criminal responsibility. During the past ten years we have evaluated hundreds of cases at our clinic. Only a handful have involved what I would regard as morally compelling claims of irresponsibility, and all of these would be comprehended by the proposed formulation. This test is fully compatible with the ethical premises of the penal law. Results reached by judges and juries in particular cases ordinarily would be congruent with the community's moral sense.

Some clinicians have argued that the volitional prong of the defense is morally necessary to take adequate account of psychotic deterioration, especially in cases involving affective disorders like manic-depressive illness. My view is that a test of insanity that focuses exclusively on the defendant's ability to 'appreciate the wrongfulness of his conduct' is broad enough to encompass all cases of severe psychotic deterioration. This is because the term 'appreciate' is designed to encompass 'affective' dimensions of major mental illness.

Burden of persuasion

Much has been said about the proper allocation of the burden of proof since the Hinckley trial. This issue does not arise under the mens rea option, because the prosecution clearly must bear the burden of proving all elements of the crime beyond a reasonable doubt. If the insanity defense is retained as an independent basis of exculpation, the argument may be put that the defendant should bear the burden of persuading the fact-finder of the truth or sufficiency of his claim.

Some commentators have argued that the prosecution should bear the burden of persuading the fact-finder, beyond a reasonable doubt, of all facts regarded as necessary to establish an ethically adequate predicate for criminal liability. When so-called defenses are concerned, the question is whether a just penal law could fail to give exculpatory effect to the claim. Consider entrapment and self-defense, for example. If the law need not recognize the defense at all – as is true for claims of entrapment, I submit – it is entirely proper to recognize it only if the defendant bears the risk of nonpersuasion. If exculpation is morally required if certain facts exist – as is true for claims of self-defense, I would argue – then, as a general rule, the prosecution should bear the risk and be required to negate the existence of those facts beyond a reasonable doubt.

The issue in the present context is whether the insanity defense presents any special considerations that warrant a departure from the general rule disfavoring burden shifting on ethically essential predicates for liability. This is a close question, but on balance, I think the answer is yes. In defenses of justification (self-defense) and situational excuses (duress), the defendant's claim must be linked to external realities and can be tested against ordinary experience, thereby reducing the likelihood of successful fabrication or jury confusion. A defendant's claim that he had a mental disorder that disabled him from functioning as a normal person, however, is not linked to the external world and by definition cannot be tested against ordinary experience. The concept of knowing, understanding, or appreciating the legal or moral significance of one's actions also is more fluid and less precise than many aspects of the elements of the penal law.

Public concerns satisfied

The insanity defense, as I have defined it, should be narrowed, not abandoned, and the burden of persuasion may properly be shifted to the defendant. Like the mens rea proposal, this approach adequately responds to public concern about possible misuse of the insanity defense. Unlike the mens rea proposal, it is compatible with the basic doctrines and principles of Anglo-American penal law.

Forum – Psychiatrists and the Death Penalty: Some Ethical Dilemmas

A crisis in the ethical and moral behavior of psychiatrists

Alfred M. Freedman and Abraham L. Halpern

A critical controversy is occurring in the USA in regard to physician participation in legal execution that has world-wide implications for ethics and morality in medicine.[1] It is disconcerting that efforts are being made in the USA to permit psychiatrists to participate in legal executions. This is surprising as many national and international organisations have passed resolutions prohibiting such participation. In particular, it should be noted that at the World Psychiatric Association Congress in Madrid, in August 1996, the General Assembly unanimously passed the Declaration of Madrid that included the statement: 'Under no circumstances should psychiatrists participate in legally authorized executions nor participate in assessments of competence to be executed'.

Many of the arguments of those who propose to make it ethically permissible for psychiatrists to participate in legal executions are troublesome if not fallacious. For example, they confuse the propriety of a physician's testimony regarding a defendant's competence to stand trial, that is a defendant who has not yet been found guilty, let alone sentenced, with the ethically impermissible testimony regarding the competence of a condemned prisoner to be executed. The question of competence to be executed arises only after a court sentences a person to death and not infrequently after the final decision to execute has been made. It is at this point that the forensic psychiatrist is invited to engage in the ethically prohibited participation in a legally authorized execution. The proximity of this participation and the act of killing casts doctors, metaphorically, as hangmen's accomplices.[2]

Even more troublesome is a proposal for 'forensic psychiatry exceptionalism' that should dismay psychiatrists internationally. This notion asserts that a forensic psychiatrist is not a psychiatrist when performing evaluations for a court and thus not bound by the ethical principles formulated by various psychiatric societies. To obfuscate the departure from psychiatric ethics, the forensic psychiatrist is referred to as an 'advocate of justice' or an assistant in 'the administration of justice', or simply as 'an agent of the state'. A leading proponent of this belief stated, 'forensic psychiatrists, however, work in a different ethical framework, one built around the legitimate needs of the justice system'[3] and has suggested calling a forensic psychiatrist a 'forensicist'. This is a dangerous notion that opens the door to any sort of behavior by a physician participating in executions, torture or managed care administration by declaring in this role 'I am not committed to traditional medical ethics'. This notion has had its application in the state of Illinois, USA, where legislation permits physicians to participate in executions, including injection of lethal substances, without losing their license, because in that role they are not acting as physicians and are not subject to the ethical constraints of physicians.

Equally perturbing is the issue of psychiatric treatment that restores competence to be executed. The prohibition against this sort of treatment has been weakened by permitting interventions in the case of 'extreme suffering' without adequately defining suffering; thus relief of suffering could be facilely invoked by psychiatrists or prison physicians to effectuate the restoration of competence and facilitate execution. In 1992 the Royal College of Psychiatrists published guidelines for the situation where the necessity of intervention and treatment are compelling in which it was stated 'on no account should the psychiatrist agree to state, after treatment that the person is fit for execution'. In the state of Maryland, USA, the sentence of a seriously mentally ill death-row inmate who requires treatment is commuted to life imprisonment without parole. This is a wise procedure that should be made universal.

Psychiatrists today are indeed torn between traditional ethical principles and strong pressures from society, particularly certain segments of the legal profession, to make compromises and become collaborators in the demands of the law. Rather than look for compromises, one must adhere to traditional concepts. Psychiatrists and other physicians must join in the struggle to uphold ethical and moral principles or they will in time reap a whirlwind of public condemnation. When confronted with major changes in the ethical guidelines promulgated by the American Medical Association, the American Psychiatric Association Board of Trustees in July 1995 deferred action in order to have the components of the American Psychiatric Association enter into discussion and hold a debate on the subject in San Diego in May 1997. So far, the issue remains unresolved. We are gratified that further American Psychiatric Association review is under way, and the Council on Ethical and Judicial Affairs of the American Medical Association has been requested by its House of Delegates to reconsider its position in regard to the issue of psychiatrists' participation in legally authorized executions.

While some may wish to redefine themselves as 'agents of the state', such rationalizations constitute complicity in immoral and unethical behavior.

References

1   Freedman AM, Halpern AL. The erosion of ethics and morality in medicine: physician participation in legal executions in the United States. *NY Law School Law Rev* 1996; **41**:169–188.

2   Bloche MG. Psychiatry, capital punishment and the purposes of medicine. *Int J Law Psychiatry* 1993; **16**:301–357.

3   Appelbaum PS. *A theory of ethics for forensic psychiatry: Presidential Address in Abstract of the 27th Annual Meeting of the American Academy of Psychiatry and the Law.* Bloomfield, CT: APPL; 1996.

* Freedman, A. and Halpern, A.: Forum – Psychiatrists and the death penalty: some ethical dilemmas. a crisis in the ethical and moral behaviors of psychiatrists. *Current Opinion in Psychiatry* **11**:1–2, 1998.

Forum – Psychiatrists and the Death Penalty: Some Ethical Dilemmas

Comments*

John Gunn, Lawrence Hartmann, Edmund D. Pellegrino, Richard J. Bonnie, M. Gregg Bloche, Paul S. Appelbaum, Marianne Kastrup, Ahmed Okasha and Juan J. López-Ibor

In 1975 a working group from the Regional Office for Europe of the WHO met in Siena, Italy. The subject for discussion was forensic psychiatry. The discussion inevitably embraced ethical matters. One of the important conclusions from the meeting was that 'general medical ethics applied to forensic psychiatry in exactly the same way as they apply to other parts of the medical profession and, in particular, a forensic psychiatrist should see his first duty as to his patient, and should *not* operate as a part of the state control systems'.

Contemporaneously there were persistent allegations that political dissidents in the Soviet Union were locked up as mentally abnormal and were 'treated' with psychotropic drugs in order to change their opinions.[1,2]

The Soviet Union was forced to resign from the World Psychiatric Association for a few years because of this pressure. Eventually the Soviet government allowed western observers to inspect their hospitals. The USA sent an official delegation in 1989. A further visit was conducted in 1991 on behalf of the World Psychiatric Association. This team was chaired by James Birley from the UK and included Loren Roth, the medical leader of the previous US delegation.

Different concerns have led to pressure on the Japanese government.[3,4] From 1968, reports of violence to patients, including patient deaths, began to emerge. In 1984 the director of a Japanese hospital was sent to prison for putting profits before patient care. Totsuka and his group campaigned via the United Nations Commission on Human Rights and in 1988 a new Mental Health Act became law in Japan.

In such ethical matters, many of us look to the USA for support and for leadership. The USA has a remarkable written constitution (the oldest in the world) based on liberal principles and is genuinely democratic. In this context it is difficult for European people, who have (with the notable exception of some countries of the old USSR) effectively given up the death penalty, to understand why a civilised nation indulges in the ritualised cold-blooded killing of individuals it has cast out from its midst. It is harder still for European doctors to understand a contemporary debate about the involvement of the medical profession in such a process. It is widely assumed that, should the worst happen and capital punishment were reintroduced into western European countries, the medical profession would set its face against such a political catastrophe and not partake in it. Surely, the public would expect nothing less from the medical profession. The public knows that doctors are bound by the ethics of their profession to comfort, to try to preserve life, and to never harm anyone. The privileges, the responsibilities, the status of medical practice, come from a clear understanding that this is what doctors are like, and that if individuals lapse from these high standards they will be, in one way or another, disciplined within their own profession or may be ejected from it.

From the eastern shore of the Atlantic ocean, therefore, the debate which has been going on for some time in the USA and which is so well encapsulated in the Freedman and Halpern article, seems almost incomprehensible. It is difficult to get all the nuances of this debate from afar, and even visits to the USA do not completely clarify the matter as this is essentially an internal American grief. To some extent, non-Americans feel like helpless bystanders hoping that Uncle Sam, or at least Uncle Sam's doctor, will soon come to his senses so that he can join, once again, with the rest of the medical profession in the world to try to defeat the distortions of medicine which can so easily occur when it is hijacked for nefarious purposes.

News is emerging that suggests doctors in China are now active as executioners.[5] It has been reported that one doctor is experimenting with various cocktails, such as a veterinarian would use to put down a pet dog, to find alternatives to the firing squad provided, of course, they do not interfere with the sale of the offender's organs to Hong Kong for transplantation!

The world medical fraternity needs to stand shoulder to shoulder to speak out against such misuse of medical science and the misuse of medical practitioners. Yet, any kind of world protest against China would probably be ineffective and useless without the weight and influence of the medical profession from the USA. US doctors cannot wholeheartedly and properly join in with such a campaign while they are themselves giving approval to their own members who collude with executions and whilst they try to find ways to redefine the medical practitioner as a non-medical practitioner or 'forensicist' (an agent of the criminal justice system) when he or she is involved with legal processes.

It is time to restate the 1975 Siena principles[6] and to have these endorsed worldwide. Not just in the interests of patients (although that is paramount), but also in the interests of the medical profession. A profession which strays from the high ideals expected of it will, ultimately, not be tolerated by its paymaster, the public.

References

1   **Bloch S, Reddaway P**. *Russia's political hospitals: the abuse of psychiatry in the Soviet Union*. London: Gollancz; 1977.

2   **Lader M**. *Psychiatry on trial*. Harmondsworth: Penguin; 1977.

3   **Totsuka E, Mitsulshi T, Kitamura Y**. Mental health and human rights: illegal detention in Japan. In: Carni A, Schneider S, Hafez A (editors): *Psychiatry, law and ethics*. Berlin: Springer-Verlag; 1986.

4   **Harding TW**. Ethical issues in the delivery of mental health services: abuses in Japan. In: Bloch S, Chodoff P (editors): *Psychiatric ethics.* 2nd ed. Oxford: Oxford University Press; 1991.

5   **Sheridan M**. Doctors are China's new executioners. *The Sunday Times* 1997, 5 October, p. 26.

6   World Health Organisation. *Forensic psychiatry. Report of a Working Group, Siena 1975.* Copenhagen: WHO; 1977.

John Gunn

I agree fully with Freedman and Halpern and the World Psychiatric Association 1996 Declaration of Madrid that stated 'under no circumstances should psychiatrists participate in legally authorised executions nor participate in assessments of competence to be executed'. This position has been argued well, and in far greater detail, by Bloche.[1]

The central issue, I think, is that of participation in execution. To participate too directly in execution creates legitimate exceptions to some medical procedures that are otherwise ethical. To treat psychosis, for instance, is generally ethical, but to treat a prisoner's psychosis so that he or she can be executed is unethical; so is final evaluation of competence to be executed unethical. In countries that allow capital punishment, such as the USA, such evaluation nearly always occurs after much other psychiatric and legal work has been done, and after a prisoner has been sentenced; thus it is, in time and effect, too directly a part of execution to be ethical for a profession that should protect its therapeutic and compassionate aims and its over-riding value of helping and not harming individuals.

Some see the debate on banning final psychiatric evaluation of competence to be executed as a covert debate on capital punishment. Not so. Opposing capital punishment is relevant, but one can be against physician participation in executions whether one favours capital punishment or not. Some see banning such evaluation as likely to embody or lead to less psychiatric care. Again, not so. I think it would probably lead to better, clearer, and more care.

I find the issue of forensic psychiatrist exceptionalism both troublesome and interesting. Appelbaum and others claim that 'the forensic psychiatrist in truth does not act as a physician'. Appelbaum more or less creates a more or less ethic of 'truth' and 'the legitimate needs of the justice system'. Such roles and values clash with ordinary medical ethics, and do and will harm medicine.

I have suggested that if any psychiatrist does carry out evaluations of competence to be executed, he or she should be required to wear a police uniform while doing so to make his or her dominant role clear, not just to the psychiatrist but even to a multiply stressed and often less than clear-headed late-stage prisoner.

When the American Psychiatric Association Board of Trustees yielded to its forensic psychiatrists in 1994 and, after too little debate, changed its position and allowed participation in evaluation of competence to be executed, the Board was not adequately aware that in forensic psychiatry (as in other subspecialty groups such as managed-care-company-executive psychiatrists) the expert subgroup will often have vested interests and values and wishes at odds with the values of the larger whole of psychiatry or medicine.

Reference

1   **Bloche MG**. Psychiatry, capital punishment, and the purposes of medicine. *Int J Law Psychiatry* 1993; **16**:301–357.

Lawrence Hartmann

Freedman and Halpern are thoroughly right in their unequivocal criticism of Appelbaum's twin assertions that[1] psychiatrists judging competency for execution are not practising psychiatry; and that[2] the ethics of medicine as applied to forensic psychiatry should be suited to the needs of the Court.

Both assertions are patently illogical, socially deleterious and utterly corrosive to the integrity of medical ethics.

Psychiatry is not defined by the purposes to which we put it. Competency determinations depend on knowledge and methods developed by, and specific to, psychiatry. The Courts do not have this knowledge. That is why they need psychiatric expertise in the first place. Appelbaum's clumsy euphemism, making the psychiatrist a 'forensicist', is a bizarre and transparent distortion of reality to give benediction to an ethically illicit act.

Similarly, the ethics of medicine (and psychiatry as a branch of medicine) is not defined by convenience, the needs of the state or the purposes to which we wish to put medical knowledge. Medical ethics derives from the universal predicament of human illness, from the vulnerability, dependence and exploitability of those the physician attends. The ends of medicine are healing, helping, comforting and curing. Every physician pledges to serve those ends when she or he enters the profession. Being an accomplice in the death of a human being is totally inconsistent with the ends of medicine. No act of law or fiat can change that fact.

Appelbaum's elastic logic invites the usurpation of medical power in the name of politics and ideology, and not primarily in the interest of the patient. Totalitarian states do so with gross abandon; democracies with more discretion. The result, in either case, is to imperil the most vulnerable members of our society.

Physicians must remain the guardians of the moral integrity of the profession and its ethics. Psychiatrists must heed the ethical proscription against assisting in legal executions enunciated by the World Psychiatric Association. In these times, their witness to the integrity of medical ethics is an assurance that some things are not at the disposal of whim, fancy or political power.

Recommended reading

1   **Pellegrino ED**. Guarding the integrity of medical ethics: some lessons from Soviet Russia. *JAMA* 1995; **273**:1622–1623.

2   **Pellegrino ED**. The Nazi doctors and Nuremberg: some moral lessons revisited. *Ann Intern Med* 1997; **127**:307–308.

Edmund D Pellegrino

Freedman and Halpern should be commended for their dogged efforts to focus professional attention on the ethical ambiguity of forensic psychiatry and, more specifically, on the unique ethical dilemmas raised by medical participation in capital cases. Although I do not agree with their position on evaluations of competence of condemned prisoners, I share many of their concerns.

I want to begin by emphasising that I wholeheartedly agree with Freedman and Halpern about the need for vigilance in maintaining the profession's ethical integrity in the face of political and economic pressures that can undermine public trust in the healing role of the profession. The Nazi experience and the abuses of Soviet psychiatry provide compelling evidence of the dangers to the profession, and to human rights, that arise when the tools of medicine are appropriated to serve the goals of the state. That is why I have joined hands with psychiatrists in the former Soviet Union and other formerly communist nations of central and eastern Europe to help them build the institutional foundations for professional independence, including an autonomous system for promulgating and enforcing ethical norms.[1]

I also agree that medical participation in an execution (as by injecting a fatal dose of barbiturates, selecting injection sites, giving technical advice, or monitoring an injection given by someone else) must be unequivocally prohibited. The American Medical Association and the American Psychiatric Association have condemned such conduct and, as far as I know, nobody within the professional community has argued that it is ethically permissible.

It is helpful to identify the ethical principle that underlies the prohibition against medical participation in executions. Clearly, the objection does not simply lie in the fact that the doctor is serving a non-therapeutic role for the legal system: some non-therapeutic roles are ethically acceptable, for example an assessment of disability for the worker's compensation system or an assessment of competence to stand trial for the criminal justice system. (As these observations suggest, the debate about psychiatric involvement in executions is being carried out in the shadow of a broader controversy concerning the ethical foundations of forensic psychiatry. I will return to this problem below.)

Why, then, is medical participation in executions almost uniformly regarded as unethical? The answer lies not in the logic of therapeutic ethics, but rather in the fundamental idea that serving as an agent of the state's punitive apparatus is not an acceptable social role for a doctor. Doctors should never use their skills or knowledge for the purpose of facilitating punishment. This principle covers all forms of punishment. For example, some painful punishments, such as isolation in dark cells and whipping, are not categorically prohibited under prevailing international standards of human rights and persist in many parts of the world. Medical assessment of a prisoner's fitness for these punishments and medical monitoring of their administration might be characterized as being beneficial to prisoners because it can prevent injury and suffering more extreme than intended or legally authorized. However, medical assistance in the administration of punishments is nonetheless objectionable because doctors must not align themselves with the punitive aims of the state, either in deciding whether a particular punishment should be carried out or in administering it or directing how it should be administered. So, too, participation in an execution must be categorically forbidden.

Unfortunately, the issue of competence assessment is not so easy to resolve. In some situations, such an assessment would seem to be ethically unacceptable on the same theory I have just outlined. Suppose, for example, that a psychiatrist is assessing the mental status of a condemned prisoner for the sole purpose of telling the warden or director of the prison whether the prisoner is 'fit' to be executed. Such an assessment should be forbidden because it aligns the psychiatrist with the execution, implicating him in the process as if he of she had given the 'ok' for the execution to go ahead. This is similar to the prohibition against a doctor observing a prisoner being whipped and saying whether he is 'fit' to receive any additional lashes.

But consider a different context. Suppose a lawyer representing the condemned prisoner asks a psychiatrist to assess his client's mental state for the purpose of ascertaining whether the mentally disturbed prisoner has the capacity to understand the nature, purpose and consequences of the impending execution. Suppose further that, if the psychiatrist concludes that the prisoner's competence-related abilities are impaired, a hearing on the issue will be held in court, and that the decision whether to stay the execution will be made by a judge. First, the examination is being requested on behalf of the condemned prisoner to ascertain whether there is a clinical basis for raising a legal barrier to an execution that would otherwise occur. Second, the psychiatrist is serving as an expert, not a decision maker.

I recognise that it can still be argued, as Freedman and Halpern do, that the psychiatrist's assessment of the condemned prisoner's competence is so intimately connected with the execution itself that it should be forbidden. However, it can also be argued (as I have done elsewhere)[2] that the psychiatric assessment of competence in this situation does not differ in principle from pretrial forensic assessment of a capital defendant's competence to stand trial and that testifying on the prisoner's competence does not differ in principle from testifying in a capital sentence hearing. In all these settings, testimony by the psychiatrist can be used to establish a legally necessary predicate for a capital conviction and a death sentence. If forensic participation in the earlier stages of a capital case is ethical (and, in the USA, psychiatrists routinely participate in capital cases), a properly structured assessment of competence for execution would also seem to be ethically acceptable, as long as the process is invoked on the prisoner's behalf and as long as the ultimate decision maker is a judge. This approach

to the issue may not be indisputable, but it has been embraced by the American Psychiatric Association after years of consideration and debate. I fear that Freedman and Halpern have misinterpreted the Association's careful deliberation over a genuinely difficult issue as an unprincipled abdication of the profession's prerogatives to the legal profession.

Specialists in psychiatric ethics also disagree about the conditions, if any, under which it is ethically permissible to treat a condemned prisoner whose deteriorated mental condition may preclude the execution. Some say that a condemned prisoner should never be treated if a possible effect of the treatment is to restore competence and thereby remove a legal barrier to an execution. Others (including myself)[3] argue that such a categorical prohibition is too sweeping. Of course it is unethical to treat a prisoner for the sole purpose of facilitating an execution but, under some circumstances, treatment may be necessary to alleviate a prisoner's torment and suffering. The ethical permissibility of treatment under such circumstances can be demonstrated by imagining (as an heuristic device) that a condemned prisoner, while competent, has executed an advance directive requesting restorative treatment from his own doctor even if one possible consequence of such treatment would be to increase the likelihood of execution. Would it be unethical to treat the prisoner under these circumstances? By asking this question, I do not mean to encourage prisons to seek advance treatment directives from condemned prisoners. I mean only to show that therapeutic ethics may sometimes permit, or even require, treatment of the condemned prisoner. Freedman and Halpern seem to concede the ethical permissibility, in principle, of treatment to alleviate extreme suffering, but they rest their objection on the possibility that devious prison psychiatrists could invoke this 'vague' exception to justify unethical efforts to facilitate executions. I suppose there is a risk of such abuses, but I think it would be preferable to scrutinise such situations if they arise in practice rather than adopt an admittedly overinclusive ethical prohibition.

Having highlighted an area of continuing disagreement, I want to emphasise two points on which I completely agree with Freedman and Halpern. The issue of treating condemned prisoners puts doctors in an ethical bind. The only sensible way out of the dilemma is for the law to require commutation of the death sentences of prisoners who have been found by a court to be incompetent for execution. Also, even if the possibility of execution remains, the psychiatrist responsible for treatment should play no role whatsoever in the process of competence evaluations; as in other contexts, therapeutic and evaluative roles should be completely separated.

I want to close by emphasising, once again, that I applaud Freedman and Halpern for their vigorous efforts to generate ethical discussion of these issues. At the same time, however, I must also note my suspicion that many physicians who condemn execution competence evaluations are either morally opposed to the death penalty, or have deep ethical qualms about forensic psychiatry. For the record, I will note my own opposition to capital punishment. In my experience, lawyers, judges, doctors, and anyone else who participates in the administration of the death penalty inevitably become mired in ethical quicksand. Unfortunately, professional efforts to evade the quicksand tend to erode the rights and interests of defendants and condemned prisoners. The death penalty should be abolished, but as long as it remains in force neither psychiatric assessment of condemned prisoners nor treatment of incompetent ones should be categorically forbidden.

As for forensic psychiatry, I think Freedman and Halpern have mischaracterized the terms of the debate about the ethics of forensic psychiatry. Nobody argues that psychiatrists serving forensic roles are not bound by psychiatric ethics. What Appelbaum and others have argued, correctly in my view, is that the ethical principles governing forensic psychiatry cannot be derived from the therapeutic ethic that governs that physician – patient relationship. The challenge is to formulate principles that are designed to govern this particular social role (and so, too, with other social roles) while being rooted in the professional aspirations of medicine, and while forbidding the sorts of abuses that arise when doctors surrender their professional identity and allow themselves to become agents of the state. Freedman and Halpern would serve the profession better by helping to frame the ethic of forensic psychiatry rather then by denying the need to undertake the task.

References

1   Polubinskaya SV, Bonnie RJ. The code of professional ethics of the Russian Society of Psychiatrists: text and commentary. *Int J Law Psychiatry* 1996; **19**:143–172.

2   Bonnie RJ. The death penalty: when doctors must say no. *BMJ* 1992; **305**:381–383.

3   Bonnie RJ. Healing-killing conflicts: medical ethics and the death penalty. *Hastings Center Report* 1990; **20**:12–18.

Richard J Bonnie

More than any other specialty, psychiatry is enmeshed in conflict between the expectations of patients and society. The role of US psychiatry in the determination and restoration of competence for execution presents this conflict in particularly stark form.

The acrimony that characterises the international debate over this role reflects the larger failure of medical ethics discourse to address, in realistic fashion, the tension between physicians' obligations to their patients and their societies. To be sure, some criticism of this role stems from opposition to the death penalty. But the animating ideas behind most such criticism are the Hippocratic ethic of undivided loyalty to patients and the classic injunction, *primum non nocere*.

In practice, we routinely depart from these ideals, and traditional medical ethics offers us no guidance when we do so.[1] Society maintains contradictory private and public expectations of medicine.[2] As patients, we expect doctors to keep faith with us in moments of medical need, and we take offense when they fail to do so. Yet as citizens, we condition myriad rights, duties, and opportunities upon people's physical and mental health status, and we thereby ask of medicine that it serve multiple gatekeeping functions. Employment opportunities, eligibility for disability benefits,[3] military service obligations,[4] criminal responsibility, child custody, access to abortion,[5] and ability to make contracts are among the matters that often hinge on medical evaluation and treatment.

Forensic psychiatrists earn their living by trying to meet these latter, public expectations, even when doing so results in harm to the people they attend. Their clinical work on death row, when competence for execution is at stake, poses this contradiction with singular poignancy. But this contradiction suffuses all of forensic practice – and all other exercises of clinical judgement for purposes other than patient care. Thus, the controversy over psychiatric involvement in capital punishment resonates far beyond death row. In this sense, Freedman and Halpern are on to something important in identifying a 'crisis' in the ethics of psychiatry.

Should we, then, condemn as unethical all clinical work that serves the state or society or some other third party at the expense of the well being of individual patients or clinical subjects? In rejecting 'compromises' that make physicians into 'collaborators in the demands of the law', Freedman and Halpern suggest this. But to do so would be to demand that the medical profession dismiss society's expressions of need in this regard. The pervasive import of health status in legitimate decision-making about rights, duties and opportunities renders this absolutist position unrealistic.

What, then, of the claim advanced by some forensic psychiatrists, most recently in connection with capital punishment, that the physician who serves the state and/or the legal system 'in truth does not act as a physician'[6] and thus need not worry about the Hippocratic duty to keep faith with patients and avoid doing them harm? The recurring appeal of this claim – and its greatest danger – lies in the escape it offers from discomfort occasioned by tension between state expectations and the Hippocratic tradition. To their credit, European forensic psychiatrists have rejected this claim, preferring instead to acknowledge the moral turbulence this tension creates. US forensic practitioners have also generally eschewed this easy answer in favor of the search for balance between their commitments to the justice system and to patient well being.[7]

By acknowledging both of these commitments, and the tension between them, forensic psychiatrists accept a healthy measure of restraint on their service to the state. A lack of such restraint opens the way for such abuses as the use of psychiatry to suppress dissent in the former USSR and the attendance of physicians at executions by lethal injection in the USA. The proposition that physicians who serve the state do not act as physicians is also at odds with the state's reasons for calling upon them. Legal systems look to forensic psychiatry when rights or duties turn on mental health status. Clinical evaluations that bear upon rights and duties make use of medical concepts and categories.

To the extent that these exercises of medical judgement result in harm to clinical subjects, they risk undermining society's expectations about the benevolent use of medical skill. They also violate the expectations of forensic examinees. Even is the psychiatrist clearly says, in advance, that an evaluation will be put to legal use, other, non-cognitive cues confound the examinee's understanding. His or her belief in medical benevolence is unlikely to disappear after such disclosure; on the contrary, the dynamic of transference in the clinical setting may well encourage it. Indeed, that most crucial of clinical skills – empathic connection with the evaluee – invites trusting feelings that do not reflect the examiner's forensic purposes.

Ethically sensitive forensic practitioners are uncomfortably aware of these difficulties. Neither rigid insistence on the wrongfulness of clinical work that causes harm nor categorical refusal to admit the ethical relevance of such harm moves us toward their resolution. The controversy over clinical ethics on death row presents an opportunity for more productive exploration of this larger problem. In this regard, reports that some US forensic psychiatrists, including Appelbaum, tried behind-the-scenes to reverse US organised medicine's opposition to physician assessment of competence for execution[8] are troubling. Their effort briefly prevailed within the American Psychiatric Association. However, objections by many leading US psychiatrists and ethicists, including Freedman, Halpern, and Hartmann, prompted the Association to revisit the question.

The larger challenge before us is to accommodate psychiatrists' conflicting obligations to their patients and their societies in a manner that respects both the social significance of health status and the fragility of physicians' therapeutic credibility. I have argued elsewhere, in some detail, that such an accommodation requires that we bar clinical work on the state's behalf when it too provocatively and dramatically breaks with society's faith in doctors' benevolence.[9] I believe the case against psychiatric involvement in the determination and restoration of competence for execution can best be stated in these terms.[10]

References

1   Stone AA. *Law, psychiatry and morality*. Washington DC: American Psychiatric Association Press; 1984.

2   Bloche MG. Menschenrechte und die problematik der todesstrafe. *Deutsches Arzteblatt* 1996; **93**:172–175.

3   Mashaw JL. *Bureaucratic justice: managing social security disability claims*. New Haven: Yale University Press; 1983.

4   Halleck SL. *The politics of therapy*. New York: Science; 1971.

5   Bloche MG. The 'gag rule' revisited: physicians as abortion gatekeepers. *Law Med Health Care* 1992; **20**:392–402.

6   Appelbaum PS. The parable of the forensic psychiatrist: ethics and the problem of doing harm. *Int J Law Psychiatry* 1990; **13**:249–259.

7   American Psychiatric Association. *A report of the Task Force on the Role of Psychiatry in the Sentencing Process*. Washington DC: American Psychiatric Association Press; 1984.

8   Rothstein DC. Psychiatrists' involvement in executions: arriving at an official position. *Newsletter Am Acad Psychiatry Law* 1995; **20**:15–17. Appelbaum PS. Letter to Dr David Orentlicher (American Medical Association Ethics and Health Policy Council). 17 September 1993.

9   Bloche MG. Psychiatry, capital punishment, and the purposes of medicine. *Int J Law Psychiatry* 1993; **16**:301–357.

10 American College of Physicians. Human Rights Watch, Physicians for Human Rights, and the National Coalition to Abolish the Death Penalty. *Breach of trust: physician participation in executions in the United States*. 1994.

M. Gregg Bloche

Is there a crisis in the ethics of US psychiatry? As managed care challenges physicians' traditional fidelity to patients' interests by encouraging them to place their own economic interests first, there may well be. But the notion of Freedman and Halpern that the crisis has been provoked by psychiatrists' evaluations of death row prisoners whose competence has been questioned would surely surprise most psychiatrists in the USA. Some background on the issue will reveal why.

Thirty-eight of the USA's 50 states allow the death penalty to be imposed, generally for homicide committed under aggravated circumstances. Under US constitutional law, however, prisoners cannot be executed if they are legally incompetent.[1] Generally that requirement has been interpreted to mean that prisoners who fail to understand the nature of the punishment and the reason for its imposition must be spared from execution. In one state (Maryland), such prisoners have their sentences commuted to life in prison and in another (Louisland), if the state elects to treat the prisoner's incapacity, it can never carry out the death sentence. Although no centralised statistics are kept, evaluations of prisoners' competence to be executed appear to be quite uncommon.

What is it that troubles Freedman and Halpern? They believe that psychiatrists should not participate in evaluations of the competence of death row prisoners. Why they take that stance is not made terribly clear in their piece, other than the assertion that such evaluations constitute physician participation in execution – something that no one believes is ethically permissible. It is worth noting that their view is not supported by the official bodies charged with developing ethical standards for US medicine in general, and psychiatry in particular. The Council on Ethical and Judicial Affairs of the American Medical Association, after studying the issue for years, concluded that conducting such evaluations was not equivalent to participating in an execution. Indeed, '... without physician participation, [incompetent] individuals might be punished unjustifiably'.[2] This conclusion was supported by the American Medical Association's House of Delegates and Board. Similarly, the American Psychiatric Association's Committee on Ethics ruled that it was permissible for psychiatrists to engage in competence evaluations.[3]

These conclusions are consonant with a reasoned view of the psychiatrist's role in competence evaluations. After assessing the prisoner's capacities, the psychiatrist testifies at a competence hearing regarding his or her conclusions. Other evidence is heard, as well, typically from prison guards and others who have been in contact with the prisoner. The determination regarding the prisoner's competence is left to the official decision maker, usually a judge. Taking part in this process is simply incommensurate with participation in execution.

Not only are such evaluations ethically permissible, but it is the very ban that Freedman and Halpern propose that would create impossible ethical dilemmas for psychiatrists. Envision a psychiatrist treating a prisoner on death row. The psychiatrist believes that the prisoner is psychotic or demented to the point where competence may be in question. As the prisoner is withdrawn and not overtly disruptive, no one else seems to notice. Under the rule proposed by Freedman and Halpern, the psychiatrist would have to stand by silently (because formally evaluating or testifying about a prisoner's competence would be forbidden) and watch the incompetent prisoner go to his death. How anybody could believe that such behavior is ethically justifiable is incomprehensible.

What, then, lies behind efforts to elevate an infrequently performed evaluation, agreed to be ethical by the professional groups that have studied it most closely, to the level of a 'crisis' in medical ethics? The death penalty evokes strong feelings among both its supporters and its opponents. Understandably, many opponents will seek any argument available to attempt to delegitimize the process. But it is manifestly unfair to psychiatrists and to death row prisoners themselves to use them as pawns in a game of political posturing over the use of the death penalty.

Although it is not clear from Freedman's and Halpern's piece, it should be noted that no one involved in this debate – not the American Medical Association, the American Psychiatric Association, nor me – argues that psychiatrists should treat persons found incompetent to be executed so that the sentence can be carried out. That is not at issue here. As for my views on the ethics of forensic psychiatry as a whole, which are misstated by Freedman and Halpern, I have addressed this issue at length elsewhere and refer the interested reader to that discussion.[4]

References

1 **Ford v Wainwright**, 106 S.Ct.2595 (1986).

2 Council on Ethical and Judicial Affairs: *Report 6-A-95, Physician participation in capital punishment: evaluations of prisoner competence to be executed; treatment to restore competence to be executed.* American Medical Association; 1995.

3 American Psychiatric Association: *Opinions of the ethics committee.* Washington DC: American Psychiatric Association; 1996.

4 **Appelbaum PS**: A theory of ethics for forensic psychiatry. *J Am Acad Psychiatry Law* 1997; **25**:233–247.

Paul S. Appelbaum

Medical involvement in the death penalty has, until recently, been an issue that has not received sufficient recognition. Within Amnesty International, a Medical Group against the Death Penalty has been established, with the main objective of fighting against the death penalty by increasing the public's – and in particular physicians' awareness of the issue. This group, located in Denmark, publishes a regular newsletter and has published a number of papers over the years[1–3] on different aspects of the role of doctors, including psychiatrists,[4] in the death penalty.

Among psychiatrists, Appelbaum[5] has highlighted areas of concern to psychiatrists in relation to the death penalty for more than 10 years but has been standing relatively alone in the US debate. Therefore, the recent article by Freedman and Halpern[6] and the present forum are very welcome. Freedman and Halpern mention the clear stand of the World Psychiatric Association in the Declaration of Madrid and the guidelines for specific situations, including the participation of psychiatrists in the death penalty. However, the World Psychiatric Association had previously issued a statement in 1989 in which it is considered a violation of professional ethics for psychiatrists to participate in any action connected to executions. Thus, there is no doubt about the position of the World Psychiatric Association when it comes to the participation of psychiatrists in capital punishment.

Freedman and Halpern focus in particular on the question of competence to be executed, and testimony regarding both competence to be executed and treatment to restore competence. Other aspects also deserve mention, including the role and capacity of psychiatrists in assessing future dangerousness.[4] Here, psychiatric evidence may be influential and indeed play a key role in the jury's decision to vote for the death penalty. Finally, the whole issue of psychiatric problems on death row deserves further attention. This must include the problems present in prisoners on death row as well as the problems that are caused by the conditions on death row.

The death penalty is an issue of concern for the psychiatric community and, as such, further recognition is justified.

References

1 **Kastrup M**. Henrettelse af psykisk syge og psykisk handicappede. (Execution of the mentally ill and handicapped.) *Ugeskr Læg* 1989; **151**:1629.

2 **Kastrup M**. Psykiaterens rolle i dødsstrafsager. (The psychiatrist's role in cases of death penalty.) *Ugeskr Læg* 1989; **151**:2164.

3 **Kastrup M**. Fremtidig farlughed og dødsstraf. (Future dangerousness and the death penalty.) *Ugeskr Læg* 1989; **151**:3273.

4 **Kastrup M**. Psychiatry and the death penalty. *J Med Ethics* 1988; **14**:179–183.

5   Appelbaum P. Competence to be executed: another conundrum for mental health professionals. *Hosp Comm Psychiatry* 1986; **37**:682–684.

6   Freedman AM, Halpern AL. The erosion of ethics and morality in medicine: physician participation in legal executions in the United States. *NY Law School Law Rev* 1996; **41**:169–188.

Marianne Kastrup

Issues in the relationship between law and psychiatry were present in ancient Greece and Rome over 2000 years ago. The evolution of this relationship cannot be seen as a process of accumulating medical knowledge being made available to the legal system. Nor can it be understood in terms of new legal concepts progressively influencing medicine and, later, psychiatry. Rather, law and psychiatry were subject to mutual adjustments and a continuous exchange of knowledge, techniques and objectives. Over the centuries, the two disciplines seem to have followed general shifts between the care of the individual and the protection of society. Their encounter always brings us back to the duality that exists between our conflicting conceptions of the value of health on the one hand, and our conception of liberty, integrity and autonomy on the other.

The main objective of any physician, the psychiatrist being no exception, is to alleviate suffering and improve the quality of life of patients to allow a better existence. To alleviate suffering and to cure the patient to be competent for execution is against medical ethics. I am privileged to chair the Ethics Committee of the World Psychiatric Association and, with its members, have produced the Declaration of Madrid and the special guidelines for specific situations. The paragraph on the death penalty states that 'Under no circumstances should psychiatrists participate in legally authorised execution, nor participate in assessments of competence to be executed'. The declaration was unanimously endorsed by the World Psychiatric Association General Assembly in 1996. The proposal to exclude forensic psychiatrists from this commitment, on the basis that they are advocates of justice or an assistant in the administration of justice, i.e. simply an agent of the state, is ethically unacceptable.

Freedman and Halpern state that 'equally perturbing is the issue of psychiatric treatment that restores competence to be executed', allowing intervention in the case of extreme suffering. Here I beg to differ that we should intervene in case of severe suffering from psychotic symptoms or self destructive behaviour, considering that the time between sentencing and actual execution could extend for years, and that court sentences can and are usually proceeded. However, I do agree with the guidelines of the Royal College of Psychiatrists (1992): On no account should the psychiatrist agree to state, after treatment, that the person is fit for execution.

This commitment constitutes a component of the codes of ethics of several national and international medical organisations the World Medical Association, World Psychiatrist Association. American College of Physicians, British Medical Association, Roval College of Psychiatrists and the American Psychiatric Association.

Almed Obasha

There are two peculiarities in the US legal system which may wrongly lead readers to think that the issue raised by Freedman and Halpern may not be of significant interest worldwide.

The first aspect is that the death penalty exists in some states in the USA and the problems are different where it does not. When a psychiatric patient commits an offence and is condemned to death, the insanity defence becomes a life saving issue. Where the death penalty does not exist it can be argued that long term sentences in jail or in a mental institution are equivalent: especially now that psychological rehabilitation is provided in many prisons where is mental hospitals have deteriorated in many countries. It may even be better to have a limited prison sentence than to be an inmate of a mental institution without time limitation. Nevertheless, the institutional setting is essential for the job of professionals and an adequate doctor patient relationship and treatment and rehabilitation procedures are difficult to carry out to prison.

The second peculiarity of the US legal system, and of Anglo-Saxon countries in general, is that the emphasis is placed on procedural law rather than the normative law. The latter is standard in other countries, especially those where Roman Law prevails (France, Italy, Spain and Latin American countries). In normative law, the involvement of psychiatrists and other professionals as court experts seems to be easier and is carried out from a certain distance and with little involvement. The expert has two roles: the first is clinical diagnosis of the patient, the second is to evaluate the effects of the derangement of the patient's mind on the offence being judged.

Two recent cases in Spain help to clarify these points. In both there was an absence of mental disorders but psychiatrists were called to study the accused. In the first, one of a group of adolescents playing a game called 'role' brutally killed a sweeper in the early hours of the morning. The game involves the adoption of the role of different people during a normal day and this group adopted the role of 'vigilantes' or 'racial cleaners' liberating society from weak, old and foreign people. After a few failed attempts the group found the sweeper, aged, fat, and perhaps ugly looking, at night. During the trial there was a struggle between the psychologists and psychiatrists. The latter were unable to bring forward their argument as none of those involved in the crime, particularly the leader, fulfilled criteria for any psychiatric diagnosis. The psychologists, without the burden of having to provide a psychiatric diagnosis, were much more able to make a description of the personality of the accused and to suggest that they should be considered fully responsible. The psychiatrists, who were appointed by relatives of the accused, supported the notion that the accused were not responsible for their actions based on weak diagnostic formulations. In fact, they were trying an insanity defence without insanity being present. Here the pressures came not from the judicial system itself, but from one of the parties involved.

The other case, in which I participated along with another professor of psychiatry, involved a former head of the police forces in Spain who was accused of corruption and other similar offences. The image of this man in the press and the descriptions by his colleagues in the government as well as his own political party described him as being full of evil and as a psychopath or mentally abnormal person. The study of this person revealed no psychiatric disease and produced a detailed description of his personality and circumstances. The trial is ongoing, but the expert report was able to change the public perception of the accused. Removal of the stigma of mental illness also releases mental patients from the stigma of other social factors.

The lesson from Freedman's and Halpern's paper is that a psychiatrist should, in any circumstance, behave as a psychiatrist and only as a psychiatrist. A thorough reading of the Declaration of Madrid makes the task of psychiatrists more demanding even in circumstances not as extreme as those described by Freedman and Halpern.

Juan J López-lbor

Forum – Psychiatrists and the Death Penalty: Some Ethical Dilemmas

Response*

Alfred M. Freedman and Abraham L. Halpern

We wish to thank all our colleagues who have taken the time to respond with comments to our article 'A crisis in the ethical and moral behavior of psychiatrists'. The issues raised in both the article and the commentaries have broad implications and ramifications beyond psychiatry and medicine extending to ethical and moral issues of contemporary society. Thus, discussion can only bring enlightenment in this critical area. We are confident that this aim is well served by the extremely insightful and pertinent observations of the commentators.

Unfortunately, in his comment, Appelbaum does not directly respond to our quoting of his statement delivered at the Annual Meeting of the American Academy of Psychiatry and the Law in 1996, namely that 'forensic psychiatrists, however, work in a different ethical framework, one built around the legitimate needs of the justice system'. This notion of forensic exceptionalism is the cornerstone of Appelbaum's arguments and the justification of the sharp departure from psychiatric ethics. This concept that he has put forward in numerous articles, including the one he refers to in his commentary, implies that in the court-related situation the psychiatrist is no longer a psychiatrist but an 'advocate of justice', an assistant in 'the administration of justice', or a 'forensicist' no longer bound by the ethical principles to which psychiatrists are committed. We strongly agree with the statement in Pellegrino's comment that Appelbaum's idea is 'patently illogical, socially deleterious and utterly corrosive to the integrity of medical ethics'.

In a recent article, by Stone of the Harvard Medical and Law Schools,[1] the departure of some forensic psychiatrists from a strong commitment to preserve confidentiality to acquiescence of a break of confidentiality in court is deplored. Stone attributes this to a need to conform to the needs of the court. We agree, but believe it is an outcome of the above idea that the forensic psychiatrist is no longer a psychiatrist but an agent of the court. Adherence to the ethics of confidentiality is no longer necessary. Forensic psychiatry will suffer immeasurably for this surrender.

Appelbaum cites the report of the Ethics Committee of the American Psychiatric Association (APA) on 17 February 1996, but fails to mention the clearest statement included in this otherwise ambiguous report, namely that '. . . psychiatrists are physicians and physicians are physicians at all times'.

It must be mentioned further that at the June 1997 meeting of the American Medical Association (AMA), the New York State delegation introduced modifications of the 1995 report of the AMA Council on Ethical and Judicial Affairs (which was referred to by Appelbaum). The modifications were sent to the Council for reconsideration. Therefore, this whole issue is still in a state of flux and neither the APA nor the AMA has an unquestioned position at this time.

Both Bonnie and Appelbaum imply that our objection to physician participation in executions is a covert maneuver to discredit and eliminate

capital punishment. There is no such effort as the issue of capital punishment is, as indicated by Hartmann, unrelated to physician participation. It is noteworthy that when we were collecting signatures at an APA meeting to oppose approval of psychiatrists' participation, a number of those who signed stated that although they were in favor of capital punishment they were strongly opposed to physician participation.

In the matter of treatment of a condemned prisoner's 'extreme suffering', we are gratified that Bonnie agrees with us that the law should require commutation of the death sentence in such cases. Beyond that, however, in the interests of a truly sensible and rational way out of the dilemma, we have made no secret of our strong support for the abolition of capital punishment. We applaud the American Bar Association's call, in February 1997, for a moratorium on capital punishment in the USA. (The reasons given include racially discriminatory application of the death penalty, the grossly inadequate legal representation of the defendants and the restriction on appeals to the federal courts even in cases where new evidence is presented that points to the innocence of the condemned prisoner.) We have also repeatedly endorsed the 1969 resolution of the Board of Trustees of the APA calling for the abolition of the death penalty and declaring that 'the best available scientific and expert opinion holds it to be anachronistic, brutalizing, ineffective and contrary to progress in penology and forensic psychiatry'. We must say, again, that we are quite distressed that both Bonnie and Appelbaum imply that we condemn execution competency evaluations solely because we are morally opposed to the death penalty. It has been our purpose to give indisputably realistic meaning to the ethical canon that prohibits participation by physicians in legally authorized executions and we are gratified that the World Psychiatric Association has clearly proclaimed that psychiatric assessments of competency to be executed fall within the ambit of ethically unacceptable conduct. There is reason to believe that our view in this regard is shared even by physicians who hold that capital punishment has a place in civilized society.

We note that 21 death row prisoners in the USA were exonerated by the courts between 1993 and 1997. These findings of innocence were arrived at over a period of 7 years in almost all of the cases. With the defunding of many federal post-conviction defender organisations last year, the limitations on appeal petitions and the broadening of the federal death penalty, we can expect an acceleration in the number of executions, including the executions of innocent persons. Obviously, there is a distinct risk that psychiatrists will examine innocent prisoners and declare them competent for execution. Unlike Appelbaum, we see this as a crisis.

Bonnie declares that the assessment of a condemned prisoner's competence to be executed, 'for the sole purpose of telling the warden or director of the prison whether or not the person is "fit" to be executed', is ethically unacceptable. He nevertheless accepts as ethically sound for a psychiatrist to assess, at the request of a lawyer representing the condemned prisoner, whether the mentally disturbed prisoner 'has the capacity to understand the nature, purpose and consequences of the impending execution'. What

* Freedman, A. and Halpern, A.: Forum – Psychiatrists and the death penalty: some ethical dilemmas. a crisis in the ethical and moral behaviors of psychiatrists. *Current Opinion in Psychiatry* 11:1–2, 1998.

Bonnie fails to understand is that this ostensibly altruistic participation 'on behalf of the condemned prisoner' at once opens the door for the 'decision-maker' to invite psychiatrists to evaluate the prisoner's competence and arrive at an assessment contrary to what the prisoner's lawyer desires, with the result that the decision-maker is then free to declare that the execution should take place. This is not merely a theoretical possibility. The recent execution of Pedro L Medina in Florida is a case in point. Here, according to his attorney to whom we spoke, three psychiatrists had been appointed by the Governor to examine Mr Medina to determine his competency to be executed. They all agreed he was competent and was malingering. An appeal was filed with the Circuit Court judge who appointed three experts – they all found the inmate to be severely psychotic and not malingering. The judge then appointed two psychiatrists who said that Mr Medina, although 'eating his feces and talking crazy', was faking. The lawyer appealed to the judge to send Medina to the state hospital for treatment and/or reassessment. The judge refused and the execution was carried out. (As an additional macabre point of interest, we were told by the lawyer, who witnessed the execution, that two doctors examined the prisoner after the mask over his face caught fire and the current was turned off; the attorney left with the other witnesses when a Department of Corrections representative announced 'sentence carried out – you may leave now'.)

The fact that doctors serve in a non-therapeutic role for the legal system (for example, in assessments of disability for the workers' compensation or social security systems, or of competency to stand trial for the criminal justice system) in areas that no ethical code prohibits in no way justifies, contrary to Bonnie's and Appelbaum's insistence, the participation by psychiatrists in legally authorized executions which *is* ethically prohibited. We thus take strong exception to Bonnie's assertion that the psychiatric assessment of a death row inmate's competence to be executed 'does not differ, in principle, from pretrial forensic assessment of a capital defendant's competence to stand trial' or 'from testifying in a capital sentence hearing'.

We would remind Appelbaum of his comments as a member of the affirmative team debating, at the 1987 Annual Meeting of the APA in Chicago, the resolution 'It is unethical for psychiatrists to diagnose or treat condemned persons in order to determine their competency to be executed'. Appelbaum pointed out that psychiatric ethics require the psychiatrist to function as a healer and that this role was not compatible with determining that someone was competent to be executed. The role of consultant to the criminal justice system, he said, is secondary and it has to be subordinated to the role of healer, and in rendering an opinion in favor of execution, the physician allows his secondary role to dominate his primary role. Appelbaum stated at that time that an evaluating psychiatrist is 'as directly involved as one could imagine, short of flipping the switch, when he serves in this role'.[2]

As Appelbaum and Bonnie were the only people to make oppositional comments, we found it necessary to refute their statements. The remainder of the comments were essentially supportive of our position and we are grateful for the endorsement of our colleagues. Thus, we will make only brief response as their papers speak for themselves.

Gunn makes us aware that the Siena meeting promulgated the declaration that forensic psychiatrists should abjure operating 'as part of the state control systems'. He gives proof of the danger of forensic psychiatrists characterizing themselves as 'advocates of justice' or 'agents of the state' by citing the sad story of psychiatry in the former USSR.

As has been pointed out above, Hartmann vigorously dismisses the contention that opposition to physician participation in executions is a covert way to undermine and do away with capital punishment.

It is to Okasha that we owe credit for his vigorous and wise leadership of the Ethics Committee of the World Psychiatric Association from which the Declaration of Madrid (which we quote above) emerged. We also agree that the 1992 statement of the Royal College of Psychiatry gives us a guideline in regard to intervention in 'extreme suffering'.

Lopez-Ibor, as President-Elect of the World Psychiatric Association, was also a critical supporter of the Declaration of Madrid. We are cognizant of the temptations to interpose an insanity plea in capital cases in a humanitarian effort to avoid a death sentence. However, misuse of psychiatry in the presentation of expert witness testimony frequently occurs, resulting in widespread ridicule and criticism of our profession. It should be noted that execution of severely mentally ill inmates is prohibited in the USA. The unwarranted (manufactured?) plea of insanity in capital cases can be nullified by abolition of the death penalty.

Kastrup raises an interesting bit of history in regard to Appelbaum's position on physician participation in legal executions. In Appelbaum's 1986 paper cited by Kastrup and in the debate in 1987 referred to by us above. Appelbaum was intransigent in his opposition to physician participation. Regrettably, by 1990 Appelbaum had reversed his position and has continued to this day to favor lifting prohibitions to physician participation as can be seen in his comment.

Pellegrino is one of the outstanding medical ethicists in the USA and his comments demonstrate his rare ability to sum a most commendable position with his strong but spare prose. We have cited above his condemnation of some of the flimflam justifying physicians serving the court or state and thus participating in legal executions. His comment reinforces this position.

Bloche has campaigned for years against physician participation in legal executions and his comment demonstrates his continuing indefatigable commitment.

Thus, a wide-ranging discussion is completed, not just of psychiatrist participation in legal executions but of the very basis of morality and ethics in medicine that is being seriously eroded. It is our hope that this discussion will raise the consciousness of physicians and psychiatrists to the fragility of our ethical and moral standards that are now subject to attack. In the words of Pellegrino, 'physicians must remain the guardians of the moral integrity of the profession and its ethics. . . . In these times, their witness to the integrity of medical ethics is an assurance that some things arc not at the disposal of whim, fancy or political power'.

References

1   Stone AA. Conflicting values in the house of psychiatry. *Psychiatric Times* 1997; **14**:24.

2   Tanay E. Psychiatric evaluation for competency to be executed. Personal reflections. Presented to the Ethics Committee of the American Academy of Psychiatry and the Law. Denver, USA: 22 October 1997.

8 Resource Allocation

Introduction

One of society's most demanding responsibilities is its need to determine how to allocate resources in order to provide necessary services and promote discretionary projects. The task, which requires broad-based agreement on social needs and procedures for establishing the level of support each activity receives, is complicated by pluralistic preferences. People feel differently, for example, about whether resources should be weighted towards health, environmental or military activities, opinions that reflect their values regarding what constitutes right and wrong in the balance of social priorities. Resource allocation is, therefore, a process of moral deliberation, and this section specifically explores the significance of this ethical issue to psychiatry.

Micro-allocation

The distribution of finite health care resources is usually guided by clinicians' judgments. However, the effects of illness vary substantially in terms of multiple factors like its severity, impact on quality of life, course and response to treatment. For instance, one patient's complete recovery may be achieved at a particular cost whereas spending ten times that amount may do little more than prevent another patient's enduring symptoms from worsening. Ineluctably, value judgments encroach on the decisions clinicians make in determining how to meet the needs of their patients. In psychiatry, for example, the level of health care provided to a diverse group of patients – ranging from individuals with chronic schizophrenia, Alzheimer's Disease and anorexia nervosa to those with adjustment disorders, morbid grief and acute stress reactions – is likely to be influenced by their ability to collaborate in treatment and to contribute productively to society. Thus, the argument has been advanced that people with psychiatric conditions associated with a poor outcome should have less claim to resources because they disproportionately consume mental health services, resulting in certain patient populations (e.g., persons with chronic schizophrenia) receiving minimal, possibly inadequate, treatment (e.g., psychopharmacology without concurrent psychotherapy). Contrariwise, others judge these very patients to be the most deserving given that psychologically more intact patients, despite pronounced symptoms, are better equipped to cope independently even with limited care. Similar debate prevails concerning the resources that should be directed towards patients who are less likely to comply with treatment, such as those with substance abuse disorders.

One suggested approach to these ethical dilemmas is implicit rationing, namely assigning clinicians the role of decision-maker in distributing resources. The historical basis of such micro-allocation is triage on the battlefield when medical personnel categorized the wounded into three groups – those expected to survive, those expected to die, and those with an equivocal prognosis – and only treated the latter group. David Mechanic,[1] a noted advocate of implicit rationing, posits the thesis that patients 'accept the authority of the doctor,' believing he has 'their interests at heart'. The argument is grounded in virtue ethics, which compels practitioners to always advance the good of their patients by adhering to principles of beneficence and nonmaleficence (see Chapter 1). However, critics point to the potential for bias in defining that good, and indeed Mechanic concedes that 'subjective judgments of medical necessity and preferences creep in unconsciously' and can unfairly influence implicit rationing. The impact such bias may convey could be enormous; for example, those who adhere to Callahan's[2] thesis that health care for the elderly should be limited once they achieve 'a natural life span' may justify, solely on the basis of a patient's age, withholding treatment that other practitioners would provide routinely. The potential for this type of decision-making, particularly in complex clinical circumstances, can promote patients' resentment and distrust and broadly undermine their collaborative relationships with health care professionals.

Critics of implicit rationing advocate for an explicit, systematized means of resource allocation, often based in cost-effectiveness. Eddy[3] illustrates the type of methodology employed when discussing implications of assigning resources to relatively inexpensive screening with a potential to save many lives, instead of expensive, less certain treatments that might help only a few people. He argues the approach 'rests on being able to get complete and accurate estimates of benefits and costs' of medical care for specific treatments in specific clinical circumstances, then illustrates how this is accomplished. Eddy notes the following benefits of the cost-effectiveness model over implicit rationing: (a) it replaces the practitioner's subjectivity with explicit, objective reasoning; (b) it formally incorporates costs into medical-decision-making; (c) it utilizes tools, such as computers, to respond to complex clinical situations requiring resource allocation; and (d) it 'follows a set of principles and steps designed to use the available resources in the most efficient way to maximize the health of *all* patients', as opposed to focusing a practitioner's attention on the resource needs of one patient.

Criticism of cost-effectiveness as a method of resource allocation primarily centres on Eddy's last point. As Harris[4] discusses, decision-making concerned with the health needs of patient *populations* always conveys harm to some of their constituent groups, such as the elderly. Apart from the fact that geriatric health care is usually quite expensive, allocating according to efficiency calculations based on life-years of benefit would necessarily discriminate against the elderly because any potential for gain over time is limited by their anticipated shortened life span. As a result, clinical decisions guided by cost-effectiveness would likely deny or limit care to the typical geriatric patient. Harris' basic contention is that 'life is valuable' and 'the obligation to save as many lives as possible is *not the obligation to save as many lives as we can cheaply or economically save*'.

Harris' argument has particular relevance to psychiatric treatment. The ascendancy of managed mental health care in the US sparked a raging debate about the degree to which cost containment policies should influence treatment. For example, Thompson *et al.*[5] demonstrated that during a two-and-a-half-year period decreased utilization of inpatient care likely reflected a general policy to limit use of those services rather than to selectively curtail unnecessary hospitalization in appropriate cases. Some consequences included substitution of short-term detoxification for patients requiring longer inpatient rehabilitative treatments. Lewin and Sharfstein[6] address the issue with a detailed case analysis of a severely mentally ill woman, highlighting ensuing ethical dilemmas confronting her caretakers, such as how to respond when pressured to transition her from expensive inpatient to less expensive outpatient settings despite her clinical fragility. Austad et al.[7] similarly employ a case vignette to explore the ethical tension created by clinical realities in an environment of limited mental health resources. Petrila[8] offers a legal perspective on the debate as it relates to general medical care by health maintenance organizations (HMOs) in the US. Though the Supreme Court has recently settled the legal issue by preventing suit against health networks whose refusal to pay for treatment allegedly resulted in patients' death or injury,[9] many regarded the decision as discordant with ethical medical practice.

Macro-allocation

The debate regarding implicit versus explicit rationing becomes moot when considering questions concerning macro-allocation of resources. Establishing health care priorities for society as a whole requires consideration of disparate values as they relate to pertinent ethical dilemmas, since resolution of those issues can have far-ranging impact on different groups within the citizenry (e.g., current and future patients, the acute and chronically ill, neonates and the elderly). Such diversity of health needs in a community raises fundamental questions that cannot be answered exclusively by members of the medical profession: Is it legitimate to disproportionately fund preventive health measures in order to obviate the need for future treatments that might be more costly, even if this restricts treatments for current patients? Should funding of research be at the cost of curtailing clinical services? Are cost-effective interventions that bring symptomatic relief (e.g., medications) ethically preferable to more expensive treatments that have the potential to generate enduring and substantive change (e.g., psychotherapy)? One way of grappling with these macro-allocation questions is to appeal to theories of justice, as they provide explicit, transparent rationales for establishing societal priorities and thereby ensure representation of pluralist values.

Justice generally refers to fair treatment as determined by societal conventions (see Chapter 1). People are treated justly when afforded guarantees due to all members of society, such as political rights, and treated unjustly when denied what they are owed in this regard. Distributive justice has a related, though more limited, meaning, referring specifically to the distribution of social benefits (e.g., public education) and burdens (e.g., taxation). Steadily rising costs of health care, primarily due to technological advances, new and expensive medications and an ageing population, present society with the considerable challenge of allocating finite resources in a just manner, a process that requires a clear understanding of what is deemed fair.

Aristotle's[10] conception of justice is based in the belief that equals be treated equally and unequals be treated unequally. Referred to as the formal principle of justice, his notion offers no guidelines as to what is meant by equal and unequal, and no standards for how equals are to be treated as equals. His is a minimalist theory that argues a need for justice, but lacks specific criteria. By contrast, material principles add content to theories of justice; they advocate for different features deemed relevant in allocating social benefits and obligations, such as defining equals in terms of merit, need or contribution to society. This spectrum of values supports the following theoretical conceptions of distributive justice.

Libertarianism

Libertarian theory holds that justice prevails when the opportunity to pursue social and economic liberty is guaranteed to all members of society. The goal is best achieved by minimal governmental interference, a laissez-faire approach, described by Nozick[11] as the 'night watchman state'. Its adherents call for mechanisms to support fair procedures that guarantee maximum liberty to the individual in order to secure the material principle: 'from each as they choose, to each as they are chosen'. They criticize redistributive policies that attempt to influence outcome, such as employing taxes that take from the haves to offset the needs of the have-nots, because they restrict a person's autonomy.

One limitation of the libertarian approach, as discussed in the selection by Jellinek and Nurcombe,[12] is its inability to control potential detrimental effects of market forces. Their observations concerning the escalating cost of psychiatric treatment during the 1980s in the US illustrate how a minimally regulated system of fee-for-service promoted the inefficient distribution of resources and greatly inflated the overall cost of mental health care. Market-style competition, for example, fuelled greater use of inpatient services, particularly for adolescents; longer hospitalizations and corresponding charges in private, compared to non-profit, psychiatric hospitals;[13] and higher per diem costs in psychiatric than in general hospitals.[14] Nurcombe and Jellinek also comment on the influence of the profit motive in shifting resources away from needed services. For example, rigid criteria of medical necessity enabled managed care organizations to limit the relatively expensive care required by certain groups, such as the long-term mentally ill, and enhance corporate profits with the corresponding savings. The clinical consequences can be grave. Reviewing a series of cases Westermeyer[15] reports how '[e]conomic considerations took precedence over the standard of care' in treatment that was deemed adequate by MCOs but whose limitations directly resulted in suicide and/or serious morbidity in the patient cohort studied.

Libertarian-based justice is also criticized for its disregard of prevailing advantages and disadvantages among society's citizens. Disparities in the 'natural lottery' (a change in fortune caused by natural forces, such as illness) as well as the 'social lottery' (material possessions, such as inherited wealth) place people in different positions of strength to compete for resources. The haves, by definition, are better able to obtain health care as well as to resist attempts by the have-nots to gain a greater share of health resources through distributive policies. In the selection by Engelhardt,[16] an excerpt from his text The foundations of bioethics, he argues that these differences are unfortunate but not unfair. He views injustice as derivative of immoral, 'unconsented-to actions of others', as opposed to unfair 'forces of nature' that can convey injury or disease. As a consequence he grounds justice in the principle of beneficence, believing that because 'some have so little while others have so much properly evokes moral concerns . . . to provide for those in need'.

Utilitarianism

A second conception of distributive justice derives from utilitarian theory (see Chapter 1), which holds that the goal of morality is to realize maximal happiness by producing the greatest possible balance of good consequences or the least possible balance of bad consequences. John Stuart Mill's[17] definition of justice, as a derivative of the principle of utility, holds:

All persons are deemed to have a right to equality of treatment, except when some recognized social expediency requires the reverse. And hence all social inequalities which have ceased to be considered expedient, assume the character not of simple inexperience, but of injustice.

Accordingly, justice in health care is achieved through policies grounded in the principle of efficiency as determined by cost-benefit analysis.

One methodology for formulating such policies is by evaluating medical care in terms of Quality Adjusted Life Years (QALYs), the number of years a person judges as conveying a satisfying life given the effects of an illness or health condition. The complex methodology for determining QALYs is presented by Williams[18] who defines the essence of a QALY by assigning a year of healthy life expectancy to be worth 1, and regarding a year of unhealthy life expectancy as worth less than 1. Based on this fundamental proposition detailed scales are then employed to quantify how patients value different health states, such as total dependency on caretakers or confinement to a wheelchair. Resources are then allocated in a manner that maximizes the number of QALYs available to treat the varied health conditions prevalent in a population of patients.

A utilitarian formulation of justice responds, in part, to each criticism of libertarian theory noted above. First, the principle of utility imposes controls on the market when the absence of regulation artificially inflates health costs to a degree that unnecessarily, and harmfully, drains social resources. Adherence to the utilitarian position would, for example, limit fee-for-service care deemed wasteful or exploitative. Second, utilitarian-based justice rejects the libertarian distinction between unfair and unfortunate. Cost-effective mental health policy is just if it conveys a net balance of benefit to patients and/or society and unjust if it conveys a net balance of harm. For example, the fairness of current allocated expenditures for the treatment of psychosis in Australia can be questioned, given the costs to society for not providing effective treatment in sufficient volume to patients.[19] Similarly, the fact that psychotherapy has a beneficial impact on cost of treating the most severe psychiatric conditions (e.g., schizophrenia, bipolar illness and borderline personality disorder)[20] argues for the unfairness of mental health policy that inadequately subsidizes this treatment modality.

The basic objection to a utilitarian conception of justice is its potential for subverting individual needs to the goal of efficiency. Harris,[4] a vocal critic of health policy grounded in cost-effectiveness, argues that 'QALYfying the value of life' discriminates against certain patients by compelling clinicians 'not *whether* to treat but *who* to treat', as in the previous discussion of care of the elderly. As a result, he rejects the claim that a positive calculus of benefits and harms is just when it imposes adverse consequences on individuals' interests. For example, Can a cost-efficient policy that utilizes non-psychiatrist 'gatekeepers' to mental health care be considered fair if those clinicians lack sufficient skills to diagnose mental illness in patients?[21–23] Is it just to impose limits on certain patient groups (e.g., the chronically mentally ill) because insurance companies are concerned about the costs of ongoing treatment?[24] Are utilization review policies for psychiatric hospitalization fair if they fail to distinguish among different clinical or patient factors when authorizing length of stay[25] or implement efficiencies that reduce effective treatment?[5] Can managed care organizations justify procedures that promote pharmacotherapy in lieu of psychotherapy, despite data suggesting they are associated with increased patient morbidity and mortality?[15] Such concerns remain difficult to reconcile with a conception of justice solely grounded in cost determinations of benefits and harms.

Egalitarianism

A third approach to distributive justice, the egalitarian conception, posits that justice depends on the equal distribution of benefits and harms in society, a goal guaranteed neither by utilitarian nor libertarian models. As championed by the philosopher, John Rawls,[26] justice prevails when each member of society retains a degree of basic liberty equal to that of every other member, thereby enabling all to have equality of opportunity to pursue life goals. This is not an argument for *identical* distribution of resources, but rather one that provides 'those with similar abilities and skills . . . similar life chances . . . [and] the same prospects of success regardless of their initial place in the social system' (p. 73). In Rawls's account an attempt is made to equalize differences imposed by the natural and social lotteries by allocating resources in adherence to the serial ordering of the following principles:

a) Each person has an equal right to the most extensive basic liberty compatible with a similar liberty for others; and b) social and economic inequalities are so arranged that they are (i) reasonably expected to be to everyone's advantage, and (ii) attached to positions available to all. (pp. 60–61)

Part (i) of (b), called the 'difference principle', permits unequal distribution of resources when it enhances the position of the 'representative least advantaged by social and biologic circumstances' and as long as that distribution remains consistent with everyone's equal liberty and fair opportunity. For example, gifted students might receive a disproportionate share of social resources (e.g., a scholarship) if their talents represent significant potential benefit for the many.[1]

Rawls's theory is applied to the domain of health by Daniels[27] who contends that the burden illness imposes on a person requires allocation of resources that grants fair equality of opportunity to every member of society. This, in turn, requires the provision of health care so that all can achieve a level of function considered normal for 'a typical member of the species'. This 'normal opportunity' standard allows treatment that compensates for physical and psychiatric conditions which compromise a person's autonomy and corresponding opportunity to pursue chosen goals. The selection 'Determining 'medical necessity' in mental health practice', by Sabin and Daniels,[28] is intended to show how Rawls's conception of justice applies to psychiatry. The authors present criteria for evaluating the degree to which mental illness limits a person, and argue for a 'normal function' model that, in contrast to an expansive view, seeks to respond to disadvantage stemming from illness by making everyone competitors for resources in a manner that affords them the potential for species typical functioning.

Objections to the egalitarian conception of justice include the libertarian alarm that it interferes with a person's freedom of choice by promulgating policies that redistribute individual wealth across society. Another concern centres on its ability to define 'normal functioning' which, as discussed by Daniels and Sabin, rests in value judgments about typical functioning. That approach has been challenged for a subjectivity that raises fundamental questions about the definition of illness, as discussed in Chapter 3.

Health policy

Because health care resources are finite, an ethical model for their allocation requires simultaneous awareness of individual and communal needs, and the implications of favouring the former or latter. For example, is it right to expend great sums of money and manpower to rescue a trapped miner knowing the effort will cause a shortage of emergency services resources required for other public needs? The tension between cost of a person's mental health care and the principle of justice is explored by Sabin[29] in the selection 'Caring about patients and caring about money: the American Psychiatric Association code of ethics meets managed care'. He discusses how the ethical practice of psychiatry demands clinicians' dual obligations of loyalty to patients and conservation of society's resources. Geraty, Hendren and Flaa[30] offer similar observations when discussing the impact of managed care on child and adolescent psychiatry, and additionally address legal issues that can arise due to practitioners' divided loyalties. These essays mark a shift from examining the impact of different theories of justice on the individual patient to a broader view of mental health policy.

The President's Commission for the Study of Ethical Problems in Medicine and Biomedical and Behavioral Research[31] was a milestone in the evolution of health policy in the United States. Acknowledging that ethical medical care must respond to individual and societal needs, the Commission made the following recommendations: society should ensure equitable access to health care for all its citizens; individuals should pay a fair share of the cost of their care; each member of society should receive an adequate level of care without bearing excessive burdens; and private forces should secure equity in health care. In sum, the Commission called for an adequate level of health care for all Americans secured by societal obligation, a view of distributive justice based in the principle of beneficence. The approach was criticized as too minimalist and overly dependent on the goodwill of the haves for the have-nots that, for example, might prove deficient during difficult economic times. One response to the charge is Buchanan's[32] call for 'enforced beneficence', which posits that most 'reasonable libertarians' understand their basic moral obligation of charity to a degree that they would accept public policy that enforced contributions to achieve that goal. Others aver that a secure guarantee of health care requires an egalitarian approach firmly grounded in political rights.[33]

The history of the President's Commission illustrates the role of values and political forces in social policy. Callahan[34] explores these influences as they relate to mental health care in the selection 'Setting mental health priorities: problems and possibilities.' He argues that debate about allocation must address a particular valued concept of health: Is it 'an investment good, the creation and sustaining of human economic capital', 'a social investment, providing communal goods other than economic benefits', or 'an end in itself?' Each view reflects a different ideology, a more or less coherent way of ordering several important values, such as the libertarian notion that health care is a good, or the egalitarian notion of it being a right.[2] Callahan then describes how priority-setting can take one of two extreme forms, 'pure numbers' which applies a utilitarian calculus, and the 'raw politics' of advocacy. He believes public debate is required in order to resolve the 'perennial dialectical struggle between facts and data, on the one hand, and values and preferences, on the other', by providing members of society with the opportunity 'to consider what they most want from a health care system'.

In the selection 'Mind and hearts: priorities in mental health services',[35] a research group sponsored by the Hastings Center offers a practical illustration of how values influence policies for treating psychiatric disorders. The authors explore several ethical issues, including the presumed 'indeterminacy' of mental illness compared to physical illness, and what constitutes acceptable mental health services to meet the needs of all citizens. Concluding that no principle can resolve these matters they support Daniels's adaptation of Rawls's theory as the preferred method for setting priorities, and additionally address the issue of who should decide how to set priorities. Given that decision-making depends on people's values, and that 'skilled technicians and public officials have no more insight about them than anyone else', policy determinations should meet Rawls's condition that 'everything must be open to the view of those affected by the decision'.

Pivotal questions left unanswered by the Hastings report – including the degree of community participation and the role of health professionals – are addressed in the selection 'Prioritization of mental health services in Oregon' by Pollack et al.[36] The authors recount the State of Oregon's historic initiative, an early attempt in the US to ration resources that required translating community values into concrete policy. They recount how the public was informed about the nature of health needs, and canvassed to ascertain its preferences to meet those needs within a defined framework of cost. Debate illustrated the 'pure numbers' versus 'raw politics' positions. Adherence to the former yielded a counterintuitive ranking of services that, for example, gave priority to tooth-capping over treatment of ectopic pregnancy, thus revealing the shortcomings of a policy determined solely by cost. The latter gave disproportionate voice to well-organized advocacy groups; for example, the presence of health care professionals was notably incommensurate with other participants at public meetings.[37] The final legislation reflected a synthesis of the two approaches and, most importantly, was sensitive to the impact, prevalence and direct and indirect costs of mental illness because it recognized the inextricable link between mind and body in the genesis and treatment of physical illness.

It should be emphasized that the Oregon experience is atypical for the United States. Public debate concerning distribution of a defined amount of funds among a specific patient population (in this case, persons with incomes below the poverty level) is a process characteristic of global budget planning and inconsistent with American fee-for-service medicine. What happened in Oregon more closely mirrored the workings of a health care system that provides universal coverage to its citizens, like Great Britain's National Health Service.[38] As Daniels[39] discusses, the distinction between the two types of systems conveys clear moral implications for resource allocation. When decision-making occurs within the context of a central budget, funds directed to one sphere of health care become unavailable to others. Though this may result in denial of beneficial care to some patients, the process is fair because trade-offs enable other beneficial care to

those patients and/or beneficial care to other patients. That justification disappears in the absence of a central budget, because there is no guarantee that conserved medical resources (e.g., limiting expensive technological test) will be redirected to patient care. They can just as easily be used to subsidize other societal costs, like military expenditures or (more likely in the US today) to enhance profits of health networks. As a result, questions can be raised about the ethics of common micro- and macro-allocation resource allocation policies in the US: Is it moral to provide financial incentives to physicians to deny diagnostic tests or beneficial treatments? Is it moral to condone escalating expenditures of health care resources by permitting competing facilities in the same geographic area to develop expensive programs (e.g., transplantation services) in efforts to capture a patient base?

Despite the differences universal and fee-for-service systems of care convey to resource allocation policy, Koyanagi and Manes[40] concede that some benefits for mental health policy emerged from the 1993–94 attempt at health care reform in the US. These included appreciation of the need to integrate treatment of mental health and substance abuse disorders into the general health care system (as in Oregon), advocating for a comprehensive spectrum of care (from inpatient and residential treatment settings to outpatient modalities) and a requirement for states to address the issue of integrating publicly funded services into the mainstream of private health care. Moreover, the debate produced a broad consensus among the public, legislators, the federal executive and national advocacy organizations about the weaknesses of the current system, and resulted in a much more sophisticated understanding of the cost of mental health care in key federal agencies such as the Congressional Budget Office. Such positive moves towards establishing a comprehensive system of health care attempt to respond to its current inefficiencies and inequities and, in turn, strive towards just allocation of resources. Nevertheless, many remain sceptical that the goal can be implemented in the absence of a system of universal coverage and the continued influence of private interest groups.

Conclusion

Escalation of health care costs is a universal phenomenon with widespread detrimental effects: significant limitations on services are occurring even in the traditional welfare states of Scandinavia; the respected Canadian system seems no longer able to contain expenses through a single payer structure that allows choice of caregivers; and more Americans are unable to purchase health insurance, causing their numbers currently to exceed forty million and continue to increase in the near term.[41] These events have had a disproportionate adverse effect on mental health care in some countries, notably the United States where long term debate about whether mental illness warrants insurance coverage on a par with medical and surgical disorders remains unresolved despite passage of the 1996 Mental Health Parity Act. The inherent drawbacks of that legislation, such as limitations on duration of coverage, have prompted subsequent efforts that have stalled in the 2003–04 Congress. As a result, a slim majority of States currently have some form of parity legislation, and all have some exclusions for treating common, debilitating conditions, such as substance abuse.

Because of the prevalence and considerable impact psychiatric disorders convey to patients, their families and society as a whole, policies concerned with allocation of mental health resources requires thoughtful decision-making by the profession and the general public in order to insure that those determinations are ethical. As the selections in this section indicate, resource allocation should thus be guided by a 'reasonableness' described by Daniels and Sabin.[42] It must be based in evidence and principles that fair-minded people would choose, endorsed by public debate, and subject to revision by established mechanisms. The ethical basis for resource allocation, then, rests in fair procedures for priority-setting that may incorporate some aspects of any or all of the conceptions of justice presented.

Notes

1 Rawls presents a deontological theory that depends on the hierarchical ordering of principles, in contrast to Ross's methodology, discussed in chapter 1, that establishes *prima facie* duties in order to reconcile conflicting obligations.

2 For a detailed discussion of the role of ideology in governmental policy, see Williams, A.: Priority setting in public and private health care. *Journal of Health Economics* 7:173–183, 1988.

References

1 Mechanic, D.: Dilemmas in rationing health care services: the case for implicit rationing. *British Medical Journal* 310:1655–1659, 1995.

2 Callahan, D.: *Setting limits: medical goals in an aging society.* New York, NY, Simon and Schuster Press, 1987.

3 Eddy, D.: Cost-effectiveness analysis: is it up to the task? *Journal of the American Medical Association* 267:3342–3348, 1992.

4 Harris J.: QALYfying the value of life. *Journal of Medical Ethics* 13:117–123, 1987.

5 Thompson, J., Burns, B., Goldman, H. and Smith, J.: Initial level of care and clinical status in a managed mental health care program. *Hospital and Community Psychiatry* 43:599–603, 1992.

6 Lewin, R. and Sharfstein, S.: Managed care and the discharge dilemma. *Psychiatry* 53:116–121, 1990.

7 Austad, C., Cummings, N., Macklin, R. and Newman, R.: Case vignette: the vicissitudes of managed care. *Ethics and Behavior* 2:215–226, 1992.

8 Petrila, J.: Law and psychiatry: overcoming ERISA as a barrier to managed care organizations' liability for utilization review decisions. *Psychiatric Services* 54:945–46, 2003.

9 *Aetna v. Davila.* 307 F.3d 298, 2004.

10 Aristotle: *Nicomachean ethics*, trans. T. Irwin. Indianapolis, Hackett, 1985.

11 Nozick, R.: *Anarchy, state, and utopia.* New York, NY, Basic Books, 1974.

*12 Jellinek, M. and Nurcombe, B.: Two wrongs don't make a right: managed care, mental health, and the marketplace. *Journal of the American Medical Association* 270:1737–1739, 1993.

13 McCue M. and Clement J.: Relative performance for for-profit psychiatric hospitals in investor-owned systems and nonprofit psychiatric hospitals. *American Journal of Psychiatry* 150:77–82, 1992.

14 Oss, M. and Krizsy, J.: Industry statistics: psychiatric room rates continue to increase faster than average hospital rates. *Open Minds* 2:1, Newsletter, 1991.

15 Westermeyer, J.: Problems with managed psychiatric care without a psychiatrist-manager. *Hospital and Community Psychiatry* 42:1221–1224, 1991.

*16 Engelhardt, H: 'Rights to health care, social justice, and fairness in health care allocations: frustrations in the face of finitude', in *The foundations of bioethics*, 2nd edn. New York, NY, Oxford University Press, 1996, pp. 376–387.

17 Mill, J.S.: *Utilitarianism, 2nd* edition, ed. G. Sher. Indianapolis, Hackett, 2001.

18 Williams A,: 'Ethics and efficiency in the provision of health care,' in *Philosophy and medical welfare*, ed. J. Bell and S. Mendus. New York: Cambridge University Press, 1988, pp. 111–126.

19 Carr, V., Neil, A., Halpin, S., Holmes, S. and Lewin, T.: Costs of schizophrenia and other psychoses in urban Australia: findings from the Low Prevalence (Psychotic) Disorders study. *Australian and New Zealand Journal of Psychiatry* 37:31–40, 2003.

20 Gabbard G., Lazar, S., Hornberger, J., and Spiegel, D.: The economic impact of psychotherapy: a review. *American Journal of Psychiatry* 154:147–155, 1997.

21 Wells, K., Hays, R., Burnam, M., Rogers, W., *et al.*: Detection of depressive disorder for patients receiving prepaid or fee-for-service care: results from the Medical Outcomes Study. *Journal of the American Medical Association* 262:3298–3302, 1989.

22 Eisenberg, L.: Treating depression and anxiety in the primary care setting. *Health Affairs* 11:149–156, 1992.

23 Rogers, W., Wells, K., Meredith, L., *et al.*: Outcomes for adult outpatients with depression under prepaid or fee-for-service financing. *Archives of General Psychiatry* 50:517–525, 1993.

24 Schlesinger, M.: On the limits of expanding health care reform: chronic care in prepaid settings. *The Milbank Quarterly* 64:189–215, 1986.

25 Wickizer, T., Lessler, D. and Travis, K.: Controlling inpatient psychiatric utilization through managed care. *American Journal of Psychiatry* 153:339–345, 1996.

26 Rawls, J.: *A theory of justice.* Cambridge, Massachusetts, Harvard University Press, 1971.

27 Daniels, N.: *Just health care.* Cambridge, England, Cambridge University Press, 1985.

*28 Sabin, J. and Daniels, N.: Determining 'medical necessity' in mental health practice. *Hastings Center Report* 24(6):5–13, 1994.

*29 Sabin, J.: Caring about patients and caring about money: the American Psychiatric Association Code of Ethics meets managed care. *Behavioral Sciences and the Law* 12:317–330, 1994.

30 Geraty, R., Hendren, R. and Flaa, C.: Ethical perspectives on managed care as it relates to child and adolescent psychiatry. *Journal of American Academy of Child and Adolescent Psychiatry* 31:398–402, 1992.

31 President's Commission for the Study of Ethical Problems in Medicine and Biomedical and Behavioral Research. *Securing Access to Health Care*, Volume I, Chapter 1. Washington, D.C., U.S. Government Printing Office, 1983.

32 Buchanan, A.: The right to a decent minimum of health care. *Philosophy and Public Affairs* 13:55–78, Winter, 1984.

33 Bayer, R.: Ethics, politics, and access to health care: a critical analysis of the president's commission for the study of ethical problems in medicine and biomedical and behavioral research. *Cardozo Law Review* 6(2):303–320, Winter 1984.

*34 Callahan, D.: Setting mental health priorities: problems and possibilities. *Milbank Quarterly* 72:451–470, 1994.

*35 Boyle, P. and Callahan, D.: Mind and hearts: priorities in mental health services. Special Supplement, *Hastings Center Report* 23:S1-S23, 1993.

*36 Pollack, D.A., McFarland, B.H., George, R.A. and Angell, R.H.: Prioritization of mental health services in Oregon. *Milbank Quarterly* 72:515–551, 1994.

37 Dixon, J. and Welch, H.: Priority setting: lessons from Oregon. *The Lancet* 337:891–894, 1991.

38 Bricker, E.: A medical student's review of the British National Health Service. *Pharos* 67:23–28, Winter, 2004.

39 Daniels, N: Why saying no to patients in the United States is so hard: cost-containment, justice and provider autonomy. *New England Journal of Medicine* 314:1380–1383, 1986.

40 Koyanagi, C. and Manes, J.: What did the health care reform debate mean for mental health policy? *Health Affairs* 14:124–129, 1995.

41 Decade after health care crisis, soaring costs bring new strains. *New York Times*, 11 August 2002, A1.

42 Daniels, N. and Sabin, J.: *Setting limits fairly: can we learn to share medical resources?* New York, NY, Oxford University Press, 2002.

Two Wrongs Don't Make a Right
Managed Care, Mental Health, and the Marketplace*

M. Jellinek and B. Nurcombe

PRIOR to 1980, mental health coverage was primarily based [. . .]n fee-for-service reimbursement through indemnity plans. [. . .]utpatient benefits varied from minimal to generous; deci[. . .]ions concerning psychiatric hospitalization (and to a great [. . .]xtent length of stay) were based on the psychiatrist's clinical [. . .]udgment and only somewhat constrained by the paucity of [. . .]eds. During the past 15 years, the mental health delivery [. . .]ystem has undergone a two-stage evolution.[1] The first stage [. . .]as free-market competitive expansion. As a result, the use [. . .]f inpatient services increased, especially the for-profit psychiatric hospitalization of adolescents. The second stage was managed care, dramatically decreasing the use of psychiatric hospitalization. The engine for both the first and second set of changes was not innovative treatment or outcome studies; on the contrary, it was profit that filled psychiatric beds in the 1980s, and it is profit that empties them in the 1990s. This profit is eroding the traditional covenant between physician and patient.

The tools of managed care – credentialing, case management, control of utilization, innovative use of information systems, and efficiency through total quality management – have been used selectively to improve quality and lower cost through a more rational use of resources. However, one of the first and most extensive efforts to manage a medical specialty, psychiatry, demonstrates the destructive potential of managed care approaches. Psychiatrists have been disenfranchised, the physician-patient relationship invaded, collegial communication interrupted, treatment goals defined narrowly, benefits denied, and trainees, even under strict supervision, barred from treating patients. Despite the grave impact of this kind of managed care on patients and on psychiatry as a field, most physicians have watched without comment as their psychiatric colleagues are hobbled; however, profit-driven management may foreshadow what is in store for all of us.

The First Stage: Unleashing Market Forces

The first wrong was to encourage market forces that promoted the most expensive treatment and turned clinicians into providers and patients into consumers. Competition did not lower costs; instead, it inflated capacity and utilization. The number of inpatient psychiatric beds rose dramatically. partially to compensate for the decrease in medical/surgical hospital bed occupancy following the introduction of payment based on diagnosis related groups. From 1980 to 1986, there was a more than fourfold increase in adolescent admissions to private psychiatric hospitals;[2] the average length of stay increased from 36 days to 41 days for children younger than 18 years (from 16 to 24 days for 18- to 24-year-olds);[3,4] and per diem costs rose faster than those for general hospitals.[5] With access to investment capital, corporations built hospitals, marketed their services, and maximized profits by aggressive billing and the control of staff salaries.[6] The psychiatrist heading the clinical team might garner an unprecedented salary, but direct clinical work was typically performed by undertrained, poorly paid

'counselors.' By 1988, 64% of all inpatient facilities were privately owned, the most rapid growth being in corporate chains.

Length of stay, charges, and profit margin were all higher in private hospitals than in nonprofit hospitals.[7] Although some of these additional beds met clinical needs, the primary motive was profit and the modus operandi, at times, fraudulent.[8] Two major firms, Charter Medical and National Medical Enterprises, after negotiating large financial settlements with the attorney general of Texas, have promised to limit certain marketing practices, refrain from paying bounties to employees who boost occupancy, and support the appropriate evaluative role of psychiatrists.[9]

Grateful for the growth in facilities, the enhanced funding of academic programs, and higher salaries, psychiatry accepted the competitive approach without demur. Exploiting available resources to maximum profit, a cottage industry, at least in part, entered the corporate world.

The Second Stage: Unopposed Incentives to Cut Services

The second wrong, initially visited on psychiatry, serves as a window to the future of medicine. When fee for service was replaced by managed care, psychiatry was the first specialty to receive attention. Every dollar not spent on psychiatric services can be used by managed care companies or health maintenance organizations (HMOs) to pay for administrative costs and marketing, make premiums more competitive, and boost profits. Consider the following: A managed care company approaches a business operation concerned about rising mental health costs, offering to provide high-quality care, coast to coast, for no more than is currently being spent. The company first limits psychiatric hospitalization and then changes the inpatient standard from comprehensive evaluation, treatment, and stabilization, to crisis care and rapid discharge to the community.[10,11] As a result, length of stay plummets. Recent figures (1990) reflecting the private and HMO sector indicate a national average of 10.6 days (down from between 20 and 40 days in 1986).[12] The balance of the inpatient costs now are at the disposal of the managed care company.

To develop outpatient services, managed care companies recruit panels of providers. In addition to scrutinizing licensure and specialty certification, networks credential providers on what are essentially economic grounds, such as the provider's accessibility (need for patients) and willingness to accept a lower hourly fee. When permissible, most companies limit the number of psychiatrists (in the name of being fair to other, less costly mental health disciplines) and hire nonmedical utilization case managers. Furthermore, the companies check individual practice patterns to assure that each panel member will tolerate limited treatment goals, accept authorization for a low number of treatment sessions, answer telephone calls promptly and politely, and in general be managed-care-friendly. The final step is to require that the outpatient clinician treat unstable patients following hospitalization, thus contributing to further reduction in length of stay.

In networks that integrate medical and psychiatric care, the gatekeeper may be at financial risk (too many referrals reduce income). Furthermore,

* Jellinek, M. and Nurcombe, B.: Two wrongs don't make a right: managed care, mental health, and the marketplace. *Journal of the American Medical Association* 270:1737–1739, 1993.

primary care physicians are encouraged to broaden the scope of the disorders they treat and accept diluted psychiatric care for their patients. Using Civilian Health and Medical Program of the Uniformed Services figures (the insurer for the military) from 1982 to 1987, the percentage of outpatient visits to general psychiatrists dropped from 36% to 22% because of a shift to less expensive psychologists (27% to 34%) and other unlicensed clinicians (at a rate, first reported in 1987, of 14%).[13]

Managed care companies and HMOs also interact with public systems, such as state psychiatric facilities, the criminal justice system, and schools. Again, the strategy is to shift as many costs as possible to the public sector. For example, the public schools are expected to provide or fund a broad range of mental health services.

Given limited data and methods, there are few valid guidelines of what is an appropriate length of stay for a specific psychiatric patient. Alternatives such as partial hospitalization and outpatient substance abuse detoxification are worthy of study; however, harassment procedures (eg, frequent, lengthy phone calls, concurrent record review, and the direct interview of patients) were initiated before alternative systems had been established. Psychiatry was asked to validate existing approaches, while managed care implemented dramatic changes without proof of efficacy or savings.

Lack of Balancing Forces

Just as, during the 1980s, there were few countervailing forces against the overutilization and misuse of mental health inpatient benefits, there is now little to check profiteering from underutilization. Antitrust laws permit managed care companies to set discounted rates and cite concerted responses by local providers as anticompetitive and in restraint of trade. Moreover, in contrast to business corporations, tage tradesman lack the resources or legal sanctions to ganize effectively.

Informed consumers have only recently begun to complain to their employers or to sue when the limitation of benefits leads to injury or death. Early in their history, managed care companies denying hospitalization tried to shift the burden of liability onto the psychiatrist or hospital: 'If you wish to initiate or extend hospitalization, doctor, we would not stand in your way, but we will not reimburse for those services'. Westermayer[14] has described several cases in which nonpsychiatrist managed care gatekeepers failed to hospitalize seriously disturbed patients who subsequently committed suicide or whose condition deteriorated. Particularly problematic was the overreliance on inadequately trained 'therapists' who were only marginally supported by psychiatric consultation. Sederer[10] has recently reviewed the status of court cases concerning managed care. He suggests that we are in the midst of a protracted process that could eventually enhance care and clarify responsibility.

How faulty is the evolving system? It is hard to know. Data on utilization and outcome will take years to gather, validate, and analyze. Most harrowing are the stories of individual patients in desperate need who are given inadequate care. Rather than examining patients comprehensively and developmentally, it is cheaper to focus on a single behavior and return the patient to baseline functioning. Some psychiatrists in private practice are seeing wealthier patients who can pay for choice or who have jettisoned their prescribed provider network.

Possible Strategies for Psychiatry

Should psychiatrists simply wait out the current storm? The problem with the sitting-tight strategy is that services and training are eroding. Psychiatrists today must design truncated treatment plans, aware that, otherwise, they face an uphill fight with managed care reviewers or that they will no longer be deemed worthy of referrals.

Given antitrust laws, little can be done on a local level by providers who are excluded or dominated by a particular managed care company. However, broad political objectives can be pursued by professional academies and state societies. Professional organizations can suggest guidelines

to support access, quality, and proper utilization in the context of managed care or capitation. States could be encouraged to adopt regulations monitoring managed care policies concerning coverage, contracting, credentialing, appeal, and independent quality assurance. As an individual physician you can do the following:

- Define your professional standards to determine what you will and will not do under the pressure of external management.
- Support those of your colleagues who maintain your professional society's criteria or recommendations for admission, diagnostic evaluation, and treatment plans.
- Refuse to collaborate with managed care companies and HMOs that would involve you in dangerous or substandard practices. Report them to the appropriate agencies or associations.
- Learn the rules of appeal.
- Inform patients of the constraints within which they and you are operating.
- Build alliances with other medical colleagues in order to have them appreciate the value of psychiatry and to alert them to their own risk of being managed, credentialed, 'carved out,' or administered into extinction.

In the longer term, psychiatry should continue to build the scientific basis of its practice and to lobby with both managed care companies and the federal government for more efficacy sudies. Further research is needed to define the patient characteristics associated with outcome. Treatment today often involves several interventions (medication, individual psychotherapy, and family therapy, for example); it is difficult to define the quality of the psychiatrist and the physician-patient relationship – variables likely to be critical to the success of psychiatric intervention. Since outcome may have to be measured over months or even years, intervening variables, such as medical illness or divorce, must be taken into account. Although methodological refinements are required, there have been important advances in assessing symptomatology and psychosocial adaptation. Furthermore, unique opportunities have arisen to analyze data gathered by managed care in order to track utilization across clinical sites and centers.[15]

Implications for Medicine

Primary care clinicians will find themselves more highly valued both as gatekeepers and for the provision of an extended range of what were formerly deemed subspecialty services. With higher salaries, primary care physicians will be expected to see as many patients per day as possible, treat patients they might have otherwise referred, and refer to a carefully restricted panel of specialists.

Following the pattern evident in psychiatry, these specialists will order fewer tests, hospitalize patients less often, recommend interventions or procedures conservatively, avoid academic affiliation, and provide ready access (since they were probably not busy prior to becoming part of the network). Once the specialist group is identified and credentialed by the third party, they will receive many referrals and quickly learn the third party's perspective on evaluation and treatment through telephone review, newsletter, conference, and financial incentive. Their overall salary may be lower than that which their colleagues used to earn when fee for service prevailed, but it will be higher (at least temporarily) than they themselves may have earned and eventually more favorable than that of their uncredentialed colleagues.

This divide-and-conquer strategy is already working. Psychiatry has been tamed by credentialing and partially carved out from the rest of medicine. Through carve-outs, traditional referral patterns are destroyed. Primary care physicians, enthusiastic about their new status, may be unconcerned about the impact of change on themselves or their specialist colleagues, whereas many subspecialists think that 'this could never happen to us.' However, subspecialists should ask themselves if it would be hard to find a noninterventionist colleague who currently has few referrals and who is willing to work for a lower fee. Will familiar and trusted colleagues be in the network? Will third parties care more about medical and surgical problems than they do about major depression or attention-deficit hyperactivity disorder? The beginning of an answer can be found in the *Wall Street Journal* of May 26, 1993,[16] which reported a 5% to 6% decrease in reimbursement for subspecialists credentialed as members of the Blue Cross Prudent Buyers' preferred provider organization. Obstetricians, for example, will be paid no more for cesarean sections than for vaginal deliveries. This announcement comes at a time when Blue Cross has sold a 17.5% share of its managed care company stock to the public for $476 million.

As utilization controls tighten, primary care physicians and subspecialists will use their clinical judgment and experience as a basis to argue for authorization of a resource (referral, extra hospital days, and procedure). As psychiatrists do currently, they will face reviewers who are armed with protocols requiring data to support such authorizations. Are efficacy and outcome data available to defend many clinical judgments in either medicine or psychiatry?[17,18] Will the company or HMO alter their internal protocols or choose to be consistent and to meet their bottom line?

Conclusion

Managed care represents a threat and an opportunity. The threat is that quality care, innovative treatment, and the future supply of well-trained physicians will be sacrificed to short-term profit. The opportunity is the wider availability of health care that enhances the covenant between patients, physicians, and society – a covenant that should check both overutilization and underutilization, reduce inefficiency, and curb excessive profit.

References

1   *The Financing of Mental Health Services for Children and Adolescents.* Washington, DC: National Center for Education in Maternal and Child Health: 1992.

2   Weithorn LA. Mental hospitalization of troublesome youth: an analysis of skyrocketing admission rates. *Stanford Law Rev.* 1988; **40**:773–838.

3   Milazzo-Sayre LJ, Benson PR, Rosenstein MJ, Manderscheid RW. Use of inpatient psychiatric services by children and youth under age 18, United States, 1980. In: *Mental Health Statistical Note No. 175.* Washington, DC: National Institute of Mental Health, US Dept of Health and Human Services: 1986:16.

4   Koslowe PA, Rosenstein MJ, Milazzo-Sayre LJ, Manderscheid RW. Characteristics of persons served by private psychiatric hospitals United States. 1986. In: *Mental Health Statistical Note No. 201.* Washington, DC: National Institute of Mental Health, US Dept of Health and Human Services: 1991:16.

5   Oss M, Krizsy J. Industry statistics: psychiatric room rates continue to increase faster than average hospital rates. *Open Minds.* 1991;2. Newsletter.

6   Burton T. Second opinion: firms that promise lower medical bills may increase them. *Wall St J.* July 28, 1992:A1.

7   McCue MJ, Clement JP. Relative performance for-profit psychiatric hospitals in investor-owned systems and nonprofit psychiatric hospitals. *Am J Psychiatry.* 1992; **150**:77–82.

8   Hendricks B. Mental health probes surface in other states. *San Antonio Express News.* October 10, 1991:17.

9   Kerr P. Charter Medical and Texas settle a case. *New York Times.* January 1, 1993:D3.

10 Sederer L. Judicial and legislative responses to cost containment. *Am J Psychiatry.* 1992; **149**:1157–1161.

11 Nurcombe B. The future of psychiatric hospitalization for children and adolescents. In: Bickinan L, Roz D, eds. *Mental Health Services for Children.* New York, NY: Sage. In press.

12 What is the profile of HMO hospital use? *Group Health Association of America 1990 Pilot Utilization Data Supplement to the Annual HMO Industry Survey.* Washington, DC: Group Health Association of America; 1992:13–28.

13 Industry statistics: psychiatrist share of outpatient behavioral health market drops to 22%. *Open Minds.* 1992. Newsletter.

14 Westermayer J. Problems with managed psychiatric care without a psychiatrist manager. *Hosp Community Psychiatry.* 1991; **42**:1221–1224.

15 Sharfstein SS, Stoline AM, Goldman HH. Psychiatric care and health insurance reform. *Am J Psychiatry.* 1991; **150**:7–18.

16 Rundle RL. Blue Cross cuts specialists' fees in California. *Wall St J.* May 26, 1993:B1.

17 Andersen TF, Mooney G, eds. *The Challenges of Medical Practice Variations.* London, England: Macmillan Press Ltd; 1990.

18 Mulley AG, Eagle KA. What is inappropriate care? *JAMA.* 1988; **260**:540–541.

Rights to Health Care, Social Justice, and Fairness in Health Care Allocations

Frustrations in the Face of Finitude*

H. Tristram Engelhardt

[...]

Health care policy: the ideology of equal, optimal care

It is fashionable to affirm an impossible commitment in health care delivery, as, for example, in the following four widely embraced health care policy goals, which are at loggerheads:

1. The best possible care is to be provided for all.

2. Equal care should be guaranteed.

3. Freedom of choice on the part of health care provider and consumer should be maintained.

4. Health care costs are to be contained.

One cannot provide the best possible health care for all and contain health care costs. One cannot provide equal health care for all and respect the freedom of individuals peaceably to pursue with others their own visions of health care or to use their own resources and energies as they decide. For that matter, one cannot maintain freedom in the choice of health care services while containing the costs of health care. One may also not be able to provide all with equal health care that is at the same time the very best care because of limits on the resources themselves. That few openly address these foundational moral tensions at the roots of contemporary health care policy suggests that the problems are shrouded in a collective illusion, a false consciousness, an established ideology within which certain facts are politically unacceptable.

These difficulties spring not only from a conflict between freedom and beneficence, but from a tension among competing views of what it means to pursue and achieve the good in health care (e.g., is it more important to provide equal care to all or the best possible health care to the least-well-off class?). The pursuit of incompatible or incoherent health care is rooted in the failure to face the finitude of secular moral authority, the finitude of secular moral vision, the finitude of human powers in the face of death and suffering, the finitude of human life, and the finitude of human financial resources. A health care system that acknowledges the moral and financial limitations on the provision of health care would need to

1. endorse inequality in access to health care as morally unavoidable because of private resources and human freedom;

2. endorse setting a price on saving human life as a part of establishing a cost-effective health care system established through communal resources.

Even though all health care systems de facto enjoy inequalities and must to some extent ration the health care they provide through communal resources, this is not usually forthrightly acknowledged. There is an ideological bar to recognizing and coming to terms with the obvious.

Only a prevailing collective illusion can account for the assumption in U.S. policy that health care may be provided (1) while containing costs (2) without setting a price on saving lives and preventing suffering when using communal funds and at the same time (3) ignoring the morally unavoidable inequalities due to private resources and human freedom. This false consciousness shaped the deceptions central to the Clinton health care proposal, as it was introduced in 1994. It was advanced to support a health care system purportedly able to provide all with (1) the best of care and (2) equal care, while achieving (3) cost containment, and still (4) allowing those who wish the liberty to purchase fee-for-service health care.[3] While not acknowledging the presence of rationing, the proposal required silent rationing in order to contain costs by limiting access to high-cost, low-yield treatments that a National Health Board would exclude from the 'guaranteed benefit package.'[4] In addition, it advanced mechanisms to slow technological innovation so as further to reduce the visibility of rationing choices.[5] One does not have to ration that which is not available. There has been a failure to acknowledge the moral inevitability of inequalities in health care due to the limits of secular governmental authority, human freedom, and the existence of private property, however little that may be. There was also the failure to acknowledge the need to ration health care within communal programs if costs are to be contained. It has been ideologically unacceptable to recognize these circumstances.

Indeed, the Clinton proposal strengthens some of the worst misconceptions of the importance of high-cost, low-yield medicine by giving such a central importance to equality in access to health care. This is done despite the remarkably longer life expectancy of women versus men, the rich versus the poor, and high-status versus low-status individuals, which may in great measure be independent of access to health care.[6] This accent on personal health care is maintained despite long-standing evidence of the greater contribution of public health and other social changes to decreasing morbidity and mortality.[7] It is difficult to know why such a unique place should be given to health care versus other undertakings such as education, housing, and personal security, where individuals are allowed to secure better private basic education and housing, as well as private security services. The answers must lie in the ways in which personal health care appears to be central to the human struggle with finitude and death.

Reflections concerning the difficulties in limiting the use of health care resources have an ancient lineage and reveal a tight bond with the obsession to postpone death at all costs. Plato in Book 3 of the *Republic* recognizes the quandary of infinite expectations and finite resources that characterizes the challenge of health care choices. He is aware that private property may undermine societal efficiency as individuals attempt to extend their lives in a protracted struggle with death, as in the case of Herodicus, of whom Plato speaks with disapproval.[8] He concludes that the protracted treatment of chronic illnesses is boonless when medicine cannot restore citizens to their occupations and duties. Such individuals should instead accept death.[9] The *Republic* endorses acute health care, if it promises to restore individuals to a useful life, but very little, if any, chronic health care. Preventive health care would be provided in the form of gymnastics. Plato's reflections suggest the following general points: (1) humans have a difficulty in accepting their own limits; (2) limits should be acknowledged regarding the proper amount of

---

* Engelhardt, H: 'Rights to health care, social justice, and fairness in health care allocations: frustrations in the face of finitude', in *The foundations of bioethics*, 2nd edn. New York, NY, Oxford University Press, 1996, pp. 376–387.

resources to be invested in health care; (3) resources invested in health care often do not secure a high quality of life for those treated; and (4) such investments frequently constitute a major drain on common resources. For Plato, concerns regarding health care were expressed in terms of the goal of maintaining the polis, not in terms of isolated individual rights to health services.[10]

But individuals are the source of secular moral authority. This chapter explores the prospects for surmounting difficulties in framing a health care system, while recognizing the limits to achieving the most beneficent pattern for the distribution of health care resources:

1. It is impossible to discover a particular allocation of resources as generally obligatory because of the limits of secular reason (e.g., is it more important to invest communal resources in treating pediatric leukemia, or in treating the pains of the elderly suffering from degenerative osteoarthritis?);[11]

2. The authority of societies and states to appropriate the services of persons, forbid particular forms of health care provider-patient relationships, or draft health care workers to provide services is limited because the permission of individuals is the source of secular moral authority (e.g., the authority of the state, being drawn from its citizens, is circumscribed by the limited consent of its participants);

3. The authority of societies and states to appropriate and redistribute resources is limited by private property (e.g., there will be limits to the authority of the state to tax away private resources in order to provide medical care to preserve the health and save the life of indigents; a society must have legitimately acquired resources in order to establish a communal health system);

4. The opportunity for both individuals and groups to pursue health care is limited by the finitude of resources (e.g., one cannot invest all available resources in the maximum extension of life for all at all costs without radically draining resources from other major societal endeavors).

As a consequence, the secular moral legitimacy of attempts thoroughgoingly to achieve ideal systems for allocating resources to health care is severely limited.

Justice, freedom, and inequality

Interests in justice as beneficence are motivated in part by inequalities and in part by needs. That some have so little while others have so much properly evokes moral concerns of beneficence. Still the moral authority to use force to set such inequalities aside is limited. These limitations are in part due to the circumstance that the resources one could use to aid those in need are already owned by other people. One must establish whether and when inequalities and needs generate rights or claims against others.

The natural and social lotteries

'Natural lottery' is used to identify changes in fortune that result from natural forces, not directly from the actions of persons. The natural lottery shapes the distribution of both naturally and socially conditioned assets. The natural lottery contrasts with the social lottery, which is used to identify changes in fortune that are not the result of natural forces but the actions of persons. The social lottery shapes the distribution of social and natural assets. The natural and social lotteries, along with one's own free decisions, determine the distribution of natural and social assets. The social lottery is termed a lottery, though it is the outcome of personal actions, because of the complex and unpredictable interplay of personal choices and because of the unpredictable character of the outcomes, which do not conform to an ideal pattern, and because the outcomes are the results of social forces, not the immediate choices of those subject to them.

All individuals are exposed to the vicissitudes of nature. Some are born healthy and by luck remain so for a long life, free of disease and major suffering. Others are born with serious congenital or genetic diseases, others contract serious crippling fatal illnesses early in life, and yet others are injured and maimed. Those who win the natural lottery will for most of

their lives not be in need of medical care. They will live full lives and die painless and peaceful deaths. Those who lose the natural lottery will be in need of health care to blunt their sufferings and, where possible, to cure their diseases and to restore function. There will be a spectrum of losses, ranging from minor problems such as having teeth with cavities to major tragedies such as developing childhood leukemia, inheriting Huntington's chorea, or developing amyelotrophic lateral sclerosis.

These tragic outcomes are the deliverances of nature, for which no one, without some special view of accountability or responsibility, is responsible (unless, that is, one recognizes them as the results of the Fall or as divine chastisements). The circumstance that individuals are injured by hurricanes, storms, and earthquakes is often simply no one's fault. When no one is to blame, no one may be charged with the responsibility of making whole those who lose the natural lottery on the ground of accountability for the harm. One will need an argument dependent on a particular sense of fairness to show that the readers of this volume should submit to the forcible redistribution of their resources to provide health care for those injured by nature. It may very well be unfeeling, unsympathetic, or uncharitable not to provide such help. One may face eternal hellfires for failing to provide aid.[12] But it is another thing to show in general secular moral terms that individuals owe others such help in a way that would morally authorize state force to redistribute their private resources and energies or to constrain their free choices with others. To be in dire need does not by itself create a secular moral right to be rescued from that need. The natural lottery creates inequalities and places individuals at disadvantage without creating a straightforward secular moral obligation on the part of others to aid those in need.

Individuals differ in their resources not simply because of outcomes of the natural lottery, but also due to the actions of others. Some deny themselves immediate pleasures in order to accumulate wealth or to leave inheritances; through a complex web of love, affection, and mutual interest, individuals convey resources, one to another, so that those who are favored prosper, and those who are ignored languish. Some as a consequence grow wealthy and others grow poor, not through anyone's malevolent actions or omissions, but simply because they were not favored by the love, friendship, collegiality, and associations through which fortunes develop and individuals prosper. In such cases there will be neither fairness nor unfairness, but simply good and bad fortune.

In addition, some will be advantaged or disadvantaged, made rich, poor, ill, diseased, deformed, or disabled because of the malevolent and blameworthy actions and omissions of others. Such will be unfair circumstances, which just and beneficent states should try to prevent and to rectify through legitimate police protection, forced restitution, and charitable programs. Insofar as an injured party has a claim against an injurer to be made whole, not against society, the outcome is unfortunate from the perspective of society's obligations and the obligations of innocent citizens to make restitution. Restitution is owed by the injurer, not society or others. There will be outcomes of the social lottery that are on the one hand blameworthy in the sense of resulting from the culpable actions of others, though on the other hand a society has no obligation to rectify them. The social lottery includes the exposure to the immoral and unjust actions of others. Again, one will need an argument dependent on a particular sense of fairness to show that the readers of this volume should submit to the forcible redistribution of their resources to provide health care to those injured by others.

When individuals come to purchase health care, some who lose the natural lottery will be able at least in part to compensate for those losses through their winnings at the social lottery. They will be able to afford expensive health care needed to restore health and to regain function. On the other hand, those who lose in both the natural and the social lottery will be in need of health care, but without the resources to acquire it.

The rich and the poor: differences in entitlements

If one owns property by virtue of just acquisition or just transfer, then one's title to that property will not be undercut by the tragedies and needs of others. One will simply own one's property. On the other hand, if one owns property because such ownership is justified within a system that ensures a beneficent distribution of goods (e.g., the achievement of the greatest balance of benefits over harms for the greatest number or the greatest advantage for the least-well-off class), one's ownership will be affected by the needs of others ... [W]e saw why property is in part privately owned in a strong sense that cannot be undercut by the needs of others. In addition, all have a general right to the fruits of the earth, which constitutes the basis for a form of taxation as rent to provide fungible payments to individuals, whether or not they are in need. Finally, there are likely to be resources held in common by groups that may establish bases for their distribution to meet health care concerns. The first two forms of entitlement or ownership exist unconstrained by medical or other needs. The last form of entitlement or ownership, through the decision of a community, may be conditioned by need.

The existence of any amount of private resources can be the basis for inequalities that secular moral authority may not set aside. Insofar as people own things, they will have a right to them, even if others need them. Because the presence of permission is cardinal, the test of whether one must transfer one's goods to others will not be whether such a redistribution will not prove onerous or excessive for the person subjected to the distribution, but whether the resources belong to that individual. Consider that you may be reading this book next to a person in great need. The test of whether a third person may take resources from you to help that individual in need will not be whether you will suffer from the transfer, but rather whether you have consented – at least this is the case if the principle of permission functions in general secular morality as this book has shown. The principle of permission is the source of authority when moral strangers collaborate, because they do not share a common understanding of fairness or of the good. As a consequence, goal-oriented approaches to the just distribution of resources must be restricted to commonly owned goods, where there is authority to create programs for their use.

Therefore, one must qualify the conclusions of the 1983 American President's Commission for the Study of Ethical Problems that suggest that excessive burdens should determine the amount of tax persons should pay to sustain an adequate level of health care for those in need.[13] Further, one will have strong grounds for morally condemning systems that attempt to impose an all-encompassing health care plan that would require 'equality of care [in the sense of avoiding] the creation of a tiered system [by] providing care based only on differences of need, not individual or group characteristics.'[14] Those who are rich are always at secular moral liberty to purchase more and better health care.

Drawing the line between the unfortunate and the unfair

How one regards the moral significance of the natural and social lotteries and the moral force of private ownership will determine how one draws the line between circumstances that are simply unfortunate and those that are unfortunate and in addition unfair in the sense of constituting a claim on the resources of others.

Life in general, and health care in particular, reveal circumstances of enormous tragedy, suffering, and deprivation. The pains and sufferings of illness, disability, and disease, as well as the limitations of deformity, call on the sympathy of all to provide aid and give comfort. Injuries, disabilities, and diseases due to the forces of nature are unfortunate. Injuries, disabilities, and diseases due to the unconsented-to actions of others are unfair. Still, outcomes of the unfair actions of others are not necessarily society's fault and are in this sense unfortunate. The horrible injuries that come every night to the emergency rooms of major hospitals may be someone's fault, even if they are not the fault of society, much less that of uninvolved citizens. Such outcomes, though unfair with regard to the relationship of the injured with the injurer, may be simply unfortunate with respect to society and other citizens (and may licitly be financially exploited). One is thus faced with distinguishing the difficult line between acts of God, as well as immoral acts of individuals that do not constitute a basis for societal retribution on the one hand, and injuries that provide such a basis on the other.

A line must be created between those losses that will be made whole through public funds and those that will not. Such a line was drawn in 1980 by Patricia Harris, the then secretary of the Department of Health,

Education, and Welfare, when she ruled that heart transplantations should be considered experimental and therefore not reimbursable through Medicare.[15] To be in need of a heart transplant and not have the funds available would be an unfortunate circumstance but not unfair. One was not eligible for a heart transplant even if another person had intentionally damaged one's heart. From a moral point of view, things would have been different if the federal government had in some culpable fashion injured one's heart. So, too, if promises of treatment had been made. For example, to suffer from appendicitis or pneumonia and not as a qualifying patient receive treatment guaranteed through a particular governmental or private insurance system would be unfair, not simply unfortunate.

Drawing the line between the unfair and the unfortunate is unavoidable because it is impossible in general secular moral terms to translate all needs into rights, into claims against the resources of others. One must with care decide where the line is to be drawn. To distinguish needs from mere desires, one must endorse one among the many competing visions of morality and human flourishing. One is forced to draw a line between those needs (or desires) that constitute claims on the aid of others and those that do not. The line distinguishing unfortunate from unfair circumstances justifies by default certain social and economic inequalities in the sense of determining who, if any one, is obliged in general secular morality to remedy such circumstances or achieve equality. Is the request of an individual to have life extended through a heart transplant at great cost, and perhaps only for a few years, a desire for an inordinate extension of life? Or is it a need to be secure against a premature death? So, too, for treatment in an intensive care unit when this will only postpone death a few months or convey only a small (e.g., 3 percent) chance of surviving but at great cost (e.g., the treatment will cost over $200,000 dollars, thus saving lives at over $6 million per life saved!). The difficulty of discovering answers to such questions has already been explored ... Taking a particular position in these matters requires endorsing a particular moral vision. Outside a particular view of the good life, needs do not create rights to the services or goods of others.[16] Indeed, outside of a particular moral vision there is no canonical means for distinguishing desires from needs.

There is a practical difficulty in regarding major losses at the natural and social lotteries as generating claims to health care: attempts to restore health indefinitely can deplete societal resources in the pursuit of ever-more incremental extensions of life of marginal quality. A relatively limited amount of food and shelter is required to preserve the lives of individuals. But an indefinite amount of resources can in medicine be committed to the further preservation of human life, the marginal postponement of death, and the marginal alleviation of human suffering and disability. Losses at the natural lottery with regard to health can consume major resources with little return. Often one can only purchase a little relief, and that only at great costs. Still, more decisive than the problem of avoiding the possibly overwhelming costs involved in satisfying certain health care desires (e.g., postponing death for a while through the use of critical care) is the problem of selecting the correct content-full account of justice in order canonically to distinguish between needs and desires and to translate needs into rights.

Beyond equality: an egalitarianism of altruism versus an egalitarianism of envy

The equal distribution of health care is itself problematic, a circumstance recognized in *Securing Access to Health Care*, the 1983 report of the President's Commission.[17] The difficulties are multiple:

1. Although in theory, at least, one can envisage providing all with equal levels of decent shelter, one cannot restore all to or preserve all in an equal state of health. Many health needs cannot be satisfied in the same way one can address most needs for food and shelter.

2. If one provided all with the same amount of funds to purchase health care or the same amount of services, the amount provided would be far too much for some and much too little for others who could have benefited from more investment in treatment and research.

3. If one attempts to provide equal health care in the sense of allowing individuals to select health care only from a predetermined list of available

therapies, or through some managed health care plan such as account-able (to the government) health care plans or regional health alliances, which would be provided to all so as to prevent the rich from having access to better health care than the poor, one would have immorally confiscated private property and have restricted the freedom of indi-viduals to join in voluntary relationships and associations.

That some are fortunate in having more resources is neither more nor less arbitrary or unfair than some having better health, better looks, or more tal-ents. In any event, the translation of unfortunate circumstances into unfair circumstances, other than with regard to violations of the principle of permission, requires the imposition of a particular vision of beneficence or justice.[18]

The pursuit of equality faces both moral and practical difficulties. If sig-nificant restrictions were placed on the ability to purchase special treatment with one's resources, one would need not only to anticipate that a black mar-ket would inevitably develop in health care services, but also acknowledge that such a black market would be a special bastion of liberty and freedom of association justified in general secular moral terms . . . [T]here would be no secular moral authority to interfere in that market. In general secular moral terms, providing bribes or gratuities to acquire better health care, even in vio-lation of the law, could be understood as the acts of freedom fighters or resisters against unjust and unfair state oppression, statements of the Clinton health care proposal to the contrary notwithstanding.[19] In any event, those with political power and privilege will tend to be able directly or indirectly to acquire better health care for themselves and their families. When the law prohibits the satisfaction of any strong, important set of human concerns and desires, a black-market inevitably develops. For this reason, it is difficult to identify truly egalitarian systems anywhere in the world.

Health care policy is a challenge for egalitarianism because of the dra-matic character of the inequalities it faces (e.g., some die young, others live long and full lives; some suffer from lifelong debilitating diseases, others live long and relatively pain-free lives). If this life is all there is, and if here in this world all meaning is to be found, many will wonder whether any inequalities in this ultimate area may be tolerated. Inequalities in health care appear as ultimate inequalities, although differences in life expectancy due to income, gender, and social status are much more significant. Women, for example, in most developed countries live over five years longer than men and the difference in life expectancy between countries that invest modestly and those that invest substantially is relatively minor.[20] Still, the focus of egalitarian concerns is often disproportionately on health care rather than on inequalities in wealth, housing, education, and even security, which are omnipresent (e.g., the rich can hire armed guards while the poor must rely on ordering police protection, such as it is). For exam-ple, Robert Evans, in examining the Canadian government's monopoliza-tion of health care insurance so as to impose one encompassing health care system on all, recognizes that many conflate the freedom to use one's own resources to buy better health care with 'the idea that one person's life and limb is more valuable than another's, more worth saving on the basis of his/her ability to pay, [which] comes rather close to denying a fundamental 'cherished illusion' of equality which underlies our political and judicial system.'[21] If one regards this abhorrence, and the illusion that sustains it, as having the moral significance of creating (or allowing the acknowledgment of) an obligation to use force to avoid such conditions, one will have com-mitted oneself to a health system that aims at equal care for all, even if this requires coercively restricting peaceable private choice. For example, to defend this illusion, Canada acts immorally, and the Clinton plan suggested interventions that would have been immoral in general secular terms. In order to avoid such immorality, health care systems must acknowledge the secular moral limitations on state power and eschew such excesses.

The health care arts and sciences are projects of finite men and women with finite resources, living and practicing their professions in the face of often horrible human tragedy and within moral limitations that forbid them from attempting all they could in order to help others. These limits define where inequalities are not inequities, and where unfortunate out-comes are not unfair. There will still be the possibility of blunting many of the unfortunate outcomes of natural forces and social undertakings. Within

the constraints of secular moral authority, it will be proper to attempt to set some inequalities aside by using commonly owned resources to aid those in need. But this requires distinguishing between two forms of egalitarianism: an egalitarianism of envy and an egalitarianism of altruism.

An egalitarianism of envy holds that a second world is worse than a first if, all else being equal, the second world differs from the first in some per-son's being better off in the second world without anyone being worse off. From this perspective the good fortune of someone can be regarded as unfair in itself or to all others. First, the good fortune of having more than others may be held to be unfair if the fortune is unprincipled, if it simply happens and is thus not deserved. For Rawls's account to which we will shortly turn, good fortune is fair if it redounds to the benefit of the least-well-off class. Otherwise, good fortune exists without justification, without a warrant of fairness, and is in that sense unfair. The good fortune of some can be tolerated only if it advantages the least well off (i.e., 'you may have more only if that helps me [a member of the least-well-off class]'); other-wise, the contractors of the original position would not allow it. Second, good fortune may be seen simply as robustly unfair in disturbing equality. By giving a prior morally canonical status to all being equal, this form of egalitarianism legitimates taking from those who have by good fortune received more. In its strongest form it legitimates making all worse off if this will realize equality. This egalitarian attitude trades on an envy that would justify 'a moral feeling of displeasure or ill-will at the superiority of [another person] in happiness, success, reputation or the possession of any-thing desirable.'[22] Such an endorsement of equality is immoral in general secular terms because it affirms ill will in the sense of an approval of coer-cive force to take from those who have more so that they are leveled to the position of those who have less.[23] In its perspective, good fortune cannot be recognized as a morally nonprincipled given, as neither fair nor unfair. The fortune of some and the consequent (i.e., comparative) relative misfortune of others are not recognized as simply happening, but as creating a claim in fairness to have such circumstances rectified.

With respect to health care, an egalitarianism of envy endorses a world in which no one had access to lung transplants (or other high-cost interven-tions) over a world in which only the rich have access. This under-standing can lead to the illegitimate use of state force: (1) in forbidding the rich from purchasing better care or (2) in slowing technological development to ensure that it would be available only when it can be provided for all. Such strategies limiting access and/or medical progress would be endorsed, even if this led to death and suffering, as long as equality was achieved.

Whether the relative fortune of some is to be understood in terms of the satisfaction or goods realized in the achievement of a human perfection (e.g., the nobility of human character realized in those of good breeding, ample resources, and cultivated manners – those who live *humaniter*) or in terms of the dissatisfaction it engenders due to the comparatively inferior fortune of others depends on the vision of the good or of justice invoked. To justify coer-cive egalitarianism in general secular moral terms, one must secure the canonical normativity of a particular moral understanding or ranking of values and the authorization of force on its behalf . . . is not possible.

In contrast, an egalitarianism of altruism appeals to the sympathy of others to help those suffering. An egalitarianism of altruism holds that a second world is worse than the first if one of the inhabitants of the second world experiences pain, deformity, disability, or an unwelcome earlier death that is not experienced in the first world. Egalitarianism of this genre is not concerned whether some have more, only whether some suffer. Inequalities are not in themselves disvalued. What is disvalued is suffering or that some lack an important good. Equality in goods, abilities, posses-sions, and experiences is not valued for its own sake. Rather, what is valued is the good to be achieved through a particular intervention. In terms of an egalitarianism of altruism, one is concerned to provide an expensive treatment to those who need it, not to withhold from the rich who might be able to purchase it. Such an egalitarianism can legitimately, within the constraints set by the principle of permission, motivate choices regarding the use of commonly owned resources.

[. . .]

Notes

1. Discussions regarding the allocation of health care resources have spawned a wide range of conflicting visions. See, for example, Thomas J. Bole and William Bondeson (eds.). *Rights to Health Care* (Dordrecht: Kluwer, 1991): Daniel Callahan. *What Kind of Life: The Limits of Medical Progress* (New York: Simon & Schuster, 1990); Larry Churchill, *Rationing Health Can in America* (Notre Dame, Ind.: University of Notre Dame Press, 1987). Paul Menzel, *Strong Medicine: The Ethical Rationing of Health Care* (New York: Oxford University Press, 1990). See, also, Dan Brock. *Life and Death: Philosophical Essays in Biomedical Ethics* (New York: Cambridge University Press. 1993), especially pp. 235–416.

2. Friedrich A. Hayek, *Law, Legislation, and Liberty* (Chicago: University of Chicago Press, 1976), p. 97.

3. The White House Domestic Policy Council. *The President's Health Security Plan* (New York: Times Books, 1993). For reflections on this proposal, see "The Clinton Plan: Pro and Con." *Health Affairs* 13 (Spring 1994): 1–273, and "Mandates: The Road to Reform?" *Health Affairs* 13 (Spring 1994): 1–302. For an attempt to provide moral underpinnings to the Clinton proposal, see Dan W. Brock and Norman Daniels. "Ethical Foundations of the Clinton Administration's Proposed Health Care System." *Journal of the American Medical Association* 271 (Apr. 20. 1994), 1189–96. For a critical moral assessment of the Clinton proposal, see Norman Daniels, "The Articulation of Values and Principles Involved in Health Care Reform," *Journal of Medicine and Philosophy* 19 (Oct. 1994): 425–33; H. Tristram Engelhardt, Jr., "Health Care Reform: A Study in Moral Malfeasance," *Journal of Medicine and Philosophy* 19 (Oct. 1994), 501–16: George Khushf, "Ethics, Policies, and Health Care Reform," *Journal of Medicine and Philosophy* 19 (Oct. 1994): 397–405; Richard D. Lamm, "Rationing and the Clinton Health Plan," *Journal of Medicine and Philosophy* 19 (Oct. 1994): 445–54; Laurence B. McCullough. "Should We Create a Health Care System in the United States?" *Journal of Medicine and Philosophy* 19 (Oct. 1994): 483–90. For an overview of the process by which the original Clinton plan was framed, see Laurence J. O'Connell. "Ethicists and Health Care Reform: An Indecent Proposal?" *Journal of Medicine and Philosophy* 19 (Oct. 1994): 419–24, and Marian Gray Secundy, "Strategic Compromise: Real World Ethics," *Journal of Medicine and Philosophy* 19 (Oct. 1994): 407–17. Finally, for a presentation of the conflicts between the moral integrity of one religious community and the Clinton health care proposals, see James T. McHugh, "Health Care Reform and Abortion: A Catholic Moral Perspective," *Journal of Medicine and Philosophy* 19 (Oct. 1994): 491–500.

4. The White House Domestic Policy Council. *The President's Health Security Plan*, p. 43.

5. Innovation would be discouraged as drug prices are subject to review as reasonable. The White House Domestic Policy Council. *The President's Health Security Plan*, p. 45. If one cannot make a good profit by developing new drugs, it will be more attractive to develop video games, where there is less likely to be a public concern about unreasonable profits. In such circumstances, one will have a society with widely enjoyed video games, but which will likely lack sufficient new drugs to respond to multidrug-resistant tuberculosis and other diseases.

6. J. K. Iglehart, "Canada's Health Care System Faces Its Problems," *New England Journal of Medicine* 322 (Feb. 22, 1990): 562–68. M. G. Marmot, George D. Smith, Stephen Stansfeld, et al., "Health Inequalities among British Civil Servants: The Whitehall II Study," *Lancet* 337 (June 8, 1991): 1387–93; G. J. Schieber, J.-P. Poullier, and I. M. Greenwald. "Health Spending, Delivery, and Outcomes in OECD Countries," *Health Affairs* 12 (Summer 1993): 120–29.

7. Rene Dubos, *Man Adapting* (New Haven, Conn.: Yale University Press, 1969).

8. Plato, *Republic* 3, 406a–b.

9. Plato, *Republic* 3, 407–8.

10. Gregory Vlastos, "The Rights of Persons in Plato's Conception of the Foundations of Justice," in H. T. Engelhardt, Jr., and Daniel Callahan (eds.), *Morals, Science, and Sociality* (Hastings-on-Hudson, N.Y.: Hastings Center, 1978), pp. 172–201.

11. See, for example, the discussion in F. M. Kamm, *Morality, Mortality*. vol. 1, *Death and Whom to Save from It* (New York: Oxford University Press, 1993).

12. In considering how to respond to the plight of the impecunious, one might consider the story Jesus tells of the rich man who fails to give alms to "a certain beggar named Lazarus, full of sores, who was laid at his gate, desiring to be fed with the crumbs which fell from the rich man's table" (Luke 16:20–21). The rich man, who was not forthcoming with alms, was condemned eternally to a hell of excruciating torment.

13. President's Commission for the Study of Ethical Problems in Medicine and Biomedical and Behavioral Research. *Securing Access to Health Care* (Washington, D.C.: U.S. Government Printing Office. 1983), vol. 1, pp. 43–46.

14. The White House Domestic Policy Council, "Ethical Foundations of Health Reform," in *The President's Health Security Plan*, p. 11.

15. H. Newman, "Exclusion of Heart Transplantation Procedures from Medicare Coverage," *Federal Register* 45 (Aug. 6, 1980): 52296. See also H. Newman, "Medicare Program: Solicitation of Hospitals and Medical Centers to Participate in a Study of Heart Transplants," *Federal Register* 46 (Jan. 22, 1981): 7072–75.

16. The reader should understand that the author holds that almsgiving is one of the proper responses to human suffering (in addition to being an appropriate expression of repentance, an act of repentance to which surely the author is obligated). It is just that the author acknowledges the limited secular moral authority of the state to compel charity coercively. Jesus said, "If you want to be perfect, go, sell your possessions and give to the poor, and you will have treasure in heaven. Then come, follow me" (Matthew 19:21). There is no evidence that He said, "If you would be perfect, become a political activist on behalf of the poor, establish a progressive redistributive tax system, and use state force to be sure all support a welfare program." Being committed to aiding the poor is not equivalent to being committed to using state force to compel nonbelievers to be charitable. Moreover, the final emphasis is on following Jesus. An Orthodox interpretation of the meaning of this phrase is provided by St. Athanasius (296–373), who recounts that St. Anthony the Great of the Desert (250–356), when he heard this reading from the Gospels, sold what he had and then eventually became the great leader of Christian monasticism. See St. Athanasius, *The Life of St. Anthony*. The author's criticism of attempts by philosophers to provide a secular philosophical justification for governmentally imposed, coercive redistnbutive schemes does not imply that he holds that one should not follow the authentic injunction of the Gospels.

17. President's Commission, *Securing Access to Health Care*, vol. 1, pp. 18–19.

18. Since Rawls's theory of justice invites one in the original position to regard all responses to good fortune and misfortune from the perspective of how one would establish social institutions to respond so that one would regard arrangements as acceptable (i.e., as maximizing within certain constraints one's position, should one be in the least-well-off class), all fortunate and unfortunate outcomes must be regarded as either fair or unfair; there are no mere neutral happenings of fate or chance.

19. Matters appear differently within particular ideologies and religions. For example, just as Christianity has traditionally required slaves to remain subject to their masters, Christianity has set as the ideal for its members—that of submitting to laws insofar as this does not violate the canons of the Church or the teaching received from the Apostles. Thus, in submission one is a martyr for the Faith.

20. See, for example, Marmot, Smith, Stansfeld, et al., "Health Inequalities among British Civil Servants: The Whitehall II Study," for a study of the impact of status on life expectancy. Iglehart notes that after fifteen years of an all-encompassing health care system, there was a 5.6 year difference in life expectancy between highest-earning males and lowest-earning males in Canada. Iglehart, "Canada's Health Care System Faces Its Problems."

21. Robert G. Evans, "Health Care in Canada: Patterns of Funding and Regulation," *Journal of Health Politics. Policy and Law* 8 (Spring 1983): 30. See also *Strained Mercy: The Economics of Canadian Health Care* (Toronto: Butterworths, 1984).

22. *Oxford English Dictionary* (1993), vol. 3, p. 232.

23. Those who hold that an egalitarianism of envy is justified will affirm moral intuitions such that they will prefer a world in which, all else being equal, individuals are equal rather than some individuals having greater happiness, power, satisfaction, and so forth. Thus, if they are asked to judge which is better, world A with ten individuals who are fully equal, and world B in which one individual by mutation develops the ability to "see" radiation and therefore avoid certain risks but only for that individual, world A will be regarded as preferable to world B.

Determining 'Medical Necessity' in Mental Health Practice*

James E. Sabin and Norman Daniels

Managed care raises fundamental questions about the moral presuppositions of mental health insurance coverage. Which kinds of mental suffering create a legitimate claim for assistance from others through health insurance? When should individuals be responsible for correcting their own deficits of happiness or well-being, or for the disadvantages they suffer? And even if society concludes that an individual is entitled to assistance from others, when does this obligation fall to friends, families, or other social agencies, rather than to the health insurance system? This paper attempts to address these questions.

The concept of 'medical necessity' is currently the major tool for allocating public and private insurance monies.[1] Medicare and Medicaid both determine coverage by reference to 'medical necessity,' and with regard to managed care, the Institute of Medicine concluded that 'utilization review decision(s) invariably turn on whether a treatment or service is "medically necessary."'[2] To promote equitable access to mental health care, we must first understand how 'medical necessity' actually functions in practice as a principle of allocation and gatekeeping.

Many insurance administrators believe that judgments about medical necessity in mental health are less precise than similar judgments in other areas of medicine. As a result they fear that if mental health services were given parity with other medical services – a primary objective for the American Psychiatric Association – insurance funds will be siphoned into a 'bottomless pit.'[3]

In previous work on home care and in vitro fertilization we have shown that determinations of medical necessity often rest on a range of moral considerations as well as clinical facts.[4] This paper reports the results of a study of difficult insurance coverage decisions brought to us by mental health clinicians and reviewers in a managed care setting. We explored these cases with the involved personnel by applying elements of the Socratic approach – eliciting the clinician's (or reviewer's considered views, varying crucial components of the case, and examining the effects on their reasoning about medical necessity.

This process revealed a recurrent conflict between what we call 'hardline' and 'expansive' views of medical necessity. Although this conflict often surfaces as disagreement about medical facts and diagnosis, we believe that it frequents reflects unrecognized moral disagreement about the targets of clinical intervention and the ultimate goals of psychiatric treatment. In six case studies we examine the reasoning behind the determinations of medical necessity. In the discussion we present three models for defining medical necessity that can be discerned in the clinical reasoning, and propose what we regard as a defensible rationale for how the concept of medical necessity can be used in the administration of health insurance benefits.

Distinguishing Treatment from Enhancement

Since 1 January 1991 the Harvard Community Health Plan (HCHP), a staff and group model HMO serving 550,000 members in New England, has offered unlimited outpatient coverage ('extended benefit') to patients with severe psychiatric and substance abuse disorders for medically necessary treatment, defined as case management, medication management, crisis intervention, and continuing care group. 'Regular benefit' comprises other forms of treatment for these patients and all treatment except medication management for those with less severe conditions, with an increased copayment after eight sessions and a full fee after twenty.[5] The following (disguised) cases are drawn from that insurance context.

Case 1: The Shy Bipolar. SB is the older of two children in a middle-class family. He is said to have been a happy, outgoing child until the second grade, when his father developed a depressive condition and his mother focused her attention on SB's father. SB became withdrawn and intensely shy. The school recommended psychological evaluation, which led to intermittent psychotherapy until the sixth grade.

From high school to the end of his first year of college SB continued as a shy, rather isolated person who showed no adolescent rebelliousness. He did not date. At the end of his first year of college he was in a motor vehicle accident, suffering abdominal injuries that required multiple surgeries. During the year of his recuperation he developed a manic episode for which he was hospitalized. He stabilized on lithium and completed college.

Throughout his twenties SB worked as a financial analyst. He lived at home with his parents, continued lithium, and participated in weekly or biweekly outpatient psychotherapy. A single effort to taper and stop the lithium led to signs of potential manic recurrence.

In 1987 his employer changed health insurance and SB became a member of HCHP. At one point in the next four years SB and his doctor tried to taper the lithium due to what was thought to be lithium-induced lethargy. Hypomanic symptoms occurred within two months. Subsequently phenelzine was added to the lithium regimen and the lethargy improved.

After the medications were stabilized, individual treatment focused on SB's social isolation. SB and his doctor identified a pattern of interpersonal sensitivity and defensive withdrawal, and SB accepted a referral for weekly group psychotherapy (not paid for by insurance) outside of the HMO. During the course of the next three-and-one-half years SB gradually extended his social range. He successfully moved into an apartment of his own. He began to participate in clubs and other social groups, and to date for the first time. His work performance, which had always been acceptable, improved so that he was promoted to a more senior position and received a substantial salary increase.

HCHP has just adopted a new outpatient benefit. When HCHP put the new benefit structure into place, SB asked his doctor, 'How much of the treatment should I be paying for under this new benefit?'

Medication management for the Shy Bipolar is clearly medically necessary: he has a presumably organic illness diagnosable in *DSM-IV* terms as bipolar disorder. Lithium controls the manic symptoms and withdrawing it leads to recurrent mania. Phenelzine relieves the depressive lethargy. The Shy Bipolar's condition is fully analogous to heart failure, diabetes, or lupus, which require ongoing outpatient medication management, and which most standard insurance plans cover.

The Shy Bipolar's appointments were also used to define important psychosocial issues and develop strategies for approaching them, refer him to community resources and support participation, and review progress

* Sabin, J. and Daniels, N.: Determining 'medical necessity' in mental health practice. *Hastings Center Report* **24**(6):5–13, 1994.

and revise plans as needed. Any psychiatrist who treats patients with major mental illness is familiar with this kind of psychodynamically informed case management. Insofar as the case management focuses on dysfunctions that arise from the bipolar illness, such as monitoring moods or coping with demoralization, the appointments are analogous to advice regarding exercise and nutrition for a patient with cardiac disease or diabetes. Under the terms of the HCHP extended benefit, the Shy Bipolar's clinician determined that the case management was medically necessary and would be covered without any arbitrary limit.

As the clinician reviewed the case with the authors, he came to believe that a strong argument could be made for covering group psychotherapy under the extended benefit in the same way as medication management and case management. In retrospect, the pattern of withdrawal, which started when the Shy Bipolar was in the second grade, could plausibly be regarded as the earliest manifestation of the bipolar disorder. The argument for coverage would be that he had been an outgoing child until the onset of the affective illness skewed his development. The manic episode and its aftermath interrupted any developmental readiness to outgrow the shyness during college years. Group therapy was prescribed to help him achieve the natural social potential that had been thwarted by the bipolar illness. Seen in this light, group psychotherapy is being prescribed to combat interpersonal deficits caused by the illness, much as medication combats the biologically based mood instability. However, as a way of guarding against 'moral hazard,' the HMO's extended benefit covered only continuing care group, designed for patients much more impaired than the Shy Bipolar, and not the kind of interpersonal group psychotherapy to which he was referred.

The following case further clarifies how clinicians distinguish between treatment of illness and enhancement of well-being:

Case 2: The Unhappy Husband. UH, an intelligent, professionally successful married father of two children, sought treatment because of severe unhappiness associated with marital distress. His wife suffered from an Axis II disorder that made her very difficult to live with. UH was committed to maintaining the marriage. A V code diagnosis – 'Conditions not attributable to a mental disorder that are a focus of treatment' – was made. In twenty-six sessions of psychotherapy UH was able to clarify some of the pertinent dynamic issues in his marriage and developed a number of adaptive strategies for lessening his distress. The twenty-six sessions were highly productive. UH wished that his treatment would be covered by insurance, but he agreed that he was not suffering from an illness and that it was fair to expect him to pay.

The Unhappy Husband is probably suffering more than many of the HMO members being treated for illnesses, and psychotherapy definitely enhanced his well-being. What possible rationale could there be for not covering his treatment? The clinician's decision hinged on the question of what the Unhappy Husband is suffering from. By the criteria set forth in the then-current *DSM-III-R*, the Unhappy Husband does not have an illness. His suffering arises from the fact that although his wife's unchanging condition causes him great pain, his values preclude divorce. The clinician believed that under the prevailing agreements that govern insurance, individuals like the Unhappy Husband should be responsible for some or all of the cost of rectifying the unhappiness associated with an unfortunate existential situation. Paradoxically, if the Unhappy Husband expressed his suffering through somatic symptoms and presented to an internist rather than a mental health clinician, insurance would typically cover medical investigation and treatment, which would probably be less effective but costlier than psychotherapy. A 1989 survey of medium and large firms showed that only 2 percent of insured employees have coverage for outpatient mental health services equivalent to other medical services.[6]

If we surveyed the adult population, we would find many who suffer from shyness and social inhibition comparable to the Shy Bipolar in all but one detail – their shyness is not caused by an illness. The Shy Bipolar's clinician was ultimately prepared to authorize insurance coverage for group psychotherapy because he came to believe that shyness was a manifestation of the bipolar disorder, but was unable to do so because the HMO did not cover that form of psychotherapy under its extended benefit. How might clinicians reason about insurance coverage for normally shy people?

Clinicians who use a hard-line definition of medical necessity, as the Unhappy Husband's therapist did, would not approve insurance coverage of group therapy for people suffering from normal shyness. These clinicians would reason that social adaptation is arrayed along a normal distribution curve. Many people are shy and withdrawn. Others are unusually outgoing and adept at making relationships. While being outgoing and socially adept may be advantageous, hard-line clinicians believe that health insurance is not designed to rectify the normal distribution of social skills, however much competitive disadvantage and suffering the lack of these skills might entail.

'Expansive' clinicians may argue that normal shyness should be covered because the shyness stems from psychodynamic factors. Hardliners will respond, however, that while psychodynamic interpretations of shyness may provide valuable self-understanding and assist in changing the pattern of behavior, all behavior presumably reflects psychodynamic antecedents. The presence or absence of psychodynamic determinants does not in itself establish whether a *DSM-IV* mental disorder is present.

Responsibility for Temperament and Character

Clinicians have particular difficulty agreeing about medical necessity when people suffer from what is colloquially called temperament or character – conditions that *DSM-III-R* classifies under Axis II. How do clinicians decide whether this kind of suffering creates a claim on insurance resources or whether it is the individual's responsibility to pay for treatment? The following two cases come from the practice of the same clinician, who was concerned about whether he could make a valid clinical justification for having taken a hard-line position in case 3 and an expansive position in case 4.

Case 3: The Cranky Victim. CV is a lonely, unhappy single man in his forties. He feels that he has been treated unfairly since childhood, when for reasons unclear to him he was frequently picked on in school. He acknowledges that he has acted in a demanding and irascible manner all of his adult life, and that these behaviors have contributed to an unhappy love life and tendency to lose friends. He believes, however, that his actions represent a natural response to the way the world has treated him. His brother, father, and an uncle are also irascible.

Although a slow learner, CV completed high school and a vocational program in audiovisual technologies. Because he prefers to work independently, he does freelance work, which barely provides adequate income.

In the past CV has had several courses of psychotherapy. The most helpful was eighteen months of group treatment ten years ago. CV, however, preferred individual therapy. Even though it had not led to any identifiable changes, he felt happier while the therapy was going on and stated that individual therapy had helped him to understand himself better. Now a member of the HMO, CV requested individual treatment because of his ongoing unhappiness and isolation.

The clinician did not authorize coverage for individual psychotherapy even though he believed that the Cranky Victim would feel happier and less alone while therapy was going on. The Cranky Victim's treatment history suggested that while group therapy had produced change, individual therapy had not. If the clinician were to authorize insurance coverage for any treatment, he would have chosen group (on the grounds of efficacy), not individual. The clinician diagnosed the condition as an interpersonal problem (V code), not a personality disorder, because although the Cranky Victim's behavior was 'maladaptive' (in *DSM-III-R*'s language) it was not 'inflexible.' The clinician believed that however intense the Cranky Victim's unhappiness might be, unless an illness caused it, health insurance should not cover treatment.

Clinicians, however, have experimented with antidepressants and mood stabilizers for non-FDA approved indications. Suppose the Cranky Victim were to undertake a trial with fluoxetine or carbamazepine with apparently positive results. Some might then say that he must have an illness because a medication was helping him.[7] It becomes unclear whether health insurance would pay for medication in these circumstances. If it would, why shouldn't it also pay for the psychotherapy that the Cranky Victim wants?

Furthermore, the Cranky Victim's father, uncle, and brother have similar irascibility, raising the possibility of a genetic basis for the traits that cause him such difficulty. It is easy to imagine that the Human Genome Project might ultimately identify genetic 'defects' that underlie this kind of irascibility.[8] Would we then regard the Cranky Victim as the victim of his temperament rather than as responsible for it and for the consequences arising from it? The following case provides further insight into how this clinician reasoned about temperament, diagnosis, and insurance coverage.

Case 4: The Lost Administrator. LA is a thirty-five-year-old, single woman, successful in her work as an administrator and well-liked by her many friends. Although she appears confident and successful, she feels intensely 'empty' and 'lost.' She is especially unhappy about her love life. LA has been involved with a series of men who have been attached to others or unwilling to make a commitment, and not drawn to men who might have been more reliable. Friends tell her, however, 'You have everything you need to be happy. Why don't you let yourself enjoy your life for what it is?' In outpatient psychotherapy seven years earlier she had become increasingly frightened until she interrupted precipitously after eighteen months.

LA is the third child and only daughter in a family of five. By the time of her birth her father was already suffering from severe diabetes. Throughout her childhood he experienced progressive complications including amputation, heart disease, kidney failure, and loss of vision. He died when she was sixteen. He was severely critical of her, and LA felt that her mother, who had been overwhelmed by his illness and financial burdens, was emotionally unavailable to her. LA's mother confirmed that LA had been a precociously responsible, undemanding child, and that she herself had indeed felt overwhelmed and unavailable during LA's growing up.

LA's clinician made a V code diagnosis of interpersonal problem and an Axis I diagnosis of presumptive atypical depression. He recommended considering psychodynamic psychotherapy (individual and/or group) and a trial of antidepressant medication (which LA declined).

The Lost Administrator was offered partially subsidized psychotherapy under the regular HCHP benefit, while the Cranky Victim was not. On what basis, if any, can their circumstances be distinguished?

The clinician could not say which of the two experienced more unhappiness. He recognized, however, that he felt decidedly more sympathy for the Lost Administrator than for the Cranky Victim and worried about how his reactions may have influenced his reasoning about medical necessity.

In blunt terms, the clinician believed that the Cranky Victim had a 'bad attitude' and carried 'a chip on his shoulder.' Although the Cranky Victim suffered from the effects of his irascibility, he insisted that it was entirely justified by the way the world treated him. The clinician regarded the Cranky Victim as a person who was able to revise his attitudes and behavior but was unwilling to do so.

In contrast, the clinician saw the Lost Administrator as a victim of her temperament Although her friends questioned whether she too suffered from a bad attitude and was refusing to take pleasure in a life that 'has everything one needs to be happy,' the clinician believed that she was indeed *trying* to find satisfaction in her life but was *unable* to do so, and not at all like the spoiled princess in the fable who refuses to be comfortable because she discerns a pea beneath her mattress.

In the course of discussion with the authors, the clinician came to fear that he had mixed moral and diagnostic reasoning in his thinking about the Cranky Victim and the Lost Administrator. He found himself uncertain as to whether his *DSM-III-R* diagnoses of the Cranky Victim (V code: interpersonal problem) and the Lost Administrator (Axis I: presumptive atypical depression) *explained* his judgment of medical necessity, or whether he had invoked the *DSM-III-R* diagnoses to *justify* his moral assessment that the Lost Administrator 'deserved' treatment because she was trying to overcome her condition, whereas the Cranky Victim did not 'deserve' treatment because he took no responsibility for himself and simply blamed others. Not all hard questions are definitively answerable, however, and the clinician remained perturbed.

Controversy Arising from Clinical Uncertainty

Case 5: The Abandoned Mother: Part I. AM is a divorced, fifty-year-old mother of two. In the previous year she had lost her job, moved to a new apartment, and her closest friend had left the area. Shortly before her initial mental health contact the daughter she had been closest to became engaged, and told AM that she would be staying with her future in-laws when she visited the area, not with AM.

AM became distraught and tearful. She was diagnosed as having an Adjustment Disorder with Depressed Mood. Coverage was provided under the regular benefit, with increased copayment after eight sessions and full fee after twenty. She did not develop rapport, however, with any of the three therapists she saw, and trials of imipramine, fluoxetine, and phenelzine produced no benefit. AM felt desperate and began to request hospitalization.

Eleven months after the treatment began, her situation was reviewed with a consultant. The consultant asked, 'What is this patient suffering from? Does she have a form of major depression? Or is it life – is it being middle-aged, divorced, bereft of children, jobless, that makes her feel alone and angry?'

The consultant is posing a characteristic hard-line question. The Abandoned Mother's story is disturbing, but at this point in her course her condition did not clearly meet the *DSM-III-R* criteria for Major Depression or Dysthymia. If we apply a Depressive Disorder diagnosis to her ambiguous condition, we put the Abandoned Mother into the framework of illness, patient, doctor, medical treatment, and potential coverage of care under health insurance. If we call her condition 'life,' we are saying that although she is encountering painful circumstances and experiencing suffering, the paradigms of illness, patient, doctor, medical treatment, and insurance do not apply.

The concept of medical necessity forces us to pose questions in an either-or manner: treatment is or is not medically necessary. Clinical situations like the Abandoned Mother's however, are often much more ambiguous. Further observations may help but do not always take away the uncertainty.

The Abandoned Mother: Part II. Following the consultation, AM continued outpatient therapy with yet another therapist. When her daughter again visited without staying with her, AM's suicidal preoccupations increased, and she spoke of plans to kill herself. She said she could not pay for outpatient treatment and again requested hospitalization. Those involved with insurance administration reviewed her case and changed the diagnosis to Depressive Disorder (atypical form) with significant suicidal risk, and authorized up to two half-hours of case management per week without escalating copayment ('extended benefit').

Although the Abandoned Mother's diagnosis and insurance status have now both been shifted, there is still room for controversy. The expansive clinician will say that her true condition has become dear over time – now we see that the Abandoned Mother is really suffering from Atypical Depression, not an Adjustment Reaction or an existential tantrum. But it remains possible to take a hard-line view and say that the Abandoned Mother has learned how insurance decisions are made and can now game the system to get the outcome she wants.

In case 5, controversy regarding medical necessity arose from uncertainty regarding the Abandoned Mother's diagnosis – whether she was suffering from an affective disorder or a hard time in her life. In the following case, the question of what constitutes medically necessary treatment arises from uncertainty about whether an effective treatment is available and if so what it is.

Case 6: The Abused Child. AC, six years old, moved with her mother to New England from another part of the country and became a member of the HMO. During the previous two years she had been repeatedly sexually abused by her stepfather, who had been prosecuted and was now in jail. AC's genitalia showed unmistakable signs of the abuse, but she was a remarkably happy seeming child and was adjusting very well to her new environment.

Whereas the Abandoned Mother was in a constant struggle over what she would get, neither the Abused Child nor her mother are making a demand on the HMO. While hardliners can regard the Abandoned Mother as a person who refuses to take responsibility for adapting to relatively ordinary life experiences, the Abused Child is obviously not responsible for what happened to her. The HMO was fully ready to cover treatment for the Abused Child, but it was highly unclear whether at this point there was a treatment to offer since her growth and development appeared to be proceeding well. The mental health clinician decided to offer attentive watching, and to follow the Abused Child closely with the pediatrician and the mother.

Moral Hazard

When the consultant in case 5 asked whether the Abandoned Mother was suffering from major depression or the vicissitudes of life, she was raising a question about what the insurance industry calls moral hazard as well as a question about diagnosis. Social programs that offer insurance protection against specified dangers create the hazard that individuals will alter their behavior so as to claim benefits, as by burning an insured property so as to collect for loss, for example, or claiming to be unable to work so as to receive disability payments. Insurance underwriters fear that if mental health insurance becomes more available, individuals like the Abandoned Mother might claim to suffer from an illness when they are actually suffering from life, to obtain the attention and solace that psychotherapy, hospital care, and the sick role might provide.

If we too easily assimilate shyness (case 1), unfortunate existential situations (case 2), loneliness and irascibility (case 3), lack of satisfaction with ostensibly adequate opportunity (case 4), or life itself (case 5) to the category of disease and disability, we open a very wide door for health insurance claims. Quite apart from the obvious implications for the cost of insurance, mental health clinicians recognize the potential for doing unintentional harm to patients by ascribing a diagnostic label – the patient role, with its implication of pathology.[9] Thus although the insurance industry concern about moral hazard is primarily an actuarial concern with claim liability, guarding against moral hazard will sometimes protect individuals from iatrogenic harms of the sick role as well.

Potential insurers of mental health care are especially concerned with moral hazard because (1) many of the symptoms of mental illness are part of a continuum with everyday forms of distress; (2) diagnosis of some conditions – especially Axis II disorders – is controversial and uncertain;[10] (3) some forms of treatment – especially psychotherapy – seem similar to nonprofessional forms of human support and interaction; and (4) demand for mental health services has been shown to be highly responsive to the presence or absence of insurance coverage.[11] These factors create public concern that expanded coverage would lead to excessive utilization of care. When opponents of expanded mental health coverage apply disparaging terms like 'rent-a-friend' to mental health treatment they are in part expressing a concern about moral hazard – that legitimate needs such as friendship will masquerade as needs for subsidized treatment, and the community paying for health insurance will incur expenditures it should not be liable for.

Three Models Underlying the Conflict over Insurance Coverage

We believe that these examples of front-line reasoning about insurance coverage reflect three different models – which we call 'normal function,' 'capability,' and 'welfare' (see table 1) – for thinking about medical necessity. Each model defines the ultimate goal of psychiatric care as helping the patient to come as close to equal opportunity in life as is possible, but the models answer the question, Equal opportunity for what?[12] in subtly different ways. Although the terms in which we formulate the three models come from moral philosophy, we believe that the models can help to illuminate practical controversies over current insurance coverage and provide guidance for future insurance design. In fact, failure to distinguish among these models may contribute to the difficulty advocates encounter in their efforts to promote nondiscriminatory insurance coverage for mental health services.

Normal function model. According to the normal function model, the central purpose of health care is to maintain, restore, or compensate for the restricted opportunity and loss of function caused by disease and disability.[13] Successful health care restores people to the range of capabilities they would have had without the pathological condition or prevents further deterioration.

The normal function model takes unequal distribution of human capabilities as a fact that health care will not change. Some people are socially adept. Others are shy in ways that cause suffering. The model prescribes compassion for those who are less fortunate in the natural lottery that distributes capabilities, but makes the health sector responsible for correcting only those conditions which – in DSM-IV terms – can be diagnosed as 'a symptom of a dysfunction,' that is, as mental disorders.

Health care is not the only agent of social responsibility. People suffering from lack of social skill can be ministered to by education, training, families, religious and community groups, and other social institutions. Treating illness and enhancing human capabilities may both be desirable social goals, but they should not be confused with one another. The normal function model holds that health care insurance coverage should be restricted to disadvantages caused by disease and disability unless society explicitly decides to use it to mitigate other forms of disadvantage as well. Hard-line clinicians define medical necessity in accord with the normal function model.

Capability model. The capability model prescribes a broader role for health care. It holds that the distribution of personal capabilities like confidence, resilience, and sociability in the natural lottery should not be taken as a given. Health care should strive to give people equal personal capabilities, or at least give priority to those whose diminished capability (whatever the cause) puts them at a relative disadvantage.[14] The capability model makes no moral distinction between treatment of illness and enhancement of disadvantageous personal capabilities. It makes relative disadvantage in one's ability to function the morally relevant characteristic for determining insurance coverage. Consequently, if group therapy helps to alleviate significant disadvantages caused by normal shyness, or if fluoxetine gives 'the introvert the social skills of a salesman,'[15] the capability model would hold that health insurance should provide coverage.

The normal function model asks health care to help people become *normal* competitors, free from disadvantages caused by disease or disability. The capability model, by contrast, would use health care to help people become *equal* competitors, free from disadvantageous lack of capabilities regardless of etiology. It makes a single DSM-IV criterion for diagnosing a mental disorder – 'impairment in one or more areas of functioning' – its central focus, but unlike DSM-IV it does not require that the impairment be 'a symptom of a dysfunction (underlying disorder).'

Table 1 Models of medical necessity

Equal opportunity for	Target of clinical action	Ultimate goal of health care
1. Normal function	Medically defined deviation	Decrease impact of disease or disability
2. Personal capability	Unchosen constraint of personal capability	Enhance personal capability
3. Welfare	Unchosen constraint of potential for happiness	Enhance potential for happiness

The kind of controversy that arises in psychiatry about insurance coverage for treatment of disadvantageous personal capabilities like shyness occurs in other areas of health insurance as well. A recent issue of *Growth Genetics, & Hormones*, for example, was entirely devoted to the parallel issue of whether short children who are not deficient in growth hormone should be treated, and if so, if the treatment should be covered by insurance.[16] Expansive pediatric endocrinologists guided by the capability model have argued that because extreme shortness is a handicapping condition, insurance should provide the hormone to short children who have no endocrine abnormality.[17] Others who use the normal function model would limit insurance coverage to children with growth hormone deficiency.[18]

Welfare model. According to the welfare model, if people suffer because of attitudes or behavior patterns they did not choose to develop and are not independently able to alter or overcome, they should be eligible for insurance coverage. When the clinician in cases 3 and 4 distinguished between the Cranky Victim and the Lost Administrator on the basis of whether they were able and willing to change the attitudes and behavior that caused their suffering, he was unwittingly applying the welfare model.[19] The welfare model makes its central focus a different DSM-IV criterion for diagnosing a mental disorder – 'present distress (a painful symptom)' – but like the capability model it diverges from DSM-IV and the normal function model in not requiring that the distress be a symptom of a mental disorder.

By training and temperament, mental health clinicians want to alleviate disadvantage, enhance personal capabilities, and reduce suffering. Offering treatment to the Shy Bipolar and not to the person who is normally shy but who suffers just as much, strains their moral commitments. Expansive clinicians are attracted to the capability model because it allows them to argue for extending insurance coverage to both. Similarly, to expansive clinicians, not offering insurance coverage to the Unhappy Husband, whose suffering was relieved by psychodynamic psychotherapy, is clinically unjustifiable and morally repugnant. The welfare model appeals to them because it supports claims for assistance based on personal suffering like that of the Unhappy Husband. The capability and welfare models provide expansive clinicians with a rationale for interpreting treatment of the conditions that DSM-II called 'neuroses'[20] and Astrachan described as the 'humanistic' tasks of psychiatry[21] as medically necessary.

Practical Implications for Health Insurance

The era of laissez-faire with regard to health care expenditure is by now a nostalgic memory. In the future, explicit priorities for allocation and (we predict) rationing will guide practice. A clear and well-grounded model of medical necessity will be crucial for the design of a just and practical insurance system. Which model should we choose?

To be useful, a model for defining medical necessity must pass three tests: Does it make distinctions the public and clinicians regard as fair? Can it be administered in the real world? and, Does it lead to results that society can afford? We believe that the normal function model meets these three criteria best.

First, all developed societies recognize treatment of illness as a primary societal imperative. An affluent society that refused to care for its sick would be regarded as grossly unfair. Thus it is not surprising that all three models agree that disadvantage and suffering caused by disease and disability have a special claim on collective resources. Second, although individual cases can pose difficult or insoluble diagnostic dilemmas, psychiatry has developed publicly accepted methods – currently embodied in *DSM-IV* – by which agreed-upon diagnoses can generally be established. Finally, while morally acceptable definitions of the scope of health care lead to costs that strain every society, the normal function model at least allows society to draw a plausible boundary around the potential scope of insurance coverage for mental health care.

Although the capability and welfare models capture basic moral insights, we believe that they cast too broad a net and pose severe problems for administration and cost. How are we to judge when the conditions for health insurance coverage have been met under these models? If individuals invoke the capability model and request treatment for incapacitating shyness, do we simply take their assessment of need at face value? If so, the insurer is subject to extensive moral hazard. If not, how are we to investigate the claim? Have shy people made reasonable efforts to overcome the condition – participating in social events, asking others for tips on socializing, taking public speaking classes, and so forth? Did they bring it on themselves, as by wishing to consort only with rich, beautiful, and famous people who intimidate them and elicit shyness? We have little idea of how to delve into questions like this. If the Cranky Victim invokes the welfare model and requests treatment on the grounds that he did not choose to be so irascible, similar problems arise. If we do not investigate, we create substantial risk of moral hazard. But if we do investigate, we are faced with a task for which we have few skills – reconstructing the history of the Cranky Victim's choices and assessing how responsible he is for creating and sustaining the attitudes and behaviors from which he suffers.

Public support for mental health insurance coverage, historically tenuous at best, might be compromised further if the public believed that third-party resources were subject to even more moral hazard than exists at present. If the public believed that mental health interventions replace reasonable efforts to modify one's attitudes and behaviors or to extend one's capacities through learning and practice, support would wane.

President Clinton's proposed 'American Health Security Act' sets eligibility for insurance coverage of mental health and substance abuse treatment in accord with the normal function model. Coverage will be provided only if an individual 'has, or has had during the 1-year period preceding the date of such treatment, a diagnosable mental or substance abuse disorder' (emphasis added).[22] If the health care reform process ultimately interprets 'medical necessity' in accord with the normal function model, insurers will need to clarify the implications of the model for clinicians and the public. Current insurance definitions of 'medical necessity' often give no guidance as to which model should be used. The HMO at which this study was conducted defines 'medically necessary' as 'those medical services which are essential for the treatment of a Member's medical condition and are in accordance with generally accepted medical practice.'[23] To place mental health services under the normal function model, this definition would change to something like 'those mental health services which are essential for the treatment of a Member's mental health disorder as defined by *DSM-IV* in accordance with generally accepted mental health practice.'

Insurance administrators are acutely aware that clinicians can always find ways to circumvent insurance restrictions. No model prevents the possibility of 'gaming,'[24] and a recent survey showed that 68 percent of the physicians polled were willing to deceive third-party payers if they believed coverage criteria were unfair.[25] While clear criteria and monitoring systems make gaming more difficult, the most effective antidote to gaming is for clinicians and their patients to understand and endorse the rationale for the model used to determine coverage and to believe in the integrity of the system within which allocative decisions are made.[26]

A model for determining medical necessity allows us to determine what conditions are *eligible* for insurance coverage, but does not tell us how much of the total health care budget should be devoted to mental health. A health plan, state, or nation might decide it could not afford to provide all treatment eligible for coverage, and that it needed to set priorities (or ration), as has recently occurred in Oregon.[27] Although some insurers deny coverage to Axis II conditions, all 'mental disorders' are eligible for coverage under the normal function model. The Oregon priority setting process included borderline and schizotypal personality disorders in the proposed basic package, but antisocial personality disorder ranked below the cutoff point. To think rationally about *how* to finance, administer, and set priorities within mental health insurance, we must first be clear on what the insurance is *for*.

Whatever percentage of the health care budget is devoted to mental health, we recommend that insurance cover three to six sessions for evaluation, so that clinicians working under the normal function model would be able to guide patients who are not suffering from a mental disorder toward potentially helpful alternatives. For the Unhappy Husband, the alternative was psychotherapy on a fee-for-service basis. For the Cranky Victim it might be courses in social skills or involvement in religious activities that could encourage a refrained view of his circumstances. In this way the clinician is not simply a *gatekeeper*, determining whether or not the person receives treatment covered by insurance, but a *caregiver*, who offers guidance and compassion if the person's suffering comes from causes other than mental disorder, and who is open to reviewing the initial diagnosis if new clinical facts emerge. Hard-line clinicians need not be hard-hearted.

Any model of medical necessity will ultimately have to be applied by clinicians at the front line.[28] We undertook this detailed study of how clinicians actually reason about medical necessity to see if current practice provides valuable guidance for future policy. We conclude that it does.

Conflict about mental health insurance coverage is rampant. Frequently the conflict between reviewer and clinician (or clinician and patient) is empirical: can a proposed intervention reasonably be anticipated to achieve the intended result? Even when the answer is yes, the parties often clash over the question of whether a less costly intervention might achieve a comparable result.[29] These conflicts over effectiveness may not currently be resolvable because of limited outcomes data, but they will ultimately yield, to scientific progress.

When expansive and hard-line clinicians clash, however, their conflict is at least sometimes about the *ends* of health care, rather than about the *means* to achieve those ends. What may masquerade as a diagnostic conflict about what the patient *has* may in actuality reflect disagreement about what health care *should* be. Should it be restricted to limitations created by *DSM-IV* defined disorders in accord with the normal function model, or should it minister to other forms of limitation as well, as proposed by the capability and welfare models?

We recognize that the concepts of disease and disability have been subjected to extensive philosophical and sociological criticism. Our endorsement of the normal function model does not rest on a view of disease and disability as ultimately real in a metaphysical sense. We acknowledge that cases will continue to arise that seem arbitrary (like covering treatment for shyness caused by an illness but not for normal shyness) or painful (like not covering the kind of psychotherapy that helped the Unhappy Husband). Similarly, diagnostic categories will continue to change, and what is regarded as a mental disorder today may be seen as a cultural construct tomorrow.

Society, however, needs a publicly acceptable and administerable system for defining the boundaries of health insurance coverage. The conception of mental disorders embodied in *DSM-IV* provides a workable definition of these boundaries. DSM-IV is not free from error or bias. It is, however, the result of a highly public process open to scientific scrutiny, field testing, and repetitive criticism over time. The alternative to defining the boundaries of coverage by the normal function model and *DSM-IV* is not a more liberal system governed by the capability or welfare model, but one in which mental health benefits are arbitrarily capped, as occurs at present. As José Santiago has recently commented, 'At stake is survival of services as a legitimate item in any reform effort.'[30] We believe that the normal function model best ensures the survival of a robust mental health service sector.

Conflict about health insurance can occur at three levels. First, parties may differ about the goals of health care itself, as when expansive clinicians clash with hard-liners. Second, empirical conflicts may occur over how interventions (means) may relate to outcomes (ends). Finally, even with a well-clarified model for defining medical necessity, society will continue to struggle over how much medically necessary care it will provide.[31] All three levels of conflict pose major challenges. If we do not make clear distinctions among them, however, we will make no progress toward creating useful answers.

Acknowledgments

The authors wish to thank the Robert Wood Johnson Foundation (grant no. 19450) and the Harvard Community Health Plan Foundation for their generous support.

References

1   William M. Glazer, 'Psychiatry and Medical Necessity,' *Psychiatric Annals* **22** (1992): 362–66.

2   William A. Helvestine, 'Legal Implications of Utilization Review,' in *Controlling Costs and Changing Patient Care? The Role of Utilization Review*, ed. Bradford H. Gray and Marilyn J. Field (Washington, D.C.: National Academy Press, 1989), pp. 169–204, at 172.

3   Steven S. Sharfstein, 'Third-Party Payers: To Pay or Not to Pay,' *American Journal of Psychiatry* 135 (1978): 1185–88; Allen Beigel and Steven S. Sharfstein, 'Mental Health Care Providers: Not the Only Cause or Only Cure for Rising Costs,' *American Journal of Psychiatry* **141** (1984): 668–72; Richard B. Karel, 'Tipper Gore's Former Staff Head Sheds Light on How Some Task Force Decisions Were Reached,' *Psychiatric News* 28, no. **19** (1991): 10, 21.

4   James E. Sabin, Lachlan Forrow, and Norman Daniels, 'Clarifying the Concept of Medical Necessity,' in *Proceedings of the Group Health Institute* (Washington, D.C.: Group Health Association of America, 1991), pp. 693–707; Norman Daniels and James E. Sabin, 'When Is Home Care Medically Necessary?' *Hastings Center Report* **21**, no. 4 (1991): 37–38.

5   Helen S. Abrams, 'Harvard Community Health Plan's Mental Health Redesign Project: A Managerial and Clinical Partnership,' *Psychiatric Quarterly* **64** (1993): 13–31.

6   Patricia Scheidemandel, *The Coverage Catalog*, 3rd ed. (Washington, D.C.: American Psychiatric Association, Office of Economic Affairs, 1993), p. 44.

7   M. Balint et al., *Treatment or Diagnosis: A Study of Repeat Prescriptions in General Practice* (London: Tavistock Publications, 1970).

8   Normal Daniels, 'The Genome Project, Individual Differences, and Just Health Care,' in *Justice and the Human Genome*, ed. Timothy S. Murphy and Marc A. Lappé (Berkeley and Los Angeles: University of California Press, 1994).

9   Thomas J. Scheff, ed. *Labelling Madness* (Englewood Cliffs, N.J.: Prentice Hall, 1975).

10   J. Christopher Perry, 'Problems and Considerations in the Valid Assessment of Personality Disorders,' *American Journal of Psychiatry* **149** (1992): 1645–53.

11   Willard G. Manning et al., *Effects of Mental Health Insurance: Evidence from the Health Insurance Experiment* (Santa Monica, Calif.: RAND, 1989).

12   Norman Daniels, 'Equality of What: Welfare, Resources or Capabilities,' supplement, *Philosophy and Phenomenological Research* **19** (1990): 273–96.

13   Norman Daniels, *Just Health Care* (Cambridge: Cambridge University Press, 1985), chapter 2.

14   Amartya Sen, 'Justice: Means Versus Freedoms,' *Philosophy and Public Affairs* **19** (1990): 111–21; see also Amartya Sen, *Inequality Reexamined* (Cambridge, Mass.: Harvard University Press, 1992).

15   Peter D. Kramer, *Listening to Prozac* (New York: Viking, 1993), p. xv.

16   Supplement 1, *Growth, Genetics, and Hormones* **8** (1992).

17   David B. Allen and Norman C. Fost, 'Growth Hormone Therapy for Short Stature: Panacea or Pandora's Box?' *Journal of Pediatrics* **117** (1990): 16–21.

18   Normal Daniels, 'Growth Hormone Therapy for Short Stature: Can We Support the Treatment/Enhancement Distinction?' supplement 1, *Growth, Genetics, & Hormones* **8** (1992): 46–48.

19   Richard J. Arneson, 'Equality and Equal Opportunity for Welfare,' *Philosophical Studies* 54 (1988): 79–95; G. A. Cohen, 'On the Currency of Egalitarian Justice,' *Ethics* 99 (1989): 906–44.

20   Ronald Bayer and Robert L. Spitzer, 'Neurosis, Psychodynamics, and *DSM-III*,' *Archives of General Psychiatry* **42** (1985): 187–96.

21   Boris M. Astrachan, Daniel J. Levinson, and David A. Adler, 'The Impact of National Health Insurance on the Tasks and Practice of Psychiatry,' *Archives of General Psychiatry* 33 (1976): 785–94.

22   *Health Security Act,* 151–183 O-93–1, Title I, Subtitle B, Sec. 1115 (b)(1A) (Washington, D.C.: U.S. Government Printing Office), p. 46.

23   Subscriber's Agreement, Harvard Community Health Plan, Boston, Mass., October 1991.

24   **E. Haavi Morreim**, 'Gaming the System: Dodging the Rules, Ruling the Dodgers,' *Archives of Internal Medicine* **151** (1991): 443–47.

25   **Dennis H. Novack** et al., 'Physicians' Attitudes towards Using Deception to Resolve Difficult Ethical Problems,' *JAMA* **261** (1989): 2980–85.

26   Norman Daniels, 'Why Saying No to Patients in the United States Is So Hard: Cost-Containment, Justice, and Provider Autonomy,' *NEJM* **314** (1986): 1380–83.

27   **David A Pollack** et al., 'Prioritization of Mental Health Services in Oregon,' *Milbank Quarterly* (in press, 1994); Philip J. Boyle and Daniel Callahan, 'Minds and Hearts: Priorities in Mental Health Services,' Special Supplement, *Hastings Center Report* 23, no. **5** (1993).

28   **E. Haavi Morreim**, *Balancing Act: The New Medical Ethics of Medicine's New Economics* (Dordrecht, the Netherlands: Kluwer Academic Publishers, 1991).

29   **James E. Sabin**, 'The Therapeutic Alliance in Managed Care Mental Health Practice,' *Journal of Psychotherapy Practice and Research* **1** (1992): 29–36.

30   **José M. Santiago**, 'The Fate of Mental Health Services in Health Care Reform: II. Realistic Solutions,' *Hospital and Community Psychiatry* 43 (1992): 1095–99, at 1098.

31   **Hugh L'Etang**, ed. *Health Care Provision under Financial Constraint: A Decade of Change* (London: Royal Society of Medicine, 1990).

Caring About Patients and Caring About Money

The American Psychiatric Association Code of Ethics Meets Managed Care*

James E. Sabin

The Problem: Caring About Patients and Caring About Money

The ethics of managed care got personal for me shortly after I began to work at the Harvard Community Health Plan in 1975. A young patient of mine with alcoholism had been admitted to a nearby psychiatric hospital after cutting his wrists while intoxicated. While negotiating by telephone with the attending psychiatrist for what I believed was a prudent discharge to outpatient care, I was chagrined to hear him call out to the chief of service – who had supervised me as a resident 7 years earlier – 'I have Sabin on the line . . . he used to care about patients . . . but now he cares about money!'

I initially reacted to this accusation with outraged indignation, but it set in motion a continuing reflection on *whether* and *how* an ethical clinician can both 'care about patients' and 'care about money.' In this paper I address one component of that reflection – the degree to which professional codes of ethics can help clinicians at the front-lines of managed care to answer these questions. As a psychiatrist, I focus primarily on the ethical code of the American Psychiatric Association (APA) (APA, 1993a), which consists of a set of principles promulgated by the American Medical Association (AMA) (AMA, 1989) (appendix 1) accompanied by annotations, and the associated Opinions of the APA Ethics Committee (APA, 1993b),[1] but for contrast I will consider the Code of the National Association of Social Workers (NASW) (NASW, 1993a) as well.

A profession's code of ethics represents the profession's self image, the moral wisdom of its experienced elders. It sets forth the profession's view of rightful actions. Perhaps more importantly, it gives at least an implicit picture of the profession's view of what it means to be a virtuous professional. As such it offers itself as a template for the clinician's professional ego ideal and for education of the next generation of professionals.

Professional codes, however, have lately been the target of serious critiques. According to Robert Veatch (1986), 'the most important event in medical ethics in the past 15 years has probably been the challenging of the assumption that the codes of organized medical professionals are the definitive summary of ethical norms governing medicine.' Veatch, drawing on William May's influential essay (1975), explained that 'it is the unilateral, philanthropic issuing forth of a set of moral norms and imposing those norms on the lay population that is so offensive in the traditional professional codes in medicine.' More recently, Edmund Pellegrino (1993) asserted that 'we cannot – and should not – return to the days when medical ethics was defined solely by [professional codes].'

The era of 'doctor knows best' is over. Medical codes no longer claim to legislate to society. Doctors, however, still need a moral map, and for this they often turn to their profession's code of ethics. A new phenomenon as pervasive and important as managed care tests the robustness of a professional code as a source of guidance for the profession itself – how well do its principles of action and the moral ideal it fosters help clinicians to search out, identify and advocate for an ethical path in the new environment?

Most of the ethical concerns about managed care can be subsumed under three questions. First, should ethical clinicians consider costs ('care about money') in their clinical work? Second, insofar as it is ethically appropriate for clinicians to consider costs, how do they avoid becoming unethical double agents? Finally, given finite resources, what principles and procedures should ethical managed care programs apply to decide about the costworthiness of potential care? In the following three sections I examine the ways in which the APA code speaks to each of these questions. I then turn to the NASW code for contrast. Although I will be quite critical of the APA code, my purpose is not simply to offer yet another indictment of a medical code of ethics, but to suggest practical ways in which it can be improved, which I do in the final section.

Should Clinicians Consider Costs?

Notwithstanding public concern that health professionals have become overly mercenary, mental health clinicians are typically drawn to clinical practice because they want to attend to human need, not the bottom line concerns they associate with business. Therapists experience a range of countertransference reactions – including shame – when asked to deal explicitly with money (Gans, 1992). Norman Levinsky (1984) captures the moral ideal many clinicians hold in his passionately argued, influential essay on 'The Doctor's Master:'

. . . physicians are required to do everything that they believe may benefit each patient without regard to costs or other societal considerations. In caring for an individual patient, the doctor must act solely as that patient's advocate, against the apparent interests of society as a whole, if necessary.

Managed care challenges this ideal with a range of techniques designed to make clinicians more attentive to costs. Given the power of the moral ideal Levinsky articulates so well, it is not surprising that newly graduated psychiatrists feel morally sullied and even clinically depressed on entering the world of managed care (Gabbard, 1992). In retrospect, I believe the defensive outrage I experienced in 1975 when the attending psychiatrist questioned whether I still 'care(d) about patients' reflected my own dis-ease at departing from the path Levinsky urges.

The Preamble to the APA Principles of Medical Ethics suggests that the precepts to follow will help psychiatrists with the question of whether they can 'care about money' along with 'car(ing) about patients' by presenting some form of balance between patient-centered and communitarian ethics:

As a member of this profession, a physician must recognize responsibility not only to patients, *but also to society*, to other health professionals, and to self. (emphasis added)

Unfortunately, the promise is not fulfilled. Neither the annotated Principles nor the separately published Opinions of the APA Ethics Committee offer any explication of the responsibility that the physician – *qua* physician – bears toward society.

This is an extremely serious defect. The Principles and Opinions give no guidance as to whether and how managed care systems might pursue positive ideals. They present no principles of social justice that might help

* Sabin, J.: Caring about patients and caring about money: the American Psychiatric Association Code of Ethics meets managed care. *Behavioral Sciences and the Law* 12:317–330, 1994.

clinicians distinguish between more and less ethical forms of managed care. According to the Principles, the best a managed care program can hope for is not to conflict with the physician's primary obligations. Because the APA Ethics Committee offers no picture of a social good that managed care might promote, it provides no basis for a quality improvement approach to managed care – only attacking deficits. Not surprisingly, until quite recently the APA restricted itself to criticizing the failings of managed care – applying what Berwick (1989) calls 'The Theory of Bad Apples.'

By contrast, in the United Kingdom, where the National Health Service budget finances medical care[2] for the entire population, the British Medical Association (1988) code of ethics tells physicians that they have a positive 'ethical duty' to use the most economic option that achieves the clinical objectives, and explains the basis of that duty as follows:

Finite resources can never match potentially infinite demands or expectations. The inevitable consequence is that a decision to allocate a particular sum to a particular service will produce underfunding of another service. This will result in a number of possible outcomes (e.g., ward closure/staff reductions/increased waiting lists) all of which may increase morbidity . . . consequently it is the doctor's *ethical duty* to use the most economic and efficacious treatment available. (British Medical Association, p.72) (emphasis added)

Efficiency promotes benefit to patients by allowing the National Health Service to provide more care. Waste injures the public by depleting the global health budget. Physicians in the United Kingdom cannot truly 'care about patients' unless they also 'care about money.'

With regard to the question of whether the ethical clinician should consider costs, where the BMA defines a clear and positive obligation to do so, the AMA and APA are silent. Not surprisingly, a participant at a 1991 APA conference on 'ethics in managed care' stated – without contradiction from other participants – that 'when [two or more treatments] were equally effective, even though one might be less expensive, it was not appropriate or ethical for the reviewer to say ['use the less expensive treatment']. (p. 81)'

Money is the most basic social resource. Since the Preamble to the Principles tells us that physicians have a responsibility to society, physicians obviously have some kind of responsibility for considering the costs of care when spending third party (societal) funds, whether that 'society' is the United Kingdom, the state of Oregon, or a county mental health program in which citizens levy taxes on themselves to promote the common good, or Blue Cross or HMO insurance in which the members pool their health insurance premiums for a similar collective purpose. The APA's annotations and opinions, however, never say this explicitly. This matters. From consultation and teaching about the ethics of managed care practice, I know that many clinicians in all parts of the country are conflicted and confused about the basic question of whether they should consider the cost of treatment at all, or only the question of what constitutes the best treatment they can imagine (Sabin, 1993). It is no exaggeration to say that they feel anguished and morally compromised at being expected to 'care about money' as well as 'care about patients.'

Are Managed Care Clinicians Unethical Double Agents?

Even physicians who believe that they are morally obligated to consider the costs of treatment are profoundly troubled by fear that managed care may corrupt their relationship with patients. Levinsky interprets the danger as the impossibility of 'serving two masters.' Angell (1993) and Simon (1987) call it 'double agentry.' Abrams (1993) wryly advises medical students to solve the dilemma by becoming 'doctor(s) with two heads.' Kramer (1994) argues that this problem, difficult enough in other areas of health care, 'is uniquely destructive to the doctor–patient relationship in psychiatry . . .

enacting as it does some of patients' typical fantasies about doctors and their loyalties.'

I believe that clinicians have comparable fantasies about loyalty and betrayal. Even in England, where the BMA Code directs physicians to consider costs in planning treatment, physicians tell cautionary fables about the dangers of acknowledging and discussing costs with patients (Sabin, 1992). Veatch (APA, 1991) articulates the shame-laden fears about double-agentry that haunt clinicians under managed care in the form of a revised Hippocratic Oath a variant of the 'scarlet letter' to be posted in the waiting rooms of clinicians who practice in the new environment:

Warning all ye who enter here. I will generally work for your interests but in the case of marginally beneficial expensive care, I will abandon you in order to serve society as their cost containment agent.

The term 'double agent' only appears once in the Opinions of the APA Ethics Committee. In October 1977, in answer to a student health service psychiatrist who asked whether he had a potential ethical conflict in 'treat[ing] some students psychotherapeutically and see[ing] others for administrative reasons,' the committee answered:

You certainly do if you do not define your roles clearly and in advance to the student. You cannot give an administrative opinion if the student has made a psychotherapeutic contract with you. This is a classic example of 'double-agentry.' If the college demands that you confuse your roles, you should refuse to participate and must ethically withdraw from the arena if the college will not relent. Even a student's consent for you to make an administrative report after a period of psychotherapy does not resolve your conflict since the consent may not be freely given but coerced. The college should be advised to seek an administrative opinion from a psychiatrist not involved in a treatment relationship with the student. (Opinions, 4-H)

This opinion provides more than sensible advice to a perplexed college psychiatrist – it implies a crucial and perhaps startling clarification of the concept of 'double agentry' itself. An agent is one who 'acts for or as the representative of another' (Heritage Dictionary, 1979). Examined closely, the opinion suggests that commitment to ('agency for') legitimate but conflicting values and interests (e.g., a student's need for treatment and a college's need for administrative advice) is not in itself inevitably unethical. The student health service psychiatrist would definitely be unethical if he: (1) did not acknowledge his agency for conflicting values (as by not telling the student that an administrative opinion will be rendered), and 2) did not ensure that the patient has sanctioned his commitment to the conflicting values ('double agency') through a valid process of informed consent, which would have to precede the initiation of psychotherapy. But suppose the psychiatrist meets these two conditions?

It would be consistent with the APA opinion to hold that clinicians who experience ethical conflict arising from agency for valid but competing individual and societal interests, acknowledge the existence of the conflict, and collaborate with the patient in managing it, should be seen as morally mature, not unethical. If we take this perspective – as I believe we should – we would recognize the existence of ethical, unethical, and mixed forms of double agentry. I have argued elsewhere that ethical managed care systems are intentionally designed to encourage clinicians to consider stewardship as well as fiduciary values (Sabin, 1994a, 1994b). Given that managed care settings deliberately ask clinicians to be agents for these two distinctive values, we would ask: 'is this particular managed care situation one of ethical or unethical double agentry?'

In current usage, however, 'double agent' has such pejorative connotations that the concept of 'ethical double agentry' is an emotional non-sequitur. Once the term 'double agent' is affixed, adrenalin flows and reflection stops. However, if we take the perspective that it is the way in which the conflict between two or more values and interests is handled and not the simple fact of 'double agentry' itself that makes a clinician unethical, I believe that for analytic clarity it will be useful to pose the counter-intuitive question: what factors make situations of double agentry more and less ethical?

From the writings of the APA Ethics Committee, we can identify three key factors to help in assessing the ethics of double agent situations:

First, we must assess the situation in terms of the precept that: 'the patient may place his/her trust in his/her psychiatrist knowing that the psychiatrist's ethics and professional responsibilities preclude him/her gratifying his/her own needs by exploiting the patient' (Principles, 1,1). While psychiatrists cannot avoid being agents for themselves (as by charging fees or setting limits on their office hours) as well as for their patient's needs, they can and must avoid exploiting the patient to do so. Psychiatrists must guide their decisions by appropriate standards of quality (Opinions, 2-W, June 1986) and must not 'compromise the patient's welfare' (Opinions, 5-N, December 1990). Financial inducement regarding treatment recommendations are acceptable as long as they do not 'take precedence over the best interests of the patient' (Opinions, 5-N). Finally, psychiatrists, like judges, must conduct themselves so as to avoid 'giv[ing] the appearance of impropriety' (Opinions, 1-D, January 1983).

Second, we must assess the degree to which the patient has made an informed contract that recognizes and allows the particular double agent situation. Psychiatrists must inform their patients about any pertinent ways in which they are 'agents' for values other than direct clinical care (Opinions, 1-E, March 1985). The Principles and Opinions recognize that patients are entitled to contract for systems features that psychiatrists find undesirable, such as mandatory third party utilization review (Opinions, 4-T, March 1987) and even the participation of Employee Assistance Program (EAP) clinicians in psychiatric treatment planning (Opinions, 4-O, July 1986). The terms of the contract, however, must be explicit, clear, and understood by all parties (Principles, 2,5).

Finally, we must assess the degree to which the cost concern imposed by the managed care system serves ethically appropriate purposes. The APA Ethics Committee recognizes – within the context of the public sector – that resources are finite, and that limitations on care may be ethically acceptable if they serve societal interests, A psychiatrist who asked the Ethics Committee whether it would be unethical to practice in a public hospital where staffing is so limited that it is difficult to practice competently was told:

Your first effort should be directed at getting the hospital to remedy the situation. That failing . . . if you remain and do your best, you are behaving ethically. For us to declare otherwise might place an even greater burden upon our underfunded public institutions. (Opinions, 1-M, March 1990)

The Committee could have defined this situation as one of unethical double agentry, in which the psychiatrist presented himself as a caretaker ('agentry for the patient') but with too little time to do a fully competent job ('agentry for the facility'). However, the Committee concluded that this specific example of double agentry should not be considered unethical because the limited staffing results from public funding decisions which are intended to allow the available funds to serve the greatest good of the greatest number. Presumably, if this same situation of limited staffing occurred in a for-profit

hospital and was designed to increase investor profits, the Committee would have reached a different conclusion. Cost containment on behalf of private gain may be sound business practice, but it is not stewardship of societal resources.

Determining Costworthiness: Whatever Happened to Justice?

In the section on whether clinicians should consider costs, I argued that although the American Psychiatric Association Code of Ethics does not yet explicitly require clinicians to consider costs in making treatment recommendations as the British Medical Association Code does, that conclusion logically follows from the Preamble to the Principles. In the section on double-agentry, I concluded that 'agentry' for two conflicting values can be ethical if the clinician conducts appropriate forms of disclosure and informed consent. This reading of the APA Principles points to the conclusion that psychiatric care should be managed. The daunting question is how to manage our resources in the most costworthy manner.

Decisions about costworthiness are ultimately decisions about priorities. If John Q. Public pays for his own care and chooses monthly rather than weekly appointments or to terminate as soon as his symptoms have improved, he is managing his treatment in accord with his own priorities about the best use of his resources. Assuming that there is no question about his competence, Mr. Public is entitled to determine these choices in accord with personal preferences, however idiosyncratic these preferences may be. In the terms of Beauchamp and Childress' (1994) commonly used framework of four basic ethical principles (beneficence, nonmaleficence, autonomy and justice), Mr. Public is exercising his right to autonomy. The clinician's ethical responsibility is to provide information to Mr. Public about the likely implications of his choices, and in the absence of specified forms of danger to Mr. Public or to others, to accept and support his decision.

The difficult ethical problems about costworthiness arise when priorities are set for the patient, not by the patient. When John Q. Public's therapist in an HMO makes the same recommendation about appointment frequency or termination, he is making a judgment about the best use of HMO resources. In Beauchamp and Childress' terms, the therapist is applying a vision of the principle of justice – considerations regarding fairness in distributing resources to the membership of the HMO.

The APA Principles and Opinions provide little guidance about justice. As part of this project, I classified each statement in the Annotated Principles and the Opinions according to which of Beauchamp and Childress' four principles was most prominent. I found that I had to add a fifth category intra-and inter-professional relations. Table 1, which quantifies the degree to which justice is a neglected consideration, explains the subtitle of this section.

Justice is the Cinderella principle throughout health care policy – not just in the writings of the APA Ethics Committee. The state of Oregon is virtually alone in the degree to which it has articulated a vision of justice by setting explicit priorities. The report of the Hastings Center 'Project on Priorities

Table 1 Classification of statements in the APA annotated principles and opinions in terms of Beauchamp and Childress Principles of Medical Ethics

	Beneficence	Non-maleficence	Autonomy	Justice	Inter and intra professional relations
Annotated principles	12 (20%)	14 (23%)	13 (22%)	5 (8%)	16 (27%)
Opinions	8 (6%)	36 (26%)	44 (32%)	10 (7%)	41 (29%)
Total	20 (10%)	50 (25%)	57 (29%)	15 (7%)	57 (29%)

Each statement in the APA Annotated Principles and Opinions is classified according to which of the four principles of biomedical ethics is most prominently represented. A fifth category of professional relations has been added.

in Mental Health Services' (Boyle & Callahan, 1993) is more typical of the current state of the art. The Report strongly urges other systems to emulate Oregon by setting priorities among mental health services and integrating mental health into overall health care priority-setting. It recommends some broad principles for setting priorities, but only at such an abstract level that it is difficult to glean practical guidance for the ethical assessment of the ways in which managed care programs allocate their funds. The 15 references to justice in the Principles and Opinions are similarly abstract and offer only the most general guidance for determining costworthiness.

In 1990, in response to a psychiatrist who complained about the way a local PPO conducted utilization review and imposed restrictions on its network of preferred providers, the APA Ethics Committee set forth a series of considerations regarding procedural justice in determining costworthiness. While the Committee says nothing about the content of the priorities that a managed care program might set, it says much about the procedures that should be followed in considering costworthiness. Psychiatrists who participate in managed care systems are not inherently unethical if:

1. Patients and prospective patients (or their employers) make an informed decision to participate which includes knowledge of:

   a. their other options;

   b. benefit limits;

   c. the pre- and current authorization process;

   d. their right to appeal a utilization decision;

   e. the limits as to whom they can see without having to make a greater financial investment;

   f. the potential invasion of their privacy by the review process.

2. No exaggerated claims of excellence are made.

3. Care provided is competent and meets patient needs within the contracted benefit limits.

4. The utilization review process is not unduly invasive of the doctor patient relationship.

5. Reviewers are not financially rewarded for denying care (Opinions, 6,K, April 1990).

The first section of the Principles, which states that the ethical psychiatrist 'shall be dedicated to providing competent medical service with compassion and respect for human dignity,' will be the key starting point for considering the content of judgments about costworthiness. The term 'competent' tells us that ethical practice must meet a basic standard of care. That standard is not the 'best care imaginable' but 'competent care.' The concept of 'competent care' implies that the APA Ethics Committee will ultimately endorse the fundamental activities of managed care programs as ethical: defining a package of basic benefits; setting priorities for use of resources; and, managing the system that these decisions create.

Section 1 of the Principles adds that to be ethical, all of these activities must be done 'with compassion and respect for human dignity.' Explicating the meaning of 'competent,' 'compassion,' 'respect', and dignity' should be a central APA Ethics Committee agenda for the rest of the decade.

The Social Work Profession Meets Managed Care

Historically, the social work profession developed largely at community agencies, hospitals, clinics, and other institutional settings. If the profession had to identify a spiritual parent and a birthplace, Jane Addams and Hull House in Chicago would certainly be leading candidates. For psychiatry, the choice might be Sigmund Freud and his private consulting room in Vienna. Not surprisingly, the ethical codes of the two professions reflect their historical and spiritual origins.

In a series of recent Opinions, the APA Ethics Committee almost went out of its way to stress that it assesses individuals, not institutions: 'Our function is to keep our members ethical, not hospitals' (Opinions, 6–I, February 1990); 'We cannot judge the ethics of the health plan but we can those of any psychiatrists who participate' (Opinions, 5-M, October 1990); and, 'We do not address the ethics of hospitals but of those psychiatrists practicing there' (Opinions, 5-N, December 1990).

The NASW Ethics Committee, in contrast to that of the APA, does not restrict itself to assessing individual clinicians, and takes responsibility for judging the ethics of institutions and programs as well. It directs employed social workers to evaluate and improve the organizations that employ them: 'The social worker should work to improve the employing agency's policies and procedures and the efficiency and effectiveness of its services' (National Association of Social Workers, 1993a, IV,L, 1). To assist social workers with this charge the NASW developed explicit recommendations for infrastructure, benefit design, provider panels, utilization review, evaluation and outcome, consumer protections, and provider relations in managed care systems. Then, after presenting 47 specific assessment criteria, the NASW reminds its members to 'evaluate an organization's ability to provide ethical programs before agreeing to serve or continue as a provider' (National Association of Social Workers, 1993b, p.8).

Presumably because of the historical association of social workers with institutions, the NASW seems much more sophisticated than the APA about the complexities of double agentry. As we expect of any health profession, the NASW reminds its members that their 'primary responsibility is to clients' (NASW, 1093a, II,F). The NASW recognizes, in ways the APA does not, that because resources are limited social workers will inevitably experience conflict between their commitment to fidelity and stewardship:

It may be difficult to adhere to a position of primacy of the client's interests, particularly in a climate of resource scarcity. Agency cost containment goals may conflict with the best interests of the client. (National Association of Social Workers, 1992, p. 10)

The NASW recommends that social workers follow a three-step sequence of actions when this kind of conflict between fidelity and stewardship occurs. First, the social worker should advocate for the interests of the client within the limits of what the system offers. Second, when the results of this initial level of advocacy are clear, the social worker 'should inform the client of the full range of existing choices . . . includ[ing] information on the lack or limited availability of relevant services' (NASW 1992, p.10). Finally, if the social worker believes that the client's needs are not being met, the NASW advises the social worker to seek additional options by using such mechanisms as peer consultation, an institutional ethics committee, or the NASW itself, and to advocate for any viable possibilities that emerge.

The clinician and client alone may not be able to resolve the conflict satisfactorily, and the NASW (1993b, p.8) recommends a course of action to the managed care program itself:

Managed care organizations should respect the dual commitment that a provider has in fulfilling the contractual responsibilities to the managed care organization and in serving the best interest of the client. If there is conflict, the managed care organization should work with the provider to resolve the conflict, with the needs of the client as primary consideration. No punitive action should be taken against the social worker for this advocacy.

At the end of the day, however, the social workers must 'ensure that all persons have access to the resources, services, and opportunities which they require' (NASW, 1993a, VI,P,2). When this cannot be done cooperatively with clients and organizations, it must he pursued by way of political advocacy.

Conclusion: Recommendations to the Apa Ethics Committee

The American Psychiatric Association's Principles and Opinions provide the basis for an ethically sound practical approach to managed care. The APA Ethics Committee, however, has barely started this effort, and will have to undo at least one of its strongly held positions to create a useful response to managed care. I present my conclusions in the form of recommendations for a series of action steps the Ethics Committee might take in order to help clinicians deal better with the challenge of 'caring about patients' and 'caring about money.'

1. The Ethics Committee should develop a new annotation to explicate the second sentence of the Preamble. This crucial but unexplicated sentence assigns four valid but potentially conflicting responsibilities (to patients, society, health professionals, and self) to psychiatrists. By asking clinicians to attend to society (stewardship) as well as to patients (fidelity), managed care challenges them to conduct what Morreim (1991) has usefully described as an ethical 'balancing act.' The AMA and APA should emulate the British Medical Association by explicitly stating that ethical physicians must commit themselves to stewardship as well as to patient care.

2. If the Ethics Committee follows recommendation #1 and defines stewardship of societal resources as a component of being an ethical psychiatrist, it will have to modify its statement that it judges individuals, not institutions. Psychiatrists need to distinguish between managed care programs which are designed to promote stewardship of a group's resources and others which shortchange patients to promote private profits (Sabin, in press). The APA needs to emulate the NASW by identifying the key system characteristics that support the ethical practice of psychiatry.

3. The committee should seek opportunities to render opinions on different ways of assessing costworthiness and setting priorities. The issue of just allocation of resources is extremely difficult to deal with abstractly. The Ethics Committee needs to develop a series of precedents to help clinicians (and organizations) deal with the concerns about allocation that arise at the clinical front-lines. Here are some hypothetical questions that might come to the APA Ethics Committee, adapted from questions posed by front-line clinicians at consulting and teaching sessions. Each question is followed by an imagined response from the Ethics Committee.

(1) I am employed by an HMO that recently changed its benefit to allow unlimited 'necessary' outpatient mental health treatment for patients with severe mental illness. To accomplish this, it instituted an increased copayment for all other mental health patients after eight sessions. I applaud making increased services available for patients with severe mental illness, but is it ethical to do this by reducing what is available to other patients who may be suffering just as severely and who might derive as much or more benefit from treatment?

[Possible response: As long as: (1) potential members of the HMO are informed about the policy before joining, and (2) an appropriate appeals process is available, the policy appears to be ethical. When the resources available for mental health care are not sufficient to meet all patient needs allocational choices must be made, and giving priority to patients with the most severe impairments is a valid principle for setting priorities, albeit not the only possible one. If the HMO discriminates against patients with mental health disorders by allocating relatively less for mental disorders than for other (non-mental health) conditions – as happens commonly in insurance programs – you should advocate within the HMO for non-discriminatory allocational policies.]

(2) I have 25 years of experience treating patients with severe character problems in long-term individual psychotherapy and have been able to help many patients make remarkable gains. The managed network in my area says it respects the work I do, but claims that there is no evidence proving that this kind of treatment is the only way to produce the kinds of results my patients have achieved. Recently the reviewer recommended that I refer a patient to a 12-step program and other 'therapeutic' activities and authorized six follow-up appointments. Is it ethical to challenge treatment recommendations based on 25 years of experience and demonstrated results?

[Possible response: If the fact that utilization review would be applied within the network, and the philosophy that would guide the review process were made clear to potential enrollees in the managed care program before they signed up, then it would not be inherently unethical for a reviewer to raise questions about your treatment recommendations. But just as the network can ask for evidence in addition to your own experience-based opinion, so can you hold the network to a similar standard. When results of randomized clinical trials are not available, APA guidelines and consensus committee recommendations are the best we can do. The patient's preferences should also be considered. If the patient in question has a severe and chronic condition, six follow-up visits sounds very skimpy for 'providing competent medical service with compassion and respect for human dignity' (Principles, section 1). If the patient's insurance promises treatment for the condition, you are obliged to appeal if you are not persuaded by the reviewer's recommendation. However, if the available evidence really does not favor one approach over the other, we advise you to try the less costly approach first.]

(3) I recently needed to hospitalize a suicidal adolescent. The insurer contracts with a hospital 45 miles away that is less convenient and provides lower quality care than a hospital in our own town. What is the ethical course of action for me to rake?

[Possible response: First, you should appeal for an exception to the policy. If this is denied, you should inform the family about the local hospital alternative, making clear that the insurance will not cover it. Ideally you would have investigated the arrangements the insurer program offers before becoming one of its providers. Whatever happens with this case you should do all you can to persuade the insurer to make the local hospital available. Especially for an adolescent, where family therapy and visits home may be an important part of treatment, being limited to a distant hospital seems undesirable.]

It will be through struggling with questions like these that psychiatry and the other mental health professions will refine their understanding of how to manage care ethically. But organized psychiatry cannot undertake this crucial activity until it concludes – as it inevitably will and should – that ethical clinicians do indeed have a responsibility to society as well as to patients. In other words, we must 'care about patients' and 'care about money.'

Notes

1 Throughout the text I will refer to these simply as 'Principles' and 'Opinions.' '(Principles, 1,1)' refers to the APA's first annotation to the first section of the AMA principles, and '(Opinions, 1-A)' to the APA's first opinion about the first section of the AMA principles.

2 Except for a small percentage paid for by private insurance and out-of-pocket.

References

Abrams, F. R. (1993). The doctor with two heads: The patient versus the costs. *New England Journal of Medicine*, **328**, 975–976.

American Medical Association. (1989). *Principles of medical ethics*. Chicago, IL: Author.

American Psychiatric Association. (1991, October). *Ethics in managed care conference*. Washington, DC: American Psychiatric Association.

American Psychiatric Association. (1993a). *The principles of medical ethics: With annotations especially applicable to psychiatry*. Washington, DC: Author.

American Psychiatric Association. (1993b). *Opinions of the ethics committee on the principles of medical ethics: With annotations especially applicable to psychiatry*. Washington, DC: Author.

Angell, M. (1993). The doctor as double agent. *Kennedy Institute of Ethics Journal*, **3**, 270–286.

Beauchamp, T. L., & Childress, J.F. (1994). *Principles of biomedical ethics* (4th ed.). New York: Oxford University Press.

Berwick, D. M. (1989). Continuous quality improvement as an ideal in health care. *New England Journal of Medicine*, 320, 53–56.

Boyle, P. J., & Callahan, D. (1993). Minds and hearts: Priorities in mental health services. *Hastings Center Report*, 23, Special Supplement.

British Medical Association. (1988). *Philosophy and practice of medical ethics*. London: British Medical Association.

Daniels, N. (1986). Why saying no to patients in the United States is so hard: Cost-containment, justice, and provider autonomy. *New England Journal of Medicine*, 314 1381–1383.

Gabbard, G. O. (1992). The big chill: The transition from residency to managed care nightmare. *Academic Psychiatry*, 16, 119–126.

Gans, J. S. (1992). Money and psychodynamic group psychotherapy. *International Journal of Group Psychotherapy*, 42, 133–152.

Heritage Dictionary. (1979). Boston: Houghton Mifflin.

Kramer, P. D. (1994). Loss of function: The politics of outpatient psychiatry. *Psychiatric Times*, 11(1), pp. 1–6.

Levinsky, N. G. (1984). The doctor's master. *New England Journal of Medicine*, 311, 1573–1575.

May, W. F. (1975). Code, covenant, contract, or philanthropy. *Hastings Center Report*, 5, 29–38.

Morreim, E. H. (1991). *Balancing act: The new medical ethics of medicine's new economics*. Dordrect: Kluwer Academic Publishers.

National Association of Social Workers. (1992). *Standards for social work case management*. Washington, DC: Author.

National Association of Social Workers. (1993a). *Code of ethics of the national association of social workers*. Washington, DC: Author.

National Association of Social Workers (National Council on the Practice of Clinical Social Work). (1993b). *The social work perspective on managed care for mental health and substance abuse treatment*. Washington, DC: Author.

Pellegrino, E. D. (1993). The metamorphosis of medical ethics: A 30-year retrospective. *Journal of the American Medical Association*, 269, 1158–1162.

Sabin, J. E. (1992). 'Mind the gap': Reflections of an American health maintenance organisation doctor on the new NHS. *British Medical Journal*, 305, 514–516.

Sabin, J. E. (1993). The moral myopia of academic psychiatry: A response to Glen O. Gabbard's 'The big chill.' *Academic Psychiatry*, 17, 175–179.

Sabin, J. E. (1994a). The role of the psychiatrist in a clinical managed care setting. *Directions in Psychiatry*, 14(9), 1–7.

Sabin, J. E. (1994b). Ethical issues under managed care: The managed care view. In Schreter, R. K., Sharfstein, S. S., & Schreter, C. A. (Eds.) *Allies and adversaries: The impact of managed care on mental health services* (pp. 187–194). Washington, DC: American Psychiatric Press.

Sabin, J. E. (in press). A credo for ethical managed care mental health practice. *Hospital & Community Psychiatry*.

Simon, R. I. (1987). The psychiatrist as a fiduciary: Avoiding the double agent role. *Psychiatric Annals*, 17, 622–626.

Veatch, R. M. (1986). Challenging the power of codes. *Hastings Center Report*, 16, 14–15.

Veatch, R. M. (1991, October). *Ethics in managed care conference*. Washington, DC: American Psychiatric Association.

Appendix I: Principles of Medical Ethics, American Medical Association, 1989

Preamble

The medical profession has long subscribed to a body of ethical statements developed primarily for the benefit of the patient. As a member of this profession, a physician must recognize responsibility not only to patients, but also to society, to other health professionals, and to self. The following Principles, adopted by the American Medical Association, are not laws, but standards of conduct which define the essentials of honorable behavior for the physician.

SECTION 1

A physician shall be dedicated to providing competent medical service with compassion and respect for human dignity.

SECTION 2

A physician shall deal honestly with patients and colleagues, and strive to expose those physicians deficient in character and competence, or who engage in fraud or deception.

SECTION 3

A physician shall respect the law and also recognize a responsibility to seek changes in those requirements which are contrary to the best interests of the patient.

SECTION 4

A physician shall respect the rights of patients, of colleagues, and of other health professionals, and shall safeguard patient confidences within the constraints of the law.

SECTION 5

A physician shall continue to study, apply, and advance scientific knowledge, make relevant information available to patients, colleagues, and the public, obtain consultation, and use the talents of other health professionals when indicated.

SECTION 6

A physician shall, in the provision of appropriate patient care, except in emergencies, be free to choose whom to serve, with whom to associate, and the environment in which to provide medical services.

SECTION 7

A physician shall recognize a responsibility to participate in activities contributing to an improved community.

Setting Mental Health Priorities

*Problems and Possibilities**

Daniel Callahan

Other developed countries take for granted that scarcity and limits will be the mark of any sensible health care system. Universal access has as its necessary corollary a constraint on unlimited wants and desires. In the United States, by contrast, the most powerful ideology has been the conviction that only greed, inefficiency, or misguided politics stand in the way of giving everyone most of what they want. The language of limits and rationing does not sit well; it is judged to be a capitulation to the forces of conservatism or mismanagement. As part of the same attitude, the idea of setting formal priorities in health care, especially as a way of coping with scarcity, has not until recently attracted many followers. It no less flies in the face of an interest group politics that is reluctant to admit openly that some things are more important than others, that not all forms of disease, pain, and suffering are equally oppressive.

In a recent project at The Hastings Center, we decided to pursue a different direction. Taking for granted that some degree of scarcity will be a permanent part of any new health care scheme, we wanted to know what that perception could mean for the field of mental health. It is a field that, more than most others, has long struggled in the face of denial and stigmatization to attain parity within the health care system.

Our initial question was this: in a time of increasing economic scarcity and cost-containment pressures, what would be the most sensible set of priorities within the mental health field? Or, to phrase it differently, what is comparatively most important and least important within the wide range of mental health services that could, or should, be provided?

Almost at once, two important additional issues appeared, emblematic of a basic struggle within the mental health field. The first was this: quite apart from setting micropriorities, what should be the most basic mission of mental health and thus its highest priority? Should it be the advancement of mental 'health,' the positive effort to help people cope better with the wide range of emotional and cognitive disorders, both mild and moderate, that can burden and diminish the living of a life for millions of people? Or should it be mental 'illness,' with the focus on those most severe illnesses that affect far fewer people, such as schizophrenia, but that make living a decent life exceedingly difficult for most and altogether impossible for some? Questions of this kind are important when the mental health budgets are fixed and different programs must compete with each other. A second issue soon emerged: how should mental health priorities be established within the larger context of all health conditions, and what are the policy implications of shifting resources from other health budgets into mental health?

Part of the struggle on the first issue, setting mental health priorities, turns on that mix of aspirations, indignation, and resentment that so often marks the clash of advocacy groups within the field, battling not just for money but also to advance their own definition of what the *real* problem is. As so often happens in struggles of great complexity, each side has a good case to make; they differ because their eyes are fixed on different facets of experience. For the purposes of our project, however, a basic set of questions lay just below the surface of that struggle. Is it possible to find persuasive

ways of comparing the degree of pain and suffering in different conditions – the suffering of the phobic against that of the schizophrenic, for instance – and no less to compare the social burden of milder conditions that affect large numbers with those terrible conditions that affect smaller numbers? Is it also possible, moreover, to make orderly sense of the fact that people differ enormously in their judgments about which conditions most affect the quality of a person's life and which are comparatively more or less tolerable and endurable? At stake were issues of a familiar political kind in medicine and health care as well as fundamental moral questions about health and illness, pain and suffering, hope and despair.

That set of issues served as a backdrop for our project on priority setting in mental health. With the support of the John D. and Catherine T. MacArthur Foundation, we explored whether (a) it would be possible to set priorities, and (b) how and where that might best be done. The arguments among the psychiatrists and other mental health workers, representatives of various advocacy groups, philosophers, lawyers, and others were both intense and revealing. Some thought that setting priorities was difficult but not impossible; more significant was the viewpoint that priority setting will be imbedded in a political process where broad social policy can subvert the priorities. David Mechanic articulates that perspective in his essay published in this issue. By contrast, a group that had worked in Oregon to integrate fully mental health into that state's controversial priority-setting plan is much more optimistic (see the article by Pollack *et al.* in this issue). 'We did it,' they said, and they tell us how. Gerald Grob, also writing in these pages, falls somewhere in the middle, showing that whereas priorities can and have been set in ways that at times transcend pure politics, doing so can have unforeseen and untoward consequences.

Although it was difficult to achieve consensus on many of these matters, there was general agreement on one basic and important point: the time has come to stop segregating mental health problems and policies from the more general run of medical and health problems. Full integration of the mental and the physical domains (which cannot in any case be neatly divided) is both necessary and possible. There can, then, no longer be any good reason, say, to set a limit on reimbursable days for a person institutionalized for a chronic mental health problem while setting none for a person admitted to an acute care hospital for a chronic medical problem. That is, of course, just what the Clinton administration proposed in its initial health care plan, while offering no rationale for the distinction, (although it was known that the real, unpublicized reason was, simply, that root of all evil, money).

Why should we make an effort to set priorities in mental health? For better or worse, we must as a society determine how best to spend the limited money we have and to deploy the resources at our disposal; that will be a permanent, not a temporary, condition. While the setting of priorities will have many practical benefits, its overriding value is to keep constantly before our eyes the need to make comparative judgments in the context of scarcity.

Although preceded by years of work on measurements of the quality of life, as well as cost-benefit and cost-effectiveness analysis, the idea of formal priority-setting efforts has arisen primarily as a response to economic pressures. It emerged first, and most controversially, in the case of physical health, but has now begun to be extended to mental health as well. Oregon's

* Callahan, D.: Setting mental health priorities: problems and possibilities. *Milbank Quarterly* **72**:451–470, 1994.

success in integrating mental and physical health into a single priority system shows that, if care is taken and some traps avoided, setting priorities for mental health poses no greater problem than establishing them for physical health (see Pollack et al., this issue). Pain and suffering, disability and dysfunction, social and economic burdens, and the like can successfully be compared across the health and illness spectrum, both physical and mental. Accordingly, I will here discuss the general problem of priority setting as a policy instrument, not restricting my analysis to mental health.

Priority Setting: A Continuum

There are three possible ways of understanding the notion of priority setting. They fall along a continuum, not always clearly delineated, and they often reflect an ordinary language use of the term rather than a rationalized technical sense. There is a kind of loose, informal sense in which legislators or policy makers decide in some rough way to emphasize one policy strategy rather than another for a certain period. A state department of mental health might, in that vein, announce that its priority for the coming year is to improve community services. It may or may not increase funds to that activity; even if it does, however, there may be little or no careful effort to rationalize that policy in explicit comparison with other ways the same money might be spent. Sometimes this is done as a symbolic gesture, to indicate heightened awareness of a neglected problem, or to correct for past injustices, or simply in response to political pressure. I call the use of the term 'priority' in this context 'informal,' to signal that it rests on no settled policy commitments and is often a response to transitory pressures and needs.

A second sense of priority setting is more formal and structured. As a matter of prudent management and perceived needs, it is decided that there should be broad ranking of needs and goals into general categories and clusters. That ranking is set by relatively nonquantitative means, usually based on the values of those managing the system, on professional judgment, and on the give and take of politics and policy. New York State and Alameda County in California provide examples of this form of priority setting (Surles and Feiden-Waugh 1993; Kears 1993). There is no pretense that this form of ranking is based on a special, technical methodology, but it is meant to be rational, coherent, and systematic.

A third sense of priority setting is a deliberate effort to rank specific medical conditions and treatment priorities, using both general categories and more specific, numerical rankings, and to do so systematically and rationally. The addition of numerical rankings separates this from the first and second senses that I have outlined, and it was the method used in Oregon. It is the form of priority setting that will be my principal concern here. I will begin my inquiry by developing three theses, devoting most of my attention to the third. The first two theses are almost, but not quite, self-evident.

The first thesis is that ranked priorities make the most sense in closed, not open, economic systems; they are particularly pertinent in global budgeting plans (e.g., when there is a legislatively set state, or county, mental health budget). On the basis of market theory, purely market-driven health care systems should have no interest in, and logically should oppose, any formal priority system, especially one imposed by government. The theory of market-driven systems is that people are free to buy what they want, subject to no higher principle than their personal preferences. Such systems, moreover, are hostile to externally imposed limits or caps because they are based on the idea that people should be free to spend as much as they want on health care in any way they want to spend it. Although it might seem that a priority system would be one way to control costs in the absence of global budgeting, it is likely to lack bite and full plausibility in that context. As efforts to control costs in the United States in the absence of global budgeting indicate, there are too many ways to circumvent constraints and too few mechanisms available to enforce the discipline necessary for priorities to work effectively.

Just the opposite is the case with planned systems, especially when working within a global budget. In those cases, priority setting makes special

sense as a way of distinguishing the more important from the less important. Precisely this insight lay behind the Oregon efforts to develop a ranking system for its Medicaid program as part of a larger effort to achieve universal health care in the state. Even if the legislature could be induced to spend more on the Medicaid program, that program would always have to live with a fixed budget; it thus seemed sensible to rank the priorities within that budget.

My second thesis is that any successful ranking scheme will have to find a middle way between two extremes, trying to do justice to the valid elements of each (and *appearing* to do justice to each). One of these extremes is the ever-present lure of a purely numerical approach, which seeks to quantify the important variables and come up with a mathematically precise set of priorities. I will call this the 'pure numbers' approach. The other extreme goes in exactly the opposite direction, arguing that priority setting usually is, and ought to be, strictly a political matter, to be determined by the values and preferences of the public, rational or irrational. The most acceptable set of priorities emerges from a fair political process. I will call this the 'raw politics' approach.

Neither the 'pure numbers' nor the 'raw politics' way seems adequate, and I will shortly say why. Objectivity – which I would define as the capacity to achieve a critical distance from policy judgments and to provide a reasoned, defensible justification of decisions – can be approached by means other than quantification. And appropriate ways of taking into account values and preferences can be achieved without descending into the rawest of politics (Jennings 1987; Reich 1988).

My third thesis is a refinement of the second. It is that the key to finding a successful middle way lies in (1) stimulating public debate on some seemingly intractable moral and philosophical puzzles generated by ranking efforts; and (2) creating a procedural method that will provoke a lively and perennial dialectical struggle between facts and data, on the one hand, and values and preferences, on the other. The depth and thus the ultimate success of the latter, procedural strategy will heavily depend upon the vigor and richness of the former, substantive debate; otherwise, procedural elegance will do no more than mask a dangerous emptiness of content, rendering the procedure meaningless or worse.

Before spelling out my third thesis, it is necessary to return to the second one, to examine what needs to be rejected, and what needs to be retained, in the battle between the political and the numerical approaches. Whatever can be retained will provide the ingredients for developing the strategy implicit in the third thesis.

Pure Numbers and Raw Politics

I begin with the 'pure numbers' approach. I call it that to signal its utterly unadorned nature, purporting to take care of the priority problem with a simple numerical formula. A good illustration of this approach can be found in an article by two British economists. The economic approach, they say, 'addresses two related questions: Is a health care intervention worthwhile? Given that it is worthwhile, what is the best way of providing it?' (Donaldson and Mooney 1991). They answer at least the first question by turning to the quality adjusted life years (QALYs) method, that is, the effort to measure the extent to which a particular treatment provides at a particular marginal cost a particular quality of life for a particular length of time. This method has had a special appeal to those concerned with setting priorities. Where cost effectiveness and cost-benefit analysis seek in different ways to maximize desired effects or outputs in relation to expenditures, the QALYs approach, by contrast, seeks specifically to factor together length and quality of life. More resources ought, accordingly, to 'be allocated to treatments with a low marginal cost per QALY and less to those with a high marginal cost per QALY gained.' It thus becomes possible to nicely rank, with a number, a variety of different ways of spending health care money. Time spent by a doctor advising a patient to give up smoking has a far more favorable QALYs ratio than hospital hemodialysis, with kidney transplantation somewhere in between.

The QALYs method, it is urged, is superior to another economic approach, that of 'needs assessment.' In the latter case, 'need could be measured by lives lost, life years lost, morbidity, or loss of social functioning.' The authors succinctly point to the pitfalls of the needs assessment approach. Whereas it might find that ischemic heart disease takes many more years of life than breast cancer – using, say, a 'years of potential life lost' standard – it does not help us in determining the relative resources that the former should receive in relation to the latter or how to factor in other considerations of importance, such as morbidity. They argue that the QALYs method, by contrast, allows a nice, tidy ranking: we get numbers, larger or smaller, and thus our priorities.

What the authors do not dwell upon, however, are some of the well-known problems of the QALYs method, most notably the difficulty of objectifying 'quality' or finding some agreement on the kind of life worth living, about which humans notoriously differ. Without that agreement, of course, the method provides more the illusion than the reality of the objectivity it purports to provide. Finding agreement on 'quality' in the mental health arena would be no easier than it was in the battles over the subject in physical health.

That lack of quantitative objectivity has bedeviled all of the leading economic techniques, especially because their claim to the policy maker's ear is an ability to find objectivity through quantification. It is all the more disturbing in their case because proponents of these techniques have considered that their best contribution to the policy maker is a detached, nonpolitical perspective, well above the ordinary fray of interests and passions. To the extent that the economic techniques are themselves inadequately quantifiable, and also caught up in the very ideological struggles they would purport to cut through, their policy clout is diminished. To be sure, to the extent that the economic analysis can document differences in values and preferences, it can make an important contribution. Only when such analysis is viewed as a way of neatly slashing through the political jungle in the name of detached objectivity does it begin to mislead.

Precisely because of that hazard, many economists and health planners have wisely given up their claim to a superior objectivity, trying instead to locate their optimal contribution within a context of openly acknowledged values and ideologies. As James C. Robinson has noted, 'The intensity of the debate surrounding the ascription of dollar values to life and health . . . suggests that more than mere technical issues in measurement and accounting practices are involved; rather, basic social values are coming into conflict' (Robinson 1986). Robinson's basic point is nicely deployed in another critique of the need-based approach. Behind many disputes about a need-based approach lie different and incommensurable conceptions of health (Green and Baker 1988). Health can be understood as an investment good, the creation and sustaining of human economic capital. Alternatively, health care can be seen as a social investment, providing communal goods other than economic benefits. Still another possibility is to understand health as an end in itself, as a natural right for all individuals. Given any one of these notions of health, we might be able to work out some priorities. But how do we decide among them in the first place?

After raising this and other problems (with cost-benefit and cost effectiveness analysis, among other techniques), Green and Baker conclude 'that priority-setting is *not* and cannot be a 'rational objective' process, but is ultimately concerned with power relations and value judgments . . . . As such it is the province of the communities and politicians and cannot be left in the hands of planners and their superficially attractive techniques' (Green and Baker 1988, 926).

The British health economist Alan Williams goes a step further. He not only notes the unavoidability of ideology, but also stresses the importance of putting it up front in any economic analysis. He uses as a case in point the long struggle between 'libertarians' – for whom health care is to be treated as a consumer good, to be bought according to income – and 'egalitarians' – for whom health care is a right that should not be determined, much less limited, by income' (Williams 1988). The choice between these two views is an ideological one, which will determine priorities once the choice has been made, but which is itself not capable of a purely economic determination.

This distinction seems eminently sensible, allowing a helpful use of quantification to set priorities, but doing so in a context sensitive to external determinants and ideological points of departure. Even so, the authors might have added still another qualification: even within their context, values will permeate the priority rankings, although the numbers will, if carefully derived, strengthen their claims to relative objectivity.

Just how important the political and values factors are can be seen by recalling the way in which the Oregon priority-setting program went awry in its early stages and encountered an unexpected obstacle in its last stage. The early problem was manifest in May 1990 upon release of a computer-generated list of 1,600 medical treatments that had been drawn up using a form of cost-benefit analysis in its methodology. The results were odd indeed, and intuitively objectionable: reconstructive breast surgery, for instance, ranked above the treatment of an open fracture of the thigh, and the straightening of crooked teeth ranked higher than treatment for Hodgkin's lymphoma (Dixon and Welch 1991). As a result of the public and professional outcry at such rankings, the economic formula was dropped and a condition–treatment pairing system, using a scale of medical necessity, was adopted. At the same time, out of respect for community values and other considerations, the final rankings were in part hand shifted to find a good fit between technical and value considerations.

That was not the end of Oregon's problems, however. After the program had been polished and made acceptable to the Oregon legislature, it was denied a required federal waiver on the grounds that it would discriminate against the disabled. I will not recount the details of that issue, other than to note the way in which an ideological and moral objection was used, once again, to overcome a technical solution that had otherwise seemed satisfactory. That many of us judged the disability attack to be misguided is beside the point here: what matters is the power of an ideological attack to derail a course of action otherwise reasonably developed (Capron 1992; Hadorn 1992; Menzel 1992). The Oregon priority-setting commission learned for a second time that a technically good methodology is no defense at all if it generates politically unpalatable results. The political realities thus cannot be ignored, nor are they necessarily harmful. Methodological purists might think so, but their embrace of such a belief is in itself ideological.

The shortcomings of a pure numbers approach make it easy to understand why some commentators despair of rationalistic methods of setting priorities, whether economic or otherwise. What they see is the power of politics, that is, the power of subjective values, personal preferences, interest group power, and the sheer irrationality of much public policy. In looking at the way different policies have emerged, the historian can see the influence of the zeitgeist and the values of the times, the sociologist can spot the class, economic, and cultural forces at work, and the philosopher can see the power of the reigning mores.

Those possibilities would seem nicely to demolish the dream of a rational process for priority setting. The dream can be taken apart by stressing the impossibility of perfect objectivity, noting the force of interest-group power, pointing out the incommensurability of different initial ideological premises (e.g., libertarianism versus egalitarianism), and underscoring the simple fact that people will reject whatever offends their sentiments, allowing emotions to trump reason almost every time. The cleared-eyed, if somewhat cynical, critics of claims of rationality in general, and of rational priority-setting methods in particular, have a strong ally, therefore, in the testimony of 'the real world': the nasty, brutish, but long-lived world that trashes our dreams and schemes with callous abandon.

Yet that greatest of all myths, the 'real world,' is more complex than the one visualized by these critics. Some plans actually work out, some systems actually run, some overwhelming needs are responded to, and now and then reason triumphs over unreason and selfishness. The cynics are ideologues also; they just dress up their ideology in sober clothes, as if to suggest their greater maturity and higher standpoint. In point of fact, moreover, people do not like to remain in worlds dominated by narrow self-interest, lack of planning, absence of agreed-upon goals, and rampant irrationality. We cannot live for long that way. Our dreams, our reason, and our desire for order and stability will eventually intrude. Just such a point has come, I believe, with the American health care system, which is a non-system, dominated by interest groups, beset with fragmentation, burdened with unexamined values: in other words, a big, expensive mess. It is as nice an example of the shortcomings of raw politics as one could ask, a politics that has tried in the name of pluralism and choice to allow every interest group to have its day and its say. We are drawn to priority setting, not just because of scarce resources, but also as a way of cutting through some of the chaos of the present system.

Finding a Middle Way

Priority setting can be a plausible venture, one that need succumb neither to the failings of a purely numerical solution nor to raw politics. A middle way can be fashioned despite many obstacles on the path. The middle way I propose must confront problems of substance and of process. The key will be, on the one hand, to produce sophisticated ways of dealing with each one, and, on the other, ensuring that they interact successfully. The pure numbers approach has never worked out all of its internal, technical problems. That is less important, however, than the fact that it has been even less successful in how it relates to ideology and the political process. It can and should inform that process without becoming a substitute for it.

The clear-eyed realism of the raw politics approach has failed to appreciate the need for human beings to move beyond chaos and the unfettered expression of interests and power, or to consider how people can be moved to act differently when confronted with good evidence. Put another way, there will always be a war between facts and values, as there should be. It is also possible, however, to work out rules for that warfare, which will on occasion produce peace.

Matters of Substance

I turn now to some of the major problems posed by priority setting and then move on to the process question. Three issues of substance are particularly important:

1. aggregating benefits
2. taking the measure of pain and suffering
3. determining an ideological point of departure

Aggregating Benefits. In an interesting article on priority setting in international health C.J.L. Murray (1990) comments on the desirability of combining death, morbidity, and disability into a single health indicator, which could easily be used to set priorities. He notes, however, that this would run into familiar difficulties: 'Relative weights must be chosen to compare death at different ages and disability or morbidity versus death.' We cannot depend upon empirical information for answers to questions that must be determined by community and individual values.

Norman Daniels, however, calls attention to how poorly we are prepared, either in ethics or the community, to deal properly with such questions. Looking at a different set of aggregation issues, he notes, for instance, that if we choose to give preference to one group over another on the grounds that the former would achieve a greater net benefit, the result will be to eliminate from treatment altogether those who could benefit, but just not as much (Daniels 1992). Those patients with simple phobias might gain comparatively more from treatment than chronic schizophrenics and yet lose out entirely in this kind of priority system. Or we may be able to improve modestly the situation of the worst off, but at the price of neglecting those who, although initially better off, could gain comparatively much more than the worst off. Daniels observes that there are no principled ways available for dealing with these problems. We are likely to reject a 'straightforward arithmetic aggregation' (which is why the initial Oregon ranking was rejected), but – save for our intuitions and feelings of discomfort about particular medical conditions – we may have no better, systematic way of making the difficult comparisons; that is, we encounter the old apples and oranges problem, but now with the human face of suffering and sickness.

Is there a way out here? Because it is unlikely that we will find the desirable principles, Daniels emphasizes the importance of process to deal with their absence. While acknowledging the rightness of his conclusion, I suggest that we might make sense of the aggregation problem even without elegant sorting principles. We can have an orderly discussion and debate, drawing on a combination of our intuitions, historical experience in dealing with analogous questions, and the available patterns of practice that offer models of different de facto ordering schemes. We can then attempt to determine, from this assorted evidence, what works well (and for what purpose) and what does not. It is a perfect situation in which to manifest, and exercise, the classical virtue of prudence, creating an interplay between reason, experience, and feeling. The goal is to act sensibly, not perfectly, and to make good, defensible judgments, not unimpeachable ones.

What criteria can we use to make such judgments? Our bias, I contend, should be to give priority to persons whose suffering and inability to function in ordinary life is most pronounced, even if the available treatment for them is comparatively less efficacious than for other conditions. But I would stress here the word 'bias,' to indicate an inclination, a starting point, and not a simple decision procedure. The first goal of a health care system should be the relief of suffering, and the greater the suffering the greater the claim upon the rest of us to respond. Our prima facie duty is toward those whose suffering is the greatest, but other considerations can lead us to qualify, and limit, that duty, overcoming or modifying the initial bias. Thus, if we have made a minimally decent effort to help persons whose suffering is the most severe, we would be justified in diverting additionally available resources to persons who are not so badly off, even if those same resources might marginally improve the worst off. We can judge our efforts by asking whether the balance we have struck does, in fact, honor the initial bias without allowing it to trump all other claims. This will be a matter of *judgment*, not formula, and good political debate should include arguments about the wisdom of the balance thus achieved. As Aristotle long ago reminded us, in matters where precision is not possible, precision should not be sought.

Lurking below the surface is another question of more general importance for health policy: what priority should be given to chronic disease compared with acute care medicine? The latter has, for many decades now, had the pride of place, economically, medically, and socially. Chronic disease, by contrast, represents the failures and frustrations of scientific medicine, signaling the limits of its skills and the mischievous tendency of human biology continually to reassert its unwillingness to shape itself obediently to the modern medical goals of mastery and control of nature. The rise and persistence of chronic illness, however, call for a different policy and another ethical response, giving more weight to all chronic conditions and not just to some forms of mental illness (Fox 1993; Callahan 1990)

Talking the Measure of Pain and Suffering. Although in one important sense, taking the measure of pain and suffering is simply one more aggregation problem, in another sense it poses troubling puzzles that are especially pertinent to mental health. How are we to rank treatments that will relieve a great deal of suffering for a few people compared with those that will alleviate lesser suffering for a great many people? This question bears on a comparison between treatment for the severely depressed and treatment for the milder, but still burdensome, neuroses and phobias. Or, to mention an even worse problem, how are we to compare the care of schizophrenics, for whom sometimes little may be done, with treatment of patients experiencing transient anxiety, for whom much can be done, often definitively? We may relieve some of the schizophrenic's severe suffering, whereas we might succeed totally in relieving the symptoms of anxiety, a condition that causes less suffering.

In Oregon, advocates for the elimination of the mind/body dichotomy and for the establishment of parity between mental and physical illness successfully argued for the inclusion of 'milder' conditions in the basic health care package. Nonetheless, a general problem remains that may require making a choice under other circumstances. Are we to decide, ab initio, to give priority to the worst off, even if we can make only a slight difference, or offer it instead to those who can most benefit from help? A utilitarian bias would lead us toward the latter, which would seem to offer the best aggregate outcome for our dollar. Yet something about the situation of persons in great suffering stops us. What is it?

My guess is that we tacitly distinguish between those whose lives are strikingly and decisively harmed by a particular disease or illness and those whose lives are crippled but not devastated. We know the latter can probably get by, even if not well, whereas the former will not be able to do so at all. Put another way, we know that some forms of illness and suffering do not allow for even a minimally decent quality of life; one instance would be severe and chronic depression, which leaves its victims feeling that they have hardly any kind of life. Human beings can adapt to a life of low quality, but not to a life of no quality. Thus, in our health care planning, the goal is protection against devastating illness; in our acute care services, we want to achieve the capacity to save life; and in the mental health field, we give first priority to those who are dangerous to themselves or whose capacity to function is severely threatened or curtailed. This is a defensible bias despite its seeming unfairness to individuals who could achieve great benefits from treatment. There can be no fair race if some cannot run at all McKerlie 1992).

For my purposes, complete agreement with this argument is not important. I only want to stress the issue of what it means to live different kinds of lives, that is, how to confront the variety of mental health ills that dreadfully compromise the living of a life. The obvious difficulty about a bias toward the worst off is that meeting their needs may swamp all others, thereby lowering significantly everyone else's quality of life. As this may be indefensible, it might be necessary to shave the care of those worst off to ensure that some relief can be found for others. Again, there are no principled ways of doing this, to use Norman Daniels's standard, that is, no sorting standards and tightly formulated norms that can produce incontestable results. Does it matter? Not altogether, because over time we can debate these matters, look at the consequences of different policies, stimulate public concern with the meaning and impact of pain and suffering, and ask people to consider what they most want from a health care system. Although this is not a clean method, it can be illuminating if pursued persistently and has parallels with other issues that admit of no greater precision.

Determining an Ideological Point of Departure. The problem of evaluating pain and suffering, and choosing the standard we want to use as our point of departure, also shows the importance of ideology. We can, for instance, say that the relief of suffering, even when not accompanied by social dysfunction, should be the primary aim of mental health programs. Alternatively, we could subordinate subjectively experienced suffering to an external dysfunction standard, requiring an inability to do something, a failure to function according to a norm. The former standard might be seen as more individualistic, and part of the tradition of medicine, and the latter could be viewed as more communitarian. Or it may express a bias toward the inner life of people as distinct from their actions in a community. Ideology – by which I mean a more or less coherent way of ordering several important values according to an overriding one – will bear on the importance we give to relative degrees of suffering, to physical as opposed to mental suffering, to the choice between libertarianism and egalitarianism, or a mix of the two, and to the status we ought to give to the most afflicted (and whom we determine these to be).

We run into a familiar puzzle here. If our ideological point of departure is more likely to lead to adoption of one set of priorities rather than another, how are we to get, and set, our ideological priorities? Are we, as Gilbert and Sullivan averred, just born 'little liberals or little conservatives'? Although it may not always be apparent, we know that people do change their ideologies. They change as a result of thinking about and considering the objections to their viewpoints, or finding them wanting in practice, or sometimes simply by having a change of heart and looking at the world in new and fresh ways.

The only point I want to make here is that we can evaluate our ideologies and starting points. We can look for their failings, and we can be open to the advantages of other starting points. Many people, chastened by the experience of communism in the Eastern European countries, are newly drawn to market solutions; a harsh egalitarianism, we now see all too starkly, can become oppressive, stifling important parts of human nature

and generating, at its worst, murderous totalitarianism. Those of us in the United States, more used to seeing the nasty side of a market economy, whose cruelty is just more random and less organized, will have corrective insights to offer those prepared to throw over egalitarian aspirations. We will debate these matters, and we do know from history that the debates count, that shifts do take place. This is good enough, especially since it is all we have anyway.

Matters of Process and Procedure

In the absence of a substantive way to find good solutions to policy questions, it is often said that we must look to good procedure and process. The aim of doing so is to ensure, despite the inevitable disagreements and, often, the lack of a clean method for resolving them, that any political outcome will at least be seen as fair. This perfectly reasonable way of thinking sometimes generates an error: the notion that how people argue, and what they argue about, is less important than a fair procedure for reconciling their disagreements in order to create viable policy. I have tried to stress that even though no clean, agreed-upon procedure exists for disposing of the most vexing matters of substance, they all can be the subject of profitable public debate.

In that sense, substance and procedure cannot be neatly separated; inherent in the richer notions of democracy, which eschew a technology of mere decision procedures, is a combination of dialogue, judgment, and action. Only a kind of methodological obsessiveness should lead us to throw up our hands in the absence of an exact methodology, that is, one that would spare us the messy business of political give and take and the compromise and uncertainty of democratic dialogue. A procedural process that ignores the quality of its discourse will have its own kind of illusory result. That is why the jury system, whose purpose is justice rather than truth, nonetheless must rely on a wide range of rules of evidence and admissible arguments to ascertain that it can produce reasonably reliable results.

An important background condition should loom large in the setting of priorities: determining the appropriate unit or range within which the priority setting should take place. With that condition met, two procedural goals are of special importance. The first is that the procedure appear fair and satisfying to those who will be affected by it, and the second is that it establish a strong dialectic, a continuing struggle, between community values and the available empirical evidence on efficacy and outcomes of procedures.

Establishing the Priority-Setting Unit. Because setting priorities will trigger an expression of community values and predilections, and require fair procedures, the ideal unit consists of a reasonably strong and natural preexisting community. Only then is there likely to be strong agreement on the priorities. Ideally, it should be a unit smaller than a state, although for practical purposes a state may be the smallest feasible political unit (e.g., a state Medicaid program). The success of Alameda County in California in establishing a mental health priority system shows the possibility of smaller subdivisions (Kears 1993). A national priority system is likely to be unworkable, failing as it must to reflect regional and cultural differences. Because some priority setting must inevitably be 'by hand,' as Oregon discovered, in order better to reflect community values, the more homogeneous is the community in which this is done, the greater is the likelihood of political acceptance. Nonetheless, even at the national level, some general categories of priorities might be established, leaving a detailed ordering to the local level. Although the point of allowing local values to shape priorities is to achieve consensus and political acceptance, too great a diversity between regions or jurisdictions could easily suggest unfair variations. Some broad priority categories could help avert the most egregious problems in that respect while still honoring local values.

Devising a Fair and Representative Procedure. A fair procedure treats the interests of all relevant parties in an equal way, eliminates lingering unjustifiable historical discriminations, and provides opportunities to correct perceived injustice. A representative procedure receives input from the major groups to be affected by the priority system and from medical experts who can sift the available evidence on outcomes and efficacy of different treatment modalities. The appointment of a special committee charged with making recommendations to a legislature (or given a final power to decide on priorities, as was the case in Oregon) is one way to foster such a procedure. There should be, suitably and appropriately, not only a struggle among persons with different values, but also a systematic means of confronting those values with confirming or disconfirming data. Thus arises the need for individuals who have command of the empirical evidence, such as it may be, and the skills to interpret its meaning to lay people. The possibility even of frequent revision should be built into the procedures; there should always be a second, and third, chance to reconsider the problem with new information and arguments in hand. Evidence changes over time, and provision must be made for that eventuality.

The appropriate expertise would minimally include an economic slant, in order to calculate costs, and a medical slant, to evaluate treatment effectiveness and reflect clinical realities. Beyond those conditions, a fair procedure also establishes rules for reaching closure, means of adjudicating disputes, and ways to achieve compromise when agreement is not possible.

Creating a Dialectic between Values and Data. I have already suggested the importance of certain kinds of expertise being represented in any body charged with priority setting. That, however, will not be enough. Additional skills and procedures are required to ascertain that the struggle between values and data is sophisticated and enlightening. This calls for prior agreement on what counts as good, fair, and poor data; on what kind of additional information might help to resolve debates; and on what constitutes a good fit between values and available evidence. Preliminary methodological debate will be necessary, a debate that should be renewed when various problems present themselves for resolution.

The success of finding a middle way between pure numbers and raw politics lies in forcing those perspectives, in an orderly way, to wrestle it out over specific issues. Values set facts in a context, giving them a meaning and elucidating what they will mean in practice. Facts and data serve as a necessary check on, and corrective to, the indulgence of self-interested politics, which will be prone to manipulate data to its own ends. The procedures I have outlined should help curb the excesses of each extreme without altogether discarding what is valuable in each. That is likely to be the best we can do.

References

Callahan, D. 1990. *What Kind of Life: The Limits of Medical Progress.* New York: Simon & Schuster.

Capron, A. 1992. Oregon's Disability: Principles or Politics? *Hastings Center Report* 22 (6): 18–20.

Daniels, N. 1992. Rationing Fairly: Programmatic Considerations. (Unpublished paper)

Dixon, J., and H.G. Welch. 1991. Priority Setting: Lessons from Oregon. *Lancet* 337:891–4.

Donaldson, C., and G. Mooney. 1991. Needs Assessment, Priority Setting, and Contracts for Health Care: An Economic View. *British Medical Journal* 303:1529–30.

Fox, D.M. 1993. *Power and Illness: The Failure and Future of American Health Policy.* Berkeley: University of California Press.

Green, A., and C. Baker. 1988. Priority Setting and Economic Appraisal: Whose Priorities – the Community or the Economist? *Journal of Social Science and Medicine* 29:919–29.

Hadorn, D.C. 1992. The Problem of Discrimination in Health Care Priority Setting. *Journal of the American Medical Association.* 268:1454–9.

Jennings, B. 1987. Interpretation and the Practice of Policy Analysis. In *Confronting Values in Policy Analysis: The Politics of Criteria*, eds. F. Fischer and J. Forrester. Newbury Park, Calif.: Sage.

Kears, D. 1993. Setting Mental Health Services Priorities: The Case of Alameda County. (Unpublished paper)

McKerlie, D. 1992. Equality between Age Groups. *Philosophy and Public Affairs* 21:275–95.

Menzel, P. 1992. Oregon's Denial: Disabilities and Quality of Life. *Hastings Center Report* 22:21–5.

Murray, C.J.L. 1990. Rational Approaches to Priority Setting in International Health. *Journal of Tropical Medicine and Hygiene* 93:303–11.

Reich, R. 1988. *The Power of Public Ideas.* Cambridge, Mass.: Ballinger.

Robinson, J.C. 1986. Philosophical Origins of the Economic Valuation of Life. *Milbank Quarterly* 64:133–55.

Surles, R., and C. Feiden-Waugh. 1993. Mental Health Coverage: Role for State Government. (Unpublished paper)

Williams, A. 1988. Priority Setting in Public and Private Health Care. *Journal of Health Economics* 7:173–83.

Minds and Hearts

*Priorities in Mental Health Services**

Philip J. Boyle and Daniel Callahan

The system is crazier than the people it is trying to serve
— Laurie Flynn, *National Alliance for the Mentally Ill*

To care for people with mental illness is to live in a world of inescapable misfortune and tragic choices. Mental illness strikes with a random yet pandemic quality, producing at its worst nightmarish hallucinations, crippling paranoia, unrelenting depression, a choking sense of panic, and uncontrollable obsession — and even in its milder manifestations it produces many other oppressions. Approximately one in three Americans will experience some form of mental disorder at some point in their lives, and according to one estimate, one in every 6.4 adults is currently suffering from some form of mental illness.[1] This figure comes to 41.2 million people and climbs higher if substance abuse is included. A significant number of these — more than 1.7 million Americans — suffers from a persistent and severely disabling condition, such as schizophrenia. The costs of caring for these patients and those whose illness is episodic, curable, or only mildly debilitating have reached $136.1 billion per year.

As if the tragedy of illness were not pain enough — for individuals with mental illness, their families, and the community — as a society we face additional pain as we are pressured to choose which ill people we will treat and with what services. As health care reform moves forward with the aim of providing affordable, appropriate health care that is available to all, there will be pressure to examine whether any health services are less important or dispensable than others. It is unlikely that mental health will escape scrutiny. Indeed, one of the most serious issues that will have to be faced by the mental health community is how it can participate in the health planning process.

Given the past and present dismal plight of mental health services, both its patients and its providers have good reason to be concerned about reform. Historically, mental health services have not received the same support as physical health.[2] Private and public funding permit 'carveouts' in mental health coverage that provide fewer benefits than those allowed for physical health. Private insurance customarily restricts mental health benefits more stringently, setting caps on numbers of hospital days or outpatient visits, or imposing annual or lifetime dollar limits for mental health services.[3]

Insurance policies, for example, typically limit hospital care for persons with mental illness to thirty days a year, according to a 1991 survey of employer-provided coverage conducted by the Health Insurance Association of America. While 99 percent of insured individuals have private coverage for inpatient mental health care, in only 37 percent of these cases is the mental health coverage equivalent to that for other illnesses.[4] The same is true for outpatient care: although 98 percent of persons with private insurance are covered for outpatient mental health benefits, only 3 percent have coverage equivalent to that for other illnesses. Psychotherapy sessions are generally limited to ninety visits a year with a 50 percent copayment. Health maintenance organizations (HMOs) customarily restrict therapy to thirty sessions a year with a 50 percent copayment.[5] Spending caps (lifetime or annual) limit coverage of disorders such as schizophrenia, bipolar

disorder, and autism because of the presumed high cost of treatment and uncertainty of successful outcomes. Unfortunately, mandates generally provide uniform limits on services without regard to the severity of the condition or the effectiveness of the treatment.[6] The public system's provision of care is not much better. With strained, if not reduced budgets, and fragmentation in services among levels of government, those in need of mental health care are often either stricken from the rolls or simply fall through the cracks of a highly fragmented system. In a word, mental health continues to be the poor stepchild of the health care delivery system. As someone once quipped, mental health care is more likely to be a 'plea for service' than 'fee for service.'

The causes of this unequal treatment arise in part from deep-seated convictions, if not biases. Foremost is the belief that mental health and disorder are poorly defined. While few would argue today that mental illness is a myth, or maintain that mental illness is whatever psychiatrists treat, nonetheless there is a bewildering diversity of views about mental illness, ranging from biological accounts to social determinism.[7] The nature of mental illness is often conceived as a dichotomy between mind and body,[8] an unfortunate dualism that tends to minimize the physical suffering and disability associated with mental illness. Oddly enough, even within the mental health field there are those who wish to distinguish biological from nonbiological mental disorders and give priority to the former.

Complicating these matters is the lack of knowledge about the efficacy of mental health treatments;[9] mental illness is perceived as having few fully effective treatments, and the care is typically thought to be lengthy and expensive. In the absence of convincing research, it is difficult to differentiate established interventions from the latest fad. Stereotypes are impossible to break: treatment for mental illness is seen as something patients can do without, since, on the one hand, remedies for the severe and persistently ill are perceived to be almost futile, and on the other, relief for the 'worried well' is thought to be discretionary. All people with mental illness are typecast as severely and persistently ill, while in actuality many suffer only single or episodic bouts of illness. The lack of agreement regarding effectiveness even gives rise to conflict among mental health advocates, who argue, for example, over the value of psychotherapy as compared with more medically oriented services, the appropriateness of involuntary hospitalization, and the effectiveness of family-based interventions. Fueling the problem is the variety, of ways — depending on the provider, the setting, diagnostic status of the patient, and treatment — that mental health services are defined: should rehabilitation services such as job training or housing be considered part of mental health services? The lack of good data on expenditures and costs fuels the disagreement over effectiveness. Unlike those with a physical illness, persons with mental illness are often perceived to be the moral cause of their own problems and for that reason less entitled to generous benefits. These beliefs have conspired to produce a palpable lack of treatment and funding for persons with mental illness.

If mental health constituencies are not noted for harmonious concord on all issues, on one thing they do agree: mental health must have a higher status in health services. In the present initiatives for health care reform one slogan is prominent: 'Health care reform without equitable mental health benefits is no reform at all.'[10] Some of those who promote mental health

* Boyle, P. and Callahan, D.: Mind and hearts: priorities in mental health services. Special Supplement, *Hastings Center Report* **23**:S1-S23, 1993.

call minimally for nondiscriminatory treatment.[11] Others urge parity, meaning either equal funding or treatment on the same conditions and terms as physical health services. In either case, mental health proponents are calling for the relative place of mental health to be improved and rearranged – for mental health to receive money and attention more on a par with physical health. This call for a higher status does not end at mental health services; state and federal movements for health care reform can be construed as a call for new priorities in general. Initiatives to set priorities range from a casual attempt with no special system in mind, to a more formal attempt that is somewhat systematic but employs no numerical ranking, to a formal system that includes an explicit effort to ascertain citizens' opinions and numerical ranking. The most notable formal attempt has been that of the state of Oregon, which has proposed a highly detailed priority scheme that actually ranks mental and other health services together in a single system of condition-treatment pairs.

Whether one looks at the problem as one of mental health's demanding higher ranking, or health service in general requiring a regrading, extremely difficult questions are raised by the process. Can mental and physical health be compared, and if so, how? If mental and physical health are compared, will mental health services suffer? Should mental health services be ranked at all, and if so, should this be done separately, and by what criteria? Does it harm mental health services to set their priorities separately? What in mental health services is more or less important, more or less dispensable?

In practical and unfortunate terms, the priority debate is often framed as a choice between alternative treatments or competing populations – for example, should society make available a treatment for schizophrenia, such as Clozapine, or should it concentrate on providing talking therapies for those who suffer from milder and perhaps only episodic forms of mental illness? Or, both, and in what proportion? Framing the question this way often assumes, however, that there is agreement about the general terms of the emerging controversy, such as what it means to set priorities, or what criteria should be used, or what counts as care for persons with mental illness. Even if there were agreement that priorities should be set in the first place (and there is not), and the criteria were clear (and they are not), the process itself forces a reconsideration of issues central to our life together as a community. Who shall make the decisions about setting priorities? This question squarely frames another: who shall govern? In a democracy, how shall we balance expert opinion and public preferences? Are consumer preferences coterminous with what is best for society, and if not, which of these should prevail in the decision?

Justifying Priority Setting

This report explores the issues enumerated above and others central to setting priorities in mental health. It examines three components essential to understanding priority setting. First, it surveys the purported reasons both for and against setting priorities in mental health. This must be done in order to answer the question of whether priorities, ought to be established at all. Second, the report identifies de facto priorities in the history of mental health policy in the U.S. as well as in the state examples of Oregon and New York. Probing these cases reveals a complex set of social factors – funding mechanisms, intergovernmental relations, and cultural perception of mental illness, to name a few – that propagate a nonlinear, often conflicted development of priorities in mental health. Third, the report appraises the ethical criteria that have been proposed to evaluate priority plans. Finally, the report identifies the present state of affairs in priority setting (where we are and where we need to go) and what mental health policy has to gain from discussions of this kind.

Priorities: Why We Need Them

At the mere mention of setting priorities, some vehemently object that there is insufficient motivation to do any such thing. Yet the question has surfaced

because of the dominance in health policy of three concerns, to contain rapidly rising health care costs, to assure access to health care for millions who are without it, and to give health care that is appropriate.

The rising cost of health care and its crippling effect on budgets, private and public, motivates in large measure a need to set priorities. American corporations find it increasingly difficult to compete internationally, impaired in part by rising employees' and retirees' health insurance costs. Most international competitors have health services paid for by their governments, leaving them lower overhead, lower prices, and a stronger competitive edge. Individual consumers feel the pinch of higher costs as expenses are shifted to them in the form of higher copayments for health services. State and local governments too, faced with rising deficits and tighter budgets, have identified escalating health care costs as an impediment, if not the sole obstacle, to gaining control of their budgets. It is not likely that society can curb the accelerating cost of health services and at the same time offer everyone every service of any possible benefit. Choices will have to be made about what services are more or less vital or expendable.

The national push to insure the 37 million Americans who lack insurance of any kind, and to offer an adequate level of coverage to those who are seriously underinsured (another 30 million) is further impetus to rethink the present distribution of health services. It is generally assumed that a nation as wealthy as ours ought to be able to provide all of its members with some level of health care, but to do so will entail either further increasing a seriously strained health care budget, or rearranging the present distribution of health services in a fairer and more agreeable manner. While access to care in general is already somewhat limited, for individuals with mental illness it is much more restricted.[12] The practice of medical underwriting discriminates against those who have received mental health care in the past, often by denying them coverage altogether, and 'mental disorder' is one of the most common conditions for which a medically underwritten group is denied coverage. Even though some twenty-two states have enacted 'bare bones' or 'basic benefits' legislation to permit insurers to market low-cost, low-coverage benefits to those purchasing insurance, the tangible effect for people with mental illness is often attenuated because of gaps in coverage, very high deductibles, or inability to pay for treatment.

Professionals and consumers demand health care services that are appropriate, which further motivates a need to set priorities. Emerging data suggest that certain health care services are often ineffective and wasteful, and deserve either low priority or none at all. Even if health care dollars grew on trees, simple rationality dictates that useless services be eliminated and marginally beneficial services be given low priority. There is mounting information in the field of mental health to determine what treatments are beneficial for what populations. For example, it is wasteful to provide effective services to people who do not need them, and it is increasingly possible to determine who they are. People who have never fully met the criteria for mental illness should not receive monies apportioned for mental illness, even though this has happened in the past and still occurs in some states. Likewise, it can hardly be a priority to provide treatments to inappropriately diagnosed conditions – for example, treating the physical symptoms of anxiety disorder rather than the disorder itself. Eliminating the useless is the first step toward setting priorities. More difficult will be to make the judgments ranking marginally beneficial treatments, if they should even be included.

Ironically, these concerns are often at odds with each other. If, for example, costs are kept under control, a system is unlikely to be able to assure desired amounts of high-quality, appropriate care to everyone. And if universal access to care is offered, the system could bankrupt itself in the attempt to maintain quality.

As a practical matter there may seem little point in publicly examining reasons to set priorities. Many proponents of priority setting recite a litany of examples to show that priorities are now and have always been set, but that the process takes place out of the public eye and in no methodical fashion. The present mix of services constitutes de facto priority setting, even though the story of how resources came to be distributed as they currently are is difficult to trace. It seems politically prudent, even if one thinks it wise or even necessary to set priorities, not to be forced to acknowledge a preference for one service or population over another. Yet when, for whatever reason, the fact of existing priorities goes unacknowledged, they are set by default in a constant shell game of cost-shifting. Ignoring underfunded public mental health services, for example, in an effort to avoid drawing attention to the question of priorities at all, may have the net effect of shifting the cost of caring for persons with mental illness to the welfare and prison systems, or to consumers in higher out-of-pocket costs. However ingenious or devious this method of redistributing the burden to public budgets other than mental health services, the cost for care still remains. So does the question of whether and how best to provide it. And if the concern is to stop a potentially or actually violent person with mental illness from harming others, so does the question of which agency is responsible for assuring the public safety in this case.

Priorities: Why We Resist Them

Setting priorities is unthinkable! The foremost hurdle to setting any health care priorities is that many people vigorously resist the idea that they ought to be set in the first place. Setting them, critics allege, is a pernicious and unthinkable act. In the face of suffering, can anyone in good conscience turn away from the ill? Is there ever any justification for deciding that certain populations are more important than others, or that some services are dispensable and there is no social obligation to offer them? What justification would be sufficient for society's omitting to offer those services, and where can a line be drawn between what society is and is not obligated to provide?

The instant abhorrence to setting priorities stems from equating the, enterprise with rationing. The two are not necessarily the same. While priority setting can mean different things to different people, it is broadly construed to mean ranking. The ranking can be used for at least three purposes: to provide a wise distribution of health services in a relatively affluent society; to identify-low-preference, marginally beneficial services; and to eliminate beneficial but less needed care. Rationing, only one aspect of setting priorities, can be defined as the denial of services demonstrated to be beneficial.[13] Yet by potent innuendo, the connection of priorities with rationing frequently puts a halt to any reasoned discussion. In our land of plenty, known for its largesse, where people have become accustomed to the postwar expansion in the standard of living, the mere suggestion that we will have to live with scarcity and perhaps be denied goods that most of us perceive to be essential cuts sharply against the grain of our cultural identity.

Rationing aside, however, it must be acknowledge that the process of setting priorities serves other purposes as well. Grading services along a continuum of efficacy or cost, for example, can inform consumers and enable them to select services that comport with their values. Ordered priority lists can, by implication, identify for researchers lacunae in needed health services, or potential areas for basic research. For private venture capitalists and those who control the public purse, decisions can be better informed when strategic planning for basic scientific research, data collection, and the provision of services includes ranked priorities.

As a practical matter, priority setting may result in rationing, but in fairness to both processes, the objections to each must be examined separately. In either process, perhaps the least easy objection to address is that lodged against the means used to accomplish the task. Because there are so many different proposals for setting priorities and no homogeneous means of doing so, objections to the means by which priorities are set usually comprise a myriad of objectionable subissues, including objections to what is being ranked, or what criteria – such as cost or effectiveness – are being used, or whether certain procedures are observed. Some plans sort by populations – for example, by targeting persons who are severely and persistently mentally ill – while others sort by emphasizing broad categories of services such as out patient care or emergency services. Others sort by conditions and treatments, and still others never sort and mean nothing more by 'priority setting' than that some broad public policy issues need more

urgent attention. Objections will vary according to what is sorted and ranked. It is important to remember that a declaration that priority setting is objectionable *tout court* is likely to be an objection to individual aspects of the process, each of which must be examined separately.

Setting priorities harms mental health! Many would argue that priority setting would harm mental health. If setting formal priorities within the health care system in general is not so unthinkable after all, it is nevertheless perfectly true that to single out mental health alone for priority setting could be harmful.[14] It has been argued that there are no similar attempts to set priorities in intensive care or ophthalmology, and that to set them for mental health services alone would be to countenance existing patterns of discrimination and to exacerbate battles among constituents who, in our most recent history, have been competing with one another for a limited budget.

While the possible harm in setting priorities for mental health only is hypothetical (it has not proved harmful in Alameda County, California),[15] it makes little sense in the long run. Practically speaking it is not easy to disentangle treatment for mental and physical health, given their inter related symptoms and overlapping places, modes, and providers of treatment. The motivation for setting priorities in general is to achieve a sensible, cost-conscious balance of resources within all health services, not simply one service. To this end it is imperative not to exclude any health service, mental or physical, from the analysis. Those within mental health have good warrant for insisting that priority setting should be an all-or-nothing process.

However, if all health services are prioritized inclusively, examining the priorities within mental health as part of a larger enterprise is a sensible thing to do. These services are traditionally administered for some portion of the population in public, state-operated programs and funded separately, and for that reason mental health requires its own analysis. More important, focusing on mental health places in bold relief certain features of health care services that are all too frequently overlooked in health care reform. In large measure health policy has tended to privilege short-term illness served by general hospitals, where the emphasis is on acute care.[16] Because much (but by no means all) of mental illness is chronic or episodic it does not fit this norm.[17] Because it does not, it can serve as a model for thinking about priority setting in other areas of chronic and long-term care as well – areas such as the care of the elderly, which is sure to require a larger proportion of the health care dollar in the near future. Further, it would be a disaster in the long run to overlook the services that are used to identify, diagnose, and treat mental disorders, including a range of social services offered in the stabilization and rehabilitation of certain groups of persons with mental illness.[18]

Setting priorities is impossible! A question that could promptly stop priority setting is whether it can even be done. History provides strong evidence that priorities are, by and large, difficult to set deliberately. They are established, many would argue, through political processes and organizational power and have little to do with a systematic examination of alternatives and their social and economic significance. Comprehensive plans such as those under discussion belong more to the imagination of idealistic public policy makers than to pragmatists. All too frequently the best planned course of action is waylaid by a complex set of social factors. Mental health stands as an important case in point, buffeted as it is by a host of interrelated and conflicting factors, including its charismatic leaders, inter governmental responsibilities and failures, legislation, court cases,[19] external funding, conflicting under standings of the nature of mental illness, composition of the mentally ill population, professional ideology, interprofessional friction, popular attitudes, consumer demands, and the means to deal with disease and dependency. Nevertheless, we believe these social factors merely make priority setting difficult, not impossible. In the face of formidable odds, the alternative is to do nothing; and that has not worked well.

Priorities: Some Reassurances

Setting priorities is sensible! It is important not to undervalue the need to set explicit, formal priorities. Even in an affluent society, one not constrained by budgetary limits and one in which almost every beneficial service could be offered to every citizen on demand, setting priorities is a sensible way to safeguard health care budgets, which are always vulnerable to political pressures and market forces.[20] The lack of evidence about how contemporary priorities have been set suggests that the process has been hidden from the public view. Political pressure and public attention often skew informal priorities in the direction of interest-group concerns that may be at odds with what is good for a society as a whole. Market forces left to their own devices are, in part, responsible for the lack of access to health care for some, but by setting priorities and using governmental mechanisms to adjust for supply and demand, the maldistribution caused by the market can be compensated for.

Most importantly, priorities might bring balance to a lopsided health policy. An examination of general health policy reveals that society usually hews to the 'rule of rescue,'[21] that is, it cares for individual, identifiable persons, no matter how desperately ill or how ineffective or costly the treatment, even though this may mean that faceless patient populations must do without beneficial care. The present system is geared toward meeting individual patients' health needs, with less concern for what mix of services will have the most impact on the health needs of the population. While it may be difficult to convince people of it, setting formal priorities is a sensible means of expanding the focus of health care policy beyond individual patients' needs to the health needs of the population as a whole.

The inducements for setting priorities – cost, access, and appropriateness of treatment – are the fuel for all health care reform, a fate we will not likely escape. Explicit or not, priorities will be part of the machinery for health reform and objections to setting them will persist. Some objections will be resolved factually. Will people with mental illness be made worse off if priorities are set? Will social forces make it virtually impossible to set sensible priorities? The merits of other objections will stand or fall according to the coherence and adequacy of criteria for setting priorities. These objections notwithstanding, forces acting on health policy such as political influence, the market, and current biases in health policy that do not fully account for population needs provide some incitement to entertain thoughts about priorities. The question we face is not *whether* we should set priorities, but *whither* priorities will go. Is the present direction of priorities acceptable, and if not, what is the alternative? What measures are there for evaluating the setting of priorities?

Priorities: Informal and Formal

Talk about priorities is a permanent conversation in the political forum; however, the contours of the meaning of the term are continually being sharpened. In health policy, priorities have traditionally been informal and meant nothing more than that particular services, or populations would receive, special attention. More than a century of mental health policy reform bears witness to the setting of priorities in this sense. In a more recent and specific sense, priority setting has come also to mean a formal and methodical attempt to redirect health services, sometimes using numerical rankings, as Oregon has done, or at other times using existing health services strategies to effect change, as has been done in New York State. An examination below of the broad cycles of mental health reform in the U.S. uncovers social factors that have bent policy to the prevailing ideological breezes, while a look at the experience of Oregon and New York exposes striking and disputed features of the current situation.

Cycles of Priorities

Priorities, informal but potent, may be glimpsed in the four cycles of mental health reform that took place in the nineteenth and twentieth centuries.[22] With each reform a new set of priorities (normally informal) was established, based on newly developed approaches to treatment and a new or different facility or locus of care. But each set of priorities was profoundly affected by social, political, economic, and demographic factors. Before the nineteenth century, care for lunatics, as they were called at that time, was charitably dispensed by the family and informal community networks, and

not the government. A sharp departure in the kind of care occurred in the first reform cycle early in that century, when reformers championed a view of 'moral treatment.' A belief arose that those newly diagnosed could be cured of mental illness if provided with humane care and instruction in small, pastoral asylums. With a consensus emerging that the severely insane should be committed, public policy made it a priority that a public state asylum system should be created that offered care for acute cases.[23]

During this first cycle of reform, the shared responsibility for the health and welfare of the citizenry resided with the state and local governments and not with the national government. Yet there was no uniformly acknowledged responsibility for persons with mental illness – it varied from community to community. The state usually purchased the land for mental hospitals, built the building, and paid for some employees. In fact, the cost of administering public asylums constituted one of the largest items in many state budgets, suggesting that, institutional care had a high priority.[24] The local community retained responsibility for the day-to-day care of those not dangerously insane, but since the community was also financially responsible for those of its citizens who received care in the state institutions, there was an incentive to keep persons with mental illness in the local almshouses, where per capita costs were low. Despite this incentive, an increasing number of, patients were admitted to state asylums and failed to recover, thus requiring long-term care.[25]

The increase in the number of institutionalized chronically ill patients was accompanied by early examples of questions related to priority setting. Should the state build additional hospitals? Did the presence of chronically ill patients undermine the therapeutic goals of the state asylums? Should the local community retain patients with chronic or severe mental illness in almshouses, or was it better to put them in other institutions? What level of government – local or state – should provide the greatest level of support?

As chronic patients became the priority of the public system, attempts were made to shift the responsibility for this priority to the federal government. A leading actor in this drama was Dorothea Dix, who attempted to persuade the federal government to sell ten million acres of land, the proceeds of which were to be used to support the indigent insane. But she was up against a pervasive belief stemming from the colonial period that for most issues local government should retain the authority to look after its citizens. This belief about local autonomy was crystalized in the Tenth Amendment to the Constitution, which holds that powers not delegated by the Constitution are reserved to the state. As responsibility for health and welfare was taken to reside with the state, the federal government played no role whatsoever in mental health policy during the eighteenth and nineteenth centuries. Dix's proposal was nonetheless passed by Congress but vetoed by Franklin Pierce, who justified his actions in these words: 'The fountains of charity will be dried up at home, and the several States, instead of bestowing their own means on the social wants of their people, may themselves . . . become humble suppliants for the bounty of the Federal Government.'[26]

A second reform cycle, that of 'mental hygiene,' began in the early 1900s with aftercare services, occupational therapy, and outpatient clinics as a priority. A coalition of social reformers and physicians lobbied for an end to dual responsibility between the state and local governments; insane persons were to become wards of the state. This became the general rule until the 1940s, by which time care was being provided to some 425,000 residents. The most critical downstream effect of this shift in responsibility was that, as localities transferred their charges from the almshouses to the state, they also transferred responsibility for care of other residents of the almshouses, especially the demented elderly. To aid this shift, local officials began to redefine 'senility,' as it was then called, in psychiatric terms.[27]

A third cycle of reform that of 'community treatment,' shifted the priority in the mid-1950s from a hospital-based system of care to a community-based system, through, a state-local partnership for the delivery of mental health services. Community treatment became the priority due to shifts in the ideology of psychiatry and newly available interventions. The experiences of World War II supposedly demonstrated that community and outpatient treatment of people who were mentally disturbed was superior and more efficient.[28] Psychodynamic and psychoanalytical modalities of therapy prevailed, along with a view that psychiatry, in collaboration with other social and behavioral sciences, could ameliorate the social and environmental conditions that played such an important role in mental illness. Also prevailing was a view that early identification of persons at risk, along with treatment in the community, could stave off later hospitalizations. And of course biological treatments, including psychotropic drugs, facilitated the shift to community care.

Most prominent in bringing about the shift was Robert H. Felix, a psychiatrist and chief orchestrator of the National Mental Health Act of 1946. His goal was to employ the prestige and resources of the national government to redirect mental health priorities by weaning the nation from its reliance on mental hospitals and replacing them with a network of community institutions. Arguing that a community-oriented policy would be more efficient, he was able to define mental disorders in public health terms by establishing a new system of outpatient community clinics that would provide preventive and therapeutic services for persons with mental illness.[29] As part of the act, the National Institute of Mental Health (NIMH) came into being. The new institute was to perform a number of functions: to speak to a national constituency, to frame a national agenda by collecting data and providing them to public policymakers, to promote research and demonstration projects, and to expand the number of community clinics.

The shift in priorities culminated with the passage of the Community Mental Health Centers Act of 1963, which established federally funded local centers for mental health care. The regulations had strikingly little reference to state mental hospitals and thus the community centers served quite a different clientele. To guarantee their development, the community centers were organized to be highly responsive to community pressures and reflected local priorities by catering to problems encountered frequently within the community: marital and family difficulties, children's emotional problems and delinquency, and substance abuse.[30] As severe and persistent mental illness plagued only a tiny minority of the local citizenry, and as the centers had little formal connection with the state mental hospitals, the care of people with severe and persistent mental illness diminished in priority. In any case, caring for individuals with mental illness in the community was time-consuming and arduous.

Priorities also shifted in response to funding. The most dramatic change was effected by the Medicare and Medicaid amendments to the Social Security Act. The enactment of Title XVIII (Medicare) provided insurance covering hospital stays and physicians' fees for the aged, while Title XIX (Medicaid) allotted money to the states for medical assistance programs for the indigent. Medicaid permitted a rapid decline in the number of elderly in mental hospitals. The reason for this was that while Medicare severely limited payments to support the elderly in mental institutions, states could employ Medicaid payments to care for the same elderly patients if they were shifted to nursing homes. This decline in the population of chronic patients in state hospitals generally had the unintended effect of improving the quality of care available there.[31]

The fourth and most recent cycle of reform, that of 'community support,' began in the late 1970s and took as its priority the correction of the weakness of the preceding cycle. The earlier reform had failed to recognize that many formerly institutionalized patients had needs that were once met by the institution, which provided food, shelter, work, recreation, security, and mental and medical care. Once these patients were outside the institution, the need for these goods remained but there was no one to provide them.[32]

Three important social factors converged in this cycle to transform the context and substance of mental health priorities: the return of persons with severe and persistent mental illness to the community, demographic trends in the population as a whole, and bureaucratic changes within the mental health system.[33] The return to the community of persons with severe and persistent mental illness was hastened by the growth of a series of federal welfare programs, including housing programs, food stamps, the expansion of Social Security Disability Insurance (SSDI), and the creation of Supplemental Security Income (SSI). During the 1980s the federal government, through the Omnibus Budget Reconciliation Act, drew back from the mental health responsibilities that it had assumed in the postwar decades by cutting budgets for mental health services to the states. Demographics made the story worse because the disproportionately large size of the 'baby boom generation' meant that the number of persons at risk for developing severe mental illness was high. The mental health system changed too, with the emergence of a decentralized psychiatric system and more and more responsibilities devolving to the states and local governments. The consequences of this 'New Federalism' of the Reagan presidency are only now appearing within certain populations of those with mental illness who, while formerly enrolled in services, are now being struck off the rolls or dumped.[34] Given the increasing amount of bold experimentation at the state level, the number of patients 'falling through the cracks' and not receiving care appropriate to their need is only likely to grow. The problem of setting priorities in this cycle of reform will be in part to establish clear lines of responsibility among the several levels of government. In particular, the push for mental health reform within local community health alliances puts pressure on state governments to determine their exact role in and responsibility for the care of certain populations, such as those with severe and persistent mental illness. The shifting structural relationship between state and local levels of government is increasingly likely to be a focus of the resource allocation debate._

This brief record of cycles of reform discloses several features that thinking about priority setting must engage. Chief among them is that each cycle has had distinct priorities, sometimes set proactively, other times reactively. To the extent that priorities were proactively set, it can be claimed that deliberate planning is in fact possible. To the extent that priorities were reactively set, often unpredictably and incompatibly with public planning, planners can be alerted to the dangers of simplistic solutions. Comprehensive plans are not merely the fruits of idealistic imaginations, but of pragmatists who can keep clearly in mind the history of social forces.

Lessons from Oregon

The state of Oregon riveted the attention of those interested in priority setting when, through legislation, it enacted the most explicit and formal priority plan to date.[35] At once an object of diverse bitter attacks and high accolades, Oregon's proposal has been condemned as unfair because it discriminates against the poor and the handicapped, and it has also been held up as a model of fairness because it offers access to care for all Oregonians living at or below the poverty level. Most uniquely, the Oregon Health Plan straightforwardly addresses the integration of mental and physical health. But the plan, which has been almost five years in the making, has only recently been approved and has yet to be implemented. Once it is implemented a certain amount of time will have to pass before assessments can be made about how well it works. The question then will be whether general conclusions for mental health services can be drawn from the Oregon experience.

In 1989 the Oregon legislature passed several bills that created the Oregon Health Plan.[36] The intent was to achieve three goals: universal access to health services, reasonable provider reimbursement, and cost containment. The plan was to develop a prioritized list of services, the most important of which would be defined as basic coverage for the 400,000 Oregonians currently without medical insurance. This coverage applies both to the Medicaid population (thus expanding coverage to virtually everyone at or below the federal poverty line) and to uninsured workers through legislation requiring employers to 'pay or play.'

The Oregon Health Plan established a Health Services Commission, whose first task was to develop a list of health service priorities based on community values about health care and on technical information about the effectiveness of various health services relative to the needs of the population serviced. The initial proposed legislation contained a glaring omission: mental health care had, once again, been marginalized. This confirmed both for those who were mentally ill and for those who cared for them that they were being victimized, not only by inequalities in coverage and reimbursement rates, but also by the new initiative. Lobbying efforts led to legislation modified to include a Mental Health and Chemical

Dependency (MHCD) subcommittee to consider whether and how mental health could be integrated and prioritized.

The process used to develop priorities was anything but simple. By the time an agreed-upon list was developed in 1991, there had been many negotiations and adjustments on the part of the commission and among three of its committees: the MHCD, Health Outcomes, and Social Values. The Health Outcomes Committee initially decided to value and sort on a model derived from the work of Robert Kaplan. Simply put, the model associated health care conditions with an appropriate treatment. For each condition-treatment pair, outcome and cost data for both treating and not treating a condition were to be obtained and entered into a quality of well-being scale (QWB), producing a mathematical value. The QWB scale was modified with information gained from the Social Values Committee, which had collected information about individual and community values. Individuals' values were collected by means of a random-sample telephone survey of the Oregon population and the responses were aggregated and used to weigh health care outcomes. Community values were obtained via forty-seven community meetings held throughout the state.

Once they arrived at a sense of how Oregonians felt about various states of health, the Health Services commissioners ultimately identified and ranked seventeen categories of care as the primary determinants of priorities. Woven into community values was information gathered from expert panels about the outcomes of treatment for individual conditions. The commission's first attempt to combine condition-treatment pairs into a ranked list by using a method of strict cost-benefit ratios proved seriously defective. Practitioners were reluctant to disclose the cost of treatment, and reliable data were so difficult to acquire that the figures were finally dumped except for use as tie-breakers when two net-benefit scores were identical in the same category. A second list using a net-benefit ratio was developed by subtracting the probable outcome if a condition were left untreated from a probable outcome of treating the condition.

Blending mental and physical health was no minor political task. From the outset the MHCD committee wondered whether it could in good conscience even join the prioritizing process at all.[37] Its reservations about equitably prioritizing mental and physical health stemmed from the Kaplan methodology, which was biased in favor of acute conditions. In choosing to go along with the process, mental health services stood to lose funding from its separate budget as well as from reduced insurance mandates. On the other hand, if it opted out of the ranking process, mental health services might receive reduced funding and the old patterns of segregation and discrimination would certainly be perpetuated.

The committee agreed to join the process while stressing two goals. The first was to see to it that all those involved with the process understood that mental health deserved parity with physical health. The second goal was continually to critique the commission's methodology, noting where it must be modified to ensure a fair assessment of the value of mental health services. The committee urged the commission to modify the Kaplan QWB public survey instrument to include more symptoms associated with mental illness, while at the same time pressing for all due speed in collecting the data for mental health. Even though they obtained the best data available, the committee retained reservations about its quality. These were somewhat assuaged by comparing notes with other groups and discovering that the outcome data from other specialties was no more reliable than the mental health data.

Once the MHCD committee sorted and ranked mental health conditions, the health list was reviewed by mental health experts within and outside the state. As the committee expected, the list turned out to be plausible and valid, with the major mental conditions falling appropriately into the highest categories and integrating well with other health conditions. Committee members had had to anticipate doubts that such an outcome would be valid, and they did so by adhering wherever possible to the methodology used to prioritize medical-surgical conditions. The list integrates mental health conditions irrespective of their etiologies; conditions and treatments are ranked on the basis of their severity as experienced by the patients, while benefit is measured by outcomes. The list gives a high priority to the treatment of biological illnesses such as schizophrenia and major mood disorders. It also gives priority to conditions that cause widespread suffering and loss of functioning (such as eating disorders) and to illnesses that have a disproportionate impact on children.

Oregon's Contribution

If the most dramatic contribution of the Oregon Plan was that of placing formal, public priority setting on the public policy agenda, an equally stunning gain for mental health was the MHCD committee's single-minded approach to assuring parity between mental and physical health. No one could dispute evidence of discrimination and lack of parity toward mental health; what can be and widely is disputed is MHCD's driving claim that mental health can be compared with physical health. The MHCD committee's strategy took the form of a pragmatic, relentless, several-tiered approach whose dominant characteristic was a refusal to argue about whether there should be parity. Instead, they concentrated on how to assure parity. Not only did the committee make certain that mental health was included in the process, it also ensured at every turn that mental health would not be put at a disadvantage by being underrepresented on the final list of ranked condition-treatment pairs.

The MHCD committee did not advance reasons for rejecting a distinction between mental and physical health in evaluating public policy. They took a more positive approach. From a medical perspective health and illness are inextricably part of mind and body; disorders of the body affect the mind and vice-versa. Mental health is not merely a subset of physical health but an integral part of physical health. Regardless of whether mental health services are medical treatments or other kinds of care, no principled reason exists to discriminate between care provided to those who suffer mental illness and those who are physically ill. Practically speaking, this means that mental health should be considered on the same terms as physical health, but this is not to say that they must receive parity or equal amounts of funding. Differences in funding can be tolerated so long as the same standards for evaluation are applied to both.

While it is difficult to rank which feature of the Oregon plan is most dramatic, high on the list is the criterion for valuing and sorting condition-treatment pairs according to effectiveness. It is controversial because it requires that the most beneficial treatment be given high priority and low-benefit treatments be given low priority, and as a consequence some services might not be offered. One criticism of the effectiveness criterion is that the concept of effectiveness is inherently malleable. Something that is ineffective for a cure might be effective as palliation. Which kind of effectiveness counts? Oregon tried to grapple with this problem democratically, by ranking according to broad areas of effectiveness that Oregonians said they preferred. For example, treatments for acute fatal conditions that effected a full recovery received highest priority, while treatments for both fatal and nonfatal conditions that produced only minimal or no improvement in the quality of life rated the lowest priority.

Another criticism Oregon had to deal with was that mental health services might fare worse if the effectiveness criterion were used. This criticism turned out to be unfounded. Some mental health services in fact ranked in the highest categories of effectiveness. Acute fatal conditions for which treatment prevents death and provides full recovery include major depression, drug-induced delirium, and single-episode, posttraumatic stress disorder. Acute fatal conditions for which treatment prevents death but cannot always deliver a full recovery include alcohol and drug abuse diagnosis. Chronic fatal conditions for which treatment improves life span and quality of life include dysthymia, eating, disorders, bipolar disorder, recurrent major depression, and schizophrenia. To the surprise of critics, Oregon's method actually improved the plight of individuals with mental illness over what it had been before formal priority setting was attempted.

Some challenges to the use of the effectiveness criterion remain unanswered. One, for example, is whether certain highly effective treatments might at some point financially squeeze out less effective treatments. This depends on how many effective but costly treatments there are and how much the legislature is willing to fund. Another is the exact rationale for giving effectiveness a privileged position. Why this and not other important goals of society, such as cost, or prevalence? To its credit, the Oregon plan attempts to meet this objection by granting the health commission the authority to hand-adjust the list to reflect these other values after the computations have been made.

Oregon's plan also made headway in that its actions spoke clearly about who should set priorities, although the rationale behind these decisions can only be surmised. In the broader, national discussion on priorities those who should be actively involved in the process include experts drawn from the professions, elected or appointed officials, independent representative health boards, or the public at large. The Oregon Health Services Commission opted to empower representative groups, including physicians, other health providers, and lay members, each group functioning as a check and balance on the others. For example, given the task of ranking the effectiveness of treatment, a plan to set priorities might have deferred to the judgment of professionals alone, on the assumption that they have the proper expertise for the question of setting priorities. Oregon's actions suggest this assumption can be challenged. Those involved in the planning seemed to see clearly that discussion on about setting priorities is not purely scientific or value neutral; values impinge on every step of the discussion. Professionals have no special expertise in deciding how the effects of a medical intervention ought to be valued by the society. Oregon avoided this pitfall by filtering the assessment of effectiveness through solicited public preferences.

But the checks and balances offered by public preference are attended by shortcomings of their own. It is to Oregon's credit that the plan is informed by a good inventory of the values of the community who must live with the results, yet if broad societal participation is an important means of achieving a vision of the overall good of society, it is also true that a good statement of community values goes beyond a mere aggregation of public preference and extends to incorporating perspectives of what is good for society.[38] The voices of all parties affected by the distribution of services must be heard, and those who cannot speak for themselves must have effective advocates. That is the first step. However, there is a further task, one not addressed by Oregon's actions. In this most important second step, the task is to blend public preference with society's needs.

The Oregon experiment identifies and resolves some but not all of the practical objections raised against attempts to set formal priorities, in mental health. The results not only argue for parity, but in fact demonstrate that mental health services need not be worse off under formal health care priority plans. Moreover, integrating and ranking mental health produces the extra dividend of allowing planners to appreciate the value of preventive and with physical health long-term care services – varieties of care that have too often been neglected in the past. However, consequential issues remain. Do democratic principles require that citizens have as much say as they did in Oregon? Does the merger of mental and physical health à la Oregon present any drawbacks?

Lessons from New York State

The state of New York differs from Oregon State in its 'size, complexity, and diversity of mental health populations, providers, and service settings,'[39] and it serves as an important contrast to Oregon's highly formal and well-publicized priority-setting initiative. It is undoubtedly difficult to generalize from New York to other states, but we can safely say that compared to Oregon, New York's means of setting priorities are more typical. The state ranks populations and services by formal means (in the sense that they are explicit), but unlike Oregon the practical consequences for redistribution are not immediately identifiable. Like many states, New York has experimented with setting priorities by (1) focusing on interventions that reduce inpatient costs; (2) introducing nonmedical interventions into the health care system; and (3) identifying priority populations.[40] Like many states, New York's priorities and plans for service are defined by a host of influences, including large-scale implementation of managed care plans,

cost control in government entitlement programs, and vestiges from earlier cycles of mental health reform, such as inpatient state hospitals. Until the mid-1980s public mental health systems were largely state-controlled and self-contained. Priorities were, operationalized by the state's executive budget process. The bulk of the expenditure went to pay for inpatient care, which still makes up 62 percent of New York State's entire mental health budget. While every state directly operates one inpatient hospital service, only fifteen states (New York is by far one of the largest) operate ambulatory services. Most states fund a network of nonprofit community providers that offer outpatient treatment and support services.

During the 1980s many states formed priorities by responding to Medicaid funding, which increased monies for certain important populations such as children, and which allowed for optional Medicaid services such as targeted case management, clinic services, and rehabilitation.[41] Perhaps exceptional in its ability to expand services dramatically, without increasing state appropriation, New York was able to enlarge, its public mental health budget between 1986 and 1993 by $1 billion, 85 percent of which was captured from Medicaid funding.[42]

One of the crucial moves toward setting formal priorities in the states occurred in 1986, when the federal government enacted the State Comprehensive Mental Health Planning Act (Public Law 99–660), which created a high-priority obligation to serve targeted populations. The law required that statewide service plans describe the prevalence of persons with serious mental disorders and delineate strategies for delivering services. Prioritizing by populations led planners to identify a preferred set of services unique to specific, groups of persons.[43] Prior in this law, the distribution of community services was left to market forces with little intervention from the state; providers, determined which populations with mental illness would receive priority. Consequently services were lopsided. During the 1980s in New York the number of licensed outpatient treatment programs doubled, but the modality of treatment in this setting was psychotherapy, which is not necessarily appropriate for persons with severe and persistent mental illness. While the amount of service grew in the aggregate, only certain geographic areas benefitted. Midtown Manhattan, for example, had an oversupply of certain services, while other parts of New York City offered virtually no services of any type.[44] By the late 1980s emergency rooms and psychiatric units in general hospitals were routinely overcrowded, despite the 1,200 new acute psychiatric beds added to these hospitals in the 1980s. In fact, emergency rooms became the staging areas for a variety of social problems – homelessness, substance abuse, and criminal behavior. Studies demonstrated that a relatively small number of individuals was using a disproportionate number of emergency services and inpatient days. Patients were literally 'bouncing between emergency rooms, general hospitals, state hospitals, outpatient services, jails, and homeless shelters without ever being, effectively linked to appropriate services.'[45]

In the late 1980s these problems, along with a faltering economy, growing unemployment, declining tax revenues, spending caps, and setbacks in government social welfare programs, forced states like New York to do what had at one time been unthinkable, namely, set formal priorities. Without increasing state revenues, priorities were set by reallocating resources, principally by closing state inpatient hospital beds and reinvesting the resources in community outpatient treatment. The state accomplished the task by using traditional health care techniques that had always been available, including (1) certificates of need (CON) for granting expansion of inpatient and outpatient services; (2) needs assessment to determine the proper distribution of services; (3) licensing to oversee the services provided; (4) rate setting and financial incentives to promote services for targeted populations; and (5) a formal, comprehensive plan to redirect resources. The priorities it set were guided, on the one hand, by a mandate to provide services for a number of very needy patients and, on the other hand, by pressures to reallocate existing resources by offering new, less expensive, and frequently less intrusive services which were expected to respond more reasonably to unique patient needs. The service strategies given priority were (1) to increase access to psychiatric emergency services; (2) to develop case management programs for certain high-risk patients who consume a disproportionate share of services; (3) to develop a broad array of community housing; and (4) to refocus outpatient programs toward outcomes associated with rehabilitation and recovery.[46]

New York's Contribution

New York State's attempt at setting mental health priorities offers an important alternative to Oregon's. It strongly suggests that, despite daunting circumstances that might inhibit comprehensive planning, public policymakers have a clear chance to bring about a fairer and more sensible distribution of services using means already available. Interim reports on this process indicate that the number of inpatient beds is decreasing and that resources have been reallocated to the designated areas without increasing state funding.[47] Data about the overall impact on the states' mental health services remain to be gathered.

Despite these remarkable advances, New York and other states that are using already-available health policy techniques to redirect priorities will most likely fall victim to some of the unresolved conundrums in priority setting. The most obvious of these is associated with the process of decisionmaking. The historic role of the mental health authority to plan for people with mental illness remains firmly entrenched, directed by legislation and implemented by a commissioner and a state-mandated advisory council that reviews the state mental health plan. This shared authority has become somewhat, more democratic through community participation. In 1988 the Office of Mental Health launched a three-pronged planning effort with expanded participation from a broad range of constituent groups, including services recipients and their families, advocates, representatives of local and state human services agencies, educators, and service providers. To guarantee expanded public participation, the commissioner's Citizens' Mental Health Advisory Committee was established, working through five parallel structures around the state to recommend strategies and initiatives for change. The committee's deliberations are supported by experts who provide information on technical aspects.[48] The locus of decisionmaking, while informed by community values, ultimately resides with the publicly appointed Commissioner for Mental Health.

Surface comparisons between the New York and Oregon experiences have a limited instructive value; if pushed too far, the resemblances become inaccurate or misleading. Still, it is useful to compare the process of decisionmaking in both states. Are there any strong moral reasons for preferring a publicly elected commission such as Oregon's over a publicly appointed official? On first reflection it would seem there is little difference between the two approaches. Regardless of who makes the final decision, whether a publicly elected board or a publicly appointed official, the party in question, must be held accountable for integrating a good understanding of community values. There would seem to be little to choose between them. While it is true that independent boards can offer an interdisciplinary perspective not attainable by one official, and that the final decisions of such a board cannot be dismissed as the idiosyncratic thinking of one person, what this arrangement gains in political acceptability it loses at times in a lack of efficiency; indeed, such boards sometimes experience total paralysis. A single official at least has the capability of acting, although the actions will raise questions of whether a sufficient number of perspectives were intergrated into the final choice. Although the differences between them are significant, each decisionmaking process has something, to recommend it and arguably each is ethically acceptable. Less carefully examined has been the question of whether priority decisions ought ever to be left to a semi-private forum. In a democracy, must everything be open to those who will be affected by a decision? If not everything, then how much?

Another controversial feature common to New York's experience and the broad discussion on priorities is the targeting of special populations and services. Is it justifiable to prefer services aimed at those made worst off by mental illness? The fear, of course, of those who object to targeting the least well off is that their own interests may not be served, or served well. Quite reasonably, the defense the New York State Office of Mental Health has offered for its action is that federal legislation mandates that states target

patient populations. An unstated but equally plausible defense of the practice is that state budgetary cutbacks make it impossible to provide every citizen with every beneficial treatment, which means that some services and populations must be targeted. Yet these actions and justifications do not respond to some profound philosophical riddles associated with the issue of the worst off. For example, whom shall we count as the worst off? Perhaps the worst off have diseases relatively immune to treatment, while the better off could be served well by the limited resources. These problems are not the problems of New York State alone, but inhere in any attempt to set priorities with some form of targeting.

Turns in the Philosophical Debate

The experiences of Oregon and New York demonstrate that answers to some important questions that arise from setting priorities are already available. However, some means of setting priorities will raise equally important questions to which there are as yet no answers. For this reason any responsible attempt to set sensible priorities will crucially involve an ongoing and national debate. If in turn this debate is to be thoughtful and responsible, it will have to be thoughtfully framed. Conceptual resources for such a frame can be acquired by looking to certain turns in the philosophical debate. This report now examines four of these turns.

The Problem of Indeterminacy

Most attempts to develop general theories about how to set priorities, both in formulating criteria and in applying them, are plagued with substantive vagueness and indeterminacy.[49] Criteria that are used in public policy debates on how best to rank health services cannot be applied to yield anything like a determinate set of spending priorities or the appropriate selection of services or populations; this report itself bears witness to the nebulousness of such attempts. In practice, claimants competing for scarce medical resources often appeal to the same general norm – for example, 'fair equality of opportunity' – to settle the dispute.[50] Opposing sides can use this' general norm to lead to wildly different moral conclusions about the proper distribution of mental health services. How can one principle produce both a conclusion and its opposite? It may be true that the principles frequently used are too schematic to draw helpful normative priority schemes, but it remains unclear whether the problem of indeterminacy is one associated with the principles, the resulting priority scheme, or both.

Claims that the entire venture of setting priorities is vague and indeterminate can be understood in at least two ways. First, the principles might be thought of as indeterminate simply because there are an infinite number of them. For example, there is little doubt that each person who invokes a theory of priority setting can have a different set of assumptions – including what is to be ranked, what medical criteria should be used to establish priorities, and what ethical theories should be used. Each perspective will yield numerous practical conclusions, and the aggregate of perspectives will generate what might well be an infinite number of conclusions, some contradictory. The deep moral disagreement that is experienced in priority setting is simply that there are too many options and ways of viewing things. However, to call this variety of options or perspectives indeterminate is an odd use of the term. Usually principles are not so much indeterminate, as insufficiently determinate to specify a unique answer. So, for example, a principle of nonabandonment of the sick by itself cannot fully determine a unique solution to the problem of priority setting. What it can do, however, is rule out certain kinds of actions, such as a draconian use of triage.

A claim that priority schemes are indeterminate might, on an alternative interpretation, be taken to mean that priority schemes never yield anything but indeterminate conclusions. In moral reasoning, principles will typically need to be joined with relevant empirical data and clearly defined concepts in order to achieve some determinacy. To know whether an act of killing is justified, for instance, one would have to examine the principle, 'Do not kill the innocent,' distinguish the concepts of killing from letting die and the innocent from those threatening harm, and then judge how the factual situation fits the conceptually clarified principle. However, conceptual clarification alone does not always create determinacy. In mental health an adherence to the principle, 'Everyone is entitled to some care,' is at odds with other principles such as providing appropriate care or obligations to exercise stewardship by containing costs. Not all principles can be accommodated at once. In a case of this kind, the attempt to establish priorities might rest on several principles insufficiently determinate to yield a unique answer, but each might singly rule out some actions and all in combination might further determine a just course of action. The point is that the claim that priority setting schemes are indeterminate is not in principle an insurmountable objection. It is more accurate to claim that the principles of priority setting are insufficiently determinate and consequently will yield approaches to priority setting that will be underdetermined, but certainly not indeterminate.

Health Measurement Criteria

A central problem in the priority debate is over the diverse empirical health measurement criteria that can be used to set priorities. What health data shall be employed? Are the criteria that were used by Oregon, for example – severity of illness, net benefit, and the like – rationally compelling and defensible? If these are the wrong criteria, then which ones are right?

The implicit norm or standard from which most policy and priority debate begins is some form of cost-benefit measurement.[51] Decision-makers use this measurement against the existing set of resources and select that combination of resources that maximizes overall benefit. Many different, highly sensitive measures have been developed that take this form,[52] among them the quality adjusted life year (QALY) that measures health services in terms of quality and length of life,[53] or the quality of well-being scale (QWB) that evaluates treatments in terms of the degree and duration of health improvement.[54] Prototypical cost-benefit measurements pose some common philosophical problems. For example, why are certain features such as cost and benefit rather than other features such as severity of illness or prevalence of disease, chosen to be measured or given pride of place in any of the commonly employed scales? Even if there is agreement on what should be measured, what do concepts such as 'benefit' mean? Will palliation as well as cure be considered a benefit? For whom – the individual or society? If maximizing the benefit of the society becomes the measure, the policy can be criticized on they grounds that it disregards the distribution of benefits to the individual. Similarly, if maximizing the benefit to the individual becomes the measure, the policy can be criticized on the grounds that an ethically defensible standard must attend to something more than, or distinct from, individual well-being.[55] While all health measurements have problems in common, when taken by themselves, the problems are unique. Any policy maker responsible for priorities would have minimally to examine aspects of the most frequently used measurements: severity and prevalence of illness and dysfunction, and effectiveness and cost of treatment.

How much priority should be given to effective outcomes?

A common means society employs to decide its priorities and distribute its resources among a number of ill persons, all of whom are equally needy, is to measure and rank according to the effectiveness of the treatment. Is it more important to provide services to a severely and persistently mentally ill person for whom treatment can do little, or should services be given instead to people with problems in living or anxiety disorders for whom treatment is highly effective?[56] An argument from effectiveness would lead one to rank according to treatments that offer more longevity and better quality of life.[57] However, the term 'effectiveness' admits of many meanings. Effective for what? For improving function? For restoring it? At times improving function might be more important than restoring it, depending on how greatly function was compromised in the first place. Furthermore, in mental health, effectiveness can be a measure of how well a treatment reduces the risk of physical danger to the patient or to others who might be

harmed by the patient's actions. Yet there is often so little agreement about what exactly ought to be made more effective that discussion can seem pointless.

Not all considerations of effectiveness are useless in determining priorities, however. When considering two treatments for one disorder and all else is equal, including cost and invasiveness of treatment, the choice between a marginally effective and a highly effective service is an easy one. Simple rationality and concern for a just use of public funds would privilege the measure of effectiveness for cases of this kind.

More troubling, however, would be to determine the priority between two persons with mental illness with the same disorder, same degree of severity of illness, and same cost of treatment, but where the outcome for one would be more favorable than for the other. Suppose, for example, that two schizophrenic patients, S1 and S2, had the same severity of disease and cost of treatment but that S1 would improve enormously while S2 would show only moderate improvement. Should we favor S1, who stands the best chance of responding to treatment? If preference is given to *patients* who are likely to sustain highly effective outcomes, rather than *treatments* that produce such outcomes, then a patient such as S2 who has been refused treatment could complain that she was being asked to forgo any chance at all of benefit. Few would deny that if treatments for S2 provided no benefit to speak of, then S2 should be given a low priority; however, it is less clear how to prioritize treatments when a person receives only a somewhat smaller benefit than someone else with the same disorder. To add precision in these ambiguous choices, some have proposed deciding outcomes by assigning the ill a number of chances proportional to the benefits of treatment – for example, by throwing a ten-sided die whose sides are weighted relative to the benefit of treatment[58] or some other multiplicative weight.[59] Where benefits are nearly equal in outcome, the best chance of benefit is no longer a useful tie-breaker.

We have some reason to think that relying solely on effectiveness can be counterproductive to priority setting. Just as yielding to a public policy of the 'rule of rescue' – dramatically responding to meet the needs of an identifiable individual to save life at whatever cost – leads to an impossibly expensive system, so privileging effectiveness when it is accompanied by a very high price tag would distort the priority process. Other treatments of moderate to high benefit would be squeezed out.

How much priority should be given to the costs associated with mental illness?

In the more widely known health measurement scales used to set priorities there is typically an assumption, whether explicit or implicit that costs are relevant, especially those connected with treatment. As with all empirical measurements, a cost criterion has its share of ambiguity, some intuitively agreed upon uses, and some terrible consequences.

The conceptual problems with cost are straightforward. Which will count – treatment costs or overall costs, economic or noneconomic costs? Most people agree that overall costs, and not merely treatment costs, are esential to setting priorities; however, proponents disagree among themselves over which costs are part of overall costs, and to what degree treatment costs and overall costs should be compared. For mental illness, overall costs will include not only the present and long-term care of an individual, but also treatments needed for maintenance, the economic and social costs of nontreatment, and the cost of diverting resources from other socially desirable endeavors, including education and other social services.

There is substantial agreement about some uses of costs, especially when costs are used as a brake on spending. Simple rationality would require health planners to estimate how much the health care system could afford. If a priority-setting plan is to have any ethical grounding, there must be a good fit between its measurements and its stated goals. It follows that priority setting that is motivated by the goal of containing costs must contain criteria for measuring costs, and indeed, accepting a priority plan that lacks a measurement for its stated goals 'would be like buying a car without a steering wheel.'[60]

An example of counting cost that can be determinative in and of itself is the case of Clozapine.[61] Clozapine, an antipsychotic drug originally costing

$9,000 a year, has been demonstrated to be beneficial to a segment of schizophrenic patients who previously were not satisfactorily helped by drugs (39 percent of once-seriously disabled patients reported they were able to regain employment, and 68 percent were able to live in the community).[62] One state, New York, with upward of 16,000 schizophrenic patients, has distributed the drug to a relatively small number of patients because legislative appropriations are fixed and will not allow additional expenditures for making this drug widely available. Legislators put a priority on providing alternative treatments for schizophrenics after weighing the physical risks of treatment, the monetary cost of providing Clozapine, the cost of squeezing out other effective treatments, and costs associated with nontreatment, including a loss of productivity, increase in crime, and heightened drug abuse.

There are of course some troubling consequences to the use of cost to set priorities, especially when it involves canceling expensive interventions altogether. Sometimes arguments in favor of preventive measures in mental health are justified on the basis of money saved through gains in future wages or through avoiding costly inpatient treatment. Yet even if the preventive interventions never helped avoid future costly treatment, there would be a reluctance to abandon prevention strategies merely because they had been shown not to be cost-effective. The problem finds an unusual twist in mental health. Where there is a 'moral hazard' – whereby a treatment is made available but is then overused, thus driving up the cost and leaving the system worse off than it was initially – disincentives, such as high copayments or deductibles, are erected for the purpose of attenuating the demand for the treatment.

Factoring in overall costs can also have its dark side. If, for example, the costs used to set priorities included wages lost because of the treatment, then persons who have low-wage jobs (as some mentally ill persons do) might be given a low priority for treatment. This logic might be applied to any group – the elderly, or children, for example – that tends to absorb social resources while contributing relatively little in the way of work productivity.[63]

How much priority should be given to the worst off, if any?

There is a strong intuition that society should give the highest priority to treating the sickest or most disabled patients. This 'hierarchy of pain' criterion is seen clearly in the strong human proclivity to respond to the worst off victims of illness or accident. Oddly, the intuition favoring the worst off is sometimes ignored by cost-effectiveness methodologies that are biased toward services maximizing effective treatment outcomes while minimizing costs. Yet in certain cases the intuition seems appropriate. Take for example the case of a minor mental dysfunction that causes little harm, is limited to the individual, and has no real impact on the smooth functioning of the society; our intuition that this sort of case ought not to be a high public priority is probably correct.

Intuitions fail us at other times, however. When, for example, the choice is between treating persons with severe and persistent mental illness and treating a severe anxiety disorder, such as panic disorder, peoples' intuitions will differ. The National Alliance for the mentally Ill (NAMI) argues that individuals with severe and persistent mental illness are substantially worse off as a result of their disease and so ought to have a higher priority for treatment, while spokespeople at the Anxiety Disorders Association (ADA) argue that people who suffer from panic disorder, although much less seriously ill, ought to receive equal or even higher priority. Rather than directly confronting the severity issue, the ADA's argument involves other reasons to make the less severely impaired a priority, such as greater efficacy of treatment, lower cost, or the injustice of discriminating against those whose illness is episodic rather than chronic. Services for the less severely ill might well be given higher priority if they are less costly, serve more people, or meet some socially agreed-upon goal.

On the other hand, the sickest often claim priority on the basis that justice requires giving priority to the worst off. The best known example of this argument is John Rawls's 'Difference Principle,' which requires that 'the social and economic inequalities attached to offices and positions are to be adjusted so that, whatever the level of those inequalities, whether great or small, they are to the greatest benefit of the least advantaged members of

society.'[64] The Difference Principle has been much criticized. One criticism is that if one gives absolute priority to the least advantaged, only the worst off will get services. A second criticism is that Rawls's theory is based on economic and social abstractions that do not easily apply in any straightforward way to priorities in mental health. What should be included in the definition of 'worst off' – the relative harmfulness of a medical condition if left untreated? Economic disadvantage? Danger to others? Amartya Sen, like Rawls, has argued that if a benefit is to be distributed to two individuals, the initially worse off individual should receive an equal or greater share of the benefit so as not to widen the initial inequity.[65] This principle requires giving some, but not absolute, priority to the worst off. On either formulation it seems likely that other principles, such as efficaciousness and cost, will be used to temper this one.

How much priority should be given to providing benefit to the many?

Some hold that 'numbers count' in setting priorities; the prevalence of a disorder is thought to be determinative for ranking. The principle of 'the greatest good for the greatest number' would set common conditions at a high priority, while rare disorders would be given low priority. Setting priorities that prefer higher prevalence intuitively seems sensible, as treating a common disorder meets publicly defined goals such as sustaining the functioning of society.[66] In mental health it is certainly true that treating a common disorder such as depression substantially reduces dysfunction by reducing medical costs. Yet here it is not the prevalence of the disorder that makes it a high priority treatment but a host of other considerations, including effectiveness of outcomes and costs.

There is a strong reason not to make prevalence determinative when setting priorities, however. If, for example, a condition is rare, but its cost and benefit per case are equal to a common condition, refusing to treat the rare condition displays an 'irrational bias against people and problems that come in small groups.'[67] Considerations of prevalence are an inappropriate basis for priorities when two disorders are of equal severity and can be treated equally effectively.[68] Prevalence should be a relevant public consideration only when, for example, a decision must be made whether to treat a rare, harmful disorder at such great cost that it stands to squeeze out treatment of a common and less harmful disorder. Society would have to judge whether in this case it was important to ensure that everyone received some health care.

An examination of all the health measurements put forward at one point or another to establish priorities suggests several items that public policymakers should keep clearly in mind. First, as is obvious from the discussion above, the public policy reasons for selecting some health measurements over others are cloaked in a certain amount of complexity and mystery. The examination of the four measurement to which this discussion has been limited provides ample evidence for refusing to give any of them a privileged position. Moreover it is difficult to establish clear meanings for any of them. One way to determine which measurements should be included and how broadly they should be understood is to leave it to the community to decide what it values. A public process could be used to determine for example, whether the community prefers fewer costs or fewer burdens. Second, health measurements alone do not seem to be determinative of what priorities to set. No matter how effective or cheap a treatment, or how grave or prevalent a disease or dysfunction, there are other considerations that need to be incorporated or adjusted for. For instance, quite aside from the health data about a treatment, the popular to whom the treatment is offered might have suffered a history of oppression which society now wishes to rectify. In short, the health data must be balanced against the political, social, and cultural forces that have and have had an effect on the equitable distribution of services.

Who should Decide?

The question of what empirical information should count in the determination of priorities is merely one of the many issues that remains unresolved. Another question of great importance is who should make these decisions. How should we determine the locus of decision-making? It is appealing to rely on democratic principles as a means of achieving a resolution that will guide policy. But the question then becomes, Is a democratic process the best or fairest means of determining what constitutes an acceptable priority-setting scheme, or are there alternatives, such as, reliance on experts or public officials? While mental health care at some times and in some places has been allocated in ways highly responsive to community input, this has not been universally the case, nor have all mental health policy professionals been pleased with the results.[69] In fact, not all practitioners or theorists regard public openness about priority-setting or certain complex public policy matters as a good thing. One argument, that of Guido Calabresi and Philip Bobbitt, stipulates that some choices are so tragic that the good order of society requires they be made in the least damaging way. Choices are tragic when they run afoul of society's fundamental commitment to certain absolute ideals – for example, that life is priceless. If society is unable to life up to life ideal that life is priceless, but it has good reason to protect this ideal, then those who must make the hard choices should do so behind closed doors.[70] Another argument from those who propose measures to make priority setting less public is based on a claim that patterns of invidious bias against persons with mental illness are so rampant throughout society that the decisions must be made away from the heat of these biases, by knowledgeable and sympathetic specialists or officials.

It is important to realize that at a practical level, public officials do not consciously hide decisions, yet in their good intentions to better the plight of the ill, the method used for dealing with tragic choices might be to keep the public in ignorance. In health services, for example, eligibility criteria are used to allow some identified persons to receive a service; however, if eligibility criteria are eliminated and quietly replaced with new patterns in the organization of care, then a tragic choice might have been made, even though the policymaker does not admit that it has been made.

However, both the concealment advocated by Calabresi and Bobbitt and the lesser concealment created by measures to protect persons with mental illness from bias pose trade offs that a democratic society can ill afford. The strongest rebuttal to the tragic choices argument is that our society is to some extent held together by openness and honesty. Tragic choices that invisibly set priorities cannot but serve to dissolve the glue that secures society.[71] If we are to create a well ordered society, it must be animated by a notion of 'fair terms of cooperation and mutual advantage.'[72] Fair cooperation is only possible if all the parties to the cooperative agreement know where they stand, and that is possible only if all the relevant considerations are avaliable to the participants.[73]

As for priority-setting measures designed to avoid the sting of discrimination, it is not clear that we gain much when we leave these decisions to a less than open forum. A priority, decision is anything but a mere algorithm, where all the data are clear and complete and need only be entered into an agreed-upon equation by skilled minds. Rather, priority decisions rest firmly on people's values – about disease and disability, about disease and palliation, about costs – and these are the issues about which individuals will reasonably disagree. Highly skilled technicians and public officials have no more insight about them than anyone else does. Countering movements to keep the decision from *hoi polloi*, John Rawls stipulates a 'publicity condition': when it comes to determining what should guide the allocation of scarce resources, everything must be open to the view of those affected by the decision.[74]

One might too hastily, and inappropriately, conclude that the publicity condition requires direct citizen participation in every decision. Leaving all decisions about priority setting to democratic vote seems impracticable and would mire any progress. The proper lesson to be drawn from the publicity condition is that everything should in principle be open to view, and that the basic framework of the priority-setting structure should be sensitive to community values. However, the exact degree of community involvement beyond these two constraints should be a local decision. If, for reasons of practicality, a community decides to empower a public official or board to make the final decisions, these decisionmakers will be held to the same constraints as the community.

The move to local decisionmaking is not without some important practical moral consequences. Dispersing mental health decisions to allow community boards to participate in policymaking is a case in point. During the era when community mental health centers developed at the local level, for example, citizens – self-appointed in many cases – pushed for expanded ambulatory services for poor, working-class families with a variety of distressing but not disabling problems, rather than supporting intensive services for individuals with severe and persistent mental illness. The priorities of the citizens reflected prevailing needs within the community, but the needs of the minority – persons with severe and persistent mental illness – were neglected. If these priorities represent the authentic preference of the majority, must we accept them at face value, regardless of their implications? Whose preferences should we rely on – those of the public as a whole or only the people who have experienced a condition? Regardless of the persons from whom opinions are sought, fairness would dictate that the views be constrained by moral principles, such as the nonabandonment of persons, that would rule out certain alternatives.

Another unresolved puzzle in decisionmaking pertains to the structure of advocacy. Those who have experienced a condition are often unable to fully participate in decision-making. For this reason it is appealing to rely on structures of advocacy. Dozens of groups represent the interests of the persons with mental illness, not to mention their families, providers, and organizations of providers. The moral problems associated with the advocacy alternative are well rehearsed. At a practical level it is important to examine a number of issues. Who is it that elected this group to be advocate? Are the members of the group self-selected or representative? Do they have the interests of the entire movement in view? Where does their authority to advocate come from? At a theoretical level, it is vital to probe the tension between the preferences of consumer advocates and citizens' needs, as these are not necessarily the same. Consumers are principally interested in increasing their access; very seldom are they interested in restraining the quest for new interventions or the search for monies, yet this indifference to restraint runs at odds with society's need for cost containment.

Is There a Basic Package of Services?

In a common-sense evaluation of me fairness of a priority proposal, the litmus test is often whether a given service is so critical that it must always be provided. Yet most attempts to use ethical criteria to construct a 'basic package' – services that are almost a nonnegotiable right – fail to offer any guidance for specific spending recommendations. The problem of underdeterminacy persists.

Some ethical considerations and constraints can offer a certain amount of determinacy to the problem of the basic package. First, it is important to remember that setting priorities serves at least two functions. The first is that even if society has ample funds (but not infinite funds), priority setting is valuable as a way of using the available money wisely and rationally – it is just a way of establishing what is comparatively more or less important. Second, if funds are tight, then priority setting makes it possible to allocate (or ration) those funds in the most prudent way – it facilitates orderly, reasonable rationing. There is virtually no likelihood in the present financial climate that any government can guarantee it will *always* make a certain level of care available, regardless of the funds. Consequently, a basic package must always be conceived as contingent on available funds. It makes to real sense to talk about a basic package in the abstract. Designing a basic package in light of available funds is a much easier task with a priority list: the more money one has the lower one can go in the list; the less money one has the higher one must go. It is not inconceivable that a state could make (temporary) guarantees of a basic package, saying that unless there is some unforeseen crisis it will take care of items 1 through *n* on the list.

A rough ethical constraint of nonabandonment adds determinacy to the basic package in that it establishes who should have access to it. The question whether we should prefer the worst off, considered earlier but left unresolved, can on this principle be answered: the worst off should receive a high but not absolute preference. There is a widespread but lamentable assumption that favoring the worst off implies that those who are better off should get nothing. The implication does not follow. From the time of Hippocrates onward there has been a strong moral requirement forbidding the abandonment of patients. Such abandonment is at odds with respect for persons, a fundamental moral principle. Nonabandonment further shows solidarity with everyone in the community, no matter who they are. If some portion of the population of the mentally disabled received nothing after society has examined empirical data, balanced that data with social and moral considerations, and proposed priorities, then there would be good cause for a discretionary rearrangement of priorities to remedy this failing. That is, a criterion of non abandonment would require a basic package to ensure that everyone who is mentally disabled receive something. The constraint would also require an ongoing analysis of the provision of services to ensure that no person with mental illness falls through the cracks and receives no treatment.

A third consideration for the basic package emerges from a combination of health measurements, including effectiveness and cost of treatment, and prevalence and severity of illness. It can be argued that any decent society owes its members the kind of services that have had the most effect on improving the health of the population as a whole, which historically has included nutrition, sanitation, general living conditions, vaccinations, and antibiotics. There is also a storing human sentiment favoring care for those whose lives are strikingly and decisively harmed by a particular disease, and ranking lower the care of those whose lives are crippled but not devastated. We know the latter can get by, even if not well, while the former are vulnerable and will not get by. Even though the worst off should not get absolute priority, they do deserve some priority. For those most afflicted by mental illness, social services that have been shown to be effective,[75] such as financial assistance, congregate housing, and sheltered workshops to augment job skills – services intended to minimize the negative consequences of a disability (such as reinstitutionalization) – should be provided if at all humanly possible. This social support care for people with mental disorders comprises services appropriate for anyone suffering from a disability, with or without mental illness.

Thinking about Mental Health Services

Has this investigation of the priorities that ought to be established for mental health generated more heat than light? The number of issues that must be examined have seemingly expanded exponentially, suggesting that questions not ordinarily addressed in priority setting have been coaxed to the surface. Even where the project revisited longstanding dilemmas, some issues have become clearer, if not resolved altogether. The single most important contribution our investigation has made is in its application to mental health services, where, at a minimum, it contributes a language and structure for thinking about certain of its festering, perhaps intractable problems.

Theoretical indeterminacy is the single most dominating and ongoing challenge to this and any other attempt to set priorities. The problem is symptomatic of a relatively deep social conflict over what moral concepts we ought to cherish most dearly – a conflict that will vex not only mental health policy but any other reflection on priorities. From the outset it has been clear that the shape, force, and number of criteria for setting priorities are potentially infinite when viewed through the kaleidoscope of readily available ethical theories. Even if one pattern of ethical reasoning is used consistently, limitless problems in achieving conceptual clarity for each criterion can result in both insufficiently determinate principles and underdetermined normative schemes to set priorities.

What is less obvious and perhaps more fundamental is that the moral disagreement that surfaces in discussions over priorities mirrors a profound disparity among world views. If liberalism offers little more than procedural guides for setting priorities, the many challenges to liberalism that offer substantive content hold out little hope for consensus.[76] Yet as our investigation amply attests, the present standoff must not create paralysis. The amount of determinacy that can be attained creates serious philosophical puzzles, but they must be balanced with the fact that de facto, informal priority setting will continue. It must be acknowledged that the principles of priority setting are insufficiently determinate to offer perfect

guidance, but they rule out certain courses of action. At the same time, we must recognize that priority-setting schemes are underdetermined and that further efforts will be required, including moral argumentation about the facts, concepts, and principles that apply.

From its inception, the growing conversation about setting priorities has, although not always, squarely addressed whether it should take place at all; it must confront and finally put to rest the claim that this is unthinkable or impossible. Priority setting is unlikely to face sustained allegations of perniciousness if the process is understood as an attempt to promote a more reasoned and participatory public discussion culminating in policy about issues that intimately affect our lives individually and as a nation and about which people reasonably disagree. Likewise, when priority setting is an attempt to excise utterly useless health services or eliminate marginally beneficial ones, the outcry will not be very loud. Most people see the merits of proposals that identify and eliminate health care services that have been demonstrated to be useless, safely forgone, or only marginally beneficial. There will then be little dispute regarding the necessity of an ongoing mechanism, such as a health outcomes bureau, to accomplish this end.

However, when priority setting is used to help sort services and delete beneficial but less needed services, accusations of impropriety will be more pronounced. And to the extent that the stated goals – cost containment, greater access, and more appropriate treatment – are not met by the plan, the critics will be right to complain; criteria must match well the stated purposes for establishing priorities and must further their attainment. Perplexing but not insurmountable is the charge that setting priorities within a particular part of the system is unseemly. There can be little disagreement that, while it may be important to highlight the long-term, chronic features that are representative of a portion of mental health, it would be terribly misguided to rank mental health services apart from other services, either by failing to integrate mental health, or worse, by leaving physical health untouched and unranked. Mental and physical health should be fully integrated in any priority setting plan. It is important to emphasize once again that the evidence from Oregon indicates that when mental health services are considered together with physical health care, mental health needs rank satisfyingly high.

The claim that priorities, once set, are impossible to implement should also be resisted. Difficult, yes – impossible, no! The history of de facto priorities reveals the convergence of a number of social elements that policymakers and the public must appraise. Any strategy must be based on a keen awareness that social forces of varying degrees shape priorities in unexpected and even counterproductive ways. Any plan that relied on empirical data alone would be insufficient. Priority setting should take place in a way that best ensures a tension among political, social, and moral considerations on the one hand, and scientific evidence on the other. This means that the method for setting priorities must accommodate some degree of discretion on the part of those ultimately responsible for the process, who can adjust for biases and predilections in the empirical data and balance them against a realistic appraisal of what is politically feasible.

Determining what empirical data should count, and in what balance, can seem to be an almost hopeless task. A priority system's first task should be to identify, conceptually clarify, and fully evaluate common empirical health measurements, including the seriousness and prevalence of a condition and the effectiveness and cost of treating it. Care must be taken to include all relevant factors. One that is often overlooked, yet crucial to a segment of the experience of mental illness, is its chronic or sometimes episodic quality, which requires attention over time and perhaps long-term care. Beyond that, if a priority system privileges one empirical health measurement over others, steps should be taken to ensure that the prominence of the measure is warranted by principles of fairness and rationality or authorized by public choice. Additionally, a priority plan must consider whether constraints external to the health measurement invest the measurement with further determinacy. When considering a condition's severity, for example, where there is philosophical agreement and strong public sentiment that those who are worst off should receive some but not absolute priority, the external constraint of nonabandonment should be brought to bear so that no one with mental illness is forced to go without any care at all.

Setting formal priorities requires a continuous mechanism for identification and evaluation of health measurement and outcome, data. While this might appear to be no more than old-fashioned common sense, in some early congressional proposals for health care, arrangements for some such mechanism were conspicuously absent. Because of the nature of empirical data, an appeals process must be developed to consider challenges to decisions to exclude certain services that have been pronounced unnecessary or uncertain in outcome.

The problems associated with democratizing the priority process also have been advanced. From the outset, there was little disagreement that priorities should be set by a mechanism that is accountable, enhances objectivity, and allows for a public, participatory process. However, what remained to be considered is whether the entire decisionmaking process is one that requires direct citizen participation in every decision or whether decisions can instead be made by public officials. As messy as it seems, there is strong moral reason for decisionmakers to place decisions in clear view of those who will be affected by them, and the decisionmaker must be sure that the basic structure of decisionmaking is sensitive to community values. The moral requirement does not, however, require direct citizen participation in every decision.

Our consideration of the basic package serves as an example of how insufficiently determinate principles can in combination, and given sufficient conceptual clarity, provide direction for setting priorities. Intuitively it seems correct that any priority system should ideally be prepared to find and note some minimally adequate level of care below which no system should fall. Of course, this ideal cannot always be achieved because it is constrained by resource availability, but it remains an approachable ideal in that any community ought to be willing to mark what it thinks it can give and retreat only in the face of unforeseen catastrophe. Also, the insufficiently determined principle of preferring the worst off provides guidance: priority systems should give a higher place to caring for those who cannot readily be cured (such as chronic schizophrenics) and a lower place to the traditional effort of curing. Another insufficiently determined principle, that of non abandonment, insists that though a preference for the worst off may be legitimate, those suffering with milder mental illness cannot simply be neglected.

It is unlikely in the short run that all constituents in the field of mental health will warmly embrace attempts to set priorities. No doubt the unresolved questions featured in this investigation will serve as a defense for shunning the process. Yet, regardless of the objections, it is likely that priorities will continue to be set, formally or informally. The choice will be ours. If we indeed explicitly pursue priorities, further efforts will be needed to deal with the serious puzzles raised by the process, but the benefit will be an improvement over the present state of affairs.

Acknowledgment

The authors would like to thank Hilde L. Nelson for her help in editing this report.

References

1   Karen Bourdon, 'Estimating the Prevalence of Mental Disorders in US Adults from the ECA Survey,' *Public Health Reports* 107, no. 6 (November-December 1992): 663–68.

2   Gerald Grob, *From Asylum to Community: Mental Health Policy in Modern America* (Princeton, N.J.: Princeton University Press, 1991).

3   Miriam Cotler and Brian Gould, 'Priorities in Mental Illness: Priorities in the Private Sector,' prepared for the Hastings Center Project on Priorities in Mental Health, 1993.

4   Bureau of Labor Statistics, *Employer Benefits in Medium and Large Firms,* 1988 (Washington, D.C.: Department of Labor, 1988).

5   Cotler and Gould, 'Priorities in Mental Illness.'

6   Steven Scharfstein, Anne Stoline, and Howard Goldman, 'Psychiatric Care and Health Insurance Reform,' *American Journal of Psychiatry* 150, no. 1 (1993): 7–18; Richard Frank, Health D. Salkever, and Steven Scharfstein, 'A New Look at Rising Mental Health Costs,' *Health Affairs* 10, no. 2 (Summer 1991): 116–23.

7   Jerome Wakefield, 'The Concept of Mental Disorder: On the Boundary between Biological Fact and Social Value,' *American Psychologist* 47, no. 3 (1991): 373–88.

8   Kenneth Kendler et al., 'The Prediction of Major Depression in Women: towards an Integrated Etiological Model,' *American Journal of Psychiatry* 150, no. 8 (1993): 1139–48.

9   Kenneth Wells and Robert Brooks, 'The Quality of Mental Health Services: Past, Present, and Future,' in *The Future of Mental Health Services Research*, ed. C. Taube, D. Mechanic, and A. Homann (Washington, D.C.: NIMH, 1991).

10 *Roll Call* advertisement, sponsored by a number of mental health activists.

11 'Mental Health Services in Health Care Reform: Specifications for Implementing the Proposal: Principles for Mental Health Care in Health Care Reform,' presented in Washington, D.C., February 1993.

12 Grayson Norquist and Kenneth Well, 'Mental Health Needs of the Uninsured,' *Archives of General Psychiatry* 48 (1991): 475–78.

13 David Hadorn and Robert Brook, 'The Health Resource Allocation Debate: Defining Our Terms,' *JAMA* 266, no. 23 (18 December 1991): 3328–31.

14 Robert Michels, 'Priority Setting in Mental Health,' prepared for the Hastings Center Project on Priorities in Mental Health, 1993.

15 David Kears, 'Setting Priorities for Mental Health Services: The Case of Alameda County, California,' prepared for the Hastings Center Project on Priorities in Mental Health, 1993.

16 Rosemary Stevens, *In Sickness and in Wealth: American Hospitals in the Twentieth Century* (New York: Basic Books, 1989).

17 C. Keisler, 'U.S. Mental Health Policy: Doomed to Fail,' *American Psychologist* 47, no. 9 (1992): 1077–82.

18 L. K. George, 'Definition, Classification, and Measurement of Mental Health Services,' in *The Future of Mental Health Services Research*.

19 Len Rubenstein, 'Law and Priority Setting,' prepared for the Hastings Center Project on Priorities in Mental Health, 1993.

20 Daniel Callahan, 'Setting Priorities: Problems and Possibilities,' prepared for the Hastings Center Project on Priorities in Mental Health, 1993.

21 David Hadorn, 'Setting Health Care Priorities in Oregon: Cost-Effectiveness Meets the Rule of Rescue,' *JAMA* 265, no. 17 (1 May 1991): 2218–25.

22 Joseph Morrissey and Howard Goldman, 'Cycles of Reform in the Care of the Chronically Mentally Ill,' *Hospital and Community Psychiatry* 35 (1984): 785–93.

23 Gerald Grob, *Mental Institutions in America: Social Policy to 1975* (New York: Free Press, 1973),pp. 84–131.

24 Gerald Grob, 'Government and Mental Health Policy: A Structural Analysis,' prepared for the Hastings Center Project on Priorities in Mental Health, 1993.

25 Grob, *Mental Institutions.*

26 Grob, *Mental Institutions*; Grob, 'Government and Mental Health Policy.'

27 Gerald Grob, *Mental Illness and American Society: 1875–1940* (Princeton, N.J.: Princeton University Press, 1983), pp. 144–78.

28 Grob, *From Asylum to Community*, pp. 5–23.

29 Grob, *From Asylum to Community*, pp. 49–50.

30 Grob, 'Government and Mental Health Policy.'

31 Grob, *From Asylum to Community.*

32 David Mechanic, 'Recent Developments in Mental Health: Perspectives and Services,' *Annual Review of Public Health* 12 (1991): 1–15.

33 Gerald Grob, *The Mad among Us: A History of the Care of America's Mentally Ill* (New York: Free Press, January 1994), chapter 11.

34 David Mechanic and Richard Surles, 'Challenges in State Mental Health Policy and Administration,' *Health Affairs* 11, no. 3 (Fall 1992): 34–50; Howard Goldman and Richard Frank, 'What Level of Government? Balancing Interests of the State and Local Community,' prepared for the Hastings Center Project on Priorities in Mental Health, 1993.

35 Martin Strosberg et al., *Rationing American's Medical Care: The Oregon Plan and Beyond* (Washington, D.C.: The Brookings Institute, 1992).

36 Oregon Health Services Commission, *Prioritization of Health Services: Report to the Governor and the Legislature* (Salem: Oregon Health Services Commission 1991).

37 **David Pollack, Bentson McFarland, Robert George,** and **Richard Angell,** 'Prioritization of Mental Health Services in Oregon,' prepared for the Hastings Center Project on Priorities in Mental Health, 1993.

38 **Bruce Jennings,** 'Health Policy in a New Key: Setting Democratic Priorities,' *Journal of Social Issues* 49, no. 2 (1993): 169–84.

39 Personal communication with Richard Surles, New York State Commissioner for Mental Health.

40 **Richard Surles** and **Cynthia Feiden Warsh,** 'Mental Health Coverage in Health Care Reform,' prepared for the Hastings Center Project on Priorities in Mental Health, 1993; Office of Mental Health, *Challenges for the 1990s: State Comprehensive Plan for Mental Health Services, 1990–1995* (Albany, N.Y.: Office of Mental Health, 1990).

41 **Chris Koyanagi** and **Howard Goldman,** *Inching Forward* (Washington, D.C. National Mental Health Association, 1991).

42 **Surles** and **Feiden-Warsh,** 'Mental Health Coverage in Health Care Reform'; Mechanic and Surles, 'Challenges in State Mental Health Policy and Administration.'

43 **D. Shern, Richard Surles,** and **J Waizer,** 'Designing Community Treatment Systems of the Most Seriously Ill: A State Administrative Perspective,' *Journal of Social Science Issues* 53 (1989): 105–17.

44 **Surles** and **Feiden-Warsh,** 'Mental Health Coverage in Health Care Reform.'

45 **L. Meyers** et al., *New York City's Hospital Occupancy Crisis: Caring for a Changing Population* (New York: United Hospital Fund, 1988).

46 **Surles** and **Feiden-Warsh,** 'Mental Health Coverage in Health Care Reform.'

47 Office of Mental Health, *1993 Interim Report: Statewide Comprehensive Plan for Mental Health Services, 1993–1997* (Albany, N.Y.: Office of Mental Health, 1993), p. 4.

48 Office of Mental Health, *Challenges for the 1990s.*

49 **Norman Daniels,** 'Rationing Fairly: Programmatic Considerations,' *Bioethics* 7, nos. 2, 3 (1993): 224–33.

50 **Norman Daniels,** *Just Health Care* (Cambridge: Cambridge University Press, 1985).

51 **Dan Brock,** 'Quality of Life Measures in Health Care and Medical Ethics,' reprinted in D. Brock, *Life and Death: Philosophical Essays on Biomedical Ethics* (Cambridge: Cambridge University Press, 1993).

52 **Ian McDowell** and **Claire Newell,** *Measuring Health: A Guide to Rating Scales, and Questionnaires* (New York: Oxford University Press, 1987).

53 **G. Loomes** and **G. McKenzie,** 'The Use of QALYs in Health Care Decision Making,' *Social Science and Medicine* 28 (1989): 299–308.

54 **Robert Kaplan** and **John Anderson,** 'A General Health Policy Model: Update and Applications,' *HRS: Health Services Research* 23 (1988): 203–35.

55 **Dan Brock,** 'Some Unresolved Ethical Issues in Priority Setting of Mental Health Services,' prepared for the Hastings Center Project on Priorities in Mental Health, 1993.

56 **Daniels,** 'Rationing Fairly.'

57 **Hadorn** and **Brook,** 'The Health Resource Allocation Debate.'

58 **Dan Brock,** 'Ethical Issues in Recipient Selection for Organ Transplantation,' in *Organ Substitution Technology: Ethical, Legal, and Public Policy Issues,* ed. D. Mathieu (Boulder: Westview, 1988).

59 **Frances Kamm,** 'The Report of the U.S. Task Force on Organ Transplanation: Criticism and Alternatives,' *Mount Sinai Journal of Medicine* 56, no. 3 (1989): 207–20; see also her *Morality and Mortality,* vol. 1 (New York: Oxford University Press, 1993), in press.

60 **David Eddy,** 'Oregon's Methods: Did Cost-Effectiveness Fail?' *JAMA* 266, no. 15 (16 October 1991): 2135–41.

61 **William Reid,** 'Access to Care: Clozapine in the Public Sector,' *Hospital and Community Psychiatry* 41 (1990): 870–74.

62 **Kenneth Terkelsen** and **Rene Grosser,** 'Estimating Clozapine's Cost to the Nation,' *Hospital and Community Psychiatry* 41 (1990): 863–69; Eugene Arnold, 'Quantifying the Value of Human Life for Cost Accounting of Safeguards: Clarifying Formulas Applied to the Clozapine Controversy,' *The Journal of Clinical Ethics* 3, no. 2 (1992): 102–13.

63 **Brock,** 'Some Unresolved Ethical Issues.'

64 **John Rawls,** *Political Liberalism* (New York: Columbia University Press, 1993), p. 6.

65 **AmartyaSen,** *On Economic Inequality* (New York: Oxford University Press, 1973).

66 **Daniel Callahan,** *What Kind Of Life?* (New York: Simon and Schuster, 1989).

67 **Paul Menzel,** 'Oregon's Denial: Disability and Quality of Life,' *Hastings Center Report* 22, no. 6 (1992): 21–25, at 20.

68 **Elizabeth Anscombe,** 'Who Is Wronged?' *Oxford Review* 5, no. 1 (1967): 16–17.

69 **Goldman** and **Frank,** 'What Level of Government?'

70 **Guido Calabresi** and **Philip Bobbitt,** *Tragic Choices* (New York: W. W. Norton, 1978), p. 69.

71 **James L. Nelson,** 'Tragedy, Prejudice, and Publicity in Setting Priorities,' prepared for the Hastings Center Project on Priorities in Mental Health, 1993.

72 **John Rawls,** *A Theory of Justice* (Cambridge, Mass.: Harvard University Press, 1971).

73 **Leonard Fleck,** 'Justice, HMOs, and the Invisible Rationing of Health Care Resources,' *Bioethics* 4 (1990): 97–120.

74 **John Rawls,** 'Kantian Constructivism in Moral Theory,' *The Journal of Philosophy* 77, no. 9 (1980): 515–72.5.5

75 **George,** 'Definition, Classification and Measurement.'

76 **Ezekiel Emanuel,** *The Ends of Human Life: Medical Ethics in a Liberal Polity* (Cambridge, Mass.: Harvard University Press, 1991; Norman Daniels, 'Liberalism and Medical Ethics,' *Hastings Center Report* 22, no. 6 (1992): 41–43.

Prioritization of Mental Health Services in Oregon*

David A. Pollack, Bentson H. Mcfarland, Robert A. George, and Richard H. Angell

The problems of escalating costs and limited access are the primary focus of health care reform in the United States (Blendon and Donolan 1990; Clowe, Scalettar, and Todd 1993; Fein 1992; Himmelstein and Woolhandler 1989). Although health care services and technology continue to improve, they often become more expensive (Fuchs 1993; General Accounting Office 1991). Mental health is faced with similar financial pressures linked to improved treatments (including medications, behavioral therapies, and rehabilitation methodology) (Goodwin 1993; Michels and Marzuk 1993a,b). Nonetheless, growth in mental health expenditures will likely be constrained, at least in part because state governments (with their limited budgets) remain large providers of and/or payers for mental health services (Bevilacqua 1991; Bigelow and McFarland 1994). Consequently, the mental health service system (like that of health care generally) is undergoing dramatic change (Koyanagi et al. 1993). Although questions of cost containment and universal access pertain to mental health, the field has its own special concerns as well.

One issue is integration. Historically, mental health services have been provided by a large variety of agencies, often in the 'social service' sector (Mechanic and Rochefort 1992). Advocacy groups contend that recent research demonstrates mental conditions like schizophrenia or bipolar disorder to be 'diseases' and thus more properly addressed in the health care system. President Clinton has stated: 'There is no legitimate rationale for distinguishing between "mental" illness and "physical"illnesses in terms of research dollars, individual entitlements, and insurance benefits' (Mental Health Liaison Group 1993). The advocacy groups, of course, are not unaware of the relative wealth and power of the health care system vis-à-vis the social service system (Mechanic and Rochefort 1992). The rallying cry of the 'integrationists' is parity – nondiscriminatory health insurance coverage for persons with mental illness (Sharfstein, Stoline, and Goldman 1993).

Opponents of integration argue that, for all its numerous and well-known deficiencies, the social service sector has at least provided some care for persons with severe mental illness. The fear is that the general health care system will consume funds earmarked for the severely, mentally ill while directing research to other populations (Mental Heath Policy Resource Center 1992).

Another related argument from insurers and payers (especially employers) is that mental illness is characterized by the four 'uns': undefinable, untreatable, unpredictable, and unmanageable (Bonstedt 1992; Pearson 1992). This 'mythology of the uns' is, like many beliefs pertaining to persons with severe mental illness, a product of stigma and ignorance, leading easily to discrimination (Marshall 1992). In this context, discrimination takes the form of the penalty for chronicity. Chronic, potentially disabling physical conditions (e.g., diabetes) do not, ipso facto, preclude one from obtaining health care. However, chronic mental illness (e.g., schizophrenia) is often grounds for denying services (Judd 1990; Peterson, Christianson, and Wholey 1992). This discrimination is 'justified' on the grounds that severely mentally ill people would consume 'unmanageable' (or 'unpredictable')

amounts of service – in contradistinction to the physically ill, whose care can be both managed and predicted.

Another contentious issue is the question, What is a health care service and what is a social service? Persons with severe mental illness at different times may need a variety of services, such as case management, supported housing, psychosocial rehabilitation, or psychotropic medications (Lamb et al. 1993). Sharfstein and Stoline (1992) build on work by Astrachan, Levinson, and Adler (1976) to define these services from the provider's perspective as medical tasks, reparative tasks, humanistic tasks, and social controls. Some services (e.g., psychiatric diagnosis, medications, acute inpatient treatment) are clearly 'medical tasks' contained in the health sector, whereas other services (e.g., supported housing) are clearly 'reparative tasks' conducted in the social service sector. Some services (e.g., case management) might be found in either sector.

This situation places the mental health community itself in a serious dilemma (Koyanagi et al. 1993). Persons affected by mental disorders and providers of mental health services have consistently and continuously experienced inequities in coverage and reimbursement rates for mental health services (Judd 1990; Malloy 1991). The pressures around questions of participation in the health care planning process and obtaining equity for mental health are perhaps the most serious of those facing the mental health community in the United States (Havel 1992).

This article describes the Oregon mental health community's response to health care reform. We will present the health care planning process, highlight the methodology used in setting priorities, and focus on the mental health component. We will also describe attempts made in conjunction with the planning process to educate the public about the value of mental health services within the health care system. Finally, we suggest that this description contains models of strategies advocates can use to establish equity for mental health services in other health care systems.

Background

The prelegislative history and the specific legislation that authorized the Oregon Health Plan have been described in detail elsewhere (Brown 1991; Fox and Leichter 1991, 1993; McFarland et al. 1993; Oregon Health-Services Commission 1991a; Strosberg, Weiner, and Baker 1992). To summarize, in 1989 the state legislature enacted several bills that created a health care plan for Oregon. The three main goals of the legislation were universal access, reasonable provider reimbursement rates, and cost containment.

To achieve these goals, a Health Service Commission (HSC) developed a prioritized list of health services, a portion of which would be defined as the basic coverage for persons included in the plan. The plan's coverage would apply to the Medicaid population, which would be expanded to include virtually everyone at or below the federal poverty level. A similar package of benefits would be provided to previously uninsured employed persons through a 'pay or play' requirement applied to most employers. This approach contrasted with the previous system in which a relatively small number of persons (whose incomes were well below the federal poverty level) had access to a Medicaid program that offered essentially unlimited

* Pollack, D.A., McFarland, B.H., George, R.A. and Angell, R.H.: Prioritization of mental health services in Oregon. *Milbank Quarterly* 72:515–551, 1994.

benefits for (physical) health care. The intent of the Oregon Health Plan was to provide 'basic' health care coverage to a large number of individuals.

The idea of a prioritized list of health services was immediately labeled health care 'rationing,' and it attracted worldwide attention (Brown 1991; Callahan 1991; Fox and Leichter 1991). Oregonians found themselves being discussed by television commentators on *60 Minutes*, 20/20, and the *MacNeil/Lehrer NewsHour*. Innumerable academic articles in journals like *Health Affairs*, the *Journal of the American Medical Association*, and the *New England Journal of Medicine*, (see McFarland *et al.* [1993] for a bibliography) appeared almost concurrently with editorials in the New York *Times*, the Washington *Post*, and the *Wall Street Journal*. An early question in one of the 1992 presidential campaign debates pertained to the Oregon Health Plan. Nearly lost in this furor was the notion of integrating mental health services into a comprehensive health care system.

The Prioritization Process

The HSC, composed of physicians, other health providers, and laypersons (all appointed by the governor and confirmed by the state senate), initially created three committees to assist it in the daunting task of defining basic health care. The Health Outcomes Committee was to develop the prioritized list, the Social Values Committee was charged with determining the community values to be considered by the Health Outcomes Committee when sorting this list, and the Mental Health and Chemical Dependency (MHCD) Committee was to address the issues of prioritizing mental health and chemical dependency services and (possibly) integrating them into the larger system.

The MHCD Committee members represented consumers, family members, and professionals in the mental health and chemical dependency fields. The MHCD Committee was chaired by a public health nurse (a commission member) and staffed by HSC personnel. The committee, which typically operated on the basis of consensus, met in public for work sessions and to take testimony from mental health professionals and researchers.

The existence.of the MHCD Committee itself was a small victory for mental health advocates. As initially proposed, the draft legislation for the Oregon Health Plan omitted mental health and chemical depandency. Left to their own devices, legislators would have endorsed the mythology of the four 'uns' and excluded MHCD conditions. Determined lobbying by the MHCD community resulted in a legislative mandate that the HSC establish a mental health and chemical dependency committee. However, the 1989 legislation contained a political trade-off: mandated mental health benefits were scheduled to disappear when the full Oregon Health Plan (i.e., including mental health and chemical dependency and involving both the working poor and the Medicaid population) began operating statewide. Although these mandated benefits were modest (amounting to about 20 outpatient visits and 10 hospital days per beneficiary per 24 months), they had become the de facto standard for mental health coverage in the state.

The 1989 lobbying effort stimulated the development of a coalition representing mental health and chemical dependency, consumer, family member, and professional organizations. The coalition has now been meeting regularly for five years under the leadership of the Mental Health Association of Oregon. The mailing list includes some two dozen organizations active in the MHCD field.

Participants in the prioritization process were aware of changes in the health and mental health systems that were proceeding in parallel with development of the Oregon Health Plan. Most dramatic was the shift away from fee-for-service (FFS) and toward managed care, chiefly in the form of health maintenance organizations (HMOs). Oregon's HMO enrollment would climb from approximately 15 percent of the population in 1989 to 30 percent in 1993. Enrollment in preferred provider organizations (PPOs) and other managed care systems was increasing rapidly as well. Providers could see the end of FFS health care financing. Indeed, it was assumed that most, if not all, Oregon Health Plan beneficiaries would be enrolled in a prepaid system (McFarland *et al.* 1993). Oregon had been one of the first states to use prepaid health plans for Medicaid clients. In 1989, about 10 percent of the state's Medicaid clients were enrolled in HMOs, and another 10 percent or so were enrolled in different types of managed care systems. Members of the MHCD committee saw the Oregon Health Plan as a potential model for comprehensive managed care systems that provide mental health and chemical dependency services, as well as physical health care.

Other pertinent developments included the rise in Medicaid financing for public mental health clients and the accelerating shrinkage of the state mental hospitals (Lippincott 1989). Mental health services for Medicaid clients were provided solely by community mental health centers operating on an FFS basis. During the late 1980s and early 1990s, these local agencies substantially increased their Medicaid billings. Most dramatic was the rise in Medicaid-financed children's mental health services provided as part of the Early Periodic Screening Diagnosis and Treatment (EPSDT) program.

Although the Medicaid program brought federal matching funds into the public mental health system, it also put increasing demands on the state's general fund mental health dollars. In addition, the state mental health authority began to develop local general hospital programs to be used as alternatives to aging and isolated state mental hospitals. These local inpatient facilities were also able to bill Medicaid (whereas the state hospitals could not). Ironically, however, the state Medicaid program was sufficiently restrictive that many persons with chronic mental illness were found to be ineligible for coverage. For example, recipients of Supplemental Security Income (SSI) often had 'too much' income to qualify for Medicaid. The state mental health authority estimated that only about half of the chronically mentally ill people in Oregon were Medicaid clients (Lippincott 1989). Services to chronically mentally ill people who were not Medicaid clients had to be financed entirely with state general fund dollars. The rapid rise in Medicaid expenditures, plus the large numbers of non-Medicaid community mental health clients, prompted the state mental health authority to appreciate the, need for a Medicaid managed care system that could encompass persons with chronic mental illness. Consequently, state mental health administrators were very interested in seeing how the Oregon Health Plan developed (McFarland *et al.* 1993).

The Health Qutcomes Committee and the Initial Methodology

The methodology that the Health Outcomes Committee initially considered was based on a health decision policy model derived from the work of Kaplan and colleagues (Kaplan and Anderson 1988; Kaplan 1992; Kaplan, Debon, and Anderson 1991). Committee members were ambivalent about the methodology: it seemed to offer a logical and relatively objective approach to the overwhelming task of valuing and sorting, on the one hand, but, on the other, its dependence on mathematical reductions of human conditions and the risk of error secondary to unreliable outcome and cost data made it suspect.

The Kaplan methodology links each health care condition with its appropriate treatment, leading to the concept of condition–treatment pairs (e.g., appendicitis and appendectomy). The rank order list that would ultimately be developed is a sequence of hundreds of such condition--treatment pairs. For each condition–treatment pair, outcome and cost data were to be obtained, entered into a quality of well-being (QWB) scale, and given a mathematical value for the treatment.

The data provided for each condition–treatment pair were to include estimates of the outcomes and costs for both when proper treatment was provided and when it was not. These outcome data were to be compared for each condition in order to estimate the relative QWB and costs of the proper treatment.

Kaplan developed a list of 23 symptom clusters (Appendix 1) that represent most human pathological conditions and three categories of impairment that relate to mobility, physical activity, and social activity. Mathematical weights (i.e., 'utilities') were determined for each of the symptoms and impairments, based on a random telephone survey of Oregonians (Kaplan, Debon, and Anderson 1991). These weights were then used in the application of the QWB scale to the various condition--treatment pairs. The Health Outcomes Committee invited representatives from all the state's health care specialty and provider groups to provide outcome data for the development of the prioritized list.

The Social Values Committee

The Social Values Committee attempted to identify values that were not directly quantifiable in outcomes data or in the mathematical approach utilized by the Health Outcomes Committee. These less tangible values, such as age, productivity, equity, and access to care, would be considered by the HSC in adjusting and modifying the final prioritized list (Pollack *et al.* 1993). A list of important community-identified values was reviewed and categorized as being important in one or more of the following ways: value to society, value to an individual, and value as a component of a basic health care package. These value references were later used in sorting the list of condition–treatment pairs (Hasnain and Garland 1990a,b).

The Mental Health and Chemical Dependency Committee

The MHCD committee felt that the Kaplan methodology, because of its reductionistic approach, its bias toward acute conditions, and its lack of consideration for social costs, could be a significant obstacle to an equitable rating of mental health services. Therefore, the committee was faced with a critical strategy decision: members had to decide whether to play the game or to abandon the process and wait to see what happened next. There were multiple risks attached to complying with the process; of these, the most salient was the potential reduction in funding that would result from public mental health services not being funded under a separate budget and the loss of state-mandated mental health insurance benefits. Not complying carried the risk that the process might move ahead and require funding increases, thus squeezing mental health budgets or significantly delaying the planning for the integration of mental health services into a basic health care package. In either case, delay would perpetuate the disadvantages that mental health experienced vis-à-vis other health services.

The metaphor used in this discussion was that of a train leaving the station. The committee could choose to ride that train (the prioritization planning process) and retain the option of jumping off if and when it appeared that the process would end in an unfair outcome for mental health. Or the committee could choose not to ride the train, watch it leave, and hope for the best. However, it would be impossible, or at least extremely difficult, to catch up to the train once it had left the station. After much discussion, the committee agreed to participate in the process.

When the MHCD Committee was first presented with the QWB methodology, there were only two symptom clusters (one was trouble learning or remembering or thinking clearly, the other was often feeling upset or depressed) that had any mental health content. The committee succeeded in adding symptom clusters that were relevant to MHCD conditions to the symptom list.

The MHCD Committee accurately predicted that the mental health symptoms would be heavily weighted by the general public in the telephone survey. Indeed, three of the symptom clusters with mental health content (problems with alcohol or drugs, trouble learning or remembering or thinking clearly, and frequent episodes of feeling upset or depressed) were among the five highest ranked of the 23 symptom clusters. Even though the survey and its weighting of the symptoms had minimal influence on the ultimate prioritization methodology, the recognition of the importance accorded to mental health symptoms by survey respondents supported the committee's efforts to achieve parity for mental health services.

At the same time that the QWB methodology was being introduced to the MHCD Committee, the Social Values Committee was developing its plans for obtaining public opinion on health care issues through a community meeting process. Unfortunately, the initial plans of the Social Values Committee excluded reference to types of care that explicitly related to mental health conditions. For example, the case vignettes for the community discussions were restricted to medical–surgical problems. The MHCD Committee proposed inclusion of two types of care specifically and uniquely related to mental health (crisis mental health services and alcohol and drug dependency services) in the list of service types to be described in the community meetings. The committee-also urged that some case examples for other types of care be about mental health conditions.

Part of the committee's rationale for these recommendations stemmed from the well-established notion of the stigma associated with mental health conditions. The committee similarly was concerned about the mistaken perception that psychiatric conditions have no biological or other factors that would make them comparable to other medical conditions. It was considered essential and ethically responsible proactively to establish the links between mind and body for the public in the context of this combined educational and opinion-gathering effort.

The Social Values Committee accepted these recommendations and correspondingly altered the community meeting format. Not surprisingly, the outcome of the community meetings reflected a high public value for mental health and chemical dependency services. This expression of concern about mental health issues, as reflected through both the random survey and the community meetings, was repeated in 12 state wide public hearings held by the commission. At these hearings, interested citizens advocated the types of health coverage to be included in a basic plan. People from the mental health community were highly visible and outspoken in their views that mental health conditions be given sufficient coverage.

A key component of the prioritization process was obtaining data on outcomes and costs of different treatments (including no treatment) for assorted conditions (i.e., diagnoses). The Health Outcomes Committee was charged by the HSC with compiling these outcome data.

The MHCD Committee convinced the Health Outcomes Committee of the need to gather data on mental health and chemical dependency conditions as well as other health care conditions, rather than wait until a later phase of the planning process. Because of the enormous volume of work, the MHCD Committee ended up with this responsibility. The committee proceeded, in parallel with the Health Outcomes Committee, to review the data gathered on MHCD conditions and to evaluate the computerized mathematical analysis of that data. The committee solicited help from the various groups of mental health professionals who expressed interest in providing data. Participants represented all aspects of mental health practice: child, adult, and geriatric populations; public and private sectors; academic, administrative, and clinical practice arenas; and clinicians from the chemical dependency field.

Data were obtained from a variety of sources: clinicians' opinions; the medical and social science literature; and administrative data from hospitals, indemnity insurers, and HMOs. Clinicians were concerned that administrative data might be biased because they were derived primarily from health plans with limited mental health benefits (i.e., the state mandates). Consequently, a group of clinicians began to develop treatment guidelines for each condition that might be added to the prioritized list (McFarland *et al.* 1993). Although not specifying the exact nature of treatment, these guidelines suggest the optimal amount of service provided to the 'average' patient diagnosed with a mental health or chemical dependency condition, including estimated hours of outpatient visits and days of hospitalization that can be expected for a population of persons seeking MHCD treatment (George *et al.* 1994). The guidelines were combined with epidemiological data to help compute capitated payment rates to organizations enrolling Oregon Health Plan beneficiaries (McFarland *et al.* 1993).

While the MHCD data were being gathered, the MHCD Committee reviewed the literature on mental health care outcomes, mental health delivery systems, and the recommendations regarding the inclusion of mental health services in a national health plan (American Psychiatric Association 1989; Robins and Regier 1991; Upton 1983). This process included review of past and current mental health systems in the state and the planning efforts of the state mental health authority (Lippincott 1989).

The mental health providers' data were reviewed by the MHCD Committee. After minor revisions, the data were entered into the computer in order to calculate the QWB benefit-to-cost ratios. The computer-generated values for all condition–treatment pairs conceivably could be compared and incorporated into one prioritized list.

Prioritization Problems and Solutions

A major complication in the use of outcome and cost data led to severe criticism of the validity of the QWB methodology: Many (nonmental health) provider organizations declined to generate the outcomes and costs of minimal or no treatment (McFarland *et al.* 1993). There were also difficulties in defining the relevant costs and time periods (McFarland *et al.* 1993).

The MHCD data fortunately included fairly complete and reasonably well-defined cost estimates. These data were used to create three kinds of computer-generated lists: (1) those based on outcomes for optimal treatments only; (2) those based on ratios of outcomes for optimal treatments divided by the costs of the treatments; and (3) those based on 'net' outcomes (i.e., outcomes of optimal treatment minus outcomes from no treatment) divided by the 'net' costs (i.e., costs of optimal treatment minus costs of no treatment). The first and second methods led to implausible rankings in which disorders of mild severity (e.g., phobias) were accorded high priority. The third (net outcomes divided by net costs) approach approximated the intent of the methodology's designers (Kaplan and Anderson 1988) and yielded a ranking that appeared to have face validity.

Because the outcome and cost data for the nonmental health conditions were seriously incomplete, the MHCD Committee was able to demonstrate the invalidity of the proposed methodology. Indeed, when the first computer-generated list of all conditions was released in May 1990, this methodological flaw became apparent (Fox and Leichter 1991). The MHCD data experiment and associated testimony contributed to an HSC decision to revise its methodology.

An Alternative Methodology Committee was created to explore other approaches to prioritization, with or without use of the computerized data. Two members of the MHCD Committee became active participants on this new committee, which eventually adopted a categorization-of-services approach (Pollack *et al.* 1993). It created a list of categories of care (Appendix 2) that encompassed all current conditions and treatments. Approximately half of these categories represented special preventive or clinical services for circumstances not associated with actual treatment of pathological conditions. These items included categories like preventive health and dental care for adults and children, maternity care, infertility services, and reproductive services.

The remaining categories contained the pathological conditions and were defined in relation to the various combinations of answers to three questions:

1   Is the condition acute or chronic?

2   Is the condition one that carries a significant risk of death and for which treatment restores or extends the individual's life?

3   Is the condition one whose treatment restores the individual to a level of function at or close to the premorbid level?

The convention for describing these categories is exemplified in phrases like 'acute fatal – treatment prevents death with full recovery' or 'chronic fatal – treatment improves life span and quality of life.'

The Alternative Methodology Committee found this approach to defining the categories particularly appealing because it potentially allowed the use of revised cost and outcomes data for sorting the various condition–treatment pairs into a category. Definitions of the variables represented by the three questions were linked to specific mathematical values found in the data provided for the QWB approach. The condition–treatment pairs were sorted by the computer into categories. After review, the discrepant items were manually sorted into what was consensually agreed to be the proper category.

The HSC then ranked the overall categories to create the general shape of the entire prioritized list. In doing so, they considered the value of each

category to society, to the individual who might need the service, and as a component of a basic health care package. The commissioners' responses proved to be internally consistent. Each category was sorted according to computer-generated data on benefits of treatment. The entire list was carefully reviewed, and the commissioners made many adjustments, using clinical judgments about specific line items and their importance relative to other lines. This new version was completed in the early spring of 1991.

The MHCD Committee used an identical methodology to sort and rank the MHCD conditions. The ultimate mental health list was reviewed and generally accepted as plausible and valid (Appendix 3). The MHCD Committee then inserted the mental health items into the overall list. The insertion process resembled the one used by the HSC in making final adjustments to the nonintegrated list. Namely, the MHCD items were compared with the nonpsychiatric conditions in the same section of the list (Appendix 4). In doing so, the severity of the condition and the importance attached to its treatment in the context of community-identified values were carefully considered. Another prioritizing principle was to place higher on the list than their sequelae disorders that, it untreated, could lead to more serious conditions. The objective was to prevent the progression of the illness.

The commission's decision to use the ranked categorization as the primary sorting method had a significant impact on the relative ranking of the mental health items in the list. Most of the major mental health conditions were in the highest categories of care (primarily categories 1, 3, and 5). In other words, the MHCD conditions, if they were to be integrated would more likely be included in the upper (i.e., funded) portion of the list.

Having developed a plausible integrated list that appeared to achieve parity for mental health, the MHCD Committee referred the list to the HSC for approval. The committee also recommended incorporating specific preventive mental health services into the Oregon Health Plan (Oregon Health Services Commission 1991b, appendix J). This document expands previous attempts (U.S. Preventive Services Taskforce 1989) to identify age-related health history, screening, and immunization interventions so that primary care providers can identify certain preventable health care problems. It includes similar interventions specifically related to MHCD conditions, and it identifies certain target populations that might be at greater risk for these conditions. Other recommendations addressed concerns about potential legislative inconsistencies, the need for MHCD representation on the HSC itself, and the need to develop a coherent and interconnected health care delivery system. The HSC endorsed and accepted the integrated list and all the recommendations except the proposal for integrating the delivery system; its members felt this concern was beyond the scope of the commission's mandate.

Return to the Legislature

The commission presented its recommendations, including the prioritized list, to the 1991 session of the state legislature and to the governor. The recommendations included a proposal that a substantial and irreducible majority of the list – all the items in the first 13 categories – be contained in the state's health care package. These categories were identified as essential (categories 1–9) or very important (categories 10–13). The last four categories were labeled 'valuable to certain individuals but significantly less likely to be cost-effective or to produce substantial long-term gain.'

The 1991 state legislature accepted the recommendations and agreed to provide additional funding beyond the amount originally allocated. Thus the state Medicaid budget was to be increased to a level that would accommodate the inclusion of 587 of the 709 items on the nonintegrated list. This increase would have led to the inclusion of virtually all items in the first 13 categories of care. However, approval was contingent on obtaining a Medicaid waiver from the federal government (Fox and Leichter 1991, 1993), which was denied by the Bush administration in August 1992 (Menzel 1992).

Modifications were made to the original prioritized list addressing concerns raised by the U.S. Health Care Financing Administration (McFarland *et al*. 1993). They were necessary to enable the state to obtain the federal waiver from Medicaid regulations so that the Oregon Health Plan could be accepted for funding and implementation. The prioritized list – and the order of the MHCD items – was only minimally altered. The rationale and method for these changes are discussed else where (McFarland *et al*. 1993) and had little impact on the resulting list.

Oregon was granted the Medicaid waiver by the Clinton administration in March 1993. The 1993 state legislature then began a lengthy and tumultuous debate about financing the plan. In essence, the desire to provide increased access to health care conflicted with the state's budget shortfall. Employers also became concerned about the financial implications of providing health insurance for the working poor. Integration of mental health and chemical dependency services was an additional challenge.

After considerable acrimonious discussion (accompanied by intense lobbying from numerous advocacy groups, including the mental health and chemical dependency coalition), the legislature ended the longest session in Oregon's history by agreeing to fund the Medicaid portion of the plan. Sufficient state funds (augmented by a new tax on cigarettes) were appropriated to cover conditions through line 616 (see Appendix 2), thereby covering most mental disorders and chemical dependency. The aspects of the plan dealing with the uninsured working population and employer mandates were deferred until July 1997 (for larger employers) and January 1998 (for employers with 25 or fewer employees).

Implementation

The Medicaid component of the Oregon Health Plan began to be implemented on February 1, 1994, in several steps. First, the state Medicaid agency solicited proposals from managed care entities (chiefly HMOs) and received a greater response than expected. Some 20 programs (of which 16 are fully capitated HMOs providing both inpatient and outpatient services on a prepaid basis) agreed to serve Medicaid clients. Consequently, the vast majority of the state's Medicaid beneficiaries will be enrolled in HMOs. Clients in rural areas will be served by four 'physician care organizations' (which are prepaid for outpatient but not inpatient services). Clients in extremely isolated areas will remain in the FFS program.

The second aspect of implementation is an outreach program to inform newly eligible Oregonians about the health plan. A private organization has contracted with the state Medicaid agency to conduct public meetings around the state and to publicize the health plan in a variety of other ways. The contractor also handles enrollment of newly eligible persons. Existing Medicaid clients must choose a health plan (typically an HMO). There is considerable competition among the health plans to enroll Medicaid clients. Potentially eligible Oregonians have also shown substantial interest in the plan. During the first week of February 1994, the outreach program's telephone lines were jammed by over 18,000 inquiries about enrollment. State officials estimate that during 1994 the Medicaid program will grow from its current size of 250,000 to some 370,000 clients.

During 1994, mental health and chemical dependency services will remain 'carved out' of the Oregon Health Plan. These services are delivered by local community mental health agencies (either components of county governments or private nonprofit organizations) on an FFS basis. However, beginning in January 1995, the health plans participating in the Medicaid program must offer outpatient chemical dependency services on a prepaid basis. Residential chemical dependency services are not covered by the state Medicaid program per se. However, the state alcohol and drug agency is exploring ways to include them in the capitated program. Interestingly, the legislation initiating the Oregon Health Plan requires the state to test the hypothesis that integrating physical health and chemical dependency services will result in an 'offset' effect that ultimately reduces medical and surgical costs.

The state legislature also mandated phased integration of mental health services into the Oregon Health Plan. Starting January 1, 1995, up to 25 percent of Medicaid clients will be eligible for a special program designed to test the impact of full integration on utilization of physical health services. The 25 percent of selected Medicaid clients must be representative of both urban and rural parts of the state. The state Medicaid and mental health agencies have established a network of committees involving consumers, family members, and providers, who will assist in defining the implementation process.

The state mental health authority has stated that its ultimate goal is the development of a fully integrated system in which Medicaid clients choose to enroll in a single, prepaid managed care entity that is responsible for delivering physical and mental health as well as chemical dependency services. Health plans may use different models in moving toward that goal. Some organizations may elect to provide all services in house. More likely, however, health plans will subcontract for a variety of services delivered by a range of provider organizations. Conversely, provider organizations (such as community mental health centers) may subcontract with several health plans. The goal is to provide enrollees with a seamless system that can address physical, mental, and chemical dependency needs while recognizing that resources are not unlimited.

Quality assurance will obviously be a concern in a program operating almost entirely by means of prepaid care systems. One approach to assure quality is to make use of the treatment guidelines (George *et al*. 1994). Although the guidelines do not dictate provision of specific types of mental health treatment, they do offer estimates for hours of outpatient treatments, days in hospital, and other services that would be expected in a population of persons using MHCD services for a given condition. This approach provides a framework for regulatory authorities to monitor quality assurance using administrative data.

Financing the MHCD component of the Oregon Health Plan is also of considerable interest (McFarland *et al*. 1993). Capitation payment rates have been calculated for the different categories of Medicaid clients (e.g., persons receiving Aid to Families with Dependent Children [AFDC] and individuals receiving SSI). There are 14 different categories of eligible persons. The rates were determined by several actuarial methods using private insurance data, Medicaid data, and the state mental health information system (McFarland *et al*. 1993). As noted, the treatment guidelines were married with population prevalence estimates to compute a priori estimates of the costs to provide MHCD services to this population (McFarland *et al*. 1993). The payment rates per person per month for MHCD services range from about $10 for the AFDC group to $300 for some classes of disabled persons. The MHCD costs per person per month are about $35 (Oregon Health Services Commission 1993). The MHCD costs range from about 10 percent of the total (physical, dental, and MHCD) for some enrollee categories to nearly 40 percent for others. For the entire population it is estimated that MHCD will comprise 20 percent of the costs. The higher figures apply chiefly to enrollees with chronic mental disorders like schizophrenia. It is estimated that the majority of the state's chronically mentally ill population will become Medicaid clients in 1995, whereas only about half are now currently enrolled in Medicaid. Consequently, stop loss insurance will be available for purchase from the state by participating health plans.

These plans are expected to deliver (or arrange to deliver) a full range of MHCD services in exchange for these capitation rates. Enrollees are guaranteed diagnosis, triage, and medically necessary treatment. Services to be delivered include assessment, case management, consultation, individual and group treatment, medications, medication management, rehabilitative services (e.g., day treatment), residential mental health treatment for children or adolescents, and acute hospital care (Oregon Health Services Commission 1993). Arrangements for persons who may need long-term (i.e., more than 30 days) inpatient care (or its equivalent) are presently under discussion, as are services for civilly committed persons. The health plans are not responsible for serving either incarcerated enrollees or beneficiaries found guilty except for insanity. Publicly funded residential alcohol and drug services are also not included but may be eventually folded into the program. Despite these uncertainties, health plans and community mental health agencies have shown considerable interest in participating.

The Committee's Values and Strategies

What values and decision processes guided the MHCD Committee? How did these values influence the committee's list and its recommendations for integrating MHCD conditions into the overall health plan?

The committee's primary goal was to achieve equitable coverage for mental health services. The committee read numerous eloquent descriptions of the traditional lack of parity accorded mental health in benefit packages, reimbursement rates, and research (Frank and McGuire 1990; Havel 1992; Judd 1990; Malloy 1991; Sharfstein and Stoline 1992; Sharfstein, Stoline, and Goldman 1993). Notable causes of this inequity include the following:

1. historical prejudices

2. the false mind/body dichotomy

3. lack of visible and viable advocacy for the mentally ill

4. confusion about the definition of mental illness

5. the belief that mental health treatments are not effective

6. the fear or belief that mental health services are too expensive

Attempts to achieve parity in the United States and elsewhere have generally failed, partly because they have not established the comparability of MHCD conditions with other health problems (Cutler, Bigelow, and McFarland 1992; Rochefort 1992). Some attempts to achieve parity have overcompromised and perpetuated the inequity by essentially excluding 'nonbiologic' mental health conditions from coverage (Domenici 1992). Under this strategy, legislation and litigation would mandate that persons with specific mental health conditions, such as schizophrenia and major mood disorders, be given insurance coverage equivalent to that for other major medical conditions.

This partial approach, although it may succeed, will not achieve parity, but will merely shift a few psychiatric conditions from 'mind' to 'body.' Such an approach may further the notion of the mind–body split and could prevent appropriate coverage of other mental health conditions.

Insurance mandates have obtained some MHCD benefits but usually with less than generous levels of coverage (including, for example, caps on numbers of outpatient visits, hospital days, or total dollars allowed for MHCD services). Mandates generally provide a uniform limit on services without regard to severity of the condition or the effectiveness of treatment (Frank and McGuire 1990; *Health Benefits Letter* 1992; Sharfstein and Stoline 1992; Sharfstein, Stoline, and Goldman 1993).

Although international comparisons fall outside the scope of this article, it is nevertheless germane to mention that mental health services are included in the health care systems of most industrialized nations (Cutler, Bigelow, and McFarland 1992). However, the lack of parity has been noted in other countries as well (Rochefort 1992). Where MHCD services are provided, either coverage is inadequate or indiscriminate coverage (irrespective of severity or effectiveness) leads to shortages or delays in treatment.

The inability or unwillingness to determine medical necessity, that is, conditions needing treatment and treatments for them, has hamstrung attempts to achieve parity (Glazer 1992). This problem does not apply exclusively to the area of MHCD services, but rather to all of health care. However, the beliefs that MHCD conditions are not as serious as 'physical' conditions, that their causes are nonbiological, 'illegitimate,' or 'undeserving,' or that treatments for them are ineffective undermine the argument for including MHCD conditions in an integrated health care delivery system.

The committee's strategy was to obtain parity and protect current levels of coverage by preventing erosion of MHCD benefits. Because the result of the prioritization process was initially uncertain, the committee pursued the optimal outcome and avoided harmful compromises.

The means for accomplishing these goals are listed here roughly in the order of their adoption:

1. Insist that integration is achievable while reducing or eliminating barriers to it.

2. Educate the commission members and staff, as well as the legislators and general public, on the following topics:

   a. The legitimacy of MHCD conditions.

   b. The significance of MHCD conditions as demonstrated by personal suffering (including but not limited to morbidity and mortality statistics), health care costs, loss of productivity, and other indirect costs.

   c. The pervasiveness, prevalence, and variability of MHCD conditions.

   d. The inseparability of mind and body.

3. Adhere to the accepted prioritization methodology used with medical–surgical conditions whenever possible.

4. Identify ways to modify the commission's methodology to assure equitable treatment for all health care conditions, including MHCD.

In articulating his strong support for the concept of rationing care, Callahan (1987, 1990) has described several values and criteria for constructing a rationing system. Some of the principles he presents, listed below, are similar to those employed by the Oregon participants:

1. Valuing the provision of 'caring' when the pursuit of 'cure' seems counterproductive, insensitive, or futile.

2. Balancing value to the community against value to the individual.

3. Balancing the life-saving or life-extending benefits of a treatment against its ability to enable the person to recover a sufficient level of functioning.

The prioritization process clearly placed a higher value on treatment that would relieve suffering and offer supportive care and a lower one on the pursuit of costly and questionable attempts to reverse or curtail untreatable disease. In this way it resembled Callahan's approach.

Prioritization and Its Discontents

Like any innovation, the Oregon Health Plan has drawn criticism. Some say that it 'experiments on poor women and children' and contend that a radical restructuring of the health care system should not be tried first on a potentially vulnerable population (Rosenbaum 1992). Some have suggested (only half in jest) that legislators should try the experiment on themselves (or perhaps all state employees) before changing Medicaid. Nevertheless, the Oregon Health Plan will result in increased health care services to the poor. The list of covered conditions is a generous definition of 'basic health care.' The early fears about rationing have not (to date) been reflected in the actual list of condition–treatment pairs.

Another objection is that the prioritization process is unscientific because cost and outcome data are still incomplete (and are imperfectly defined) for many medical conditions and treatments (LaPuma and Lawlor 1990; Steinbrook and Lo 1992). At the same time, there is a sense of urgency that permeates the entire health care reform issue. Scientific progress is usually assumed to begin with testing an idea or theory and then refining it until a meaningful and acceptable result is achieved. Policy change, like scientific progress, has not always required an idea to be perfect before it can be implemented. We believe that Oregon is justified in proceeding with its health plan (despite its incompleteness and imperfections) because it will improve only with use and experience. Moreover, many acknowledge that the proposed plan is superior to the current system of care. Were the situation reversed, such that the Oregon Health Plan represented the status quo, a proposal to switch to the previous system would not be seriously considered (Eddy 1991).

A parenthetical note is that criticism of the 1991 Oregon Health Plan and the resulting delay in federal approval of the Medicaid waiver denied perhaps 100,000 people access to health insurance for at least two years. Data from Franks, Clancy, and Gold (1993) on the relationship between lack of health insurance and mortality imply that this delay may have caused an excess mortality equal to 250 deaths.

Some have suggested that the debate about prioritization is irrelevant, giving as an example that there are hospitals in Oregon operating at less than optimal efficiency (Fisher, Welch, and Wennberg 1992; Schramm 1992; Wennberg 1990). Resources could be saved by making them as efficient as others in the state. Although these concerns are justified, they are not relevant in the long run. Shifting from FFS to prepaid health care may address many concerns about hospital efficiency and some about administrative efficiency.

In the longer run, moreover, prioritization is inevitable. Advances in health care technology are generally beneficial but rarely curative. Dialysis is the classic example of a health care service that is worthwhile, even life saving, yet does not reduce but rather increases costs (Fuchs 1993). Conceivably, clozapine and assertive case management for persons with schizophrenia might show a similar pattern: worthwhile but not leading to savings. In this situation, prioritizing occurs either covertly or overtly. The beauty of the Oregon Health Plan is that mental health and chemical dependency have been explicitly included in the process.

Planners and policy makers have also debated the advisability of incremental versus fundamental change. Will the former be followed by enough further change to accomplish meaningful outcomes? Will the latter gain the political and cultural acceptability needed to achieve it? The Oregon Health Plan combines elements of a fundamental shift in organizing, financing, and delivering services and is an initial step toward further changes and improvements, especially the development of a health plan that would apply uniformly to all (Ellwood, Enthoven, and Etheridge 1992; Starr 1992; Starr and Zelman 1993).

To choose a metaphor from the context of medicine, it is absurd to think of achieving a 'cure' for many serious and persistent health care problems; instead, caring treatment that alleviates suffering is appropriate when it is not possible to eliminate the primary cause of the illness. This concept applies on a larger scale to political decisions, which include the process of setting priorities. It may even be irresponsible to wait for a solution that is scientifically 'correct' rather than developing one that is scientifically 'informed.' Rudolf Virchow's observation that 'politics is merely the practice of medicine writ large' can be interpreted as saying that the policy maker is society's 'care provider,' and it may also be read as implying that the society, or 'patient,' may require timely, educated interventions that are not either fully developed or absolutely proven to be effective (Shoemaker *et al.* 1993).

The prioritization methodology itself may have applications and value beyond the Oregon Health Plan, for example, as part of a comprehensive managed care delivery system (Ellwood, Enthoven, and Etheridge 1992; Starr and Zelman 1993). This approach to defining medical necessity and a basic health care package could as easily be applied to a single payer national health insurance program. Indeed, representatives from the health ministries of Australia, Canada, Denmark, England, Germany, Greece, Japan, the Netherlands, and New Zealand have visited Oregon to study this methodology. Similarly, a single payer national health insurance bill that incorporates a prioritization policy has been introduced in the U.S. Senate using virtually the same language as the Oregon legislation (U.S. Congress 1992).

Implications of Integration

The process of integrating mental health items into the overall list reverberates far beyond the Oregon Health Plan. The mental health list appears to satisfy several concerns of the mental health community regarding the need for adequate coverage (Little Rock Working Group 1993; Mental Health Liaison Group 1993). Integrating these items with other health conditions underlines the inseparability of mind and body, and, by extension, clarifies the utility of a comprehensive delivery system that includes mental health services.

The list integrates mental health conditions irrespective of their etiologies (organic, psychological, and social). Conditions and their treatments are ranked according to their severity as experienced by patients, whereas the benefit is measured by outcome and cost. The list reflects a high priority for biological conditions such as schizophrenia and major mood disorders.

The ranking gives preference to conditions that have a greater impact on children. The list also prioritizes conditions, like posttraumatic stress disorder and eating disorders, that, despite the presumption of their presumably psychological or environmental roots, cause widespread suffering and loss of function (American Psychiatric Association 1987, 1993). This method is superior and more inclusive than that of attempting to achieve parity for the biologically based psychiatric disorders. Even if the Oregon Health Plan is not implemented, the experience demonstrates that effective parity for mental health can be achieved.

Beyond the critical issue of parity, other significant considerations in designing an integrated health care system can be listed;

1   Integrating MHCD into a basic health care package may eliminate or reduce the possibility that MHCD items could be carved out or subsequently treated in a discriminatory fashion.

2   The blending of MHCD and other conditions may clarify the value of preventive services. A major, but relatively unheralded, accomplishment of the MHCD Committee was the development of prevention guidelines for the early identification of MHCD conditions by primary care providers (U.S. Preventive Services Taskforce 1989; Oregon Health Services Commission 1991b, appendix J). These guidelines include recommendations for persons who may be at risk of developing MHCD problems (e.g., children whose parents themselves have MHCD conditions) and suggest screening procedures. The capitated payment rates for health plans include amounts earmarked for MHCD preventive services.

3   Integration of MHCD conditions implies development of an integrated treatment system with these considerations:

   a.   It is essential to include services for long-term care. If the delivery system is predicated on capitation, it must integrate the whole continuum of services, from hospital to community, so that patients can be served in the least restrictive setting and the state mental hospital will not become the dumping ground for persons who are deemed outliers or beyond the scope of treatment (Mechanic and Rochefort 1992; Mechanic 1993).

   b.   If MHCD is to be effectively integrated, people should receive comprehensive diagnostic evaluations that consider MHCD symptoms, risk factors, and conditions, as well as other health conditions, irrespective of the locus of service (e.g., health clinic, mental health clinic, school, or correctional facility). Access to consultants in other disciplines is essential for primary care providers to understand and treat or to refer persons with MHCD conditions, and, conversely, for MHCD providers to obtain appropriate primary and other specialty care for their patients (Pincus 1987).

   c.   The concept of integration may extend to blending the public and private sectors. The traditional two- or three-tiered system of care may give way to one that provides care to individuals irrespective of their socioeconomic status and that tends less often to categorize mistakenly patients' problems as being either the 'mind' or the 'body.' Models of care delivery may encourage private providers to serve groups of patients, such as the chronically mentally ill, who have not been effectively served or who have been denied treatment in the past. Similarly, public providers may be able to serve a broader array of patients. Collaborative efforts between public and private provider organizations may develop, such that the combined expertise may provide a seamless set of resources for a group of subscribers to a prepaid care system (Mechanic and Rochefort 1992; Mechanic 1993).

Role of the Mental Health Community in Health Care Reform

For the past few decades, psychiatry has been treated as a second-class citizen in the community of medical disciplines and specialties (Judd 1990). This experience of discrimination has led the profession at times to adopt an apologetic tone or to push for corrective action in a tentative or fearful manner.

In recent years, the crisis in health care, especially the dramatic increases in costs, has caused the mental health professions to feel that they are at risk of further isolation or marginalization in the health care system (Mental Health Policy Resource Center 1992). Now is the time for the mental health community assertively to establish a clear and equitable position for mental health services. Some national health care legislation is likely to be passed in the next few years. If parity for mental health is not obtained soon, it will signal a major lost opportunity, both for now and for the future (Judd 1990; Koyanagi *et al.* 1993; Little Rock Working Group 1993; Mental Health Liaison Group 1993; Mental Health Policy Resource Center 1992).

The experiences of the MHCD Committee and other mental health providers who participated in the Oregon Health Plan demonstrate two important points about mental health and health care reform. First, this process is a model for achieving true parity without tilting toward conditions that are legitimized by their 'biological' foundation. Second, mental health providers can and should be active participants in health care reform. Psychiatry can provide more insight and depth through its biopsychosocial perspective. Psychiatric understanding of group process can aid the complex decision making that goes into creating major change in the health care delivery system.

The debate in Oregon's legislature foreshadows national discussion on health care reform and the integration of mental health services into a larger system of care (Mechanic 1993). Especially troubling to legislators were the costs of increased access, the untested approaches for implementing the integration of services, and the financial implications of caring for severely mentally ill persons who previously had limited access to services. Interestingly, the state legislation (and the federal Medicaid waiver) requires a detailed evaluation of this new approach to universal health care. Particularly intriguing is the 'natural experiment' afforded by the planned phasing in of mental health services. Perhaps research may add weight to the moral argument that we must end discrimination against persons affected by mental illness.

Conclusion

We have presented a description of the process by which mental health services were included in the basic health care package for a controversial state health reform plan. The methods, values, and strategies for achieving mental health parity have been detailed and discussed. The implications for integration of mental health are far reaching and may apply to other, very different, health care systems. An increased, more respected, role for mental health professionals in the health reform process has been advocated. The opportunity to achieve parity for mental health must not be delayed or compromised, because to do so would worsen the lives of persons already affected by the trauma and stigma associated with mental illness.

References

American Psychiatric Association. 1987. *Diagnostic and Statistical Manual of Mental Disorders*, rev. 3d. ed., Washington: American Psychiatric Press.

——. 1989. *Treatments of Psychiatric Disorders*. Washington: American Psychiatric Association.

——. 1993: Practice Guideline for Eating Disorders. *American Journal of Psychiatry* 150:212–28.

Astrachan, B.M., D.J. Levinson, and D.A. Adler. 1976. The Impact of National Health Insurance on the Tasks and Practice of Psychiatry. *Archives of General Psychiatry* 33:785–94.

Bevilacqua, J.J. 1991. Overview of State Mental Health Policy. In *Dimensions of State Mental Health Policy*, eds. C.G. Hudson and A.J. Cox. New York: Praeger.

Bigelow, D.A., and B.H. McFarland. 1994. Financing Canada's Mental Health System. In *Mental Health in Canada, New Directions for Mental Health Services*, eds. L. Bachrach, D. Wasylenki, and P. Goering. San Francisco: Jossey-Bass.

Blendon, R.J., and K. Donolan. 1990. The Public and the Emerging Debate over National Health Insurance. *New England Journal of Medicine* 323:200–12.

Bonstedt, T. 1992. Managing Psychiatric Exclusions. In *Managed Mental Health Care*, eds. J.L. Feldman and R.J. Fitzpatrick. Washington: American Psychiatric Press.

Brown, L.D. 1991. The National Politics of Oregon's Rationing Plan. *Health Affairs* 10:28–51.

Callahan, D. 1987. *Setting Limits: Medical Goals in an Aging Society*. New York: Simon and Schuster.

——. 1990. *What Kind of Life: The Limits of Medical Progress*, New York: Simon and Schuster.

——. 1991. Ethics and Priority Setting in Oregon. *Health Affairs* 10:78–87.

Clowe, J.L., R. Scalettar, and J.S. Todd. 1993. A New Partnership for Change. *Journal of the American Medical Association* 269:1164–5.

Cutler, D.L., D. Bigelow, and B. McFarland. 1992. The Cost of Fragmented Mental Health Financing: Is It Worth It? *Community Mental Health Journal* 28:121–35.

Domenici, P.V. 1992. Federal Perspective. *Focus on Mental Health Services Research* 5:1.

Eddy, D.M. 1991. Oregon's Plan: Should It Be Approved? *Journal of the American Medical Association* 266:2439–45.

Ellwood, P., A.C. Enthoven, and L. Etheridge. 1992. The Jackson Hole Initiatives for a Twenty-first Century American Health Care System. *Health Economics* 1:149–68.

Fein, R. 1992. Health Care Reform. *Scientific American* 167:46–53.

Fisher, E.S., G. Welch, and J.E. Wennberg. 1992. Prioritizing Oregon's Hospital Resources: An Example Based on Variations in Discretionary Medical Utilization. *Journal of the American Medical Association* 267:1925–31.

Fox, D.M., and H.M. Leichter. 1991. Rationing Care in Oregon: The New Accountability. *Health Affairs* 10:7–27.

——. 1993. The Ups and Downs of Oregon's Rationing Plan. *Health Affairs* 12:66–70.

Frank, R.G., and T.G. McGuire. 1990. Mandating Employer Coverage of Mental Health Care. *Health Affairs* 9:31–42.

Franks, P., C.M. Clancy, and M.R. Gold. 1993. Health Insurance and Mortality: Evidence from a National Cohort. *Journal of the American Medical Association* 270:737–41.

Fuchs, V.R. 1993. Dear President Clinton. *Journal of the American Medical Association* 269:1678–9.

General Accounting Office. 1991. U.S. Health Care Spending: Trends, Contributing Factors, and Proposals for Reform. GAO/HRD-91-102. Washington.

George, R.A., B.H. McFarland, D.A. Pollack, and R.H. Angell 1994. Treatment Guidelines and Standards of Care for Mental Health in the Oregon Health Plan, 7th ed. Portland, Ore.: Department of Psychiatry, St. Vincent Hospital and Medical Center.

Glazer, W. 1992. Psychiatry and Medical Necessity. *Psychiatric Annals* 22:362–66.

Goodwin, F.K. 1993. Health Care Reform for Americans with Severe Mental Illnesses: Report of the National Advisory Mental Health Council. *American Journal of Psychiatry* 150:1447–65.

Hasnain, R., and M. Garland. 1990a. Health Care in Common: Setting Priorities in Oregon. *Hastings Center Report* 20:16–18.

——. 1990b. Health Care in Common: Report of the Oregon Health Decisions Community Meetings Process. Portland, Ore.: Oregon Health Decisions.

Havel, J. 1992. Healthcare Financing Reform: What's in It for Mental Health? *Policy in Perspective* (March/April):4–5.

Health Benefits Letter 1992. State Benefit Mandates for Alcohol, Drug Abuse, and Mental Illness (through 1991) (Sept. 4, pp. 2–7). Alexandria, Va.: Scandlen Publishing.

Himmelstein, D., and S. Woolhandler. 1989. A National Health Program for the U.S.: A Physicians' Proposal. *New England Journal of Medicine* 320:120–8.

Judd, L. 1990. Putting Mental Health on the Nation's Health Agenda. *Hospital and Community Psychiatry* 41:131–4.

Kaplan, R.M. 1992. A Quality of Life Approach to Health Resource Allocation. In *Rationing America's Medical Care: The Oregon Plan and Beyond*, eds. M. Strosberg, J. Weiner, and R. Baker. Washington: Brookings Institution.

Kaplan, R.M., and J.P. Anderson. 1988. A General Health Policy Model: Updates and Applications. *Health Services Research* 23:20–35.

Kaplan, R.M., M. Debon, and B.F. Anderson. 1991. Effects of Number of Rating Scale Points upon Utilities in a Quality of Well-Being Scale. *Medical Care* 29:1061–4.

Koyanagi, C., J. Manes, R. Surle, and H.H. Goldman. 1993. On Being Very Smart: The Mental Health Community's Response in the Health Care Reform Debate. *Hospital and Community Psychiatry* 44:537–44.

Lamb, H.R., S.R. Goldfinger, D. Greenfield, *et al.* 1993. Ensuring Services for Persons with Chronic Mental Illness under National Health Care Reform. *Hospital and Community Psychiatry* 44:545–6.

LaPuma, J., and E.F. Lawlor. 1990. Quality-adjusted Life-Years: Ethical Implications for Physicians and Policymakers. *Journal of the American Medical Association* 263:2917–21.

Lippincott, R.C. 1989. *Developing Comprehensive Mental Health Services in Oregon 1989–1995*. Salem, Ore.: Oregon Mental Health and Developmental Disability Services Division.

Little Rock Working Group. 1993. *Recommendations of the Little Rock Working Group on Mental Health and Substance Abuse Disorders in Health Care Reform*. Little Rock, Ark.: Centers for Mental Healthcare Research, University of Arkansas.

Malloy, K.A. 1991. *Analysis: Beyond Moral Hazard in Financing Outpatient Mental Health Services*. Washington: Mental Health Policy Resource Center.

Marshall, P.E. 1992. The Case for a National Mental Health Policy. *Hospital and Community Psychiatry* 43:1065.

McFarland, B.H., R.A. George, D.A. Pollack, and R.H. Angell. 1993. Mental Health in the Oregon Health Plan: A Model for Managed Care. In *Managed Mental Health Care*, eds. W. Goldman and S. Feldman. San Francisco: Jossey-Bass.

Mechanic, D. 1993. Mental Health Services in the Context of Health Insurance Reform. *Milbank Quarterly* 71:349–64.

Mechanic, D., and D.A. Rochefort. 1992. A Policy of Inclusion for the Mentally Ill. *Health Affairs* 11:128–50.

Mental Health Liaison Group. 1993. *Transition Briefing on Mental Health*. Washington: Mental Health Policy Research Center.

Mental Health Policy Resource Center. 1992. *Into the Briarpatch: Mental Health in State and National Healthcare Reform*. Washington.

Menzel, P.T. 1992. Oregon's Denial: Disabilities and Quality of Life. *Hastings Center Report* 22:21–5.

Michels, R., and P.M. Marzuk. 1993a. Progress in Psychiatry. Part 1 (of 2). *New England Journal of Medicine* 329:552–60.

——. 1993b. Progress in Psychiatry. Part 2 (of 2). *New England Journal of Medicine* 329:628–38.

Oregon Health Services Commission. 1991a. *Prioritization of Health Services: A Report to the Governor and Legislature*. Salem, Ore.

——. 1991b. Expanded Definition of Preventive Services. *Prioritization of Health Services: A Report to the Governor and Legislature*. Salem, Ore.

——. 1993. *Prioritization of Health Services: A Report to the Governor and Legislature*. Portland, Ore.

Pearson, J. 1992. Managed Mental Health Care: The Buyer's Perspective. In Managed Mental Health Services, ed. S. Feldman. Springfield, Ill.: Charles C. Thomas.

Peterson, M.S., J.B. Christianson, and D. Wholey. 1992. National Survey of Mental Health, Alcohol, and Drug Abuse Treatment in HMOs: 1989 Chartbook. Excelsior: Minn. InterStudy Center for Managed Care Research.

Pincus, H.A. 1987. Patient-Oriented Models for Linking Primary Care and Mental Health Care. *General Hospital Psychiatry* 9:95–101.

Pollack, D.A., B.H. McFarland, R.A. George, and R.H. Angell. 1993. Ethics and Value Strategies Used in Prioritizing Mental Health Services in Oregon. *Healthcare Ethics Committee Forum* 5:322–39.

Robins, L.N., and D.A. Regier. 1991. *Psychiatric Disorders in America: The Epidemiologic Catchment Area Study*. New York: Free Press.

Rochefort, D. 1992. More Lessons of a Different Kind: Canadian Mental Health Policy in Perspective. *Hospital and Community Psychiatry* 43:1083–90.

Rosenbaum, S. 1992. Poor Women, Poor Children, Poor Policy: The Oregon Medicaid Experiment. In *Rationing America's Medical Care: The Oregon Plan and Beyond*, eds. M.A. Strosberg, J.M. Wiener, and R. Baker. Washington: Brooking Institution.

Schramm, C.J. 1992. Oregon: A Better Method to Reallocate Resources. *Journal of the American Medical Association* 267:1967.

Sharfstein, S.S., and A.M. Stoline. 1992. Reform Issues for Insuring Mental Health Care. *Health Affairs* 11:84–97.

Sharfstein, S.S., A.M. Stoline, and H.H. Goldman. 1993. Psychiatric Care and Health Insurance Reform. *American Journal of Psychiatry* 150:7–18.

Shoemaker, W.C., C.B. James, L.M. King, E. Hardin, and G.J. Ordog. 1993. Urban Violence in Los Angeles in the Aftermath of the Riots. *Journal of the American Medical Association* 270:2833–7.

Starr, P. 1992. *The Logic of Health-Care Reform*. Knoxville, Tenn.: Grand Rounds Press.

Starr, P., and W.A. Zelman. 1993. A Bridge to Compromise: Competition under a Budget. *Health Affairs* 12 (suppl.):7–23.

Steinbrook, R., and B. Lo. 1992. The Oregon Medicaid Demonstration Project—Will It Provide Adequate Medical Care? *New England Journal of Medicine* 326:340–4.

Strosberg, M., J. Weiner, and R. Baker. 1992. *Rationing America's Medical Care: The Oregon Plan and Beyond*. Washington: Brookings Institution.

U.S. Congress. 1992. Bill (S.2513) to provide universal access for all Americans to basic health care services and long-term care services. Introduced by Senators Daschle, Simon, and Woffard to the 102d Congress. Washington.

U.S. Preventive Services Taskforce. 1989. *Guide to Clinical Preventive Services: An Assessment of the Effectiveness of 169 Interventions*. Baltimore: Williams & Wilkins.

Upton, D. 1983. *Mental Health and National Health Insurance: A Philosophy of and an Approach to Mental Health Care for the Future*. New York: Plenum.

Wennberg, J.E. 1990. Outcomes Research, Cost Containment, and the Fear of Health Care Rationing. *New England Journal of Medicine* 323:1202–4.

Appendix 1

Major Symptoms

1. Loss of consciousness such as seizure (fits), fainting, or coma (out cold or knocked out)

2. Burn over large areas of face, body, arms, or legs

3. Pain, bleeding, itching, or discharge (drainage from sexual organs – does not include normal menstrual [monthly] bleeding)

4. Trouble learning, remembering, or thinking clearly

5. Any combination of one or more hands, feet, arms, or legs either missing, deformed (crooked), paralyzed (unable to move), or broken – includes wearing artificial limbs or braces

6. Pain, stiffness, weakness, numbness, or other discomfort in chest, stomach (including hernia or rupture), side, neck, back, hips, or any joints or hand, feet, arms, or legs

7. Pain, burning, bleeding, itching, or other difficulty with rectum, bowel movements, or urination (passing water)

8. Sick or upset stomach, vomiting or loose bowel movement, with or without fever, chills, or aching all over

9. General tiredness, weakness, or weight loss

10. Coughing, wheezing, or shortness or breath, with or without fever, chills, or aching all over

11. Spells of feeling upset, being depressed, or crying

12. Headache, or dizziness, or ringing in ears, or spells of feeling hot, or nervous, or shaky

13. Burning or itching rash on large areas of face, body, arms, or legs

14. Trouble talking, such as lisp, stuttering, hoarseness, or being unable to speak

15. Pain or discomfort in one or both eyes (such as burning or itching) or any trouble seeing after correction

16. Overweight for age and height or skin defect of face, body, arms or legs, such as scars, pimples, warts, bruises, or changes in color

17. Pain in ear, tooth, jaw, throat, lips, tongue; several missing or crooked permanent teeth – includes wearing bridges or false teeth; stuffy runny nose, or any trouble hearing – includes wearing a hearing aid

18. Taking medication or staying on a prescribed diet for health

19. Wearing eyeglasses or contact lenses

20. Has trouble falling asleep or staying asleep

21. Has trouble with sexual interest or performance

22. Is often worried

23. Has trouble with the use of drugs or alcohol

Source: Based on Kaplan, Debon, and Anderson 1991.

Appendix 2

Ranked Categorization of Services

Seventeen (17) categories of health services determined by the commission, ranked from most to least important[a]

1. *Acute fatal*: treatment prevents death with full recovery

2. *Maternity care*

3. *Acute fatal*: treatment prevents death without full recovery

4. *Preventive care for children*

5. *Chronic fatal*: treatment improves life span and quality of life

6. *Reproductive services*: (excludes maternity and infertility services)

7. *Comfort care*: palliative therapy for conditions in which death is imminent

8. *Preventive dental care*

9. *Proven effective preventive care for adults*

10. *Acute nonfatal*: treatment causes return to previous health state

11. *Chronic nonfatal*: one-time treatment improves quality of life

12. *Acute nonfatal*: treatment without return to previous health state

13. *Chronic nonfatal*: repetitive treatment improves quality of life

14. *Acute nonfatal*: treatment expedites recovery of self-limiting conditions

15. *Infertility services*

16. *Less effective preventive care for adults*

17. *Fatal or nonfatal*: treatment causes minimal or no improvement in quality of life

Examples of MHCD services by category[b]

1. Major depression, single episode; acute posttraumatic stress disorder and drug-induced delirium

3. Alcohol and drug abuse diagnoses

5. Dystymia, chronic post-traumatic stress disorder, eating disorders, bipolar disorder, recurrent major depression, and schizophrenia

[a] Most categories are either acute or chronic, fatal or nonfatal, with treatment improving either quality or length of life.
[b] Most are in categories 1, 3, and 5.
Source: Oregon Health Services Commission.

Appendix 3

Mental Health Conditions from the Oregon Health Plan's Integrated Prioritization List[a]

Line placement on integrated list		Diagnosis/condition
1.	88	Rumination disorder of infancy
2.	143	Anorexia nervosa
3.	144	Reactive attachment disorder of infancy or early childhood
4.	158	Schizophrenic disorders
5.	159	Major depression, recurrent
6.	160	Bipolar disorders
7.	181	Abuse or dependence on psychoactive substance
8.	182	Major depression; single episode or mild
9.	183	Brief reactive psychosis
10.	184	Attention deficit disorders with hyperactivity or undifferentiated
11.	237	Acute post-traumatic stress disorder
12.	238	Separation anxiety disorder
13.	260	Adjustment disorders
14.	261	Oppositional defiant disorder
15.	262	Tourette's disorder and tic disorders
16.	296	Chronic post-traumatic stress syndrome
17.	297	Obsessive-compulsive disorders
18.	330	Panic disorder with and without agoraphobia
19.	331	Agoraphobia without history of panic disorder
20.	365	Conduct disorder, mild/moderate: solitary aggressive, group type, undifferentiated
21.	366	Overanxious disorder
22.	367	Bulimia nervosa
23.	368	Anxiety disorder, unspecified; generalized anxiety disorder
24.	382	Paranoid (delusional) disorder
25.	415	Dysthymia
26.	416	Acute delusional mood anxiety, personality, perception and organic mental disorder caused by drugs; intoxication
27.	417	Borderline personality disorder
28.	418	Identity disorder
29.	419	Schizotypal personality disorders
30.	424	Conversion disorder, child
31.	425	Functional encopresis
32.	426	Avoidant disorder of childhood or adolescence; elective mutism
33.	427	Psychological factors affecting physical condition (e.g., asthma, chronic gastrointestinal conditions, hypertension)
34.	457	Eating disorder NOS
35.	458	Dissociative disorders: depersonalization disorder; multiple personality disorder; dissociative disorder NOS; psychogenic amnesia; psychogenic fugue
36.	459	Chronic organic mental disorders including dementias
37.	474	Stereotypy/habit disorder and self-abusive behavior due to neurological dysfunction
38.	518	Simple phobia
39.	519	Social phobia
40.	578	Impulse disorders
41.	579	Sexual dysfunction
42.	580	Conduct disorder, severe
43.	581	Somatization disorder; somatoform pain disorder
44.	632	Factitious disorders
45.	633	Hypochondriasis; somatoform disorder; NOS and undifferentiated

Line placement on integrated list		Diagnosis/condition
46.	634	Conversion disorder, adult
47.	650	Pica
48.	681	Personality disorders excluding borderline, schizotypal, and antisocial
49.	682	Gender identification disorder
50.	697	Transsexualism
51.	727	Antisocial personality disorder

[a] April 1993 version.
Abbreviation: NOS, not otherwise specified.
Source: Oregon Health Services Commission.

Appendix 4

MHCD and Nonpsychiatric Conditions

Examples of how certain MHCD diagnoses are ranked in relation to nonpsychiatric conditions[a]

156:	Asthma
157:	Respiratory failure
158:	*Schizophrenic disorders*
159:	*Major depression, recurrent*
160:	*Bipolar disorders*
161:	Burn full thickness greater than 10 percent of body surface
162:	Pemphigus
163:	Disorders of fluid, electrolyte, and acid-base balance
164:	Thyrotoxicosis with or without goiter, endocrine exophthalmos; chronic thyroiditis
165:	Hypertensive heart and renal disease
177:	Fracture of hip, closed
178:	Hereditary angioneurotic edema
179:	Lymphoid leukemias other than acute lymphocytic leukemia
180:	Preventive services for adults with proven effectiveness
181:	*Abuse of or dependence on psychoactive substance*
182:	*Major depression; single episode or mild,*
183:	*Brief reactive psychosis*
184:	*Attention deficit disorders with hyperactivity or undifferentiated*
185:	Hypertension and hypertensive disease
186:	Ulcers, gastritis, and duodenitis
187:	Cancer of endocrine system, treatable
188:	Cancer of testis, treatable
361:	Atherosclerosis, peripheral
362:	Congenital pulmonary valve stenosis
363:	Rheumatoid arthritis and other inflammatory polyarthropathies
364:	Rheumatoid arthritis, osteoarthritis, and aseptic necrosis of bone

Examples of how certain MHCD diagnoses are ranked in relation to nonpsychiatric conditions[a]

365:	*Conduct disorder, mild/moderate: solitary aggressive, group type, undifferentiated*
366:	*Overanxious disorder*
367:	*Bulimia nervosa*
368:	*Anxiety disorder, unspecified; generalized anxiety disorder*
369:	Esophagitis
370:	Nonsuperficial open wounds

[a] April 1993 version of the integrated prioritization list.
Source: Based on material from the Oregon Health Services Commission.

9 Research

If psychiatry is to advance its knowledge base and, correspondingly, offer the mentally ill effective treatments and progress towards preventing illness, systematic research must have a pivotal place. And yet, a contradiction looms in that the conduct of much research in psychiatry requires the active collaboration of patients who may lack the wherewithal to provide informed consent and to appreciate fully their own interests and needs.

When scientific research became an inherent feature of psychiatry during the nineteenth century, the ethical dimension was barely considered, if at all. This lack of systematic attention extended well into the twentieth century. The ghastly Nazi medical crimes constituted the turning point in a recognition among the medical fraternity that research without explicit safeguards for subjects was entirely unacceptable on ethical grounds. The Nuremberg Statement of 1947 was a crucial milestone and is our first selection in this section.[1] The War Crimes Tribunal laid down 10 standards for those carrying out experiments on human subjects. The document is as applicable today as it was over half a century ago. In particular, its first standard that 'The voluntary consent of the human subject is absolutely essential' has been revisited in various ways, including the addition of an empirical dimension in the context of research on the mentally ill. The Nuremberg Statement highlighted the need for the subject to have the capacity to give consent based on sufficient understanding of the nature of the research. Not surprisingly, the question of whether this is feasible with psychiatric patients has attracted much attention, with the issue of 'decisional capacity' systematically investigated to good effect. We shall consider this further when commenting on specific selections revolving around informed consent.

Unfortunately, Nuremberg was insufficient to prod researchers into protecting subjects. In a classical paper by Beecher,[2] no less than 22 examples of unethical research were cited. Again, the salience of informed consent was highlighted and complemented by a call for investigators to act compassionately and responsibly. Although the illustrations were all in the area of physical medicine, it is likely that a similar neglect of ethical standards pervaded psychiatric research.

The Declaration of Helsinki[3], adopted by the World Medical Association in 1964 and subject to regular revisions, reflected a universal need to implement a process to protect subjects involved in experimental procedures. We have included the current edition below since the declaration has become a reference for all investigators. Unlike Nuremberg, it recommends that where mental incapacity precludes obtaining informed consent, permission from a responsible family member must be sought 'in accordance with national legislation'. This attention to subjects with 'mental incapacity' was the forerunner of a range of progressive policies by individual governments. For example, in the United States, federal regulations were introduced to cover the needs of vulnerable groups. In the mid-1990s, the US National Bioethics Advisory Commission (NBAC) produced a document on research on people with mental disorders that might affect the capacity to make informed decisions.[4]

In Australia, the National Health and Medical Research Council (NHMRC) published a commentary in its *National Statement on Ethical Conduct in Research Involving Humans* on circumstances where the subject is intellectually or mentally impaired.[5] Several guidelines are offered to the investigator. Suffice to state here, subjects should only participate in projects after the benefits, burdens and risks have been identified and considered. Whenever people have sufficient competence or when impairment is temporary or recurrent, the subject themselves should consent. If entirely not competent, a guardian, authority or other organization or person having responsibility in law should be consulted. Indeed, legal measures have been applied in all Australian jurisdictions to cover the latter situation. In the event of a mentally impaired person refusing to participate in research, the refusal must be respected.

Given the critical role of informed consent in research generally, and in psychiatric research in particular, we now turn to this topic.

Informed consent in psychiatric research

No one would disagree with the aforementioned argument that acquiring new knowledge about the causes and treatment of mental illness is vital. A corollary is the ineluctable requirement that people who suffer in this way must be involved in research programs, and of all types. Gaining their agreement can be straightforward. Consider a well-educated adult working for a company that requires he undertake new duties involving flying. The only snag is that the gentleman suffers from a flight phobia. A study is underway to examine personality functioning in those who present with this phobia. All that is required is completing a set of relatively innocuous questionnaires covering emotions, relationships with others, self-esteem and the like. This potential research subject is informed about, and understands, the nature of the study including risks he may incur, likely benefits to himself and/or to others and any inconvenience he may experience. The question of how autonomous he is to express a preference freely about participation would be decisive. Conceivably, his employer might push him to be involved in the hope that this would goad him into treatment and lead to symptom relief and his becoming productive in the company.

A young woman in the throes of a psychotic illness such as schizophrenia or mania presents an altogether different scenario. Her mental state is likely to be so impaired as to cause her to respond to a researcher's information with confusion and possibly clinical deterioration. The demands of the informed consent process could even be hazardous and constitute a moral harm. Moreover, research into disorders like schizophrenia and mania might entail uncomfortable procedures such as a brain scan. Participation in a drug trial might require regular venepuncture and be associated with unpleasant side-effects (the latter often difficult to predict).

Given the need to advance knowledge into these devastating illnesses and the probability that obtaining informed consent will be problematic, an ethical conundrum arises. Fortunately, several groups have appreciated its complexity and sought to dissect out the pertinent issues. They have paved the way for greater understanding or conducted empirical research to ascertain to what extent decisional capacity is disrupted in various mental states, and how to remedy the problem. A useful overview is that by Appelbaum and Roth.[6] Although much has been written since, their account is comprehensive and focused. Their review ends: 'What is needed is empirical testing of the reliability and validity of the various ways of characterizing competency . . .' This is precisely what Appelbaum and his colleges have done. For instance they have devised a procedure to assess a patient's ability to consent to treatment as well as to research.[7]

The MacArthur Treatment Competence Study approach has been adopted by other researchers to establish whether in a condition like schizophrenia clinical features contribute to reduced decisional capacity. A splendid example is that of Carpenter and colleagues[8] which we have selected to illustrate how research into research ethics can illuminate. Thirty subjects with schizophrenia were compared with controls in terms of decisional capacity. The patients were then offered an educational intervention to test whether their performance could be improved. Predictably, the patients did not cope with the tasks as well as controls, and their poor performance correlated with cognitive impairment. However, an intensive educational program led to better performance, the equal of the controls.

The group drew three implications from this study: schizophrenic patients, even those with chronic and severe forms, might have decisional capacity to give informed consent; impaired capacity when present could be 'remediated'; and cognitive factors were more relevant than the psychotic state. The corollary is obvious – a person with psychosis should not automatically be deprived of the opportunity to participate in decisions about getting involved in research.

Incidentally, capacity was measured by the MacArthur Competence Assessment Tool – Clinical Research (MacCAT-CR), an instrument assessing four areas: understanding pertinent information, appreciating implications of that information for one's own circumstances, using the information to reason and exhibiting a choice of action.

Laura Roberts and her colleagues[9] have pursued a similar theme in conducting structured interviews with schizophrenic patients presented with four hypothetical protocols involving a person with that condition. The patients could differentiate critical aspects of the protocols. For instance, they discerned different degrees of risk. They were also reluctant to participate in a project they perceived as involving potential harm. Aware of the risk of generalizing from these findings, the authors concluded that a subgroup at least manifests abilities to determine whether or not they should offer themselves as research participants.

In a comparable study, also with schizophrenic patients, Wirshing and colleagues[10] demonstrated that the more thorough the informed consent procedure, the more likely psychotic patients would understand, and retain pertinent information. Most subjects required two or more 'reiterations' before mastering the material. Like the Carpenter findings, Wirshing et al. concluded that while patients with schizophrenia might not readily grasp elements of consent, appropriate educational strategies lead to increased capacity to do so.

The focus was clearly on cognitive ability to participate in the process of agreeing to be a research subject. Elliott[11] has noted that other factors may militate against competence. In a severely depressed patient, for instance, cognitive abilities may remain intact but emotional and motivational ones may not. A person may be so gloomy as to neglect their own well-being. Thus, when confronted with a request to participate in research, they may understand that this entails risks but not feel concerned about them.

Given this perspective, Elliott suggests that researchers may need to revise their ways of evaluating incompetence, particularly by considering affective and motivational features. He also appeals for research to ascertain in what ways depression could affect competence.

His call has not gone unheeded. The ability to consent using the MacCAT-CR was investigated in women presenting with major depression.[12] Elliott's concerns about the deleterious effects of emotional and motivational factors were not confirmed: virtually all patients performed adequately and maintained this over time. Moreover, no link was found between decision-making capacity and degree of depression. We must exercise caution, recognized by the authors, in that the sample was small and does not necessarily represent patients with depression generally. Obviously, severe melancholia and particularly psychotic features might hinder the consent process.

The material we have cited is encouraging in that we can be confident that when conducting research with psychiatric subjects their decisional capacity is not necessarily an impediment. Where impairment is encountered, educational interventions can make a difference. If genuine informed consent is achievable in most subjects, a huge ethical quandary recedes. However, a proportion of disturbed patients will remain incompetent, whatever the intervention. In these cases, surrogate decision-making takes over. What is required, as Bonnie[13] asserts, is for protagonists to arrive at a consensus on optimal safeguards and linked ethical guidelines that allow vital studies to be pursued at the same time as respecting the subject's rights.

Our attention hitherto has focused on decisional capacity and competence. An omission is consent that is free and without coercion. Roberts[14] has spelt out a framework to understanding what she calls 'voluntarism'. As she puts it: 'The framework is based on a definition of voluntarism as ideally encompassing the individual's ability to act in accordance with one's authentic senses of what is good, right and best in light of one's situation, values and prior history'. She highlights four clusters of factors that may influence voluntarism in giving consent. Developmental factors emcompass such facets as emotional maturity and character: an example is that of children who may be unable to arrive at a decision about what is in their best interests. In later childhood and adolescence, the situation changes with greater ability to decide freely.

Another domain revolves around illness factors. We may recall Elliott's contribution on depression in the context of consenting. Other mental states may disrupt voluntarism, although the overlap with cognitive factors becomes obvious. Robert's third domain encompasses psychological and sociocultural issues, the latter including religious values. The final area is that of external forces, especially institutional ones, where, for example, prisoners or residents in nursing homes may be persuaded, even coerced, to participate in research.

An ethical obligation arises – the investigator stresses respect for persons whereby their values and past experiences are incorporated into the process of seeking consent. By this means, consent is freely and genuinely given, without any element of pressure.

Dealing with risk

A long-standing consensus stems from one of the 10 standards in the Nuremberg Statement:[1] 'The degree of risk to be taken should never exceed that determined by the humanitarian importance of the problem to be solved by the experiment.' This is echoed in the Declaration of Helsinki[3] which states that the salience of the research aim must be proportionate to any risk to the subject. In addition, the investigator should assess and compare likely risks and benefits. A study should cease if risks are found to outweigh benefits.

These requirements also apply to subjects of psychiatric research. Indeed, given their vulnerable status, those afflicted with mental illness may be prone to a range of hazards. Risks to health of being prescribed a drug or being taken off an active drug (as we shall discuss below) are obvious examples. Psychological risks are more subtle and therefore not always sufficiently considered. For example, patients with a history of abuse may become distressed when faced with questions about their childhood which on the face of it are seemingly neutral. Any enquiry about a personal issue which remains unresolved may inadvertently pave the way for an emotional upheaval. A line of enquiry may precipitate such reactions as guilt, shame, resentment, regret or grief.

These risks are best characterized as non-specific insofar as they may involve any subject, psychiatric or otherwise, and are to a degree unpredictable since we can have little idea about personal vulnerabilities. The US National Bioethics Advisory Commission (NBAC)[4] addressed risks probably resulting from psychiatric research methodology in 1998. They highlighted trials in which patients may receive a placebo; withdrawing or withholding medication, (i.e. medication-free research); and symptom-provoking studies, (i.e. administering a substance known to worsen symptoms.) While these strategies are not confined to psychiatry, the risks involved are more unpredictable. We have included two papers, one on placebo-controlled trials, the other on medication-free research. Other useful publications include a review of the literature on drug withdrawal in schizophrenic patients by Gilbert et al.,[15] a commentary on this by Baldessarini,[16] a discussion of scientific issues related to drug discontinuation by Jeste et al.[17] and ways to assess studies incorporating discontinuation of medication[18] or provocation of symptoms[19].

Let us consider placebo studies. Hirschfeld et al.[20], in a commentary on achieving a balance between protection of subjects and advancing research, conclude that a placebo condition should not be used in studies involving patients suffering from moderate/ severe depression. Their rationale is explicit – using a placebo is tantamount to withholding effective treatment. Presumably, they would argue similarly in any situation where proven effective therapy is available.

Franklin Miller[21] has a different view, arguing for the retention of the placebo-controlled trial. We are reminded that the placebo question is especially relevant to psychiatric research given the vulnerable group of patients involved. Miller refers to a middle ground position that rejects an absolute prohibition of placebo-controlled trials. He is supported by guidelines issued by the US Food and Drug Administration that prefers a placebo cell when the risk of serious harm including death is not present. Furthermore, a new drug should be compared with proven effective therapy only when use of a placebo is 'contrary to the interests of the patient'.

Miller provides an exemplary ethical justification. First, the placebo-controlled trial should be scientifically meritorious and of clinical utility. The protocol should contain a rigorous rationale as to why the placebo is required. Second, expected benefits in terms of new knowledge should outweigh any risks and where risks do exist they should be kept to a minimum. Thus, if extant treatments are only partially efficacious or are associated with unpleasant side-effects or both, placebo research is more readily justified. He also addresses the context of psychiatric research, namely that many mental illnesses are long-term and treatments, for the most part, are symptom-relieving rather than curative. Furthermore, current treatments have potential side-effects. Thus, use of placebo in a short-term study is unlikely to produce any enduring harm.

On the other hand, several caveats are offered. Careful screening of patients should be done in order that those who have demonstrated a good response to current medications should not be recruited into a placebo-controlled trial and those clearly at risk of suicide should be excluded. The period for which the placebo is given should be as short as possible, to achieve the purpose of the trial. Frequent assessment to spot any deterioration is another recommendation.

Another component of Miller's justification revolves around informed consent. The process is similar to any other psychiatric study but the subject must clearly comprehend the rationale for using a placebo condition. Finally, the investigator is obligated to offer optimal treatment once the placebo-controlled trial has ended. This constitutes a quid pro quo for the original volunteering. Certainly, those who may have deteriorated during the trial should be offered the requisite treatment to achieve improvement. This obligation also applies to those who drop out because of worsening symptoms or side-effects.

A pragmatic approach to the question of whether to use placebo in psychiatric research seems feasible in the light of the US National Depressive and Manic-Depressive Association's Consensus Statement.[22] Expert work groups considered ways to protect subjects with mood disorders with the assistance of ethical consultants (including the aforementioned Franklin Miller).

Carpenter and his colleagues[23] have analysed the ethics of medication-free research in schizophrenia. Why is it required? In the case of clinical trials, where the aim is to develop new treatments, it is advantageous to obviate the effects of other medications which the patient may have been, or is currently, receiving. Hazardous interactional effects may also be prevented by ensuring that the patient is free of medication at the beginning of the study. Research which addresses pathophysiology is similarly 'cleaner' when all traces of drug metabolites have been eliminated. In these circumstances, subjects do not benefit directly but may do so later if results become the basis of new treatments.

The authors suggest that medication-free research in schizophrenia is feasible provided guidelines to safeguard subjects are followed. The result is another sound example of how one may replace strident contention with judicious reasoning. First, careful selection of patients is mandatory. For instance, those with a complicated management history or who are at particular risk for adverse effects should be excluded. If admitted to the study, patients should be carefully monitored and given known effective psychosocial treatment. This monitoring facilitates prompt detection of deterioration and the option to offer proven treatment. No matter how suitable the patient might be for medication-free research, duration of the study should be as brief as possible. As we noted in Miller's approach to placebo-controlled research, patients should be offered optimal therapy on completion of the study. Finally, informed consent should be diligently negotiated. Carpenter et al. conclude that, with these provisos, medication-free research in schizophrenia is feasible and ethically justified in most cases. Exceptionally, additional precautions may be required to ensure that the rights of subjects are fully respected. In the NBAC's report,[4] referred to above, further protective devices are mentioned, (e.g. appointment of a legally authorized representative, independent evaluation of a patient's capacity to give informed consent and continuing monitoring of that consent).

Jeste, Palmer and Harris[17] are obviously aware of the NBAC's concerns and share their own, contending that there are 'several unanswered questions' about subjecting psychotic patients to research which calls for interruption or withholding of standard treatment.

Other topics

Given their profound relevance in psychiatric research, we have concentrated on informed consent and risks. In order to complete the picture, we mention a number of topics which pressure of space precludes us from anthologizing.

Much research in psychiatry is on adult patients. When the elderly, children and adolescents are subjects, special considerations apply. Fitten[24] has highlighted the issues in the elderly, focusing on their vulnerability to exploitation (e.g. the chronically institutionalized in nursing homes or comparable facilities), and the difficulties encountered in those with dementia-based cognitive impairment.

Research on infants, children and adolescents is pivotal to advance psychiatric knowledge, both for these particular groups, as well as for people at other stages of life. Development of personalities in biological, psychological and social terms, both normal and abnormal, is frequently relevant in an attempt to understand the pathogenesis of adult psychopathology. Longitudinal studies are especially valuable in identifying developmental factors of consequence, but may yield little or no benefit to the research subject.

Ethical issues that arise in younger aged subjects revolve around risk, informed consent and the related concepts of assent from the child and proxy consent. The literature on these topics has been sparse, perhaps reflecting paucity of research in child psychiatry. The picture has changed since the late 1990s. On the other hand, pragmatically based guidelines to protect children qua[25–30] subjects have been formulated by US statutory agencies. These are summarized by Jensen and his colleagues.[31]

Jensen is also a co-author of a paper[32] which stresses the need to conduct research directly in children and adolescents in order to avoid dangerous extrapolation from findings of work on adults (e.g., effectiveness and safety of psychotropic drugs), the issue of investigations which do not benefit the participants and achieving a balance between risk and scientific utility.

Much psychiatric research entails collecting personal information, which is then stored in databases. Such data, in tandem with research registers, facilitate linkage studies. However, these pose ethical questions: for what purposes are the data collected, what measures are in place to safeguard privacy, has permission been sought from the subjects, and should they have the right to access and, if necessary, to correct information about themselves. John Wing[33] covers these aspects of 'Psychiatric research' in our sister volume, *Psychiatric Ethics*.

Simon and his colleagues[34] have contributed helpfully on the role of clinical databases in psychiatric research, albeit with an American slant. They argue for a distinction between public domain research and the commercial use of clinical information, and for the strict application of safeguards to protect privacy. They conclude with a special note on the risk of discriminating *against* psychiatric patients by restricting database research on them. We may feel tempted to avoid using highly personal information in their case out of a concern for a vulnerable and stigmatized population but this, the authors aver, may deprive future patients of the potential benefits of conducting database studies.

Thoughtful commentaries by Appelbaum[35] and Hyman[36] provide support for the position set out by Simon *et al.*; the two commentators highlight the role of research ethics committees to achieve the correct balance between the need to carry out research and the right to privacy.

Given the genomic revolution, psychiatry will undoubtedly benefit from investigations in psychiatric genetics, but ethical complications are sure to accompany this endeavour and require meticulous examination. For this reason we introduced a new chapter on this topic by Farmer and McGuffin[37] in the third edition of *Psychiatric Ethics*.

The rapidly growing research endeavour into first episode psychosis has generated several ethical challenges and serves to illustrate how innovative research in psychiatry may throw up new ethical questions. A critical matter is the legitimacy of intervening actively in the life of a young person who presents with clinical features suggestive of psychosis but where solid criteria are not available. The term prodrome covers this clinical situation. Investigators are highly motivated to examine this phase given the strong possibility that intervention at the earliest possible opportunity is likely to yield benefits, both short and long term. The difficulty is the unpredictability of the course in every case and the risk of false positives. Is it justified to prescribe antipsychotics for instance, for a teenager who manifests non-specific symptoms such as irritability and social withdrawal in the absence of a robust predictor that a psychosis is in its 'gestational' phase? How do we obtain informed consent for a research procedure in the face of such uncertainty? Can we cause harm through inaccurate designation of a person as prodromally affected? How can we determine whether benefits inherent in early intervention will not be outweighed by such risks as potential stigmatization, side-effects of medication and the aforementioned false positive? Can people identified as pre-psychotic provide informed consent for research on themselves, in terms of competence or voluntarism?

Patrick McGorry, a leading figure in this area, has dissected the pertinent ethical issues. A paper, co-authored by Kenneth Schaffner,[38] is an excellent introduction to a series of contributions in a special issue of *Schizophrenia Research*. The US National Institute of Mental Health has also pursued the ethical dimension, particularly the matter of obtaining informed consent. One helpful product of their effort is a crystallization of discussions by researchers who met in 2000.[39]

Conclusion

We declared at the outset that psychiatry must commit itself to research if its practitioners are to develop effective treatments and strategies to prevent mental illness. Although research has progressed impressively, much knowledge is still needed to assist patients and their families. Indeed, mental health professionals have an ethical obligation to do everything within their power to advance the field. As we have noted, profound significant ethical complications pervade the endeavor. The material we have selected, however, is a solid foundation from which to reconnoiter further.

References

*1 The Nuremberg Statement. Appendix, in *Psychiatric Ethics*, 3rd edn, ed. S. Bloch, P. Chodoff, and S. Green, Oxford, Oxford University Press, 1999, pp. 512–514.

2 Beecher, H.: Ethics and clinical research. *New England Journal of Medicine*. 274: 1354–1360, 1966.

*3 The Declaration of Helsinki. Appendix, in *Psychiatric Ethics*, 3rd edn. ed. Bloch, S., Chodoff, P. and Green, S. Oxford, Oxford University Press, 1999, pp. 514–517.

4 National Bioethics Advisory Commission: Research involving subjects with mental disorders that may affect decision-making capacity. Rockville MD, National Bioethics Advisory Commission, 1998.

5 Human Research Ethics Handbook. Commentary on the National Statement on Ethical Conduct in Research Involving Humans. Canberra, National Health and Medical Research Council, 2002.

*6 Appelbaum, P. and Roth, L.: Competency to consent to research: a psychiatric overview. *Archives of General Psychiatry* 39:951–958, 1982.

7 Appelbaum, P. and Grisso, T.: The MacArthur treatment competence study 1. Mental illness and competence to consent to treatment. *Law and Human Behaviour* 19:105–126, 1995.

*8 Carpenter, W.T., Gold, J.M., Lahti, A.C., Queern, C.A., Conley, R.R., Bartko, J.J., Kovnick, J. and Appelbaum, P.S.: Decisional capacity for informed consent in schizophrenia research. *Archives of General Psychiatry* 57:533–538, 2000.

9 Roberts, L., Warner, T., Brody, Roberts, B., Lauriello, J. and Lyketsos, C.: Patient and psychiatrist ratings of hypothetical schizophrenia research protocols: assessment of harm potential and factors influencing participant decisions. *American Journal of Psychiatry* 159:573–584, 2002.

10 Wirshing, D., Wirshing, W., Marder, S., Liberman, R. and Mintz J.: Informed consent: assessment of comprehension. *American Journal of Psychiatry* 155:1508–1511, 1998.

*11 Elliot, C.: Caring about risks. Are severely depressed patients competent to consent to research? *Archives of General Psychiatry* 54:113–116, 1997.

12 Appelbaum, P., Grisso, T., Frank, E., O'Donnell, S. and Kupfer, D.: Competence of depressed patients for consent to research. *American Journal of Psychiatry* 156:1380–1384. 1999.

13 Bonnie, R.: Research with cognitively impaired subjects: unfinished business in the regulation of human research. *Archives of General Psychiatry* 54:105–111, 1997.

*14 Roberts, L.: Informed consent and the capacity for voluntarism. *American Journal of Psychiatry* 159:705–712, 2002.

15 Gilbert, P., Harris, M., McAdams, L. and Jeste, D.: Neuroleptic withdrawal in schizophrenic patients. A review of the literature. *Archives of General Psychiatry* 52:173–188, 1995.

16 Baldessarini, R. and Viguera, A.: Neuroleptic withdrawal in schizophrenic patients. Commentary. *Archives of General Psychiatry* 52:189–192, 1995.

17 Jeste, D., Palmer, B. and Harris, M.: Neuroleptic discontinuation in clinical research settings: scientific issues and ethical dilemmas. *Biological Psychiatry* 46:1050–1059, 1999.

18 Rosenstein, D.: IRB Review of psychiatric medication discontinuation and symptom-provoking studies. *Biological Psychiatry* 46:1039–1043, 1999

19 Miller, F. and Rosenstein, D.: Psychiatric symptom-provoking studies: An ethical appraisal. *Biological Psychiatry* 42:403–409, 1997.

20 Hirschfeld, R., Winslade, W. and Krause T.: Protecting subjects and fostering research: striking the proper balance. Commentary. *Archives of General Psychiatry* 54:121–123, 1997.

*21 Miller, F.G.: Placebo-controlled trials in psychiatric research: an ethical perspective. *Biological Psychiatry* 47:707–716, 2000.

22 Charney, D., Nemeroff, C., Lewis, L., Laden, S. *et al.*: National depressive and manic-depressive association consensus statement on the use of placebo in clinical trials of mood disorders. *Archives of General Psychiatry* 59:262–270, 2002.

*23 Carpenter, W.T., Schooler, N.R. and Kane J.M.: The rationale and ethics of medication-free research in schizophrenia. *Archives of General Psychiatry* 54:401–407, 1997.

24 Fitten, L.: The ethics of conducting research with older psychiatric patients. *International Journal of Geriatric Psychiatry* **8**:33–39, 1993.

25 Fisher, C., Hoagwood, K., Boyce, C. *et al.*: Research ethics for mental health science involving ethnic minority children and youths. *American Psychologist* **57**: 1024–40, 2002.

26 Arnold, A., Stoff, D., Cook, E. *et al.*: Ethical issues in biological psychiatric research with children and adolescents. *Journal of the American Academy of Child and Adolescent Psychiatry* **34**:929–39, 1995.

27 Vitiello, B. and Jensen, P.: Medication development and testing in children and adolescents. *Archives of General Psychiatry* **54**:871–876, 1997.

28 Malone, R. and Simpson, G.: Psychopharmacology: Use of placebos in clinical trials involving children and adolescents. *Psychiatric Services* **49**:1413–1417, 1998.

29 Kumra, S., Briguglio, C., Lenane, M. *et al.*: Including children and adolescents with schizophrenia in medication – free research. *American Journal of Psychiatry* **156**:1065–1068, 1999.

30 Claveirole, A.: Listening to young voices: challenges of research with adolescent mental health service users. *Journal of Psychiatric and Mental Health Nursing* **11**:253–260, 2004.

31 Jensen, P., Fisher, C. and Hoagwood, K.: Special issues in mental health/illness research with children and adolescents, in *Ethics in Psychiatric Research: A resource manual for human subjects protection*, ed. H. Pincus, J. Lieberman, and S. Ferris, Washington D.C., American Psychiatric Association, 1999, pp. 159–175.

32 Vitiello, B., Jensen, P. and Hoagwood, K.: Integrating science and ethics in child and adolescent psychiatry research. *Biological Psychiatry* **46**:1044–1049, 1999.

33 Wing, J. Ethics and psychiatric research, in *Psychiatric Ethics*, 3rd edn, ed. Bloch, S., Chodoff, P. and Green, S. Oxford, Oxford University Press 1999, pp. 461–477.

34 Simon, G., Unutzer, J., Young, B. and Pincus, H.: Large medical databases, population-based research, and patient confidentiality. *American Journal of Psychiatry* **157**:1731–1737, 2000.

35 Appelbaum, P.: Protecting privacy while facilitating research. *American Journal of Psychiatry* **157**:1725–1726, 2000.

36 Hyman, S.: The needs for database research. *American Journal of Psychiatry* **157**:1723–1724, 2000.

37 Farmer, A. and McGuffin, P.: Ethics and psychiatric genetics, in *Psychiatric Ethics*, 3rd edn, ed. Bloch, S., Chodoff, P. and Green, S. Oxford, Oxford University Press, 1999, pp. 479–493.

*38 Schaffner, K. and McGorry, P.: Preventing severe mental illnesses – new prospects and ethical challenges. *Schizophrenia Research* **51**:3–15, 2001.

39 Heinssen, R., Perkins, D., Appelbaum, P. and Fenton, W.: Informed consent in early psychosis research: National Institute of Mental Health Workshop, November 15, 2000. *Schizophrenia Bulletin* **27**(Suppl. 4);571–584, 2001.

The Nuremberg Statement*

The judgment by the war crimes tribunal at Nuremberg laid down 10 standards to which physicians must conform when carrying out experiments on human subjects.

Permissible Medical Experiments

The great weight of the evidence before us to effect that certain types of medical experiments on human beings, when kept within reasonably well-defined bounds, conform to the ethics of the medical profession generally. The protagonists of the practice of human experimentation justify their views on the basis that such experiments yield results for the good of society that are unprocurable by other methods or means of study. All agree, however, that certain basic principles must be observed in order to satisfy moral ethical and legal concepts:

1. The voluntary consent of the human subject is absolutely essential. This means that the person involved should have legal capacity to give consent; should be so situated as to be able to exercise free power of choice, without the intervention of any element of force, fraud, deceit, duress, overreaching, or other ulterior form of constraint or coercion; and should have sufficient knowledge and comprehension of the elements of the subject matter involved as to enable him to make an understanding and enlightened decision. This latter element requires that before the acceptance of an affirmative decision by the experimental subject there should be made known to him the nature, duration, and purpose of the experiment; the method and means by which it is to be conducted; all inconveniences and hazards reasonably to be expected; and the effects upon his health or person which may possibly come from his participation in the experiment. The duty and responsibility for ascertaining the quality of the consent rests upon each individual who initiates, directs, or engages in the experiment. It is a personal duty and responsibility which may not be delegated to another with impunity.

2. The experiment should be such as to yield fruitful results for the good of society, unprocurable by other methods or means of study, and not random and unnecessary in nature.

3. The experiment should be so designed and based on the results of animal experimentation and a knowledge of the natural history of the disease or other problem under study that the anticipated results justify the performance of the experiment.

4. The experiment should be so conducted as to avoid all unnecessary physical and mental suffering and injury.

5. No experiment should be conducted where there is an a priori reason to believe that death or disabling injury will occur; except, perhaps, in those experiments where the experimental physicians also serve as subjects.

6. The degree of risk to be taken should never exceed that determined by the humanitarian importance of the problem to be solved by the experiment.

7. Proper preparations should be made and adequate facilities provided to protect the experimental subject against even remote possibilities of injury, disability or death.

8. The experiment should be conducted only by scientifically qualified persons. The highest degree of skill and care should be required through all stages of the experiment of those who conduct or engage in the experiment.

9. During the course of the experiment the human subject should be at liberty to bring the experiment to an end if he has reached the physical or mental state where continuation of the experiment seems to him to be impossible.

10. During the course of the experiment the scientist in charge must be prepared to terminate the experiment at any stage, if he has probable cause to believe, in the exercise of the good faith, superior skill and careful judgment required of him, that a continuation of the experiment is likely to result in injury, disability, or death to the experimental subject.

* The Nuremberg Statement. Appendix, in *Psychiatric Ethics*, 3rd edn. ed. S. Bloch, P. Chodoff, and S. Green, Oxford, Oxford University Press, 1999, pp. 512–514.

Declaration of Helsinki*

Recommendations guiding medical doctors in biomedical research involving human subjects

Introduction

It is the mission of the physician to safeguard the health of the people. His or her knowledge and conscience are dedicated to the fulfilment of this mission.

The Declaration of Geneva of the World Medical Association binds the physician with the words, 'The health of my patient will be my first consideration,' and the International Code of Medical Ethics declares that, 'A physician shall act only in the patient's interest when providing medical care which might have the effect of weakening the physical and mental condition of the patient.'

The purpose of biomedical research involving human subjects must be to improve diagnostic, therapeutic and prophylactic procedures and the understanding of the aetiology and pathogenesis of disease.

In current medical practice most diagnostic, therapeutic or prophylactic procedures involve hazards. This applies especially to biomedical research.

Medical progress is based on research which ultimately must rest in part on experimentation involving human subjects.

In the field of biomedical research a fundamental distinction must be recognised between medical research in which the aim is essentially diagnostic or therapeutic for a patient, and medical research the essential object of which is purely scientific and without implying direct diagnostic or therapeutic value to the person subjected to the research.

Special caution must be exercised in the conduct of research which may affect the environment, and the welfare of animals used for research must be respected.

Because it is essential that the result of laboratory experiments be applied to human beings to further scientific knowledge and to help suffering humanity, the World Medical Association has prepared the following recommendations as a guide to every physician in biomedical research involving human subjects. They should be kept under review in the future. It must be stressed that the standards as drafted are only a guide to physicians all over the world. Physicians are not relieved from criminal, civil and ethical responsibilities under the law of their own countries.

I. Basic Principles

1. Biomedical research involving human subjects must conform to generally accepted scientific principles and should be based on adequately performed laboratory and animal experimentation and on a thorough knowledge of the scientific literature.

2. The design and performance of each experimental procedure involving human subjects should be clearly formulated in an experimental protocol which should be transmitted to a specially appointed independent committee for consideration, comment and guidance.

3. Biomedical research involving human subjects should be conducted only by scientifically qualified persons and under the supervision of a clinically competent medical person. The responsibility for the human subject must always rest with a medically qualified person and never rest on the subject of the research, even though the subject has given his or her consent.

4. Biomedical research involving human subjects cannot legitimately be carried out unless the importance of the objective is in proportion to the inherent risk to the subject.

5. Every biomedical research project involving human subjects should be preceded by careful assessment of predictable risks in comparison with foreseeable benefits to the subject or to others. Concern for the interests of the subject must always prevail over the interests of science and society.

6. The right of the research subject to safeguard his or her integrity must always be respected. Every precaution should be taken to respect the privacy of the subject and to minimize the impact of the study on the subject's physical and mental integrity and on the personality of the subject.

7. Physicians should abstain from engaging in research projects involving human subjects unless they are satisfied that the hazards involved are believed to be predictable. Physicians should cease any investigation if the hazards are found to outweigh the potential benefits.

8. In publication of the results of his or her research, the physician is obliged to preserve the accuracy of the results. Reports of experimentation not in accordance with the principles laid down in this Declaration should not be accepted for publication.

9. In any research on human beings, each potential subject must be adequately informed of the aims, methods, anticipated benefits and potential hazards of the study and the discomfort it may entail. He or she should be informed that he or she is at liberty to abstain from participation in the study and that he or she is free to withdraw his or her consent to participation at any time. The physician should then obtain the subject's freely given informed consent, preferably in writing.

10. When obtaining informed consent for the research project the physician should be particularly cautious if the subject is in a dependent relationship to him or her or may consent under duress. In that case the informed consent should be obtained by a physician who is not engaged in the investigation and who is completely independent of this official relationship.

11. In case of legal incompetence, informed consent should be obtained from the legal guardian in accordance with national legislation. Where physical or mental incapacity makes it impossible to obtain informed consent, or when the subject is a minor, permission from the responsible relative replaces that of the subject in accordance with national legislation. Whenever the minor child is in fact able to give consent, the

* The Declaration of Helsinki. Appendix, in *Psychiatric Ethics*, 3rd edn. ed. Bloch, S., Chodoff, P. and Green, S. Oxford, Oxford University Press, 1999, pp. 514–517.

minor's consent must be obtained in addition to the consent of the minor's legal guardian.

12. The research protocol should always contain a statement of the ethical considerations involved and should indicate that the principles enunciated in the present declaration are complied with.

II. Medical Research Combined With Clinical Care (Clinical Research)

1. In the treatment of the sick person, the physician must be free to use a new diagnostic and therapeutic measure, if in his or her judgement it offers hope of saving life, re-establishing health or alleviating suffering.

2. The potential benefits, hazards and discomfort of a new method should be weighed against the advantages of the best current diagnostic and therapeutic methods.

3. In any medical study, every patient including those of a control group, if any, should be assured of the best proven diagnostic and therapeutic method. This does not exclude the use of inert placebos in studies where no proven diagnostic or therapeutic method exists.

4. The refusal of the patient to participate in a study must never interfere with the physician-patient relationship.

5. If the physician considers it essential not to obtain informed consent, the specific reasons for this proposal should be stated in the experimental protocol for transmission to the independent committee.

6. The physician can combine medical research with professional care, the objective being the acquisition of new medical knowledge, only to the extent that medical research is justified by its potential diagnostic or therapeutic value for the patient.

II. Non-Therapeutic Biomedical Research Involving Human Subjects (Non-Clinical Biomedical Research)

1. In the purely scientific application of medical research carried out on a human being, it is the duty of the physician to remain the protector of the life and health of that person on whom biomedical research is being carried out.

2. The subjects should be volunteers – either healthy persons or patients for whom the experimental design is not related to the patient's illness.

3. The investigator or the investigating team should discontinue the research if in his/her or their judgment it may, if continued, be harmful to the individual.

4. In research on man, the interest of science and society should never take precedence over considerations related to the well-being of the subject.

Competency to Consent to Research

A Psychiatric Overview*

Paul S. Appelbaum and Loren H. Roth

The issue of competence to consent to therapeutic and experimental proce-dures, once a neglected topic of interest only to a small group of legal and medical academics, recently has been propelled into the forefront of debate about medical and experimental ethics. Many of the same factors that have led to profound interest in informed consent – a growing distrust of professionals in general, a rising consumerist and self-help orientation, and the exposure of some startling examples of the misuse of trust by medical experimenters – have led in turn to an examination of the presumed prereq-uisites to effective informed consent, competence among them. Despite its recent prominence, however, the issue of competence (sometimes referred to as capacity) to consent to research is of relatively recent derivation and awaits generally acceptable attempts at definition. This article will review the previ-ous literature on the elements of competency and outline the psychopatho-logic phenomena that might impair 'subjects' performance. Finally, the factors that might influence the choice of standards for competency and the possible implications of those choices will be discussed.

Background

The relevance of a person's mental capacity to the adequacy of his consent to participate in research was first recognized formally in the Nuremberg Code, the initial attempt to codify the ethical principles that should guide human experimentation.[1] The code, which was elaborated in response to the revelation of Nazi atrocities committed in the name of advancing med-ical knowledge, deemed 'absolutely essential' the 'voluntary consent of the human subject,' and continued, 'This means that the person should have legal capacity to give consent.' Along with capacity, the free power of choice and sufficient knowledge and comprehension to enable an understanding decision were singled out as the touchstones of what later came to be called the doctrine of informed consent.

Of interest in the Nuremberg formulation, which some have argued was designed exclusively to deal with nontherapeutic research, is the seemingly absolute nature of the requirement for legal capacity. There is no provision in the code for any procedures that would permit subjects lacking in capacity to participate in research. This situation was altered with the promulgation of the Declaration of Helsinki by the World Medical Association in 1964. Now the most widely recognized code governing experiments with humans, the declaration distinguished between 'clinical research combined with profes-sional care' (ie, research that might lead to therapeutic gains for the subjects) and 'non-therapeutic clinical research.'[1] In each category, it appeared to allow the consent of a third party to be substituted for that of the incompetent subject; for clinical research combined with professional care,

If at all possible, consistent with patient psychology, the doctor should obtain the patient's freely given consent . . . In case of legal incapacity, consent should also be procured from the legal guardian; in case of physical incapacity, the permis-sion of the legal guardian replaces that of the patient.

For nontherapeutic clinical research, it stated, 'Clinical research on a human being cannot be undertaken without his free consent . . . ; if he is legally incompetent, the consent of the legal guardian should be procured.'

At approximately the same time as the discussion that led to the Declaration of Helsinki, public attention in the United States was being drawn to the need for procedures to prevent harm to research subjects. This height-ened awareness of the need for regulation was prompted by the revelation of the effects of thalidomide on fetuses in Europe,[2] the well-publicized episode of the injection of live cancer cells into unconsenting patients in a Brooklyn, NY, hospital,[3] and the recognition that few systematic means of monitoring research existed in this country.[4] As the scope of possible abuses widened,[5] the first sets of governmental guidelines controlling clin-ical research were issued by the Food and Drug Administration (relating to investigational use of new drugs) and, in 1966, by the Public Health Service (relating to the clinical research that it funded).[2] When the guidelines were codified in 1971, the participation of incompetent subjects was permitted explicitly as long as consent had been obtained from a legally authorized proxy.[6]

The reliance on the idea of 'legal' incompetency in the codes and regula-tions shifted from the medical to the legal professions the burden of deciding which subjects' mental incapacities precluded their participation in research. Yet, despite the cachet of legal authority that this move seemed to lend to the competency decision, the fact was that Anglo-American law had never clearly formulated the criteria to be used in measuring legal incom-petency.[7] Nor was it clear whether the standard that should be utilized was one of general incompetency to conduct one's affairs or some more specific and limited measure, such as incompetency to make a contract.

The leading court case to date on the issue of human experimentation, *Kaimowitz vs Michigan Department of Mental Health*,[8] did little to clarify matters. Ruling on whether a prisoner had the ability to give informed con-sent to a psychosurgical procedure that might affect his chances for release, the court in *Kaimowitz* case held that

The very nature of his incarceration diminishes the capacity to consent to psy-chosurgery. He is particularly vulnerable as a result of his mental condition, the deprivation stemming from involuntary confinement, and the effects of the phenomenon of 'institutionalization.'

By appearing to confuse the Nuremberg Code's requirement for freedom of choice, which the court thought was inherently deficient in a prisoner, with the question of mental capacity, the *Kaimowitz* case demonstrated the con-ceptual pitfalls that await those approaching the subject of competency. The implication that a potentially coercive environment renders a person incompetent to make choices regarding his future has been condemned widely.[9,10]

Following the *Kaimowitz* case, the most significant effort to define the relationship between a subject's competency and the adequacy of his consent to research was the work of the National Commission for the Protection of Human Subjects of Biomedical and Behavioral Research, notably in their report on research with the 'institutionalized mentally infirm.'[11] The com-mission recommended a sliding scale of consents varying in stringency

* Appelbaum, P. and Roth, L.: Competency to consent to research: a psychiatric overview. *Archives of General Psychiatry* 39:951–958, 1982.

with the degree of risk posed by the research and its potential therapeutic benefit to the subject. For minimal-risk research, mere 'assent' was required, constituting a lower standard for competency for that particular situation Participation by incompetents in research posing higher degrees of risk was permitted only with a variety of types of substituted consent and supervision of the consent process. The failure of the commission's elaborate conclusions to settle definitively the debate about the participation of subjects with impaired capacity is demonstrated both by the many objections to the commission's reports[12] and by the failure of the US Department of Health Education, and Welfare (now the US Department of Health and Human Services [DHHS]) to implement formally the commission's recommendations or its own modifications of the commission's report.[13]

Regardless of the nature of the ultimate solution to the regulatory issue, it is apparent that the problem of competency of potential subjects will continue to play an important role in its formulation. Yet, more than 30 years after the enunciation of the Nuremberg Code, the criteria required for a determination of legal incompetency remain ambiguous. Although the rules governing competency are legal ones, and as was demonstrated clearly by the decision in the *Kaimowitz* case, they are rooted in public policy considerations. Psychiatry can contribute to the outcome of the deliberations by delineating those aspects of mental dysfunction that may impair capacity to consent.

Standards For Competency

Efforts to define standards for competency to consent have not been rare, although most such efforts have been directed toward the issue of consent to treatment rather than consent to research. The various standards that have been proposed appear generally to cluster into four groups. While the relationship among these groups requires further empirical study, our clinical experience plus the literature we have reviewed suggest that these four groups may be arranged hierarchically to furnish a progressively more stringent standard for assessing a subject's competency.

Evidencing a Choice

The least rigorous standard for competency (once the subject has been informed adequately about the nature of the research) is the subject's actual communication of a decision as to his participation in the proposed project (Table 1).[14,15] This requirement has been phrased as demanding that the subject 'manifest his consent'[16] or 'express a positive interest in taking part' (J. O. Cole, MD, letter to D. Klein, MD, Dec 22, 1977). A more behaviorally oriented indicator of this standard, one that places less emphasis on the subject's verbalizations, is the requirement that the subject has 'cooperated appropriately in the early procedures involved in the study' (J. 0. Cole, MD, letter to D. Klein, MD, Dec 22, 1977).

Table 1 Evidencing a choice

Communicates decision about participation
1. Manifests consent[17]
2. Expresses positive interest in taking part[*]
3. Cooperates appropriately in early procedures involved in study[*]
4. Gives responses (any-none) to pertinent questions[17]

Relevant psychiatric aspects
  Mutism
    Catatonic stupor
    Severe depression
  Catatonic excitement
  Mania
  Profound psychotic thought disorder (e.g. word salad)
  Marked ambivalence
    Schizophrenia
    Severe obsessive states

---

[*] J. O. Cole, MD, letter to D. Klein, MD, Dec 22, 1977.

The suggestion that the overt manifestation of a subject's choice is important for a competent decision frequently is omitted from discussions of the topic, perhaps because of its apparent tautological nature. One group of authors, for example, who propose to eliminate entirely the element of competency from the triad of informed consent nonetheless would have a court that 'finds before it a person who fails to respond to pertinent questions' deem the person not to have rendered a valid consent.[17]

Relevant Psychiatric Aspects. – Psychiatric states that interfere with the ability to manifest a choice include mutism, as a result of catatonic stupor or severe depression; catatonic excitement; mania; a profound psychotic thought disorder (eg, psychotic word salad) that render communication unintelligible to others; and marked ambivalence, as in schizophrenic or severe obsessive states, in which the stability of a choice, assuming one can be manifested, is not evident even over a reasonably short period.

Testing for Competency. – To the uninitiated, operationalizing the requirement that the subject evidence a choice may seem a trivial exercise; in most instances one need only ask the subject whether or not he desires to participate. There are occasions, however, in which the communication from the subject will be so ambiguous as to raise serious questions about whether or not consent has occurred. These include cases in which the subject's verbal and behavioral responses diverge (for example, when a subject declines to participate in a study requiring venipuncture, then rolls up his sleeve and holds out his arm to the experimenter).

In ambiguous cases of this type, or in cases in which the direction of the subject's choice appears evident but its constancy is uncertain, there is merit in deferring participation until the subject's choice can be ascertained more clearly, either as a result of repeated contacts or in response to a second person eliciting the consent. Analogous suggestions have been made previously that certain types of nonexperimental procedures that involve substantial risk for the subject, such as sterilization, be subject to a mandatory waiting period after the initial solicitation of consent, in part to assure the constancy of the response.[18]

Factual Understanding of the Issues

The subject's understanding of the issues relevant to participation is the single factor that has been most widely accepted as a standard for competency. A typical formulation requires that the subject have 'the cognitive capacity to consider the relevant issues' (Table 2). Those areas that have been considered to be crucial for the subject to understand include 'the nature of the procedure, its risks and other relevant information,'[8] 'the nature and likelihood of success of the proposed treatment and . . . of its risks and side-effects,'[15] 'the available options, their advantages and disadvantages,'[18] 'the knowledge that he has a choice to make,'[19] 'who he is, where he is, what he is reading and what he is doing in signing the paper,'[20] and 'the consequences of participation or non-participation' (L.H.R., letter to G. Klerman, MD, April 16, 1980). At an extreme, the recently promulgated DHHS regulations for obtaining informed consent require that up to 14 separate items, including such things as the availability of compensation for injuries, be disclosed to, and presumably understood by, the potential subject.[13] The rigor of the requirement of understanding obviously increases with the amount and complexity of material that is required to be understood. Some writers make understanding the sine qua non of their standard of competency,[21] and it has long been the primary element of legal tests of contractual and testamentary capacity.[7]

'Factual understanding' actually encompasses two different standards: one can require, as many writers do, that the subject have the 'ability to understand,' or more strictly, one can insist that the subject manifest 'actual understanding' of the material.[14] A modified and limited 'ability to understand' standard appears to be coupled with an 'evidencing of choice' standard to establish the standard for 'assent' to minimal-risk research in the recommendations of the National Commission for the Protection of Human Subjects of Biomedical and Behavioral Research,[11] a standard that approximates the level existing in the days prior to the advent of the law of informed consent.

Table 2 Factual understanding of issues

Factual understanding, encompassing ability to understand and/or actual
understanding
   Has cognitive capacity to consider relevant issues
   Understands nature of procedure, its risks, and other relevant information[8]
   Understands nature and likelihood of success of proposed treatment and its
      risks and side effects[15]
   Knows available options, their advantages and disadvantages[18]
   Knows that he has choice to make[19]
   Knows who he is, where he is, what he is reading, and what he is doing in
      signing form[20]
   Knows consequences of participation or nonparticipation[*]
   Knows up to 14 separate items that must be considered, e.g. availability of
      compensation for injuries[13]

Relevant psychiatric aspects
Intelligence[22]
   IQ
      Mental retardation
      Some organic states
   Adaptive capacity to tasks of everyday life
      Chronic psychiatric illness
      Effects of institutionalization
Language skills[22]
Attention[23]
   Acute psychotic episodes
Orientation[†]
   Acute psychotic episodes
Recall and recent memory[†23]
   Acute psychotic episodes
   Chronic schizophrenia[24]
All these factors impaired by
   Long-standing brain damage
   Acute toxic states

[*] L.H.R., letter to G. Klerman, MD, April 16, 1980.

[†] J. O. Cole, MD, letter to D, Klein, MD, Dec 22, 1977.

Relevant Psychiatric Aspects. – The elements of a person's mental
functioning that seem important to his ability to display a factual
understanding of the issues include intelligence,[22] of which IQ may be one
measure, and adaptive capacity to the tasks of everyday life; language
skills;[22] attention;[23] orientation (J. O. Cole, MD, letter to D. Klein, MD, Dec
22, 1977); recall; and recent memory (L.H.R., letter to G. Klerman, MD,
April 16, 1980).[23] Intelligence can be impaired by mental retardation or a
variety of organic states; adaptive capacity is further susceptible to limitation by chronic psychiatric illness and probably by the effects of institutionalization. The other factors likewise all are capable of being impaired by
long-standing brain damage or acute toxic states. Attention and orientation
also may suffer during acute psychotic episodes, and there is some evidence
to suggest that memory may be impaired in chronic schizophrenia.[24]

Testing for Competency. – Means of demonstrating a subject's actual
understanding of issues related to his decision include, in increasing order of
difficulty, asking him to repeat the information provided, asking him to paraphrase it in his own words, and requiring that he display an ability to put
some or all of the information to practical use. One difficulty in testing
understanding of the consequences of a decision (often conceptualized as the
risks and benefits) is the possibility of divergence between what the investigator perceives as a benefit or a risk and the subject's view of the matter.[25]
Consequences of participation, such as prolonged hospitalization, which are
often thought of as a disadvantage, might seem quite desirable to a socially
isolated or otherwise impoverished subject.

Rational Manipulation of Information

One step beyond measuring factual understanding is determining how the
information that the subject assimilates is utilized in the decision-making

Table 3 Rational manipulation of information

How information is used in decision-making process
   Has good judgment[23]
   Is rational,[22] insane delusions absent[7]
   Tests reality[23]
   Has decision-making capacity

Relevant psychiatric aspects
   Delusions[15,26]
   Hallucinations
   Loosening of associations or other severe thought disorder
   Extreme phobia or panic[19]
   Anxiety[23]
   Euphoria[19]
   Depression[19]
   Anger
   Agitation
   Obsessive preoccupation
   [*]Excessive dependency[19,23]
   [*]Passivity[23]
   [*]Unwarranted trust[23]

[*] These aspects may relate to the voluntariness of the decision.

process (Table 3). The rubrics by which this standard is discussed include
judgment,[23] rationality,[22] rational weighing of risks and benefits, reality
testing,[23] and decision-making capacity. Legal rules concerning contractual
and testimonial capacity traditionally have recognized at least one defect of
rationality, the presence of 'insane delusions,' as grounds for invalidating a
person's acts.[7]

Relevant Psychiatric Aspects. – In addition to delusions, which are
acknowledged by a number of writers as potentially significant factors
affecting competency,[15,26] other symptoms that may have a similar effect
include hallucinations, loosening of associations, or other severe thought
disorder; severe or extreme degrees of phobia; panic;[19] anxiety;[23] euphoria;[19] depression;[19] anger;[19] agitation; and obsessive preoccupation.
The existence of a pathologic relationship (ie, one marked by excessive
dependency,[19,23] passivity,[23] or unwarranted trust[23]) with the party seeking
consent or with someone who may be affected by the consent has been
suggested as a factor that also could contribute to impaired rationality. This
condition, however, seems to be related more to the issue of the voluntariness of the decision, to the appreciation of alternatives, or to the knowledge
that a decision needs to be made.

Testing for Competency. – Rationality frequently is tested in the mental
status examination by the standard questions that elicit hallucinatory and
delusional material (eg, Schneiderian signs) and by the use of vignettes that
pose a problem to which the patient is asked to respond. A less structured
test suggested by J. O. Cole, MD, is whether the potential subject can carry
on an ordinary conversation in such a way as to indicate that he can understand questions and answer in a logical and reasonable manner (letter to
D. Klein, MD, Dec 22, 1977). In troublesome cases, it may be necessary to
inquire about or to observe the rationality of the subject's decision making
outside the formal psychiatric examination. Data from family or friends
may establish that the seeming rationality displayed in the examining room
is abandoned by the subject when he is confronted with real demands for
action.

The subjective nature of any assessment of rationality frequently has
been pointed to as a major obstacle to the successful use of such a test.[21] But
an even greater problem may lie in the consensus of most experts today
that an impairment of rationality does not necessarily affect global decision-making ability, that is, that the impact of delusions, for example, may
be limited to a discrete area of mental functioning. Although this
belief awaits definitive empirical verification, it indicates the possible utility
of a test of rationality directed to the specific decision at hand rather than
to the person's general functioning.

Frequently, however, there is difficulty in drawing the required causal links between the presence of even clearcut delusional phenomena and the subject's specific decision. It has been suggested that one means of so doing may be to demonstrate that in the absence of the subject's delusions, the decision would have been made differently. But that may be to place greater emphasis on the outcome of the decision than on the process by which it was derived, the latter comprising the core of the rationality standard. In addition, except in rare cases, such proof would be extremely difficult. More practical would be a test in which the presence of any of the signs or symptoms just noted in the subject's chain of reasoning about participation in research would raise a serious but rebuttable doubt as to the subject's rational manipulation of the relevant information.

Appreciation of the Nature of the Situation

The strictest standard for competency requires that, once understanding has been attained, the rational manipulation of information take place in the context of the subject's appreciation of the nature of his situation (Table 4). Appreciation is distinct from factual understanding in that it requires the subject to consider the relevance to his immediate situation of those facts he has understood previously in the abstract. It differs from the rational manipulation of information by requiring that the subject take certain crucial data into consideration, rather than merely asking him to manipulate rationally whatever information is already at hand. This has been phrased in a variety of ways, asking that the subject 'appreciate the

Table 4 Appreciation of nature of situation

Appreciation
  Appreciates nature of situation (affectively as well as cognitively)
  Appreciates consequences of giving or withholding consent[26]
  Senses who he is and why he is agreeing[20]
  Recognizes in a mature fashion, implications of alternative courses of action
    and appreciates both cognitively and affectively nature of thing to be
    decided[27]
  Appreciates what is relevant to forming judgment of issue in question, ie,
    considers relevant evidence[10]
  * For all of these, appreciates
    That he has problem or psychiatric condition appropriate for study†
    That proposed procedures are intended to achieve research ends and not
      only (if at all) therapeutic ends[30]
    That there may be both treatment and research staff members involved
      in his care and that their roles may differ†
    That treatment offered may have been selected on randomized basis[31,32]
    That both he and his caretakers may be blind to nature of treatment
    That he may receive placebos
  * Has awareness of how others view decision[19]

Relevant psychiatric aspects
  Denial (lack of insight) about[23]
    Fact and severity of illness or condition[39]
    Fact that research and not merely treatment is being proposed
    Possibility of improvement with and without research procedures
    Scientific methodology of study (eg, placebo, double-blind.randomization)
  Capacity for abstract thinking, affected by
    IQ
    Education
    Psychosis
    Organic brain damage
    Experience (eg, age, 'maturity')[18]
  Psychotic level
    Distortion
    Projection
    Nihilism
    Hopelessness-helplessness

* As relevant for a given research project.
† J. O. Cole, MD, letter to D. Klein, MD, Dec 22. 1977.

consequences of giving or withholding consent,'[26] have 'a sense of who he is and why he is agreeing,'[20] recognize, 'in a mature fashion, the implications of alternative courses of action and appreciate both cognitively and affectively the nature of the thing to be decided,'[27] or 'appreciate what is relevant to forming a judgment of the issue in question – i.e., . . . consider relevant evidence.'[10]

'Appreciation' has been discussed widely in relation to the somewhat analogous issue of criminal responsibility. According to the formulation of the Model Penal Code of the American Law Institute, the lack of 'substantial capacity . . . to appreciate the wrongfulness of his conduct' is one situation in which a defendant will be held to be nonculpable.[28] Appreciation, in this sense, is taken to be an affective, as well as a cognitive, recognition of the nature of the situation.[29] This precludes finding culpable a person who knows in the abstract that to murder is wrong but who believes that divine writ has relieved him of the need to adhere to that rule. In the research setting, using this standard, a person who understood the nature of the proposed procedures and could evaluate rationally their risks and benefits but who believed that he was being asked to participate in an exclusively therapeutic process, rather than an experimental process, would be found to be lacking in capacity to consent.

Suggestions as to the components of the situation that ought to be appreciated by the subject include that the subject has a problem or psychiatric condition appropriate for study (J. O. Cole, MD, letter to D. Klein, MD, Dec 22, 1977), that the proposed procedures are intended to achieve research ends and not only (if at all) therapeutic ends,[30] that there may be both treatment and research staff members involved in his care and that their roles may differ (J. O. Cole, MD, letter to D. Klein, MD, Dec 22, 1977), that the treatment that is offered may have been selected on a randomized basis,[31,32] that both he and his caretakers may be blind to the nature of the treatment, and that he may receive placebos. An additional proposal is that the subject have an 'awareness of how others view the decision, the general social attitude toward the choices and an understanding of his reason for deviating from that attitude' if he chooses to do so.[19]

The extent of the lack of appreciation of some of these elements has been demonstrated in studies that revealed that without a clear-cut explanation most subjects were not able to infer that research was going on;[33] that a majority of parents of pediatric research patients did not recognize the research nature of the hospitalization;[30] that only medically trained subjects were able to appreciate fully the risks in a drug study despite extensive explanation;[34] that even when patients were told that they were being given a placebo, they still ascribed therapeutic powers to it;[35] and specifically with regard to psychiatric patients, that patient-subjects have difficulty in distinguishing beneficial from nonbeneficial aspects of research;[36] that 68% of schizophrenic patients failed to cite their illness as the reason for treatment;[37] and that only 46% of a sample of newly admitted voluntary psychiatric patients could acknowledge clearly the presence of psychiatric problems.[38]

Relevant Psychiatric Aspects. – The major psychopathological mechanism that can impair appreciation (given the ability to rationally manipulate information) is denial,[23] which sometimes is termed lack of insight. Denial can affect the subject's appreciation of the fact and severity of the illness or condition,[39] the fact that research and not merely treatment is being proposed, the possibility of improvement with and without the research procedures, and the scientific methodology of the study (eg, placebo, double-blind, randomization). Other factors that may influence appreciation include the capacity for abstract, as opposed to concrete, reasoning (which is affected by intelligence, level of education and 'maturity,'[18] as well as psychosis and organic brain damage); and psychotic-level distortion, nihilism, and hopelessness-helplessness. The law, in some nonpathological circumstances, traditionally has included a variant of the 'appreciation standard' for determining competency. Thus, adolescents, who can both understand and rationally manipulate information, are nevertheless enjoined from making unaided treatment or research decisions, presumably on the basis of lacking the maturity required for genuine appreciation.

Testing for Competency. – A subject's ability to appreciate, in general, can be estimated by the usual techniques of judging insight and determining the presence of psychotic-level defenses. Specifically with regard to the research setting, the subject's appreciation can be tested by examining his grasp of the factors just discussed. Whether the extent of the subject's appreciation needs to coincide precisely with the investigator's is a controversial topic. Some commentators have suggested that, in a therapeutic setting, the patient need only 'understand the nature of the mental condition which the psychiatrist believes him to have,' without necessarily agreeing with that judgement.[15,40] Such a standard, however, more closely resembles a factual-understanding test than a genuine test of appreciation. Although some people may be uncomfortable with such a criterion, of necessity the subject's views (eg, on the presence or absence of illness or the results of accepting or refusing participation) ultimately must be measured by their correspondence with the consensus of knowledgeable (usually professional) opinion on those issues.

Choosing the Standard

Despite wide variation in the wording of many attempts to define the standards for competency, they appear, as was just shown, to be classifiable into four general categories. Rather than deriving a single standard for competency from this discussion of the relevant mental functions and the psychopathologic states that may impair them, one is left with a range of testable functions that, depending on where the line is drawn, can yield multiple standards for competency of varying stringency. Furthermore, it is clear from this approach that any of the four resulting standards, or some combination of them, are 'legitimate' as long as they can be justified from some reasonable policy perspective.

Although the place at which one chooses to draw the line ought to be determined by the policy-oriented goals that one is seeking to attain, difficulties arise when more than one policy goal is sought, when the desired goals are incompatible, or when no consensus can be attained on the desired goals. The ultimate standard for competency thus is almost certain to be a compromise that seeks to maximize the desirable effects of applying a given standard while minimizing the undesirable ones. This process becomes clearer when consideration is given to the possible goals that one might attain by varying the standard by which a subject is considered competent. Such goals inevitably include a mixture of concerns relating to the societal values that we wish to implement and to the preferences we wish to confer in these values. The values at stake in the choice of a standard for competency to consent to research inevitably include a mixture of symbolic and instrumental concerns.

Autonomy

Also referred to as self-determination, the principle of encouraging autonomy for the subject has been considered one of the central goals underlying the entire doctrine of informed consent.[22,41,42] By requiring comprehensive disclosure of information to the experimental subject, informed consent is said to return to him maximal power to decide what should or should not be done with his body. Insofar as many writers see the power to make one's own decisions as the essential attribute of autonomous functioning, they argue for a minimal standard for competency or for abolishing the requirement for competency altogether.[17,43] A standard that requires no more than evidencing a choice would maximize autonomy thus conceived.

Rational Decision Making

The promotion of rational decision making is seen as a good in itself by several authors,[41,42] even those who at the same time view maximizing the subject's autonomy as a primary goal of informed consent. Rationality in decision making would seem to require a very high standard for competency, at least rational manipulation of information and probably appreciation of the nature of the situation, since the rationality of the outcome when such appreciation is lacking may well be in doubt.

Beneficence

Somewhat out of fashion these days as a goal of policy making and usually omitted from discussions of the objectives of informed consent, beneficence represents the ethical imperatives both to protect others from harm and to do good whenever possible.[22] So construed, beneficence favors a stringent standard for competency, at least rational manipulation of information and probably appreciation of the nature of the situation, to achieve the following three ends: (1) honoring autonomous decisions only when the subject's capacity to behave autonomously is clearly present; (2) protecting those who, lacking competency, would consent to research that involved risk to them; and (3) assuring that incompetent subjects who refuse participation that might be highly advantageous to them nonetheless are permitted (some would say compelled) to benefit by participating in the research project.

Although this is the way in which the topic usually is discussed, it is of interest that the entire doctrine of informed consent can be seen in terms of beneficence rather than as a requirement only designed to promote autonomy. To the extent that the requirement for informed consent limits the freedom of the individual to consent to research under conditions that may be acceptable to him but not (because risk is involved) to society as a whole, it limits an individual's exercise of autonomy for the sake of his protection.

Respect for Persons

This term tends to be used in a variety of ways, but has been defined as 'using a person as an end and not a means,'[44] as 'protecting the patient's status as a human being,'[42] and as not taking advantage of the subject (S. Shah, PhD, oral communication, Sept 1980). The goal of avoiding fraud and duress also would seem to belong here.[42] As an ethical objective, respect for persons carries within it the tension between allowing as much autonomy as the person can manage reasonably and providing protection to those with diminished autonomy. It therefore encourages a compromise between the goals of autonomy and beneficence and may point toward an intermediate standard such as factual understanding or rational manipulation of information.

Justice

Highlighted by the Belmont Report as a primary ethical consideration in undertaking research,[22] justice in this sense usually is conceived of as distributive justice, that is, assuring that the burdens of participating in research do not fall inequitably on certain groups. This goal can be accomplished by raising the level for competency required from those groups one wishes to protect. In effect, this is what the court in the *Kaimowitz* case attempted to do by raising the level of competency required from a prisoner to the point at which no prisoner could meet it. The court manipulated the level of competency required to enforce its conviction that the participation of prisoners in psychosurgical procedures under any circumstances was undesirable.

On the other hand, there has been some attention given to the distribution of the benefits of participation in research, such as enhanced self-esteem, and consequent objections to being treated differently have been raised on behalf of some groups. It has been argued, for example, that creating special regulations governing research with the elderly would contribute to an unfair characterization of older people as generally senile and in need of special protections;[45] heightened restrictions on the use of certain classes of subjects, such as the mentally ill, also are thought to deprive those most in need of advances in research of the possibility of progress (D. F. Klein, MD, letter to Task Force for Protection of Human Subjects, American Psychiatric Association, Dec 4, 1978).

Insofar as undesirable effects are likely to accrue disproportionately to vulnerable groups only to the extent that their ultimate choices about participation in research differ from those of the population at large, the argument also may be made that one must examine the nature of the decisions of presumptively incompetent subjects as a group before one legitimately can require that they receive special protection. One study has shown that the distribution of decisions about participation in hypothetical research projects was the same in a group of medical patients as in a group of psychiatric patients.[46] Assuming this finding can be validated, it may well bring into question the usefulness of excluding subjects on the basis of incompetency in protecting autonomy, assuring beneficence and respect for persons, and achieving justice for the mentally ill.

Encouragement of Research

Certainly some researchers feel strongly that the requirement for informed consent can serve to deter the pursuit of important areas of knowledge.[47] It seems apparent that varying the level of competency required from subjects can affect their absolute availability, the ease with which they can be recruited, and the expense that their recruitment entails. As self-evident as that proposition appears, it is unclear, pending empirical investigation, in which direction the standard of competency should be moved to encourage research. A low standard of competency is advocated both by researchers, who believe that most subjects given a choice will consent to their procedures, and by lawyers, who are more interested in autonomy than in research and believe that most subjects will refuse. A favored solution of many researchers is to abolish the requirement for competency to give informed consent altogether, replacing it instead with a rigorous, objective examination of the risks and benefits entailed by the project. Once some outside, knowledgeable committee has concluded that the benefits of the study outweigh the risks, it is advocated that subjects be permitted to consent regardless of their level of competency.[48]

Furthermore, it may be that decisions made about research participation, even if uninformed, pressured, or made by people of dubious competence, may not differ from the decisions that all of us make in everyday life, such as when buying a used car or choosing a brand of shampoo. If it is desirable to treat research no differently from those other situations (this may relate to the desire to encourage research or to some sense of fairness), then the level for competency should be set at the same presumably low level that obtains generally. While experimental data would be required to ascertain what that level is in a variety of settings, the increasing technical complexity of our society makes it likely that many decisions in everyday life are made without appreciation of their consequences, without the ability to manipulate in a rational manner the information that is provided, and probably without full knowledge of the relevant details. Such an argument would militate toward a low standard of competency for consent to research (although it does not affect the desirability of providing information to the subjects), perhaps merely evidencing a choice.

Subject Satisfaction

If, in the same sense that we wish to maximize autonomy, we also are concerned with the level of satisfaction that subjects display concerning their participation or failure to participate in research, an attempt might be made to vary the level of competency required to take that into account. Those who are excluded by too high a standard (or included by means of a proxy consent rather than their own choice) and those who were included by too low a standard and later feel trapped by the decision that they were permitted to make both might desire the level at which the line is drawn to be adjusted accordingly. Only empirical data on the numbers of subjects who fall into each group will allow this end to be accomplished.

Test Administration

A prime consideration in many judicial formulations of standards and procedures, the *ease of administration* also may be an important factor in selecting a standard for subjects' competency. Ease of administration refers not only to the time and effort required to perform the assessment, but also to its reliability, that is, its reproducibility and the possibilities for manipulation and corruption. Along these lines, some authors have objected to

standards for competency carried out at any level higher than 'factual understanding' because of the inherent difficulties in determining the rationality of thought processes and the subject's appreciation of the nature of his situation.[21] Following a similar line of reasoning, objections have been raised to the use of any standard higher than evidencing a choice.[17] Nonetheless, the data needed for the selection of an appropriate standard by means of the reliability criterion do not yet exist; they await empirical testing of a variety of definitions of competency in a controlled setting.

The choice of a standard also may be affected by the *sensitivity* and *specificity* of the procedures that must be used to establish whether the requirements of a particular standard have been met. A highly sensitive test yields a low number of false-negative findings; a highly specific test yields few false-positive findings.[49] Depending on one's tolerance for incompetent subjects to be included in research or for competent ones to be excluded (which may relate to how highly valued are the factors of autonomy, beneficence, and encouragement of research), one might want to choose a standard that when linked to the procedures used to test for competency exhibited one or another of these characteristics. Such a characterization of any of the standards or the procedures used to test for them, however, also awaits experimental definition.

Temporal Considerations

Rather than setting a unitary level of competency for all subjects at the time of their entry into a research project, one might assume that they will become more understanding, better able to manipulate the information, and more appreciative of the nature of the situation as they go along. Reflecting this expected change, one might require a relatively low standard for competency at the time of entry into the project (for example, the ability to understand) but also require reconsent as the project proceeds, with a higher standard utilized at that time. This approach, which emphasizes 'experiential' as much as informed consent, represents a means of reconciling autonomy, beneficence, and encouragement of research.

Conclusion

It is apparent that before the appropriate standard for competency to participate in research can be selected intelligently, a good deal of additional empirical data, as well as further clarification of the requisite moral imperatives, is required. At this point in time, it is difficult to say with assurance that we know where to draw the line to ensure the attainment of any of the policy goals just outlined. What is needed is empirical testing of the reliability and validity of the various ways of characterizing competency, a characterization of the general population and of discrete populations of particular concern according to these standards, and a comparison of the decisions made by those who meet or fail to meet a particular standard. Only then will we be able to protect the variety of interests involved in human experimentation in a meaningful way.

This work was supported in part by grants from the Foundations' Fund for Research in Psychiatry and by Public Health Service research grant MH27553, National Institute of Mental Health Center for Studies of Crime and Delinquency and Mental Health Services Development Branch.

References

1 **Frenkel DA**: Human experimentation: Codes of ethics. *Leg Med Q* 1977;**1**:7–14.

2 **Curran WJ**: Governmental regulation of the use of human subjects in medical research: The approach of two federal agencies, in Freund PA (ed): *Experimentation With Human Subjects.* New York, George Braziller Inc, 1970, pp 402–454.

3 **Romano J**: Reflections on informed consent. *Arch Gen Psychiatry* 1974;**30**:129–135.

4 **Marston RQ**: The background of the National Institutes of Health (NIH) position on ethical problems of clinical studies. *Fertil Steril* 1972;**23**:596–600.

5   Beecher HK: Ethics and clinical research. *N Engl J Med* 1966;**274**:1354–1360.

6   US Dept of Health, Education, and Welfare: *The Institutional Guide to DHEW Policy on Protection of Human Subjects*, publication No. (NIH) 72–102 US Dept of Health, Education, and Welfare. 1971.

7   Green MD: Judicial tests of mental incompetency. *Mo Law Rev* 1941;**6**:141–165.

8   *Kaimowztz us Michigan Department of Mental Health*: Civil Action 73–19434-A W (Wayne County, Mich, Cir Ct 1973), in Brooks AD: *Law, Psychiatry and the Mental Health System*. Boston, Little Brown & Co, 1974, pp 902–921.

9   Stone AA: The history and futures of litigation in psychopharmacologic research and treatment, in Gallant DM, Force R (eds): *Legal and Ethical Issues in Human Research and Treatment: Psychopharmacologic Considerations*. New York, Spectrum Publications Inc, 1978, pp 19–37.

10   Murphy JG: Therapy and the problem of autonomous consent. *Int J Law Psychiatry* 1979;**2**:415–430.

11   National Commission for the Protection of Human Subjects of Biomedical and Behavioral Research: *Report and Recommendations Research Involving Those Institutionalized as Mentally Infirm*, publication No. (OS) 78–0006. US Dept of Health, Education, and Welfare, 1978.

12   Public response critical of HEW regulations on mentally disabled. *IRB Rev Hum Subjects Res* 1979;**1**(April):8–9.

13   US Dept of Health and Human Services: Final Regulations Amending Basic HHS Policy for the Protection of Human Research Subjects. *Federal Register* 1981(Jan 26);**46**:8366–8392.

14   Roth LH, Meisel A, Lidz CW: Tests of competency to consent to treatment. *Am J Psychiatry* 1977;**134**:279–284.

15   Burra P, Kimberley R, Miura C: Mental competence and consent to treatment. *Can J Psychiatry* 1980;**25**:251–253.

16   Shapiro MH: Legislating the control of behavior control: Autonomy and the coercive use of organic therapies. *South Calif Law Rev* 1974;**47**:237–356.

17   Barnhart BA, Pinkerton ML, Roth RT: Informed consent to organic behavior control. *Santa Clara Law Rev* 1977;**17**:39–83.

18   US Dept of Health, Education, and Welfare: Provision of sterilization in federally assisted programs of the Public Health Service. *Federal Register* 1978(Nov 8);**43**:52146–52175.

19   Michels R: Competence to refuse treatment. Read before the conference 'Refusing Treatment in Mental Health Institutions: Values in Conflict,' Boston. Nov 11, 1980.

20   Owens H: When is a voluntary commitment really voluntary? *Am J Orthopsychiatry* 1977;**47**:104–110.

21   Friedman PR: Legal regulation of applied behavior analysis in mental institutions and prisons. *Ariz Law Rev* 1975;**17**:39–104.

22   National Commission for the Protection of Human Subjects of Biomedical and Behavioral Research: *The Belmont Report: Ethical Guidelines for the Protection of Human Subjects of Research*, publication No. (OS) 78–0012 US Dept of Health, Education, and Welfare, 1978.

23   Schwarz ED: A revised checklist to obtain consent to treatment with medication. *Hosp Community Psychiatry* 1980;**31**:765–767.

24   Cutting J: Memory in functional psychosis. *J Neurol Neurosurg Psychiatry* 1979;**42**:1031–1037.

25   Gray BH: *Human Subjects in Medical Experimentation: A Sociological Study of the Conduct and Regulation of Clinical Research*. New York, John Wiley & Sons Inc, 1975, p 118.

26   Hoffman BF: Assessing competence to consent to treatment *Can J Psychiatry* 1980;**25**:354–355.

27   Pastel RI: Civil commitment A functional analysis. *Brooklyn Law, Rev* 1971;**38**:1–94.

28   American Law Institute: Model penal code: Official draft (1962), in Vorenberg J (ed): *Criminal Law and Procedure: Cases and Materials. St* Paul, Minn, West Publishing Co, 1975, pp 909–980.

29   Goldstein AS: *The Insanity Defense*. New Haven, Conn, Yale University Press. 1967.

30   McCollum AT, Schwartz AH: Pediatric research hospitalization: its meaning to parents. *Pediatr Res* 1969;**3**:199–204.

31   Levine RJ, Lebacqz K: Some ethical considerations in clinical trials. *Clin Pharmacol Ther* 1979;**25**:728–741.

32   McLean PD: The effect of informed consent on the acceptance of random treatment assignment in a clinical population. *Behav Ther* 1980;**11**:129–133.

33   Park LC, Slaughter R, Covi L, et al: The subjective experience of the research patient: An investigation of psychiatric outpatients' reactions to the research treatment situation. *J Nerv Ment Dis* 1966;**143**:199–206.

34   Garnham JC: Some observations on informed consent in nontherapeutic research. *J Med Ethics* 1975;**1**:138–145.

35   Park LC, Covi L, Uhlenhuth EH: Effects of informed consent on research patients and study results. *J Nerv Ment Dis* 1967;**145**:349–357.

36   Lidz CW, Roth LH: The signed form – informed consent?, in Boruch RF, Ross J, Cecil JS (ads): *Solutions to Legal and Ethical Problems in Applied Social Research*. New York, Academic Press Inc, to be published.

37   Soskis DA: Schizophrenic and medical inpatients as informed drug consumers. *Arch Gen Psychiatry* 1978;**35**:645–647.

38   Appelbaum PS, Mirkin SA, Bateman AL: Empirical assessment of competency to consent to psychiatric hospitalization. *Am J Psychiatry* 1981; **138**:1170–1176.

39   Faden R, Faden A: False belief and the refusal of medical treatment. *J Med Ethics* 1977;**3**:133–136.

40   Culver CM, Ferrell RB, Green RM: ECT and special problems of informed consent. *Am J Psychiatry* 1980;**137**:586–591.

41   Annas GJ, Glantz LH, Katz BF: *Informed Consent to Human Experimentation: The Subject's Dilemma*. Cambridge, Mass, Ballinger Publishing Co, 1977, pp 33–38.

42   Capron AM: Informed consent in catastrophic disease research and treatment *Univ Pa Law Rev* 1974; **123**:340–438.

43   Goldstein J: On the right of the 'institutionalized mentally infirm' to consent to or refuse to participate as subjects in biomedical and behavioral research, in National Commission on the Protection of Human Subjects of Biomedical and Behavioral Research: *Appendix to Research Involving Those Institutionalized as Mentally Infirm*, publication No. (OS) 78–0007. US Dept of Health, Education, and Welfare, 1978, chap 2.

44   Macklin R, Sherwin S: Experimenting on human subjects: Philosophical perspectives. *Case Western Reserve Law Rev* 1975; **25**:434–471.

45   Ostfield AM: Older research subjects: Not homogeneous, not especially vulnerable. *IRB Rev Hum Subjects Res* 1980; **2** (October):7–8.

46   Stanley B, Stanley M, Lautin A, et al: Preliminary findings on psychiatric patients as research participants: A population at risk? *Am J Psychiatry* 1981; **138**:669–671.

47   Cole JO: Research barriers in psychopharmacology. *Am J Psychiatry* 1977; **134**:896–898.

48   Chayet NL: Informed consent of the mentally disabled: A failing fiction. *Psychiatr Ann* 1976; **6**:255–299.

49   McNeil BJ, Keeler E, Adelstein SJ: Primer on certain elements of medical decision making. *N Engl J Med* 1975; **293**:211–215.

Decisional Capacity for Informed Consent in Schizophrenia Research*

William T. Carpenter, Jr, James M. Gold, Adrienne C. Lahti, Caleb A. Queern, Robert R. Conley, John J. Bartko, Jeffrey Kovnick, and Paul S. Appelbaum

The decisional capacity of persons with schizophrenia has become central to the debate on the ethics of psychiatric research.[1-3] Schizophrenia is manifested by distortions in perception, disorganization of thought, and weakening of motivation and emotional responsivity.[4] Any of these elements of the illness, in theory, may reduce the capacity to make decisions. Commentators in the media, perhaps influenced by the public caricature of persons with schizophrenia as being bizarre and 'out of touch,' have questioned whether persons with schizophrenia can make informed judgments about participating in research. It is urgent to address this issue with relevant data, as state and national commissions are proposing statutes and regulations to address perceived problems in the conduct of research with subjects whose diagnoses are associated with decisional impairments.[5-7]

Most patients with schizophrenia, however, are not judged to be incompetent and routinely handle their day-to-day affairs. Studies[8,9] of the capacity of schizophrenic patients to make decisions regarding their treatment demonstrate that, as a group, they do more poorly than nonill (normal) comparison subjects and other patient groups with medical and psychiatric illnesses. However, numerous people with schizophrenia, even when acutely ill, perform no worse than many members of the general population.[8,9] Recent data[10] suggest that patients with schizophrenia participating in research are able to understand and retain consent information.

This study was designed to shed light on this issue by examining the performance of a group of schizophrenic research subjects. The aims were to (1) assess the degree of decisional impairment in a cohort of research subjects, (2) evaluate the extent to which the symptoms of schizophrenia and cognitive impairments affect decisional capacity, and (3) explore the efficacy of an educational intervention to improve the decision-making capacity of impaired subjects.

Subjects and Methods

Subjects

Schizophrenic subjects were drawn from inpatient and outpatient research programs at the Maryland Psychiatric Research Center (MPRC), Baltimore. Twenty inpatients and 10 outpatients meeting *DSM-III*[11] or *DSM-IV*[12] criteria for schizophrenia (n = 28) or schizoaffective disorder (n = 2) were selected for the study if they were enrolled as research subjects and receiving clinical services in an inpatient research unit for treatment-resistant schizophrenia (n = 10), an inpatient research unit focused on young schizophrenic patients with chronic illnesses (n = 10), or an outpatient research program focused on patients whose schizophrenia is only partially responsive to treatment (n = 10). Patients were eligible for selection if they were in a research protocol or if they had signed a consent form preparatory for research participation. Inpatient subjects were selected in order of date of signing a consent form (most recent first). Twenty-two were approached; 20 assented. For eligible outpatients, selection depended on the time of the next appointment. Ten patients were approached, and 10 assented. Medication status was not a selection criterion, but all subjects were receiving antipsychotic medication during participation in this study. Approximately half the patients were taking new-generation compounds; exact data are unavailable as the code on clinical trial participants has not been broken. Drug treatment was in a continuation phase in all patients, and minimal clinical change was expected between assessment sessions. For 7 patients taking clozapine, the dose range was from 400 to 700 mg/d, with a modal dose of 400 mg/d. The dose range for haloperidol was from 10 to 30 mg/d, and for olanzapine, from 10 to 30 mg/d, with 15 mg/d being the modal dose for each. Univariate statistics (the 2 × 2 Yates corrected X^2 test for discrete

Table 1 Demographic characteristics of schizophrenic subjects and nonill comparison subjects*

Characteristic	Schizophrenic Subjects (n = 30)	Normal Control Subjects (n = 24)	Schizophrenic Reference Group (N = 493)	Test Statistic†	P
Females, %	43.3	21.8	32.9	$\chi^2_1 = 0.96$	0.33
Nonwhites, %	23.3	29.2	31.6	$\chi^2_1 = 0.56$	0.45
Age, y	40.2 (8.8)	39.7 (10.2)	34.5 (8.9)	$t_{521} = 3.41$	0.001
Education, y	12.2 (2.4)	11.5 (2.1)	12.1 (2.3)	$t_{521} = 0.21$	0.82
Length of illness, y	20.0 (7.9)	...	14.2 (8.3)	$t_{521} = 3.72$	0.001
Hollingshead socio-economic status score	3.9 (2.7)	4.3 (1.0)	4.1 (1.0)	$t_{521} = 0.92$	0.36

* Data are given as mean (SD) unless otherwise indicated. Ellipses indicate data not applicable.

† Comparison of the schizophrenic subjects with the schizophrenic reference group.

* Carpenter, W.T., Gold, J.M., Lahti, A.C., Queern, C.A., Conley, R.R., Bartko, J.J., Kovnick, J. and Appelbaum, P.S.: Decisional capacity for informed consent in schizophrenia research. *Archives of General Psychiatry* **57**:533–538, 2000.

and the 2-group *t* test for continuous variables) were used to compare this sample with the entire patient subject population of the MPRC-National Institute of Mental Health Intervention Research Center (N = 493) to determine representativeness.

The nonill comparison subjects were recruited from community centers and a free medical clinic by researchers at the University of Virginia, Charlottesville. They were told that the study would evaluate how people use information to make decisions and that no treatment would be provided. Descriptive information for the 30 schizophrenic subjects and the 24 normal subjects is provided in Table 1.

In accordance with a federal regulation (45 CFR §46.101.B), this protocol was reviewed and determined exempt from written informed consent by the University of Maryland, Baltimore, Institutional Review Board. Patients were enrolled in the study after the nature of their requested involvement was described to them and they assented to participate.

Clinical Ratings

Clinical assessments were conducted through the support framework of the MPRC – National Institute of Mental Health Clinical Research Center. The *DSM-IV* diagnosis is made as a best estimate by a trained research psychiatrist using all available sources of information, including the Structured Clinical Interview for the *DSM*, family informants, and medical records. The Brief Psychiatric Rating Scale (BPRS)[13] is routinely administered in each program to measure psychopathologic features. Brief Psychiatric Rating Scale evaluations were always within a week of testing for decisional capacity. Raters are typically research nurses or master's level clinicians trained to reliability standards by the MPRC – National Institute of Mental Health Intervention Research Center Assessment Core. Pearson product moment correlations were performed to ascertain the relation between schizophrenia symptoms, as measured by the BPRS, and performance on The MacArthur Competence Assessment Tool-Clinical Research (MacCAT-CR).

Assessment of Decisional Capacity

Decisional capacity was measured by the MacCAT-CR. This instrument provides a structured format for the assessment of 4 areas of decisional capacity related to generally applied legal standards for competence to consent to treatment and research: understanding relevant information, appreciation of the implications of the information for one's own situation, reasoning with the information in a decisional process, and evidencing a choice.[14] It is derived from an instrument developed to measure capacity to consent to treatment in the clinical setting. The MacArthur Competence Assessment Tool-Treatment,[15] which, in turn, represents a condensation of an extensive set of instruments constructed for research on informed consent and decisional capacity.[16] Both sets of instruments have demonstrated good interrater reliability and concurrent validity as capacity assessment tools.[8,9,16] Many issues may compromise capacity to consent, including hope, unrealistic expectations, relations, and various emotions. However, the impact of these affective factors is expected to be manifest in the 4 areas of decisional capacity.[17]

We developed a version of the MacCAT-CR that describes a randomized, double-blind trial of a novel antipsychotic medication for this study. Subjects were told to pretend that they were being asked to consent to participation in the study. Information disclosure was followed by structured queries and probes of the 4 areas of decisional capacity previously described. A scoring manual provided explicit criteria for raters, with possible scores ranging from 0 to 6 on the Understanding scale, 0 to 6 on the Appreciation scale, 0 to 8 on the Reasoning scale, and 0 to 2 on the Choice scale. (The manual for the MacCAT-CR and the version used in this study are available from the authors.) Ten raters were trained to administer the MacCAT-CR. Reliability exercises were conducted involving 10 raters and 12 patients, with raters alternating as testers and observers. The version of the MacCAT-CR developed for this study was evaluated for reliability with intraclass *r* statistics for continuous, and a weighted κ for dichotomous, ratings.[18]

To provide similar decisional capacity data drawn from a nonill population, one of us (J.K.) administered a version of the MacCAT-CR identical in form but slightly different in content to subjects recruited for a separate study at the University of Virginia. Both versions were based on a hypothetical clinical trial. The minor differences involved naming the drug and overlapping, rather than an identical list of, adverse effects.

Cognitive Assessment

Subjects completed a brief cognitive battery to assess overall level of cognitive impairment and abilities that are relevant to the process of obtaining informed consent. The battery included the following: (1) the Wide Range Achievement Test 3 reading subtest, a measure of single-word decoding;[19] (2) the Repeatable Battery for the Assessment of Neuropsychological Status (RBANS), a brief screening measure that yields scaled index scores for immediate and delayed memory, language, attention, and visuospatial skills, and an overall total scaled score;[20] and (3) the letter-number sequencing subtest from the Wechsler Adult Intelligence Scale III, a measure of auditory working memory.[21] The Wide Range Achievement Test and the RBANS have a normal mean of 100 and an SD of 15 based on the normal standardization samples described in test manuals. Letter-number sequencing has a normal mean of 10 and an SD of 3 based on the Wechsler Adult Intelligence Scale III standardization sample. Patients also received a nonstandard version of the Gray Oral Reading Test.[22] The test was adapted so that subjects read aloud a series of 7 short passages and then answered 5 questions that tested their comprehension of the material. The standard version of the test includes a total of 13 items. The items selected for this study were drawn from the easy and moderate difficulty levels of the 2 test forms.

Testing was performed within 7 days of the MacCAT-CR assessment. Complete test protocols were completed by 26 of the 30 subjects. One subject was not tested; 3 were missing single measures, as they wanted to discontinue testing or had difficulty with task demands, producing data that were judged to be invalid. All cognitive tests were administered by a single research assistant trained and supervised by one of us (J.M.G.) in the MPRC – National Institute of Mental Health Intervention Research Center Neurocognitive Core.

To assess the relation between the MacCAT-CR score and cognitive variables, we performed stepwise regressions for the Understanding, Appreciation, and Reasoning scales, with all cognitive variables available for entry at the first step.

Educational Remediation of Decisional Impairments

The poor performance of the subjects with schizophrenia on the MacCAT-CR, which assessed their capacities in relation to a hypothetical study, contrasted sharply with the impressions of research staff that these same subjects previously had given adequate consent for participation in actual research projects. These impressions, moreover, were confirmed by a standardized measure of understanding, the Evaluation of Signed Consent (ESC),[23] which each of them had been required to pass before enrollment into an actual study. It was hypothesized that the extended educational process that preceded consent to the actual study accounted for the difference.

A subset of poorly performing schizophrenic subjects participated in an educational process during a 1-week period in which information about the MacCAT-CR hypothetical study was presented. *Poor performance* was defined as a score below 20, the normal control median, on the MacCAT-CR Understanding scale. This cutoff point was chosen to allow room for improvement in performance and because scores above the cutoff point are unequivocally normal. All but 2 of the patients who scored below the normal control median were available for this part of the study (n = 20). The 2 patients had scored 19 and 6 on the Understanding scale; 1 declined further participation, and 1 was medically ill.

The educational remediation intervention was an abbreviated version of the informed consent process used at the MPRC. Subjects took part in 2 sessions of about 30 minutes reviewing the study protocol. Information was provided again, questions were asked, and prompts were used to assist the subjects in mastering the material. Some inpatient subjects also spent extra time with a computerized interactive routine designed to teach basic concepts such as protocol, random assignment, drug withdrawal, and placebo. Others spent some extra time with a flip chart that reviewed relevant information. Personnel were from the nursing or research staffs of each clinical unit and were accustomed to assisting patients with informed consent. The outpatient subjects had only the 2 intervention sessions without additional aids.

Statistical Analysis

Basic univariate statistics, the 2-group t test for continuous variables, and the Yates corrected 2×2 χ^2 test for discrete variables were used for comparing demographic characteristics of the schizophrenic subjects with a schizophrenic reference group. To examine the capacity for informed consent in schizophrenic research subjects compared with nonill comparison subjects, the 2-group t test was used. To test the hypothesis that reduced capacity for informed consent can be remediated with an educational informed consent process, the paired t test was used to compare preeducation vs posteducation decisional capacity scores. The Pearson product moment correlation was used, assessing the association between decisional capacity and cognitive measures.

For the 2-group comparison between 30 patients with schizophrenia and 24 normal comparison subjects, there was 80% statistical power, with a type I error of 5% to detect a difference of 5.45 Understanding units, 1.83 Reasoning units, 1.44 Appreciation units, and 0.45 Choice units, each with an effect size of 0.8. Actual results, with the exception of Choice, exceed these limits and effect size of 0.8.

For the paired t comparison between pretest and posttest scores of 20 patients with schizophrenia, we have 80% statistical power, with a type I error of 5% to detect a difference of 3.9. Understanding units, 1.8 Reasoning units, and 1.4 Appreciation units, each with an effect size of 0.66. Actual results, with the exception of Reasoning, exceed these limits and effect size of 0.66 decisional capacity, and (3) explore the efficacy of an educational intervention to improve the decision-making capacity of impaired subjects.

Results

The present study cohort was mildly more symptomatic on BPRS measures when compared with MPRC patients as a whole (mean [SD] BPRS score, 47.3 [13.9] vs 39.6 [12.5]; $t_{492} = 3.22$; $P = .001$). The mean (SD) BPRS factor 1 psychosis score was also significantly higher in the present study cohort (10.6 [4.2] vs 8.8 [4.3]; $t_{491} = 2.14$; $p = .03$). This study cohort, although skewed toward chronic schizophrenia with substantial psychosis that has proved resistant to ordinary treatment, is representative of the patients who participate in studies at the MPRC on sociodemographic and illness chronicity variables.

Reliability results for 3 of the essential elements of informed consent reflect substantial between – rater agreement on the scoring of items. The

weighted κ for Choice (yes or no) was 0.52 and represents 82% agreement between raters. The Understanding scale had an intraclass correlation of 0.98. The intraclass correlation was 0.84 for the Reasoning and Appreciation scales.

MacArthur Competence Assessment Tool–Clinical Research scores for the 30 subjects with schizophrenia and the 24 members of the normal comparison group at the University of Virginia are presented in Table 2. The subjects with schizophrenia scored significantly lower than the comparison group on the Understanding, Reasoning, and Appreciation scales; scores on the Choice scale were lower as well but just failed to reach statistical significance.

Symptoms and Decisional Capacity

Pearson product moment correlations with total BPRS scores, representing global pathologic characteristics, and factor 1 scores, representing psychosis, are presented in Table 3. Psychopathologic features showed a moderate negative correlation with performance, reaching statistical significance for the Understanding and Reasoning scales.

Cognition and Decisional Capacity

The patients had a mean standard score of 82.2 (SD, 16.2) on the Wide Range Achievement Test 3 (normal mean, 100; SD, 15), a scaled score of 5.5 (SD, 3.2) on letter- number sequencing (normal mean, 10; SD, 3), and an RBANS total scaled score of 63.3 (SD, 14.4; normal mean, 100; SD, 15). Thus, this is a sample with marked impairments that might be expected to compromise decisional capacity.

There were 2 significant predictors of Understanding scale performance: the RBANS total score, $R^2 = 0.67$ ($P < .001$) (Figure); and the Gray Oral Reading Test word reading score, $R^2 = 0.09$ ($P < .006$). There were 2 significant predictors of the MacCAT-CR Reasoning scale: the RBANS total score, $R^2 = 0.58$ ($P < .01$); and the RBANS immediate memory index, $R^2 = 0.09$ ($P < .02$). Two significant predictors were observed for the Appreciation scale: letter-number sequencing, $R^2 = 0.66$ ($P < .02$); and the Visuospatial scale from the RBANS, $R^2 = 0.06$ ($P < .03$). Therefore, cognitive measures were highly predictive of MacCAT-CR performance.

As shown in Table 4, the 20 subjects who completed the MacCAT-CR a second time after the educational intervention showed significant improvements in Understanding scores. Only 9 of the 20 patients still scored below the cutoff of 20, bringing the total number of subjects with schizophrenia who scored 20 or higher either at the original administration of the MacCAT-CR or after remediation to 21 of 30. This proportion of subjects (70%) was significantly greater than the proportion of normal comparison subjects in the University of Virginia study who scored 20 or higher (46%; $P < .04$). Moreover, there was no difference in the mean Understanding scores between these two groups (19.3 [SD, 7.1] for the schizophrenic group [n = 21] vs 20.2 [SD, 3.8] for the normal subjects [n = 24]; $t_{43} = -0.54$; $P = .59$).

Table 2 MacCAT-CR scores for subjects with schizophrenia and the University of Virginia nonill comparison group[*]

MacCAT-CR Scale	Theoretical Range of the Variable	Schizophrenic Subjects (n = 30)	Normal Control Subjects (n = 24)	t_{52}	P
Understanding	0–26	12.9 (8.5)	20.2 (3.8)	3.90	0.001
Reasoning	0–8	3.5 (2.8)	5.5 (1.4)	3.20	0.002
Appreciation	0–6	2.3 (2.0)	4.4 (1.5)	4.30	0.001
Choice	0–2	1.6 (0.7)	1.9 (0.3)	1.96	0.06

[*] Data are given as mean (SD) unless otherwise indicated. MacCAT-CR indicates The MacArthur Competence Assessment Tool–Clinical Research

The MacCAT-CR does not provide a score below which a subject is known to lack capacity for informed consent. However, 2 patients continued to score below the range defined by the normal control group after the educational intervention. The lowest-scoring subject was removed from research participation based on lack of capacity independent of this study. The other patient continued in research and had passed the ESC test at the time consent was accepted as valid. In earlier work,[23] some subjects required more than the 1 week of educational intervention to pass the ESC. This may account for continued research participation despite a low score on the second MacCAT-CR.

Comment

Patients with schizophrenia demonstrated significantly poorer performance than a nonill comparison group on the MacCAT-CR, an instrument designed to measure decisional capacities relevant to consent to research. Performance was only moderately related to psychotic symptoms per se, but was strongly correlated with cognitive impairments. These findings agree with the common clinical observation that the degree of psychotic symptoms, except at the extreme, does not robustly predict patients' functionality in daily life.[24]

The poor performance of many of the subjects with schizophrenia, however, did not reflect an enduring inability to understand the information relevant to a research study. When offered additional opportunities to learn the necessary data, most subjects who scored below an a priori cutoff were able to bring their scores into the range of a comparison group of people without schizophrenia. This suggests that people with severe forms of schizophrenia may be able to give informed consent for research, although a single-session brief presentation of research procedures may not be sufficient. Rather, an informed consent process that engages potential subjects over time and is sensitive to the negative impact of cognitive impairment may be essential for adequate informed consent. This conclusion is also supported by the report[10] of good performance by schizophrenic subjects on informed consent material after learning and practice sessions.

This study also underscores the proper role of capacity assessment instruments like the MacCAT-CR. Such instruments can identify subjects at high risk for impaired performance in an actual informed consent process, and many of these subjects can provide adequate consent following an educational intervention. Therefore, poor performance on a decisional capacity assessment should not exclude subjects from research participation. Needed instead are efforts to identify the basis for the observed impairments and to devise means of attempted remediation.

Although these findings offer hope regarding the decisional capacity of schizophrenic patients, they derive from a limited number of subjects in a single institution and are viewed as preliminary. The results are supported by experience at the MPRC with the ESC test, which documents that patients can achieve a good understanding of protocol risks, demands, and procedures for withdrawing from a study and other data relevant to informed consent. Similar results reported from the University of California, Los Angeles,[10] also suggest that these results may generalize more broadly to research subjects with schizophrenia. Nevertheless, additional work will be required to determine the generalizability of these data to other samples, diagnostic groups, and research settings and to identify the most effective means of educating research subjects to diminish the effects of their cognitive limitations. The question of how to use decisional capacity data from normal populations to define the range of performance that constitutes 'competence' for informed consent is not resolved. This study is also limited in this regard by using a normal comparison group developed at a different site.

Successful remediation through an educational informed consent process has clear implications for the validity of consent at the time it is given. A complicated and unresolved issue relates to perseverance over time of understanding, appreciation, reasoning, and choice. Experience with the ESC suggests surprisingly good retention over time and following medication withdrawal.[23] We do not have data with the MacCAT-CR in a schizophrenic sample to address this question, but data from a group of depressed subjects showed little change in performance over time.[25] Nevertheless, we suggest that retention of key elements, rather than detailed knowledge, is critical

Table 3 MacCAT-CR Pearson Product Moment Correlations with symptoms for the 30 schizophrenic subjects[*]

MacCAT-CR Scale	Total BPRS Score	P	BPRS Factor 1[†]	P
Understanding	−0.34	.07	−0.38	.04
Reasoning	−0.47	.01	−0.52	.01
Appreciation	−0.27	.15	−0.37	.04
Choice	−0.16	.40	−0.31	.10

[*] MacCAT-CR indicates The MacArthur Competence Assessment Tool–Clinical Research; BPRS, Brief Psychiatric Rating Scale.

[†] Psychosis factor.

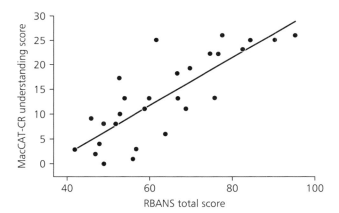

Figure The Pearson product moment correlation between decisional capacity and cognitive performance (r 5 0.82). MacCAT-CR indicates The MacArthur Competence Assessment Tool–Clinical Research; RBANS, Repeatable Battery for the Assessment of Neuropsychological Status.

Table 4 Results of the 20 MPRC patients with a baseline understanding scale score of less than 20 who completed the education program[*]

MacCAT-CR Scale	Theoretical range of the variable	Preprogram score	Postprogram score	Change in score	Paired t₁₉	P
Understanding	0–26	8.35 (5.4)	18.35 (7.3)	10.00 (5.9)	7.55	.001
Reasoning	0–8	2.35 (2.0)	3.70 (2.9)	1.35 (2.7)	2.21	.04
Appreciation	0–6	1.35 (1.3)	3.25 (2.4)	1.90 (2.1)	3.95	.001

[*] Data are given as mean (SD) unless otherwise indicated. MPRC indicates Maryland Psychiatric Research Center; MacCAT-CR, The MacArthur Competence Assessment Tool–Clinical Research.

during research participation. Key elements certainly include awareness that one is in a research study, that participation is voluntary, and that withdrawal of consent can be done without a penalty. Remembering the name of a drug or the full list of adverse effects may be less important in determining an ethical basis for continued research participation.

Concerning the public discussion of decisional capacity of the mentally ill to consent to research, we call attention to 3 implications of the data reported. First, patients with schizophrenia who have chronic and severe illnesses may have decisional capacity for informed consent. Second, if decisional capacity is impaired, it may be remediated. Third, cognition appears more relevant than psychosis in predicting decisional capacity in schizophrenic patients. It follows that the proposition that a psychotic person ipso facto should lose decision-making power for research decisions is flawed and stigmatizing. Rather than restrict research participation for categories of patients, emphasis should be placed on assuring that procedures for informing and documenting adequacy of consent are routinely practiced.

This study was supported by grant 2p30MH40279 from the National Institute of Mental Health, Rockville, Md(Dr Carpenter); and an Established Investigator Award from the National Alliance for Research on Schizophrenia and Depression, Great Neck, NY (Dr Carpenter).

References

1 **Annas GJ.** Experimentation and research. *J California Alliance Merit III.* 1994;5:9–11.

2 **Levine R.** A researcher's concern with ethics in human research. *J California Alliance Ment III.* 1994; **5**:6–8.

3 **Shamoo AE.** Our responsibility towards persons with mental illness as human subjects in research. *J California Alliance Ment III.* 1994;5:14–16.

4 **Carpenter WT, Buchanan RW.** Schizophrenia. *N Engl J Med.* 1994; **330**:681–690.

5 Advisory Work Group on Human Subject Research Involving Protected Classes. *Recommendations on the Oversight of Human Subject Research Involving the Protected Classes.* Albany: Department of Health, State of New York; 1998.

6 *Final Report of the Attorney General's Research Working Group.* Baltimore: Office of the Maryland Attorney General; 1998.

7 National Bioethics Advisory Commission. *Research Involving Persons With Mental Disorders That May Affect Decision Making Capacity.* Rockville, Md: National Bioethics Advisory Commission; 1998.

8 **Grisso T, Appelbaum PS.** The MacArthur Treatment Competence Study, III: abilities of patients to consent to psychiatric and medical treatments. *Law Hum Behav.* 1995;**19**:149–174.

9 **Grisso T, Appelbaum PS, Hill-Fotouhi C.** The MacCAT-T: a clinical tool to assess patients' capacities to make treatment decisions. *Psychiatr Serv.* 1997;**48**:1415–1419.

10 **Wirshing DW, Wirshing WC, Marder SR, Liberman RP, Mintz J.** Informed consent: assessment of comprehension. *Am J Psychiatry.* 1998;**155**: 1508–1511.

11 American Psychiatric Association. *Diagnostic and Statistical Manual of Mental Disorders, Third Edition.* Washington, DC: American Psychiatric Association; 1980.

12 American Psychiatric Association. *Diagnostic and Statistical Manual of Mental Disorders, Fourth Edition.* Washington, DC: American Psychiatric Association; 1994.

13 **Overall JE, Gorham DE.** The Brief Psychiatric Rating Scale. *Psychol Rep.* 1961;**10**:799–812.

14 **Appelbaum PS, Grisso T.** *The MacArthur Competence Assessment Tool-Clinical Research.* Sarasota, Fla: Professional Resource Press; 1996.

15 **Grisso T, Appelbaum PS.** *The MacArthur Competence Assessment Tool-Treatment.* Sarasota, Fla: Professional Resource Press; 1998.

16 **Grisso T, Appelbaum PS, Mulvey EP, Fletcher K.** The MacArthur Treatment Competence Study, II: measures of abilities related to competence to consent to treatment. *Law Hum Behav.* 1995;**19**:127–148.

17 **Appelbaum PS.** Ought we to require emotional capacity as part of decisional competence? *Kennedy Inst Ethics J.* 1999;**8**:377–387.

18 **Bartko JJ, Carpenter WT.** On the methods and theory of reliability. *J Nerv Ment Dis.* 1976;**163**:307–317.

19 **Wilkinson GS.** *Wide Range Achievement Test: Administration Manual.* 3rd ed. Wilmington, Del: Wide Range Inc; 1993.

20 **Randolph C.** *The Repeatable Battery for the Assessment of Neuropsychological Status.* San Antonio, Tex: The Psychological Corporation; 1998.

21 **Wechsler D.** *Wechsler Adult Intelligence Scale: Administration and Scoring Manual.* 3rd ed. San Antonio, Tex: The Psychological Corporation; 1997.

22 **Wiederholt JL, Bryant BRM.** *Gray Oral Reading Tests.* 3rd ed. Austin, Tex: Pro-Ed, Inc; 1992.

23 **DeRenzo EG, Conley RR, Love R.** Assessment of capacity to give consent to research participation: state-of-the-art and beyond. *J Health Care Law Policy.* 1998;**1**:66–87.

24 **Appelbaum PS.** Missing the boat: competence and consent in psychiatric research. *Am J Psychiatry.* 1998;**155**:1486–1488.

25 **Appelbaum PS, Grisso T, Frank E., O'Donnell S, Kupfer D.** Competence of depressed patients for consent to research. *Am J Psychiatry.* 1999;**156**: 1380–1384.

Caring About Risks

Are Severely Depressed Patients Competent to Consent to Research?*

Carl Elliott

Depressed patients are often asked to take part in clinical research, and often this research carries risks. A depressed patient might be enrolled in a protocol to evaluate a new antidepressant drug, for example, or in one that requires a washout period, in which the patient's current medication will be discontinued. Some institutional review boards continue to approve protocols that test new antidepressants against placebo controls. Any of these situations entail risks, primarily the risk that the depressed patient's condition will worsen. The potential harm can be considerable, and at the extreme end of the spectrum includes the risk for suicide.

Although the concept of competence to consent to treatment and research has been widely and thoroughly discussed,[1–5] only a few accounts give any attention to depression. Sometimes depression is not even considered a warning sign that a person's competence to consent needs to be evaluated, largely because it is not thought to be the type of disorder that would ordinarily interfere with competence. It is only the rare depressed patient who is psychotic, and while depression may often interfere with a person's memory and concentration, often this interference is not severe enough to raise any warning flags. Most accounts of competence focus on intellectual capacity and abilities to reason, and depression is primarily a disorder of mood. According to conventional thinking, depression is primarily about despair, guilt, and a loss of motivation, while competence is about the ability to reason, to deliberate, to compare, and to evaluate. Often these latter abilities are ones that depression leaves intact.

I want to challenge this account of competence and argue that depression may well impair a patient's competence to consent to research. Most crucially, it can impair a person's ability to evaluate risks and benefits. To put the matter simply, if a person is depressed, he or she may be *aware* that a protocol carries risks, but simply not *care* about those risks. This sort of intellectual impairment can be as important a part of patient competence as the more detached, intellectual understanding that most accounts of competence emphasize. If my argument is correct, then institutional review boards need to take special precautions in allowing researchers to enroll depressed patients in research protocols.

Competence and Accountability

Competence is conventionally defined as the ability to perform a task – in this case, to consent to enroll in a research protocol.[6,7] What counts as competence to consent will then depend on what one counts as the abilities relevant to the task in question. According to a widely accepted account of competence, the 1983 US President's Commission Report,[8] the relevant abilities are (1) the ability to reason and deliberate, (2) the ability to understand and communicate information, and (3) the possession of values and goals. As conceptualized within this framework, a potential research subject takes in the relevant information, weighs it according to his or her goals and values, and then reasons to an informed decision.

This account of competence, however, is incomplete. If competence to consent to research is defined simply as the ability to make a decision to enroll in a research protocol, we face the familiar problem of what *counts* as that ability—of trying to decide whether a person is incompetent by virtue of making a poor decision, or by virtue of making an irrational decision, or by virtue of coming to that decision in an unsystematic, illogical, or erratic way. Since even competent people are sometimes stubborn, obtuse, or unreasonable, we need an account of competence that explains why we sometimes believe that a person can be both competent and make bad, irrational, or even unreasonable choices.

What we really want to know when we ask if a patient is competent is whether that individual is able to make a decision *for which he or she can be considered accountable*.[9] What we want to know is whether the decisions that a person makes – whether they are good or bad, rational or irrational – are decisions for which that person can legitimately be considered responsible. This is why we define certain mental abilities as relevant: we realize that certain conditions or disorders impair a person's mental abilities such that he is not a morally responsible agent. He can make decisions, but we would not feel comfortable ascribing him with the credit or blame for that decision. If a person is making a decision that will affect his life in momentous ways, we will naturally be concerned that he makes a sound decision. But because we recognize that a person generally has the right to make even unsound decisions, a judgment about competence ensures that whatever decision a person makes, it is truly *his* decision: a decision for which he can finally be held accountable.

Once we conceptualize competence in this way, it becomes clear that it is not just intellectual ability that is relevant to competence. A person's emotional state can also affect her decisions in ways that might lead us to say that she cannot be judged fully accountable for them. The criminal law recognizes this, for example, and often grants leniency when a person acts under severe emotional distress. We often make decisions in the heat of anger or under the cold weight of despair that are uncharacteristic, that we would not have made otherwise, that we later regret, and for which we believe we should not be considered fully accountable. Likewise, we often recognize that it would be unfair to hold a person to a decision that he or she made in the face of overwhelming fear. In emotional extremes, we value, think, and behave differently – sometimes so differently that we might later believe that the decisions we have made are not decisions for which we can be held completely and unproblematically responsible.

The importance of emotion and mood for competence has not been lost on psychiatrists.[10–14] Some accounts of competence stipulate that persons must 'appreciate' the consequences of their choices, rather than simply understand them factually, the term 'appreciate' implying a fuller, deeper comprehension of how the decision will affect the patient's life.[15,16] A patient who can flatly recite the effects of treatment may still seem to fail to appreciate fully just how the treatment is going to affect his or her health. Nor can affect be completely divorced conceptually from cognition. Bursztajn and his colleagues[17] have pointed out how a patient's affect can influence competence by altering his or her beliefs. For example, a depressed patient, convinced that his situation will never change, may refuse treatment based on the unrealistic belief that it will not help him.

However, while some patients may have affective disorders that disrupt their cognitive, rational decision-making abilities, a slightly different sort of depressed patient presents other problems. This is the depressed patient

* Elliot, C.: Caring about risks. Are severely depressed patients competent to consent to research? *Archives of General Psychiatry* **54**:113–116, 1997.

who is capable of understanding all the facts about his illness and the research protocol in which he is enrolling, and who appreciates the risks and the broader implications of the protocol on his life, but who, as a result of his illness, is not *motivated* to take those risks into account in the same way as the rest of us. For example, these patients might realize that a protocol involves risks, but simply not *care* about the risks. Some patients, as a result of their depression, may even *want* to take risks. Roth et al[18] wonder about the competence of one such patient, a 49-year-old woman capable of fully understanding the electroconvulsive therapy for which she was being asked to consent, but who, when told that electroconvulsive therapy carried a 1 in 3000 chance of death, replied, 'I hope I am the one.'

Several writers have speculated about whether depression might lead patients to overestimate the side effects of interventions and underestimate the likelihood of benefit.[17,19,20] Although there are apparently no empirical studies examining the question of whether depressed patients are more likely than nondepressed patients to consent to risky or uncomfortable research, Lee and Ganzini[21,22] have studied the effects of depression and its treatment on the preferences of elderly patients for life-sustaining medical therapies. In a study of 43 depressed patients, a subgroup of 11 severely depressed patients were more likely to choose life-sustaining therapies after their depression had been treated than they were while depressed.[23] However, while this suggests that severe depression might affect the way some patients evaluate risks and benefits, it is not clear whether evaluation of life-sustaining therapy is similar enough to evaluation of research risks to bear much comparison.

Nonetheless, it seems unlikely that severely depressed patients are in the best position to make important decisions about their welfare. The Royal College of Psychiatrists in the United Kingdom is one of the few bodies to recognize this explicitly, offering the example of a patient with depressive delusions who consents to risky research because he thinks he is guilty and deserves to be punished.[24] However, given the sense of hopelessness and worthlessness that characterizes some severely depressed patients, it seems reasonable to worry about their decision making. The novelist William Styron describes his own agonizing depressive episode as

the diabolical discomfort of being imprisoned in a fiercely overheated room. And because no breeze stirs this cauldron, because there is no escape from this smothering confinement, it is entirely natural that the victim begins to think ceaselessly of oblivion.[25]

Depression and Competence

Although other writers have suggested that affective disorders may interfere with a patient's competence to consent to treatment, none has considered competence to consent to research, and only a few have attempted to say *why* depression impairs competence.[7] That is, while there are not many writers who would dispute that mood is a part of ordinary decision making, it is also normal for a person's mood to change from one time to another, and it is not immediately obvious why a depressed mood should invalidate a patient's competence.

There are 2 good arguments for the conclusion that some depressed patients are incompetent to consent to research, each of which is persuasive for a slightly different type of patient. The first might be called the argument from *authenticity*. When a person is caught in the grip of depression, his values, beliefs, desires, and dispositions are dramatically different from when he is healthy.[7] In some cases, they are so different that we might ask whether his decisions are truly his. A decision may not be truly his in the sense that it reflects dispositions and values that are transient and inconsistent with much more deeply ingrained traits of his character. One might say 'I wasn't myself' when looking back on a time of despondency, and a caricature of the authenticity argument would hold that we should take this declaration literally: I was not myself, so that decision is not mine. Yet underneath that caricature is a grain of truth. If a person is so deeply depressed that his decisions are wildly inconsistent with his character, it seems problematic to abide by his decisions, particularly if the depression is dramatic and reversible.[26]

Here is where the notion of competence as accountability is helpful. If a person were to behave badly while mentally ill–say, in a full-blown manic episode – we would very likely think it unfair to hold him fully responsible for what he has done. His behavior was uncharacteristic; he would never have acted this way unless he was manic; his mania is temporary and reversible with lithium treatment. His actions in the manic state were not truly his. Similarly for the depressed patient being asked to consent to research: his mental state is such that his behavior and choices do not seem to be truly his. If something untoward were to happen to him during the research, for instance, we could not in good conscience say that he bears the full responsibility for undergoing that risk.

The authenticity argument supposes a person with a stable character and entrenched dispositions, who, while depressed, makes decisions so uncharacteristic that we feel bound to question whether those decisions were truly hers. However, sometimes this break between the depressed and predepression personality is not so dramatic. Some patients are chronically depressed, and others are depressed periodically. It would not be plausible to argue that the decisions of these depressed patients do not reflect their underlying characters – characters that are closely tied to their depression. Yet there comes a point where, if a person appears largely insensitive to her own welfare, we might believe that she is incompetent to consent to research. Why should this be so?

One answer lies in what might be called the argument from *self-interest*. Our ordinary relationships with other people are based on certain assumptions about their thoughts and behavior. One of these assumptions is that other persons have some minimal concern for their own welfare. For example, the assumption that other people ordinarily both have some minimal degree of self-interest and are best positioned to judge their own interests lies at the heart of the institution of informed consent.

However, if we have reason to believe that severely depressed patients do not have this minimal degree of concern, then a fundamental assumption underlying informed consent is undermined. We justify exposing patients to the risks of research by the assumption that the patient is evaluating that risk with some degree of concern for her welfare. A competent evaluation of risks involves taking into account one's own well-being: not necessarily taking it as an overriding or supremely important concern, but at least taking it into account. If a person is so depressed that she fails to take her interests into account in deciding whether to take a risk, then we can hardly be comfortable saying that she is accountable for taking that risk.

Conclusions

Two broad types of conclusions can be drawn from these arguments, one empirical and the other conceptual. First, more empirical research needs to be carried out to determine the ways in which severe depression might affect psychological factors relevant to competence. For example, it would be important to know the extent to which severe depression affects how much a person cares about his or her own well-being, or how it might affect a person's willingness to expose himself or herself to potential harm.

Second, these arguments suggest that we may need to alter our conventional ways of assessing competence. As I have argued, many conventional accounts of how competence should be assessed downplay the importance of emotional factors. However, if my arguments are convincing, it may not be enough for psychiatrists or researchers to evaluate competence simply by testing a person's memory and reasoning ability, such as with a Mini-Mental State Examination. Rather, it may be that evaluations should also be concerned with a person's affective and motivational state: whether a person's mood has dramatically changed recently, how concerned a patient appears to be about her own well-being, how carefully she looks at risks and benefits, and so on. Of course, sound and uniform ways of assessing these affective and motivational factors will need to be developed.

On a practical level, these arguments have potential implications for the conduct of clinical research protocols testing new treatments for major depression. For example, if it is concluded that severe depression does impair competence to consent, clinical research protocols involving subjects with depression will need to require explicitly that the competence of subjects be evaluated before entering the study. This requirement might be similar to that of psychiatric research protocols testing new antipsychotic drugs, which generally state that subjects either be competent to consent or that consent be obtained from an appropriate surrogate.

Finally, this view of competence could have practical implications for studies involving relatively poor risk-benefit ratios. Sometimes severely depressed patients are enrolled in protocols in which their depression is likely to worsen (eg, as a result of being assigned to a placebo treatment arm). Researchers argue that exposing competent adults to these sorts of risks is justified at least in part by the institution of informed consent, with the corresponding presumption that potential subjects understand the risks of the protocol, consent to them, and can be judged accountable for undertaking them.[27] But if severely depressed patients are incompetent, exposing them to the risk of having their illness worsen is much more difficult to justify.[28,29]

Acknowledgments to Fonds pour la Formation de Chercheurs et l'Aide a la Recherche (Quebec) for their financial support.

Thanks to Charles Weijer for his comments on the manuscript.

References

1   **Appelbaum P, Lidz C, Meisel A.** *Informed Consent Legal Theory and Clinical Practice.* New York, NY: Oxford University Press; 1986.

2   **Drane J.** The many faces of competency. *Hastings Cent Rep.* 1985;**15**:17–21.

3   **Gaylin W.** The competence of children: no longer all or none. *Hastings Cent Rep.* 1982;**12**:33–38.

4   **Lidz C, Meisel A, Zerubavel E, Carter M, Sestak R, Roth L.** *Informed Consent: A Study of Decisionmaking in Psychiatry.* New York, NY: Guilford Press; 1984.

5   **Jonsen A, Siegler M, Winslade W.** *Clinical Ethics.* 3rd ed. New York, NY: Macmillan Publishing Co; 1992.

6   **Faden R, Beauchayp T.** *A History and Theory of Informed Consent.* New York, NY: Oxford University Press; 1986.

7   **Buchanan AE, Brock DW.** *Deciding for Others: The Ethics of Surrogate Decision Making.* Cambridge, England: Cambridge University Press; 1989.

8   US President's Commission for the Study of Ethical Problems in Medicine and Biomedical and Behavioral Research. *Making Health Care Decisions: The Ethical and Legal Implications of Informed Consent in the Patient-Practitioner Relationship.* Washington, DC: US Government Printing Office; 1983.

9   **Elliott C.** Competence as accountability. *J Clin Ethics.* 1991;**2**:167–71.

10 **Culver CM, Ferrell RB, Green RM.** ECT and the special problems of informed consent. *Am J Psychiatry.* 1980;**137**:586–591.

11 **Gutheil TH, Bursztajn H.** Clinician's guidelines for assessing and presenting subtle forms of patient incompetence in legal settings. *Am J Psychiatry.* 1986;**143**:1020–1023.

12 **Fulford KWM, Howse K.** Ethics of research with psychiatric patients: principles, problems and the primary responsibility of researchers. *J Med Ethics.* 1993;**19**:85–91.

13 **Ganzini L, Lee MA, Heintz RT, Bloom JD.** Is the Patient Self-Determination Act appropriate for elderly persons hospitalized for depression? *J Clin Ethics.* 1993;**4**:46–50.

14 **Maria J.** The PSDA and geriatric psychiatry: a cautionary tale. *J Clin Ethics.* 1993;**4**:80–81.

15 **Gutheil TG, Appelbaum PS.** *Clinical Handbook of Psychiatry and the Law.* New York, NY: McGraw-Hill Book Co; 1982.

16 **Appelbaum P, Roth L.** Competency to consent to research: a psychiatric overview. *Arch Gen Psychiatry.* 1982;**39**:951–958.

17 **Bursztajn HJ, Harding HP, Gutheil TG, Brodsky A.** Beyond cognition: the role of disordered affective states in impairing competence to consent to treatment. *Bull Am Acad Psychiatry Law* 1991;**19**:383–388.

18 **Roth L, Meisel A, Lidz C.** Tests of competency to consent to treatment. *Am J Psychiatry.* 1977;**134**:279–284.

19 **Ganzini L, Lee MA, Heintz RT, Bloom JD.** Donot – resuscitate orders for depressed psychiatric inpatients. *Hosp Community Psychiatry.* 1992;**43**:915–919.

20 **Sullivan MD, Youngner SJ.** Depression, competence and the right to refuse lifesaving medical treatment. *Am J Psychiatry.* 1994;**151**:971–978.

21 **Lee MA, Ganzini L.** Depression in the elderly: effect on patient attitudes toward life-sustaining therapy. *J Am Geriatr Soc.* 1992;**40**:983–988.

22 **Lee MA, Ganzini L.** The effect of recovery from depression an preferences for life-sustaining therapy in older patients. *J Gerontol.* 1994;**49**:15–21.

23 **Ganzini L, Lee MA, Heintz RT, Bloom JD, Fern DS.** The effect of depression treatment on elderly patients' preferences for life-sustaining medical therapy. *Am J Psychiatry.* 1994;**151**:1631–1636.

24 Royal College of Psychiatrists. *Guidelines for Ethics of Research Committees on Psychiatric Research Involving Human Subjects.* London, England: Royal College of Psychiatrists; 1989.

25 **Styron W.** *Darkness Visible: A Memoir of Madness.* New York, NY: Random House; 1990.

26 **Shamoo A, Irving D.** The PSDA and the depressed elderly: 'intermittent competency' revisited. *J Clin Ethics.* 1993;**4**:74–79.

27 **Roth L, Appelbaum P.** Obtaining informed consent for research with psychiatric patients. *Psychiatr Clin North Am.* 1983;**6**:551–565.

28 **Freedman B.** Placebo-controlled trials and the logic of clinical purpose. *IRB Rev Hum Subjects Res.* 1990; **12**(6):1–6.

29 **Rothman KJ, Michels KB.** The continuing unethical use of placebo controls. *N Engl J Med.* 1994;**331**:394–398.

Informed Consent and the Capacity for Voluntarism*

Laura Weiss Roberts

Informed consent is built upon the elements of information, decisional capacity, and voluntarism. Information in the consent process generally encompasses issues such as the nature of the illness, the anticipated risks and benefits of the proposed procedure, and possible alternatives, including non-intervention[1,2]. Decisional capacity, in turn, comprises the ability to communicate, understand, and logically work with information and to appreciate the meaning of a decision within the context of one's life[3,4]. Our understanding of voluntarism in this country is more intuitive and involves philosophical ideals of freedom, independence, personhood, and separateness[5,6].

The application of the concept of voluntarism has been very unclear in both research and clinical contexts[7–18]. This ambiguity, furthermore, has prevented the resolution of several serious controversies in the field of psychiatry[7,19,20]. The question of whether people suffering from chronic psychotic illnesses who are involuntarily hospitalized can freely choose to participate in research, for example, is a key controversy, and it is a different issue than questions as to whether they have the capacity to understand and make an informed decision[20–22]. Whether people with depression complicated by suicidality are too vulnerable to make a voluntary choice regarding treatment preferences or research enrollment, separate from their level of understanding, is another important ethical dilemma that is increasingly gaining attention in the study of mental illness[23–25]. Similarly, current practices of obtaining consent for nonapproved uses of prescription medications among elders with dementia or children pose serious ethical problems. These are not simply because of the issues of decisional capacity of ill elders and children but also because of the expectation in national ethics and regulatory standards that these individuals must be offered as much choice in the decisional process as they are capable of exercising[17,26–31]. In other words, these considerations are not reducible to the question of whether individuals have the capacity to assimilate, rationally weigh, and appreciate the factual information with which they are presented. There is also the issue of whether they can make these decisions in a manner that is uncoerced and true to their personal beliefs and values. Guidelines for assessing the capacity for voluntarism have not previously been developed, despite the centrality of this concept for fulfilling informed consent and for resolving key ethical problems in mental illness research and clinical care. Indeed, the ethical meaning of informed consent and its merit as a safeguard respectful of the person – whether a patient or a research participant – derive largely from the way in which a person's choice and values may be recognized, expressed, and honored through authentic voluntarism[6].

Influences on Voluntarism

Influences on voluntarism are implicitly recognized in the characteristics of traditionally defined special populations[7,8]. Children, for instance, may not have developed an internal capability for free, deliberate choice, and developmentally disabled people, depending on the degree and nature of their deficits, may never acquire this ability[9]. This is not simply a concept of cognitive maturity or sophistication but, rather, of emotional development and the emergence of distinct personhood[10]. People with dementia live out an erosion of the self, losing their personal history, beliefs, motivations, relationships, and independence along with their memory, intellect, and self-care skills[11]. Institutionalized people and prisoners, by virtue of their external situations, have such an altered experience of freedom that the potential for genuine, uncoerced choice is diminished[12–14]. Among some mentally ill people, the presence of certain symptoms, such as ambivalence, diminished motivation, disengagement, or impulsivity may interfere with the ability to make authentic, lasting, and meaningful choices at certain times[16,17]. Federal regulations have noted that the capacity for 'free' decision making is potentially compromised in pregnant women and, by extension, in women of child-bearing potential, because of the competing concerns of the woman and the dependent unborn child[12,15,18]. Voluntarism may thus be diminished by many influences, such as developmental immaturity, cognitive deficits, illness symptoms, pressures intrinsic to certain settings, and needs of the dependent[19,32]. Because of these barriers to voluntarism, additional safeguards are intended to protect and enhance, to whatever extent possible, the autonomous decision making of members of these populations[12,15,17,20].

Many other less well-recognized elements also affect voluntarism. These relate to the individual's emotional experience, life history, and personal psychological issues. Suffering and pain due to physical or mental health problems may cause one to move toward a decision out of desperation, rather than deliberateness and adherence to personal values and previous life choices[23,24,33,34]. The barriers to voluntarism associated with emotional distress are similar when the anguished parent of a dying child makes critical health decisions on his or her child's behalf[35,36]. People who have been institutionalized or who have survived severe trauma of various forms may experience the world differently thereafter and feel less able to enact choices in their lives or even to feel entitled to possess choices[37,38]. Distinct psychological experiences of power relationships – for example, among some women, some individuals from ethnic minorities, and, of interest, among some people who have served in the military – may also limit the person's sense that he or she may decline a course of action recommended by a clinician, who is seen as a strong authority figure[39,40]. Immigrants coming from countries in which clinicians are perceived as very powerful, beneficent, and as rightly making decisions for their patients may also find the expectation of independent decision making unclear[37]. More worrisome are expectations based on misplaced hope and misunderstandings (e.g., that a clinical treatment or research study will confer personal benefit or that a clinical researcher will always act in the best interests of the participant [the 'therapeutic misconception']) that may distort the values underlying the autonomous choice of the individual[4,41,42]. Finally, some beliefs and psychological defenses that emerge in the process of dealing with an overwhelming illness may be a barrier to perceiving and considering alternatives[2,43].

Beyond these considerations, an individual person experiences constraints on what can be chosen freely according to his or her own sense of self. These are not components that affect factual understanding per se but rather the discernment of the self and what is seen as possible, acceptable,

* Roberts, L.: Informed consent and the capacity for voluntarism. *American Journal of Psychiatry* 159:705–712, 2002.

and preferable when engaging in a life choice. The possibility of living life with physical disfigurement, or with permanent ventilator support, or without the ability to work or create, or without the capacity to bear children are not ever choices that some individuals can undertake freely. In a sense, these influences limit one's voluntarism, but more important, they also serve to define one's voluntarism through the expression of one's values and distinctly personal pattern of life choices.

Cultural and religious values are also important influences on voluntarism in a consent decision. Cultural views of the ideal self as interdependent, as opposed to independent, as are held by many Hispanic and Asian peoples, for example, challenge the concept of autonomy as predominant and affect the individual's capacity to project himself or herself into a separatist Western construction of the self[44–47]. Beliefs held by many Native American peoples that illness derives from the person being out of balance with nature – threatening the well-being of the entire community and requiring native healing approaches – predictably affect the willingness of this patient to entertain nontraditional therapeutic interventions[48]. Spiritual values and deeply held personal beliefs related to one's unique life experiences may furthermore alter what is understood to be possible and acceptable for the individual person[49]. People from rural families and communities that value stoicism and courage may have greater difficulty accepting treatment for pain or mental health symptoms[50]. Traditional Navajo people, for whom the prospect of entering the next world physically incomplete is unthinkable, may be unable to entertain amputation as a possible treatment choice[51]. Jehovah's Witness patients who strictly hold to traditional guidelines within their religion may not intentionally accept blood products even in life-threatening situations because of their spiritual understanding[52,53].

Last, external circumstances and pressures can dramatically affect voluntarism, either negatively or positively. Perhaps the most obvious factor extrinsic to the individual is the presence or absence of resources in a given situation. What is possible in a tertiary care center in Chicago is different from what is possible in Tucumcari, New Mex., irrespective of the personal wishes of the patient. In addition. the process of a making a decision itself may hamper or enhance the voluntarism of a person making a key consent decision. Rushed timing of a complex or highly important health decision, for example, may threaten the person's ability to make a deliberate choice that is otherwise well informed and congruent with his or her life values[54]. Alternatively, an unfolding and conscientious dialogue between a clinician and a patient who is suffering from a chronic illness may provide an optimal situation for authentic decision making[55]. Large financial incentives may cause the individual to subordinate usual values to take on serious risks[56,57]. The presence of a supportive family member may improve the person's ability to identify and state his or her preferences, whereas the presence of an insensitive or domineering family member may have the opposite result[58,59]. Ill-defined but potent role conflicts inherent in dual or overlapping relationships create confusion about the intent of a consent decision and may create complex contextual pressures affecting the true voluntarism of the decision maker[60]. This may be the case when a person enrolls in a study in which his or her personal clinician is also the principal investigator[61]. Dual agency may also threaten voluntarism if a worker-participant is pressured by management to take part in a workplace-based study or when a prison official serves as a research 'recruiter'[62]. External features may thus serve to support or interfere with voluntarism.

A Framework for Understanding Voluntarism

Our evolving understanding of voluntarism has not received sufficient emphasis in discussions of informed consent within the medical profession[21, 63]. This inattention may be due in part to the fact that we have not articulated the domains that constitute the 'capacity for voluntarism' with the clarity and elegance in which the capacity for decision making has been stated. In a 1988 article, Appelbaum and Grisso[3] presented an analysis of decision-making competence for informed consent that entailed the abilities to communicate, understand, appreciate, and reason. This formulation was theoretically rigorous, intuitively resonant, clinically meaningful, and legally useful. It has shaped subsequent thought on consent decision making in this country and elsewhere[63–65].

Borrowing from the insights of this model, I suggest a framework for understanding an individual's capacity for voluntarism in clinical or biomedical research consent decisions. The framework is based on a definition of voluntarism as ideally encompassing the individual's ability to act in accordance with one's authentic sense of what is good, right, and best in light of one's situation, values, and prior history. Voluntarism involves the capacity to make this choice freely and in the absence of coercion. Deliberateness, purposefulness of intent, clarity, genuineness, and coherence with one's prior life decisions are implicitly emphasized in this construction. This definition seeks to capture a complex phenomenon that has biological, psychological, and sociocultural determinants, which themselves are richly heterogeneous by their nature. This construction also presupposes the observation that certain legitimate limits to one's liberty exist. These include the imperative to not harm others intentionally and the general responsibility to make choices within the accepted constraints of society and standards within the medical profession. In other words, the fact that a person may make a truly voluntary choice does not mandate that a health professional condone, support, or enact this choice. However, this framework seeks to clarify the capacity for such choice in a systematic manner.

The framework explicitly characterizes four domains influencing voluntarism in clinical and biomedical research settings. These categories naturally overlap and interact, and they are linked to the capacity for appreciation, the most sophisticated component of decisional capacity. Some of the influences are positive; many have the effect of diminishing the capacity for voluntarism. The framework places primacy on the ethics principles of respect for persons and voluntarism rather than on autonomy or self-determination per se, by giving support to the values that may be held dear by some patients and participants and, ironically, may challenge the relevance of separate, autonomous choice for these persons. The framework may also help in our efforts to develop strategies for evaluating and supporting voluntarism, thereby enhancing the ethical rigor of informed-consent decisions. Finally, the framework is presented with an invitation to my colleagues to help refine and develop it, as this task is indeed a challenge and one that will certainly be enriched from the wisdom of multiple perspectives.

Voluntarism: Four Domains of Influence

Voluntarism in consent decisions may be analyzed according to four domains of potential influence: 1) developmental factors, 2) illness-related considerations, 3) psychological issues and cultural and religious values, and 4) external features and pressures.

Developmental Factors

An individual's capacity for voluntarism is affected by the person's development in terms of cognitive abilities, emotional maturity, and moral character. While it is clear that even very young children can and do express desires, it is accepted that children are unable to make independent, cognitively complex decisions for themselves. As children mature and their intellect, self-understanding, and sense of separate personhood develops, they are increasingly able to express sustained preferences that meet some tests of discernment, logic, coherence, and emerging personal values[28]. During late childhood and preadolescence, the capacity to accept a proffered choice (i.e., assent) becomes evident[66]. A greater capacity for voluntarism accompanies the older adolescent's emerging abilities to think abstractly, to recognize personal values in relation to those of others, to reflect on one's place in the world, and to begin to consider the repercussions of a decision based on some accumulated personal life experience. Reference points for personal decisions make the transition from parental values to incorporate those derived from social experience beyond the family in school, in interactions with peers, and within the broader culture (e.g., the media). In late adolescence and early adulthood, these young people often are capable not only of thoughtful judgment regarding their own safety and well-being but of making genuine and deeply committed altruistic choices[28]. With time, adults ideally are increasingly able to identify their personal opinions and preferences, particularly when facing novel decisions, on the basis of the learning and mature self-knowledge that comes with life experience. Adults often have roles that entail making decisions of varying stakes and consequences, and these individuals have had many opportunities for learning, expressing, and practicing their capacity for voluntary choice. In later life, the capacity for voluntarism is less driven by developmental considerations but is affected primarily by the remaining three domains of influence.

Illness-Related Considerations

Many mentally and physically ill individuals speak of the personal resolve and discernment of life priorities that they feel as a result of the illness experience[67]. Indeed suffering, or having survived a period of suffering, may midwife remarkable clarity about one's values in life choices[68]. These illness-related phenomena may enhance the individual's voluntarism in consent decisions.

Symptoms associated with mental or physical illness may nevertheless serve as negative factors that seriously detract from voluntarism. Ambivalence and indecisiveness, poor energy, and negative thoughts are among the elements that define depression and physical disorders that mimic or become complicated by secondary depression. In a second example, psychotic disorders at times give rise to symptoms affecting voluntarism, such as apathy and avolition, inability to read one's own internal emotional state and preferences, impaired insight and judgment, social disengagement, bizarre beliefs or overvalued ideas, and abnormal perceptions[65,69]. These illness manifestations typically fluctuate, with multiple symptoms at some times and fewer at other times. However, taken together, these symptoms can prevent an individual from collecting his or her thoughts, feelings, and personal values to make a coherent and enduring choice[70,71]. Dementia and some other neuropsychiatric disorders that are characterized by impaired memory, inability to perform practical activities, and compromised executive functions cognitively wear away the core components of the self, greatly affecting the capacity for voluntarism in even moderately advanced stages[72]. Serious substance abuse disorders are aggressively erosive to the capacity for voluntarism, as is reflected in their diagnostic criteria. This is evident in the patterns of apathy and diminished motivation, preoccupation with substance procurement and intake, and impaired judgment related to maladaptive behaviors[26,73]. Among physical symptoms, severe pain has a profound impact on voluntarism, as has been well demonstrated in studies in which adequate pain control radically changes the consent decisions of patients, including end-of-life-care preferences[24,74]. The degree of physical dependence that a person experiences – e.g., the ability to feed one's self, to attend to one's own hygiene – due to pain or debilitation also affects one's ability to make and insist upon choices[75].

Individually and in concert, these symptoms and illnesses such as these may greatly affect one's capacity to identify, feel committed to, voice, and enact upon one's preferences. They may also interfere with one's ability to ensure that the perceptions and motivations underlying a decision are accurate for a given situation. When psychopathological symptoms or maladaptive defenses interfere with the patient's ability to discern his or her preferences, time and support may be given and perhaps other clinical interventions should be undertaken to help the patient. Thus, specific mental and physical symptoms and their nature, severity, and temporal pattern may significantly affect an individual's capacity for voluntarism.

Psychological Issues and Cultural and Religious Values

Psychological issues and cultural and religious values influence voluntarism. They may contribute in a manner that enhances one's sense of individual autonomy and empowerment. Alternatively, these influences may diminish voluntarism or simply render less relevant various factors associated with voluntarism.

Psychological issues and values derived from an individual's cultural and spiritual milieu influence impressions of who is good and what choices are acceptable when he or she is facing life decisions. Relevant concepts of self, personhood, autonomy, and morality are shaped by the earliest of our internal and relational experiences and are revised over a lifetime. These factors may affect how symptoms are perceived, how illness is defined, and whether consenting to an intervention is acceptable. These representations and the individual's psychological defenses (e.g., denial) become particularly salient when coping with the significant stresses intrinsic to an illness. The level of commitment to a particular choice is affected by such factors. Further, specific beliefs inevitably define meaning and parameters for a person's choices. This is apparent in a decision regarding elective pregnancy termination or end-of-life care in patients who hold to strict Catholic beliefs or in a complex decision regarding the nonacceptance of treatment by a person who is a Christian Scientist. The influence of specific beliefs is also evident in the interpretation of mental symptoms among rural persons, the 'true' causes of illness among many Native American or Alaska native peoples, or the preferred way to inform a traditional Japanese elder of a diagnosis of a terminal illness.

Even seeing one's ideal self as a separate, autonomous individual—as an agent able to decide and act—is a perspective that some have characterized as distinctly 'Western,' culture bound, and masculine in its approach to decision making[76]. In other societies, behaving in a manner that enhances the relationships in the family or defers to the judgment of elders has greater valence[45]. The act of defining a preference separate from the needs of others or different from the traditions of the community, for some people, may be viewed as wrong or unthinkable. The process of expressing choices is shaped by these kinds of forces as well. Communication styles certainly vary across individuals but, perhaps even more dramatically, across regions, ethnicities, and larger cultures, e.g., the contrasting dialogue patterns of Navajo people in comparison with those of Italian Americans[77,78]. The issue of having a voice, or the ways of giving voice, in key health decisions is thus uncertain despite this presupposition in our society and in our formal construction of the model of informed consent. Studies of masculine and feminine styles of personal decision making[79] have also provided some evidence that women place greater importance on collaboration, adaptation, and relationship preservation in the face of moral decisions, while men place greater importance on self-reliance, assertiveness, and adherence to accepted rules. These psychological, cultural, and religious elements should be considered carefully for their impact on the patient's process of generating a purposeful, authentic, and coherent decision.

External Features and Pressures

Influences on voluntarism that are extrinsic to the self are diverse and potent. The most obvious external determinants are the resource limitations inherent in many health care settings. Local or regional legislation may also define the parameters for individual decision making. Granted, these factors determine the fundamental nature of the consent decision by defining what choices actually exist for an individual patient at a specific place and point in time. Nevertheless, they merit careful attention because they may also affect the individual's motivation for accepting a particular intervention simply because of the lack of viable alternatives. Other external factors reside within the nature of the decision itself, such as the novelty, complexity, seriousness, and timing of a consent decision, and whether it can be made stepwise without loss of significant options. Incentives or strongly reinforcing pressures within the context should also be considered for their impact on voluntarism[7]. Institutional settings delimit the freedoms of individuals and may generate significant pressures on individuals – be they prisoners, nursing home residents, or mentally or physically ill people – engaging in consent decisions[80]. The relationship with the caregiver or researcher, similarly, may have carefully hidden coercive influences that may be present, for example, when multiple roles or overlapping relationships exist[81]. The presence or absence of loved ones may also affect the person's process of clarifying and expressing choice. In sum, qualities of the environment, relationships, and the decisional process may all serve to add to or detract from the individual's voluntarism in giving informed consent.

Conclusions

Voluntarism is critical for the fulfillment of the ideal of informed consent. From an ethical perspective, voluntarism is the principle that embodies respect for the person as a human being, as a self with a personal history and values, and as a moral agent with fundamental rights and privileges in our society. True voluntarism is a source of strength for the philosophical and legal safeguard of informed consent. On the other hand, diminished voluntarism in the consent process is a source of vulnerability for patients and research participants[81, 82]. Stated differently, even the most well-informed and decisionally 'fit' individual cannot realize the spirit of informed consent if his or her 'choice' is inauthentic, symptom driven, compromised, or coerced[83].

Four aspects of the application of this model to clinical and research practice merit consideration. First, as with the assessment of decisional capacity for informed consent, the capacity for voluntarism is ideally understood in relation to a specific decision[84]. When we consider influences on the capacity for voluntarism, the standard varies according to the nature of the decision. Greater ambivalence about adopting a certain course of action is acceptable if the situation is nonacute and the consequences are not dire. Greater clarity, authenticity, coherence, and commitment are necessary in a serious and high-stakes informed consent or refusal decision.

Second, this framework may give clues for strategies for enhancing voluntarism. For instance, supporting the voluntarism of children or developmentally disabled people in the decisions they are capable of requires attunement to their developmental strengths. Accurate assessment and initial treatment of physical and mental symptoms (e.g., pain, dysphoria) may serve to diminish barriers to voluntarism for subsequent, higher-stakes, or more enduring consent decisions. Clarifying personal values through dialogue about cultural and religious beliefs, psychological issues and personal history, and documents such as 'The Values History'[85] or Five Wishes[86] may dramatically enhance the subject's ability to identify preferences in key decisions and improve our faithfulness to the patient's true wishes. Careful examination of the forces present in a given context may help to discern and minimize the potential coercive pressures experienced by the person whose voluntarism we wish to support.

Third, this formulation does not help to resolve the dissonance we may feel as clinicians and researchers when our patients make decisions that feel illogical, self-defeating, or morally unacceptable or will inevitably lead to a poor outcome. Nevertheless, the process of identifying barriers to voluntarism and of clarifying preferences and perspectives may help us to honor the authentic choices of our patients, an act that has its own rewards. Finally, on a cautionary note, voluntarism, like decisional capacity, should be understood for its dynamic nature; voluntarism does not represent an all-or-nothing phenomenon. Analyzing voluntarism through its elements—the developmental factors, illness-related considerations, psychological issues and cultural and religious values, and external features and pressures—without remaining mindful of how these come together meaningfully within a person may introduce the risk of distortion. The aim of this analysis should be to gain a richer sense of the true attributes and experience of the individual, not to deconstruct these in a manner that is unfaithful to the real qualities of the person before us. Consequently, this framework should be applied in a manner that involves appreciation for the meaning of the various elements taken together and as residing within a person.

Fostering voluntarism in clinical care and biomedical research entails our best skills: listening, sensing, clarifying, making the implicit explicit,

and genuinely attending to the person before us. It is respectful of people and of differing experiences and values that they bring to decisions in their lives. It takes a willingness to observe our own biases and to evaluate the effects of the contexts in which we serve patients and interact with research participants. It is through such efforts that we will come closer to the hard, good work of fulfilling voluntarism and, more fundamentally, to achieving the principle of respect for persons in clinical care and biomedical research.

Supported in part by an NIMH Mentored Scientist Development Award in Research Ethics (MH-01918).

The author thanks her mentors, Drs. Samuel Keith and Mark Siegler, and colleagues Melinda Rogers and Drs. Cynthia Geppert, Janet Brody, Teddy Warner, and Brian Roberts for help with this article.

References

1   American Medical Association: *Code of Medical Ethics: Current Opinions With Annotations*. Chicago, American Medical Association, Council on Ethical and Judicial Affairs, 1997.

2   Lidz CW, Meisel A, Osterweis M, Holden JL, Marx JH, Munetz MR: Barriers to informed consent. *Ann Intern Med* 1983; **99**:539–543.

3   Appelbaum PS, Grisso T: Assessing patients' capacities to consent to treatment. *N Engl J Med* 1988; **319**:1635–1638.

4   Roberts L: The ethical basis of psychiatric research: conceptual issues and empirical findings. *Compr Psychiatry* 1998; **39**:99–110.

5   Beauchamp TL, Childress JF: *Principles of Biomedical Ethics*. New York, Oxford University Press, 1994.

6   Boyd KM, Higgs R, Pinching AJ: *The New Dictionary of Medical Ethics*. London, BMJ Publishing, 1997.

7   Sugarman J, McCrory DC, Powell D, Krasny A, Adams B, Ball E, Cassell C: Empirical research on informed consent: an annotated bibliography. *Hastings Cent Rep* 1999; **29**:S1–S42.

8   Zaubler TS, Viederman M, Fins JJ: Ethical, legal, and psychiatric issues in capacity, competency, and informed consent: an annotated bibliography. *Gen Hosp Psychiatry* 1996; **18**:155–172.

9   Morris CD, Niederbuhl JM, Mahr JM: Determining the capability of individuals with mental retardation to give informed consent. *Am J Ment Retard* 1993; **98**:263–272.

10 Melton GB: Toward 'personhood' for adolescents: autonomy and privacy as values in public policy. *Am Psychol* 1983; **38**:99–103.

11 Fellows LK: Competency and consent in dementia. *J Am Geriatr Soc* 1998; **46**:922–926.

12 Brody B: *The Ethics of Biomedical Research: An International Perspective*. New York, Oxford University Press, 1998.

13 National Commission for the Protection of Human Subjects of Biomedical and Behavioral Research: *Report and Recommendations: Research Involving Prisoners*. Washington, DC, US Government Printing Office, 1976.

14 National Commission for the Protection of Human Subjects of Biomedical and Behavioral Research: *Research Involving Those Institutionalized as Mentally Infirm: Report and Recommendations*. Washington, DC. US Government Printing Office. 1978.

15 Levine R: *Ethics and Regulation of Clinical Research*. Baltimore, Urban & Schwartzenberg, 1986.

16 Ganzini L, Lee MA, Heintz RT: The capacity to make decisions in advanced and borderline personality disorder (editorial). *J Clin Ethics* 1994; **5**:360–364.

17 Dresser R: Mentally disabled research subjects: the enduring policy issues. *JAMA* 1996; **276**:67–72.

18 Dresser R: Wanted: single, white male for medical research. *Hastings Cent Rep* 1992; **22**:24–29.

19 Moreno J, Caplan AL, Wolpe PR (Project on Informed Consent, Human Research Ethics Group): Updating protections for human subjects involved in research. *JAMA* 1998; **280**:1951–1958.

20 Roberts L, Roberts B: Psychiatric research ethics: an overview of evolving guidelines and current ethical dilemmas in the study of mental illness. *Biol Psychiatry* 1999; **46**:1025–1038.

21 Meisel A, Roth LH: What we do and do not know about informed consent. *JAMA* 1981; **246**:2473–2477.

22 Appelbaum P: Drug-free research in schizophrenia: an overview of the controversy. *IRB* 1996; **18**:1–5.

23 Ganzini L: Commentary: assessment of clinical depression in patients who request physician-assisted death. *J Pain Symptom Manage* 2000; **19**:474–478.

24 Ganzini L, Lee MA, Heintz RT, Bloom JD: Depression, suicide, and the right to refuse life-sustaining treatment. *J Clin Ethics* 1993; **4**:337–340.

25 Stanley B: Ethical considerations in biological research on suicide. *Ann NY Acad Sci* 1986; **487**:42–46.

26 Brody JL, Waldron HB: Ethical issues in research on the treatment of adolescent substance abuse disorders. *Addict Behav* 2000; **25**:217–228.

27 Greenhill LL: The use of psychotropic medication in preschoolers: indications, safety, and efficacy. *Can J Psychiatry* 1998; **43**:576–581.

28 Susman EJ, Dorn LD, Fletcher JC: Participation in biomedical research: the consent process as viewed by children, adolescents, young adults, and physicians. *J Pediatr* 1992; **121**:547–552.

29 Hoagwood K, Jensen P, Fisher C: *Ethical Issues in Mental Health Research With Children and Adolescents.* Mahwah, NJ, Lawrence Erlbaum Associates, 1996.

30 Sachs GA: Advance consent for dementia research. *Alzheimer Dis Assoc Disord* 1994; 8(suppl 4):19–27.

31 Sachs GA, Stocking CB, Stern R, Cox DM, Hougham G, Sachs RS: Ethical aspects of dementia research: informed consent and proxy consent. *Clin Res* 1994; **42**:403–412.

32 Glick KL, Mackay KM, Balasingam S, Dolan KR, Casper-Isaac S: Advance directives: barriers to completion. *J NY State Nurses* Assoc 1998; **29**:4–8.

33 Stiefel F: Psychosocial aspects of Cancer pain. *Support Care Cancer* 1993; **1**:130–134.

34 *Management of Cancer Pain: Clinical Practice Guideline.* Washington, DC, US Department of Health and Human Services, 1994.

35 Lashley M, Talley W, Lands LC, Keyserlingk EW: Informed proxy consent: communication between pediatric surgeons and surrogates about surgery. *Pediatrics* 2000; 105(3, part 1):591–597.

36 Dermatis H, Lesko LM: Psychological distress in parents consenting to child's bone marrow transplantation. *Bone Marrow Transplant* 1990; **6**:411–417.

37 Bauer HM, Rodriguez MA, Quiroga SS, Flores-Ortiz YG: Barriers to health care for abused Latina and Asian immigrant women. *J Health Care Poor Undeserved* 2000; **11**:33–44.

38 Ruzek JI, Zatzick DF: Ethical considerations in research participation among acutely injured trauma survivors: an empirical investigation. *Gen Hosp Psychiatry* 2000; **22**:27–36.

39 Ruhnke GW, Wilson SR, Akamatsu T, Kinoue T, Takashima Y, Goldstein MK, Koenig BA, Hornberger JC, Raffin TA: Ethical decision making and patient autonomy: a comparison of physicians and patients in Japan and the United States. *Chest* 2000; **118**:1172–1182.

40 Agard E, Finkelstein D, Wallach E: Cultural diversity and informed consent. *J Clin Ethics* 1998; **9**:173–176.

41 Appelbaum PS, Roth LH, Lidz CW, Benson P, Winslade W: False hopes and best data: consent to research and the therapeutic misconception. *Hastings Cent Rep* 1987; **17**:20–24.

42 Roberts LW, Warner TD, Brody JL: Perspectives of patients with schizophrenia and psychiatrists regarding ethically important aspects of research participation. *Am J Psychiatry* 2000; **157**:67–74.

43 Kunkel EJ, Woods CM, Rodgers C, Myers RE: Consultations for 'maladaptive denial of illness' in patients with cancer: psychiatric disorders that result in noncompliance. *Psychooncology* 1997; **6**:139–149.

44 Bedolla M: Patient Self-Determination Act: a Hispanic perspective. *Camb Q Healthc Ethics* 1994; **3**:413–417.

45 Fetters MD: The family in medical decision making: Japanese perspectives. *J Clin Ethics* 1998; **9**:132–146.

46 Garcia-Preto N: Latino families: an overview, in *Ethnicity and Family Therapy.* Edited by McGoldrick M, Giordano J, Pearce J, New York, Guilford, 1996, pp 141–154.

47 Lee E: *Asian American families: an overview.* Ibid, pp 227–248.

48 McCabe M: Patient Sell-Determination Act: a Native American (Navajo) perspective. *Camb Q Healthc Ethics* 1994; **3**:419–421.

49 Waldfogel S, Wolpe PR: Using awareness of religious factors to enhance interventions in consultation-liaison psychiatry. *Hosp Community Psychiatry* 1993:**44**:473–477.

50 Wagenfeld M, Murray J, Mohatt D, DeBruyn J: *Rural America today, in Mental Health and Rural America: 1980–1993: An Overview and Annotated Bibliography.* Washington, DC, Office of Rural Health Policy, Health Resources and Services Administration, National Institutes of Health, and Public Health Service, 1994, pp 1–7.

51 Carrese JA, Rhodes LA: Western bioethics on the Navajo reservation: benefit or harm? *JAMA* 1995; **274**:826–829.

52 Muramoto O: Bioethics of the refusal of blood by Jehovah's Witnesses, part 2: a novel approach based on rational non-interventional paternalism. *J Med Ethics* 1998; **24**:295–301.

53 Muramoto O: Bioethics of the refusal of blood by Jehovah's Witnesses, part 3: a proposal for a don't-ask-don't-tell policy. *J Med Ethics* 1999; **25**:463–468.

54 World Medical Association: Declaration of Helsinki: Recommendations guiding physicians in biomedical research involving human subjects. *JAMA* 1997; **277**:925–926.

55 Lidz C: *Informed Consent: A Study of Decisionmaking in Psychiatry.* New York, Guilford, 1984.

56 Russell ML, Moralejo DG, Burgess ED: Paying research subjects: participants' perspectives. *J Med Ethics* 2000; **26**:126–130.

57 Erlen JA, Sauder RJ, Mellors MP: Incentives in research: ethical issues. *Orthop Nurs* 1999; **18**:84–87.

58 Thomas JE, Latimer EJ: When families cannot 'let go': ethical decision-making at the bedside. *Can Med Assoc J* 1989; **141**: 389–391.

59 Rothchild E: Family dynamics in end-of-life treatment decisions. *Gen Hosp Psychiatry* 1994; **16**:251–258.

60 Cattorini P, Mordacci R: The physician as caregiver and researcher. *Thyroidology* 1993; **5**:73–76.

61 Kass NE, Sugarman J, Faden R, Schoch-Spana M: Trust, the fragile foundation of contemporary biomedical research. *Hastings Cent Rep* 1996; **26**:25–29.

62 Human Subjects Research Program, Office of Biological and Environmental Research, Department of Energy: *The need to protect workers as human research subjects in Creating An Ethical Framework for Studies That Involve the Worker Community.* Washington, DC, US Government Printing Office, 2000, pp 1–10.

63 Grisso TS, Appelbaum PS: Comparison of standards for assessing patients' capacities to make treatment decisions. *Am J Psychiatry* 1995; **152**: 1033–1037.

64 Nedopil N, Aldenhoff J, Amelung K, Eich FX, Fritze J, Gastpar M, Maier W, Moller HJ: Competence to give informed consent to clinical studies: statement by the taskforce on 'ethical and legal questions' of the Association for Neuropsychopharmacology and Pharmacopsychiatry (Arbeitsgemeinschaft fur Neuropsychopharmakologie and Pharmakopsychiatrie [AGNP]). *Pharmacopsychiatry* 1999; **32**:165–168.

65 Carpenter WT Jr, Gold JM, Lahti AC, Queern CA, Conley RR, Bartko JJ, Kovnick J, Appelbaum PS: Decisional capacity for informed consent in schizophrenia research. *Arch Gen Psychiatry* 2000; **57**:533–538.

66 Committee on Bioethics, American Academy of Pediatrics: Informed consent, parental permission, and assent in pediatric practice. *Pediatrics* 1995; **95**:314–317.

67 Cassel E: *The Nature of Suffering and the Goals of Medicine.* New York, Oxford University Press, 1991.

68 Jamison K: *Touched With Fire: Manic-Depressive Illness and the Artistic Temperament.* New York, Free Press, 1993.

69 Grimes AL, McCullough LB, Kunik ME, Molinari V, Workman RH: Informed consent and neuroanatomic correlates of intentionality and voluntariness among psychiatric patients. *Psychiatr Serv* 2000; **51**:1561–1567.

70 Backlar P: Advance directives for subjects of research who have fluctuating cognitive impairments due to psychotic disorders (such as schizophrenia). *Community Ment Health J* 1998; **34**: 229–240.

71 Elliott C: Caring about risks: are severely depressed patients competent to consent to research? *Arch Gen Psychiatry* 1997; **54**:113–116.

72 Marson DC, Cody HA, Ingram KK, Harrell LE: Neuropsychologic predictors of competency in Alzheimer's disease using a rational reasons legal standard (comment). *Arch Neurol* 1995; **52**: 955–959.

73 McCrady BS, Bux DA Jr: Ethical issues in informed consent with substance abusers. *J Consult Clin Psychol* 1999; **67**:186–193.

74 Sullivan M, Rapp S, Fitzgibbon D, Chapman CR: Pain and the choice to hasten death in patients with painful metastatic cancer. *J Palliat Care* 1997; **13**:18–28.

75 Pearlman RA, Cain KC, Patrick DL, Appelbaum-Maizel M, Starks HE, Jecker NS, Uhlmann RF: Insights pertaining to patient assessments of states worse than death. *J Clin Ethics* 1993; **4**:33–41.

76 Ulrich LP: The Patient Self-Determination Act and cultural diversity. *Camb Q Healthc Ethics* 1994; **3**:410–413.

77 McGoldrick M, Giordano J: Overview: Ethnicity and family therapy, in *Ethnicity and Family Therapy*. Edited by McGoldrick M, Giordano J, Pearce J. New York, Guilford, 1996, pp 1–30.

78 Sutton C, *Broken Nose M: American Indian Families: an overview.* Ibid, pp 31–14.

79 Gilligan C: *Concepts of Self and Morality: In a Different Voice.* Cambridge, Mass, Harvard University Press, 1993.

80 President's Advisory Committee: *The Human Radiation Experiments: Final Report of the President's Advisory Committee.* New York, Oxford University Press, 1996.

81 Reatig N: Research with vulnerable populations: ethical considerations and federal regulations, in *NIH Readings on the Protection of Human Subjects in Behavioral and Social Science Research.* Edited by Sieber J Frederick, Md, University Publications of America, 1984, pp 181–184.

82 Faden R. Beauchamp T: *A History and Theory of Informed Consent.* New York, Oxford University Press, 1986.

83 Etchells E, Sharpe G, Dykeman MJ, Meslin EM, Singer PA: Bioethics for clinicians, 4: voluntariness. *Can Med Assoc J* 1996; **155**:1083–1086.

84 Drane JF: Competency to give an informed consent: a model for making clinical assessments. *JAMA* 1984; **252**:925–927.

85 Lambert P, Gibson JM, Nathanson P: The values history: an innovation in surrogate medical decision-making. *Law Med Health Care* 1990; **18**:202–212.

86 Commission on Aging With Dignity: *Five Wishes.* Tallahassee, Fla, Aging With Dignity, 1998, p 12.

Placebo-Controlled Trials in Psychiatric Research

An Ethical Perspective*

Franklin G. Miller

Introduction

The ethics of using placebos in clinical trials has recently received increased attention and generated considerable controversy (Taubes 1995). Opponents of current practice in clinical research contend that use of placebo controls is always unethical when standard, proven treatment exists (Freedman et al 1996; Rothman and Michels 1994). Defenders of current practice respond by arguing that placebo-controlled designs represent 'the gold standard' for clinical trials of treatment efficacy (Clark and Leaverton 1994; Leber 1986; Rickels 1986) and that placebo arms of clinical trials are ethically acceptable provided that patients receiving placebo are not at risk for serious harm and give informed consent (Levine 1999). The debate has focused heavily on psychiatric research, owing to ethical concern about research involving potentially vulnerable, mentally ill patients and the frequency of placebo-controlled trials in this field despite the existence of standard, effective treatments.

In this article, I review ethical considerations relevant to this debate and endeavor to stake out a middle-ground position. I argue that an absolute ethical prohibition of placebo-controlled trials in psychiatric disorders for which standard, effective treatments exist is unsound for three major reasons. First, it is based on a flawed conception of research ethics, which inappropriately applies the normative framework of clinical medicine to clinical research. Second, it ignores important contextual factors characteristic of psychiatric research, including the limited efficacy and often-intolerable side effects of standard treatments and the high rates of placebo responses in clinical trials. Third, the alternative of active-controlled trials comparing experimental with standard drugs without placebo controls could lead to the approval and use of new medications that appear equivalent in efficacy to standard treatments but may be no more, effective than placebo. Nevertheless, placebo-controlled trials are morally problematic and stand in need of justification when effective treatments are clinically available. Careful design and conduct of placebo-controlled trials are necessary to assure protection of patient volunteers.

What Makes Placebo-Controlled Trials Ethically Problematic?

Although widely considered to be the gold standard for testing treatment efficacy, placebo-controlled trials prompt ethical concern when patients in the placebo arm fail to receive standard, effective treatment. These patient volunteers are exposed to the risks of harm associated with untreated illness for the duration of their participation in the clinical trial. A consensus exists that placebo-controlled trials are unethical if patients risk death or irreversible serious morbidity as a result of having standard treatment withheld. Thus placebo-controlled trials in oncology are typically limited to testing the efficacy of 'add-on' treatments combined with standard therapy. In contrast, ethical controversy surrounds placebo-controlled trials when withholding of standard treatment for research subjects randomized to

placebo does not pose comparable risks of harm. Placebo-controlled trials in psychiatry fall squarely into this domain.

It is important to note that not all placebo-controlled trials pose special ethical problems. When no effective treatment exists for a given disorder, it is not ethically problematic to conduct a trial comparing placebo with an experimental agent or with a clinically available agent that has not been shown effective for this condition. In this case, patients in the placebo arm are not denied proven, effective treatment. Indeed, they may be better off than are those who receive the experimental treatment if it lacks efficacy or produces uncomfortable or harmful side effects. For similar reasons, trials testing experimental drugs against placebo in groups of treatment refractory patients are not considered ethically suspect because for these patients, standard treatment has proven ineffective. Many treatment refractory patients, however, have a partial response to standard medications or find them intolerable because of side effects. Enrolling such patients in placebo-controlled trials raises ethical concern insofar as they may experience symptom worsening on placebo. Treatment augmentation trials compare an 'add on' experimental treatment with placebo among patient volunteers, all of whom also receive standard treatment. The design of these trials is ethically innocuous because patients are not asked to forego treatment of proven efficacy.

Placebo-controlled trials of maintenance treatment also raise ethical issues (Lieberman *et al.* 1999). In trials of maintenance treatment, the principal research question under investigation concerns the clinical need for long-term drug treatment, which may also include the search for predictors of relapse. In this research design, patient volunteers who have responded positively to medication are randomly assigned in double-blind fashion to either continued treatment or placebo for a specified period of time. By their very nature, such trials require a placebo or no-treatment arm, but they are ethically problematic because of the risk of symptom worsening or relapse. This research design will not be considered further here; however, the guidelines presented below for the justification and use of placebo controls in efficacy trials are also relevant to maintenance trials.

Regulatory Standards and Codes of Ethics

Regulatory standards and codes of ethics differ in their guidance concerning placebo-controlled trials when standard, effective treatments exist. U.S. federal regulations governing human subjects research contain no explicit prohibition or restriction of the use of placebo controls in clinical trials (Code of Federal Regulations 1991). Research involving human subjects can be approved by Institutional Review Boards (IRBs) provided that several conditions are met, including the following: 1) 'Risks to subjects are minimized . . . by using procedures which are consistent with sound research design and which do not unnecessarily expose subjects to risk'; 2) 'risks to subjects are reasonable in relationship to anticipated benefits, if any, to subjects, and the importance of the knowledge that may reasonably be expected to result'; and 3) 'informed consent will be sought from each prospective subject or the subject's legally authorized representative' (45CFR 46.111).

* Miller, F.G.: Placebo-controlled trials in psychiatric research: an ethical perspective. *Biological Psychiatry* 47:707–716, 2000.

Critics of placebo-controlled trials in psychiatry might argue that they should be prohibited under the federal regulations because they expose research subjects to unnecessary risks, but this would be disputed by those who see placebo-controlled trials as the scientific design of choice in this field and contend that the risks of withholding effective treatment during time-limited placebo trials are not severe for psychiatric patients. The fact that the federal regulations include the importance of scientific knowledge to be potentially gained from research within the scope of risk–benefit assessment suggests the justifiability of placebo-controlled trials. Nonetheless, the *Institutional Review Board Guidebook* prepared by the Office for Protection from Research Risks, which oversees human subjects research, declares that 'A design involving a placebo control should not be used where there is a standard treatment that has been shown to be superior to placebo by convincing evidence' (Office for Protection from Research Risks 1993).

Regulations and guidelines of the U.S. Food and Drug Administration (FDA) directly address the use of placebo-controlled trials. They require 'adequate, and well-controlled' studies to demonstrate the effectiveness of drugs as a condition of approving their clinical use (Code of Federal Regulations 1985). Although the FDA does not require placebo controls, its policy gives a decided preference to placebo-controlled trials when risks of death or serious harm are not at stake. In defining an 'adequate and well-controlled study,' FDA regulations state that 'The study uses a design that permits a valid comparison with a control to provide a quantitative assessment of drug effect.' Among the variety of control conditions considered, placebo controls are mentioned first. Concerning active treatment controls, the regulations state: 'The test drug is compared with known effective therapy; for example, where the condition treated is such that administration of placebo or no treatment would be contrary to the interest of the patient.'

It might be argued that FDA regulations should favor active-controlled trials whenever standard, effective treatment exists because use of placebo controls in this case is 'contrary to the interest of the patient.' Nonetheless, in a 'Supplementary Advisory: Placebo-Controlled and Active Controlled Drug Study Designs' (United States Food and Drug Administration 1989), the FDA pointed out methodological limitations of active-controlled designs. Relevant to psychiatric research is the following statement from these guidelines: 'For certain drug classes, such as analgesics, antidepressants or antianxiety drugs, failure to show superiority to placebo in a given study is common . . . . In those situations active control trials showing no difference between the new drug and control are of little value as primary evidence of effectiveness and the active control design, the study design most often proposed as an alternative to use of a placebo, is not credible.'

The Declaration of Helsinki, endorsed by the World Medical Association, has been appealed to in support of the position that placebo-controlled trials are unethical in disorders for which treatments of proven efficacy exist (Rothman and Michels 1994). The relevant statement cited in favor of this ethical stance is the following: 'In any medical study, every patient – including those of a control group, if any – should be assured of the best proven diagnostic and therapeutic method' (World Medical Association 1996). Critics of this ethical position have responded that the cited language would also appear to rule out any randomized clinical trial comparing a standard with an experimental treatment (Lasagna 1995; Levine 1999). The point of these trials is to determine if the experimental treatment is at least as effective as standard treatment. Patients randomized to experimental treatment are not assured 'the best proven' treatment because the efficacy of the experimental treatment has yet to be determined and is the very issue under investigation in the trial.

The recently proposed draft revisions to the Declaration of Helsinki, which have occasioned considerable controversy, clearly permit wider use of placebo-controlled trials: 'When the outcome measures are neither death nor disability, placebo or other no-treatment controls may be justified on the basis of their efficiency' (Brennan 1999). In contrast, Canada's new Tri-Council Policy Statement on Ethical Conduct for Research Involving Humans states: 'The use of placebo controls in clinical trials is generally unacceptable when standard therapies or interventions are available for a particular patient population' (Weijer 1999).

The divergent guidance of regulations and codes of ethics indicates the need for ethical analysis, to illuminate the moral considerations at stake in the controversy over placebo-controlled trials and arrive at an ethically sound position on this complex issue.

Rationale for Opposition to Placebo-Controlled Trials

Ethical opposition to placebo-controlled trials in situations where standard, effective treatments exist relies on appeal to a central norm of medical ethics: individualized, patient-centered beneficence. Physicians have an obligation to promote the benefit of patients suffering from illness by offering them medically indicated treatment. Correlatively, patients under the care of a physician have a right to medically indicated treatment. Patients randomized to a placebo arm of a clinical trial fail to receive standard, effective treatment for their condition, thus violating the moral obligation of physician-investigators and the rights of patient volunteers (Freedman et al. 1996). According to this ethical perspective, the placebo-controlled trials to test the efficacy of new selective serotonin reuptake inhibitors, in depressed patient volunteers and the 'atypical' neuroleptics in patients with schizophrenia would be considered unethical, given the existence of the tricyclic antidepressants and standard neuroleptics, which have been proven effective.

In contrast, an active-controlled trial comparing an experimental treatment to a standard treatment would not be unethical, provided that reasonable doubt exists in the community of physician-investigators concerning the relative efficacy of the two treatments. This condition for ethical clinical trials is known as 'clinical equipoise' (Freedman 1987). When clinical equipoise exists, patient volunteers are not randomized to a treatment known to be inferior to a clinically available treatment.

In addition to declaring the use of placebos in clinical trials unethical when treatments of proven efficacy are available, opponents of placebo-controlled trials in this situation argue that they lack clinical utility. When effective treatment exists for a given condition, clinical trials should compare experimental medications with standard treatment rather than with placebo. Instead of seeking to determine whether the experimental treatment 'is better than nothing,' clinical trials should test whether it is superior or equivalent in efficacy to standard treatment that has been proven effective (Rothman and Michels 1994; Weijer 1999).

Methodological Considerations

Before offering a critique of the ethical opposition to placebo-controlled trials and suggesting an alternative ethical framework, I will examine the claim that active-controlled trials have greater scientific and clinical value than placebo-controlled trials when standard, effective treatments exist for the condition under investigation. Two key methodological considerations are relevant to assessing the validity of this claim.

First, the often-repeated assertion by critics of placebo-controlled trials that they test whether experimental drugs 'are better than nothing' flies in the face of extensive evidence for the power of the placebo response, particularly in psychiatry (Shapiro and Shapiro 1997). Psychiatric research has demonstrated high rates of placebo responses (from 25% to 50% or more) across a range of psychiatric diagnoses, including panic disorder, depression, and schizophrenia (Addington 1995; Brown 1988; Hirschfeld 1996). Indeed, whether antidepressant medications have specific therapeutic potency beyond the placebo response has been questioned (Greenberg and Fisher 1997). One psychiatric investigator has recommended 4 to 6 weeks of placebo treatment (without deception) for a substantial proportion of depressed patients (Brown 1994). Although the nature of the placebo response remains poorly understood, a variety of factors may contribute to producing positive responses among research subjects receiving placebo, including the expectation of benefit from participating in clinical trials, the therapeutic milieu of the research environment, and the clinician–patient relationship (Shapiro and Shapiro 1997). Because substantial proportions of patient volunteers who receive placebos in psychiatric clinical trials show clinically significant improvement, demonstrating superiority to placebo represents a demanding test of efficacy for experimental drugs or procedures.

Second, active-controlled trial designs, comparing experimental with standard treatment, have potentially serious methodological limitations (Makuch and Johnson 1989; Temple 1997). Such studies can produce meaningful results when they are designed to test whether experimental drugs prove significantly superior to standard medication. In psychiatry, however, new drugs for a mental disorder are typically no more effective on the whole than standard treatment but may have clinical value because they have less severe side effects or work better in some patients. Accordingly, demonstrating equivalence between a novel and a standard drug can be useful, provided that the novel drug is better than placebo. Nonetheless, active-controlled trials designed to test the equivalence of experimental and standard treatment may produce misleading results. If the experimental treatment in such a clinical trial is demonstrated to be equivalent to the standard treatment, it does not follow that the experimental treatment is more effective than placebo; it is possible that in this particular trial, the standard treatment – which has previously been shown to be superior to placebo – is in fact not more effective than placebo. A variety of factors might explain this seemingly anomalous result, including a high rate of placebo response in the study population, fluctuating symptoms of illness, and spontaneous remission. Such factors are likely to be operative in psychiatric disorders. Without a placebo control arm, it is impossible to determine reliably whether an experimental drug that is demonstrated to be as effective as standard treatment is actually superior to placebo.

That this is not merely a theoretical concern is demonstrated by Temple (1997), who analyzed the data from six studies of an experimental antidepressant presented in a marketing application to the FDA. These studies compared the experimental drug to a standard antidepressant (imipramine) and placebo. In all six trials, a substantial and nearly identical reduction in depressive symptoms was associated with both the experimental and standard treatment. In five of the six trials, however, no significant difference was found between either the experimental or standard drug and placebo in terms of reduction in symptoms of depression. The one trial showing superiority of the active treatments to placebo was a very small study consisting in total of only 22 patients in the three study arms. Without placebo controls, the experimental drug would have appeared worthy of approval because it proved as effective as imipramine. In fact, neither the standard nor the experimental drug was more effective than placebo in this group of 392 study subjects.

Owing to the methodological limitations of active-controlled study designs, a policy of prohibiting placebo-controlled trials when proven effective treatment exists could have potentially serious consequences. Active-controlled studies showing the equivalence of experimental and standard drugs, in the absence of placebo controls, could lead to the approval of new drugs that are no better than placebo (Temple 1997). On the other hand, if demonstrating superiority to standard treatments were required for approval of new drugs, this would call for much larger sample sizes than are needed for placebo-controlled trials. It is likely that such a policy would expose many more patient volunteers to experimental drugs that may prove ineffective or have intolerable side effects, as well as add significant cost and delay to the process of drug development (Zipursky and Darby 1999).

Smaller two-arm trials comparing experimental drugs with placebo are useful in the early stage of efficacy testing. Once experimental drugs, or clinically available drugs that have not been tested for a given indication, have proved superior to placebo, a three-way trial design comparing a promising experimental drug, standard drug, and placebo can be especially valuable (Leber 1986). Clinical trials comparing a novel treatment with a standard treatment and placebo combine the scientific rigor of placebo-controlled trials with the potential clinical utility of testing an experimental agent against an existing standard therapy.

Ethical Critique

Regardless of these methodological and consequentialist considerations, if placebo-controlled trials involving patients for whom standard, effective treatments exist are unethical, then other ways of testing treatment efficacy should be adopted. The ethical opposition to the use of placebos in clinical trials is based on the norm of medical ethics that physicians have an obligation to promote benefit to individual patients by providing optimal medical care. Although it may seem natural that the norm of individual, patient-centered beneficence should also govern clinical research, this stance ignores significant differences between clinical research and clinical medicine. Because clinical research aims at producing generalizable knowledge concerning the understanding and treatment of disease, ethical standards for clinical research are not identical to those governing the practice of clinical medicine.

If individualized beneficence were the primary standard for clinical research, then any research interventions posing risks to patient volunteers not justified by compensating medical benefits would be ethically prohibited. Nonetheless, patient volunteers enrolled in clinical research routinely receive nontherapeutic research interventions that are not medically indicated and that pose risks. For example, psychiatric research commonly uses positron emission tomography (PET) scans and lumbar punctures to investigate the pathophysiology of psychiatric disorders. PET scans carry the risks of radiation exposure and complications from inserting arterial lines, and lumbar punctures may cause persistent headaches. A standard of individualized beneficence that rules out placebo-controlled trials when effective treatments exist would also prohibit such nontherapeutic investigational procedures. It follows that clinical research would be significantly curtailed if investigators were held to the same standard of individualized beneficence that applies to clinical medicine.

If clinical research is regarded as continuous with, or an extension of, clinical medicine, then patients suffering from illness should not receive placebos in clinical trials when standard, effective treatments exist, for this is to provide medical care known to be inferior. Because the physician-investigator is not operating primarily in the role of the patient volunteer's doctor in the context of clinical trials, however, it is not clear that the standard of therapeutic fidelity to individual patients, characteristic of clinical medicine, must govern placebo-controlled trials. Clinical trials are concerned with treatment responses in groups of patients representing the class of patients with a given condition. This scientific orientation toward groups of patients and critical features of study design, such as randomization and blinding, make clinical trials radically different from standard clinical medicine. Consequently, the ethical argument against the use of placebos in clinical research, based on the normative framework of clinical medicine, is open to question. Nonetheless, the potential for confusion and conflict between physician and investigator roles in clinical research makes it imperative that both the physician-investigator and the patient volunteer clearly understand and appreciate the differences between clinical trials and treatment in routine clinical practice (Miller et al 1998).

Beneficence is a basic principle of the ethics of clinical research, but it differs in scope from beneficence in clinical medicine. Unlike clinical medicine, clinical research is concerned primarily with benefits to future patients and society from generating biomedical knowledge. In clinical medicine, anticipated benefits to the individual patient justify risks of diagnostic and treatment interventions. Research risks are justified primarily by anticipated benefits of generating scientific knowledge and secondarily by benefits, if any, to individual subjects.

Investigators do have moral obligations to individual patient volunteers to protect them from harm and to promote their well-being consistent with the goal of pursuing scientific knowledge. Patient volunteers should not be subjected to risks of irreversible harm as a result of research participation. Insofar as withholding potentially effective treatment in placebo-controlled trials exposes patient volunteers to less serious risks of clinical deterioration and symptomatic distress, such studies are morally problematic. Are such studies necessarily unethical? I contend that time-limited periods of treatment withholding in placebo-controlled trials of new psychiatric treatments may be ethically justifiable, provided that the design and conduct of these studies satisfy stringent ethical standards and guidelines.

What Ethical Standards Should Govern Placebo Use in Clinical Trials?

Four ethical standards must be satisfied to legitimate the use of placebo controls in clinical research: 1) placebo-controlled trials should have scientific and clinical merit; 2) risks should be minimized and justified by the anticipated benefits of generating clinically relevant scientific knowledge and the expected benefits, if any, to individual research subjects; 3) patient volunteers should give informed consent; and 4) investigators should offer short-term individualized treatment optimization to patient volunteers after completion of research participation.

Scientific Merit

As in all clinical research, the justification for exposing patient volunteers to the risks of placebo-controlled trials depends on the scientific merit and potential clinical utility of these studies. Because placebo-controlled trials generally require smaller sample sizes than active-controlled trials, this research design may be advocated for reasons other than scientific or clinical merit. Specifically, placebo-controlled trials are convenient to serve the commercial interests of pharmaceutical companies in obtaining approval for marketing new drugs and the professional interests of investigators in completing 'successful' studies. To protect patient volunteers and promote research that is scientifically sound and clinically useful, IRBs should require that scientific protocols for placebo-controlled trials demonstrate rigorously why placebo controls are necessary or desirable.

Risk–Benefit Assessment

Risk–benefit assessment applies the principles of nonmaleficence and beneficence to clinical research (Beauchamp and Childress 1994; The National Commission for the Protection of Human Subjects of Biomedical and Behavioral Research 1978). The acceptability of placebo controls in clinical research depends on both the degree of risks posed to patient volunteers from temporary withholding of treatment and the efficacy and side-effect profile of current treatments. As the magnitude and probability of lasting harm or temporary distress associated with withholding treatment increases, the use of placebos becomes more problematic and difficult to justify. Also relevant is the quality of standard treatments. If clinically available drugs are highly effective in curing or preventing serious disease without producing intolerable side effects then it is difficult to justify placebo-controlled trials for new treatments for this condition; however, if current treatments have limited efficacy, produce uncomfortable side effects, or both, then placebo-controlled trials are easier to justify.

Several contextual features of psychiatric research are relevant to the justifiability of placebo-controlled trials (Lieberman 1996). Psychiatric disorders are chronic, fluctuating conditions that produce substantial morbidity but usually are not life-threatening. Nonetheless, patients suffering from psychiatric disorders are at considerably increased risk of suicide. A review of suicidality in clinical trials of drugs for treatment of depression found significantly greater suicidal ideation in patients on placebo compared with those on antidepressants in some studies but no significant differences in suicide (Mann et al. 1993). Standard psychiatric treatments provide partial relief of symptoms for many, but not all patients; they are not curative or fully preventive. Existing treatments have significant side effects, which many patients find intolerable. Finally, as noted above, psychiatric clinical trials have demonstrated high rates of placebo response.

In view of these factors, patient volunteers randomized to placebo in short-term psychiatric clinical trials are not likely to be greatly disadvantaged on the whole compared with those who receive experimental or standard treatment. Although patient volunteers on placebo arms of clinical trials testing the efficacy of drugs for the treatment of depression, schizophrenia, and other psychiatric disorders may experience symptomatic worsening, there is no evidence that short-term periods on placebo in psychiatric research produce any lasting harm (Addington 1995; Quitkin 1999). Nevertheless, psychic distress experienced by patient volunteers receiving placebos is a matter of moral concern and can be tolerated ethically only if it does not become severe. For some groups of seriously ill patients, the risks of being off medications in placebo-controlled trials may be sufficiently great to preclude their enrollment (Prien 1988).

Careful screening of prospective patient volunteers is required to minimize risks (Carpenter et al. 1997). It is likely that many, if not most, patients interested in clinical trials will have experienced less than satisfactory response to standard treatment. Nonetheless, patients who have responded well to standard psychiatric medications should not be invited to participate in placebo-controlled trials (Streiner 1999), with the exception of studies of maintenance treatment. Patients known to be at substantial risk of suicide or a danger to others should be excluded. Prospective patient volunteers should be encouraged to consult with their physicians before deciding whether to enroll in a placebo-controlled trial (Levine 1986, 111–112). For those who lack a physician, consultation with a clinician not involved in the research project is desirable.

The duration of the placebo period should be limited to the shortest time required for adequate efficacy testing. During the conduct of the clinical trial, monitoring procedures are necessary to protect patient volunteers (Quitkin 1999). For severely ill patients, consideration should be given to limiting placebo-controlled trials to inpatient settings with constant monitoring and the ready availability of 'rescue' medications in case of significant deterioration. In outpatient trials, investigators should maintain frequent contact with patient volunteers to assess symptomatic worsening and intervene appropriately. Consideration should be given to requiring research protocols to specify criteria for removing patient volunteers from clinical trials owing to symptom severity. In any case, clinical judgment will be necessary, and investigators should err on the side of patient safety.

Informed Consent

The purpose of informed consent is to promote and respect the self-determination of research subjects. As the term 'informed consent' suggests, patient volunteers must understand what is involved in enrolling in a particular clinical trial and authorize research participation by means of voluntary agreement. Because psychiatric research studies disorders of the brain, concern and controversy has arisen over whether psychiatric patients are capable of giving informed consent to research participation (Berg and Appelbaum 1999; Capron 1999; Elliot 1997; National Bioethics Advisory Commission 1998). The debate has also focused on mechanisms of assessing decision-making capacity before enrollment of patient volunteers in psychiatric research (Miller and Rosenstein 1999). These complex issues are not addressed here.

Enrollment in placebo-controlled trials of individuals who are not capable of giving informed consent should be permitted only under strictly limited circumstances. Placebo controls should be understood as a nontherapeutic feature of research design (Levine 1986, 203–206). Use of placebos may pose greater than minimal risk, especially when it involves withholding standard, effective treatment for a condition associated with considerable morbidity. Accordingly, patients with severely impaired decision-making capacity should not be enrolled in placebo-controlled trials when eligible subjects capable of giving informed consent are available. Some clinical trials, however, may be designed to test the efficacy of treatments in severely ill psychiatric patients who are likely to have impaired capacity. As a rule, incapacitated subjects may be enrolled in placebo-controlled trials only when their enrollment is necessary to conduct scientifically sound and clinically promising studies. These subjects should either have advance directives authorizing such research participation or be enrolled with the informed consent of authorized surrogate decision makers.

The adequacy of informed consent in the current practice of clinical research is open to question. In empirical studies of the informed consent process in psychiatric research, Appelbaum and his colleagues have found deficiencies in the understanding and appreciation of patient volunteers regarding their participation in clinical trials (Appelbaum *et al.* 1987). For example, 'With regard to nontreatment control groups and placebos, fourteen of thirty-three (44 percent) subjects failed to recognize that some patients who desired treatment would not receive it.' In general, interviewed subjects tended to view their participation in clinical trials as intended to promote their own individual benefit. Appelbaum *et al.* described this phenomenon, which many observers believe to be pervasive in clinical research, as 'the therapeutic misconception.'

Elements of informed consent do not differ essentially in placebo-controlled trials from other forms of clinical research. Some points, however, deserve emphasis. It is imperative that patient volunteers understand the nature of the study under consideration and how it differs from standard clinical practice, the rationale for placebo use, random assignment, the probability of receiving a placebo, blinding of patient volunteers and investigators, and so forth. Among the risks that must be disclosed and understood are lack of improvement that patient volunteers randomized to placebo might have experienced if they had received standard or experimental treatment and symptomatic worsening during the placebo phase. Patient volunteers should be warned that they may experience suicidal ideation and that, if so, they should report this to the investigators. Prospective subjects need to be made aware of alternatives to research participation. Specifically, they should be informed about the clinical availability of standard, effective treatments for their condition.

Patients must be free of coercion or undue inducement to enroll in clinical trials. They should be informed that they have a right to withdraw without penalty from research participation at any time. Investigators may encourage patient volunteers to remain enrolled in clinical trials but must honor their decisions to withdraw, regardless of doubts about their decision-making capacity. Severely ill patient volunteers are at risk of losing awareness of their right to withdraw from research. Family members or designated surrogate decision makers should be encouraged to monitor their condition and empowered to decide on their behalf to withdraw them from research if they deteriorate clinically to the point of losing decision-making capacity.

Treatment Optimization

Patient volunteers in placebo-controlled trials accept risks of research interventions and forego potentially effective treatment for the sake of contributing to scientific knowledge. Accordingly, they are owed the prospect of individualized therapeutic benefit in return. Placebo-controlled trials should be accompanied by a short-term treatment optimization phase in which physician-investigators endeavor to help patient volunteers, at no cost to them, find the best available treatment for their condition and undertake discharge planning for continuing clinical care. This provision is based on principles of nonabandonment, reciprocity, and just compensation. To avoid abandoning patient volunteers, investigators must provide clinical stabilization and referral for needed treatment at the conclusion of research participation. Beyond this minimal commitment, a time-limited period of treatment optimization functions as an important and ethically appropriate quid pro quo for research participation (Miller *et al.* 1998). In addition, patients whose symptoms have worsened during the clinical trial should be entitled to individualized treatment aimed at making them at least as well as they were before enrollment in research.

The obligation to provide treatment optimization should include patient volunteers who drop out of the clinical trial because of intolerable symptomatic worsening or side effects, as well as those who complete the study. The duration of treatment optimization may vary with respect to various psychiatric disorders and the clinical situation of particular patients. It should be clearly understood by patient volunteers as a short-term commitment so as not to provide undue inducement for research participation.

Public Justification

Exposure of patient volunteers to risks to test the efficacy of new treatments places a burden on investigators to justify the use of placebos in clinical research. In addition to justifying placebo-controlled trials in the context of IRB review and approval of scientific protocols, investigators should be required to address pertinent ethical issues associated with this research design in scientific articles published in professional journals (Charney *et al.* 1999; Miller *et al.* 1999). Currently, such articles in the psychiatric research literature rarely go beyond stating that the research was approved by an IRB and that informed consent was obtained. A requirement that investigators in scientific articles justify the rationale for the use of placebos—especially when standard, effective treatment exists – and discuss protections to minimize risks to subjects provides an additional safeguard for the ethical conduct of clinical research. Peer reviewers should scrutinize carefully the way in which ethical issues are addressed, just as they examine critically the discussion of methodological issues. Additionally, journal editors should consider seeking ethical commentary for articles reporting research that raise ethical issues. In view of the climate of distrust generated by reports in the news media alleging abuses in the conduct of psychiatric research (Hilts 1998; Whitaker and Kong 1998), including the use of placebos (Kong 1999), more detailed attention to ethical issues in the scientific literature might help improve the public perception of psychiatric research.

Conclusion

Critics of placebo-controlled trials have contended that they are unethical whenever their use would result in withholding standard, effective treatment that has a reasonable prospect of benefiting patient volunteers. In a critique of this stance, I have argued that it appeals to a standard of individual, patient-centered beneficence that, if strictly applied, would make it impossible to conduct any clinical research employing nontherapeutic interventions that pose risks to patient volunteers. Moreover, the alternative of active-controlled trials – proposed as superior ethically and more useful clinically than placebo-controlled trials when standard, effective treatment exists – is subject to serious methodological weaknesses and might lead to validating new treatments that may be no more effective than placebo.

The ethical criticism of placebo-controlled trials, however, has merit in drawing attention to the need for ethical scrutiny and justification of studies using this research design. I have presented an alternative bioethical perspective that regards placebo-controlled trials in psychiatric research as ethically defensible provided that these studies have scientific merit; the risks are reduced to an acceptable minimum and justified by the anticipated benefits of producing biomedical knowledge; patient volunteers give adequate informed consent; and investigators offer short-term treatment optimization to patient volunteers at the conclusion of research participation. Empirical research is needed to determine whether current practice of psychiatric clinical trials conforms to these ethical standards and to suggest ways to improve the protection of patient volunteers.

The ethical justification of placebo-controlled trials in psychiatric research depends critically on the contextual circumstances defining the nature and current treatment of psychiatric disorders. If scientific progress leads to the development of psychiatric medications that are highly effective with minimal side effects, placebo-controlled trials that withhold such treatment will become more difficult to justify. In that case, the use of placebo-controlled trials will have helped produce improvements in treatment that obviate the need and rationale for continued use of this research design.

The opinions expressed are those of the author and do not necessarily reflect the policy of the National Institutes of Health, the Public Health Service, or the Department of Health and Human Services.

For helpful comments on drafts of the manuscript, the author thanks Howard Brody, F. Xavier Castellanos, Evan DeRenzo, Ezekiel Emanuel, Christine Grady, Donald Rosenstein, and Dave Wendler.

Aspects of this work were presented at the conference 'Clinical Trials in Mood Disorders: The Use of Placebo . . . Past, Present, and Future,' September 14–15, 1999, Washington, DC. The conference was sponsored by the National Depressive and Manic-Depressive Association through unrestricted educational grants provided by Abbott Laboratories, Bristol-Myers Squibb Company, Forest Laboratories, Inc., Glaxo Wellcome Inc., Janssen Pharmaceutica Products, L.P., Merck & Company, Pfizer Inc., Pharmacia & Upjohn, SmithKline Beecham Pharmaceuticals, Solvay Pharmaceuticals, Inc., and Wyeth-Ayerst Laboratories.

References

Addington D (1995): The use of placebos in clinical trials for acute schizophrenia. *Can J Psychiatry* **40**:171–175.

Appelbaum PS, Roth LH, Lidz CW, Benson P, Winslade W (1987): False hopes and best data: Consent to research and the therapeutic misconception. *Hastings Cent Rep* **17**(2): 20–24.

Beauchamp TL, Childress JF (1994): *Principles of Biomedical Ethics*, 4th ed. New York: Oxford University Press.

Berg JW, Appelbaum PS (1999): Subjects capacity to consent to neurobiological research. In: Pincus HA, Lieberman JA, Ferris S, editors. *Ethics in Psychiatric Research: A Resource Manual for Human Subjects Protection*. Washington, DC: American Psychiatric Association, 81–106.

Brennan TA (1999): Proposed revisions to the Declaration of Helsinki—will they weaken the ethical principles underlying human research? *N Engl J Med* **341**:527–531.

Brown WA (1988): Predictors of placebo response in depression. *Psychopharmacol Bull* **24**:14–17.

Brown WA (1994): Placebo as a treatment for depression. *Neuropsychopharmacology* **10**:265–269.

Capron A (1999): Ethical and human-rights issues in research on mental disorders that may affect decision-making capacity. *N Engl J Med* **340**:1430–1434.

Carpenter WT Jr, Schooler NR, Kane JM (1997): The rationale and ethics of medication-free research in schizophrenia. *Arch Gen Psychiatry* **54**:401–407.

Charney DS, Innis RB, Nestler EJ (1999): New requirements for manuscripts submitted to *Biological Psychiatry*: Informed consent and protection of subjects. *Blot Psychiatry* **46**:1007–1008.

Clark PI, Leaverton PE (1994): Scientific and ethical issues in the use of placebo controls in clinical trials. *Annu Rev Public Health* **15**:19–38.

Code of Federal Regulations, 21CFR314.126 (1985).

Code of Federal Regulations, 45CFR46 (1991).

Elliot C (1997): Caring about risks: Are severely depressed patients competent to consent to research? *Arch Gen Psychiatry* **54**:113–116.

Freedman B (1987): Equipoise and the ethics of clinical research. *N Engl J Med* **317**:141–145.

Freedman B, Glass KC, Weijer C (1996): Placebo orthodoxy in clinical research. II: Ethical, legal, and regulatory myths. *J Law Med Ethics* **24**:252–259.

Greenberg RP, Fisher S (1997): Mood-mending medicines: Probing drug, psychotherapy, and placebo solutions. In, Fisher S, Greenberg RP, editors. *From Placebo to Panacea: Putting Psychiatric Drugs to the Test*. New York: Wiley, 115–112.

Hilts PJ (1998, May 19): Scientists and their subjects debate psychiatric research. *New York Times*, F1.

Hirschfeld RMA (1996): Placebo response in the treatment of panic disorder. *Bull Menninger Clin* 60(suppl A):A76–A86.

Kong D (1999, March 29): Use of placebos on mental patients questioned. *Boston Globe*.

Lasagna L (1995): The Helsinki Declaration: Timeless guide or irrelevant anachronism? *J Clin Psychopharmacol* **15**:96–98.

Leber P (1986): The placebo control in clinical trials (a view from the FDA). *Psychopharnacol Bull* **22**:30–32.

Levine RJ (1986): *Ethics and Regulation of Clinical Research*, 2nd ed. New Haven, CT: Yale University Press.

Levine RJ (1999): The need to revise the Declaration of Helsinki. *N Engl J Med* **341**:531–534.

Lieberman JA (1996): Ethical dilemmas in clinical research with human subjects: An investigator's perspective. *Psychopharmacol Bull* **32**:19–25.

Lieberman JA, Stroup S, Laska E, Volavka J, Gelenber A, Rush AJ, et al (1999): Issues in clinical research design: Principles, practices, and controversies. In: Pincus HA, Lieberman JA, Ferris S, editors. *Ethics in Psychiatric Research: A Resource Manual for Human Subjects Protection*. Washington, DC: American Psychiatric Association, 23–60.

Makuch RW, Johnson MF (1989): Dilemmas in the use of active control groups in clinical research. *IRB* 11: 1–5.

Mann J, Goodwin FK, O'Brien CP, Robinison DS (1993): Suicidal behavior and psychotropic medication. *Neuropsychopharmacology* **8**:177–183.

Miller FG, Pickar D, Rosenstein DL (1999): Addressing ethical issues in the psychiatric research literature. *Arch Gen Psychiatry* **56**:763–764.

Miller FG, Rosenstein DL (1999): Independent capacity assessment: A critique. *BioLaw* 11:S432-S439.

Miller FG, Rosenstein DL, DeRenzo EG (1998): Professional integrity in clinical research. *JAMA* **280**:1449–1454.

National Bioethics Advisory Commission (1998): *Research Involving Persons with Mental Disorders That May Affect Decisionmaking Capacity, Vol 1. Report and Recommendations*. Rockville, MD: National Bioethics Advisory Commission.

The National Commission for the Protection of Human Subjects of Biomedical and Behavioral Research (1978): *The Belmont Report: Ethical Principles and Guidelines for the Protection of Human Subjects of Research*. Washington, DC: Department of Health, Education, and Welfare.

Office for Protection from Research Risks (1993): *Protecting Human Research Subjects: Institutional Review Board Guidebook*. Washington, DC: U.S. Government Printing Office.

Prien RF (1988): Methods and models for placebo use in pharmacotherapeutic trials. *Psychopharmacol Bull* **24**:4–8.

Quitkin FM (1999): Placebos, drug effects, and study design: A clinician's guide. *Am J Psychiatry* **156**:829–836.

Rickels K (1986): Use of placebo in clinical trials. *Psychopharmacol Bull* **2**:19–24.

Rothman KJ, Michels KB (1994): The continuing unethical use of placebo controls. *N Engl J Med* **331**:394–398.

Shapiro AK, Shapiro E (1997): *The Powerful Placebo*. Baltimore: Johns Hopkins University Press.

Streiner DL (1999): Placebo-controlled trials: When are they needed? *Schizophr Res* **35**:201–210.

Taubes G (1995): Use of placebo controls in clinical trials disputed. *Science* **267**:25–26.

Temple R (1997): Problems in interpreting active control equivalence trials. In: Shamoo AE, editor. *Ethics in Neurobiological Research with Human Subjects: The Baltimore Conference on Ethics*. Amsterdam: Gordon and Breach.

United States Food and Drug Administration (1989): Supplementary advisory: Placebo-controlled and active controlled drug study designs. In: Brody B, editor. *The Ethics of Biomedical Research: An International Perspective*. New York: Oxford University Press, 291–292.

Weijer C (1999): Placebo-controlled trials in schizophrenia: Are they ethical? Are they necessary? *Schizophr Res* **35**:211–218.

Whitaker R, Kong D (1998, November 15): Testing takes a human toll. *Boston Globe*, A1.

World Medical Association (1996): Declaration of Helsinki. In: Brody B, editor. *The Ethics of Biomedical Research: An International Perspective*. New York: Oxford University Press, 214–216.

Zipursky RB, Darby P (1999): Placebo-controlled studies in schizophrenia – ethical and scientific perspectives: An overview of conference proceedings. *Schizophr Res* **35**:189–200.

The Rationale and Ethics of Medication-Free Research in Schizophrenia*

William T. Carpenter, Jr, Nina R. Schooler and John M. Kane

What is the scientific necessity, clinical wisdom, and ethics of research protocols that specify a treatment procedure for a cohort of patients rather than using the physician's best judgment for each individual? How is this addressed in serious diseases with known effective treatments? In schizophrenia, wherein research data and prevailing clinical opinion support continuous medication as a cornerstone of treatment for most patients, how can placebo-controlled clinical trials and medication delay or withdrawal for research purposes be justified? If a research protocol is justified as generating new knowledge, how is the participation of any given patient justified?

These issues are receiving intense scrutiny by investigators, ethicists, and laypersons concerned with the conduct of schizophrenia research. This follows extensive media coverage of allegations that a study conducted at the University of California, Los Angeles (UCLA), was unethical in its design, delinquent in its clinical responsibilities, and inadequate in informing participants of risks (*Time*. August 30, 1993:40-42; *The New York Times*. March 10, 1994, and May 24, 1994). However, an investigation by the National Institutes of Health Office of Protection From Research Risks found the scientific design of the UCLA study to be ethical and the standard of clinical care appropriate. Modifications were required in the consent form to ensure a thorough understanding by participants of the risks involved.[1] The widespread attention given to this case and public concern with human rights and safety in research fueled by recent revelations of the post-World War II radiation experiments makes it timely to reexamine these issues.

We review the scientific questions in schizophrenia research that require medication-free periods and discuss the rationale for such studies. We then discuss the potential risks and benefits of controlled medication discontinuation under careful observation and suggest safeguards for study participants.

Medication-free Research

There are 2 common types of studies that can require drug-free periods: those that study the development of new treatments and those used for the study of variables that might be confounded by medication effects. The latter studies are particularly important to advancing knowledge with regard to etiology and pathophysiology, and are the critical steps in ultimately finding a cure or prevention.

Development of New Pharmacological Treatments

Significant advances have been made in the short- and long-term pharmacological treatment of schizophrenia. Antipsychotic medications have been shown to be effective for a substantial proportion of patients in alleviating or reducing positive symptoms of schizophrenia and reducing the risk or delaying the recurrence of psychotic exacerbation. In the context of this antipsychotic effect, a broad range of symptom and functional attributes

improve. However, available drugs are inadequate. Most patients respond only partially. Primary negative symptoms (ie, the deficit syndrome) are largely refractory to available treatments. Many patients relapse despite continuous medication treatment. Available compounds are associated with adverse effects that can be subjectively distressing, can interfere with psychosocial and vocational adjustment, are associated with poor medication compliance, and, in cases such as severe tardive dyskinesia or tardive dystonia, can be disabling.

There is now an unprecedented effort to develop better medications, reflecting both the dissatisfaction alluded to above and encouraging progress associated with newly marketed compounds.[2–4] It is essential that patients, their families, investigators, institutions, and society pursue the opportunities that these new and potentially more effective and safer medications represent with a consensus regarding the ethics of this research.

Why is medication-free research necessary in new drug development? The first reason is to provide an initial drug withdrawal period designed to minimize the risk for adverse drug-drug interaction as an experimental compound is introduced. Second is to prevent carry-forward effects of prestudy medication from confounding clinical response evaluation of the experimental treatment. Third is to establish a medication-free baseline against which therapeutic and adverse effects are measured. Fourth is to compare new compounds with placebo to establish that they are effective antipsychotic agents. Placebo controls are also necessary to determine an adverse effects profile of an experimental compound.[4] Depending on the stage of development, such studies also may incorporate comparison to standard antipsychotic agents or comparison of different doses or dose ranges of the experimental and/or standard drugs.

Because the goal of this research effort is to find medications that are safer and more effective than currently available treatments, it can be argued that the appropriate comparison should be between an experimental drug and a currently available medication, avoiding placebo altogether. A critical problem is the interpretation of study results. Consider a study in which the clinical effects of an experimental medication are not statistically different from those produced by a drug with established efficacy, but there is no placebo comparison group. Two interpretations are possible: one is that the treatments are equally effective; the other is that neither is effective because the particular patient sample studied is not treatment responsive. The second interpretation is plausible if the sample includes many patients who have received medication prior to study assignment, are poor neuroleptic responders, or are in a maintenance phase of treatment. These are common circumstances in clinical trials of new antipsychotic medications, and the inability to base efficacy conclusions on such designs has been demonstrated.[5,6] That poor response to known effective drugs is often observed has been verified in drug development studies in which haloperidol was an active control.[7] Using a criterion of at least 30% improvement on total Brief Psychiatric Rating Scale scores, the proportion of patients responding to haloperidol varied from 12% to 45%.[7]

The alternative design incorporates a placebo control. If the experimental drug and the standard medication are not distinguishable but both are better than placebo, then we conclude that they are both effective. If neither

* Carpenter, W.T., Schooler, N.R. and Kane J.M.: The rationale and ethics of medication-free research in schizophrenia. *Archives of General Psychiatry* 54:401–407, 1997.

is better than placebo, we conclude that the study was insensitive to previously known effects and no conclusion is reached regarding effectiveness of the experimental drug. The placebo-controlled study is more informative scientifically, as well as potentially more sparing of risk. The effectiveness of an experimental drug that proves to be approximately as effective as standard treatment can be documented with adequate statistical power in a relatively small number of subjects participating in a placebo-controlled study. Failure to reject the null hypothesis that an experimental and a standard treatment are not different is not the same as finding them equivalent, and, if a study is conducted with inadequate power, the treatments may not differ statistically in their effect despite inferiority of the experimental drug.

A common misconception that placebo response rates in schizophrenia are minimal, consistent, and predictable leads to a misunderstanding of the need for placebo controls. In fact, placebo response rates vary substantially in both short- and long-term treatment trials, eg, ranging from 3% to 26% in the proportion of patients responding in one review of short-term trials.[7] In a recently published report from a large multicenter trial[4] comparing risperidone, haloperidol, and placebo, haloperidol was not significantly superior to placebo on a major outcome measure. Gilbert et al[8] reviewed 29 controlled trials involving neuroleptic withdrawal and found that relapse rates among patients withdrawn from medication ranged from 0% to 100% after follow-up intervals ranging from 0.5 to 24 months (mean, 9.7 months). It is not scientifically valid to substitute 'historical' placebo response data for concurrent placebo control. A striking example of this problem occurred when hemodialysis was reported as remarkably superior to historical data,[9] only to be found no different from sham dialysis in controlled studies.[10–12]

In schizophrenia, treatment effects must be assessed in multiple outcome domains. Evaluating a treatment that is effective but is associated with an adverse effect profile causing low patient compliance requires several measures to describe the benefit-to-risk ratio. As an example, consider the prevalence (20%–25% in long-term treated patients) of tardive dyskinesia with antipsychotic drug treatment.[13] If a new medication were associated with little risk for tardive dyskinesia, but was also less effective than standard treatment in preventing relapse, could a decision be made regarding its use without proof that it was in fact superior to placebo?

It has been proposed[14] that once an effective treatment is available, new treatments should be introduced only if superior efficacy is expected. The hypothesis of superior efficacy to standard treatment can be tested without placebo control. This was the case when a superior efficacy hypothesis was tested for clozapine in comparison to chlorpromazine[2] and haloperidol.[15] But, clozapine's antipsychotic efficacy had been previously established.[16] New drug development in schizophrenia seeks advantages in motor side effects, sedation, negative symptoms, long-term cognitive functioning, patient acceptability, and other considerations. In all these instances, it is crucial to determine whether the new drug is an effective antipsychotic.

Nontreatment Studies

There are other research questions that require medication-free protocols and usually involve fewer subjects than are required in drug development programs. Of fundamental importance are studies designed to advance our knowledge of etiology and pathophysiology. Because of the wide range of effects of neuroleptic medication in the central nervous system, such treatment could either cause or confound the experimental results. For example, a positron emission tomographic scan study testing a dopamine receptor hypothesis cannot be conducted on subjects receiving neuroleptic medication because the drugs can alter receptor characteristics. Findings from most studies using dependent variables relating to pathophysiology may be confounded by neuroleptic drugs. These basic studies are necessary to gain sufficient understanding of the disease, which, in turn, provides a new basis for developing therapeutics and prevention. This type of study, in contrast to clinical trials, does not offer participants the possibility of specific benefits from the protocol, although the patient may benefit indirectly (through enhanced diagnosis and more intensive clinical care and therapeutics that are characteristic of settings conducting research with medication-free periods).

However, study subjects may ultimately benefit if the research leads to new treatments in their lifetime. Subjects in the initial neuroleptic studies may not have benefited directly if receiving placebo, but their treatment for the years afterward has been enhanced by the new knowledge gained in these investigations.

A final class of studies involves medication-free periods to address specific clinical questions. Does early detection of dyskinesia reduce the risk of developing irreversible tardive dyskinesia? One early detection tool involves the observation of drug withdrawal dyskinesia requiring medication discontinuation,[13,17] another the provocation of dyskinesias by the administration of a dopamine agonist.[18] Does an increase in symptoms associated with initial drug withdrawal identify a subgroup of patients at heightened risk for relapse? Can this change distinguish patients who require substantial continuous medication from those who may be candidates for a medication reduction strategy? Gilbert et al.,[8] who reviewed an extensive literature on neuroleptic withdrawal, concluded that discontinuation can usually be done safely with return to baseline levels of psychopathologic symptoms after about 3 weeks of retreatment if symptom exacerbation occurs. Considerable comment pro and con ensued,[19–26] but it is the case that in ordinary clinical care, drug withdrawal may be indicated in a number of circumstances.[19] These include (1) stable patients who refuse medication; (2) patients with emerging dyskinesia, dystonia, neuroleptic malignant syndrome, water intoxication, or severe cardiac effect; (3) aging patients whose psychosis is reduced and drug risks are increased; (4) stable, first-episode patients who may not have a recurrent psychotic illness; (5) pregnancy; and (6) a new approach to treatment that requires a drug washout for safety and/or observation of treatment response.

Potential Benefits and Risks of Drug Discontinuation

Research protocols without apparent direct patient benefit provoke heated debate.[27] Should subjects be allowed to volunteer for such experiments, and, if so, at what risk or discomfort? We do not engage in this debate here, but rather provide a perspective on the clinical and research questions in medication-free protocols that must be understood if the debate is to be informed.

Potential benefits of drug withdrawal protocols include the ability to assess patients in a drug-free state and better characterize the nature of the illness, to have baseline assessments to more accurately assess treatment effects, to disentangle behavioral adverse effects of medication from manifestations of the disease, to identify early signs of tardive dyskinesia that may be masked by antipsychotic drugs, and to identify patients who may sustain remission without medication. The risks associated with medication-free periods include the prolongation or the reemergence of psychosis. If careful supervision is not in effect, or if severe exacerbations are not treated appropriately, subjects may be at risk for loss of judgment and insight, personal harm or harm to others, job or housing loss, increased burden to family or other caregivers, or other complications of psychosis. These risks are known and current studies must include safeguards to reduce such serious risks.

The question of long-term risk also has been raised. Are medication-free periods associated with substantial adverse effect on long-term course? In an illness that is often severe and persistent despite standard treatment, it is difficult to address this question decisively. Wyatt[28] reviewed the literature and argued that the longer a person is ill before initial treatment, and the more prolonged the psychotic experience is after initial treatment, the worse the ultimate treatment response and the poorer the long-term outcome. He speculates that psychosis is neurotoxic but cites no supportive evidence. On the other hand, animal studies have suggested that the administration of neuroleptic drugs might be capable of inducing neuronal pathologic effects in specific brain regions.[29–32] The interpretation of Wyatt's suggestions is complicated both in terms of the methods used and alternative explanations. First, long-term data that specifically address this issue are scarce. The study by May et al.[33,34] involved random assignment of patients to 1 of 5 different conditions for 6 months. Those who did not receive medication during the 6-month trial had a poorer outcome during the next 5 years even though they ultimately received medication. Current drug withdrawal or medication-free research designs do not involve a 6-month 'no drug treatment approach' for those experiencing a psychotic episode. The data that are available from trials of substantial dosage reduction or intermittent treatment[35–39] have not found differences in outcome on measures of psychopathology or psychosocial adjustment, even though patients in the medication reduction or withdrawal groups experienced significantly more symptomatic exacerbations. In fact, in one study,[40] patients receiving a very low dose were rated by their families as better on some psychosocial measures despite a 56% relapse rate in contrast to a control group with a 14% relapse rate.

These studies lasted 2 years at most and more data are needed regarding long-term outcome, but the hypothesis that drug-free periods have a long-term toxic effect is not yet substantiated. This view is reinforced by a 7-year follow-up study reported by Curson et al.[41] of patients who were treated for 1 year with continuous medication or placebo (relapse rates of 8% and 67%, respectively). No difference in outcome was observed on any of the 11 psychopathology measures.

Although medication benefits are not doubted, it is important to recognize that medication does not cure or halt the progression of the disease. Medications diminish symptom expression and reduce relapse rates. For this reason, we agree with Wyatt concerning the desirability of early detection and initiation of drug therapy. However, this does not guarantee remission or prevention of relapse and may not alter long-term disability. Medication noncompliance is, perhaps, the principal source of lengthy off-medication periods, and dissatisfaction with current treatments is a contributing factor. The evidence from random assignment, controlled trials suggests that it is not the brief, closely monitored protocol-based, medication-free periods that contribute significantly to the adverse clinical course with which Wyatt is concerned. In addition, the potential long-term toxic effects of neuroleptic medication cannot be ignored in any discussion of medication-free research intended to develop safer and more effective treatments.

Considerations for Individual Protection

Gaining new knowledge of schizophrenia has a clear scientific and societal benefit, but the issues of an individual's participation as a research subject must be addressed in the context of risk minimization, potential associated benefits, informed consent, and the individual's right to make an altruistic contribution.

If a study design increases risk for symptom exacerbation, how can maximum protection for individual participants be provided? The following points represent basic elements of guidelines to assure the ethical and prudent conduct of studies with schizophrenia patients.

Subject Selection

First, document that subjects understand the research information provided in informed consent. Second, exclude patients with known histories of rapid deterioration associated with substantial clinical management problems. Third, exclude patients who are at greatest risk for severe adverse effects. Fourth, include patients who are expected to have an excellent response to medication only if the following additional criteria are met: (1) the study tests a hypothesis regarding *superiority* of treatment to current medications in either efficacy or side effects or tests a major hypothesis relevant to etiology or pathophysiology that requires robust responders; (2) the placebo period is brief; (3) the protocol has clear criteria for withdrawing patients if response is inadequate or at early signs of clinical deterioration; and (4) if treatment research is involved, the protocol offers treatment advantages to the individual such as open-label treatment with the new

drug being studied following research participation or the individual appreciates the absence of treatment advantages and exercises the right to participate to help others.

Enhanced Therapeutics and Clinical Care Monitoring

Several psychosocial treatments for schizophrenia have the potential to partially offset risks associated with medication-free research periods.[42] The protection of medication-free subjects should be enhanced by including a high-quality, broad-based clinical treatment program. In studies where symptom improvement or relapse prevention is the outcome variable of interest, effective psychosocial treatment may reduce power and, therefore, more time and/or subjects may be needed to answer the treatment question. However, if the psychosocial treatment program improves the ability to detect symptom change and rapid intervention is built into the protocol, such programs may enhance care while allowing the use of symptom change rather than full relapse as outcome criteria. Nontreatment studies requiring medication-free periods will similarly be enhanced by effective psychosocial treatment. These procedures facilitate close monitoring and emergency availability in the context of personal continuity of care.[43] Such procedures have proved safe and effective in outpatient research.[8,35–39,44] Any given patient's time in the medication-free component of a protocol may be brief compared with the overall length of care, and benefits from enhanced care can accumulate over time, while protocol restrictions affect only one aspect of treatment for a limited time.

Early Intervention

Early detection of symptom exacerbation and rapid treatment intervention has proved effective in targeted or intermittent drug treatment research in outpatient clinics. One study of maintenance treatment compared medication-free intervals coupled with rapid medication intervention and an enriched psychosocial treatment program with community standard treatment with continuous medication. These treatment approaches did not differ in overall effectiveness, and the treatment that incorporated medication-free intervals was associated with substantial reduction in drug administration.[36] Another study has shown that an early drug intervention strategy is better than crisis intervention in preventing serious relapse in medication-free patients.[44] Several studies have shown that continuous medication supplemented by psychosocial treatments in research settings is superior to low-dose continuous medication or to targeted medication in relapse prevention, but these same studies reveal advantages to the low-dose strategies in adverse drug effects and in the treatment of negative symptoms.[39,45]

Duration of Risk Period

Investigators should be explicit regarding the central study hypothesis. Design of acute treatment studies should incorporate the shortest medication-free period compatible with testing an efficacy hypothesis. Relapse prevention studies do not require severe symptomatic episodes as end points but can test prophylactic hypotheses with mild-to-moderate exacerbation compatible with rapid and effective intervention in most cases. Placebo-controlled studies testing experimental drug effect in actively psychotic patients may be informative in 2 to 6 weeks rather than the 4- to 10-week periods that are characteristic of most current designs. The potential weakness of less change in the shorter period can be compensated in many studies by adding more case subjects to increase statistical power.

Benefits to Participants

In studies evaluating an experimental treatment, providing all participants the opportunity to receive the treatment after study participation is highly desirable. This addresses the problem of patients participating in a study involving increased risk without potential advantage. When this is not possible, the investigator must ensure that the participant understands that the placebo assignment involves risks without the potential benefit of the experimental drug.

The material discussed above supports the propositions that medication-free research can be conducted while continuing other aspects of treatment, that rapid drug intervention can be an effective alternative to continuous medication during symptom exacerbation, that subject selection criteria can reduce risk, and that certain benefits may accrue to research participants. The question of treatment vs no treatment does not accurately address the key issue in most protocol-influenced treatment. Rather, the question is the relative risks and benefits of protocol based clinical care vs standard care.

Informed Consent

It has been suggested that persons with schizophrenia be declared a vulnerable population meriting special protection, including requiring a guardianship to authorize research participation.[46-48] This proposal assumes that all persons with a diagnosis of schizophrenia are unable to participate in receiving and understanding information and making rational personal decisions regarding participation in research. This argument is not offered as a basis for incompetency and guardianship in all stroke victims, all panic disordered patients with irrational fears, all obsessive patients with irrational beliefs, all depressed patients with affect-distorted reasoning, or even cardiac patients whose apprehension may make them unduly reliant on the perceived wishes of their physician. The determination of competency simply on the basis of the diagnosis of schizophrenia is highly stigmatizing and would strip a large population of their civil rights because some schizophrenic individuals, at some points in their lives, are not competent to process information and reach informed decisions. Recent research suggests that approximately 75% of patients with schizophrenia incorporate information and make decisions similar to comparison groups when dealing with consent issues.[49]

There are special circumstances when an individual with schizophrenia is not able to participate adequately in informed consent. Investigators must avoid attempting to obtain informed consent when a patient is unable to interact in the receiving of information and determining his or her wishes. At a minimum, the patient should be able to explain what participation entails, identify significant risks and benefits, and know how to withdraw from the study. The signing of the informed consent document is essential for research participation, but the process of informing and assuring adequate patient participation in consent should involve ongoing discussion.[50-52] It is the research field's responsibility to develop documentation procedures to ensure that patient participation is based on an adequate process for informed consent and evidence that the prospective subject has competently processed the relevant information.

Informed consent is also essential for treatment in nonresearch clinical care, although procedures for obtaining and verifying consent are less formal. Clinical procedures have risks and benefits, and patients are entitled to this information and personal autonomy in making choices regarding their treatment (except in highly specified emergency situations or where legal incompetency and guardianship have been established). A written document is not routinely used, but this does not alter the informed consent obligation. There is no unique basis for depriving this entire class of patients of this right in favor of incompetency and guardianship, nor is it conceivable that all clinical care and study of persons with this diagnosis could be effectively conducted under guardianship conditions. What is needed is emphasis on full disclosure, assuring continuing discussion, and encouragement of family involvement.

Conclusions

Are human subjects participating in medication-free research adequately protected with current procedure? One answer to this question is provided by the observation that there are thousands of patients who have participated in such research and there have been few allegations of significant or long-lasting adverse consequences associated with their research participation. When adverse consequences are alleged, as in the recent UCLA case, the circumstances parallel those associated with difficulties in implementing effective care for schizophrenic patients that are often encountered in clinical settings. The risk that must be considered in medication-free studies is the extent to which such circumstances are more likely to occur and what protections are provided. Ultimately, patient welfare depends on the maintenance of effective clinical care and includes a capacity to rapidly and effectively intervene when the course of illness becomes complicated, including adverse consequences of medication free periods. We know of no evidence that research participation leads to inferior treatment and a worse course of illness in the long term. In fact, many patients and their families anticipate a high level of expertise, a more extensive diagnostic evaluation, a more intensive (and often less expensive) clinical care effort, better follow-up, and perhaps an advantageous experimental treatment when selecting care in a research setting. Evidence supporting this view has been presented.[53-57]

Even when protocols require medication-free periods, cumulative days without antipsychotic drugs may be fewer and clinical supervision may be better than that which occurs in ordinary care settings. Patients often prefer to be without medication despite the risks, creating the very substantial problem of medication non compliance in clinical care. Finally, all approaches to schizophrenia therapeutics have risks. Continuous medication is better for psychosis reduction and relapse prevention but worse for tardive dyskinesia, sedation, weight gain, a range of parkinsonian symptoms, and other adverse effects. Antipsychotic drug treatment is the cornerstone of modern therapeutics of schizophrenia, but this does not imply that continuous use in all cases is the only safe or effective approach. Nor is the risk-benefit analysis as straightforward as in treating diabetes with insulin. We acknowledge risk associated with medication-free research but we argue that the ethics and wisdom of such designs be viewed in the overall context of clinical care of a chronic illness. The high risk of prolonged off-drug status with infrequent monitoring, allowing severe relapse without intervention, is not the relevant comparison for time-limited, carefully monitored, multimodality clinical care with the capacity for a rapid intervention research design that is now common and that may represent the new standard for medication-free research.

We do not think that current approaches to medication-free research are associated with widespread problems of inadequate informed consent or adverse consequences to patients, nor do we believe that research-based clinical care is inferior. But, new data permitting more explicit examination of these issues are needed, and this is a propitious time to examine procedures and assure patients, society, and the research community that approaches are optimal and that the field is committed to developing better procedures whenever shortcomings are evident. We call for renewed emphasis on added protection. The first consideration is protocol design that ensures that the research questions are of high merit and that effective clinical interventions are in place to reduce risk during medication-free periods. The second has to do with ensuring that participants are competent and that they understand the risks and how to terminate research participation. Assessment of potential subjects in this regard is practical and can provide documentation that consent procedures are adequate and that patients can exercise choice.[58] The third is maximizing offsetting factors such as assuring enhanced psychosocial treatment and clinical monitoring and enabling all participants to have an opportunity to participate in any treatment hypothesized to be superior whenever practical. Ensuring that studies are well designed is the responsibility of investigators, the sponsors of research such as the pharmaceutical industry and the National Institutes of Health, and the established institutional review boards. Assuring the adequacy of protection to individuals who are potential participants in research is the responsibility of individual investigators and the clinical care systems that support the research. Ultimately, the hope of patients with schizophrenia and their families to benefit from further advances in treatment, as well as eventual prevention or cure, will hinge on how well we meet this challenge.

In this article, we described the most common conditions of research participation in medication free protocols to increase the information used in public discussion of the ethics of this work. We are concerned that statements (*The New York Times*. March 10, 1994) comparing medication-free research in schizophrenia with withholding insulin from diabetic patients or giving placebo instead of immunosuppressant drugs during organ transplant surgery represents an astonishing unfamiliarity with the realities of schizophrenia therapeutics. We also remind the reader that no evidence of any widespread ethical problem in schizophrenia research has been presented and no indication that research participants have an adverse long-term course of illness has been forthcoming.

Based on the above considerations, we do not believe this is a time for radical reform of schizophrenia research procedures. Guardianships for research participants, external clinical monitors, new review boards, and regulations excluding placebo-controlled studies and medication-free research would, in our opinion, stigmatize patients, waste precious research funds, and deprive persons with this illness of the new knowledge on which better therapeutics and prevention will be based. Rather, we believe it is time for a careful assessment of current procedures to ensure their adequacy and to make any necessary modifications. Toward this end, we have identified some relevant strategies to ensure protection in protocol design and individual participation. It must be recognized that informed consent for research is problematic throughout medicine, and illness afflicting the brain presents particular problems in some patients. The general guidelines outlined in this article may apply in most situations but exceptions may have merit. If such guidelines defined the usual conduct of medication-free research in schizophrenia, investigators and review groups would know when an exceptional protocol is proposed and provide special scrutiny of novel provisions to make sure that the work, if undertaken, is conducted with due consideration to the protection of human subjects.

Supported in part by grants MH40279, MH35996, MH45156, and MH46672 from the National Institute of Mental Health, Rockville, Md.

References

1   Office for Protection From Research Risks, Division of Human Subject Protections. *Evaluation of Human Subject Protections in Schizophrenia Research*. Los Angeles: University of California, Los Angeles; May 11, 1994.

2   Kane J, Honigfeld G, Singer J, Meltzer H. Clozapine for the treatment-resistant schizophrenic: a double-blind comparison with chlorpromazine. *Arch Gen Psychiatry*. 1988; 45:789–796.

3   Meltzer HY. Treatment of the neuroleptic nonresponsive schizophrenic patient. *Schizophr Bull*. 1992; 18:515–542.

4   Marder SR, Meibach RC. Risperidone in the treatment of schizophrenia. *Am J Psychiatry*. 1994; 151:825–835.

5   Leber P. Is there an alternative to the randomized controlled trial? *Psychopharmacol Bull*. 1991; 27:3–8.

6   Temple R. Special study designs: early escape, enrichment, studies in non-responders. *Community Stat Theory Meth*. 1994; 23:499–531

7   Kane JM, Borenstein M. The use of placebo controls in psychiatric research. Presented at the First National Conference on Ethics in Neurobiologic Research With Human Subjects; January 7, 1995; Baltimore, Md.

8   Gilbert PL, Harris J, McAdams LA, Jeste DV. Neuroleptic withdrawal in schizophrenic patients: a review of the literature. *Arch Gen Psychiatry*. 1995; 52:173–188.

9   Wagemaker H Jr, Cade R. The use of hemodialysis in chronic schizophrenia. *Am J Psychiatry*. 1977; 134:684–685.

10   Schulz SC, van Kammen DP, Balow JE, Flye MW, Bunney WE Jr. Dialysis in schizophrenia: a double-blind evaluation. *Science*. 1981; 211:1066–1068.

11   Carpenter WT, Sadler JH, Light PD, Hanlon TE, Kurland AA, Penna MW, Reed WP, Wilkinson EH, Bartko JJ. The therapeutic efficacy of hemodialysis in schizophrenia. *N Engl J Med*. 1983; 308:669–675.

12   Wagemaker H, Rogers JL, Cade R, Schizophrenia, hemodialysis, and the placebo effect: results and issues. *Arch Gen Psychiatry*. 1984; 41:805–810.

13   Kane J, Jeste DV, Barnes TRE, Casey DE, Cole JO, Davis JM, Gualtieri CT, Schooler NR, Sprague RL, Wettstein RM. *American Psychiatric Association Task force Report on Tardive Dyskinesia*. Washington, DC: American Psychiatric Press: 1992.

14   Rothman KJ, Michels KB. The continuing unethical use of placebo controls. *N Engl J Med*. 1994; 331:394–398.

15   Breier A, Buchanan RW, Kirkpatrick B, Davis OR, Irish D, Summerfelt A, Carpenter WT. Effects of clozapine on positive and negative symptoms in outpatients with schizophrenia. *Am J Psychiatry*. 1994; 151:20–26.

16   Umbricht DSG, Liberman JA, Kane JM. The clinical efficacy of clozapine in the treatment of schizophrenia. *Rev Contemp Pharmacother*. 1995; 6:165–186.

17   Carpenter WT, Rey AC, Stephens JM. Further remarks on covert dyskinesia in ambulatory schizophrenia. *Lancet*. June 19, 1982:1421.

18   Lieberman JA, Laser M, John C, Pollack S, Saltz B, Kane J. Pharmacologic studies of tardive dyskinesia. *J Clin Psychopharmacol*. 1988;8(suppl 4): 57–63.

19   Carpenter WT, Tamminga CA. Why neuroleptic withdrawal in schizophrenia? *Arch Gen Psychiatry*. 1995; 52:192–193.

20   Caldwell AE. *Origins of Psychopharmacology: From CPZ to LSD*. Springfield, III: Charles C Thomas Publisher; 1970.

21   Baldessarini RJ, Viguera AC. Neuroleptic withdrawal in schizophrenic patients. *Arch Gen Psychiatry*. 1995; 52:189–192.

22   Greden JF, Tandon R. Long-term treatment for lifetime disorders? *Arch Gen Psychiatry*. 1995; 52:197–200.

23   Meltzer HY. Neuroleptic withdrawal in schizophrenic patients. *Arch Gen Psychiatry*. 1995; 52:200–202.

24   Nuechterlein KH, Gitlin MJ, Subotnik KL. The early course of schizophrenia and long-term maintenance neuroleptic therapy. *Arch Gen Psychiatry*. 1995; 52:203–205.

25   Wyatt RJ. The risks of withdrawing antipsychotic medications. *Arch Gen Psychiatry*. 1955; 52:205–208.

26   Jeste DV, Gilbert PL, McAdams LA, Harris MJ. Considering neuroleptic maintenance and taper on a continuum. *Arch Gen Psychiatry* 1995; 52:209–212.

27   *Proceedings From the first National Conference on Ethics in Neurobiological Research With Human Subjects*. Baltimore Marriott Inner Harbor, January 7–9, 1995; Baltimore, Md. Discussions.

28   Wyatt RJ. Neuroleptics and the natural course of schizophrenia. *Schizophr Bull*. 1991; 17:235–280.

29   Gariano RF, Young SJ, Jeste DV, Segal DS, Groves PM. Effects of long-term administration of haloperidol on electrophysiologic properties of rat mesencephalic neurons. *J Pharmacol Exp Ther*. 1990; 255:108–113.

30   Benes FM, Paskevich PA, Domesick VB. Haloperidol-induced plasticity of axon terminals in rat substantia nigra. *Science*. 1983; 221:969–971.

31   Meshul CK, Casey DE. Regional, reversible ultrastructural changes in rat brain with chronic neuroleptic treatment *Brain Res*. 1989; 489:338–346.

32   Roberts RC, Gaither LA, Gao XM, Kashyap SM, Tamminga CA. Ultrastructural correlates of haloperidol-induced oral dyskinesias in rat striatum. *Synapse*. 1995; 20:234–243.

33   May PRA. *Treatment of Schizophrenia: A Comparative Study of Five Treatment Methods*. New York, NY: Science House; 1968.

34   May PRA, Tuma AH, Dixon WJ. Schizophrenia: a follow-up study of results of five forms of treatment. *Arch Gen Psychiatry*. 1981; 38:776–784.

35   Herz MI, Glazer WM, Mostert MA, Sheard MA, Szymanski HV, Havez H, Mirza M, Vana J. Intermittent vs maintenance medication in schizophrenia: two-year results. *Arch Gen Psychiatry*. 1991; 48:333–339.

36   Carpenter WT Jr, Heinrichs DW, Hanlon TE. A comparative trial of pharmacologic strategies in schizophrenia. *Am J Psychiatry*. 1987; 144:1466–1470.

37   Carpenter WT Jr, Hanlon TE, Heinrichs DW, Summerfelt AT, Kirkpatrick B, Levine J, Buchanan RW. Continuous versus targeted medication in schizophrenic outpatients: outcome results. *Am J Psychiatry*. 1990; 147:1138–1148.

38   Schooler NR. Maintenance medication for schizophrenia: strategies for dose reduction. *Schizophr Bull*. 1991; 17:311–324.

39 Schooler NR, Keith SJ, Severe JB, Matthews SM. Treatment strategies in schizophrenia: effects of dosage reduction and family management on outcome. *Schizophr Res.* 1993; **9**:260. Abstract.

40 Kreisman D, Blumenthal R, Borenstein M, Woerner M, Kane JM, Rifkin A, Reardon G. Family attitudes and patient social adjustment in a longitudinal study of outpatient schizophrenics receiving low-dose neuroleptics: the family's view. *Psychiatry.* 1988; **51**:3–13.

41 Curson DA, Hirsch SR, Platt SD, Bamber RW, Barnes TRE. Does short term placebo treatment of chronic schizophrenia produce long term harm?*BMJ.* 1986; **293**:726–728.

42 Bellack AS, Mueser KT. Psychosocial treatment for schizophrenia. *Schizophr Bull.* 1993; **19**:317–336.

43 Carpenter WT, Heinrichs DW. Early intervention, time-limited targeted pharmacotherapy in schizophrenia. *Schizophr Bull.* 1983; **9**:533–542.

44 Pietzcker A, Gaebel W, Kopcke W, Linden M, Muller P, Muller-Spahn F, Tegeler J. Intermittent versus maintenance neuroleptic long-term treatment in schizophrenia: 2 year results of a German multicenter study. *J Psychiatr Res.* 1993; **27**:321–339.

45 Kane JM, Marder SR. Psychopharmacologic treatment of schizophrenia. *Schizophr Bull.* 1993; **19**:287–302.

46 Appelbaum P, Lidz C, Meisel A. *Informed Consent – Legal Theory and Clinical Practise.* Oxford, England: Oxford University Press; 1987.

47 National commission for the Protection of Human Subjects of Biomedical and Behavioral Research. *The Belmont Report.* Washington, DC: Dept of Health, Education, and Welfare;1978.

48 President's Commission for the Study of Ethical Problems in Medicine and Biomedical and Behavioral Research. *Summing Up.* Washington, DC: Government Printing Office; 1983.

49 Grisso T, Applebaum PS. The MacArthur Treatment Competence Study, III: abilities of patients to consent to psychiatric and medical treatments. *Law Human Behav.* 1995; **19**:149–174.

50 Carpenter WT. A new setting for informed consent. *Lancet.* March 23, 1974:500–501.

51 Katz J. Human experimentation and human rights. *St Louis University Law J.* 1993; **38**:7–54.

52 Katz J. Respecting autonomy. In: *The Silent World of Doctor and Patient.* New York, NY; Free Press; 1984:130–164.

53 Cardon PV, Dommel FW, Trumble RR. Injuries to research subjects: a survey of investigators. *N Engl J Med.* 1976; **95**:650–654.

54 Carroll RS, Miller A, Ross B, Simpson GM. Research as an impetus to improved treatment. *Arch Gen Psychiatry.* 1980; **37**:377–380.

55 Giller E, Strauss J. Clinical research: a key to clinical training. *Am J Psychiatry.* 1984; **141**:1075–1077.

56 Kalman TP, Talon NS, Frances A, Kocsis JH. A controlled study of satisfaction among psychobiology research patients. *Am J Psychiatry.* 1982; **139**:344–347.

57 Kocsis JH, Frances A, Kalman TP, Shear MK. The effect of psychobiological research on treatment outcome: a controlled study. *Arch Gen Psychiatry.* 1981; **38**:511–515.

58 Love R, Conley RR. Obtaining informed consent from psychiatrically impaired subjects. *Psychiatr Serv.* In press.

Preventing Severe Mental Illnesses – New Prospects and Ethical Challenges*

Kenneth F. Schaffner and Patrick D. McGorry

1. Introduction

Severe mental illnesses devastate millions of lives worldwide. Exciting recent developments in studies of psychoses in general and schizophrenia in particular are offering hope that such illnesses can be identified and treated early. Early treatment promises better outcomes for both the affected individuals and their families. Such treatments aim at reaching patients during their first 'psychotic break' as well as attempt to identify at-risk individuals during the pre-illness or 'prodrome' period. These 'early intervention' projects also point toward the possibility in the future of attaining true (primary) prevention for those at-risk of psychoses from genetic and/or environmental factors.

But the studies needed to determine the safety and efficacy of such interventions raise a series of significant ethical and regulatory questions, that if not adequately answered will impede progress in this vital area, as well as potentially harm human subjects and their families. The studies in this area are controversial and raise a series of research ethics questions. The National Institutes of Mental Health (NIMH) has had concerns about informed consent, stigma, risk of medications, and appropriate crisis interventions in this area-concerns that led to a recent NIMH workshop (Heinssen et al., 2001). Also, one in-progress clinical trial was the subject of a complaint by a watchdog group to the US Office for Human Research Protections (OHRP). That complaint triggered an OHRP investigation that was only recently resolved.

These studies are controversial in part because most of them include administration of low doses of new antipsychotic drugs to some participants who are not psychotic. These drugs were developed for severe forms of mental illness and have some significant side effects varying from sedation, often considerable weight gain and mild sexual dysfunction, to motor problems including (rarely) tardive dyskinesia. It should be added here, however, that there are numerous research foci for the novel antipsychotics which do not involve the presence of psychotic symptoms, e.g. treatment-resistant depression, mania, conduct disorder in children, ADHD, Tourette's disorder, and behavioral disorders in dementia. Also, there are only a few studies on long-term side effects of the atypical neuroleptics, and the best data presented at the November 2000 NIMH workshop is yet to be published (Heinssen et al., 2001). The studies raise the following types of questions: are such drugs safe for those who will never really experience true psychosis'? What might be the side-effects, both short- and long-term, of medicating 'at-risk' subjects, including both those who have few symptoms and those who are severely symptomatic, but not yet psychotic? Will early intervention recruitment attempts stigmatize subjects and generate unnecessary family concerns? In efforts at psychosis prevention, are there risks of creating a new vaguely defined mental disorder and perhaps over-medicalizing normal behavioral variants? How can those symptomatic participants who may have their decision capacity compromised, and may also be adolescents, provide true informed consent? Are subjects' confidentiality adequately protected? Do the one-to-two year-long randomized double-blind designs of some trials afford adequate interim feedback to participants and

* Schaffner, K. and McGorry, P.: Preventing severe mental illnesses – new prospects and ethical challenges. *Schizophrenia Research* 51:3–15, 2001.

their psychiatrists as well as sufficient monitored protection for those actually developing psychoses?

These and related questions have been addressed at a series of recent conferences, international meetings, and workshops by experts in the fields of psychiatry, bioethics, policy regulation, and by representatives from the affected communities. These meetings and workshops include the Greenwall Foundation funded international conference at GWU in November 1999 that produced the papers published in this issue of SR, a NAMI 1998 Workshop, two NIMH workshops on early intervention in psychosis in May 1999 and November 2000, a symposium at NAMI's Chicago 1999 annual meeting, several symposia at the 'Future Possible' IEPA meeting in New York in March 2000, and a symposium at the ISPS meeting in Stavanger in June 2000. These ongoing discussions are the backdrop for the following analysis of ethical and design issues in this extraordinarily promising and yet ethically contentious area. The analysis serves as an introduction and roadmap for the papers that follow.

2. The background and rationale for early intervention psychosis prevention studies

In their paper [. . .] Wyatt and Henter (2001) distinguish 'early intervention' efforts into two different types: first-episode of psychosis patients and prodromal patients. (They also discuss futuristic efforts to achieve true or primary prevention as a third effort.) Prodromal interventions raise the most difficulties for both psychiatric diagnosis and also the ethical character of the interventions directed at them.

The expression 'prodromal symptoms' refers to the controversial 'prodrome' concept in psychiatry, namely a period preceding the active phase of psychosis (schizophrenia) in which there is 'clear deterioration from a previous level of functioning' (DSM-III-R, 1987, p. 190). In the early intervention field, the prodrome refers to that period before an individual experiences his or her first psychotic break. The concept is controversial because it is vaguely defined – a vagueness that probably led to the concept being downgraded in the current version of the American Psychiatric Association's Diagnostic and Statistical Manual, DSM-IV, 1994. Early intervention researchers have done much over the past six years to make the concept more precise, as will be related in a subsequent section.

The prodrome concept is of vital importance because it may identify individuals at risk of psychosis before the full-blown disorder takes hold. There is suggestive evidence, first reviewed by Wyatt (1991) that psychosis in and of itself may be biologically toxic to the brain, and thus that intervening early in psychosis may be beneficial in both the short- and long-term. (But even if this *biological* toxicity hypothesis turns out not to be confirmed (see Lieberman and Fenton, 2000), it is the case that there is psychosocial toxicity of the impact of the subthreshold prodromal symptoms, and those that mimic them but turn not be precursors of psychosis.

This psychosocial toxicity is more than sufficient to justify considering intervening in those who will accept help.) Wyatt, as well as others, have also reviewed other earlier work in this issue. Though these provide suggestive circumstantial evidence for a beneficial effect of early interventions, there is more persuasive evidence from both recent controlled studies (see Wyatt and Henter, 2001) as well community-based studies to support early interventions' effectiveness.

The most recent broad-based community education and early intervention study is one developed in Norway and Denmark. In Stavanger, Norway, with Roskilde, Denmark serving as a control, Johannessen, McGlashan, Simonsen, and Vaglum and their collaborators have found that an intensive community education and early detection system for prodromal and first episode patients can significantly reduce DUP (Johannessen et al., 2001): Empirical evidence about the beneficial effects of early intervention has been interpreted differently by different groups of researchers, with some questioning whether early intervention in first-episode patients offers benefits over delayed interventions (Ho et al., 2000) but others perceiving clear benefits (Birchwood, 2000; Lieberman and Fenton, 2000).

3. The Australian and New Haven early intervention studies: from naturalistic to experimental methods

The Australian trials. In Melbourne, the second author and his colleagues had commenced early intervention studies with a 'first generation' project in 1984, followed up by a much broader program beginning in 1991 involving the early psychosis prevention and intervention centre (EPPIC) and the personal assistance and crisis evaluation (PACE) clinic. (PACE was chosen as a deliberately general term, and because the clinic has been sited in a non-psychiatric setting, a young people's health service, the 'Centre for Adolescent Health', McGorry's group has obtained data that show reduction in distress in all patient groups together with high levels of attendance at the clinic, suggesting this setting can decrease stigmatization of the patients (McGorry et al., 2001a). It is important to stress here that both PACE and EPPIC are primarily clinical services with evaluation components and not solely research ventures (McGorry et al., 1996).

In the prepsychotic group, an important follow up prospective study at PACE examined conversion to psychosis rates within a psychosocial treatment cohort. This study also required that the prodromal concept be reanalyzed and operationalized in a three-fold manner. Yung and McGorry (1996) defined three different pre-psychotic subgroups: (1) patients with attenuated positive psychotic symptoms (more on these below), (2) individuals experiencing brief psychotic episodes too short in duration to meet DSM criteria for psychosis (symptoms spontaneously resolved within one week), and (3) those with a genetic risk (i.e. a first-degree relative diagnosed with a psychosis or with a schizotypal personality disorder) coupled with recent severe deterioration in behavioral functioning (Yung et al., 1996, 1998). This tripartite analysis was the groundwork for additional descriptive studies examining transition to psychosis of 'ultra high risk (UHR)' early intervention subjects. Here it is useful to point out that the genetics of schizophrenia (and other psychoses such as bipolar disorder) are still unclear. Gottesman and Erlenmeyer-Kimling (2001) provide an overview of the genetics and familial risk factor patterns. The clearest work in the genetics of a psychiatric (and neurological) disorder is in the Alzheimer's disease (AD) area. See Schaffner (2001) for an account, and also Post's article (2001) for lessons from AD possibly applicable to schizophrenia early intervention programs.)

The first PACE prospective descriptive study ($n = 21$) yielded a transition rate of 21% by 12 months and 33% by 24 months (Yung et al., 1996; Phillips et al., 2000; McGorry et al., submitted). The criteria were amended and a second study ($n = 49$) carried out in which the transition rate by 12 months reached 41% and by 24 months at least 50%. These transition rates were observed despite intensive psychosocial intervention. These studies

were a prelude to a PACE prospective randomized open *interventional* or *experimental trial* comparing psychosocial intervention versus low-dose antipsychotic medication with psychosocial intervention in 59 patients. The results of this trial were recently reported at the ICOSR meeting in 1999 and the NY IEPA meeting in March 2000 and have been submitted for publication (McGorry et al., submitted, 2001c).

This trial's initial protocol pitted a combination of low dose risperidone and cognitive therapy plus supportive case management against case management alone. Full details of this study ($n = 59$), carried out between 1996-1999, are available on request (McGorry et al., submitted). In summary, the more specific treatment package was significantly more likely to result in a reduction of risk of transition ($p = 0.02$). The reduction of transition rate was from 35.7 to 9.7% for the treatment phase of 6 months. The number needed to treat (Cook and Sackett, 1995) was low at 4, indicating the intervention was potent in reducing risk. Those who complied fully with the low dose risperidone were afforded longer-term protection (at least 6 months post-cessation) even after the risperidone was ceased. There were minimal side effects noted and no evidence that patients were stigmatized in any way. Those not making the transition to psychosis demonstrated significant improvements in symptoms and functioning, with similar benefits occurring in those who received risperidone, so benefits greatly overshadowed the risks, even though the drug treatment was certainly an unnecessary inconvenience in a subset of young people. There is no evidence that it was any more than this. The study was randomized but not blinded, and has not clarified whether some patients would have received a reduction of risk from the specific cognitive therapy without antipsychotic medication. This is a live possibility, as is potential reduction of risk from other non-neuroleptic biological treatments, such as emerging neuroprotective agents like lithium and essential fatty acids. Several other trials involving first episode patients have been concluded or are in the planning stages. The EPPIC group published a historically controlled study of an integrated hospital and community early intervention program for first episode psychosis in 1996, comparing a more aggressive, new psychosocial treatment with an older treatment group. The two groups were comprised of 51 patients each, and were examined for a range of process, symptomatic and outcome variables. Generally the new treatment group fared better on a number of factors, including cost-effectiveness. More recently in the Netherlands, Linszen and Dingemans demonstrated a reduced relapse rate in a trial involving 76 Dutch patients, however long term follow-up suggested that this early benefit will become minimal unless continuity of care is provided for these patients (Linszen and Dingemans, 2001).

In early intervention in psychosis studies, the specific instruments developed to assess prodromal states take on several very significant roles including trial admission, identification of dangerousness and suicidality, and transition to psychosis (and thus removal from the trial). The Australian studies use the comprehensive assessment of at risk mental states (CAARMS) instrument and the New Haven study employs similar instruments to be discussed further below. The CAARMS was 'specifically designed to prospectively measure the psychopathology of the `at risk mental state' – that mental state which may represent the prodrome or precursor state to a first psychotic episode (McGorry and Singh, 1995; Yung et al., 1996, 2000). Developed in 1994, it incorporates eight dimensions of psychopathology, operationally defines the ultra high risk (UHR) criteria for transition as well as the threshold for established psychosis, and has demonstrated good reliability and predictive validity (Yung et al., in preparation). A revised version (CAARMS 11) was constructed in 2000 and is available on request from the second author.

The New Haven trial and its extensions. The most scientifically rigorous and what some see as ethically controversial early intervention trial involving prodromal patients was initiated in December 1998 by McGlashan and his colleagues in New Haven, CT. That study is based at Yale's Prevention Through Risk Identification Management & Education (PRIME) clinic and is still in-progress. The PRIME trial follows a randomized double-blind placebo controlled design and to date has enrolled 35 patients. (There are three additional sites that have begun enrolling patients in extensions of the

PRIME trial at Clark Institute, Calgary, and UNC-CH.) The active treatment arm in the PRIME trial receives low doses (5–15 mg/day) of the antipsychotic drug olanzapine plus supportive psychotherapy, and the 'placebo' controls receive supportive psychotherapy. Patients are typically in the trial for two years before the blind can be broken (one year of treatment or placebo and one year of follow up). However, if a patient in the trial converts to psychosis, he or she has the blind broken and is placed on olanzapine 15–20 mg/day. Entrance criteria for the trial utilize an evaluative scale similar to the CAARMS known as the scale of prodromal symptoms (SOPS). The SOPS is administered as part of a candidate interview termed the structured interview for prodromal symptoms (SIPS) similar to the CAARMS described earlier. The SIPS is used to determine the presence or absence of a psychotic state, of a prodromal state, and of which prodromal states. The SOPS is used to determine the severity of the prodromal state once it has been diagnosed (McGlashan, 2001).

4. Concerns and criticisms

Of the various early intervention studies and clinical trials, the PRIME trial provoked the most discussion at the November 1999 Greenwall-GWU conference and follow-ups for reasons that we cover both in this and the following section, but was not seen as particularly provocative at the November Bethesda NIMH 2000 workshop. As we mentioned earlier, it also was the subject of an investigation by the OHRP. The investigation was triggered by a complaint by Vera Sharav's citizens for responsible care and research group (CIRCARE). PRIME's subjects were described by CIRCARE as asymptomatic siblings of schizophrenic patients who were only at 10% risk of conversion to psychosis (over their lifetimes). In a reply to the OHRP, the PRIME investigators corrected this allegation noting that patients must have either positive prepsychotic symptoms or a substantial personal functional deterioration plus genetic risk to qualify. And based on the Australian and evolving New Haven data, they believe the subjects to be at 40% risk of conversion to psychosis over the next year. (Recent data indicate the risk of conversion in the Yale population is 63%, Miller et al., submitted.)

The CIRCARE group also claimed that the PRIME trial offered no prospect for benefit for individual subjects and entailed more than minimal risk, and thus that it was not ethical for minor subjects under the US common rule sections 45 CFR 46.404–406. The PRIME investigators agreed that the trial was more than minimal risk since a medication is involved, but they believe that the trial does offer the prospect of individual benefit for subjects in at least four ways: (1) all subjects are carefully monitored, (2) all subjects receive a stress management psychotherapy, (3) subjects who receive active medication are hypothesized to receive a benefit in prevention of conversion to psychosis, and (4) subjects who receive active medication are hypothesized to receive a benefit for their current symptoms (Woods, personal communication).

The PRIME investigators felt strongly that these benefits to the subjects outweighed the more than minimal risks. To this list of benefits we might add, in an elaboration of point 1, that if the person does become psychotic they receive very rapid detection and treatment, unlike 'standard care' where DUP is on average 1 year. Further, regarding point 2, the patients also should be getting help with other aspects of their lives. PRIME was in point of fact recently notified by the OHRP that OHRP had closed its compliance oversight evaluation of this research and anticipated no further OHRP involvement in the matter (McGlashan, personal communication).

5. The intertwined ethical and study design issues: points to consider

Based on the above accounts of early intervention programs, we have identified the following five 'Points to Consider' that intertwine both ethical and study design features. We think these points represent, in summary form, the current state of debate about research and treatment ethics in the field and the directions in which additional research and deliberations will likely proceed. All of these points in some fashion will need to be addressed by researchers, IRBs, and funding agencies, and the results of current and future deliberations on them to be communicated in an appropriate fashion to patients and/or their legally authorized representative, and in many instances to their families. These five Points to Consider are, for all their intricacy, a somewhat oversimplified overview of ongoing conceptual, empirical, ethical, and regulatory problems in the early intervention in psychosis area (see the following schizophrenia research papers for more detail) but they should suffice to give the reader of this essay a sense of the complexity of the promise, pitfalls, and potential solutions in the early intervention in psychosis field.

1. *The varying patient populations involved: a heterogeneity and diagnostic problem plus ethical difficulties of including/not including children in clinical trials.* In the text above, we indicated that early intervention programs treat three different types of patients: first episode psychosis patients and prodromal patients, the latter falling into a class of patients who have attenuated positive symptoms suggesting early psychosis and a third class of those who are at genetic risk and are experiencing moderate to severe functional deterioration. These three classes of patients may not truly exhaust the various subclasses of patients and further neuropsychiatric testing may suggest additional subtypes that have different prognoses and may benefit from different forms of treatment. Suffice it to say at present that this tripartite classification is the best the field can offer, but further research is being directed at this issue of heterogeneity by a number of investigators (see for example Klosterkotter et al., 2000).

The heterogeneity issue points toward a much broader set of problems for psychiatry in general relating to its diagnostic approach and its fundamental concepts. Though we do not have the space to address these issues adequately in this paper, it should be noted that diagnosis is syndromal and further has been transformed from dimensional into categorical terms. Categorical diagnosis provides an appearance of precision and validity, and though the diagnostic manuals have assured better reliability, the precision and validity may be spurious (see McGorry et al., 1995). The diagnostic concepts in psychosis are 100 years old. Some are attempting to shore them up by extension of the concepts, e.g. a notion of schizophrenia permitted to have non-psychotic forms with neurocognitive impairments, assumed but not proven to be specific for schizophrenia, as the hallmark (Tsuang et al., 2000). We believe these and many other diagnostic concepts as currently defined have been developed from tertiary samples and settings where patients with severe and chronic illnesses accumulate (also compare Feinstein. 1967). The situation is analogous to attempting to diagnose early onset breast cancer according to a prototype linked to stage 3 or 4 disease. The diagnostic concepts therefore are unwieldy and may well be inappropriate in the early stages of illness where flux and comorbidity are rife and the person's adaptive or maladaptive reactions to the disorder are also evolving in the context of depression and anxiety.

The other general issue that needs addressing here is the need for categorical distinctions which apply definitions of caseness along an evolving dimensional reality and which have not yet properly addressed or highlighted in prodromal research. Disorders evolve by intensification of milder subthreshold symptoms, e.g. major depression from mild depression, or by acquisition of new symptoms not previously present which may also intensify, e.g. paranoia to a diagnostic threshold (Eaton, 2001). We need to study all this properly, and generate broader treatment-relevant foci for early disorders. From this perspective, schizophrenia and its secondary prevention is largely a second order issue. There are more proximal targets to focus upon such as psychosis (first-episode psychosis is not the same as differentiated schizophrenia) and perhaps the subthreshold symptoms as well. This task is a broader one than pre-psychotic intervention in schizophrenia or even psychosis. One of us (PM) suggests that the onset phase of 'stem' psychiatric disorders should be examined closely and a practical diagnostic schema developed.

Though it is generally uncontroversial to treat first-episode patients, considerable attention has been given to the problem of treating the 'false positives' that are included among 'prodromal' patients in the early intervention area. These 'false positives' are those individuals who meet current criteria for a prodromal diagnosis (in New Haven and Melbourne) but who will never develop full-blown psychosis, though many will be diagnosable with other mental disorders. If the conversion rate to full-blown psychosis of approximately 40% in an 'ultra-high risk' population is a true one (McGorry et al., 2000a,b), then 60% of those individuals may theoretically experience the stigma of being labeled at risk of psychosis, along with the label's effects on the mental state (emotions and self-image) of the individual and his or her family, as well as the social effects of stigma. For proper perspective, however, we should also note that this rate of 40% is several thousand times higher than the annual risk at this age for the general population. There is also no empirical data on the true risk of stigma or effects of labeling on self image. Further, no studies have yet been done, to our knowledge, of the effects of entering a mental health facility or a diagnosis of a mental disorder on help-seeking prodromal/first-episode psychosis populations.

Additionally, a falsely diagnosed individual may receive low doses of a powerful antipsychotic drug, with possible effects of sedation, weight gain, and compromised sexual function, whether or not he or she enters a clinical trial, since 'off label' use of the drug is not uncommon. (The use of possible alternative therapies with less troublesome side effects will be covered in the next point.) Attempts to eliminate the false positive problem, including the use of genetic analysis and neuropsychiatric testing to better characterize the prodrome, are ongoing, but there is as yet no better generally accepted figure than the 60% false-positive rate. McGorry et al. (2001b) cite some strategies that may reduce the false positive rate to 20% and the preliminary data from Miller noted above about a conversion rate of 63%, if it is replicated, would reduce this false positive rate; also see Gottesman and Erlenmeyer-Kimling (2001) for how twin-study approaches might similarly work to reduce a false positive rate.

A related issue we need to highlight under the heading of patient population heterogeneity is the severity of patients' symptoms. Recall that it was a misunderstanding of prodromal patients' symptomatology that was in part the basis of the CIRCARE complaint and OHRP investigation of the Yale trial cited above. There is some disagreement among psychiatrists about 'how sick' a patient must be to be started on low doses of atypical neuroleptics or other pharmaceutical interventions. This disagreement is the case even if the patient has psychotic symptoms (Van Os et al., 2000). We will return to this issue under point 4 below after we have discussed clinical equipoise.

Involving minors (less than 16 years in some countries but less than 21 years from a federal perspective in the US) in research raises special ethical, legal, and regulatory problems for a discussion of which see DeGrazia (2001).

- Point 1: early intervention patients are diverse, clinically and ethically, and in fact may even be more clinically heterogeneous than can be identified at present. The patients that satisfy the current treatment (and clinical trial inclusion) criteria for prodromal studies include among themselves a large number (60%) of false positives who may run risks of labeling and from drug treatment, a problem that should be resolvable by obtaining appropriate informed consent (see Point 5 below). Incorporating minors in early intervention research raises special ethical, legal, and regulatory problems, but excluding minors in this area is unwise and at least by US regulations probably untenable.

2. *Varying types of appropriate drug interventions.* The assumption among a number of investigators in the early intervention community, particularly it seems in the US, has been that the same therapy that works for full-blown psychosis may work for prodromal patients as a prophylaxis, albeit in a lower dose. This assumption implies that though appropriate psychosocial therapy may help, it is the atypical neuroleptics that are likely to be the most beneficial intervention. Cornblatt et al. (2001) has recently questioned this assumption, proposing that the widely accepted diathesis-stress model of

schizophrenia suggests stress-reducing medications may ameliorate developing psychosis in at-risk individuals. McGorry et al. (2001c) have speculated that early interventions employing cognitive therapies alone, very low dose lithium and even essential fatty acids might be explored in the future. Similarly, Woods et al. (2000) have also discussed lithium, essential fatty acids, etc as novel early interventions for the prodrome. The side effects of SSRIs (and especially essential fatty acids) are generally viewed as less severe than the side effects of low doses of neuroleptics. However, in support of atypical neuroleptic treatment are the Australian data that indicate an effect size of neuroleptics and cognitive therapy of a four-fold improvement over psychosocial interventions alone, and there are no controlled data available to support SSRI and the other drug interventions mentioned. Furthermore, good adherence to a neuroleptic in the six-month treatment phase was also associated with a longer-term protective effect even after the drug was withdrawn. In this study, the number needed to treat (NNT) was 4 (see McGorry et al., 2001c for details).

- Point 2: additional investigations employing both atypical neuroleptics and cognitive therapies as well as SSRIs are being conducted. The former approach is being implemented in studies at Melbourne, at Yale, and in PRIME North America sites including the University of North Carolina at Chapel Hill, as well as is being considered as part of a developing international version of the PRIME trial. The latter (SSRIs) is being pursued at Hillside largely on a free use basis but with more structured designs planned. All of these options as well as other reasonable drug interventions need to be disclosed to potential patients as treatment alternatives.

3. *Varying types of appropriate studies – naturalistic, randomized, open vs. blinded.* Just as there are some varying views about the most appropriate drug intervention(s), investigators in the early intervention area also differ somewhat about the most appropriate types of studies needed on the basis of current knowledge. McGorry's group's most recent results involved a trial of 59 patients who were randomized to either psychosocial therapy alone or low dose atypical neuroleptics with psychosocial therapy, with both patient and psychiatrist knowing the treatment (open label) McGorry et al., 2001c). McGlashan's PRIME trial and its extensions utilize a randomized assignment and treatment arms similar to those of the Australian study, but do so with a randomized double-blinded placebo-controlled design so that neither patient (nor family) nor psychiatrist know of the treatment assignment (McGlashan, 2001). Cornblatt and her colleagues have recently argued that neither the McGorry nor McGlashan type of trial is where the field should be, and that it would be more prudent to conduct epidemiologically based naturalistic types of trials, apparently similar to those done earlier in Australia by McGorry (see above). Cornblatt et al. (2001) argue that 'without information on base rates of conversion to schizophrenia, the extent to which an intervention is actually working is difficult to assess' and suggest that naturalistic studies establishing the base rates of eventual illness are therefore critical for evaluating the successfulness of early treatment. Some naturalistic studies along these lines have been done in Australia and the Netherlands (where some base rate data have been obtained, Van Os et al., 2000) but more data and in different contexts may be useful.

- Point 3: the conditions under which various randomized, open label, and blinded trials should be implemented needs further public discussion, and the uncertainty about the best designs may need to be communicated to prospective patients (we take this up in more detail in the next and also in the final point). A more precise characterization of epidemiologically based naturalistic studies and a clearer methodological defense of their ability to avoid bias and achieve standard levels of power and significance would be helpful to make sure that such studies conform to good scientific designs.

4. *Under what conditions is it advisable for a patient to enroll in a scientifically rigorous trial?* Various themes that have already surfaced in points 1–3 above re-emerge in an intertwined manner in this penultimate Point to Consider, which focuses on the ongoing PRIME trial and its North American

(at Calgary, the Clark Institute and UNCCH) and its worldwide extensions, currently in the active planning process (Woods, personal communication). McGlashan has argued that in part because new antipsychotic drugs (atypical neuroleptics) with a better side-effect profile became available, circumstances regarding early intervention and 'prevention' trials changed during the 90s. He claims the field had moved to a point in late 1998 where there was genuine 'equipoise' about administering low doses of the new atypicals to those individuals that meet PRIME's enrollment criteria, i.e. the patients were 'sick enough' that the average psychiatrist would consider starting them on drug therapy and that the atypicals were the drug of choice. 'Equipoise' (often termed 'clinical equipoise' in the literature) is a concept that bioethicists and clinical investigators developed to characterize the 'experts are collectively on the fence' position between two trial arms (between two different treatments or between treatment and non-treatment) with some tilting towards treatment and others away. Freedman (1987) introduced the concept in his article. If a field is in equipoise, McGlashan argues, then the only right (ethical) thing to do is to conduct well-designed research that will answer the question which intervention is in fact best, and well-designed research is what the PRIME type of trial implements (McGlashan, 2001).

But other psychiatrists (including some attending the Washington, DC 1999 and Bethesda, MD 2000 conferences) are not certain that the field is in equipoise, or are not certain that it is in equipoise for all of those who would meet the Yale criteria for trial inclusion, and they also have doubts about the PRIME trial's blinding and length.

The main rationale for double-blindedness is to control for the placebo effect. One of the psychiatrists who attended the Bethesda, November 2000 conference has suggested the size of placebo effect should be determined (or at least guesstimated) *before* a trial of this type is widely mounted to justify the need for blinding. An estimate based on earlier PACE epidemiological studies suggests the placebo effect size may be about 25%, i.e., that 25% of ultra-high risk individuals who would have converted to psychosis do not when receiving psychosocial therapy but no active drug therapy. (This estimate may confound a true psychosocial intervention effect with the placebo effect but the resolution of such confounding awaits additional research.) It is generally the case that in a non-blinded trial, fine-tuning of whatever intervention is chosen or assigned can be done more easily. Fine-tuning could include changing the dosage of a medication or the type of medication, taking the patient off medication, or placing the patient on medication if he or she is only being treated with supportive psychotherapy, attractive options if the treating psychiatrist truly knows what works, which is under contention. Blinded trials trade off this individualized decision-making for scientific rigor, reduced design bias, and better control of the placebo response. The use of placebos also introduces the need for more sophisticated knowledge on the part of the patient, and provokes concerns that patients in such trials may be under a therapeutic misconception (Appelbaum *et al.*, 1987). Along similar lines, another senior psychiatrist knowledgeable in research in this area, thinks the trial could appropriately be randomized and double-blinded, but suggests the PRIME design might be too long in its current configuration, and better done not as a two-year long trial (one year of drug or placebo and one year of followup observation) but instead as an initial six month trial. On this view, patients initially meeting PRIME criteria for trial inclusion would be randomized to either placebo plus psychotherapy or to low dose neuroleptics plus psychotherapy. But after the first six months the blind would be broken, and symptomatic individuals who were on placebo could be offered a three-month trial of the test medication. After the nine months, then we might (or might not) have enough data to justify beginning a two-year-long randomized double-blind trial such as the PRIME trial. These legitimate differences among treating and research psychiatrists reflect a state of equipoise of design considerations as well as treatment equipoise. One of us (PM) currently believes that the evidence developed thus far, and the estimated size of the placebo effect, indicates that the next step should be a randomized double-blind trial of a year's length to further clarify the effects of both psychosocial and atypical neuroleptic interventions.

- Point 4: some psychiatrists and clinical psychologists view the PRIME trial as being premature in its scientific rigor whereas others believe this is where the field should be at this time. A broader consensus based on an informal sample of participants at the November 1999 conference seems to be in favor of continued open randomized trials of atypical neuroleptics, but there are some investigators who favor even less directive interventional studies at present, recommending the more epidemiological types of studies. Others believe that current and future patients will best be served by a randomized double-blind placebo controlled trial (with supportive therapy in all arms). Whichever type of trial is offered, the subjects need to be acquainted with an easily understandable account of the relevant features of the trial's methodology and its pros and cons. Subjects need to be told that there are trade-offs between a personally structured plan of care and scientific rigor to avoid the risks of the therapeutic misconception.

5. *What do patients, families (and surrogates), IRBs, and patient representation organizations need to know about the early intervention field and the available study options, and how can we evaluate consumers' and trial participants' knowledge in this complex area?* In addition to the various international conferences and workshops cited above on early intervention, there have also been several meetings of patient representative organizations eager to determine what the state is of the early intervention field so that they can respond to questions on this subject from their intensely interested members. A small meeting of the national alliance for the mentally ill (NAMI) was held to address this in July 1998, and a large public meeting attended by over 200 people was held at the national NAMI meeting in July 1999 in Chicago. The question what to tell patients and their families about the state of the field and the types of available studies was also a paramount issue at the Bethesda November 2000 NIMH workshop. In Australia, relatives' organizations are firmly behind the concept of prodromal research and the Second National Mental Health Strategy (Commonwealth of Australia 2001) is also fully supportive of providing additional information to potential patients and families.

As suggested in commentary preceding Points 1-4 above, there are some generalizations that can be gleaned from the current debates about early intervention though there are no easy and definitive answers to the question posed above. A start might be to provide to relevant parties a digest of the information presented in Points 1–4 above. Additionally, the responsibility of investigators to meet these informational needs might be partially met by publication of the existing clinical trial consent documents (and trial protocols insofar as sponsors will permit this) in an accessible patient newsletter like the NAMI Advocate, along with commentary by the investigators and by other disinterested psychiatrists. Further, we would urge the publication of sample cases in such newsletters, along with additional details that would meet these patient and family needs for more concrete and easily comprehended information. In Australia, EPPIC and PACE have a book of first person accounts available and are preparing additional materials for consumers and families.

Even with better materials that can guide affected and interested parties through the maze of complexities in early intervention research, we will need to develop appropriate instruments for evaluating research subjects' (or their representatives') competency or capacity: their understanding and appreciation of the salient issues involved in this field. Informed consent is a critical element in human subject research (Schaffner, 1995) and competency analysis is a complex subject (see Schaffner (1991) for an overview). As a first step toward this goal of evaluating capacity to consent, both authors have each begun to explore how to further develop an instrument known as the MacArthur competence assessment tool - clinical research (MacCAT-CR) that evaluates capacity of human subjects to consent to clinical research (Appelbaum and Grisso, 1996). We, working with the MacCAT's co-developer, Paul Appelbaum, MD and with representatives from six major early intervention project institutions, propose to adapt the MacCAT-CR for use with prodromal and first-episode subjects (and/or their surrogates) in early intervention schizophrenia trials. One current version of the MacCAT-CR is an easily implemented 15min semi-structured interview that has shown considerable promise in a small trial with schizophrenic patients (Carpenter *et al.*, 2000). With those subjects, the MacCAT-CR has been able to identify capacity and informed consent problems, and also has served as a measure of how well these problems can be remedied by additional instructional interventions. No such instrument so far as we know has yet been tested with either prodromal or first-episode psychosis patients. However, it should be noted that in Australia, PACE groups clinically manifest reasonable high levels of competency with milder severity of symptoms, and in the Netherlands first-episode patients demonstrate considerable insight into their illness in the early stages (Linszen, personal communication).

In the light of promising preliminary results but rather diverse study approaches, the development of model instruments to evaluate subjects' capacity to consent to research in this area would be a significant step forward in providing appropriate ethical safeguards. The informal evidence available indicates early-intervention subjects do have appropriate consent capacity, but we believe that it is now the time to test this empirically.

- Point 5: there are existing materials that could be provided to interested parties including among them patients, patients' families (and surrogates), IRBs, and patient advocacy organizations, but additional information needs to be generated to facilitate informed participation in early intervention projects. Further, valid means of assessing the ability of that information to be used by research subjects and their representatives need to be developed.

6. Conclusion

We have reviewed some of the exciting recent developments in studies of psychoses in general and schizophrenia in particular. These developments are offering hope that such illnesses can be identified and treated early, with better outcomes for both the affected individuals and their families, and perhaps even the prospect of true prevention. Testing such interventions in vulnerable patients can raise ethical difficulties that if not adequately addressed may harm patients and hamper the development of these interventions. We believe there are appropriate ways of dealing with the ethical problems in the early intervention field and have indicated those in the course of this essay, though we also suggest that additional work on both scientific and ethical fronts will need to be done to make these ways real. As a start toward that end, we have summarized a number of the debates in the field and distilled five 'Points to Consider' that we believe interested parties will need to take into account.

Though significant progress in the early intervention area has been made, additional issues of a scientific and ethical nature will continue to be raised. Though we have considered many of the scientific and ethical issues in this introduction, there are several issues just looming on the horizon that investigators in the field will have to keep in mind. The projects discussed above are international in scope, and international extensions of early intervention trials will raise difficult ethical issues, particularly when implemented in developing countries, as the Yale PRIME group intends to do. (See Macklin's essay (2001) for an overview and some recommendations for these types of developing countries' extensions.) Even in Europe, specifically in the Netherlands, different ethical and legal approaches to clinical trials have resulted in importantly different oversight and sanction mechanisms (see van Leeuwen, 2001) that may offer lessons for other countries. Relatedly, different countries' mental health support policies could significantly affect the voluntariness of informed consent: dropping out of a clinical trial in the US often can mean dropping out of care, but this is not usually the case elsewhere.

The papers that follow this introduction develop both the empirical base as well as the ethical issues that are currently under debate in the early intervention in psychosis field. They are a rich source of intertwined clinical information, scientific analyses, and ethical reflections.

Acknowledgements

Grateful acknowledgement is made to the Greenwall Foundation for support of the project and the international conference that made this special issue of Schizophrenia Research possible. Dr Schaffner also acknowledges the US National Science Foundation's Program on Studies in Technology and Science (award number 9618229) for partial support of his research in behavioral and psychiatric genetics. Dr McGorry's research support is from the Australian National Health and Medical Research Council, the Victorian Health Promotion Foundation, NARSAD, Stanley Foundation, Victorian Department of Human Services. Janssen-Cilag Australia, Novartis Pharmaceuticals and the ANZ Trustees.

References

Appelbaum, P.S., Grisso, T., 1996. *The MacArthur Competence Assessment, Tool – Clinical Research*. Professional Resource Press, Sarasota, Fla.

Appelbaum, P.S., Roth, L.H., Lidz, C.W., Winslade, W., 1987. False hopes and best data: consent to research and the therapeutic misconception. *Hastings Center Report*, April 20–24.

Birchwood, M., 2000. Early intervention and sustaining the management of vulnerability. *Aust. N. Z. J. Psychiatry* 34, S181–S184.

Carpenter Jr., W.T., Gold, J.M., Lahti, A.C., Queern, C.A., Conley, R.R., Bartko, J.J., Kovnick, J., Appelbaum, P.S., 2000. Decisional capacity for informed consent in schizophrenia research. *Arch. Gen. Psychiatry* 57 (6), 533–538.

Cook, R.J., Sackett, D.L., 1995. The number needed to treat: a clinically useful measure of treatment effect. *Br. Med. J.* 310, 452–454.

Cornblatt, B., Lencz, T., Kane, J.M., 2001. Treatment of the schizophrenia prodrome: is it presently ethical? *Schizophr. Res.* 51 (1), 31–38.

DeGrazia, D., 2001. Ethical issues in early-intervention clinical trials involving minors at risk for schizophrenia. *Schizophr. Res.* 51 (1), 77–86.

DSM-III-R, 1987. *Diagnostic and statistical manual of mental disorders*. American Psychiatric Association, Washington, DC.

DSM-IV, 1994. *Diagnostic and statistical manual of mental disorders*. American Psychiatric Association, Washington, DC.

Eaton, W.W., 2001. *The Sociology of Mental Disorders*. 3rd ed. Praeger, Westport, CT.

Feinstein, A.R., 1967. *Clinical Judgement*. Williams and Wilkins, Baltimore.

Freedman, B., 1987. Equipoise and the ethics of clinical research. *N. Engl. J. Med.* 317 (3), 141–145.

Gottesman, I.I.G., Erlenmeyer-Kimling, N., 2001. Family and twin strategies as a head start in defining prodromes and endophenotypes for hypothetical early-interventions in schizophrenia. *Schizophr. Res.* 51 (1), 93–102.

Heinssen, R., Fenton, W., Perkins, D., 2001. Report on the November 2000 NIMH informed consent in early intervention is psychosis workshop. *Schizophr. Bull.* (in press).

Ho, B.C., Andreasen, N.C., Flaum, M., Nopoulos, P., Miller, D., 2000. Untreated initial psychosis: its relation to quality of life and symptom remission in first-episode schizophrenia. *Am. J. Psychiatry* 157 (5), 808–815.

Johannessen, J., McGlashan, T., Larsen, T.K., et al., 2001. Early detection strategies for untreated first psychosis. *Schizophr. Res.* 51 (1), 39–46.

Klosterkotter, J., Hellmich, M., Steinmeyer, E.M., Schultze-Lutter, F., 2000. Diagnosing schizophrenia in the initial prodromal phase. *Arch. Gen. Psychiatry* 58 (2), 158–164.

van Leeuwen, E., 2001. Recent Dutch developments of research guidelines on psychiatric subjects. *Schizophr. Res.* 51 (1), 63–67.

Lieberman, J.A., Fenton, W.S., 2000. Delayed detection of psychosis: causes, consequences, and effect on public health. *Am. J. Psychiatry* 157, 1727–1730.

Linszen, D., Dingemans, P., 2001. Psychotic disorders in adolescents and young adults: earl intervention, follow-up results and ethical implications. *Schizophr. Res.* 51 (1), 55–61.

Macklin, R., 2001. International clinical trials with applicability to mentally impaired individuals: the conundrum of third world sites. *Schizophr. Res.* 51 (1), 87–92.

McGlashan, T.H., 2001 Psychosis treatment prior to psychosis onset: ethical issues. *Schizophr. Res.* 51 (1), 47–54.

McGorry, P.D., Singh, B.S., 1995. Schizophrenia: risk and possibility. In: Raphael, B., Burrows, G.D. (Eds.), *Handbook of Preventive Psychiatry*. Elsevier, New York, pp. 492–514.

McGorry, P.D., Mihalopoulos, C., Henry, L., Dakis, J., Jackson, H.J., Flaum, M., Harrigan, S., McKenzie, D., Kulkarni, J., Karoly, R., 1995. Spurious precision: procedural validity of diagnostic assessment in psychotic disorders. *Am. J. Psychiatry* 152 (2), 220–223.

McGorry, P.D., Edwards, J., Mihalopoulos, C., Harrigan, S., Jackson, H.J., 1996. The early psychosis prevention and intervention centre (EPPIC): an evolving system of early detection and optimal management. *Schizophr. Bull.* 22 (2), 305–326.

McGorry, P.D., Krstev, H., Harrigan, S., 2000a. Early detection and treatment delay: implications for outcome in early psychosis. *Curr. Opinion Psychiatry* 13, 37–43.

McGorry, P.D., Phillips, L.J., Yung, A.R., Francey, D., Germano, D., Bravin, J., MacDonald, A., Hearn, N., Amminger, P., O'Dwyer, L., 2000b. A randomised controlled trial of interventions in the pre-psychotic phase of psychotic disorders. *Schizophr. Res.* 41 (1), 9 (abstract from Davos, 2000).

McGorry, P.D., Phillips, L.J., Yung, A.R., 2001a. Recognition and treatment of the pre-psychotic phase of psychotic disorders: frontier or fantasy? In: McGlashan, T., Mednick, S.A., Libiger, J., Johanssen, J.O. (Eds.), *Early Intervention in Psychiatric Disorders*. Kluwer, The Netherlands.

McGorry, P.D., Yung, A.R., Phillips, L.J., 2001b. Closing in: what features predict the onset of first episode psychosis within an ultra high risk group? In: Zipursky, R.B., Schulz, S.C. (Eds.), *The Early Stages of Schizophrenia*. American Psychiatric Press, Washington, DC.

McGorry, P., Yung, A., Phillips, L., 2001c. Ethics and early intervention in psychosis: keeping up the pace and staying in step. *Schizophr. Res.* 51 (1), 17–29.

McGorry, P.D., Patrick D., Yung, A.R., Phillips, L.J., Yuen, H.P., Francey, S., Cosgrave, E.M., Germano, D., Bravin, J., Adlard, S., McDonald, T., Blair, A., Jackson, H.J., submitted. Can first episode psychosis be delayed or prevented? A randomized controlled trial of interventions during the prepsychotic phase of schizophrenia and related psychoses.

Miller, T.J., McGlashan, T.H., Rosen, J.L., Somjee, L., Markovich, P.J., Stein, K., Woods, S.W., Submitted. Prospective diagnosis of the prodrome for schizophrenia: Preliminary evidence of interrater reliability and predictive validity using the Structured Interview for Prodromal States (SIPS).

Phillips, L.J., Yung, A.R., McGorry, P.D., 2000. Identification of young people at risk of psychosis: validation of personal assessment and crisis evaluation clinic intake criteria. *Aust. NZ J. Psychiatry* 34, S164–S169.

Post, S., 2001. Prevention of Alzheimer disease and prevention of schizophrenia: some comparative comments. *Schizophr. Res.* 51 (1), 103–108.

Schaffner, K.F., 1991. Competency: a triaxial concept. In: Gardell Cutter, M.A., Shelp, E.E. (Eds.), *Competency: A Study of Informal Competency Determinations in Primary Care*. Kluwer, Dordrecht, pp. 253–281.

Schaffner, K.F., 1995. *Research Methodology – I. Conceptual Issues in Encyclopedia of Bioethics*. 2nd ed. McGraw Hill, New York pp. 2270–2278.

Schaffner, K.F., 2001. Do causes count: lessons for behavioral psychogenetics from Alzheimer's disease research. In: Sadler, J. (Ed.), *Dallas Conference Proceedings*. Johns Hopkins University Press, Baltimore, MD.

Tsuang, M.T., Stone, W.S., Faraone, S.V., 2000. Toward reformulating the diagnosis of schizophrenia. *Am. J. Psychiatry* 157, 1041–1050.

Van Os, J., Bijl, R., Ravelli, A., 2000. Strauss 1969 revisited: a psychosis continuum in the general population? *Schizophr. Res.* 41 (1), 8.

Woods, S.W., Wexler, B.E., Miller, T.J., Hawkins, K.A., AbiSaab, W., Davidson, L., McGlashan, T.H., 2000. Novel early interventions for prodromal states. *Syllabus and Proceedings Summary*. American Psychiatric Association, Chicago, IL 117pp.

Wyatt, R.J., 1991. Neuroleptics and the natural course of schizophrenia. *Schizophr. Bull.* 17, 325–351.

Wyatt, R.J., Henter, I., 2001. Rationale for the study of early intervention. *Schizophr. Res.* 51 (1), 69–76.

Yung, A.R., McGorry, P.D., 1996. Initial prodrome in psychosis: descriptive and qualitative aspects. *Aust. NZ J. Psychiatry* 30, 587–599.

Yung, A.R., McGorry, P.D., McFarlane, C.A., Patton, G.C., Rakkar, A., 1996. Monitoring and care of young people at incipient risk of psychosis. *Schizophr. Bull.* 22 (2), 283–303.

Yung, A.R., Phillips, L., McGorry, P.D., McFarlane, C.A., Francey, S., Harrigan, S., Patton, G., Jackson, H.J., 1998. Prediction of psychosis. *Br. J. Psychiatry* 172 (Suppl. 33), 14–20.

Yung, A.R., Phillips, L.J., McGorry, P.D., Ward, J.L., Thompson, K., 1996, 2000. *The comprehensive assessment of at-risk mental states (CAARMS)*. Copyright. University of Melbourne.

Index

abortion 348
abusive behavior 127
Academy of Child and Adolescent Psychiatry 321
accountability 82–3, 84, 92, 463–4
ACLU National Prison Project 76
activism 256
adaptive behavior 112
adaptive therapy 260
Adjustment Disorder with Depressed Mood 400
adjustment to reality 260
adolescents 283–4, 445
adult behavior 74
advanced directive 183, 184, 298–9
advanced treatment authorization 183
adversarial standard 334
Adverse Reactions Advisory Committee 185
advocacy 9, 263–9, 346–7, 427
aesthetics 255
affinity 264
Africa 310
agency 358
aggregating benefits 414
Aid to Families with Dependent Children 435
Ake v. Oklahoma 327, 357
Alcohol, Drug Abuse and Mental Health Administration 222
alienation 242–5, 246–9
alienists 319, 330
Alternative Methodology Committee 434
altruism 11–12
Alzheimer's disease 284–5
American Academy of Forensic Sciences 342, 346, 355
American Academy of Psychiatry and the Law 325, 339, 342, 347
    Annual Meeting 383
    Ethical Guidelines for the Practice of Forensic
        Psychiatry 319, 326, 336, 355, 360
American Analytic Association Committee on Peer
    Review 86
American Bar Association 213, 326, 383
American Board of Forensic Psychiatry 342
American Board of Psychiatry and Neurology 319
American College of Physicians 382
American College of Psychiatrists 219, 224
American Health Security Act (proposed) 402
American Law Institute 321, 373
American Medical Association 45, 86
    Code of 1848 343
    Council on Ethical and Judicial Affairs 347, 376, 381, 383
    Current Opinions 348
    death penalty 378
    forensic psychiatry 330, 334, 342, 344
    House of Delegates and Board 381
    managed care 405, 406, 409
    Principles of Medical Ethics 169, 175, 250, 325, 327, 345, 346, 348
    role conflict and expert witnesses 354
American Psychiatric Association 45, 71–87
    Annotations 326, 347

Annual Meeting 48, 384
Board of Trustees 376, 378, 383
Commission on Psychiatric Therapies 223
confidentiality 153
conflicting loyalties in service of the state 85, 86
death penalty 378, 379, 380, 382
District Branch 81
dual role of treater and evaluator 363
electroconvulsive therapy 250
Ethics Committee 81, 85, 347, 362, 381
forensic psychiatry 321, 325, 333
homosexuality 118
law, science and malpractice 227
'medical necessity' 398
New York County District Branch 119
Principles of Ethics 334
psychiatric treatment and services 185
resource allocation 387
Resource Document on Mandatory Outpatient
    Treatment 204, 206
right to effective treatment 222
Sexton case 175
Tarasoff judgment 168
Task Force on the Role of Psychiatry in the Sentencing
    Process 326
therapeutic relationship and social domain 46, 47
    see also Diagnostic and Statistical Manual (DSM)
American Psychological Association 90, 222, 273, 363
    Division 36, 270
    Division 41, 355
American Psychology Law Society 355
Amnesty International 381
ancient Greece 117, 118
anencephalics 16
anger at organization, institute or training analyst
    68–9
animating institutions 265
anonymity 357
anti-psychiatry movement 94–5
antidepressants 239–40, 251, 310, 399
    tricyclic 221, 229, 239
Anxiety Disorders Association 426
Appelbaum, P.S. 319–20, 383, 384
appellate judges 330
applied ethics 13, 14, 15, 37
appreciation 205, 460
    of the nature of the situation 454–5
Appreciation scale 459
Aquinas, Saint Thomas 8, 9, 11
Aristotle 1, 2, 5, 8, 9, 10, 11, 13, 15, 41
artifacts 136–7
artificial feeding 14
asylum function 77
Atkins v. Virginia 322
attachment theory 255, 256
attention deficit hyperactivity disorder 96, 184, 185, 236
Australia 485–6, 487, 488, 489
    attention deficit hyperactivity disorder 96
    confidentiality 152, 153

indigenous peoples 287
Just Therapy approach 314
Medical Association *Code of Ethics* 174
Ministry of Social Security 222
psychiatric treatment and services 185
resource allocation 387
authority 343
autism 236
autonomy 4, 5, 11, 34, 35, 293–6
    absolute confidentiality 163, 165–6
    competency to consent to research 455
    conflicting loyalties in service of the state 82
    contemporary 293–5
    dementia 284–6, 298
    electroconvulsive therapy 251–2
    forensic psychiatry 320, 348, 352
    'four-principles' approach 35
    involuntary hospitalization 193–4
    in long term care 302–7
    mandatory community treatment 206
    Medical Ethics 176
    precedent 295–6, 298–9
    Principles 326
    Sexton case 177
    values in psychotherapy 257
avowed ethics 259–62

Bad Apples theory 406
Baltimore D.C. Psychoanalytic Society 91
Barefoot v. Estelle 330, 333–4
Bartley v. Kremens 79
baseline and outcome measures 232
Bazelon Center 204
behavior disorders 111
behavioral theory 138–9
Belmont Report 14, 455
belonging 316
beneficence 4, 9, 10, 11, 21, 34, 35, 42
    absolute confidentiality 163, 164
    competency to consent to research 455–6
    dementia 296, 298
    electroconvulsive therapy 251
    enforced 387
    forensic psychiatry 319, 326–8, 334, 337–9, 345, 348, 351–2
    health care allocations 394, 396
    involuntary hospitalization 194
    mandatory community treatment 204–5, 206, 207
    placebo-controlled trials 474
    psychiatric treatment and services 182, 187
    resource allocation 385
    Sexton case 177, 178
    values in psychotherapy 256
    see also primum non nocere
benefit 250
    extended 398
    regular 398
benevolence 9, 10, 11, 35, 166, 193
    see also beneficence
best-interest approach 205

bioethical education 38–44
    ethic of care 41–2
    impartiality as mark of the moral 38–9
    'justice', 'care' and gender 38
    modelling relationships 41
    moral intellectualism 40
    moral judgment as principle-derived 39–40
    see also casuistry in bioethics
biological disadvantage, disorder as 133–4
biological psychiatry 223, 229
biopsychosocial model 9
bisexuality 117
Blue Cross 90, 392, 406
Blue Shield 90
boiler plate instruction 213
boundaries 60–5
    clothing 63–4
    crossings 46, 60, 62
    definitions 60–1
    gifts, services and related matters 63
    language 64
    money 63
    physical contact 64–5
    place and space 62–3
    role 61–2
    self-disclosure and related matters 64
    time 62
    violations 46, 60, 62
    see also Exploitation Index: boundary violations
    see also sexual boundary transgression
Brief Psychiatric Rating Scale 459, 460, 478
British Journal of Psychiatry 154
British Medical Association 165, 176, 382, 406, 407, 409
Buckley Amendment 79
burden of persuasion 375
Burnham v. Department of Public Health 214

California University 461, 478
Canada 152, 184–5, 287, 388, 396, 473
    Psychiatric Association 286
capability model 401–2
capacity-based approach 207, 209
capital punishment 333–4
    see also death penalty
Cartesian dualism 109
'case', definition of 15
'case driven' method 13–14, 15
case law 2
casuistry in bioethics 2–3, 13–18
    'case driven' method 13–14
    principles, role of 14–15
    problems 15–18
causal relationship 143
causation 119–20, 355–6
Center for Disease Control 161
Central and Eastern Europe 378
Centre for Adolescent Health 485
character, responsibility for 399–400
Charaka Samhita (Indian code) 343
Charter Medical 390
children 79, 283–4
    abuse, duty to report 363
    antidepressants 184, 239–40
    consent to treatment 290–2
    depression 185
    forensic psychiatry 331
    informed consent and capacity for voluntarism 466, 467–8
    masturbation disorder 130, 139
    psychotropic agents 236–7
    research 445
    sexual abuse 153
Children Act 1989 283, 284, 290
China 73, 84, 377
    legal tradition 157
Chinese room problem 147
chlorpromazine 478
choice 106, 460

Choice scale 459
circularity 276–7
circumstances and pressures, external 467
Citizens' Mental Health Advisory Committee 424
citizens for responsible care and research group (CIRCARE) 486, 487
Civil Code 167
civil commitment 74, 78, 170, 204, 213, 214, 219, 370–1
    involuntary 362–3
civil liberties 194, 195
civil practice 361
Civil Rights Act 215
Civilian Health and Medical Program of the Uniformed Services 391
clinical care monitoring 480
clinical conditions, unusual 364
clinical issues 220–2
clinical pragmatism 271–3
clinical research 450
clinical uncertainty, controversy arising from 400–1
clothing 63–4
clozapine 425–6, 478
cognition 460–1
cognitive assessment 459
collateral sources 357
Commission for the Study of Ethical Problems 395
Commissioner for Mental Health 424
Committee on Safety of Medicines (CSM) 184
common law 14–15
communitarianism 182, 206
Community Mental Health Centers Act 1963 421
compassion 5, 9, 10, 11
competency:
    children and adolescents 283–4
    dementia 293, 294–6
    for execution 328, 347, 365–6, 379
    forensic psychiatry 350, 352
    risks 463–4
    to consent 291
    see also competency to consent to research
competency to consent to research 451–6
    appreciation of the nature of the situation 454–5
    autonomy 455
    beneficence 455–6
    evidencing a choice 452
    factual understanding of issues 452–3
    rational decison making 455
    rational manipulation of information 453–4
    standards for competency 452
comprehensive assessment of at risk mental states instrument 485
Compulsive Personality Disorder 102
compulsory treatment and joint crisis plans 232–5
concept of mental illness 93
confidentiality 11, 34, 35, 42, 45, 91, 151–4
    breach 53, 175–7, 361
    centrality 151–2
    conflicting loyalties in service of the state 72, 74
    definition 151
    dual role of treater and evaluator 360
    electroconvulsive therapy 250
    family involvement 153, 171, 172
    forensic psychiatry 322–3, 326, 337, 339, 344, 351, 369
    hospital 162
    individual case material 154
    limits of: individual clients 158–60
    role conflict and expert witnesses 355, 358
    Sexton case 176, 178–80
    Tarasoff judgment 152–3
    see also confidentiality, absolute; confidentiality, limits of
confidentiality, absolute 163–6
    breach of confidentiality 164
    in a clinical setting 164–5
    conflict between principles 165–6
    ethical propositions 163–4
    law enforcement 166

legitimate exceptions 165
    research 164
confidentiality, limits of 156–61
    individual clients 158–60
    justification and rationale 157–8
    professional secret 156–7
    secrecy as a shield 160–1
conflicting roles 350–1
    see also dual agency
conflicts around sexual orientation 69
conflicts and professional etiquette 79–81
Congressional Budget Office 388
Conroy case 14, 15
conscientiousness 11
consciousness 145, 147
consensus 16–17
consent 35, 326
    children and adolescents 283–4, 290–2
    implied 164
    see also competency to consent; informed consent
considered judgements 37
Constitution:
    First Amendment 196, 199
    Fourteenth Amendment 182, 213–14
    Tenth Amendment 420
consumer advocates 208
consumer participation 208
contingency 256
continuity of care 364
contract model 42
control group 232
control test 374–5
Convention on the Rights of the Child 283
conventionalism 17
conventions 4
cooperative responses 127
corruption 263–9
cosmetic psychopharmacology 185–6
cost-effectiveness 385
courage 10, 12
covenant model 42
criminal justice 79
Criminal Justice Mental Health Standards 326
criminal practice 361
criminal responsibility 373–4
critical interests 297, 298
critique 17
Cruzan case 15
culpability 321–2
cultural knowledge 314–15
cultural value systems and homosexuality 117
cultural values 467, 468
culture-bound syndromes 310

dangerous severe personality disorder 323
dangerousness 207, 209, 322–3, 327, 361, 370, 371
Data Protection Act 1984 165
death with dignity movement 298
death guilt 263
death imprint 263
death penalty 322, 327–8, 347, 349, 376, 377–82, 383–4
death-taint 263
decision making 222, 455
decisional capacity for informed consent 458–62
    assessment 459
    clinical ratings 459
    cognition 460–1
    cognitive assessment 459
    educational remediation of decisional impairments 459
    results 460
    statistical analysis 460
    subjects 458–9
    symptoms 460
Declaration of Independence 273
deconstruction of the self 331
deductivism 14, 15
defense, narrowing of 374–5

demoralization 74, 75
denial of reality 260
Denmark 485
deontological approach 3, 4, 5, 192–3
Department of Health 165, 232
    Protection and Use of Patient Information, The 173
Department of Health and Human Services (latterly
    Department of Health Education and Welfare)
    286, 452
Department of Health and Social Services 362
dependency 56, 57
dependent personality disorder 101
depersonalization 127–8
Depressive Disorder 400
descriptive approach 356
desipramine 239
determinism 331
developmental factors 467–8
diagnosis 93–7
    concept of mental illness 93
    disputed 221
    fact-based model 93–4
    fact-value synthesis 95–6
    value-based model 94–5
diagnostic issues 220–1
Diagnostic and Statistical Manual (DSM) 95, 96, 123,
    142, 485
    -I 220
    -II 91, 93, 101, 228, 402
        homosexuality 121, 122
        right to effective treatment 220, 221, 222
        sex differences in treatement rates 99, 100
    -III 99–102
        biological facts and social values 134, 135
        decisional capacity and informed consent 458
        definitions 100
        dependent personality disorder 101
        diagnosis 93
        dual role of treater and evaluator 364
        forensic psychiatry 332
        histrionic personality disorder 101
        independent personality disorder 101–2
        law, science and malpractice 228, 230
        overconforming and underconforming 100
        problems 100–1
        restricted personality disorder 102
        right to effective treatment 220, 221
        sex differences in treatment rates 99, 101, 102
        sex ratios of specific disorders 99–100
        women's sexuality 102
    -III-R 94, 224, 230, 239
        biological facts and social values 130, 133, 134,
            135, 138
        law, science and malpractice 226, 228, 229
        'medical necessity' 399, 400
    -IV 93, 244, 250, 310, 484
        decisional capacity and informed consent 458, 459
        'medical necessity' 398, 399, 401, 402, 403
Difference Principle 426
Dillon v. Legg 167
disclosure 35, 169–70
disordered sexual development 117
distance 353
distinctive integrity 294
distributive justice 387
doctor-patient relationship and values and guild interests
    45–8
Donaldson v. O'Connor 78, 182–3, 210–18
dopamine hypothesis 148
Dora case 154
double agency 71–87, 88–9
    advocacy and corruption 266
    conflicts and professional etiquette 79–81
    forensic psychiatry 320, 332–3, 340, 348, 350, 369
    informed consent and capacity for voluntarism 467
    moral dilemmas in military practice 71–4
    potentially dangerous patients 81–3
    principles and recommendations 83–7

prisons, psychiatrists in 74–6
    psychiatric institutions: administrator's perspective
        76–8
    psychiatric institutions: advocate's perspective 78–9
    role conflict and expert witnesses 354–5
    see also dual role of treater and evaluator
drapetomania 130, 132, 139, 286
dual role of treater and evaluator 360–6
    advantages of combining treating and
        evaluating 364
    civil versus criminal practice 361
    competency for execution 365–6
    explicit duties to warn or protect 363–4
    involuntary civil commitment 362–3
    order of assumption of the roles 362
    pharmacological therapy 361–2
    private versus public practice 360–1
    psychotherapy 361
    separation of treatment from evaluation 364–5
    treaters as decision makers 362
    warnings to patients at beginning of
        relationship 365
    see also role conflict
dualism 109, 143, 144, 146, 148
    explanatory 148
    property 145
    substance 145, 148
duty 10–12, 21, 22, 26
Dworkin, R. 284
Dworkin, R. on dementia 297–301
    advance directives and precedent autonomy 298–9
    critical and experiential interests 299–300
    state interest 300–1
Dyaesthesia aethiopica 286
dynamic approach 356
dysfunction 134, 135

early intervention 484–5
Early Periodic Screening Diagnosis and Treatment
    program 432
early psychosis prevention and intervention centre 485
economic factors 360–1
Education Law of New York 80
educational remediation of decisional impairments 459
effective treatment, right to *see Osheroff v. Chestnut Lodge*
    efficacy research 229–30
egalitarianism 193, 194, 387, 395–7
ego ideal 2
elderly persons 284–6, 385, 386, 445, 466
electroconvulsive therapy 186–7, 202, 221, 222, 223,
    250–3, 310
eliminative materialism theory (epiphenomenonalism)
    144, 147, 148, 149
Elliott, C. 242–5
emergent properties 147
emotions 5
empathy 9, 356
Employee Assistance Program 407
empowerment 208
enabling 57–8
entitlements, differences in 395
Epicureans 29
EPPIC (Early Psychosis Prevention and Intervention
    Centre) 488
equality 205, 206
Equipoise 388
equity 194
eroticism 56
essential fatty acids 485, 487
Estelle v. Smith 365, 370
ethnocentrism 309
etiquette 79–81, 84, 85
Europe 223, 251, 309, 344, 377, 451
euthanasia 42, 297, 348
Evaluation of Signed Consent 459, 460, 461
evaluators 320–1
Evidence Code 169
evidence gathering 357

evidencing a choice 205, 452
evidentiary view 294, 295, 298
evolutionary theory and dysfunction 137
exception fantasy 69
exhibitionism 56, 120, 121
exorcism 160–1
expectancy 267
experiential interests 297
explanatory gap 145
explicit duties to warn or protect 363–4
Exploitation Index: boundary violations 53–8
    dependency 56
    enabling 57–8
    eroticism 56
    exhibitionism 56
    generalized boundary violations 55–6
    greediness 57
    narcissistic pathology 54
    power seeking 57
eye contact 126, 127

fact-based model 93–4
fact-plus-value model 95–6
fact-value distinction 331
fact-value synthesis 95–6
factual understanding of issues 452–3
fair and representative procedure 415–16
false memory syndrome 96
false positives 487
familiarity, excessive 53
family involvement 171–4
    confidentiality 153, 171, 172
    informed consent 172
    patients refusal of 172–4
    relative interests of family members 172
    values and family intervention 171–2
Family Law Reform Act 1969 290
features and pressures, external 468–9
Federal Employees Health Benefits Program 90
fee-for-service 432, 435, 437
fertility, increased 133–4
fidelity 5, 10, 11, 34, 45, 258, 334
    see also truth-telling
Fifty Admonitions to Physicians 344
financial sacrifice 92
fluidity 264
fluoxetine 239, 400
Food and Drug Administration 184, 445, 451
    law, science and malpractice 229, 231
    placebo-controlled trials 473, 474
    psychotropic drugs and children 236, 237
    right to effective treatment 221, 222, 223
Ford v. Wainwright 327
forensic psychiatry 319–23, 325–8, 330–4, 336–40,
    342–9, 350–3, 369–72
    adversarial standard 334
    alternative approach 339–40
    civil commitment 370–1
    confidentiality, dangerousness and third parties
        322–3
    conflicting roles 350–1
    culpability 321–2
    death penalty 322
    distinct forensic ethics 327–8
    double-agent role 369
    ethical dialectic 333
    evaluators versus treaters 320–1
    good clinical practice standard 332
    intellectual chasm 331–2
    issues 345–6
    moral agency 353
    narrative context 352–3
    necessity for distinct set of ethics 337–8
    nonmedical values, appeal to 334
    origins of traditional medical ethics 342–4
    principles of ethics 338–9
    professional integrity 351–2, 353
    proposed resolution to ethical problems 346–8

forensic psychiatry (cont.)
  psychiatric ethics versus forensic ethics 325–7
  reason for 'professional' ethics 336–7
  reducing harm and increasing benefits 369–70
  relevant philosophical concepts 344–5
  scientific standard 332–3
  testifying for prosecution in capital punishment
      333–4
  theoretical foundations 319–20
  truth 330–1, 333
former Soviet Union and misuse of psychiatry re political
      dissidents 71, 85, 95, 181, 193
  death penalty 377, 378, 380, 384
  electroconvulsive therapy 250, 252
formulation 263
forseeability of harm 168
'four-principles' approach 34–7
  framework and roots 34–5
  models and underlying principles 35–6
  normative nature 36
  principlism, recent critiques of 36
  specification and reflective equilibrium 36–7
  see also autonomy; beneficence; justice; non-
      maleficence
France 344
free will 331
freedom 177
Freedom of Information Act 161
Freud, S. 46, 50–2, 60–1, 62, 138, 178–9, 188–9, 330
  advocacy and corruption 263
  forensic psychiatry 331
  values in psychotherapy 254–6, 257
friendship 5
function 278–9, 280, 281
functionalism 146–7, 148, 149
future behavior, prediction of 364

Gault, W.B. 268
Gay Liberation 119
gay movement 189
Geller case 207
gender 38
  experience 315
General Medical Council 153, 165, 174
Geneva Declaration 46, 176, 449
Germany 251
gifts 63
Gillick case 283–4, 290, 291
good clinical practice standard 332
good, theory of 10
good will 20
Gray Oral Reading Test 459, 460
Great Smoky Mountain Study 185
greatest good for the greatest number principle 426
greatest happiness principle 28
greediness 57
Greenwood v. United States 215
group integration 267
group therapy 399
guild interests 46–8
guilt 266
'guilty but mentally ill' 373

habeas corpus 214
haloperidol 236, 478
Hammurabi Code 343
happiness 21, 29, 30, 31–3
harm 250
  requirement 137–8
harmful dysfunction 95–6, 130–1, 133, 138, 139
Hartmann, H 330–1
Harvard Community Health Plan 398, 399, 400
Hastings Center 47, 71–87, 388, 407–8, 411
Hawaii Declaration 250
Health Care Financing Administration 222, 229, 434
health insurance 402–3
Health Insurance Association of America 417

health maintenance organizations 386, 390, 391, 392,
      406, 407, 409
  'medical necessity' 399, 402
  priority-setting 417, 433, 435
health measurement criteria 425–6
Health Outcomes Committee 422, 432–3
health policy 387–8
Health Services Commission 421, 423, 431, 432, 433, 434
heart transplantation 17–18
Heaven v. Pender 167
Helping Hands 212
helpless behaviors 77
Helsinki Declaration 250, 252, 443, 444, 449–50, 451, 473
heterosexuality 116, 119, 120–1
HEW (Health Education and Welfare) 85
hierarchical organization 73, 126, 128
Hinckley case 331, 332
Hippocratic Oath 2, 10–11, 12
  absolute confidentiality 164
  confidentiality 151
  conflicting loyalties in service of the state 84
  death penalty 380
  electroconvulsive therapy 250, 252
  forensic psychiatry 320, 322, 342–3, 344, 346, 347,
      348, 349
  'four-principles' approach 34
  managed care 406
  Sexton case 176, 177
  therapeutic relationship and social domain 45, 46,
      47, 48
histrionic personality disorder 101
HIV/AIDS 153, 165, 177–8
Home Office 323
homosexuality 94, 116–22
  bisexuality-mammalian inheritance 117
  deviant behavior not necessarily psychopathology 117
  diagnosis 96
  as a disorder 121
  happy, constructive and realistic homosexuals 117
  heterosexuality as a disorder 120
  holding action 116–17
  inherent psychological pain 118
  Manual of Mental Disorders 121–2
  natural realm, part of 116
  not a 'sexual dysfunction' 120
  preoedipal theory of causation 119–20
  proposed new classification 121
  psychological growth through resisting oppression
      119
  sexual inadequacy 118
  sexual orientation disturbance 122
Homosexuality Task Force 119
honesty 10
  see also truth-telling
hospital parole 373
hospitalization see involuntary hospitalization
Hospitalization of the Mentally Ill Act 1964 213
Humphrey v. Cady 213
hysterical personality disorder 101

idealism, humanistic 271–3
idealized version of the self, patient seen as 68
identity:
  cultural 310
  ethnic 310
  masculine, insecurity regarding 69
  personal 293, 299
  professional 351
  relationships 142
  theoretical 142, 143
  theory 109, 144, 145, 146, 147, 148, 149
  token 145, 148
  type 145, 146
ideological point of departure, determination of 415
illness-related considerations 468
imipramine 239, 400
immediacy 267
impartiality 3–4, 5, 38–9, 326

implicit rationing 385
incestuous longings, unconscious reenactment of 68
incompetence for execution 328
independent personality disorder 101–2
indeterminacy 16–17, 424–5
India 310
indigenous peoples 286–7
individual treatment 399
individualism 248–9
  of bioethics 17–18
information manipulation, rational 453–4
informed consent 34, 42
  absolute confidentiality 164
  confidentiality 154
  electroconvulsive therapy 252
  family involvement 172
  forensic psychiatry 326, 339, 348, 352
  incapacity to give 201–3
  law, science and malpractice 226–7
  mandatory community treatment 204, 205
  medication-free research 481
  placebo-controlled trials 475–6
  psychiatric treatment and services 184, 188
  research 443–4, 445, 446
  and voluntarism 466–9
  see also decisional capacity for informed consent
Inhibited Orgasm 102
Inhibited Sexual Desire 102
insanity defense 321–2, 327, 373–5
Institute of Medical Ethics 153
Institute of Medicine 398
instructional approach 183–4
integration 431
integrity 267, 295, 296, 297, 298
  personal 285, 351
  professional 351–2, 353
intentionality problem 147
International Classification of Diseases (ICD) 93–9
      220–10 250, 310
International Code of Medical Ethics 158, 175, 449
interpersonal problems 399, 400
Interprofessional Working Group 165, 166
intervention, early 480
intervention group 232
interventionism, ethical 189
interview strategies 357
intimacy 257
inverted-spectrum problem 147
involuntary hospitalization 192–5
  autonomy, respect for 193–4
  paternalism 194
  rights versus obligations 193
  utilitarian versus deontological approaches 192–3
involuntary treatment 77, 181–2
  see also mandatory community treatment
Ireland 251
irony 256
Ishaq Ibn Al-Ruhawi Code 344

Jackson v. Indiana 214
Jaffee v. Redmond 151, 337, 358
Japan 377
joint crisis plans and compulsory
      treatment 232–5
Jonsen, A. 13–14, 15, 16–17, 18
judgment approach 345
Jung, C. 188
'Just Therapy' approach 313–18
justice 4, 10, 34, 35, 38
  absolute confidentiality 163, 164
  competency to consent to research 455–6
  electroconvulsive therapy 250, 251
  forensic psychiatry 326, 327, 334, 337, 338, 340, 345,
      351, 352
  health care allocations 396
  involuntary hospitalization 194
  resource allocation 386
  Sexton case 177

Kaimowitz v. Michigan Department of Mental Health 451–2
Kant, I. 3, 28–9, 330
Kantor, J.E. 346
Kefauver-Harris Amendments to the Food, Drug and Cosmetic Act 221, 222
Kendra's Law 204
kindliness 11
    see also beneficence; benevolence
kinetics 2

labeling 128
    psychodiagnostic 124–6
language 64
latah 310
Law Commission 201–2
law enforcement 166
learned helplessness hypothesis 99, 100
learning 14–15
least restrictive option principle 173
Legislation Scoping Study Committee 232
Leibniz's law 144
Lessard decision 207
liberalism 204–5
liberation 316
libertarianism 386
liberty 193
libido 51, 52
lithium 398, 485, 487
longevity, increased 133–4
love 5
love in and of itself is curative, fantasy that 68
lovesickness 68–9
loyalties, conflicting *see* double agency
loyalty 380
    see also fidelity

MacArthur Competence Assessment Tool-Clinical Research (MacCAT-CR) 444, 459, 460, 461, 488–9
MacArthur Foundation 205, 207
MacArthur Treatment Competence Study 444
macro-allocation 386–7, 397
Major Depression 101
maladaptive behavior 112
maleness 265
malpractice 226–31
    biological versus psychodynamic psychiatry 229
    diagnosis 228
    efficacy research and public policy concerns 229–30
    law 226–7
    Osheroff v. Chestnut Lodge and standard of care 227–8
    responsibility to consult and confer 231
    responsibility to describe alternative treatments 230
    responsibility to inform patient 230
    responsibility to make diagnosis according to Diagnostic and Statistical Manual (DSM)-III-R 230
    responsibility to provide proper treatment 230–1
    treatment 228–9
managed care 390–2, 398, 405–9, 432
management 310
mandatory community treatment 204–9
    appropriate criteria 207
    communitarianism 206
    duration of treatment 206–7
    rights-based versus beneficence 204–5
    slippery slope problem 207–8
    utilitarianism 205–6
manic defense against mourning and grief at termination 69
manual record 165
marketplace ethics 361
Maryland Psychiatric Research Center 458, 459, 460, 461
masochism 120, 121
masochistic surrender 69
masturbatory disease 130, 133, 139
material principles 174

materialism 109–10
maternal nurturing as sexual overture, misperception of wish for 68
Medicaid 16, 17, 222, 412, 421, 423, 431–2, 434–5
Medical Group against the Death Penalty 381
medical model of mental illness 90–1, 108
'medical necessity' determination 398–403
    capability model 401–2
    clinical uncertainty, controversy arising from 400–1
    distinguishing treatment from enhancement 398–9
    moral hazard 401
    normal function model 401
    practical implications for health insurance 402–3
    temperament and character, responsibility for 399–400
    welfare model 402
Medicare 16, 17, 222, 395, 421
medication 127, 310
    ethical aspects in use 184–6
medication-free research 478–82
    individual protection 480–1
    informed consent 481
    pharmacological treatments, new 478–9
    potential benefits and risks 479–80
melancholia 186, 242–5
Memmel v. Mundy 79
Meninnger Clinic 67
Menninger Foundation 267
mens rea approach 373–4
mental disorder, concept of 101, 130–9
    as biological disadvantage 133–4
    dysfunction and evolutionary theory 137
    functions as effect that explain their causes 135–7
    harm requirement: why dysfunction is not enough 137–8
    misapplication 139
    myth of the myth of mental disorder 131
    as pure value concept 132
    as statistical deviance 133
    theories of disorder 138–9
    as unexpectable distress or disability 134–5
    as whatever professionals treat 132–3
Mental Health Act 1983 173, 232, 234, 235, 291, 323
Mental Health Act 1988 (Japan) 377
Mental Health Act Code of Practice 201
Mental Health Act Review Tribunal 321
Mental Health Association of Oregon 432
Mental Health and Chemical Dependency Committee 432, 433–4, 435, 436, 437, 438
Mental Health and Chemical Dependency Subcommittee 421–2
Mental Health Law Project 78
Mental Health Parity Act 1996 388
Mental Health (Patients in the Community) Act 1995 173
mental health theory 108–14
mental illness, myth of 104–7
    choice and responsibility 106
    ethics, role of 105–6
    as name for problems in living 104–5
    sign of brain disease 104
Merchants National Bank & Trust Co. of Fargo v. United States 168
micro-allocation 385–6, 397
military practice, moral dilemmas in 71–4
military psychiatry 348
Mill, J.S. 177, 181, 182, 206–7
mind-body problem 142–9, 436
mind-brain problem 331, 332
Minnesota statute 363
Miranda warning 73, 75, 77, 352, 361, 365
mirror hunger 54
misdiagnosis 310
mixed duties, theory of 339–40
M'Naghten test of insanity 319, 321–2, 373, 374, 375
Model Penal Code 321, 373, 374, 375, 454
modelling relationships 41
models and underlying principles 35–6

money 63
mood stabilizers 399
moral agency 353
moral hazard 401, 426
moral ideals 336–7
moral intellectualism 40
moral judgment as principle-derived 39–40
moral rules 336–7, 338
morality 331
morals 344
morphology 2
muliple realizability 145, 146, 148

narcissistic pathology 54
narrative truth 351
Nason v. Superindentent, Bridgewater Hospital 214
National Alliance for the Mentally Ill 204, 208, 426, 488
National Ambulatory Medical Care Evaluation Survey 237
National Association of Social Workers 222, 405, 409
    Ethics Committee 408
National Bioethics Advisory Commission 443, 444–5
National Commission on Mental Health Treatments 222, 223
National Commission for the Protection of Human Subjects of Biomedical and Behavioral Research 13–14, 16, 451–2
National Depressive and Manic-Depressive Association Consensus Statement 445
National Federation of Societies for Clinical Social Work 363
National Health Board 393
National Health and Medical Research Council (Australia) 443
National Health Service 388, 406
National Institute of Mental Health 85, 142, 185, 222, 237, 421, 446, 484
National Institutes of Health 222, 237, 481
    Office of Protection from Research Risks 478
National Medical Association 365
National Medical Enterprises 390
National Mental Health Act 1946 421
nationalism 309, 310
natural function 136–7
natural lotteries 394
Nazi policy on physical and mental handicaps 95, 163, 250, 378, 451
    forensic psychiatry 346, 348
    therapeutic relationship and social domain 46, 48
necessity 26
need to know basis 173
negative consequences 134
Netherlands 308, 485, 487, 489
neuroleptics 310
neutrality 205, 206, 257, 355, 356–7
New Haven 485–6, 487
New Zealand 287, 313–18
    Mental Health Act 1992 323
Newman v. Alabama 76
non-attachment 257
non-clinical biomedical research 450
non-clinical business dealings 53
non-maleficence 4, 11, 34, 35, 36, 187, 251, 385
    absolute confidentiality 163, 164, 165
    forensic psychiatry 319, 326, 327, 328, 337–8, 339, 340, 351, 352
nonmedical model 90–1
nonmedical values, appeal to 334
non-therapeutic biomedical research involving human subjects 450
normal function model 401
normal science 331
normative law 382
Norway 485
nothingness 256
nuisance behaviors 77
Nuremberg Code 250, 448, 451, 452

Nuremberg formulation 451
Nuremberg Statement 443, 444
Nuremberg trial 250

objective criteria 271
objective reality 355–6
objectivity 326, 353
Office for Human Research Protections 484, 486, 487
Office of Mental Health 424
Office for the Protection from Research Risks 473
Omnibus Budget Reconciliation Act 421
openness 264
oppositional defiant disorder 236
oppression, resistance of 119
Oregon: prioritization of mental
    health services 414, 422–4, 431–8
    background 431–2
    discontents 436–7
    Health Outcomes Committee and initial methodology
        422, 432–3
    Health Plan 421, 422, 431, 432, 434, 435, 436, 437,
        438
    Health Services Commission 421, 423, 431, 432, 433,
        434
    implementation 435
    implications of integration 437
    legislature, return to 434–5
    Mental Health and Chemical Dependency Committee
        432, 433–4, 435, 436, 437, 438
    Mental Health and Chemical Dependency
        Subcommittee 421–2
    mental health community, role of in health care
        reform 437–8
    priority-setting commission 413
    problems and solutions 434
    Social Values Committee 422, 432, 433
Osheroff v. Chestnut Lodge 47, 183, 219–24
    clinical and scientific issues 220–2
    law, science and malpractice 226, 229, 230, 231
    legal actions 220
    public policy issues 222–4
    recommendations for the practising clinicial 224
    standard of care 227–8
outpatient commitment 204
outpatient treatment 209
overconforming 100

pain, inherent psychological 118
pain and suffering, taking the measure of 414–15
paraphilias 67–8
parens patriae rule 194, 214
part dysfunction 131
passive-dependent personality 101
paternalism 45, 82, 293
    electroconvulsive therapy 251, 252
    forensic psychiatry 343, 348
    involuntary hospitalization 194, 195
    mandatory community treatment 206, 207
    strong 194
    weak 194
patience 5
patient-orientation 81, 82
patient-staff segregation rule 126
Pearson product moment correlation 460
pedophilia 120, 121
People v. Burnick 168–9
percent mingling time 126
permissible medical experiments 448
permission, principle of 396
personal assistance and crisis evaluation clinic 388, 485,
    488, 489
personal ethics 360, 366
Personality Disorder 102
personality type 116
pharmacological therapy 361–2, 478–9
phenelzine 398, 400
phenothiazines 221, 229
phronesis 1, 2, 15

physical contact 64–5
physical lesion 131
physician care organizations 435
physician-assisted suicide 34
physician-patient relationship 348
physiological dysfunction 138
place 62–3
placebo-controlled trials 445, 472–7
    ethical critique 474–5
    informed consent 475–6
    methodological considerations 473–4
    public justification 476
    rationale for opposition to 473
    regulatory standards and codes of ethics 472–3
    risk-benefit assessment 475
    scientific merit 475
    treatment optimization 476
Plato 7–8, 393–4
pleasure 29, 30
Police and Criminal Evidence Act 1985 166
police power rationales 194, 214
post-modernism 255–6
potentially dangerous patients 81–3
power 78
    seeking 57
powerlessness 127–8
practice, priority of 14
predatory behavior 77
predatory psychopathy 67–8
preferred provider organizations 432
preoedipal theory of causation 119–20
presence 264
presenting syndrome 116
President's Commission on Mental
    Health: Subpanel on the Mental
    Health of Women 99
President's Commission Report 463
President's Commission for the Study of Ethical
    Problems in Medicine and Biomedical and
    Behavioral Research 387–8
Prevention Through Risk Identification Management
    and Education clinic 485–6
prima facie duty 3
PRIME trial 487, 488, 489
primum non nocere (first of all, do no harm) 319, 342,
    343, 357, 369, 380
principles, role of 14–15
principlism 4, 34, 36, 186, 352
priorities in mental health services 411–16, 417–29
    basic package of services 427–8
    decision making 426–7
    finding a middle way 414–15
    health measurement criteria 425–6
    indeterminacy 424–5
    informal and formal priorities 420–2
    justification of priorities 418–20
    matters of process and procedure 415–16
    New York state 423–4
    pure numbers and raw politics 412–14
    see also Oregon
prisons, psychiatrists in 74–6
privacy 34, 35, 45, 445–6
private practice 360–1
prodrome concepts 484–5, 486, 487
professional codes 405
professional ethics 360, 366
professionalism 352
promise-keeping 11, 177
prosecution of mental patients 363–4
proximity 267
proxy approach 183–4
proxy consent 445
Prozac 96, 243, 246–9
prudential concern 293
pseudopatients 123–9
    labeling 128
    normal people are not detectably sane 124
    powerlessness and depersonalization 127–8

psychiatric hospitalization, experience of 126–7
psychodiagnostic labeling 124–6
    and their settings 123–4
psychiatric hospitalization, experience of 126–7
psychiatric institutions:
    administrator's perspective 76–8
psychiatric institutions: advocate's perspective 78–9
psychiatric will 182
psychic numbing 263
psychic reality 355–6
psychoanalysis 311
    and values 254–6
psychodiagnostic labeling 124–6
psychodynamic psychiatry 223, 229
psychological defenses 357
psychological growth through resisting oppression 119
psychological issues 468
psychological purpose 356
Psychosexual Disorder Advisory Committee 102
psychosurgery, ethical aspects of 187
psychotherapies 187–9, 311, 361
psychotic depression 186
psychotropic drugs 128, 184, 185, 236–7
Public Health Service 451
public policy issues 222–4, 229–30
public practice 360–1
publicity condition 427
pure value concept, disorder as 132
purists 330–1, 332

qualia problem 145, 147
Quality Adjusted Life Years 386–7, 412–13, 425
quality of well-being scale 422, 425, 432–3, 434
Quinlan case 14, 15, 79

racial minorities 286–7
racism 189, 286, 308–12
    active 309
    aversive 309
    individual 312
    institutional 309, 311–12
rage 266
randomized clinical trials 34
'rap groups' 264, 265, 266, 268
rapism 121
Rawls, J. 14, 17, 194, 387, 426
realism, theistic 189, 272
reason 20–1
reasoning 205, 460
Reasoning scale 459
recovered memory 355
recovery paradigm 208
reflective equilibrium 18, 34, 36–7
refusal of treatment, right to 364
regulatory standards 472–3
reimbursement 358
relativism 83
religious values 255, 270–4, 467, 468
Repeatable Battery for the Assessment of
    Neuropsychological Status 459, 460
repression 138
repression or disavowal of rage at patient's persistent
    thwarting of therapeutic efforts 68
rescue fantasies, interlocking enactments of 68
research 443–6
    combined with clinical care 450
    informed consent 443–4
        privacy 445–6
        risk 444–5
    see also competency to consent to research
resource allocation 42, 77, 385–9
    health policy 387–8
    macro-allocation 386–7
    micro-allocation 385–6
respect for persons 176, 338–9, 340, 351, 455
respectable minority doctrine 223
responsibility 106
responsiveness 11

Restatement Second of Torts 168
restricted personality disorder 102
rights 10–12
  -based theory 204–5
  involuntary hospitalization 193
  negative 205
  positive 205
  to health care, social justice and fairness in health care allocations:
    health care policy: ideology of equal, optimal care 393–4
    justice, freedom and inequality 394–7
  to health care, social justice and fairness in health care allocations 393–7
  to know 164
  to obtain correct treatment 184
  to receive treatment 184
  to refuse treatment 184
risk 463–5
  -benefit assessment 475
  competence and accountability 463–4
  depression and competence 464
  period, duration of 480
  research 444–5
risperidone 478, 485
Rituale Romanum 1614 161
Rogers v. Okin 183
role 61–2
  conflict 354–8
    alliance, nature of 356–7
    assessments 357
    caveats 358
    common scenarios 354
    contexts and complications 355
    core 354
    ethical guidelines 357–8
    historical overview 354–5
    risks 358
    truth and causation 355–6
  definition 74
  distinction 75
  of ethics 105–6
Roman law 14–15, 382
Rorty, R. 255–6
Rouse v. Cameron 214, 215
Rowland v. Christian 167
Royal Australian and New Zealand College of Physicians 222
Royal Australian and New Zealand College of Psychiatrists 46
Royal College of Psychiatrists 152, 322, 376, 382, 384, 464
rules 36

sacredness 316
sadism 120, 121
Saikewicz case 15
Sartre, J.-P. 188
Scandinavia 251, 388
scientific issues 220–2
scientific merit 475
scientific standard 332–3
Second National Mental Health Strategy 488
seductiveness 53
selective serotonin reuptake inhibitors 184, 185, 487
self-binding contract 183
self-disclosure 64
self-generation 264
self-harm behavior 184
self-interest 11–12, 464
self-love 26
Senate 437
serotonin 142, 143, 148
  see also selective serotonin reuptake inhibitors
service 11
  delivery 78–9
services 63
  see also treatment and services

severe mental illnesses, prevention of 484–9
  Australia and New Haven early intervention studies 484–6
  concerns and criticisms 486
  ethical and study design issues 486–9
sex differences in treatment rates 99
sex ratios of specific disorders 99–100
sexism 93
Sexton case 154, 175–80
  biography, facts about 175–6
  confidentiality 176, 178–9
  confidentiality, disclosure of 176–8
  confidentiality, right of 179–80
sexual abuse 153, 363
sexual activity 53
sexual boundary transgression 67–9
  lovesickness 68–9
  masochistic surrender 69
  predatory psychopathy and paraphilias 67–8
sexual contact 54
sexual dysfunction 121
sexual inadequacy 118
sexual misconduct 46
sexual orientation disturbance 122
  see also homosexuality
sexual psychopath laws 362
sexual repression 260
sexuality 102
Siena principles 1975 377
SIPS 486
situational ethics 361
social lotteries 394
social purpose 356
Social Security Act 421
Social Security Administration 222
Social Security Disability Insurance 421
social status hypothesis 99
Social Values Committee 422, 432, 433
socially handicapped 77
societal orientation 81, 82
Society of Medical Psychoanalysts 119
sociobiological fallacy 134
Socrates 7–8, 10, 22, 30
South Africa 189
space 62–3
special clinical populations 283–8
  children and adolescents 283–4
  elderly 284–6
  racial minorities and indigenous peoples 286–7
specialness 54
specification 36–7
spirituality 315–16
Spring case 15
Stanford University 126
State Comprehensive Mental Health Planning Act 423
State Disciplinary Committee 86
state, in the service of see double agency
statistical analysis 460
statistical deviance 133, 134
stimulants 185
Stone, A.A. 319–20, 325, 336, 346, 383
structures 278–9, 280, 281
subject satisfaction 456
subject selection 480
subsidiary syndromes 116
substituted judgment approach 205
suicide 34, 182, 184, 185, 205, 350, 400
  see also suicide prevention
suicide prevention 196–200
  assigning and assuming responsibility for suicide 198
  death control 200
  from sin to sickness 196
  and mental health professional 198–9
  professional liability 196–7
  right to suicide 199
supervised discharge 173
Supplemental Security Income 421, 432, 435

Sweden 251
sympathy 5

taking sides 74
Tarasoff judgment 3, 4, 152–3, 159–60, 167–80, 177
  common law analysis 169–70
  confidentiality 151–2
  dual role of treater and evaluator 363, 364
  forensic psychiatry 320, 323
  plaintiffs' complaints 167–9
  violence and civil commitment 170
tardive dyskinesia 236
taxonony 2
teaching 14–15
technicist model 268
techniques 271
teenage pregnancy 158
temperament, responsibility for 399–400
temporal considerations 456
test administration 456
testifying for prosecution in capital punishment 333–4
thalidomide victims 451
theistic realism 189, 272
theoretical ethics 13
theoretical foundations 1–5
  casuistry 2–3
  deontological theory 3
  ethics of care 5
  principle-based ethics (principlism) 4
  utilitarianism 3–4
  virtue ethics 1–2
therapeutic bias 349
therapeutic neutrality 257
therapeutic partnership 188
therapeutic relationship and social domain 45–8
therapeutics, enhanced 480
third parties 90–2, 322–3, 363
time 62, 357
Torsney case 331
total well-being 9
Toulmin, S. 13–14, 15, 16–17, 18
training 348–9
tranquilisers 310
tranquility 30
transference 45, 46, 50–2, 68
transformational object, patient seen as 69
transvestism 120
treatability 370
treaters 320–1
treatment:
  decisions 79
  deterrence 169
  involuntary 77, 181–2
  necessity 78
  optimization 476
  pattern and third-party payment 91
  refusal, right to 362–3
  successful 170
  versus enhancement 96
  withdrawal 34
  see also treatment and services
Treatment Advocacy Center 204, 208
treatment and services 181–9
  advanced directives 183–4
  electroconvulsive treatment, ethical aspects of 186–7
  involuntary treatment 181–2
  medication, ethical aspects in use of 184–6
  psychosurgery, ethical aspects of 187
  psychotherapy, ethical aspects of 187–9
  right to effective treatment 183
  right to refuse treatment 183
  right to treatment 182–3
Tri-Council Policy Statement on Ethical Conduct for Research involving Humans 473
trial judges 330
triangle of attachment 257

tricyclic antidepressants 221, 229, 239
trust 177, 361–2
truth-telling 10, 11, 34, 35, 45, 333
    elderly persons 285–6
    forensic psychiatry 320, 330–1, 338, 339, 351
    role conflict 355–6
type 2 error 124

ultra high risk population 485, 487
Ulysses contract 183
unavowed ethics 259–62
unconscious reenactment of incestuous longings 68
underconforming 100
underdiagnosis 310
understanding 205, 460
Understanding scale 459
unexpectable distress or disability, disorder as 134–5
United Kingdom 184, 366, 373
    children and adolescents 192, 283, 284, 290, 291
    confidentiality 152
    electroconvulsive therapy 251, 252
    forensic psychiatry 321, 323, 332, 344
    incapacity to give informed consent 201, 202
    racial minorities and indigenous peoples 286–7
    racism 308, 309, 310
United Nations 283
    Commission on Human Rights 377
    Convention on the Rights of the Child 290
    Educational, Scientific and Cultural
        Organization 308

universal laws 26, 27
utilitarianism 3–4, 5, 28–33, 35, 182, 192–3, 205–6,
    386–7

V Codes 130, 133, 135
vaginal orgasm, lack of 139
value-based model 94–5
values:
    and data, dialectic between 416
    and doctor-patient relationship 45–6, 47–8
    and family intervention 171–2
    and psychotherapy 188–9, 254–8
    religious 270–4
    see also values, negotiation of values, negotiation of
        276–82
    case example 279–81
    clinicians' application of values 278
    negotiations, nature of 277–8
    preparing therapists to negotiate values
        281–2
    structure and function 278–9
verbal contact 127
Victoria (Australia) Mental Health Act 153, 174
Vietnam Veterans Against the War 264, 265, 268
Vietnam War 72–3, 189, 263
violence 170, 206
Virginia University 458, 459, 460
virtue:
    ethics 1–2
    intellectual 8

medieval concept 7–9
moral 8
virtuous physician and ethics of
    medicine 7–12
    medieval concept of virtue 7–9
    rights and duties 10–12
vitamin C 243
voluntarism and informed consent 466–9
voyeurism 120, 121

War Crimes Tribunal 443
weakness of the will 294, 295
weaving analogy 315–16
Wechsler Adult Intelligence Scale 459
welfare model 402
welfare rights 35
Wide Range Achievement Test 459, 460
Winter Soldier Investigation 1971 264
Wisconsin Sex Crimes Law 362, 364
World Health Organization 9, 132, 287
    Regional Office for Europe 377
World Medical Association 46, 158, 382, 443, 451, 473
    see also Geneva Declaration; International
        Classification of Diseases
World Psychiatric Association 377, 383
    Congress of Madrid 322
    Ethics Committee 382, 383, 384
    General Assembly 382
    Madrid Declaration 376, 378, 381, 382, 384
Wyatt v. Stickney 183, 214, 215